DONATED BY

SCANNER APPEAL

PROPERTY OF

X RAY DEPARTMENT

DO NOT REMOVE

COMPUTED TOMOGRAPHY OF THE BODY

ALBERT A. MOSS, M.D.

Professor of Radiology
University of California, San Francisco
School of Medicine
San Francisco, California

GORDON GAMSU, M.D.

Professor of Radiology
University of California, San Francisco
School of Medicine
San Francisco, California

HARRY K. GENANT, M.D.

Professor of Radiology, Medicine and
Orthopaedic Surgery

University of California, San Francisco
School of Medicine
San Francisco, California

W.B. Saunders Company

PHILADELPHIA   LONDON   TORONTO   MEXICO CITY   RIO DE JANEIRO   SYDNEY   TOKYO

W. B. Saunders Company: West Washington Square
Philadelphia, PA 19105

1 St. Anne's Road
Eastbourne, East Sussex BN21 3UN, England

1 Goldthorne Avenue
Toronto, Ontario M8Z 5T9, Canada

Apartado 26370—Cedro 512
Mexico 4, D.F., Mexico

Rua Coronel Cabrita, 8
Sao Cristovao Caixa Postal 21176
Rio de Janeiro, Brazil

9 Waltham Street
Artarmon, N.S.W. 2064, Australia

Ichibancho, Central Bldg., 22–1 Ichibancho
Chiyoda-Ku, Tokyo 102, Japan

Library of Congress Cataloging in Publication Data

Moss, Albert A.
    Computed tomography of the body.

    1. Tomography.   I. Genant, Harry K.   II. Gamsu, Gordon.   III. Title.
RC78.7.T6M68   1983   616.07'572   83-2976
ISBN 0-7216-6574-8

Computed Tomography of the Body   ISBN   0-7216-6574-8

Last digit is the print number: 9   8   7   6   5   4

This work is dedicated to our wives,
Marla, Lynn, and Gail,
and to our children,
Jennifer and Jeffrey
Jessica
Laura, Justin, and Jonathan

CONTRIBUTORS

DOUGLAS P. BOYD, Ph.D.

Professor of Radiology (Physics), Department of Radiology, University of California, San Francisco, School of Medicine, San Francisco, California

ROBERT C. BRASCH, M.D.

Associate Professor of Radiology, Department of Radiology and Pediatrics, University of California, San Francisco, School of Medicine, San Francisco, California

CHRISTOPHER E. CANN, Ph.D.

Associate Professor of Radiology, University of California, San Francisco, School of Medicine, San Francisco, California

NEIL I. CHAFETZ, M.D.

Assistant Professor of Radiology, University of California, San Francisco, School of Medicine, San Francisco, California

LAWRENCE E. CROOKS, Ph.D.

Associate Professor of Electrical Engineering, Assistant Director, University of California Radiologic Imaging Laboratory, University of California, San Francisco, School of Medicine, San Francisco, California

PETER L. DAVIS, M.D.

Assistant Professor, Department of Radiology, University of California, San Francisco, School of Medicine, San Francisco, California

MICHAEL P. FEDERLE, M.D.

Associate Professor of Radiology, University of California, San Francisco, School of Medicine; Chief, Sections of Gastrointestinal Radiology and Computed Body Tomography, San Francisco General Hospital, San Francisco, California

GORDON GAMSU, M.D.

Professor of Radiology and Chief, Pulmonary Radiology, University of California, San Francisco, School of Medicine, San Francisco, California

HARRY K. GENANT, M.D.

Professor of Radiology, Medicine, and Orthopaedic Surgery; Chief, Skeletal Radiology, University of California, San Francisco, School of Medicine, San Francisco, California

HENRY I. GOLDBERG, M.D.

Professor of Radiology and Chief, Gastrointestinal Radiology, University of California, San Francisco, School of Medicine, San Francisco, California

CLYDE A. HELMS, M.D.

Assistant Professor of Radiology, University of California, San Francisco, School of Medicine, San Francisco, California

ROBERT J. HERFKENS, M.D.

Assistant Professor of Radiology, Department of Radiology, University of California, San Francisco, School of Medicine, San Francisco, California

R. BROOKE JEFFREY, M.D.

Assistant Professor of Radiology, Department of Radiology, University of California, San Francisco, School of Medicine, San Francisco, California

LEON KAUFMAN, Ph.D.

Professor of Physics; Head, Experimental Nuclear Instrumentation; Director, University of California Radiologic Imaging Laboratory, University of California, San Francisco, School of Medicine, San Francisco, California

MARTIN J. LIPTON, M.D.

Professor of Radiology and Medicine; Chief, Cardiovascular Imaging Section; Member Cardiovascular Research Institute, University of California, San Francisco, School of Medicine, San Francisco, California

JOHN R. MANI, M.D.

Associate Clinical Professor, Department of Radiology, University of California, San Francisco, School of Medicine; Radiologist, Ralph K. Davies Medical Center, San Francisco, California

ANTHONY A. MANCUSO, M.D.

Associate Professor of Radiology, University of Utah, School of Medicine, Salt Lake City, Utah

ALEXANDER R. MARGULIS, M.D.

Professor and Chairman, Department of Radiology, University of California, San Francisco, School of Medicine, San Francisco, California

ALBERT A. MOSS, M.D.

Professor of Radiology, Chief, Computed Body Tomography; Department of Radiology, University of California, San Francisco, School of Medicine, San Francisco, California

DENNIS L. PARKER, Ph.D.

Asisstant Professor of Radiology (Physics), Department of Radiology, University of California, San Francisco, School of Medicine, San Francisco, California

RUEDI F. THOENI, M.D.

Associate Professor, Department of Radiology, University of California, San Francisco, School of Medicine; Chief, Gastrointestinal Radiology, Letterman Army Medical Center, San Francisco, California

W. RICHARD WEBB, M.D.

Associate Professor of Radiology, Department of Radiology, University of California, San Francisco, School of Medicine, San Francisco, California

PREFACE

This book evolved as the product of the experience, expertise, and dedication of the radiologists and physicists engaged in computed tomography at the University of California, San Francisco. It is presented as a comprehensive state-of-the-art text on computed body tomography. Although the concept of writing such a text had been considered for several years, we felt it prudent to delay its implementation until the rapid technologic advancements of the early years had reached a plateau. Rather than present early experiences and potential uses of computed tomography, we waited until our experience had matured and a more inclusive text could be written.

The contents of this text are organized so that basic anatomy and computed tomographic techniques are discussed for each region of the body. The computed tomographic features of disease entities are described and illustrated, and the relationship of computed tomography to other imaging techniques is presented. Recommendations are offered as to the role of each modality in specific clinical situations. The book presents an integrated approach that reflects our current standard of practice. Obviously, knowledge of computed body tomography is still expanding, and undoubtedly, recommendations, techniques, and patterns of utilization will change. Certainly, the introduction of nuclear magnetic resonance will have an impact on computed body tomography. Consequently, we have devoted a chapter to this new method of obtaining cross-sectional images of the body.

In the writing of this book, there have been many people without whose support, guidance, insight, and help this work could not have been completed. We thank our colleagues who contributed their time and case material, and acknowledge the secretarial support of Susan Hilary, Ann Tso, and Denise Nakano; the illustration department at UCSF; and the editorial services of Steven Ordway and Jo Wheeler. We particularly thank Dr. Alexander R. Margulis for his continuous encouragement and support.

ALBERT A. MOSS
GORDON GAMSU
HARRY K. GENANT

ix

CONTENTS

1 BASIC PRINCIPLES OF COMPUTED TOMOGRAPHY

Douglas P. Boyd
Dennis L. Parker

Computed body tomography (CT) has become the diagnostic procedure of choice for most neurologic diseases, and new applications are developing rapidly. At this point, a short review of the basic principles of CT should be useful in aiding the reader in gaining an appreciation for the complexity of disciplines involved and in developing an intuitive understanding of the nature, limitations, and artifacts of the images of the various types of CT scanners.

The first part of this chapter illustrates the concepts of CT for the ideal situation. Errors in measurement and problems resulting from sampling techniques, for example, are omitted. The fundamental problems, physical limitations, and general effects of the actual implementation of CT that are true for all CT scanners are then considered. The added difficulties that arise in body CT compared with head CT are discussed.

The second section discusses the history of developments in computed tomography, including many important technologic breakthroughs.

The various geometries of CT scanners as given by the relative arrangement of x-ray source and detectors are discussed in the third part.

The fourth section describes image noise, artifacts, and image quality as defined in terms of numerical descriptors such as spatial resolution, contrast resolution, and CT number accuracy. The tradeoffs between image quality and patient dose are considered.

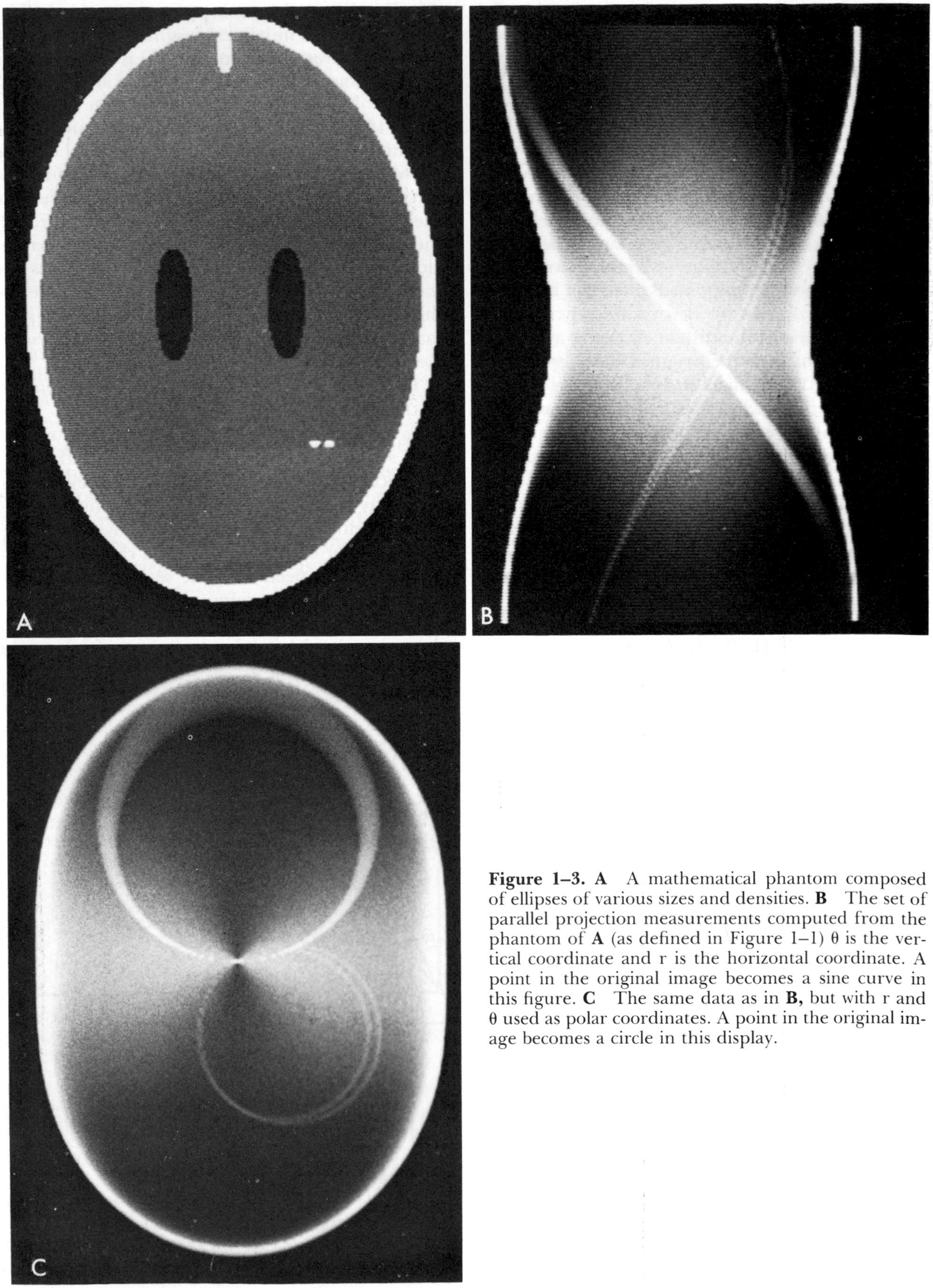

Figure 1–3. A A mathematical phantom composed of ellipses of various sizes and densities. **B** The set of parallel projection measurements computed from the phantom of **A** (as defined in Figure 1–1) θ is the vertical coordinate and r is the horizontal coordinate. A point in the original image becomes a sine curve in this figure. **C** The same data as in **B,** but with r and θ used as polar coordinates. A point in the original image becomes a circle in this display.

traverse: A separate profile is obtained for each angle.

Examples of a radon transformation are shown in Figure 1–3. In Figure 1–3*A* a simple diagram composed of ellipses of different "densities" is shown. Two high-density "calcified" points are at the lower right. If the set of all projections is computed, it can be displayed as shown in Figure 1–3*B* with θ as the y-axis and r as the x-axis. It can also be displayed using r and θ as polar coordinates as in Figure 1–3*C*. Displays of the radon transformation in the format of Figure 1–3*B* are generally referred to as *sinograms* because a point in object traces out a sine curve in the display as seen for the pair of points. In the the polar coordinate display, a point in the object becomes a circle.

The objective of the computer reconstruction program is to convert or transform a series of profiles into a CT image. This procedure is illustrated in Figure 1–4. In Figure 1–4(a) the profiles of a point object in the scanned slice of four view angles separated by 45° steps are shown. One approach to reconstruction would be to simply project the profiles back across the CT image as

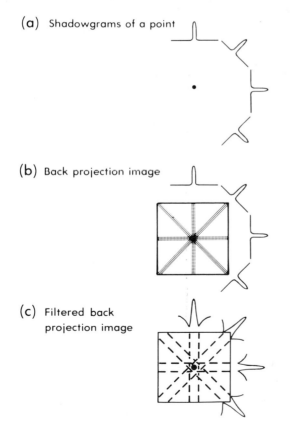

(a) Shadowgrams of a point

(b) Back projection image

(c) Filtered back projection image

Figure 1–4. Principle of filtered back-projection reconstruction.

shown in Figure 1–4(b), similar to the principle of axial tomography. This procedure produces a starlike reconstruction. If a large number of views were used, the radial streaks would merge together and the point reconstruction would become a smooth image with a peak at the center and falling off as l/r, where r is the distance from the center of the point. Such streaks may occasionally appear in scanners in which the number of views are only marginally adequate and are referred to as angular "aliasing streaks" or the "angular undersampling" artifact.

One method of accurate reconstruction would be to mathematically remove the l/r blurring from the back-projected image. Such a technique is referred to as "unfolding" or "deconvolution." If the profiles are accumulated at equal angular intervals from 0 to 180°, this process of deconvolution may be accomplished by first modifying the profiles prior to their back projection. The modification is produced by applying a mathematical "filter" or "convolution" function to the profile so that the resulting reconstructed image more closely resembles the original object from which the original, unmodified profiles were obtained. The modified profiles and resulting modified backprojected image are indicated in Figure 1–4(c). This technique of modified or filtered back projection is essentially the image reconstruction process used by all modern CT scanners.[2] Thus the principle of CT rests on the premise that it is possible to accurately reconstruct a two-dimensional object from many angles of view. Similarly, a three-dimensional image may be reconstructed from a series of two-dimensional projections.

PRACTICAL IMPLEMENTATION OF COMPUTED TOMOGRAPHY

As might be inferred, the ideal implementation of computed tomography would reconstruct a continuous distribution of attenuation coefficient measurements within a plane or slice through the object of interest. The distribution would be known accurately and precisely at all points within the two-dimensional object plane. The reconstruction of a continuous distribution requires that measurements be made of all possible projections, along lines of negligible width, through the object within imaging plane. Because the lines are of negligible width, this requires a very large (infinite) number of projection measurements. The negligible width requirement also means that the x-ray source and detector elements must all have negligible width. Thus, the reconstruction of a

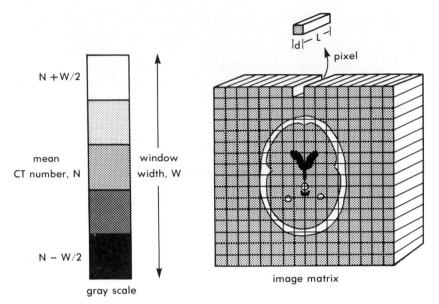

Figure 1–5. Gray scale CT image matrix.

continuous distribution (at very high resolution) is impractical both from the consideration of the large amount of measurements required as well as the constraints on smallness of the x-ray source and detectors.

The reconstructed CT image is represented by a two-dimensional matrix of CT numbers. Because of the practical limitations of finite beam width and the finite number of projection measurements, the spatial resolution possible in the reconstructed image is compromised. Intuitively, this is seen to happen because of the blurring effect of scanning very fine details by a rather coarse beam. Typically, the effective width of the beam created by the geometry of the source, detector, and associated collimators varies from about 3 mm down to less than 0.5 mm among various commercially available CT scanners. The number of individual projection measurements varies between about 25,000 and 1 million. It is generally true that the number of elements in the final display matrix should not be greater than the number of individual projection measurements which gives the number of resolution elements that can be determined. This would mean that the final reconstruction matrix should be between 160 × 160 and 1000 × 1000. The matrix size of commercial CT scanners is found to vary between 160 × 160 and 512 × 512 picture elements. In general, the picture elements are referred to as "pixels." High-resolution reconstructions of local regions (target reconstructions) can generally be obtained to utilize the full resolution when the number of display elements is significantly less than the number of measurements.

Another geometric limitation in CT scanners is the fact that the beam does not have negligible width in the direction perpendicular to the scan plane. In order to obtain sufficient x-ray signals, this width is generally between 2 to 20 mm and can often be varied under operator control. Thus the CT number corresponds to the mean value of density or, more accurately, the linear attenuation coefficient within the volume of tissue denoted by a particular pixel. This volume element has a depth, L, which is the CT section thickness or slice thickness indicated in Figure 1–5.

LIMITATIONS INHERENT IN BODY COMPUTED TOMOGRAPHY

In addition to geometric considerations, there are other limitations that are directly related to the number and energy distribution of the photons within the beam. These affect the accuracy and precision of the measurements and lead to artifacts, which are discussed later.

The number of photons that are detected directly affects that precision with which the attenuation coefficient can be measured. For example, the total attenuation of an x-ray beam that passes through the thicker parts of the body is considerably greater than that of beams used in head scanning. The practical implementation of whole body CT is thus much more difficult than that of head CT because of this greatly increased constraint on the dynamic range that is observed by the detection system. Also, because the body is larger, either more detectors or longer scan times (or both) are required to produce images of contrast and spatial resolution comparable to those of head CT. Finally, internal motion of organs (lung, heart, digestive tract) is much more problematic in body CT than in head CT.

DEFINITION OF NUMBERS IN COMPUTED TOMOGRAPHY

As mentioned, the linear attenuation coefficient of any medium is a strong function of x-ray energy. In order to determine a tissue characteristic (such as density) using the values of reconstructed linear attenuation coefficient, it is necessary that the energy spectrum of the x-ray beam be known. Since the spectrum varies from scanner to scanner as well as for various points along the penetrating beam path of each measurement of a given scanner, an approximation based on the use of "CT numbers" is commonly used. In this method the measured linear attenuation coefficients for air and water using a specific scanner are used to transform the measured attenuation coefficient of the object into a standard, relative unit called the CT number. The CT number is generally defined by the relationship:

$$CT\ number = K\frac{\mu - \mu_{water}}{\mu_{water} - \mu_{air}}$$

which assigns water the CT number 0 and air the value $-K$. Early CT scanners used a scale where K was given the value 500. Air then had the value of -500 and dense bone was between 500 to 1000. In this early scale, most soft tissues fall in a range of $+20$ to $+30$. A change of five CT numbers represents approximately a 1 per cent change in linear attenuation coefficient. At the present time, nearly all manufacturers have adopted the convention that assigns K the value 1000. In this case, air has the value -1000; dense bone, between 1000 to 2000, and soft tissue, in the range of $+40$ to $+60$. This latter scale is referred to as the *Hounsfield scale*, the units as *Hounsfield Units* (H). It is evident that a change of one Hounsfield Unit corresponds to a change of 0.1 per cent in linear attenuation coefficient relative to water.

A number of excellent articles summarize the important principles and physical concepts in computed tomography.[3–7]

HISTORY OF COMPUTED TOMOGRAPHY

The almost sudden success of computed tomography has been due to the fact that highly developed technologies from various branches of the sciences were simultaneously acquired. Thus, although the commercial development of CT began in the early 1970s, a complete history of CT must include many developments in various technologies during the many decades preceding the first implementation. These include the mathematical achievements of Radon[1] and others, the development of x-ray technology—specifically medical x-ray technology—as well as general radiology, and the introduction of inexpensive mini- and microcomputers and array processors. Developments in each of these areas occurred in such a way that by the late 1960s, all the necessary technical elements required for the invention of CT scanning were in place.

From the early discovery of x-rays, it was soon apparent that transmission images of the human body could yield an immense amount of interesting and often diagnostically useful information. However, because a three-dimensional structure was being "projected" onto a two-dimensional display, much information about a specific internal structure was masked by the shadows of overlying and underlying structures. In order to eliminate the unwanted structure detail in the final image, various "tomographic" techniques were developed. In conventional linear tomography, a tomographic section or plane of interest is held in focus while overlying and underlying layers are blurred, owing to relative motion of the source and film receptor. Thus noise (i.e., unwanted structure information) caused by superimposed layers is converted to a background noise similar to that caused by scattered radiation.

The radiation dose can be quite high for a complete examination, since the planes above and below the focal plane are exposed to the full x-ray beam for each exposure. This problem is avoided by the technique of axial tomography as introduced by Takahashi.[8] In axial tomographic systems a fan x-ray beam rotates around the body, exposing only a single transverse axial cross section of the body. A radiographic film cassette on the opposite side of the body rotates together with the source. The film is nearly parallel to the x-ray fan but is tilted slightly so that the transmitted fan beam exposes the entire film at each angle of rotation. This causes the fan beam projection to be smeared or "back-projected" across the film during the scan. The final image is an approximate representation of the density distributions of the scanned section but contains considerable blurring that limits the utility of this method. The blurring results from the fact that an axial tomographic or back-projection image is only a first-

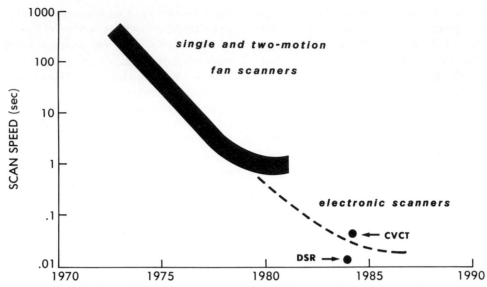

Figure 1–6. The evolution of CT scanner speed. The solid curve indicates the advances made using mechanical scanning systems by increasing the numbers of detectors and x-ray fan angle. The dashed curve indicates projected future advances based on millisecond motion, electronic scanning techniques.

order approximation to the true density cross section. The solution to this problem of blurring would require a computer program specifically designed to accomplish the required deblurring. Such a technique would then be referred to as *computed axial tomography.*

Since Radon's contribution,[1] a variety of mathematical techniques for reconstruction have been developed by many authors. These methods are sometimes jointly referred to as the inverse radon transformation. During the 1950s and 1960s, these techniques were applied to scientific problems in many fields including radio astronomy and electron microscopy.[9, 10]

Cormack first applied the techniques of image reconstruction from projections to radiography and carried out demonstration experiments using "phantoms."[11] Kuhl and Edwards[12] applied these principles to nuclear medicine and developed computed emission tomography. Hounsfield[13] developed the first clinically viable CT scanner, the EMI neuroscanner, which became an immediate success during the early 1970s. Cormack and Hounsfield later shared the Nobel prize for medicine in 1980.

Shortly after the tremendous diagnostic capabilities of CT were recognized, a dozen or more x-ray equipment manufacturers joined EMI in the production of CT scanners. The performance and technical sophistication of CT equipment evolved rapidly in this competitive atmosphere. For example, the introduction of fan beam scan-

ning techniques led to scan time reductions from 300 seconds to 2 seconds in just 4 years (Fig. 1–6), and further improvements in scanning speed are expected. The intense competition caused technical developments to be made rapidly, and the proprietary nature of the technical information resulted in the need for duplication of technical research by each of the interested companies. At the same time, government regulations designed to eliminate overpopulation of these expensive medical devices quickly reduced the total market available. For these and other related reasons, many of the early CT scanner manufacturers (including EMI, the originators) yielded to the fierce competitions and discontinued their own production and development of CT scanners. However, by 1982, more than 5000 scanners had been installed worldwide, with several hundred scanners now being sold annually. Aggressive new companies began to enter the field and introduced competitive technical approaches to scanner design. In June 1982 the federal "certificate-of-need" regulations designed to limit the number of CT scanners installed were dropped as a result of studies that proved the cost effectiveness of CT scanning.

DESIGN OF CT SCANNERS

GENERAL CONSIDERATIONS

A modern CT facility consists of a scanning gantry that includes the collimated x-ray source and detectors, the computer data acquisition and reconstruction system, a motorized patient-handling table, and a CT viewing console. The major technical difference between various commercial scanners lies in the gantry design and involves the number and type of x-ray detectors used as well as their scanning motion. These differences are discussed later in this chapter.

Data acquisition and reconstruction systems consist of one or more minicomputers and related peripheral equipment, such as a magnetic tape unit for archival storage, a line printer for printing CT numbers in regions of interest, an operator's control keyboard and display, data acquisition electronics, and special processors to speed the reconstruction computations. The complexity of this system is related to the size of the detector array, scanning speed, and the required speed of image reconstruction. In CT scanners with slow scan time (1 to 5 minutes), image reconstruction is performed during scanning and the CT image becomes available for viewing after the end of the scan. In faster scanners (2 to 20 seconds), image reconstruction cannot presently be performed during scanning and the additional computation time can become a limiting factor in patient throughput. Therefore, fast scanners often employ fairly complex special hardware and array processors that produce reconstructions in as little as 6 seconds.

The patient-handling table is usually motorized, with horizontal and vertical drives. The couch may be automatically indexed in the horizontal direction under computer control to position a series of adjacent tomographic sections. Laser-produced light beams are used initially to localize the patient with respect to markers recorded on a projection radiograph. Either the gantry or the couch may be designed for tilting to about 20° from the horizontal.

CT display systems offer a great range of options for quantifying regions of interest, image processing, radiation therapy treatment planning, and production of hard copies. Regions of interest are selected by electronically outlining the selected region on the television display monitor using a manually controlled cursor such as a brightened dot or cross. The cursor is moved by manipulating a velocity-sensitive joystick, a position-sensitive track ball, or an electronic tablet. A computer program displays the outlined region's area and calculates the mean CT number and various statistical parameters. With the image in digital format, various image manipulation routines can be applied digitally in order to increase the visibility of desired information.

One very useful image-processing option appears to be spatial smoothing to enhance the low-contrast detectability of larger lesions having a CT number very similar to surrounding tissue. Alternatively, some benefits of spatial smoothing can be accomplished by viewing the CT image with a minifying lens, by stepping back a fair distance from the image, or by using a smaller auxiliary television monitor. Many manufacturers offer software and hardware options for computing radiotherapy treatment planning using the CT image. Hard copies of CT images and related analyses are produced with Polaroid cameras, 70-mm roll-film cameras, or multiformat cameras that record several CT images on a single sheet of large format x-ray film. CT images may also be stored in digital format on inexpensive magnetic floppy disks that have a capacity of up to several images.

TYPES OF SCANNING GANTRIES

There are currently three types of scanning gantries in common use. All employ a fan of x-ray beams that are used in combination with a position-sensitive detector array. X-ray fan angles range from 3° to greater than 90°, with the wider angles providing greater utilization of the total flux of x-radiation produced at the x-ray tube anode. Detector arrays contain from three to more than 1000 discrete detector elements. The more detectors that are simultaneously recording transmitted x-ray intensities, the faster the scanning sequence may be completed. In addition, larger detector arrays typically permit the size of an individual detector element to be minimized, leading to significant improvements in spatial resolution. The use of large detector arrays can be costly. Such systems are typically several times more expensive than their simpler counterparts.

For detector arrays of up to about 90 elements, the *translate-rotate* scanning sequence, similar to that of the original EMI brain scanner, is used. Scintillation-crystal detectors coupled to photomultiplier tubes or xenon ionization chambers are used to detect and record the x-ray beam intensities. During each traverse, each detector records a parallel ray profile at successive angles within the x-ray fan. Following the traversing motion, the system rotates by an amount equal to the width of the fan; for example, a system with 30 detectors at one third–degree intervals requires

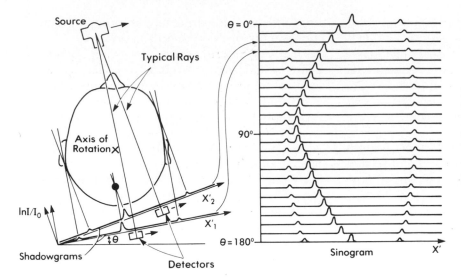

Figure 1–7. Basic principles of translate-rotate fan scanning. Profiles produced by two representative detectors of detector array are indicated. Typical sinogram indicating peaks caused by skull and dense lesion is illustrated.

18 translations at 10° steps to obtain 180 degrees of projection data for a total of 540 profiles. In such systems, mechanical considerations limit the ultimate scanning speed obtainable to about 10 seconds.

If 300 to 600 detectors can be used, it is possible to eliminate the need for a linear traverse by measuring all the sample points in a given profile simultaneously. In such systems, only pure rotary motion is required and scanning speeds of 2 seconds or faster can be achieved. Because both the detector array and x-ray source rotate, this geometry is often referred to as a *rotate-rotate* geometry.

A third type of scanning system (*rotate-station-*

ary) uses a stationary ring detector array with 600 or more detectors arranged in a circle about the patient. A rotating fan of x-radiation produces the scan.

These three configurations lead to important differences in performance characteristics. Figures 1–7 through 1–9 illustrate the basic differences. Transmission data recorded by the detectors may be plotted as a profile in which the x-axis represents the position of a particular measurement and the y-axis represents the log of the detected intensity divided by the incident intensity. In the following sections we compare the sequence of data collection and some inherent properties of the three scanning geometries.

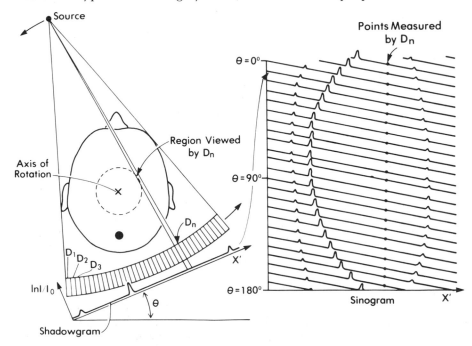

Figure 1–8. Principle of rotary fan-rotary detector fan scanning. Profile is generated by simultaneous outputs of all detectors in curved detector array. Typical rotary scanner is illustrated along with location of points measured by single detector element, D_n. Measurements of each detector describe vertical line in sinogram that should be compared to horizontal lines measured by individual detectors in translate-rotate systems. Dashed circle illustrates location of ring artifact that would be produced by an error in detector D_n.

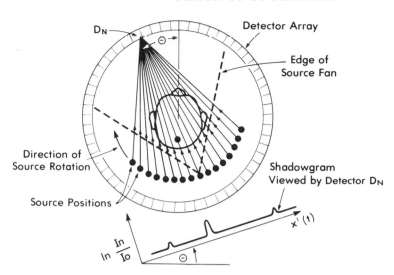

Figure 1–9. Basic principle of data acquisition for stationary detector ring systems. Each profile is produced by recording serial outputs from each detector during scan; such measurements are referred to as *detector-fan profiles*. Measurements recorded by individual detector elements describe nearly horizontal lines in sinogram similar to example of translate-rotate systems.

Translate-Rotate

Figure 1–7 illustrates the projection data recorded by two particular detectors of a translate-rotate fan system. The detectors and source traverse linearly from left to right at a particular gantry rotation angle or view angle θ. Peaks caused by the skull and a radiographically dense lesion are illustrated. Each detector in the fan measures a profile at a slightly different angle, providing multiple views within the fan angle. The gantry rotates, using angular steps equal to the fan angle until a complete set of profiles covering 0 to 180° is obtained.

The completed scan data represented may be plotted as a series of profiles in a two-dimensional $\theta - x'$ graph or matrix form similar to the format of Figure 1–3B.

θ is the view angle of a particular measuring ray, and x' is the distance of each ray from the axis of rotation. This graph is often called a *sinogram* because the locus of points described by an object point, for example, the dense lesion illustrated, describes a sine curve whose amplitude and phase are related to the polar coordinates of the object point. The computer reconstruction program can be considered a two-dimensional transformation of the sinogram into the CT image. The data organization of Figure 1–7 is ideally suited to the requirements of fast-modified back-projection reconstruction methods.

For a translate-rotate fan system with n detectors, every n^{th} line or profile of the sinogram represents data gathered by a particular detector. If that detector malfunctions, only the corresponding profiles are disturbed and image degradation may be minimal because back projection smoothly

distributes the error over the entire image. The detectors may be easily calibrated at the left- and right-hand edges of the profile where the rays bypass the outer contours of the body. Thus long-term detector stability is not required, and inexpensive photomultiplier tube-based detectors are suitable.

Rotate-Rotate

Pure rotary fan systems are illustrated in Figure 1–8. In this case, a profile at a particular angle θ is recorded simultaneously by a large number of individual detector elements. Only pure rotation of the source and detector is required to form a complete set of profiles. The sinogram consists of slanted lines, since adjacent measurements within the diverging fan beam are at slightly differing angles. Reconstruction may be accomplished by reorganizing the set of fan rays into equivalent sets of equally spaced parallel rays and using standard methods. This process is often referred to as reordering and rebinning.[14] Alternatively, direct divergent beam reconstruction algorithms may be employed.[15]

The locus of points corresponding to a particular detector is now along a vertical line in the sinogram, as illustrated by the dots in Figure 1–8. An error along this line transforms to a circle in the reconstructed image, as illustrated by the dashed curve in the CT image. Thus small-detector errors tend to produce circular or "ring" artifacts in pure rotary fan systems. In addition, the detectors cannot be continuously calibrated during the scan as in translate-rotate systems. Calibration is accomplished at infrequent intervals using a known absorber such as a cylindric water phantom. Thus the requirements for detector accuracy and stability are very high in a rotary fan system. Fortunately, xenon ionization chambers and solid-state detector arrays can be built to perform within these requirements.

Rotate-Stationary

The stationary ring detector-rotary fan (Figure 1–9) produces a sinogram similar to that of Figure 1–8. Here the divergent ray profiles are obtained by recording the output of a particular detector as the source moves on its circular path on the opposite side of the body. Such profiles are sometimes referred to as *detector fans*. The number and angular spacing of detector profiles depend on the number and spacing of detectors. The locus of points in the sinogram recorded by a particular detector is a slanted, nearly horizontal line. Thus detector errors in stationary ring designs propagate as in translate-rotate systems, and the same advantages of insensitivity to small errors of a few detectors and the ability to perform continuous detector calibrations are inherent in the design. A disadvantage is that many times more detectors are required by this system, since only a fraction are recording data at any one time.

The ability to obtain good spatial resolution and high quantum detection efficiency simultaneously can be difficult in stationary designs. Spatial resolution is strongly dependent on the width of detector elements, but if detector element width is minimized, it is sometimes necessary to leave gaps between the detectors in the ring. Since the source x-ray fan is continuous, x-ray photons falling in the gaps between detectors contribute to patient dose but are not utilized by the scanner. Increasing the number of detectors is helpful, but the number of profiles to be reconstructed also increases thereby and this can necessitate expensive additional computer hardware. One approach to this problem is to minimize the diameter of the detector array. This approach has been developed in one commercial scanner in which the source rotates outside of the detector ring. In this system, the detector ring wobbles or "nutates," so that the near portion of the ring does not block the source fan.

The technical tradeoffs among the various scanner types are difficult to evaluate. In general, rotary scanners have faster scan speed and fewer motion streak artifacts than the translate-rotate type. The stationary detector array version requires more, but less accurate, detectors than do the rotary detector designs. Slow scanners (1 to 2 minutes) may be suitable for brain scanning when patient volume is low because the head can usually be effectively immobilized. Body scanning, particularly in the thorax and upper abdomen, usually requires a scan time of less than a breath-holding interval (20 seconds). Faster rotary scanners (2 to 5 seconds) are less apt to be affected by streaks caused by peristaltic motion of the bowel.

Important commercial competitive factors currently include image quality and dose, scan speed, processing speed, and economic considerations. Other features that appear to be of value are variable-slice thickness, variable field size (by direct magnification or through software), high- and low-sensitivity scan selection, advanced reconstruction algorithms that correct the beam-hardening effect, cursors for outlining regions of interest, sagittal and coronal reconstructions, dual-energy scans, and so forth. All of these features are already available on many commercial scanners.

The assessment of comparative image quality and dose is often a complex task. Some manufacturers can provide contrast-detail graphs at various dose levels that provide a rather complete description of the detection capability of the scanner as a function of object size. Many phantoms are available that can be scanned in a given machine to produce similar information in semi-quantitative form. Any study of image quality must include consideration of the occurrence of image-degrading artifacts, particularly the streak artifacts. Perhaps the best "phantom" for evaluating the frequency and intensity of streaks is the body of an actual patient that contains the necessary high-contrast, streak-producing edges and moving structures. When evaluating patient CT images, it is important to know whether the images are selected as the "best" or whether they are representative of a typical series of clinical images.

Cost is an important consideration that must take into consideration the patient load and expected throughput as well as the initial installation and maintenance charges. Patient throughput depends on a number of factors that vary considerably among the various scanners. These include:

1. Image processing time.
2. Scanning time (including the tube-cooling cycle).
3. Image display, analysis, storage, and retrieval.
4. Facilities for patient preparation and staging.

IMAGE NOISE, ARTIFACTS, AND IMAGE QUALITY

The evaluation of image quality in computed tomography can proceed at various levels. In the ideal (but impractical) situation, each number in the CT image will be directly related to the average linear attenuation coefficient within the corresponding volume element in the original object. Further, the relationship would be identical for each picture element. For a variety of reasons and in various ways, the picture elements of the final image will not be consistently related to the original distribution through the object. Generally, such variations in the final image are referred to as artifacts and are often given names that relate to their appearance in the image or their cause. In this section we describe several of the more common sources of artifacts and the manner in which they may be manifested in the final image.

The sources of artifacts may be divided into several classes:

1. Random noise, such as that due to quantum statistics and electronic noise.
2. Periodic noise, such as x-ray intensity ripple.
3. Geometric limitations, such as finite numbers of detectors, and the width of the x-ray source and detector elements.
4. Polychromatic x-ray spectra.
5. Instrument deficiencies and failures.
6. Object-related artifacts, such as x-ray scatter, x-ray opaque regions, and object motion.

RANDOM NOISE

Because the dose to the patient is directly related to the number of photons incident on the patient, it is desirable to obtain the best image quality for the fewest number of photons. It is therefore best that the major source of artifact in the CT image be due to the number of x-ray photons detected and that all other sources of image artifact and degradation be kept below this level. When counting photons, the variance in the measurement is about equal to the number of photons counted. The measured intensity can thus be considered as the expected number of photons (the value consistent with the "true" attenuation experienced) plus some random error. Because of the reconstruction process, the random noise becomes correlated in the final image, generating characteristic CT noise.[16]

In addition to random noise resulting from photon statistics, there is also random noise from other sources, such as current detection electronics and digitizing electronics, which are also present and which result in noise in the final image essentially identical to photon noise.

GEOMETRIC ARTIFACTS

As suggested earlier, ideal image quality requires an infinite number of views and samples (rays) per view in such a manner that measurements are made along every possible line through the plane of the object. If some compromises are made in the size of object that can be resolved and in the amount of fine structure that can exist in the object, it is possible to achieve reasonable image quality with a finite number of views and a finite number of rays per view. Generally, with a finite number of rays per view, streaks will occur in the final image and will be found to emanate from sharp (high-contrast) edges and small structures of high density. These artifacts are often referred to as aliasing artifacts and related directly to the ability of the scanner to resolve fine detail with a finite sample spacing.

The number of views necessary relates directly to the desired spatial resolution, the number of rays per view, and the angular symmetry of the object. If insufficient numbers of views are used, streaks will be found to occur at large distances from very dense points.

Many other sources of geometric error can exist. If the center of rotation is not the same as that used by the reconstruction program, the image in a full 360-degree scanner will be blurred. In 180-degree scanners, this error causes an artifact that resembles a tuning fork around dense points. Imprecise or inaccurate detector positioning can result in streaks. The positioning of individual detector elements must be very accurate in rotate-rotate geometries or rings will result. Streaks can also result if the x-ray fan beam profile is not uniformly thick, thus causing some dense, out-of-plane structures to be included in only part of the scan.

NONLINEAR ARTIFACTS

There are several sources of image degradation that occur because the physical implementation of CT deviates from the assumed simple mathematics.

Edge Gradient and Partial Volume Artifacts

The reconstruction mathematics assumes that measurements are made along lines of negligible thickness. If strips are used, the mathematics still applies if the projected density (i.e., attenuation coefficient) is averaged over the strip width. Unfortunately, the intensity is averaged over the strip width. Taking the logarithm of the averaged intensity ratio does not yield the average projected attenuation coefficient. The difference is largest in the presence of dense edges or small points that are only partially included within the strip width. This inconsistency results in streaks from edges and small, dense, points.[17]

X-ray Spectral Artifacts

The reconstruction mathematics assumes also that the attenuation coefficient at each point is constant for all radiation beams that sample that point. This is not the case for the broad diagnostic x-ray spectra used in CT x-ray tubes. Because the linear attenuation coefficient is a function of x-ray energy, it is found that more of the lower-energy x-ray photons are removed from the beam during the traverse of an object. In this manner, the farther a beam passes through an object, the more penetrating it becomes. Because those rays that pass through the edges of the object are hardened less than those passing through the center, the apparent attenuation coefficient is less at the center than the edges. Thus a cupping or decrease in CT numbers is found to occur near the center of the reconstructed image. This result is sometimes referred to as the *beam-hardening artifact.* In the case of soft tissues that are all similar in attenuation coefficient energy dependence, it is possible to correct this artifact using a simple table look-up procedure.[18]

Polychromatic artifacts are caused by the fact that bone attenuation differs considerably in energy dependence from soft tissue. Streaks tend to occur between dense, high atomic number structures such as bones. This artifact can often be superimposed on partial volume streaks originating from the same bones.

X-ray Intensity Fluctuations

Fluctuation in x-ray intensity appears to be a problem in rotate-stationary geometries. The rotation of the anode can cause a periodic fluctuation in the x-ray intensity that appears in the image as circular moire pattern.[19] For scanner fan angles less than about 39°, this artifact can be completely eliminated by adjusting the scan speed or anode rotation speed. If a transient spike occurs in the x-ray intensity, it is likely that streaks may occur in the final image.

X-ray Scatter

Scattered radiation that originates from photons removed from the primary beam in the object results in an artifact that is similar to beam hardening and can lead to cupping or streaks.[20] Scattered radiation can contribute several per cent of the signal recorded by detectors that are exposed to the more highly attenuated beams. Rotate-rotate scanners have much more efficient scatter collimation than rotate-stationary scanners and hence less artifact.

INSTRUMENT FAILURES

Many severe problems can occur when the CT machinery is not functioning properly. When a detector channel does not function or when the detector does not respond uniformly, the resulting inconsistency will appear as an artifact in the image. In translate-rotate or rotate-stationary designs, the artifact is generally minimal, appearing only as a low-level shift in CT numbers, similar to beam hardening. In rotate-rotate geometries, the artifact is a "ring" in the final image.

OBJECT MOTION

If any part of the object moves during the course of the scan, "tuning fork"-like streaks can occur, depending upon how the motion occurred relative to the scan sequence. The intensity of this streak is dependent on the speed of the scanner relative to the speed of motion.[21] The accumulated motion between the start and end of the scan causes an inconsistency between 0-degree and 180-degree profiles leading to the most common motion streak. A small number of additional projections (i.e., overscan to 230° or so) is used to provide data that blend or "feather" the inconsistencies over a range of angles and thus reduce the intensity of this artifact.[22]

IMAGE QUALITY

The quality of the CT image can be described in terms of spatial resolution and contrast resolution. *Spatial resolution,* or "sharpness," describes the amount of blurring of a point, line, or edge in the object. The detailed character of the blurring of a point or line is indicated by the point-spread function (PSF) or line-spread-function (LSF). For most current CT scanners, these functions are approximately gaussian shaped and have a full width at half maximum of 1 to 3 mm. Spatial resolution as defined in this way is independent of x-ray intensity and dose.

Spatial resolution is sometimes confused with

the term *resolving power*. Resolving power is a measure of the minimum separation distance between two objects such as line pairs for which the separation can be resolved. Resolving power depends not only on spatial resolution but also on object contrast and noise or contrast resolution.

Contrast resolution (sometimes referred to as *density resolution*) depends on the amount of variability or scatter in the CT numbers of a uniform object and is strongly dependent on x-ray intensity and dose. This scatter arises from random photon statistical noise, such as grain, and from artifactual structured noise, such as streaks. Contrast resolution in all imaging systems depends on the object size, since the magnitude of noise fluctuations can be reduced in large areas by spatial averaging.

Contrast resolution depends on the random fluctuations or noise in the background averaged over areas comparable in size to the object of interest. This noise may be estimated by computing the standard deviation of the mean for square area elements of width, w, using a CT image of a uniform phantom such as a cylinder of water. When w is equal to the pixel size $\sigma_m(w)$ is the standard deviation of the pixel values or the pixel noise, an often quoted number. However, the pixel noise is not a good indicator of the noise or contrast resolution for large areas. The function $\sigma_m(w)$ for a typical scanner is plotted in Figure 1–10 as the dashed curve. Theoretical treatments[23] indicate that $\sigma_m(w)$ varies as the $w^{-3/2}$ due to a unique short-range noise correlation in CT scanning.

In order to take advantage of the improved contrast resolution for larger objects, we must depend on the observer's eye to perform the necessary averaging. For example, an observer whose eyes have an LSF equivalent to 1 milliradian will optimally view a CT image if viewing distance is 1000 times greater than the size of the object to be detected. A typical CT image recorded as a Polaroid picture is reduced by about a factor of 6 from the original. If we wish to detect a 1 cm lesion in the liver, for instance, the optimal viewing distance would be $1000/6 = 170$ cm. Alternatively, a minifying lens can be used to stimulate the effect of an increase in the viewing distance.

A convenient way to express the contrast resolution or detectability of CT as a function of object contrast and size is in terms of the contrast-detail diagram. This diagram is a graph of the

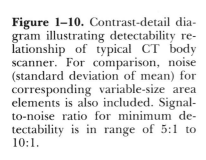

Figure 1–10. Contrast-detail diagram illustrating detectability relationship of typical CT body scanner. For comparison, noise (standard deviation of mean) for corresponding variable-size area elements is also included. Signal-to-noise ratio for minimum detectability is in range of 5:1 to 10:1.

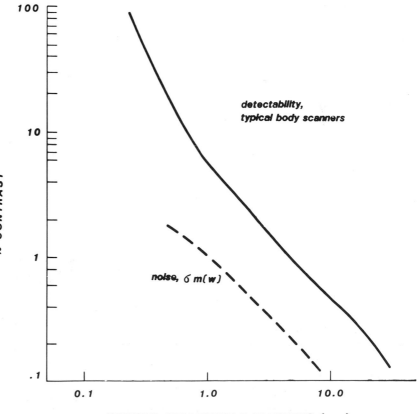

diameter of a minimum detectable object as a function of object contrast. A typical body scanner detectability curve is illustrated in Figure 1–10. The meaning of contrast is in this case as follows:

$$\frac{\mu_L \text{ (object)} - \mu_L \text{ (background)}}{\mu_L \text{ (object)}},$$

where the μ_L is the linear attenuation coefficient of the object and background. The detectability curve is approximately five times higher than the $\sigma_m(w)$ curve for the same scanner, indicating a signal-to-noise ratio of 5:1 at optimal detectability. This implies that a signal-to-noise ratio of greater than about 5:1 is necessary for object detection in this scanner. A similar detectability curve for a conventional radiographic system would be several times higher than this CT example for thick body parts in the region of w greater than 2 mm. However, for very small details (w less than 1 mm), conventional radiographic systems are generally superior, reflecting the high spatial resolution of such systems, compared with CT.

A convenient rule for remembering the contrast-detail characteristics of a given scanner is to recognize that the product of $\sigma_m(w)$ times w is nearly a constant in the region of a few millimeters to a few centimeters.[24] In the example of Figure 1–10, $\sigma_m(w) \times w \approx 1.5$ per cent mm. Thus $\sigma_m(10$ mm)≈ 0.15 per cent and we may expect to detect 10-mm lesions with a contrast of 5×0.15 or 0.75 per cent. Similarly, detectability would be 0.37 per cent at 20 mm. The function $\sigma_m(w) \times w$ is referred to as the noise granularity and ranges from about 0.5 to 2 per cent mm for many commercial scanners.[25]

If the scanned projection data contain no inconsistencies or errors of the type that produce artifacts, the noise levels in the CT image depend on the total number of detected photons, n, and vary according to the $\sqrt{n}$ law of Poisson statistics. For example, contrast resolution can be improved by a factor of 2 by increasing the number of photons and hence the absorbed dose by a factor of 4. In one body scanner, an optional slow scan—some four times slower than normal—is available for this purpose. In most CT scanners, the amount of the dose can be varied by adjusting tube current to produce the minimum acceptable level of contrast resolution required for a particular examination. Typical CT examination doses are in the range of 0.5 to 5 rads. Since contrast resolution depends on the number of detected photons, ideally all the radiation would be detected after exiting the body with no additional loss because of postpatient collimators, attenuators, or poor detector efficiency. Such a scanner would make maximal use of the photon beam and could be thought of as having a dose efficiency of

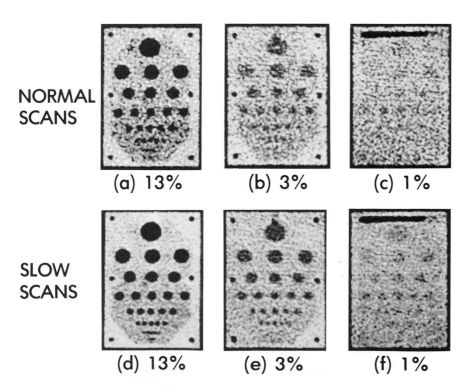

NORMAL SCANS

(a) 13%   (b) 3%   (c) 1%

SLOW SCANS

(d) 13%   (e) 3%   (f) 1%

Figure 1–11. EMI-5000 phantom scans. CT images of rods of 13 per cent or 3 per cent contrast (lowered density relative to background). Rod diameters are 15, 12, 9, 6, 4, 2, 1, and 0.5 mm. These comparisons indicate dependence of detectability and resolving power on size, contrast, and noise.

100 per cent. Current scanners appear to operate below 50 per cent dose efficiency, but a definite trend toward higher efficiencies exists.

Because spatial and contrast resolution are independent imaging characteristics, we do not need to seek an optimum tradeoff between the two as in collimators used in nuclear medicine gamma cameras or as in the selection of various film-screen combinations in ordinary radiography. In CT, spatial resolution is controlled by selecting the total number and spacing of independent samples in the projection data. In practice this may be accomplished by providing a sufficient number of detector elements in the detector array. By increasing the number of detectors (and reducing their size) with no change in collimation or total number of photons, spatial resolution may be improved independent of contrast resolution. In practical systems, spatial resolution is often determined by the limited capacity of the computer to store and process large data and image matrices economically.

Some examples of CT images of a resolving power phantom are given in Figure 1–11. As previously mentioned, the resolving power depends on both spatial and contrast resolution. In the four examples given, object contrast and noise were varied and the effect on resolving power is evident. The phantom in Figure 1–11 consists of fluid-filled holes in Lucite ranging from 8 to 1

mm in diameter. A 13 per cent contrast fluid (water) was used on the left and a 3 per cent contrast fluid was used on the right. The lower two images were low-noise in the high-contrast, low-noise examples.

Similarly, resolving power is a strong function of spatial resolution or sharpness. Figure 1–12 schematically illustrates the effect of varying spatial sharpness and noise amplitude on resolving power. The two systems represented in the lower left and upper right have comparable resolving power. An example of images from two such systems using two actual commercial scanners is included in Figure 1–13. Here a phantom consisting of water-filled holes in acrylic (13 per cent contrast) ranging from 3 to 1 mm was used. The system on the lower left has low noise but poor sharpness. The system at the upper right has good sharpness but a high noise level.

PRECISION AND ACCURACY

A further aspect of CT image quality is reflected in the numerical precision and accuracy of the measured CT numbers. These values are important in tissue characterization studies and bone mineral quantitation. *Precision* describes the ability of a CT scanner to reproduce the same mean CT number in the same region of the same patient at a later scan. *Accuracy* refers to our ability to relate a given mean CT number to the true

Figure 1–12. Schematic illustration of effect of noise and sharpness on resolving power. Curves represent CT numbers of pixels along path passing through two nearby holes in CT image of resolving power phantom. As noise increases, fluctuations in CT number increase, tending to decrease ability to resolve nearby peaks. However, width of peaks decreases as spatial sharpness increases, and peaks may be readily resolved even in presence of rather substantial noise fluctuations. Computed tomographic images of resolving power phantom using sharp but high-noise CT scanner and less sharp, low-noise scanner are included as examples. Resolving powers of these two scanners are comparable, as indicated in corresponding schematic illustrations.

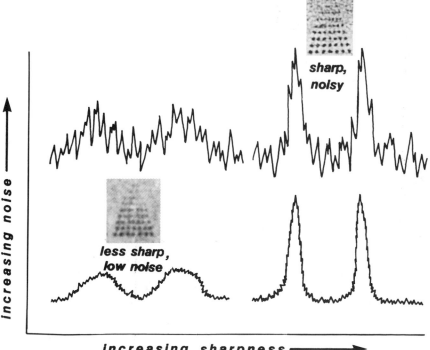

increasing noise

sharp, noisy

less sharp, low noise

increasing sharpness ⟶

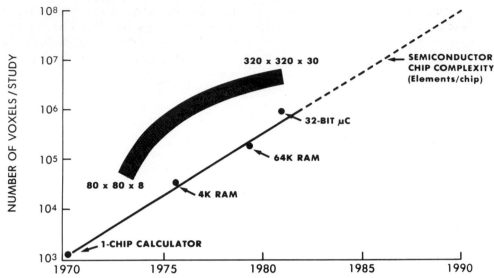

Figure 1–13. Comparison of CT picture resolution with semiconductor chip complexity. The number of elements or the most complex single chip doubled every year for the past decade, (1970–1980) and this trend is expected to continue in the future. Computed tomographic scanners use chips in the detector arrays, data acquisition systems, reconstruction processors, and display memory. The number of picture elements reconstructed in a typical CT study has tended to follow this trend, since CT manufacturers are quick to adopt the latest available semiconductor circuits. The original CT scanner used a matrix size of 80×80 in a slice, and typically eight slices were used per study. Today, matrices of 320×320 or even 512×512 are used, and often 30 or more slices are scanned. This represents a factor of a 64-fold increase in 8 years.

linear attenuation coefficient at a mean photon energy. The advent of the "air" scan, which replaces the water bag of the original head scanners, has often been accompanied by a serious loss of both precision and accuracy. Precision is important when a particular patient needs to be followed during therapy, such as for bone mineral loss. Accuracy is important for identifying specific tissues, such as in the distinction between a cyst and a solid mass—often a difference of less than ten CT numbers. Factors affecting the accuracy of CT scanners include the beam-hardening artifact, detector inaccuracy (nonlinearity), motion artifacts, partial volume effects, calibration errors, and scattered radiation.

FUTURE DEVELOPMENT OF COMPUTED TOMOGRAPHY

The rapid acceptance of CT scanning as a primary tool in x-ray diagnosis is based primarily on its ability to image soft-tissue pathologies without the need for invasive interventions such as catheterization. At each stage of CT development, new applications have been introduced as improvements in speed and resolution have been achieved. Scanning speed is important to reduce

motion blurring and motion artifacts resulting from involuntary patient motion. Resolution aids in differentiating smaller anatomic structures or detecting edges.

CT has already improved in scan speed by a factor of 300 based on the introduction of fan beam and linear detector array technology to replace the initial two-motion scanners with one-motion rotary machines. Future developments will involve the replacement of the mechanically scanned rotary source with either an electron-beam sweep (CVCT) scanner[26–28] or electronic triggering of a series of fixed sources (DSR).[29] Dynamic scanning capability has increased in a similar fashion since increasing the x-ray fan width provides increased source utilization and reduces heat loading. However, future advances in scan speed and rate of repetition will need to be based on increasing the amount of tungsten in the source, either by using larger x-ray tubes or multiple tubes.

CT scanner resolving power has been increasing as well and stood at approximately 0.8 mm in 1982 with a value of 0.1 mm projected by 1990. Resolving power and resolution depend fundamentally on the number of ray samples obtained during a scan, which in turn depend on the numbers of detectors and their sampling rate; this is heavily dependent on advances in semiconductor

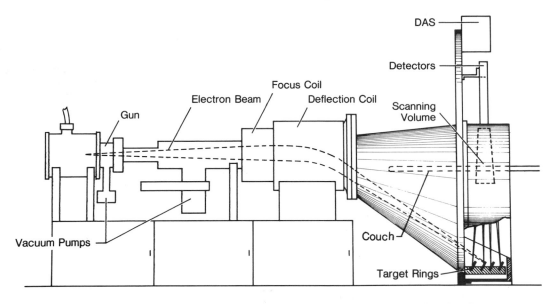

Figure 1–14. Illustration of a millisecond, multislice, beam CT scanner under development. Up to eight slices within the indicated scanning volume can be obtained without the use of mechanical motion of either scanner or patient. The basic scanning time of any pair of slices is 33 or 50 ms.

technology. Since semiconductor technology is expected to continue advancing at a rapid pace (Fig. 1–13), CT can be expected to follow. The startling conclusion is that CT may approach the capabilities of current angiographic techniques in both speed and spatial resolution within the next decade. This fundamental ability of CT to improve substantially in performance is the basis for viewing CT as a promising three-dimensional approach to noninvasive diagnosis.

The principal new application of future, high-speed multislice scanners is in cardiac diagnosis, one of the most important medical problems to-day. The goal of such devices is to improve the screening of heart disease patients who are asymptomatic or who have early symptoms, to improve the management of acute cardiac patients, and to provide an interval screening method to evaluate the effectiveness of therapeutic interventions.

The full applications of cardiac CT procedures await the demonstration of an economic CT scanner with the following "minimum" specifications:

1. A 30- to 50-ms scan speed.
2. An eight-section volume scan in 100 to 200 ms.

Figure 1–15. Cardiovascular CT (CVCT) scanner during construction at the University of California, San Francisco, in March 1982. The electron gun at the far right injects an intense electron beam into a vacuum chamber. The beam is steered around the semicircular target rings contained within the partial-cone vacuum chamber at the left, using focus and deflection coils at the center. Multiple levels of fan beam penetrate the thin window in the cone and are collimated and detected in a collimator system and detector array that will be mounted on the large flange (360°) that surrounds the patient.

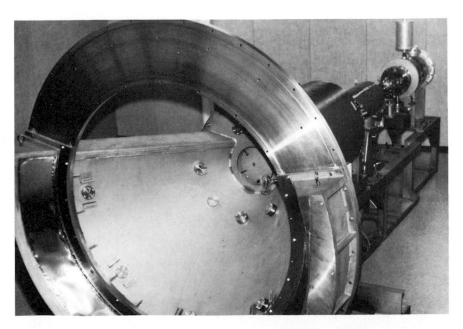

3. Volume scans repeatable at one per second.

4. Spatial and density resolution comparable with current CT body scanners.

Several scanners have been proposed or built that satisfy some of these specifications but not all of them simultaneously. Gated CT scanners meet the first and fourth requirements but not the second and third.[30] The Mayo Clinic DSR scanner meets and exceeds the first, second, and third specifications for limited-angle scanning but does not have the performance required by the fourth. Such scanners are valuable research tools and can perform many types of imaging studies but do not have the broad capability required for general-purpose cardiac CT clinical use.

The cardiovascular CT (CVCT) under development at the University of California, San Francisco, is a good example of an advanced scanner that addresses the requirements of cardiac imaging. The CVCT system (Fig. 1–14) consists of an electron-beam scan tube, a stationary detector array, and a computer data acquisition, reconstruction, and display system. An electron beam is accelerated and focused along the axis of the machine. A bending magnet deflects the beam and rapidly sweeps it along a curved tungsten target of 210° in 33 or 50 ms. Four target rings are available and are typically scanned serially to obtain a multiple-section examination. Ring collimators near the source confine the x-ray beam to a wide fan 2 cm thick directed at the patient. A fan-shaped sector of this beam (approximately 30°) is detected by a curved detector array, and the signals are utilized to reconstruct the tomographic image. The detector array consist of two rings of scintillation crystals coupled to multielement photodiodes. A single scan will thus produce a pair of side-by-side tomographic sections. For each target sweep, a pair of sections 1 cm thick are scanned. The collection of eight sections covers a region approximately 9 cm deep, large enough to cover all of the left ventricle and most of the heart of typical patient, even with only approximate positioning. A high-speed data-acquisition and 32-megabyte fast memory will permit cine-CT scanning sequences at a speed of 25 frames per second. Since two side-by-side slices are acquired simultaneously, the CVCT will generate more than 50 CT images per second.

The completed CVCT prototype was undergoing initial tests late in 1982, after the cone vacuum chamber had been installed (Fig. 1–15). The multiple-target ring, 840-element detector system, sequence and scan controller, and data acquisition system were developed by Imatron Associates, South San Francisco, California. These components were installed in the fall of 1982 and tested and debugged during the following months. The CVCT is undergoing extensive evaluation studies at the University of California, San Francisco Medical Center.

REFERENCES

1. Radon J: Über die Bestimmung von Funktionen durch ihre Integralwerte längs gewisser Mannigfaltigkeiten. Saechsische Akademie der Wissenschaften, Leipzig, Berichte über die Verhandlungen 69:262–277, 1917.
2. Shepp LA, Logan BF: Reconstruction in interior head tissue from x-ray transmissions. IEEE Trans Nucl Sci NS-21:228, 1974.
3. Brooks RA, DiChiro RA: Theory of image reconstruction in computed tomography. Radiology 117:561, 1975.
4. Brooks RA, DiChiro G: Principles of reconstructive tomography, Phys Med Biol 21:5, 1976.
5. Herman GT: Image Reconstruction from Projections: The Fundamentals of Computerized Tomography. New York, Academic Press, 1980.
6. Newton TH, Potts DG (eds): Radiology of the Skull and Brain, vol V: Technical Aspects of Computerized Tomography. St. Louis, CV Mosby, 1981.
7. Ter-Pogossian MM, et al (eds): Reconstruction Tomography in Diagnostic Radiology and Nuclear Medicine. Baltimore, University Park Press, 1977.
8. Takahashi S: Rotational radiography. Tokyo, Tokyo Japan Society for the Promotion of Science, 1957.
9. Bracewell RN: Strip integration in radio astronomy, Aust J Phys 9:198, 1956.
10. DeRosier DJ, Klug A: Reconstruction of three-dimensional structures from electron micrographs. Nature 217:130, 1968.
11. Cormack AM: Representation of a function by its line integrals with some radiological applications. J Appl Physiol 34:2722, 1963; 35:2908, 1964.
12. Kuhl DE, Edwards RQ: Cylindrical and section radioisotope scanning of the liver and brain. Radiology 83:926, 1964.
13. Hounsfield GN: A method of an apparatus for examination of the body by radiation such as X or gamma radiation. British patent No. 1283915, 1972.
14. Dreike R, Boyd DP: Convolution reconstruction of fan beam projections. Computer Graphics and Image Processing 5:459, 1976.
15. Lakshminavayanan AV: Reconstruction from divergent ray data. Buffalo, Department of Computer Science, State University of New York at Buffalo, Technical Report 92, 1975.
16. Hansen KM, Boyd DP: The characteristics of computed tomographic reconstruction noise and their effect on detectability. IEEE Trans Nucl Sci NS-25:160, 1978.
17. Joseph P: Artifacts in CT. In Newton TH, Potts DG (eds): Radiology of the Skull and Brain, vol V. St Louis, CV Mosby, 1981.
18. McCullough EC: Photon attenuation in computed tomography. Med Phys 2:307, 1975.

19. Parker DL, Couch JL, Peschmann KR, Smith V: Structured noise in computed tomography: Effects of periodic error sources. Med Phys 9:722, 1982.
20. Joseph PM, Spital RD: The effects of scatter in x-ray computed tomography. Med Phys 9(4):464, 1982.
21. Boyd DP, Korobkin MT, Moss A: Engineering status of computerized-tomographic scanning. SPIE Applied Optical Instrumentation in Medicine V 96:303, 1976.
22. Parker DL, Smith V, Stanley JH: Dose minimization in computed tomography overscanning, Med Phys 8:706, 1981.
23. Chesler DA, Riederer SJ, Pelc NJ: Noise due to photon counting statistics in computed x-ray tomography. J Comput Assist Tomogr 1:64, 1977.
24. Boyd D, Margulis AR, Korobkin M: Comparison of translate-rotate and pure rotary body scanners. SPIE Applied Optical Instrumentation in Medicine VI 127:280, 1977.
25. Cohen G: Contrast-detail-dose analysis of six different computed tomographic scanners. J Comput Assist Tomogr 3:197, 1979.
26. Boyd DP: Future technologies: Transmission CT. In Newton, TH, Potts DG (eds): Radiology of the Skull and Brain, vol V. St Louis, CV Mosby, 1981, pp 4357–4371.
27. Boyd DP: Computerized-transmission tomography of the heart using scanning electron beams. In Higgins C (ed): CTT of the Heart: Experimental Evaluation and Clinical Application. Mt Kisco, New York (in press).
28. Boyd DP, Gould RG, Quinn JR, Sparks R, Stanley JA, Herrmannsfeldt WB: A proposed dynamic cardiac 3-D densitometer for early detection and evaluation of heart disease. IEEE Trans Nucl Sci NS-26:2724, 1979.
29. Ritman EL, Kinsey JH, Robb RA, Harris L, Gilbert BK: Physics and technical considerations in the design of the DSR: A high temporal resolution volume scanner. AJR 134:369, 1980.
30. Berninger W, Redington R, Leue W, Axel L, Norman D, Brundage B, Carlsson E, Herfkens R, Lipton M: Technical aspects and clinical application of CT/X, a dynamic CT scanner. J Comput Assist Tomogr 5:206, 1981.

2 COMPUTED TOMOGRAPHY OF THE NECK

Anthony A. Mancuso

ANATOMY

The neck is separated from the floor of the mouth by the mylohyoid muscle, which originates from the myloid line of the mandible and runs obliquely and inferiorly to insert into the hyoid bone.[1] The inferior extent of the neck is the thoracic inlet, which is in an oblique plane from the suprasternal (jugular) notch to the first thoracic vertebra. For description purposes and the interpretation of computed tomography (CT) images, it is useful to divide the neck into several compartments (Fig. 2–1).

The visceral compartment of the neck is the most anterior and contains the structures of the aerodigestive tract, including the larynx, hypopharynx, trachea, and esophagus. The thyroid and parathyroid glands also lie within the visceral compartment. The infrahyoid strap muscles arise from the laryngeal skeleton and insert on the anterosuperior chest wall, forming the anterior boundary of the visceral compartment. More laterally, the sternocleidomastoid muscles extend from their relatively posterior origin on the mastoid process of the temporal bone to insert on the sternum and clavicle. The sternocleidomastoid muscle is a prominent landmark in cross sections of the neck, and although its course is quite oblique, it is for the most part seen laterally. Most important, it overlies the carotid sheaths, which are the major components of the paired compartments lateral to the viscera of the neck.

The cervical spinal cord, the spine, and the surrounding musculature form a fourth compartment posteriorly. The submandibular salivary glands are divided by the mylohyoid muscle and therefore are contained within both the floor of the mouth and the upper neck. The parotid glands also traverse the boundaries between the head and neck.

VISCERAL COMPARTMENT

In the upper neck, the larynx and hypopharynx occupy the visceral compartment. (These structures are described in detail in Chapter 3.) Figures 2–2A–E and 2–3A–D show the CT appearance of normal variations in the anatomic relationships of structures in the visceral compartment of the lower and upper neck.

The cricoid cartilage is a major landmark for several of these structures. The rounded, somewhat elliptic soft-tissue density just posterior to

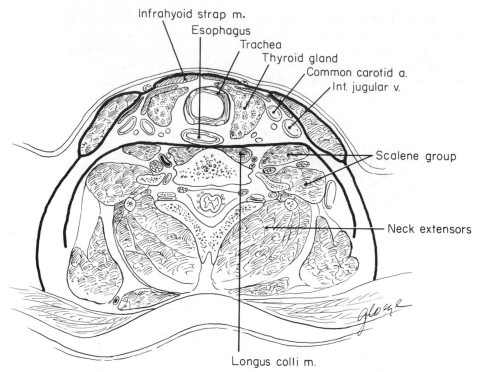

Figure 2–1. Schema of the neck. Heavy black lines show investing layer of deep cervical fascia and prevertebral fascia. Topographically, the neck is separated into the visceral compartment, which is located around the midline anteriorly; two lateral compartments, which contain mainly structures of carotid sheath; and the posterior compartment, which contains the cervical spine and its surrounding muscles. (From Mancuso AA, Hanafee WN: Computed Tomography of the Head and Neck. © 1982, The Williams & Wilkins Company, Baltimore. Reprinted by permission.)

the middle portion of the cricoid lamina represents the cricopharyngeal muscle and upper cervical esophagus (Fig. 2–2C,D). Inferiorly, the esophagus is visible as a slightly smaller soft-tissue density posterior to the trachea in the midline (Fig. 2–2A,B). At the thoracic inlet the esophagus frequently deflects very slightly to the left of the midline. The lower margin of the cricoid cartilage forms a complete ring; below this, the incomplete rings of the upper trachea are a prominent landmark in the center of the visceral compartment. The tracheal rings themselves may not be visible if they are incompletely mineralized. The posterior wall of the trachea is usually slightly convex anteriorly because the cartilaginous rings are incomplete posteriorly. The trachea normally remains midline in position through the lower neck and into the thoracic inlet and upper mediastinum.

The thyroid and parathyroid glands are at the level of and immediately below the lower margin of the cricoid cartilage. The lobes of the thyroid gland are usually seen as wedge-shaped areas of increased CT density on either side of the trachea in the lower neck (Fig. 2–2B). The upper poles of the thyroid gland can usually be seen along the posterolateral margins of the cricoid cartilage

near its articulations with the inferior horns of the thyoid cartilage (Fig. 2–2C). During intravenous infusion of iodinated contrast medium, the thyroid gland becomes much more dense than on unenhanced images. The normal parathyroid glands are not visible on CT scans of the neck; however, the inferior thyroid arteries and veins can usually be seen in the fat posterior to each lobe of the thyroid gland and anterior to the longus colli muscles (Fig. 2–2B). These tiny vessels (less than 5 mm in diameter) represent the anatomic location of the normal parathyroid glands.

LATERAL COMPARTMENT

The carotid sheaths and their surrounding fat form the two lateral compartments of the neck. The internal jugular vein lies posterior to the carotid artery in the upper neck, becomes progressively more lateral to the artery in the middle neck, and lies somewhat anterior to the artery in the lower neck (Figs. 2–2B–E and 2–3A–D). The jugular fossa lies posterior to the carotid canal at the base of the skull, whereas the venous structures lie superficial to the brachiocephalic arteries in the lower neck and upper mediastinum, where the arterial structures arise from the more posteriorly situated aortic arch. The common carotid artery bifurcates at approximately the level of the hyoid bone. Numerous tributaries enter the jugular veins, and CT scans show these as rounded densities around the carotid sheath. They are indistinguishable from enlarged nodes unless the vessels are opacified.

The deep cervical lymph nodes are divided into three groups: upper, middle, and lower (Fig. 2–4A). The most prominent node in the upper deep cervical group is the jugulodigastric node,

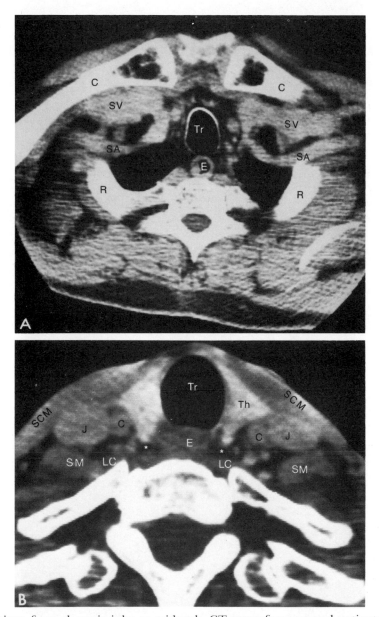

Figure 2–2. Sections from thoracic inlet to midneck. CT scans from several patients during intravenous contrast infusion. **A**   Section through thoracic inlet shows subclavian vein (SV) and subclavian artery (SA) as they enter thorax below the clavicle (C) and above first rib (R). Visceral compartment of neck is represented by trachea (Tr) and esophagus (E) in the midline. Brachiocephalic vessels surround airway. **B**   Sections at level above thoracic inlet. High CT density thyroid gland (Th) is distinguished from surrounding tissues. Esophagus (E) lies behind trachea (Tr). Small enhancing structures behind thyroid gland and in front of longus colli muscles (LC) are thyrocervical vessels. Parathyroid glands are located within small fatty space just lateral to esophagus and behind thyroid gland (asterisks). Common carotid artery (C) and jugular vein (J) lie lateral to thyroid gland and anterior to scalene muscle (SM). Sternocleidomastoid muscle (SCM) lies anterolaterally.

Illustration continued on following page

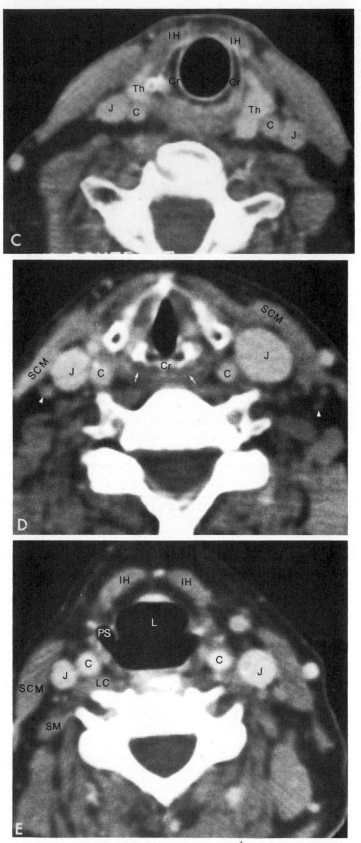

Figure 2–2. *See legend on opposite page*

which is located where the posterior belly of the digastric muscle crosses the internal jugular vein.[1] The jugulo-omohyoid node is located at the crossing of the jugular vein and omohyoid muscle[1] and is therefore at the junction of the upper and middle deep cervical groups. The nodes of the posterior triangle lie behind the internal jugular vein. The retropharyngeal lymph nodes are not accessible to physical examination. They lie above the level of the jugulodigastric node, medial to the internal carotid artery, and extend to the base of the skull.[1]

Three other groups of nodes in the neck are less often studied by CT. The submental nodes are usually palpable. The submandibular nodes surround the submandibular gland and lie just below and lateral to the plane of the mylohyoid muscle; their territory extends from the middle of the mandibular ramus to the mandibular angle. The intraparotid and periparotid nodes lie within and around the parotid gland.

Normal deep cervical nodes appear on CT scans as discrete, nonenhancing densities near the internal jugular vein and carotid artery (Fig. 2–4B).[2] They are usually 5 mm or less in diameter, with the exception of the jugulodigastric node, which normally can be up to 1.5 cm in diameter. Normal submandibular, submental, and periparotid nodes lying near the mandible or their respective salivary glands have a CT appearance similar to that of deep cervical nodes. Normal lymph nodes do not show central or peripheral (capsular) enhancement after intravenous infusion of contrast medium.[2]

Cranial nerves accompany the carotid sheaths from the base of the skull, and some remain with the vessels throughout their course in the neck. The ninth through the twelfth cranial nerves remain with the carotid sheath for at least part of its course through the neck, but they cannot be identified on CT scans. The recurrent laryngeal nerve travels with the minor neurovascular bundle (inferior thyroid artery and vein) to pierce the cricothyroid membrane and enter the lower portion of the larynx. The articulation of the inferior horn of the thyroid cartilage with the cricoid ring marks the location of the recurrent laryngeal nerve. The phrenic nerve lies near the scalene muscle group and is therefore considered with the posterior compartment of the neck.

POSTERIOR COMPARTMENT

The cervical vertebrae are surrounded by two major muscle groups. There is a group of extensor muscles that are mainly posterior to the transverse processes of the cervical vertebrae and a much smaller flexor group anterior to the transverse processes. The flexor muscles include the longus colli, longus capitis, rectus capitis, and scalene muscles (Fig. 2–1). The longus colli and longus capitis muscles lie anterior to the vertebral bodies and should not be mistaken for vascular or lymphatic structures on CT scans of the upper neck. These small muscles are symmetric and form elliptic densities that contact the anterolateral aspect of the vertebral bodies. Lower in the neck, their position assists in identifying the minor neurovascular bundle on CT scans.

The parathyroid glands lie along the course of the minor neurovascular bundle in the fat space bordered by the thyroid gland anteriorly, the longus colli muscle posteriorly, and the carotid artery laterally (Figs. 2–1 and 2–5). The scalene muscles arise from the transverse processes of the cervical vertebrae and sweep laterally with a gradual posterior curve. The levator scapulae muscles lie posterior to the scalene muscles and the phrenic nerve is anterior to the anterior scalene muscle.

A detailed knowledge of the fascia is not required to interpret CT scans of the neck. It is sufficient to understand that all of the musculature already described lies within a compartment that is limited anteriorly by the prevertebral fascia (Fig. 2–1). Posteriorly, the extensor muscle group is surrounded by the trapezius muscle, which is

Figure 2–2. *Continued* **C** Section through infraglottic larynx shows upper pole of the thyroid gland (Th) lateral to cricoid cartilage (Cr). Carotid artery (C) and jugular veins (J) are well opacified. Infrahyoid strap muscles (IH) form densities anterolateral to cricoid cartilage. **D** Section through level of true vocal cords. Visceral compartment is composed of larynx and postcricoid portion of cervical esophagus. Cricopharyngeal muscle (arrows) is posterior to cricoid cartilage (Cr). Sternocleidomastoid muscles overlie paired lateral carotid sheaths. Asymmetry in size of jugular veins is common and can be marked. Small nonenhancing densities posterior to jugular vein (J) and carotid artery (C) are normal lymph nodes (arrowheads). **E** Section through midneck at level of midsupraglottic larynx. Visceral compartment is formed by supraglottic larynx (L) and piriform sinuses (PS). Small normal nodes are found around carotid sheath. Infrahyoid strap muscles (IH) border larynx anteriorly. Longus colli muscles (LC) occur anterior to lateral masses of the cervical spine; scalene muscle group (SM) is directly lateral.

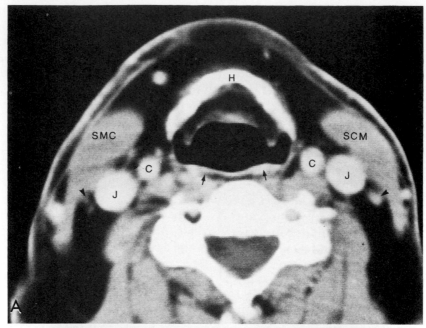

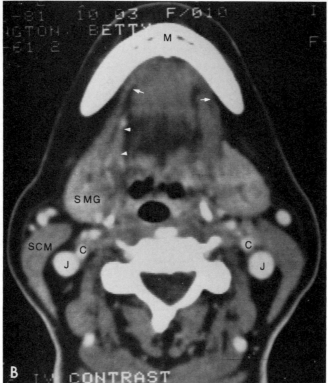

Figure 2–3. Sections from midneck to lower face. Scans illustrate normal anatomy of both neck and parotid and submandibular salivary glands. **A**   CT scan through supraglottic larynx at level of hyoid bone (H). Visceral compartment comprises supraglottic larynx and piriform sinuses. Fat within prevertebral space lies between cervical spine and pharyngeal constrictor (arrows). Carotid sheath structures are visible within the fat beneath the sternocleidomastoid muscle (SCM). Small nodes (arrowheads) are visible near carotid artery (C) and jugular veins (J). **B**   CT scan through lower oropharynx and floor of mouth. Mandible (M) is anterior. Mylohyoid muscle (arrows) separates the mouth from the upper neck. Jugular vein (J) has changed from lateral and anterior location low in neck to posterior to the carotid (C) artery higher in the neck. Small posterior triangle node visible on right behind jugular vein. Submandibular glands (SMG) enhance homogeneously and to slightly greater degree than surrounding muscles. Lingual vessels lie medial to submandibular gland within floor of mouth (arrowheads).

Illustration continued on opposite page

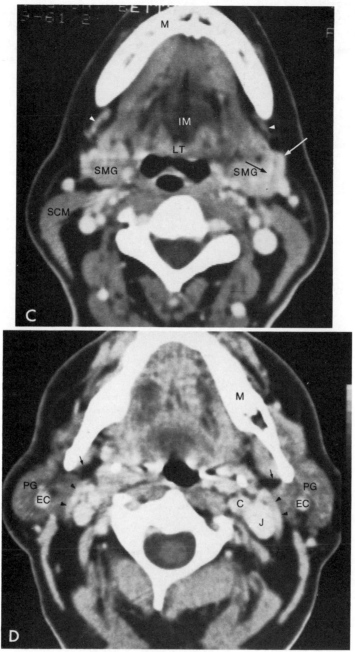

Figure 2–3. *Continued* **C**   CT scan, slightly higher than in **B** shows numerous branches of facial artery and vein coursing through and around submandibular gland (SMG), especially on left (arrows). Non-enhancing structures anterior to glands probably represent small, normal-sized lymph nodes (arrowheads). Submandibular glands enhance fairly homogeneously. The interface between base of the tongue and submandibular glands is usually visible as a result of differences in contrast medium enhancement. Normally enhancing lingual tonsil (LT) extends into intrinsic muscles (IM) of base of tongue. **D**   CT scan through the midoropharynx. Parotid glands (PG) wrap around angle and ramus of mandible (M). Their deep lobes abut a region of low CT density indicating parapharyngeal space (arrows). Mandibular vein and external carotid artery (EC) are within the substance of the gland. Digastric muscle (arrowheads) separates the parotid gland from the jugular vein (J) and carotid artery (C).

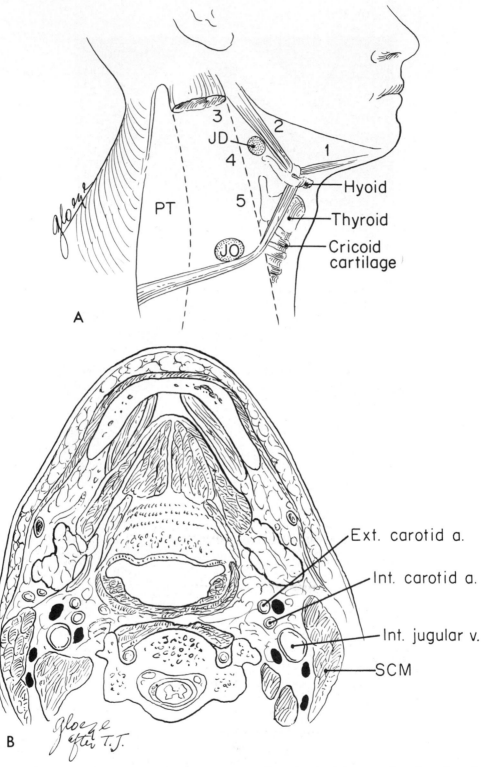

Figure 2–4. Lymph nodes of lateral compartments of neck. **A** Schema of various lymph node groups: (1) submental; (2) submandibular; and (3–5) upper, middle, and deep cervical groups. Jugulodigastric (JD) and juguloomohyoid (JO) nodes represent nodes of specific interest. The jugulodigastric node is below the posterior belly of digastric muscle. The posterior triangle (PT) nodes lie along spinal accessory nerves. **B** Typical locations of deep cervical lymph nodes (in black) in relation to the carotid sheath and surrounding muscles. SCM = Sternocleidomastoid muscle. (From Mancuso AA, Hanafee WN: Computed Tomography of the Head and Neck. © 1982, The Williams & Wilkins Company, Baltimore. Reprinted by permission.)

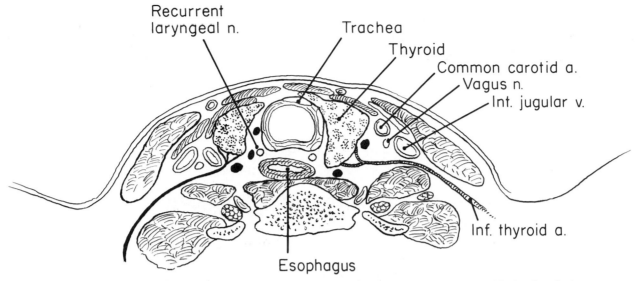

Figure 2–5. Cross section through lower neck. Anatomy of thyroid and parathyroid glands relative to structures in visceral compartment. Usual parathyroid locations (in black) are shown relative to inferior thyroid artery and recurrent laryngeal nerve. (From Mancuso AA, Hanafee WN: Computed Tomography of the Head and Neck. © 1982, The Williams & Wilkins Company, Baltimore. Reprinted by permission.)

surrounded by the investing layer of deep cervical fascia. Anteriorly and laterally, the investing layer of deep cervical fascia envelops the sternocleidomastoid muscle and courses anterior to the strap muscles (Fig. 2–1). The platysma can be seen on CT scans as a thin layer within the subcutaneous fat. Although it has no clinical significance, it should not be mistaken for normal or abnormally thickened fascia within the neck.

The cervical vertebrae, epidural space, dural sac, and cervical spinal cord are regularly visible on CT scans of the neck (Fig. 2–6). Intravenous injection of contrast medium usually produces enhancement of the epidural venous plexus, the venous plexus within the extensor muscle groups, and the vertebral arteries. CT scans with high spatial resolution can clearly define the relationship of lesions in the neck to the cervical neural

Figure 2–6. Posterior pharyngeal wall carcinoma. CT scan at level of hyoid bone shows relationship of the vertebral artery (arrow) to lateral masses. Contrast enhancement within epidural space is not prominent. (Higher in neck normal epidural enhancement, between bony spinal canal and dural sac, is more pronounced.) Also shown is relationship of neural foramina to soft tissues of the neck and various vessels.

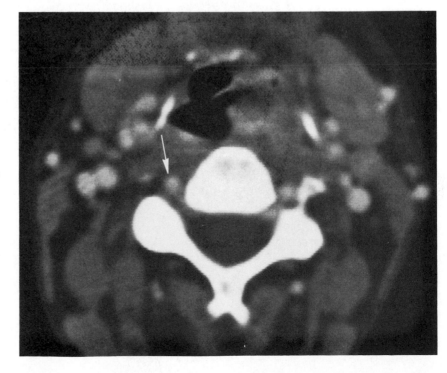

foramina, the cervical vertebral bodies, and the epidural space and cervical spinal cord. Abnormalities arising from any of these structures can often be identified and distinguished from secondary involvement.

SALIVARY GLANDS

The parotid and submandibular salivary glands bridge the anatomic compartments of the neck. Because of this unique relationship to the anatomy of the neck and because the lesions involving these glands are varied, their anatomy is considered separately. The parotid gland in most patients contains a considerable amount of fat mixed with glandular tissue and is intermediate in CT density between subcutaneous fat, muscle, and vessels (Fig. 2–7A–D). The gland wraps around the condyle and angle of the mandible, its deep lobe projecting medial to the mandible and abutting the parapharyngeal space lateral to the nasopharynx and oropharynx (Fig. 2–3D). CT scans through this region show the external ca-

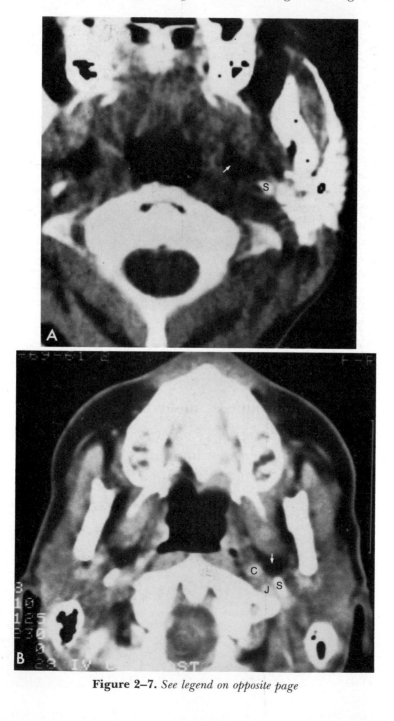

Figure 2–7. *See legend on opposite page*

rotid artery and retromandibular vein as two rounded, relatively high density structures running through the gland posterior to the mandible.

Immediately below the mastoid tip, the posterior belly of the digastric muscle is visible as an oblong density running anteriorly and medially, lateral to the carotid sheath. The digastric muscle marks the course of the facial nerve as it leaves the stylomastoid foramen to enter the parotid gland. The facial nerve is not normally visible on CT scans, but the plane of the facial nerve sepa-

rates the gland into deep and superficial portions. The parotid gland can be studied by CT combined with sialography by injection of contrast medium into Stensen's duct[3–5] or by CT after injection of intravenous contrast medium. (See the following section on examination technique.)

The submandibular gland is split by the mylohyoid muscle and therefore is partly in the floor of the mouth and partly in the upper neck (Fig. 2–3B,C).[1] The major portion of the gland lies below the mylohyoid muscle in the neck. The sub-

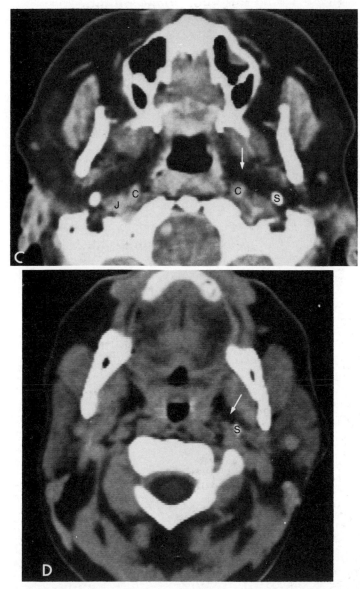

Figure 2–7. Variable appearance of normal parotid gland, depending on its fat content. **A** CT scan after left parotid duct has been filled with contrast material, which shows gland in greater detail than without contrast. **B–D** Appearance of parotid gland varies with its relative content of fat and glandular tissue. Even without injection of contrast material into parotid duct, the gland is seen. Difference in CT density between the deep lobe and the parapharyngeal space (arrows) is sufficient to distinguish the two. S = Styloid process; J = jugular vein; C = internal carotid artery.

mandibular glands are visible on CT scans from approximately the angle of the mandible to the level of the hyoid bone, and one gland is usually larger than the other. These glands are more homogeneous and denser than the parotid glands because they contain less fat.[1] Normally, the CT density of the submandibular glands approaches that of the surrounding musculature.

After intravenous injection of contrast medium, the submandibular and parotid glands both show capsular enhancement. With a bolus or rapid-drip infusion of intravenous contrast material, some internal architecture of both the parotid and submandibular glands becomes visible. This enhancement may be from opacification of the branching vessels in the gland, concentration of the iodine in the glands, or excretion of iodine into the ductal systems. A ramifying pattern can be seen with CT within the gland during peak intravascular concentrations of contrast medium and for approximately 5 to 10 minutes afterwards. This has not been shown to assist in diagnosis but does identify the normal glandular architecture. The branching pattern is usually more prominent in the submandibular gland, but can be seen within the fatty CT density of the parotid gland. The retromandibular vein and external carotid artery are visible as prominent high CT density structures in the parotid gland after either a bolus or rapid infusion of contrast material.

TECHNIQUES OF EXAMINATION

For CT examination of the neck excluding the larynx, the head should be in a neutral (slightly extended) position. For standardization, the canthomeatal line may be brought perpendicular to the scanner table by a slight tucking in of the chin. Hyperextension of the head does not seem to produce clinically significant alterations in the anatomic display. Extreme flexion or hyperextension of the neck should be avoided. For CT examination of the larynx, the neck should be moderately hyperextended, to bring the central axis of the larynx perpendicular to the plane of the scan. A digital or projection radiograph obtained in the lateral position is extremely useful for accurate localizing of the levels of the CT scans. The patient's shoulders should be relaxed, and the technician should pull them as far down as possible. The head should be immobilized. A molded radiographic sponge placed beneath the

head and upper neck can maintain a satisfactory position.

With CT scan times under 5 seconds, it is usually satisfactory to allow the patient to breathe quietly during the examination; however, suspending respiration can reduce scan artifacts in the neck and the floor of the mouth. The patient must not move or swallow while scanning is in progress.

The neck can be adequately surveyed by obtaining scans 1 cm thick at 1.0 to 1.5-cm intervals. The examination should include the abnormal area as well as areas into which the disease might extend. If more than a survey study is required, thinner sections at close intervals should be obtained through the region of interest. For example, in studying the parotid or submandibular salivary glands, sections should be 5 mm thick or less, at increments of 5 mm or less. Similar intervals and scan thicknesses should be used for detailed studies of the thyroid and parathyroid glands. Thinner sections and closer intervals may be used if the findings on a survey examination indicate the need for more refined detail.

Direct coronal scans are sometimes used to study the submandibular and parotid glands. A preliminary digital projection radiograph is especially useful in planning direct coronal examinations. It is usually necessary to tilt the gantry so that the plane of scanning is as nearly coronal as possible. CT examination of the parotid gland in the direct coronal plane will often avoid dental fillings, which can render transaxial CT scans of the parotid region uninterpretable. Direct coronal scans are rarely required, but they may be helpful for studying the submandibular glands; the same localizing and gantry-tilting maneuvers are necessary for a high-quality study. Sagittal and coronal reformations are, in general, cumbersome to perform and contribute little diagnostic information that is not apparent on the transaxial scans. Occasionally, reformations can show the superior and inferior extent of a lesion that extends from the neck through the thoracic inlet into the upper mediastinum.

Most CT studies of the neck require the injection of intravenous contrast medium. A rapid drip infusion or bolus injection provides the highest intravascular concentration of iodine.[6, 7] Contrast medium opacifies the many branching vessels in the neck, and they can be distinguished from enlarged lymph nodes or masses.[2, 8, 9] Opacification can also provide important information about the boundaries of masses, their vascularity, and their relationship to surrounding structures.[2, 3, 8, 9] The thyroid gland is enhanced after intravenous injection of contrast material, which helps to localize it precisely.

A simple bolus injection offers no advantage over rapid-drip infusion, and in fact may produce nausea, which generally delays the examination during the time of maximal intravascular opacification. Our technique is to infuse 150 ml of 60 per cent contrast medium as rapidly as possible. This requires that a 19-gauge needle be placed in a large antecubital vein and that the bottle of contrast material be elevated maximally. Scanning begins after approximately 25 ml of contrast material has been infused. Opacification of the intravascular space is maximal from the time at which 50 ml of the contrast material has been given until 5 to 10 minutes after the entire 150 ml has been given. The examination should be timed so that the area of interest is being studied during this time. Infusion of additional contrast material may be needed; however, this is done only if there is no contraindication to increasing the load of contrast material (e.g., decreased renal function or diabetes). The rapid-drip infusion can be augmented by injecting a 30 to 40 ml bolus and rescanning a particular area. It is seldom necessary to augment the initial rapid drip infusion if the area of interest is studied during maximal opacification.

Our indications for contrast infusion include suspected or known lymphadenopathy; delineating the extent of mass lesions within the neck, especially with respect to the carotid sheath; determining the vascularity of a neck mass; determining the extent of thyroid gland masses; searching for parathyroid adenomas in the neck or the anterior mediastinum; and examining the parotid or submandibular salivary glands.

Several investigators have shown that injection of contrast material into the ducts of the submandibular or parotid salivary glands before CT is useful for evaluating suspected masses in these glands.[2, 5] CT combined with sialography has been particularly helpful in distinguishing intra- from extraparotid masses and is of similar value in the submandibular salivary glands. Most currently available scanners, however, do not show the ducts of these glands in sufficient detail to allow inflammatory conditions to be evaluated. Routine sialography should be performed in patients with symptoms of inflammatory ductal disease and parenchymal disease.

CT scans after rapid intravenous infusion of contrast medium can show masses both inside and outside the salivary glands. However, CT combined with sialography can more accurately delineate masses of the parotid gland and is the preferred technique for this gland.[2-5] In the future, CT scans after intravenous infusion of contrast material will possibly prove sufficient for studying both parotid and submandibular masses. To avoid artifacts from dental fillings, which often make images through the lower portion of the parotid gland nondiagnostic, a projection digital radiograph should be obtained. The patient's head and the scanner gantry should be angled to as near a coronal plane as possible before infusing the contrast material. If that study is not helpful, contrast material can be injected into the parotid duct to show the gland in greater detail (Fig. 2–7A). Injection of the submandibular gland duct is often tedious and excessively time consuming. These patients can be studied either by the rapid drip infusion technique or by conventional sialography.

To perform CT in combination with sialography, water-soluble contrast material and various cannulas are used. Because of variations in the opening of Stensen's duct, it is useful to have Bowman lacrimal dilators and cannulas with tips of various shapes. A cannula with a tapered tip (W. Mueller, Division of American Hospital Supply Company) usually provides a snug fit and allows good filling of the ductal system and parenchyma. Even with careful dilatation, it may be necessary to use a cannula with a smaller tip than the one already described. In this case, the malleable lacrimal needle or a Rabinov sialography catheter may be used. An oily contrast medium such as Ethiodol, Pantopaque, or Lipiodol, all of which opacify the gland for an extended period of time, may also be used. In fact, scans done on the day after conventional sialography can show opacification if oily contrast media have been used.[2-4] We avoid oily contrast medium because this prolonged retention may cause granuloma formation. An advantage of oily contrast medium is that the gland can be injected outside the CT scanner room and the patient can be studied later.

PATHOLOGY

Mass lesions of the neck can originate in several areas. We will consider these lesions according to the compartment in which they are found or the organ from which they arise rather than according to an etiologic classification.

VISCERAL COMPARTMENT

Thyroid Gland

The thyroid gland anlage descends from the base of the tongue (foramen cecum) to the base of the neck. Persistence of a portion of this tract results in a thyroglossal cyst. Thyroid tissue may occur anywhere along this tract. Approximately 65 per cent of thyroglossal cysts are infrahyoid, 20 per cent are suprahyoid, and 15 per cent occur at the level of the hyoid bone.[10] These masses usually occur on or near the midline, are firm but somewhat fluctuant, and can often be correctly

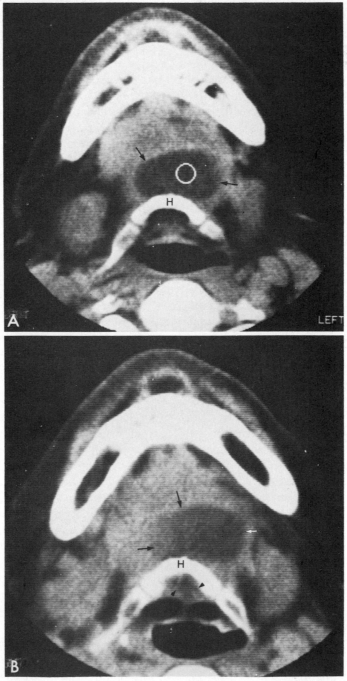

Figure 2–8. Thyroglossal duct cyst. **A** CT scan shows rounded area of low CT attenuation representing thyroglossal duct cyst (arrows) limited to soft tissues of tongue base and floor of mouth. No extension posterior to hyoid bone (H) is visible. **B** CT scan at slightly higher level shows mass anterior to the hyoid bone (H) and a component of the cyst posterior to hyoid bone (arrowheads).

Illustration continued on opposite page

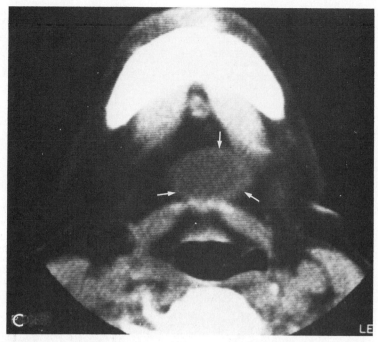

Figure 2–8. *Continued* **C** CT scan 2 cm caudad shows continuation of cyst (arrows) below hyoid. (Courtesy of Dr. Michael H. Reid, Sacramento, Cal.)

diagnosed from the physical findings. The diagnosis is confirmed by CT when a well-circumscribed, thin-walled, fluid-containing structure is localized either directly in the midline or in a paramedian position anterior to the thyroid cartilage or infrahyoid strap muscles (Fig. 2–8A–C).

One of the most important functions of CT is to detail the extent of the cyst relative to the hyoid bone and base of the tongue. Frequently, the cyst extends up and through the hyoid bone. This extension must be removed to prevent recurrence. Rarely, other cystic lesions of the neck occur anteriorly. CT scans can distinguish the origin of some of these masses and differentiate thyroglossal duct cysts from branchial cleft cysts or external components of laryngoceles.

The thyroid gland is usually examined by ultrasound rather than by CT. In patients with thyroiditis, ultrasound can show the diffusely abnormal texture of the thyroid gland, which can be distinguished from other diffuse benign or malignant masses only from the patient's history.

Benign masses of the thyroid gland are very common, and imaging of such lesions is sometimes pivotal in their treatment. Most masses of the thyroid gland are benign. Ultrasound remains the mainstay of anatomic imaging of the thyroid gland, and radionuclide imaging provides useful functional data. In patients with a large, adenomatous thyroid gland causing obstruction of the

airway (Fig. 2–9A), CT scans can show its extension behind the trachea and into the superior mediastinum (Fig. 2–9B–D). This information is valuable to the surgeon in planning resection. Rarely, the origin of a lower neck mass is unclear; CT can show whether it is a thyroid mass.

CT may be valuable in planning surgery for a thyroid malignancy. Aggressive thyroid malignancies can invade the trachea, larynx, and esophagus. Invasion may not be suspected clinically or may not be demonstrated by other imaging studies (Fig. 2–10A,B). CT scans can show invasion of these viscera, as well as regional nodal metastases. However, if ultrasound and physical examination show that the malignancy is clearly limited to the thyroid bed, there is little reason for preoperative CT.

Parathyroid Glands

Congenital lesions of the parathyroid glands are rare. Parathyroid cysts are usually visible posterior to the lower pole of the thyroid gland and are probably best evaluated by ultrasound.

Adenomas are by far the most common lesions of the parathyroid glands that require treatment. Parathyroid carcinomas are rare, and because their clinical presentation does not differ significantly from that of parathyroid adenomas, they may be considered in the same discussion. Non-invasive localization of cervical parathyroid ade-

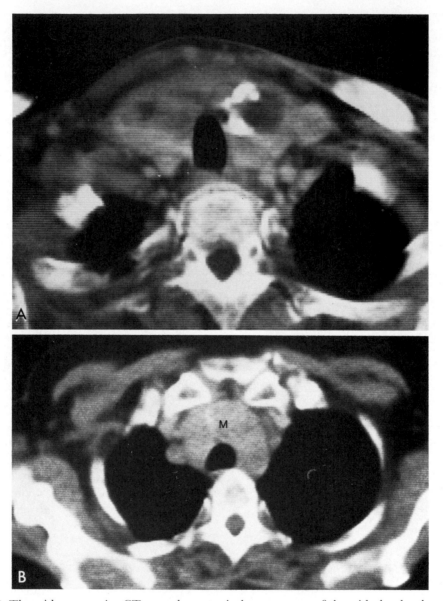

Figure 2–9. Thyroid masses. **A** CT scan shows typical appearance of thyroid gland enlarged by multiple adenomas in various states of degeneration and calcification. **B–D** Scans show thyroid goiter extending into mediastinum. Scan **B** shows mass (M) at thoracic inlet.

Illustration continued on opposite page

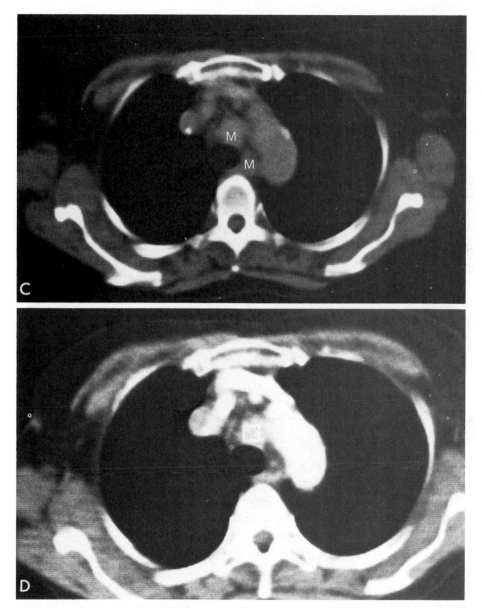

Figure 2–9. *Continued* **C** and **D** Scans before and after contrast medium infusion show exact extent of caudad extension of enlarged thyroid gland (M) into middle mediastinum. **D** Area-of-interest box showed thyroid had intense contrast enhancement but less than that of vessels.

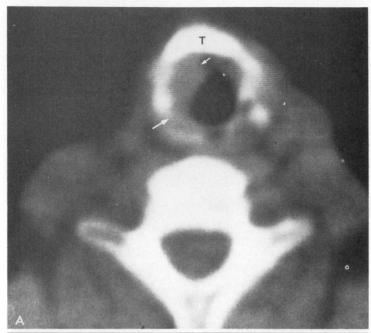

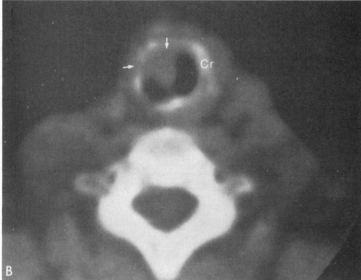

Figure 2–10. Thyroid carcinoma 15 years after bilateral radical neck dissections and total thyroidectomy. **A** CT scan through subglottic region shows mass within infraglottic larynx (arrows). Visualization of thyroid cartilage (T) at this level is abnormal and due to distortion of larynx. **B** Scan shows the mass (arrows) extending to junction of larynx and trachea. Cricoid cartilage (Cr) or upper tracheal rings are visible. Surgery confirmed recurrent tumor.

nomas can permit unilateral neck dissection in patients with primary hyperparathyroidism. High resolution ultrasonography can detect 71 to 78 per cent of parathyroid adenomas,[11–14] whereas CT can localize 50 to 77 per cent.[15, 16]

The ease of examination and accuracy of ultrasonography make it the preferred initial technique for examining the parathyroid glands (Fig. 2–11A,B). If ultrasound examination does not demonstrate a mass in the usual parathyroid locations, CT scans of the lower neck and the superior and anterior mediastinum may show a parathyroid mass (Fig. 2–12A,B). Ultrasonography often fails to demonstrate parathyroid adenomas at the upper pole of the thyroid gland,

probably because of their proximity to the laryngeal skeleton.[14] CT might help localize adenomas in this region (Fig. 2–12C), as well as in the mediastinum. When CT is used to detect parathyroid adenomas, a bolus injection of contrast material and care with the procedure are essential.[16–18] Cervical lymph nodes, tortuous vessels, thyroid masses, and even a collapsed esophagus can be mistaken for a parathyroid tumor. Streak artifacts, limited spatial resolution of some scanners, and image unsharpness from magnification can all cause difficulties with interpretation of the CT scans.[19] About 20 per cent of parathyroid adenomas enhance after a bolus injection of contrast material (Fig. 2–12C).

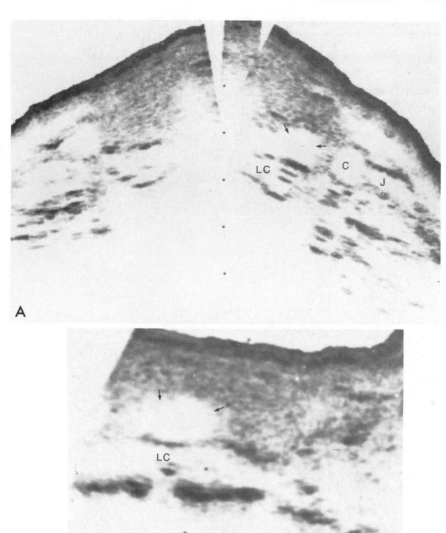

Figure 2–11. Ultrasonograms showing parathyroid adenoma. **A, B** Transverse **(A)** and longitudinal **(B)** images through the thyroid and parathyroid regions. Adenoma of left lower parathyroid (arrows) is present medial to the carotid artery (C) and jugular vein (J), and anterior to the longus colli muscle (LC).

Esophagus

Abnormalities of the cervical esophagus are seldom studied by CT. Occasionally, a Zenker's diverticulum mimics a lateral neck mass, for which CT might be indicated (Fig. 2–13). Usually the symptoms of a Zenker's diverticulum clearly relate to swallowing, and the presence of this lesion is confirmed with an esophagogram. CT is valuable for assessing malignancies of the cervical esophagus or hypopharynx that have extended inferiorly to involve the postcricoid region. CT scans can show the extent of the lesion and the presence of either cervical or mediastinal adenopathy.

Larynx

Recurrent laryngeal nerve palsies and, less commonly, phrenic nerve dysfunction, can be due to a variety of causes. Often, a specific cause is not discovered, and the dysfunction is considered idiopathic. A structural lesion causing paresis of a vocal cord or diaphragm is usually sought before the diagnosis of idiopathic dysfunction is accepted.

Before CT became available, the course of the recurrent laryngeal or phrenic nerve low in the neck could not be studied effectively. At present, the lower neck, the thoracic inlet, and the upper mediastinum can be evaluated by CT even if the nerves themselves cannot be seen. The path of the vagus nerve as far as the base of the skull can be seen on CT scans. Because CT occasionally demonstrates structural lesions, a search seems warranted in most patients (Fig. 2–14A,B). Careful imaging along the course of the minor neurovascular bundle and scrutiny of the fascial planes around the scalene muscles are important. In the mediastinum and thoracic inlet, the aortopulmonary window region on the left and the or-

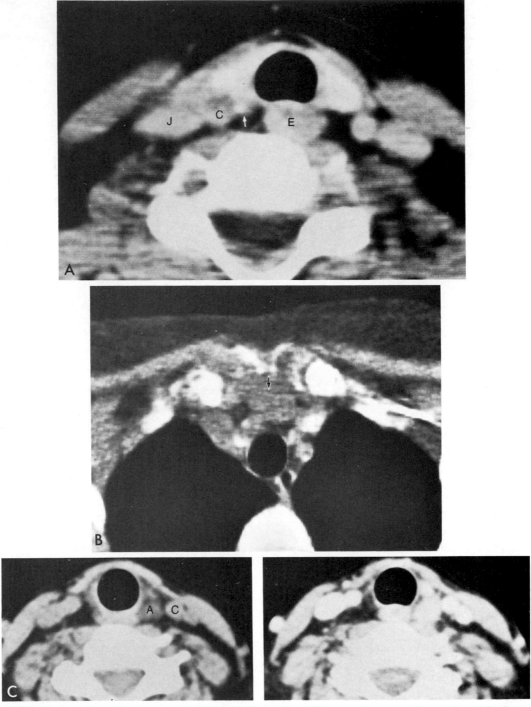

Figure 2–12. Parathyroid adenomas in three patients. **A** CT scan shows small parathyroid adenoma (arrow) medial to carotid artery (C) and jugular vein (J), and lateral to esophagus (E). **B** CT scan shows an ectopic, mediastinal adenoma (arrow). Ultrasound examination of the neck was normal in this patient. **C** CT scan at level of cricoid cartilage, before contrast medium infusion (left) shows parathyroid adenoma (A) medial to carotid artery (C). During bolus injection of contrast (right), adenoma has enhanced markedly. (**C** courtesy of Dr. D. D. Stark, San Francisco, Cal.)

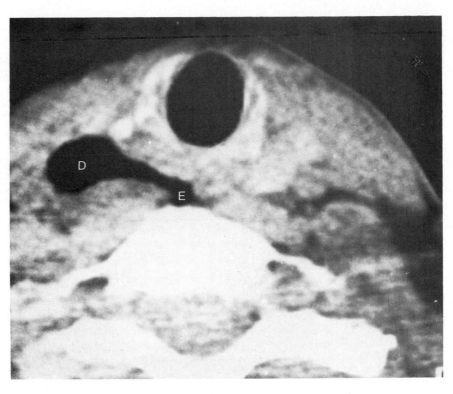

Figure 2–13. Zenker's diverticulum. CT scan shows Zenker's diverticulum (D) extending from region of cricopharyngeal muscle and upper cervical esophagus (E) into lateral soft tissues of the neck.

igin of the right subclavian artery on the right are important regions to examine. In recurrent laryngeal nerve paralysis, CT scans through the larynx will show that the affected true vocal cord lies in a paramedian position. This finding should not be mistaken for pathology of the true cord.

In our experience, CT has proved most useful in studying patients with known malignancies and recent onset of symptoms consistent with phrenic or recurrent laryngeal nerve dysfunction. Nonpalpable metastatic disease in the neck has been found to be the cause in several instances (Fig. 2–14B).[16]

LATERAL COMPARTMENT

Branchial Cleft Cyst

The branchial arches consist of five mesodermal bars separated by clefts covered by epithelium. Each cleft is in intimate contact with a pharyngeal pouch. As the embryo develops, the arches and clefts form the muscles, nerves, and cartilages of the lower face and neck. The second arch grows caudad to overlap the third and fourth arches. The second, third, and fourth clefts open into a common chamber called the cervical sinus. Branchial cleft cysts in the lateral compartment are all from the second branchial cleft or the cervical sinus. Cysts of the first branchial cleft are rare, and they present as parotid or periparotid masses.

Congenital masses in the anterolateral compartment of the neck are most often branchial cleft cysts and can usually be correctly diagnosed from the history and clinical examination.[10] Patients with such lesions have a long history of a slowly enlarging, fluctuant neck mass. Pain in region of the mass is unusual unless there is superimposed inflammation.

CT scans show branchial cleft cysts as very well circumscribed, usually thin-walled masses (Fig. 2–15A–C). Their appearance and the CT density measurements of their fluid content suggest a cyst. They neither obliterate the surrounding tissue nor invade surrounding structures. Large cysts may displace the carotid sheath, the sternocleidomastoid muscle, or the larynx. Irregularity and excessive thickness or marked contrast enhancement of the wall suggest inflammation in the cyst. Rarely, branchial cleft cysts have malignancies in their walls.[10]

All branchial cleft cysts should have a fistulous tract that extends to the hypopharynx and usually opens into the piriform sinus, valleculae, or glossopharyngeal sulcus. Most of the tract is usually not visible on CT scans, but its extension between the internal and external carotid artery can sometimes be seen. Clinically, it may not be possible to differentiate between a laryngocele extending from the appendix of the laryngeal ventricle and a branchial cleft cyst. This distinction is easily

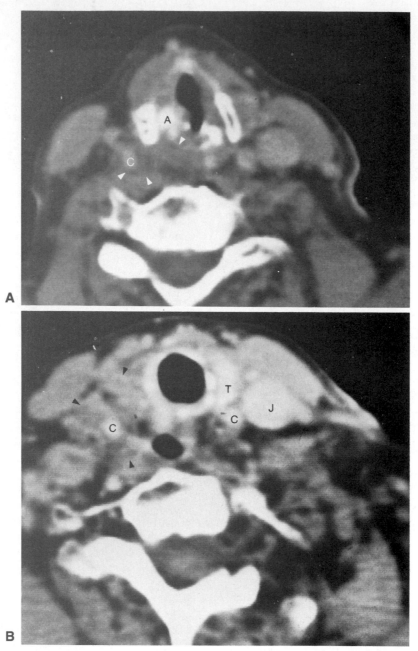

Figure 2–14. Paralyzed vocal cord. CT scans through the lower neck in a patient with metastatic breast carcinoma. **A** CT scan through true vocal cord shows superior and medial displacement of right arytenoid cartilage (A) and relatively paramedian position of true cord and base of aryepiglottic fold. Marked asymmetry in soft tissues of postcricoid region and surrounding right carotid sheath is visible, with obliteration of tissue planes (arrowheads). **B** Scan 15 mm caudad, at level of cricoid cartilage; marked asymmetry in deep soft tissue planes is seen. Carotid artery (C) is surrounded by abnormal tissue, and right jugular vein (J) does not opacify (arrowheads). Planes between carotid sheath and esophagus are obliterated, and the esophagus is retracted to right. The thyroid lobe (T) on the right side is replaced by abnormal tissue. Metastatic disease was not clinically evident.

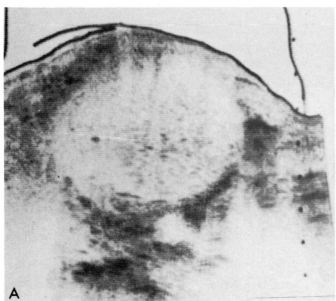

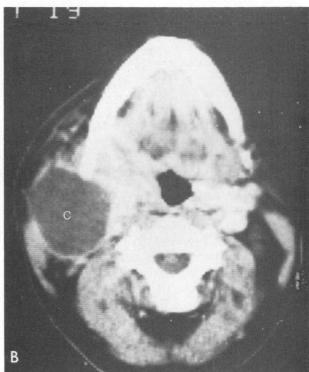

Figure 2–15. Branchial cleft cyst. **A** Ultrasonogram shows a large, primarily cystic mass, characterized by strong back wall and enhanced through transmission. Medium-level and occasional high-level gray tones within the mass represent debris within the cyst. **B** CT scan shows typical branchial cleft cyst (C) in lateral compartment of the neck. Extent of the mass and relationship to surrounding structures are demonstrated. **C** Angiogram shows arterial displacement but no increased vascularity. Angiography is not indicated for evaluation of most cystic neck masses. (Courtesy of Dr. D. Norman, San Francisco, Cal.)

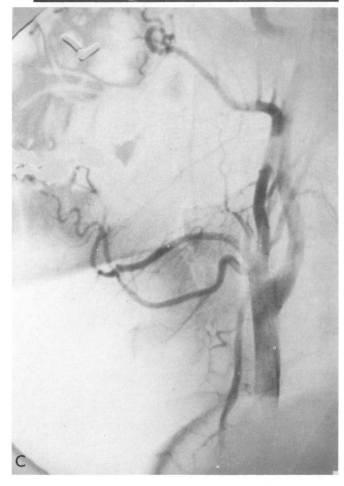

made by CT, which can demonstrate the internal component of a laryngocele within the paralaryngeal space and its extension through the thyrohyoid membrane.

Cystic Hygroma

The other common congenital cystic mass in the neck is a cystic hygroma. They are formed of dilated lymphatic channels and are a type of lymphangioma. Cystic hygromas are almost exclusively seen in children, although in rare instances they are first diagnosed in adulthood. Therapy is primarily surgical and aimed at cosmesis or relieving airway obstruction. These lesions are diffuse and appear as a lacy network of intermittent areas of high and low density on CT scans. Their diffuse and insinuating characteristics make it difficult to distinguish the normal fascial planes within the neck.

Cystic hygromas can become extremely large and can extend superiorly to the parotid region or inferiorly to the axilla. Extension within the deep planes of the neck to the parapharyngeal space can reach to the infratemporal fossa and the base of the tongue. The tumor can also extend into the thoracic inlet and superior mediastinum. Extent of cystic hygroma is best evaluated by CT, which can define the relationship of the tumor to the airway and the severity of airway encroachment.

Other Cysts

Thymic cysts are rare, and can appear identical to isolated branchial cleft cysts. Branchial cleft cysts, however, seldom extend to the clavicle, whereas this is a common characteristic of thymic cysts.[10] Parathyroid cysts are rare and typically located posterior to the thyroid gland. Thyroglossal duct cysts should not be mistaken for branchial cleft cysts on CT scans, and the course and location of thyroglossal duct cysts differ from those of branchial cleft cysts.

Hemangioma

Benign hemangiomas involving the head and neck have a distribution similar to that described for cystic hygromas. In fact, cystic hygromas may have hemangiomatous elements, and the converse is true. Most hemangiomas are present at birth or develop during infancy. Hemangiomas may be located in the skin or deep tissues. Deep hemangiomas especially are frequently not well circumscribed and are locally invasive. CT scans after infusion of intravenous contrast material may show the extent of the lesion if a significant vascular component is present (Fig. 2–16A,B). Treatment of lesions is for cosmesis and to relieve airway obstruction.

Suspected inflammatory masses of the lateral compartment are seldom studied by CT, and most often these are related to the lymph nodes. The CT appearance of enlarged, inflamed lymph nodes is indistinguishable from that of enlarged neoplastic nodes.[20, 21] Rarely, inflammation spreading from a retropharyngeal abscess or from an infectious process in the salivary glands obliterates the tissue planes in the neck, but CT rarely adds to the diagnosis or management of these problems.

Benign Neoplasms

Benign neoplastic lesions in the lateral compartment are rare and usually arise from the structures in and about the carotid sheath or from the mesenchymal elements that surround them. Carotid body tumor is probably the most common benign tumor in the lateral compartment. The diagnosis is usually suspected clinically; however, differentiation from other anterior and lateral neck masses is important in determining the need for further evaluation by angiography or neck exploration. CT scans of a carotid body tumor typically show a well-circumscribed mass at or above the carotid bifurcation; and infusion of contrast material can show a very well circumscribed, homogeneously dense pattern of enhancement (Fig. 2–17A–C). Occasionally, it may be difficult to distinguish a carotid body tumor from a paraganglioma. Both tumors can extend both caudad and cephalad in the spaces around the carotid sheath and the parapharyngeal space. Carotid body tumors rarely extend to the base of the skull, whereas tumors of the glomus jugulare and glomus vagale commonly do involve the base of the skull, in and about the carotid bulb.[10]

Neuromas and neurofibromas can present anterolaterally in the neck. The neck mass can also be a neurogenic tumor that has originated near the base of the skull, and extended inferiorly in the parapharyngeal space. On CT scans, these masses will be less intensely enhanced than paragangliomas and will sometimes have a relatively low density center (Fig. 2–18A–C). Other benign tumors in the lateral compartment are very rare. Fibromas or low grade malignancies such as fibrous histiocytomas can rarely present in this compartment. CT can demonstrate the extent of

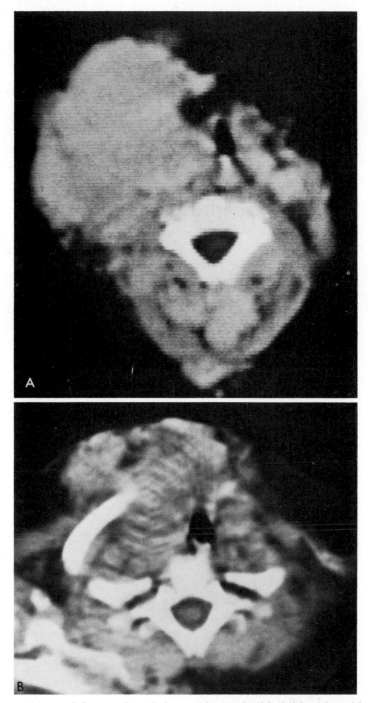

Figure 2–16. Hemangioma of face and neck in an 18-month-old child with stridor. **A** CT scan at level of larynx shows large right-sided mass displacing larynx to the left. **B** After intravenous infusion of contrast medium, at level of right clavicle, mass is still visible. Enhancement of mass has occurred. Ring densities are artifacts.

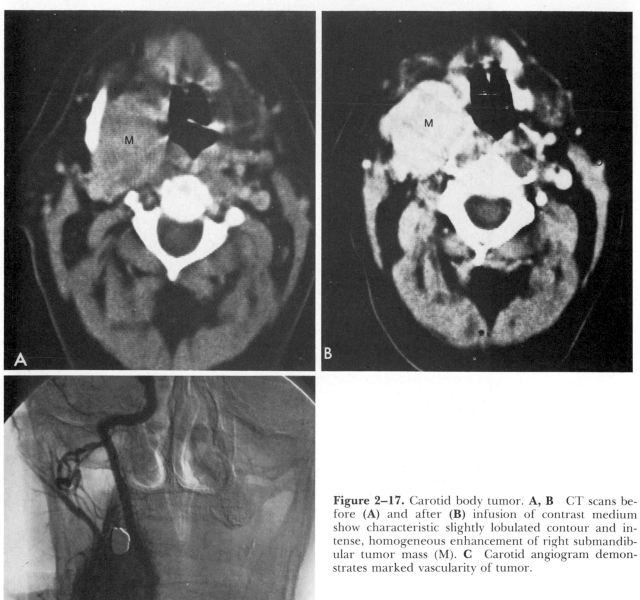

Figure 2–17. Carotid body tumor. **A, B** CT scans before (**A**) and after (**B**) infusion of contrast medium show characteristic slightly lobulated contour and intense, homogeneous enhancement of right submandibular tumor mass (M). **C** Carotid angiogram demonstrates marked vascularity of tumor.

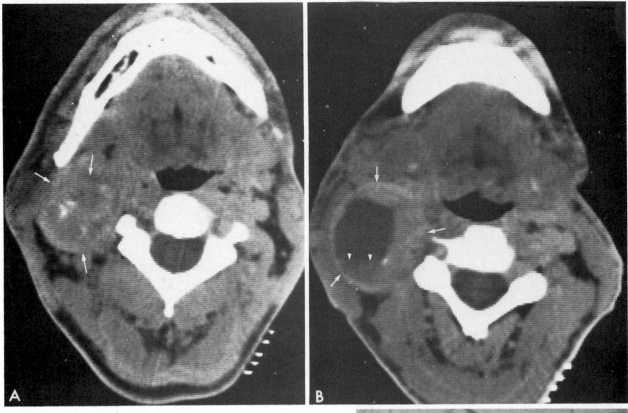

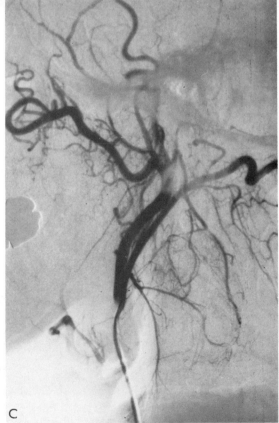

Figure 2–18. Vagus nerve neurilemoma. Patient is a 37-year-old man with neck mass for four years. **A, B** CT scans show well-circumscribed mass with peripheral enhancement. Punctate areas of calcification and central necrosis surround carotid sheath (arrows). In **B,** fluid-debris level is visible (arrowheads). These findings are nearly pathognomonic of a neurilemoma. **C** Arteriogram shows hypovascular mass displacing internal and external carotid artery branches.

these lesions and distinguish them from more common neck masses.

Lymphadenopathy

Malignant lesions involving the carotid sheath are most often metastases to the cervical nodes (Fig. 2–19). Lymph node metastases in the neck can be staged more accurately by CT than by physical examination.[2, 8, 16, 17] CT scans can demonstrate nodal metastases as large as 2 to 2.5 cm that are not clinically palpable (Fig. 2–19). CT can also demonstrate the absence of cervical nodes thought to be clinically present.[8] Moreover, it can show nodes that are beyond the normal range of physical examination, such as the high lateral and retropharyngeal groups (Fig. 2–20A,B).[2, 20, 21]

Tentative criteria for diagnosing pathologically enlarged nodes have been suggested.[2, 20–22] These criteria are as follows:

1. A nonenhancing mass at least 1.5 cm in transverse dimension. Pathologic data indicate that neck nodes of this size are likely to contain tumor.[22]

2. Obliteration of the normal tissue planes around the carotid sheath in the absence of prior surgery or radiation therapy. This criterion presupposes that adequate fat is present in the deep tissue planes and that comparison with the contralateral side can be made.

3. For patients with squamous cell carcinoma, a node of any size that shows focal low density, suggesting necrosis.

Intravenous contrast medium should always be used to distinguish nodes from the numerous branching vessels within the neck. Contrast enhancement may also help determine whether capsular or extranodal extension of the tumor is present (Fig. 2–19).[2, 8, 20, 21] Some nodes less than 1.5 cm in diameter may show a very thin rim of contrast enhancement during rapid-drip infusion (Fig. 2–21). This finding has not been adequately correlated pathologically, and it may also represent capsular enhancement in reactive nodes. A thick rim of contrast enhancement in an enlarged node usually indicates capsular or extracapsular extension of tumor. Obliteration or edema of the surrounding fat planes and swelling of the adjacent neck muscles also indicate extracapsular extension of tumor (Fig. 2–22A–G). Once the tumor has extended beyond the lymph node capsule and into the soft tissues of the neck, it may become attached to the carotid artery. If a cleavage plane between the nodal mass and the carotid artery is visible, attachment to the carotid artery can be ex-

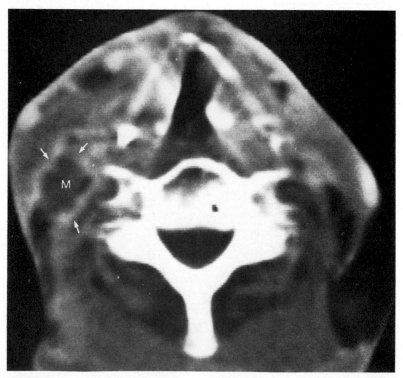

Figure 2–19. Metastasis to cervical lymph nodes. Contrast-enhanced CT scan at level of glottis shows mass (M) posterior to carotid sheath. Peripheral enhancement is present (arrows). At surgery, mass proved to be occult metastatic tumor to cervical nodes.

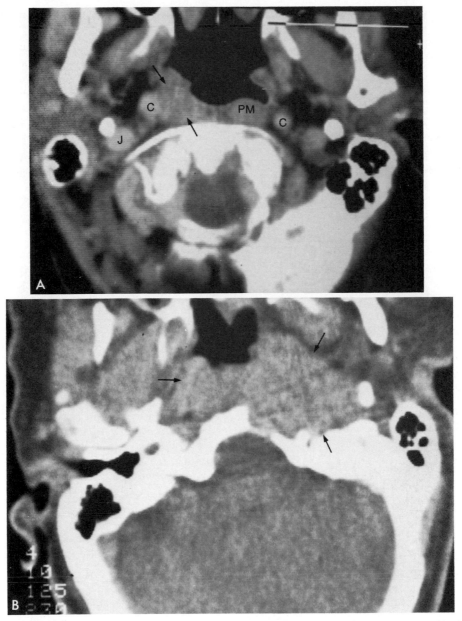

Figure 2–20. Retropharyngeal adenopathy in two patients. **A** Patient with lymphoma. Undetectable retropharyngeal adenopathy is visible on CT scan as obliteration of tissue planes between carotid artery (C) and the prevertebral muscles (PM). J = Jugular vein. **B** Patient after total laryngectomy and radical neck dissection for carcinoma of larynx, with high neck pain. Contrast-enhanced CT scan shows large nodal mass (arrows) involving retropharyngeal nodes and extending into skull base.

cluded. Unfortunately, if the tissue planes between the carotid artery and nodes are not visible, it cannot be ascertained whether the tumor abuts on, adheres to, or has invaded the carotid artery. When a nodal mass obliterates these tissue planes, a carotid artery graft may be needed during surgery. Nodal masses can also obliterate the tissue planes overlying the scalene muscles, which implies fixation to the brachial plexus; however, it is frequently difficult to determine whether the tu-

mor mass merely adheres to or encases these neural elements (Fig. 2–22A–G). This distinction is important because tumor encasement of the brachial plexus by a nodal mass is a definite contraindication to radical neck dissection. The larger the mass, the more likely is fixation to these important structures; but proximity and obliteration of tissue planes does not necessarily imply that the tumor is attached to an adjacent structure.

One of the important contributions of CT to

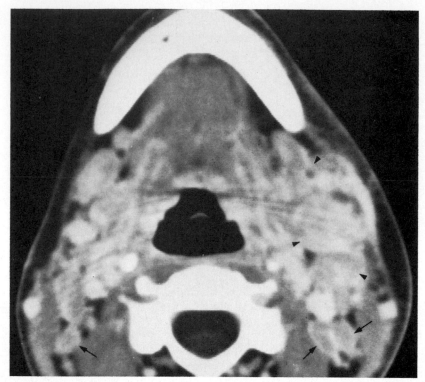

Figure 2–21. Lymphoma with large bilateral submandibular nodal masses. CT scan after intravenous contrast infusion shows multiple discrete nodes on right and large nodal mass (arrowheads) on left, indistinguishable from left submandibular salivary gland. Smaller nodes on the left and right (arrows) show a thin rim of enhancement.

the evaluation of cervical lymph nodes is assessment of the high lateral and retropharyngeal lymph nodes (Fig. 2–20A,B), which are beyond the range of physical examination or other imaging techniques. These nodes are most often enlarged in patients with recurrent tumors after initial treatment.[10] Strict criteria for evaluating these nodes are not available because it is difficult to obtain pathologic confirmation of their involvement. CT-guided fine-needle aspiration may make pathologic correlation possible in the future. We have been using the same criteria as described for evaluation of the deep cervical lymph nodes in the carotid sheath, although strict size criteria cannot be applied. The degree of asymmetry between the two sides is important in evaluating high lateral and retropharyngeal nodes. Adenopathy in these regions often presents as obliteration of the tissue planes around the internal carotid artery and jugular veins rather than as discrete mass lesions. Once tumor has involved these lymph nodes, it may extend cephalad to the base of the skull.[10]

CT has proved especially valuable in patients who have been treated with either surgery or ra-

diation for lymphoma or carcinoma involving the head and neck and who return with either neck pain or neurologic symptoms referable to the cervical cord or brachial plexus.[20] CT scans can show recurrent tumor in the lateral and retropharyngeal node groups in some of these patients (Fig. 2–20), as well as direct extension into the soft tissues of the neck and to the epidural space (Fig. 2–23A,B).

The lymph nodes in the posterior compartment of the neck lie posterior to the jugular vein and can project into the space between the sternocleidomastoid and trapezius muscles. Metastases to these lymph nodes occur infrequently, except with nasopharyngeal carcinoma. Up to 30 per cent of these tumors metastasize to the posterior compartment (Fig. 2–24). Lymphomas are the next most common group of malignancies that involve the nodes of the posterior compartment. Metastasis from squamous cell carcinoma that arises elsewhere in the upper aerodigestive tract is less frequent.[10]

Occasionally, malignancies arising in the upper aerodigestive tract will extend directly into the region of the carotid sheath, and it may be impossible to distinguish direct extension of tumor from nodal disease. Direct extension tends to stay medial to the carotid sheath, whereas nodal metastasis is often lateral and slightly anterior or posterior to the jugular vein. Direct extension of tumor into the lateral neck compartment is most commonly seen in carcinomas of the piriform sinus (Fig. 2–25) and the postpharyngeal wall but may also occur in tumors arising in the larynx and from the base of the tongue. Thyroid and cervical esophagus malignancies also occasionally extend into the lateral compartment of the neck. Surprisingly, large extensions of these tumors may not be detectable on physical examination, or they may be palpable only as a "vague fullness" in the neck. Other primary malignancies of the neck are rare and usually arise from mesenchymal elements. Low-grade fibrous histiocytoma and malignant fibrous histiocytoma are the more common of these infrequent primary tumor malignancies.

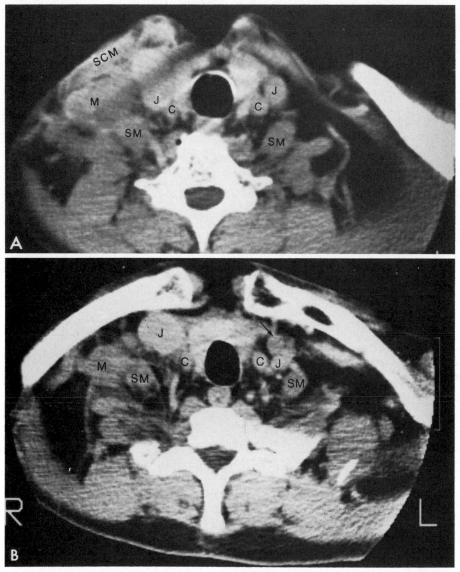

Figure 2–22. Cervical adenopathy with fixation. Three patients with carcinomas involving upper aerodigestive tract and cervical adenopathy. Each patient has extranodal extension and various degrees of attachment to surrounding structures (confirmed at surgery). **A, B** CT scans through lower neck show nodal mass (M) that is hypovascular compared with carotid artery (C) and jugular vein (J). Tissue planes surrounding the mass are indistinct, although cleavage plane is visible between mass and sternocleidomastoid muscle (SCM). The plane between the mass and the scalene muscle (SM) is lost. Mass is clearly free of the common carotid artery (C). In **B,** small contralateral node is present (arrow). (At surgery an extranodal extension with tumor adhered to scalene muscle and jugular vein was found. Carotid artery was free of tumor.)

Illustration continued on following page

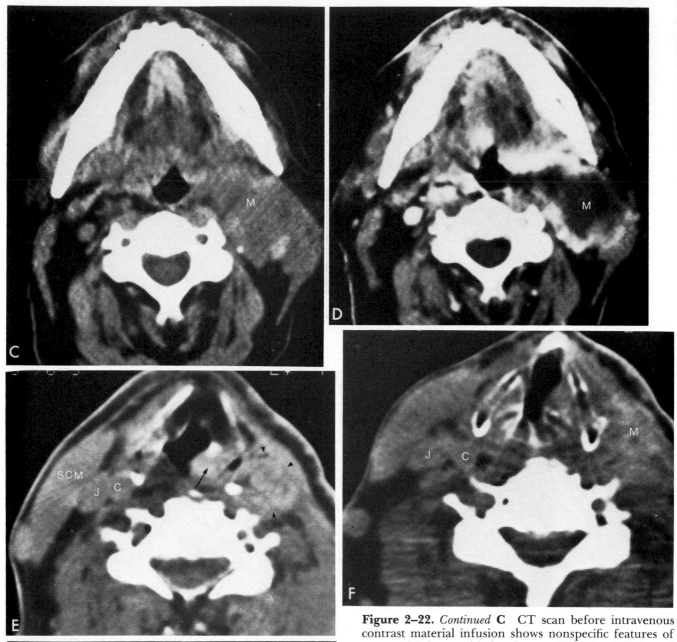

Figure 2–22. *Continued* **C**   CT scan before intravenous contrast material infusion shows nonspecific features of a mass (M) in carotid sheath area. **D**   After infusion of contrast medium wall of the mass (M) is irregular and enhanced. No definable plane between mass and surrounding muscles or vascular structures is visible. (Mass represents recurrent nodal metastases after radiation therapy. Extranodal extension and attachment to the carotid artery and the sternocleidomastoid muscle are present.) **E**   Contrast-enhanced CT scan shows thickening of left aryepiglottic fold (arrow), absent left sternocleidomastoid muscle (SCM), and enhancing nodal mass (arrowheads). **F**   CT scan demonstrates paresis of left vocal cord and ill-defined left mass (M) inseparable from surrounding deep muscles. Left carotid artery is not visible, and the left jugular vein has been resected. **G**   CT scan through undersurface of true cord shows normal opacification of right carotid artery (C), jugular vein (J), and scalene muscle (SM). On left mass is inseparable from the scalene muscles. (Surgical exploration showed recurrent nodal disease, extensive extranodal spread, and attachment to surrounding muscles.)

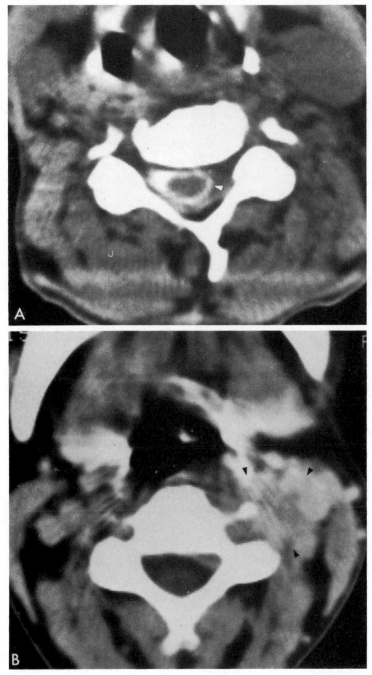

Figure 2–23. Two patients with lymphoma. **A** CT scan at level of the thyroid cartilage shows obliteration of the epidural space and displacement of the opacified dural sac and spinal cord (arrowhead). No evidence of direct extension from neck nodes or bone is seen. **B** CT scan after intravenous administration of the contrast material shows a clinically occult nodal mass (arrowheads).

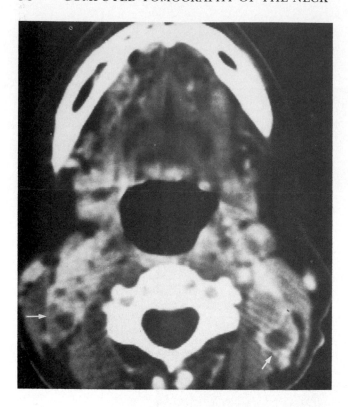

Figure 2–24. Carcinoma of the nasopharynx. CT scan shows metastasis to both deep cervical nodes and the posterior triangle (spinal accessory) nodes (arrows).

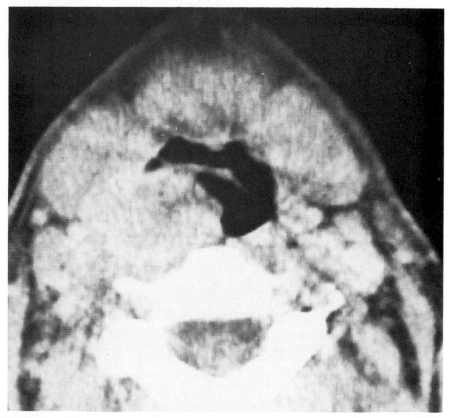

Figure 2–25. Large piriform sinus carcinoma. CT scan shows right-sided primary tumor and bilateral enlarged lymph nodes. On the right side the nodes cannot be separated from the primary tumor and could represent direct extension of tumor.

POSTERIOR COMPARTMENT

Masses in the posterior compartment are unusual and are most often of bony or neural origin. They may mimic abnormalities arising in other compartments of the neck, and CT scans can clearly identify their site of origin. Likewise, malignant lesions can extend from the other compartments of the neck to involve the neural and bony elements in the posterior compartment. These extensions may not be apparent from the clinical evaluation and will radically alter the therapeutic approach (Fig. 2–23*B*).

Experience with lesions in this compartment is largely anecdotal. We have seen several patients with expansile lesions of the cervical vertebral column, either aneurysmal bone cysts or osteoblastomas, involving the lateral masses of the cervical vertebrae and mimicking other neck masses or tumors of salivary gland origin. Perhaps the most common benign lesion in the posterior compartment of the neck is the neurofibroma, which involves the spinal cord and extends through the neural foramina into the neck or arises from the brachial plexus (Figs. 2–18*A–C* and 2–26*A–C*). In patients with malignant lesions involving cervical nodes who have neurologic symptoms or neck pain after treatment, CT can demonstrate occult nodal disease with extranodal extension or spread directly to the epidural space (Figs. 2–20 and 2–23).

SALIVARY GLAND LESIONS

Parotid Gland

Computed tomography of the parotid gland is used to evaluate suspected parotid masses and to determine whether a mass is intrinsic or extrinsic to the gland.[2–5] CT can also determine the relationship of an intrinsic mass to the facial nerve and at times suggest whether the mass is benign or malignant.

Frequently masses suspected of being within the parotid gland are external to the gland. The location of the mass in relation to the parotid gland markedly alters the diagnostic and therapeutic approach to the lesion. The surgical procedure for an intrinsic parotid mass external to the facial nerve is a superficial parotidectomy, which encompasses the mass completely and places the facial nerve at least risk. A mass medial to the plane of the facial nerve places the facial nerve at greater risk for surgical injury.

Masses medial to the parotid gland, within the parapharyngeal space, displace the parotid gland and may create the mistaken impression of an intrinsic parotid lesion. CT can often show the origin of these masses. A mass arising primarily in the parapharyngeal space is most likely to be a benign pleomorphic adenoma of accessory salivary tissue (Fig. 2–27). Paragangliomas or neuromas arising from the carotid sheath region can also cause lateral displacement of the gland. Nasopharyngeal or oropharyngeal carcinomas that are primarily submucosal occasionally extend into the parapharyngeal space and similarly displace the gland. The diagnostic approach to each of these lesions and their management differ from those for an intrinsic parotid mass.

Masses extrinsic and lateral to the parotid gland are usually enlarged periparotid lymph nodes. Enlargement is usually due to inflammation and is related to infections in the scalp and face. When CT shows that the mass is clearly extrinsic and lateral to the gland, the patient can usually be managed conservatively with observation and antibiotics. Most masses regress and require no further therapy. When the benign nature of the lesion is uncertain, excisional biopsy will be necessary.

A detailed discussion of the pathology of intrinsic parotid lesions is beyond the scope of this text; the pathology text by Batsakis is an excellent resource.[10] Approximately 85 per cent of parotid mass lesions are benign. Benign mixed tumors (pleomorphic adenomas) and Warthin's tumors are the most common benign tumors, whereas mucoepidermoid carcinoma is the most common malignancy. Adenoid cystic carcinoma is the next most common malignancy.[10]

The CT signs of malignancy include irregular margins or extension of tumor masses beyond the confines of the gland and obliteration of surrounding tissue planes (Fig. 2–28*A,B*). Associated adenopathy may also be present. Benign lesions are usually smooth and well circumscribed (Fig. 2–29), although a specific tissue diagnosis should never be attempted from CT appearances alone.

Lymphoma may present as either intraparotid or periparotid adenopathy or diffuse infiltration of the gland. When lymphoma is strictly nodal, it is usually associated with regional or disseminated disease. An infiltrating pattern is seen in the rare primary salivary gland lymphoma.

Submandibular Gland

The patient with a suspected submandibular gland mass presents the same diagnostic problem as the patient with a suspected parotid mass. The mass can be intrinsic or extrinsic to the gland, and

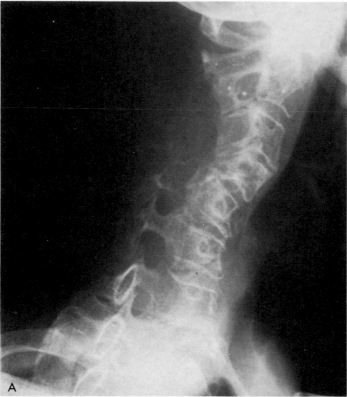

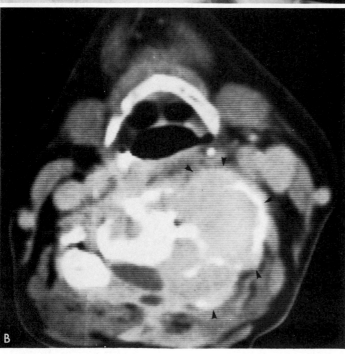

Figure 2–26. Cervical neurofibroma. **A** Oblique radiograph of the cervical spine shows combined effects of large neurofibroma and prior surgery. **B** CT scan shows extent of the neurofibroma (arrowheads), its relationship to dural sac, and its growth through the neural foramina. Expansion and destruction of skeletal structures is from progressive tumor growth. **C** Left vertebral artery angiogram shows moderate vascularity, which correlates with opacification visible on CT scan. (Courtesy of Dr. T. H. Newton, San Francisco, Cal.)

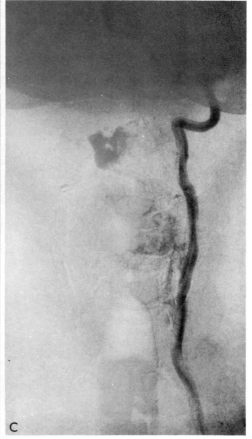

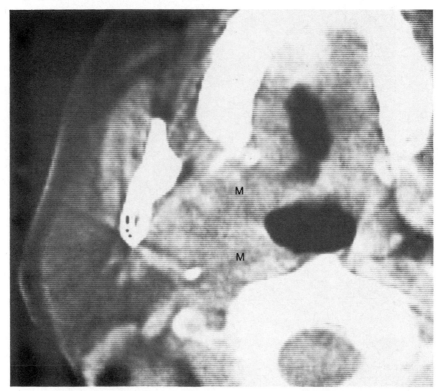

Figure 2–27. Mixed parapharyngeal tumor. CT scan shows normal deep lobe of parotid gland separate from tumor mass (M).

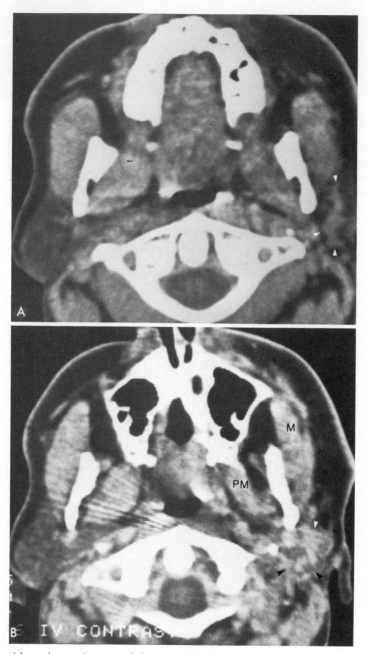

Figure 2–28. Adenoid cystic carcinoma of the parotid gland. **A**   CT scan at level of soft palate shows left parotid is abnormal (arrowheads) compared with normal right side. **B**   Two centimeters higher, CT scan through lower nasopharynx shows left periparotid region diffusely infiltrated (arrowheads). Decrease in bulk of the pterygoid (PM) and masseter (M) muscles reflects abnormality in motor division of fifth cranial nerve. (Surgery showed tumor extension to skull base at foramen ovale, stylomastoid foramen, and jugular fossa.)

the diagnosis and management differ accordingly. Extrinsic masses originate almost exclusively in periglandular lymph nodes (Fig. 2–30). The submandibular lymph nodes abut on the gland. CT after intravenous infusion of contrast medium can, however, differentiate between nodes and an intrinsic submandibular gland mass. Intrinsic submandibular gland masses are usually malignant.[10] Rarely, bony lesion of the mandible or lesions arising from the base of the tongue will present clinically as submandibular gland masses, and CT can readily diagnose these abnormalities. Enlarged periglandular lymph nodes are frequently excised because the surgical approaches to intrinsic and extrinsic masses of the submandibular gland are similar and the CT findings

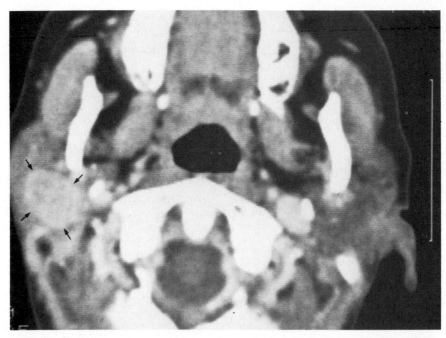

Figure 2–29. Benign mixed tumor of the parotid gland. CT scan shows well-circumscribed mass (arrows) in medial portion of superficial lobe of right parotid gland. Deep lobe is normal.

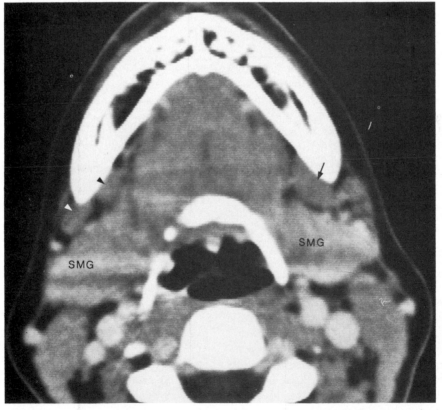

Figure 2–30. Enlarged submandibular lymph node. CT scan shows typical diffuse enhancing pattern of submandibular gland (SMG). No intrinsic masses are present. Enlarged lymph node is visible anterior to left gland (arrow), and smaller nodes are present on right side (arrowheads).

Table 2–1. INDICATIONS FOR COMPUTED TOMOGRAPHY OF THE NECK

Determination of the extent of primary and secondary neoplasms of the neck
1. Mass of unknown origin—for preoperative differential diagnosis
2. Suspected benign tumors
   a Neuromas
   b. Branchial cleft cysts
   c. Laryngocele
   d. Paragangliomas
3. Thyroid masses
   a. Extent of benign masses (goiter)
   b Stage known malignancy (nodes and deep invasion)
4. Parathyroid adenomas
   a. Usual location (complementary to ultrasound)
   b. Ectopic
5. Malignancies of the aerodigestive tract and nodes
   a. Stage primary tumor
   b. Stage cervical metastases
   c. Detect recurrent tumor
   d. Search for unknown primary neoplasms presenting as nodal metastases

Evaluation of bony abnormalities of the cervical spine, including neoplasms, fractures, dislocations, and congenital anomalies

Localization of foreign bodies in the soft tissues, hypopharynx, or larynx and assessment of airway integrity after trauma
1. Foreign body localization
2. Laryngeal trauma

Evaluation of retropharyngeal abscesses

may not alter treatment. When CT demonstrates that the lesion is an enlarged lymph node, a conservative approach similar to that followed in periparotid adenopathy may be indicated (Fig. 2–30). The combination of an intrinsic submandibular gland lesion and enlarged nodes suggests malignancy.

INDICATIONS FOR COMPUTED TOMOGRAPHY OF THE NECK

The Society for Computed Body Tomography formulated a summary statement in 1979 regarding indications for computed body tomography, including a section on the neck.[23] These general guidelines are still applicable, although in summarizing this chapter it might be useful to consider the indications for CT of the neck in more detail (Table 2–1). In the table, the Society's recommendations are given in boldface type. The subcategories provide additional detail. CT is usually unnecessary for localizing foreign bodies; conventional radiographs are usually sufficient.

The evaluation of retropharyngeal abscesses is an unusual indication for CT, but in a few instances, the extent of spread can be optimally defined by CT.

Several areas of computed tomography of the neck require further investigation. The criteria for tumor encasement of vessels and nerves need to be better defined. The CT criteria for malignant involvement of lymph nodes also warrant confirmation.

REFERENCES

1. Last RJ: Anatomy: Regional and Applied, 5th ed. Edinburgh, Churchill-Livingston, 1972.
2. Mancuso AA, Hanafee WN: Computed Tomography of the Head and Neck. Baltimore, Williams & Wilkins, 1982.
3. Carter B, Karmody CS: Computed tomography of the face and neck. Semin Roentgenol 13:257, 1978.
4. Som PM, Biller HF: The combined CT sialogram. Radiology 135:387, 1980.
5. Stone D, Mancuso AA, Rice D, Hanafee WN: CT parotid sialography. Radiology 138:393, 1981.
6. Ono N, Martinez CR, Fara JW, Hodges FJ III: Diatrizoate distribution in dogs as a function of administration rate and time following intravenous injection. J Comput Assist Tomogr 4:174, 1980.
7. Young SW, Noon MA, Marincek B: Dynamic computed tomography time-density study of normal human tissue after intravenous contrast administration. Invest Radiol 16:36, 1981.
8. Mancuso AA, Maceri D, Rice D, Hanafee WN: CT of cervical lymph node cancer. AJR 136:381, 1981.
9. Miller EM, Norman D: The role of computed tomography in the evaluation of neck masses. Radiology 133:145, 1979.
10. Batsakis JG: Tumors of the Head and Neck. Clinical and Pathological Considerations, 2nd ed. Baltimore, Williams & Wilkins, 1979.
11. Van Heerden JA, James EM, Kasell PR, Charboneau JW, Grant CS, Purnell DC: Small-part ultrasonography in primary hyperparathyroidism. Ann Surg 195:774, 1982.
12. Simeone JF, Meuller PR, Ferrucci JT, Van Sonnenberg E, Wang CA, Hall DA, Whittenberg J: High resolution real-time sonography of the parathyroid gland. Radiology 141:745, 1981.
13. Scheible W, Deutsch AL, Leopold GR: Parathyroid adenoma; Accuracy of preoperative localization by high-resolution real-time sonography. J Clin Ultrasound 9:325, 1981.
14. Kalovidouris A, Mancuso AA, Sarti D: Parathyroid ultrasonography. Br J Radiol (in press).
15. Sommer B, Welter HF, Spelsberg F, Scherer U, Lissner J: Computed tomography for localizing enlarged parathyroid glands in primary hyperparathyroidism. J Comput Assist Tomogr 6:521, 1982.
16. Whitley NO, Bohlman M, Connor TB, McCrea ES, Mason GR, Whitley JE: Computed tomography for localization of parathyroid adenomas. J Comput Assist Tomogr 5:812, 1981.
17. Reed D: Personal communication, May 1981.
18. Stark DD, Moss AA, Gooding GAW, Clark OH: Advances in parathyroid CT scanning. Radiology (in press).

19. Adams JE, Adams PH, Mamtora H, Isherwood I: Computed tomography and the localization of parathyroid tumors. Clin Radiol 32:251, 1981.

20. Harnsberger HR, Mancuso AA, Muraki A: Computed tomographic evaluation of recurrent and residual tumors of the upper aerodigestive tract and neck. Radiology (in press).

21. Mancuso AA, Harnsberger HR, Muraki A, Stevens M: CT of the cervical lymph nodes: Normal, variations of normal and applications in staging head and neck malignancies. Radiology (in press).

22. McGavran MH, Bauer WC, Ogura JH: The incidence of cervical lymph node metastases from epidermoid carcinoma of the larynx and their relationship to certain characteristics of the primary tumor: A study based on the clinical and pathologic findings for 96 patients treated by primary en bloc laryngectomy and radical neck dissection. Cancer 14:55, 1961.

23. Society for Computed Body Tomography: Special report. New indications for computed body tomography. AJR 133:115, 1979.

3 COMPUTED TOMOGRAPHY OF THE LARYNX AND PIRIFORM SINUSES

Gordon Gamsu

Computed tomography (CT) is a unique method for evaluating the larynx, and it is rapidly gaining widespread application. Before the use of computed laryngeal tomography, accurate assessment of the deep tissues and cartilages of the larynx could be achieved only by surgical exploration. Laryngoscopy, laryngography, and conventional tomography demonstrate the mucosal surface of the larynx and can only indirectly suggest abnormalities of the deep structures. Several studies[1–4] have shown that CT complements and extends these methods of visualizing the cavity of the larynx. In the clinical assessment of patients, CT is usually performed in conjunction with direct or indirect laryngoscopy and should not be expected to compete with laryngoscopy in the detection of mucosal lesions of the larynx.

Interpretation of CT scans of the larynx is difficult. A detailed knowledge of laryngeal anatomy and its appearance in the transverse plane is essential. Rigorous attention must be paid to detail in performing the examination. Misdiagnoses can be made if the patient's head is tilted or incorrectly extended. Detection and characterization of pathologic processes in the larynx require careful observation and experience. An understanding of the therapy for various laryngeal diseases and of the potential impact of CT results on patient management is also important.

ANATOMY

The larynx with its delicate cartilages, finely controlled muscles, and intricate joints and ligaments is really only a modified sphincteral valve at the entrance to the airway.[5] Suspended from above and continuous with the mobile trachea below, the larynx is capable of considerable vertical movement and rotation. It consists of an articulated cartilaginous skeleton surrounding the laryngeal airway, with many ligaments supporting the cartilages. Numerous muscles control movement of the cartilages, ligaments, and joints. Surrounding the entire larynx is a second group of muscles and ligaments that suspend the larynx from above and stabilize it from below.

LARYNGEAL SKELETON

Three large single cartilages (thyroid, cricoid, epiglottic) and three small paired cartilages (arytenoid, corniculate, cuneiform) comprise the laryngeal skeleton (Fig. 3–1). In men, the larynx measures only 4.4 by 4.3 by 3.6 cm (length, coronal diameter, and sagittal diameter); in women, it is about 25 per cent smaller.[6]

Thyroid Cartilage

The thyroid cartilage is the largest of the laryngeal cartilages and is shaped like the prow of a ship facing forward (Fig. 3–1). It is easily palpable beneath the skin and fascia of the neck. The cartilage is formed by two quadrangular plates or laminae (alae), fused in the midline at an angle of about 90° in the male and 120° in the female. A large V-shaped notch interrupts the superior margin in the midline and projects downward for about one third of the vertical height of the cartilage. The apex of the V projects slightly forward as the laryngeal prominence, or Adam's apple. The superior margin curves down posteriorly and then turns upward to become the superior horns, or cornua. The strong thyrohyoid membrane attaches to the superior margin.

During swallowing or a Valsalva maneuver, the thyroid cartilage ascends to within the horseshoe arch of the hyoid bone as far as the level of the thyroid notch, while the superior thyroid horns may ascend to between or behind the greater hyoid horns. The rounded posterior borders of the laminae terminate below to become the inferior thyroid horns, which provide attachment for

the longitudinal pharyngeal muscles. The short, thick inferior thyroid horns have small medial facets for articulation with the cricoid cartilage. The cricothyroid ligaments attach to the midportion of the inferior borders of the laminae, and the cricothyroid muscles attach to the remainder of the inferior border. The thyrohyoid, sternothyroid, and inferior constrictor muscles are obliquely attached to the outer surface of each slightly convex lamina. Thus, the thyroid cartilage is stabilized from above, below, and posteriorly by muscle and ligamentous connections.

The inner surface, near the midline, below the level of the notch, has attachments for the three ligaments and two muscles that form the bulk of the internal structures of the larynx. From superior to inferior, they are the thyroepiglottic, ventricular (false cord), and vocal (true cord) ligaments. The thyroepiglottic and thyroarytenoid muscles attach close to the ligaments.

The thyroid cartilage is sufficiently well calcified in most adults over the age of 30 years to be visible on CT scans. The degree of thyroid calcification varies among patients, but generally, it increases with age. The symmetry of calcification of the two laminae assists in the interpretation of CT scans. The posterior third of the thyroid cartilage invariably calcifies earlier than the anterior two thirds. Additional sites of dense calcification are the anterior midportion below the thyroid notch and the anterior portion of each laminae above the level of the notch. In older adults, the laminae frequently ossify and the cavity contains medullary tissue. The appearance of the thyroid laminae on CT scans depends on the spatial resolution of the scanner. Scanners with a pixel size of 1 to 1.5 mm show the laminae to be solid in about 50 per cent of older adults. In the other half, a central lucency is evident with inner and outer calcified margins. High-resolution scanners can differentiate between cortex and medulla in most older people.

Cricoid Cartilage

The "signet ring" cricoid cartilage forms the only complete cartilaginous ring in the airway (Fig. 3–1). It is smaller, thicker, and stronger than its superior neighbor. The posterior quadrate lamina, 2 to 3 cm in height and the narrower anterior arch, 5 to 7 mm in height, form the posterior and anterior boundaries of the lower larynx, respectively.[7] The cricoid is supported from above by the cricothyroid and inferior constrictor muscles attached to the outer surface of the arch

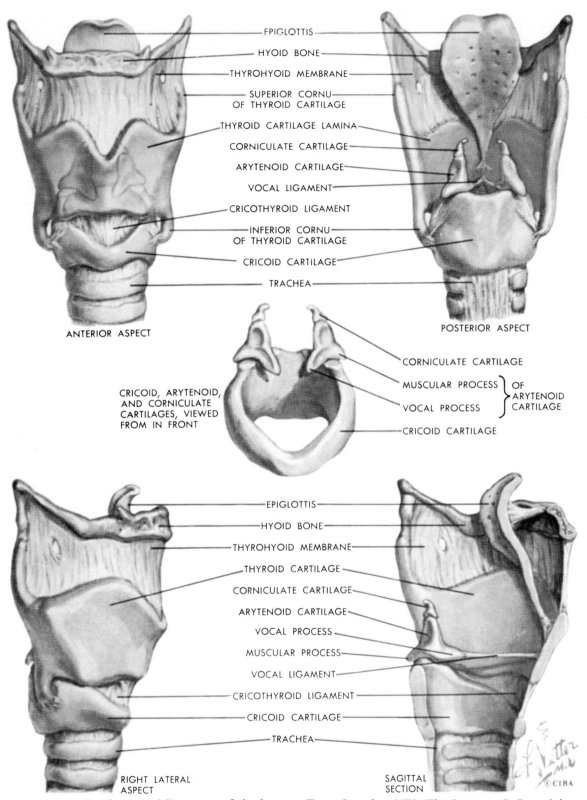

Figure 3–1. Cartilages and ligaments of the larynx. (From Saunders WH: The Larynx. © Copyright 1964, CIBA Pharmaceutical Company, Division of CIBA-GEIGY Corporation. Reprinted with permission from CLINICAL SYMPOSIA. Illustrated by Frank H. Netter, M.D. All rights reserved.)

and by the cricothyroid ligament attached to the upper rim. The lower rim provides attachment for the stabilizing cricotracheal ligament. At the junctions of the arch and the lamina are facets for articulation with the inferior thyroid horns. The ridges of the lamina afford attachment to the paired longitudinal fibers of the esophagus and a hollow for the origin of the posterior cricoarytenoid muscles. On the upper edge of the lamina are small facets for articulation with the two arytenoid cartilages. The inner surface of the cricoid is smooth and in contact with the mucosal lining of the airway. On CT scans, soft tissue is not normally visible between the inner margin of the cricoid cartilage and the airway below the vocal cords. In older adults, the cricoid cartilage is usually calcified. On CT scans, the lamina appears to have a densely calcified margin and a nonmineralized center. As with the thyroid cartilage, the cricoid cartilage can ossify and surround a marrow-containing cavity.

Epiglottic Cartilage

The mobile epiglottis is strengthened by a thin, curved paddle of elastic cartilage that projects upward and backward behind the root of the tongue (Fig. 3–1). Together with the aryepiglottic folds, the epiglottis forms the inlet to the laryngeal vestibule. Only about one third of the epiglottis has a free margin; this third is covered with mucous membrane both in front and in back. The other two thirds of the epiglottis is within the anterior wall of the laryngeal vestibule. The anterior surface of the free portion of the epiglottis faces the base of the tongue and attaches to it by a median glossoepiglottic fold and to the pharynx by two lateral pharyngoepiglottic folds. The two depressions formed by these three folds are the valleculae. The anterior wall of the inferior two thirds of the epiglottis forms the boundary of the adipose-containing pre-epiglottic space, which is behind the hyoid bone, thyrohyoid membrane, and upper portion of the thyroid cartilage. The smooth laryngeal surface of the epiglottis is concave from side to side and convex from top to bottom. The curvature is maintained by the anterior midline hyoepiglottic ligament and the posterior aryepiglottic ligaments. The stalk of the epiglottis is firmly attached by the thyroepiglottic ligament to the inner margin of the thyroid cartilage below the notch.

Calcification is not a prominent feature of the epiglottic cartilage. With high-resolution scanners, discontinuous plaques of calcium can some-

times be seen immediately inside the anterior surface of the laryngeal vestibule. The position of the epiglottic cartilage must otherwise be inferred from its anatomic location.

Arytenoid, Corniculate, and Cuneiform Cartilages

The two pyramidal arytenoid cartilages sit on and articulate with the superior surface of the lamina of the cricoid cartilage (Fig. 3–1). Their flat medial surfaces are covered with mucosa. Their concave posterior surfaces give origin to the oblique and transverse arytenoid muscles. The ridged anterolateral surface provides origin for the vocal muscle, thyroarytenoid muscle, and vestibular ligament. Toward the base of each pyramid is an anterior projection called the vocal process, from which the vocal ligament arises. Identification of the level of the vocal process of the arytenoid cartilages is of prime importance in viewing CT scans of the larynx because it precisely identifies the level of the true vocal cords. With the patient in the relaxed state, such as during quiet breathing, the arytenoid cartilages are in an abducted position less than 2 mm from the inner margin of the thyroid laminae (Fig. 3–2A). Demonstration of the vocal processes of the arytenoid cartilages is dependent on the spatial resolution of the CT scan. With intermediate resolution scanners, they are identifiable in over 50 per cent of normal adults. With thin scans and high resolution scanners, they can be identified in most people. During phonation or a Valsalva maneuver, the arytenoid cartilages adduct and rotate medially, approaching the midline (Fig. 3–2B).[8, 9]

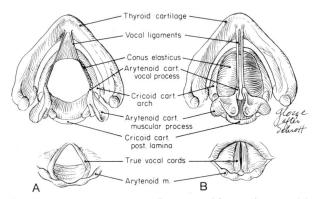

Figure 3–2. Movement of arytenoid cartilages with phonation. **A, B** Views from above of the cricothyroid complex (upper panels) and the endoscopic appearance (lower panels) during quiet breathing (**A**) and phonation (**B**). Arytenoid cartilages adduct and rotate medially during phonation. (From Mancuso AA, Hanafee WN: Computed Tomography of the Head and Neck, p 4. © 1982, The Williams & Wilkins Company, Baltimore. Reprinted by permission.)

In adults, the arytenoid cartilages are usually densely calcified. Their degree of calcification is moderately asymmetric, and on CT scans one cartilage appears larger than the other in about 10 per cent of adults. Arytenoid cartilages display three calcification patterns: they can appear as dense, round disks, or they can be comma-shaped or triangular.

The apex of each arytenoid cartilage is pointed upward and inward and bears the small nodular corniculate cartilages. On CT scans, these are normally inseparable from the arytenoid cartilages. The apex, or superior process, of the arytenoid cartilage defines the approximate level of the false vocal cords. On CT scans, the laryngeal ventricles are infrequently demonstrated, and therefore differentiation between the true and false vocal cords is not possible in most people.

The insignificant, paired, cuneiform cartilages are small, strengthening rods within the aryepiglottic folds. They are occasionally visible on CT scans as small densities within the aryepiglottic folds anterior and slightly above the arytenoid cartilages.

Hyoid Bone

The hyoid bone is not anatomically part of the larynx; but because its intimate contact with the upper airway (Fig. 3–1) makes it clinically important, it should be included in any discussion of the larynx. The hyoid is tripartite; it has a central body and two wings, each containing a greater and lesser horn. The quite massive bar of bone forming the body lies transversely in front of the pre-epiglottic space and valleculae.[10] The greater horns extend posterolaterally to encompass the lower hypopharynx and the entrances to the piriform sinuses. The larynx is suspended by the thyrohyoid membrane, which attaches the thyroid cartilage to the hyoid bone, and by the hypoepiglottic ligament, which attaches the epiglottis to the hyoid bone. They hyoid bone is in turn stabilized by attachments to the mandible and skull by the stylohyoid ligament and the digastric, stylohyoid, mylohyoid, hyoglossal, and geniohyoid muscles.

LARYNGEAL JOINTS

The larynx is capable of considerable vertical movement as a whole and also intrinsic movement by virtue of the cricothyroid and cricoarytenoid joints. Both joints are enclosed in well-formed capsules. The cricothyroid joint is synovial and allows the thyroid cartilage to tilt, rotate, and glide with reference to the cricoid cartilage. The cricoarytenoid joint allows for two directions of movement. It allows the arytenoids to rotate vertically, opening and closing the space between the true vocal cords (the rima glottidis), and it allows them to glide toward or away from each other. These two movements are coordinated so that medial rotation is accompanied by adduction and lateral rotation, by abduction.

LARYNGEAL MEMBRANES AND LIGAMENTS

The ligaments of the larynx can be considered extrinsic, connecting the laryngeal cartilages to adjacent structures, and intrinsic, connecting the laryngeal cartilages to one another.

Extrinsic Ligaments

The broad thyrohyoid membrane with its medial and lateral condensations of tissue attaches to the superior border of the thyroid cartilage and passes up behind the hyoid bone (Fig. 3–1). It is separated from the hyoid by a midline bursa, which facilitates upward movement of the larynx. On its outer surface, the thyrohyoid membrane is immediately behind the infrahyoid strap muscles. Its inner surface forms the anterior boundary of the pre-epiglottic space toward the midline, and posterolaterally the inner surface is contiguous with the upper lateral part of the piriform sinuses. The thyrohyoid membrane cannot be seen on CT scans, but its position is easily identified—between the low-density pre-epiglottic space and the higher-density strap muscles.

The epiglottis is loosely tethered by the glossoepiglottic fold and by the elastic hyoepiglottic ligament, which runs from the anterior surface of the epiglottis to the upper border of the body of the hyoid bone. The hypoepiglottic ligament is usually visible on CT scans, traversing the pre-epiglottic space in the midline.

The cricotracheal ligament forms the inferior attachment of the larynx. The fibrous membrane of this ligament connects the tracheal cartilages and continues upward to attach to the lower border of the cricoid cartilage.

Intrinsic Ligaments

The major intrinsic ligament of the larynx is the cricovocal ligament, also known as the cricothyroid membrane or conus elasticus (Fig. 3–2). It is formed by two strong, but flexible, fibroelastic sheets in the shape of a tent open at the back and slit at the top. The strong anterior portion attaches the upper edge of the cricoid arch to the inferior border of the thyroid cartilage. The midportion of this part of the membrane is subcutaneous. The more delicate lateral extensions of the conus elasticus also arise from the superior margin of the cricoid cartilage, but then they arch upward and inward to blend into the vocal ligaments and form the superior free margins of the conus elasticus. The medial surface of the conus elasticus is lined with mucous membrane continuous with that of the trachea. The lateral surface is immediately within the cricothyroid, lateral cricoarytenoid, and thyroarytenoid muscles.

The vocal ligaments stretch from the vocal processes of the arytenoid cartilages posteriorly to the inner angle of the thyroid cartilage, a little below the midpoint between the upper and lower borders. Above and parallel to the vocal ligaments are the paired ventricular, or vestibular, ligaments. These ligaments lie within the false vocal cords and are less well defined than the vocal ligaments; they extend from the tubercles on the arytenoid cartilages to the angle of the thyroid cartilage, slightly below the notch. The single, cordlike, thyroepiglottic ligament is an elastic prolongation of the epiglottic cartilage. It attaches the stem of the epiglottis to the back of the angle of the thyroid cartilage immediately above the attachment of the ventricular ligaments.

In the posterior larynx, the capsule of the cricoarytenoid joint is strengthened by a posterior cricoarytenoid ligament, which extends from the cricoid cartilage to the medial and dorsal surfaces of the base of the arytenoid cartilage.

INTRINSIC MUSCLES OF THE LARYNX

The intrinsic muscles of the larynx perform two functions: They adjust the aperture of the rima glottidis and close the larynx from the hypopharynx.

The adjuster muscles are grouped around the arytenoid cartilages and the cricoarytenoid joints to affect length, tension, and the degree of adduction of the true vocal cords (Fig. 3–3).[8] Each lateral cricoarytenoid muscle passes from the cricoid cartilage to the muscular process of the ipsilateral arytenoid cartilage, pulling it forward and downward. The posterior cricoarytenoid muscles arise from the posterior surface of the cricoid lamina to the back of the arytenoid cartilage and abducts the vocal cords. The transverse and oblique arytenoid muscles form a sling between the two arytenoid cartilages, adducting them and, hence, the true vocal cords.

The vocalis muscles, formed by the lower fibers of the thyroarytenoid muscles, are the only muscles spanning the endolarynx. Each arises from the angle of the thyroid cartilage and the conus elasticus as a broad, thin band within the true vocal cord and paralleling the vocal ligament. It passes backward to insert into the vocal process, the base, and anterior surface of the arytenoid cartilage (Fig. 3–3). By a complicated mechanism, the vocalis muscle can both shorten and adduct the vocal cord. With the present density resolution of CT, the vocalis muscle cannot be separated from the vocal ligament and paraglottic tissues.

The muscular connection between the cricoid and thyroid cartilages is the triangular cricothyroid muscle. It passes from the anterolateral outer surface of the cricoid to the inferior border of the thyroid lamina. By tilting the cricoid cartilage backward, the cricothyroid muscle causes elongation and increases tension of the vocal cords.

The sphincter muscles of the larynx are the aryepiglottic, thyroepiglottic, and thyroarytenoid (Fig. 3–3). Together they form a sling between the epiglottis, thyroid, and arytenoid cartilages. Acting in unison, they constrict the laryngeal inlet by shortening the aryepiglottic folds and pulling the arytenoid cartilages forward and upward against the posterior aspect of the epiglottis.[11]

LARYNGEAL CAVITY

The laryngeal cavity extends from the laryngeal inlet above, through the vestibule, false cords, ventricles, true cords, and subglottic space as far as the inferior border of the cricoid cartilage. The inlet of the larynx is a triangular ovoid set obliquely in the anterior wall of the hypopharynx. The anterior margin (base of the triangle) is formed by the free edge of the epiglottis, the sides by the aryepiglottic folds, and the truncated apex of the triangle by the arytenoid cartilages and the interarytenoid notch.

For clinical purposes and for the staging of laryngeal cancers, the laryngeal cavity is divided into three regions: the supraglottic, the glottic, and the subglottic (Fig. 3–4).[12]

Supraglottic Region

This region consists of the posterior surface of the epiglottis, including its tip; the aryepiglottic folds; the arytenoid cartilages; the ventricular folds (false cords); and the ventricular cavities. The vestibule of the larynx is within the supraglottic region and is bounded by the epiglottic

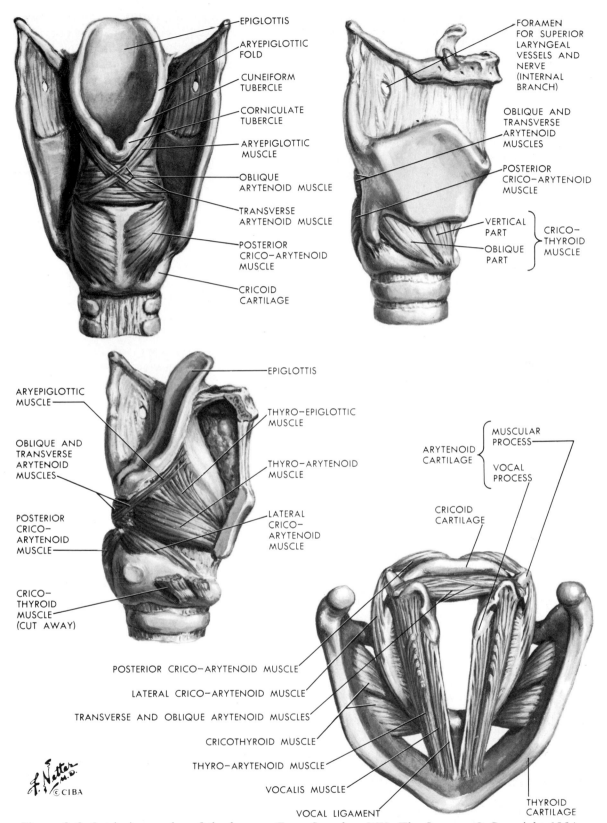

EPIGLOTTIS

ARYEPIGLOTTIC FOLD

CUNEIFORM TUBERCLE

CORNICULATE TUBERCLE

ARYEPIGLOTTIC MUSCLE

OBLIQUE ARYTENOID MUSCLE

TRANSVERSE ARYTENOID MUSCLE

POSTERIOR CRICO–ARYTENOID MUSCLE

CRICOID CARTILAGE

FORAMEN FOR SUPERIOR LARYNGEAL VESSELS AND NERVE (INTERNAL BRANCH)

OBLIQUE AND TRANSVERSE ARYTENOID MUSCLES

POSTERIOR CRICO–ARYTENOID MUSCLE

VERTICAL PART

OBLIQUE PART

CRICO–THYROID MUSCLE

ARYEPIGLOTTIC MUSCLE

OBLIQUE AND TRANSVERSE ARYTENOID MUSCLES

POSTERIOR CRICO–ARYTENOID MUSCLE

CRICO–THYROID MUSCLE (CUT AWAY)

EPIGLOTTIS

THYRO–EPIGLOTTIC MUSCLE

THYRO–ARYTENOID MUSCLE

LATERAL CRICO–ARYTENOID MUSCLE

ARYTENOID CARTILAGE

MUSCULAR PROCESS

VOCAL PROCESS

CRICOID CARTILAGE

POSTERIOR CRICO–ARYTENOID MUSCLE

LATERAL CRICO–ARYTENOID MUSCLE

TRANSVERSE AND OBLIQUE ARYTENOID MUSCLES

CRICOTHYROID MUSCLE

THYRO–ARYTENOID MUSCLE

VOCALIS MUSCLE

VOCAL LIGAMENT

THYROID CARTILAGE

Figure 3–3. Intrinsic muscles of the larynx. (From Saunders WH: The Larynx. © Copyright 1964, CIBA Pharmaceutical Company, Division of CIBA-GEIGY Corporation. Reprinted with permission from CLINICAL SYMPOSIA. Illustrated by Frank H. Netter, M.D. All rights reserved.)

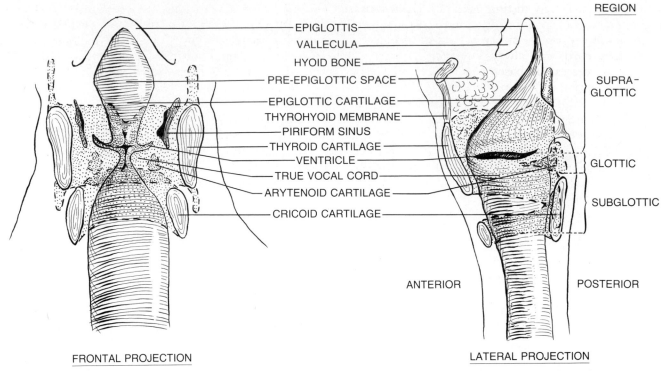

FRONTAL PROJECTION   LATERAL PROJECTION

Figure 3–4. Soft tissues and cavity of the larynx. The larynx is divided into three anatomic regions. The largest is the supraglottic region and the smallest is the glottic region.

cartilage anteriorly and the aryepiglottic folds laterally. The vestibule is smallest posteriorly, where it is limited by the fold of mucosa between the arytenoid cartilages. During swallowing, the aryepiglottic folds shorten and the arytenoid cartilages rise to the posterior wall of the epiglottis, closing the upper portion of the vestibule. The ventricular folds form two soft bumpers running from the angle of the thyroid cartilage to the arytenoid cartilages. The ventricular folds have less variety of movement than the true cords because they do not have many muscle fibers. Inferiorly they merge with the roof of the laryngeal ventricle.

The most inferior extent of the supraglottic region is the keel-shaped laryngeal ventricle between the false and true cords. Immediately beneath the mucosa of the laryngeal ventricle is the thyroarytenoid muscle. Arising as a narrow opening from the anterior recess of the ventricle is the appendix of the laryngeal ventricle. This blind sac of variable size lies between the inner surface of the thyroid cartilage and the ventricular fold. At times, it can be large, extending to the upper border of the thyroid cartilage or even through the thyrohyoid membrane to present in the neck as a laryngocele. The appendix of the laryngeal ventricle can be demonstrated in about 40 per cent of laryngograms.[13] On CT scans obtained during

phonation, it is seen in about 10 per cent of people as an air-containing structure immediately within the anterior third of the thyroid cartilage.

Glottic Region

This region comprises the true vocal cords (vocal folds), and the anterior and posterior commissures. The inferior extent of this region is not clearly defined, but it is 4 to 10 mm below the free margin of the vocal cords. The vocal folds are tightly bound to the vocal ligaments, which stretch between the junction of the lower third and upper two thirds of the thyroid cartilage at the thyroid angle and the vocal processes of the arytenoid cartilages. The anterior three fifths of the true cords form the membranous portion and the posterior two fifths form the cartilaginous portion, enveloping the vocal processes of the arytenoid cartilages. The upper surface of the true cords borders on the supraglottic region, and the lower surface merges with the subglottic region. Posteriorly the glottic region is bounded by the mucosa between the arytenoid cartilages (the interarytenoid notch, or posterior commissure).

Lateral and parallel to the vocal ligament is the amazing vocalis muscle (Fig. 3–3), which controls tension, elasticity, and rigidity of the vocal cords. During quiet breathing, true vocal cords cannot always be precisely distinguished on CT scans. In their abducted position, they blend with the soft tissues of the lateral laryngeal walls. The level of the true cords can always be inferred when the vocal processes, or bases of the arytenoid cartilages, are seen. CT scans obtained during phonation will demonstrate the normal true cords apposing at the midline.

The anterior commissure is not well defined anatomically. It is the area between the anterior junction of the true and false vocal cords. It is of great clinical significance because malignant neoplasms tend to cross the midline and to gain access to the subglottic region at this site.

Subglottic Region

This region extends from the glottis above to the lower margin of the arch of the cricoid cartilage. In transverse cross section, the airway is almost perfectly round at these levels. Anteriorly the subglottic region is limited by the mucosa over the lower third of the thyroid cartilage, the cricothyroid membrane, and the anterior arch of the cricoid cartilage. The lateral borders are formed by the portion of the cricothyroid membrane known as the conus elasticus and by the lateral arch of the cricoid cartilage. Posteriorly the large signet portion of the cricoid cartilage limits the subglottic space.

SOFT TISSUES OF THE ENDOLARYNX

Computed tomography precisely reflects the soft tissues contained within the laryngeal cartilages. The amount of soft tissue demonstrated is dependent on the level of the image, the phase of respiration or phonation, and the orientation of the larynx relative to the plane of the scan. For reproducible CT images, the vocal cords should be parallel to the plane of scanning (see the section on techniques of examination).

The most inferior extent of the subglottic region is within the ring of the cricoid cartilage, approximately 15 mm below the level of the true vocal cords. The mucosa of the airway is closely applied to the perichondrium of the underlying cartilage, and no soft tissue is visible at this level on CT scans (Fig. 3–5).[14] Over the next higher 1 cm, the more massive, posterior, signet portion of the cricoid cartilage maintains its intimate connection to the airway, without intervening soft tissue (Figs. 3–6 and 3–7). The thyroid cartilage appears anteriorly 5 to 10 mm below the level of the true cords.

Soft tissues of the endolarynx start to appear on CT scans of the glottic region (Fig. 3–8). During quiet breathing, the true vocal cords are triangular, bordered by the airway medially, the thyroid cartilage anteriorly and laterally, and the arytenoid cartilage and thyroarytenoid tissues posteriorly (Fig. 3–9A,B). As indicated previously, the base and the vocal process of each arytenoid cartilage precisely define the level of each true vocal cord. During quiet breathing, the abducted true vocal cords usually appear symmetric. The distance from the medial margin of the vocal process to the inner margin of the thyroid cartilage is only 5.5 to 9.5 mm, this distance representing the lateral thickness of the normal tissues of the cords.[14] The posterior portions of the undersurfaces of the true vocal cords are often visible for 5 mm below the level of the vocal processes of the arytenoid cartilages (Fig. 3–8). They invariably appear symmetric and should not be mistaken for a subglottic mass.

At the anterior commissure between the anterior extent of the true vocal cords, the airway is usually bordered by the inner margin of the thyroid angle. When the thyroid angle is acute, 1 to 2 mm of soft tissue is normally seen at the anterior commissure (Fig. 3–9A,B). As mentioned earlier, the posterior commissure is above the cricoid lamina between the arytenoid cartilages. Soft tissue is not usually visible in this region when the larynx is in a relaxed state.

Phonation, a Valsalva maneuver, or holding the breath with the glottis closed, causes apposition of the true vocal cords and therefore markedly changes the soft tissues of the glottis (Fig. 3–10A,B). The vocal processes of the arytenoid cartilages move medially an average of 4 to 5 mm, reflecting their abduction and medial rotation.[14] On CT scans at low window levels and wide window width, the true vocal cords can be seen spanning the glottis with a small, slit-like space between them (Fig. 3–11). During phonation, the interarytenoid portion of the airway is circular (Fig. 3–10B). Both the anterior and posterior commissures frequently show compressed soft tissues, which should not be mistaken for masses at these sites.

The laryngeal ventricles are only occasionally visible on high-resolution CT scans (Fig. 3–12A,B), and the true and false cords frequently cannot be separated. Mancuso and Hanafee[15] refer to the region 5 to 10 mm above the base of the arytenoid cartilages and their vocal processes as the transitional zone of the larynx. At this level, the anterior larynx is still characterized by the airway

Text continued on page 80

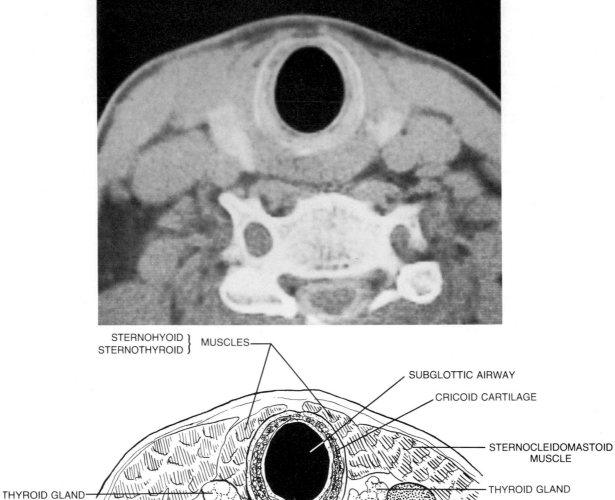

Figure 3–5. Low subglottic level of the normal larynx. CT scan (top) accompanied by a labeled schema (bottom) at the same level.

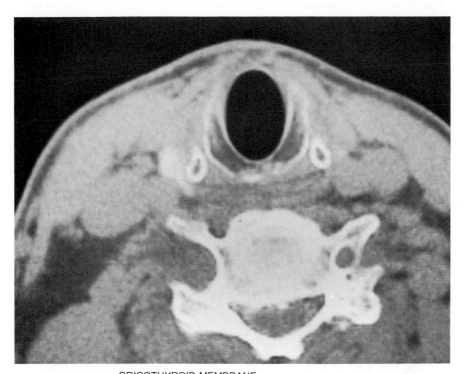

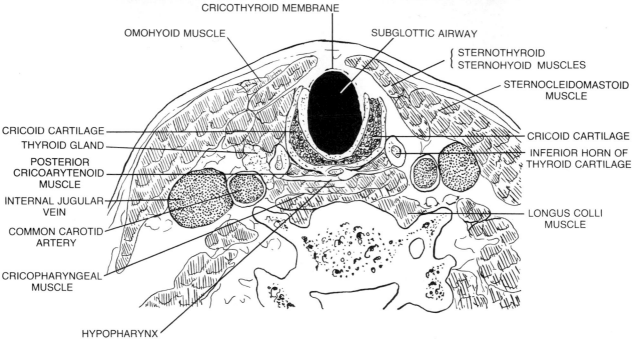

CRICOTHYROID MEMBRANE

OMOHYOID MUSCLE

SUBGLOTTIC AIRWAY

{ STERNOTHYROID
STERNOHYOID } MUSCLES

STERNOCLEIDOMASTOID
MUSCLE

CRICOID CARTILAGE

THYROID GLAND

POSTERIOR
CRICOARYTENOID
MUSCLE

INTERNAL JUGULAR
VEIN

COMMON CAROTID
ARTERY

CRICOPHARYNGEAL
MUSCLE

CRICOID CARTILAGE

INFERIOR HORN OF
THYROID CARTILAGE

LONGUS COLLI
MUSCLE

HYPOPHARYNX

Figure 3–6. High subglottic level of the normal larynx. CT scan (top) accompanied by a labeled schema (bottom) at the same level.

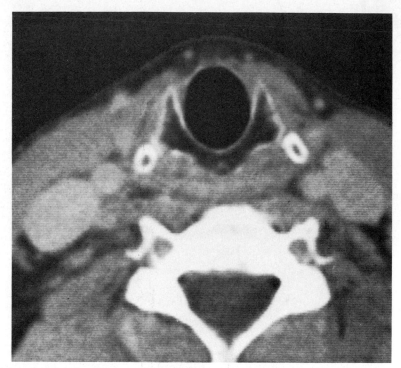

Figure 3–7. High subglottic level of the normal larynx. CT scan in a different patient than in Figure 3–6 shows the lamina of the cricoid cartilage with normal, irregular posterior border.

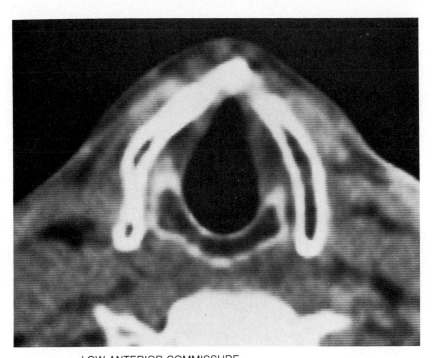

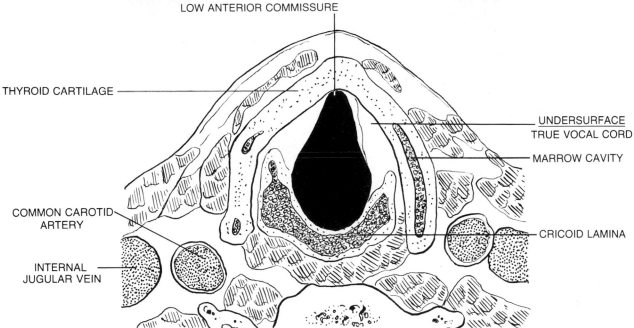

LOW ANTERIOR COMMISSURE

THYROID CARTILAGE

UNDERSURFACE
TRUE VOCAL CORD

MARROW CAVITY

COMMON CAROTID
ARTERY

CRICOID LAMINA

INTERNAL
JUGULAR VEIN

Figure 3–8. Normal larynx. CT scan (top) and labeled schema (bottom) at the same level show soft tissues of the undersurfaces of the true vocal cords and conus elasticus. The anterior commissure is immediately behind the thyroid angle.

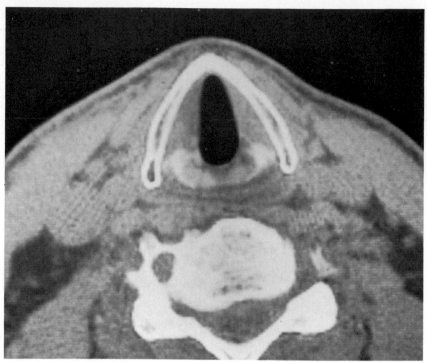

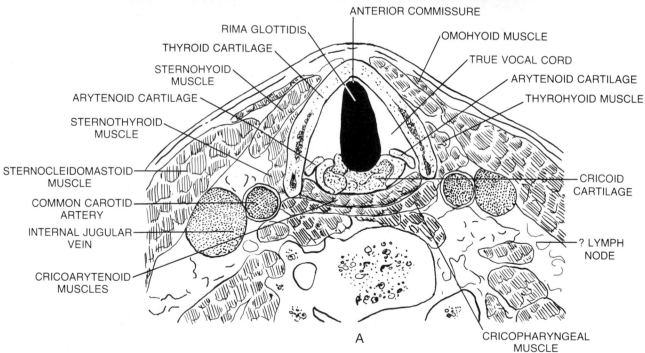

Figure 3–9. Relaxed normal larynx at the level of the glottis. **A** CT scan shows true vocal cords anterior to the arytenoid cartilages.

Illustration continued on opposite page

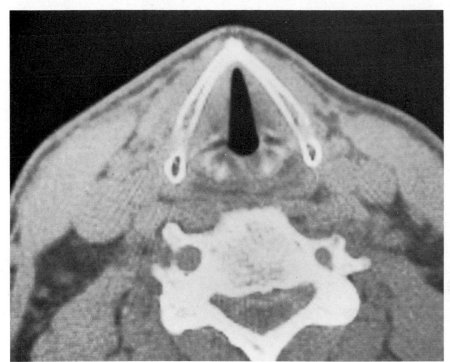

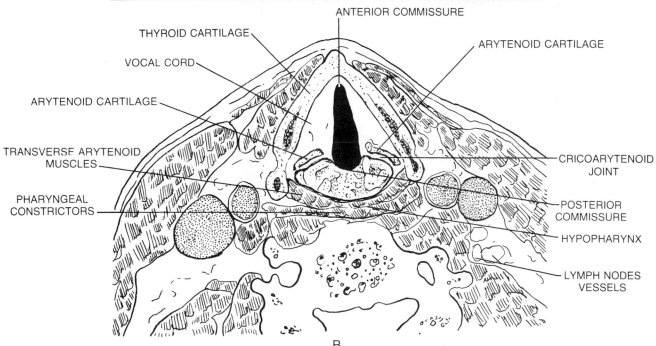

B

Figure 3–9. *Continued* **B**   Scan 3mm cephalad to **A,** the posterior surface of the partially calcified posterior wall of each arytenoid is still visible. Each scan (top) is accompanied by a labeled schema (bottom) at the same level.

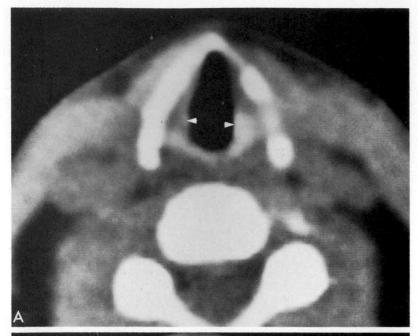

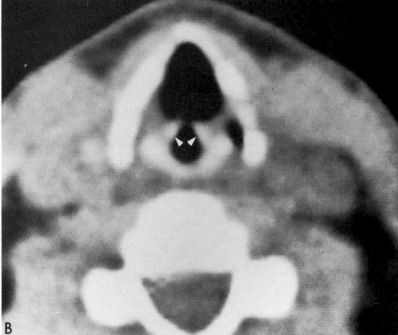

Figure 3–10. Normal glottis. **A** CT scan at a window level of 50 H and a window width of 500 H obtained during quiet breathing shows that the arytenoid cartilages (arrowheads) are abducted. **B** During phonation, arytenoid cartilages rotate and adduct (arrowheads).

remaining close to the inner margin of the thyroid cartilage. Laterally the tissues forming the false vocal cords are moderately varied in depth. They maintain a triangular shape and are symmetric from side to side. The CT density of the lateral soft tissues in the transitional zone is relatively low. These tissues are composed of fat, connective tissue, and a few muscle fibers. The density of the paralaryngeal tissues at this level may also be affected by partial CT volume-averaging of the soft tissues with air in the nonvisible laryngeal ventricle. Occasionally one or both piriform sinuses extends as far inferiorly at the transitional zone. The air-containing apex of the piriform sinus will be visible posterolaterally, immediately within the thyroid cartilage.

Posteriorly at the level of the false cords, the upper portions of the arytenoid cartilages are still evident (Fig. 3–12B). The posterior soft tissues of the larynx blend with the collapsed hypopharynx and the prevertebral tissues. The distance between the airway and the spine is about 10 mm.

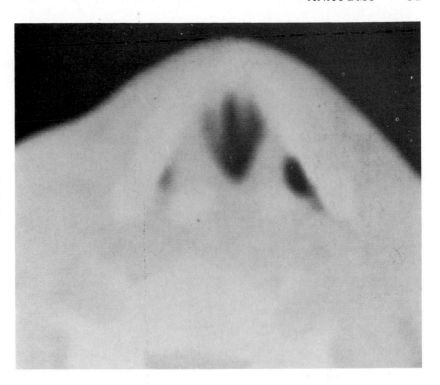

Figure 3–11. The normal glottis during phonation. CT scan at a window level of − 210 H and a window width of 1000 H shows vocal cords in adduction.

The bulk of the endolaryngeal soft tissue is found above the true and false cords. Anteriorly the pre-epiglottic space first becomes apparent 10 to 15 mm above the level of the true vocal cords (Fig. 3–13).[14] The pre-epiglottic space is limited posteriorly by the epiglottic cartilage and anteriorly by the thyroid cartilage, thyrohyoid membrane, and hyoid bone; it extends vertically for 10 to 20 mm. Inferiorly, it is narrow, but its antero-posterior diameter rapidly increases to 10 to 15 mm (Fig. 3–14). The space is triangular inferiorly and assumes a crescent shape at the level of the thyrohyoid membrane (Fig. 3–15).

More important than the dimensions of the pre-epiglottic space is its fatty density, which is readily apparent on CT scans. In the midline, the thyroepiglottic ligament can be seen as a higher CT density, ill-defined structure. On either side, the uniform low density of the pre-epiglottic space measures − 20 to − 60 H.[14] The fatty tissues of the pre-epiglottic space extend laterally into the anterior third of the aryepiglottic folds.

The lateral soft tissues of the supraglottic larynx are formed by the aryepiglottic folds. On CT scans, the lower 10 to 15 mm of each fold appears as an obliquely orientated band, between the laryngeal vestibule and the piriform sinus. Inferiorly the aryepiglottic folds cannot be separated from the false vocal cords. Posteriorly they merge with the collapsed lower hypopharynx in front of the spine. Demonstration on CT scans of the lower aryepiglottic folds as distinct structures depends on the piriform sinuses containing air. Each fold is about 5 mm thick in its inferior portion and is appreciably thinner during phonation when the piriform sinuses are distended (Fig. 3–16A,B). The difference in thickness of the aryepiglottic folds between the two sides can be up to 1.5 mm, which is readily appreciated on CT scans. Anteriorly, the folds are continuous with the pre-epiglottic space. The upper portion of each aryepiglottic fold protrudes into the airway from the sides of the epiglottis (Fig. 3–15). At this level, their free margins form the lateral boundaries of the entrance to the larynx. Cephalad, the aryepiglottic folds are continuous with the free margin of the epiglottis. In front of the epiglottis are the valleculae and the hyoid bone (Fig. 3–17).

The piriform sinuses are between the aryepiglottic folds medially and the inner margin of the posterior half of each thyroid lamina. In the transverse plane, their shapes vary from triangular to circular to elliptical, but they are generally similar from side to side. The entrance to each sinus is from the hypopharynx and is lateral to the laryngeal vestibule (Figs. 3–14 and 3–15). The lateral margin of each sinus is in intimate contact with the inner margin of the thyroid cartilage (Figs. 3–12B, 3–16A,B). The presence of any soft tissue between air in the piriform sinus and the inner wall of the thyroid cartilage is abnormal. The inferior extent of each piriform sinus varies

Text continued on page 88

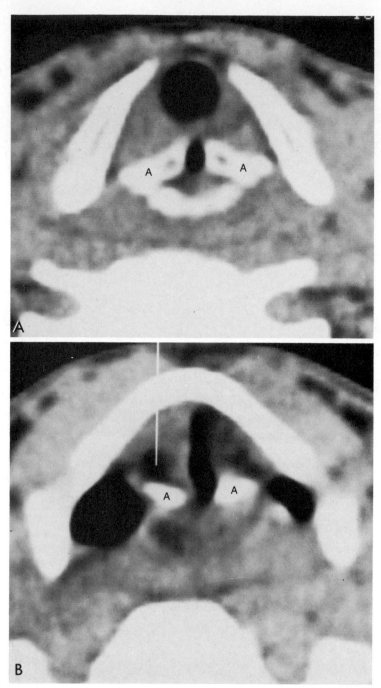

Figure 3–12. Normal glottis and laryngeal ventricle. **A** CT scan at the level of the true vocal cords shows arytenoid cartilages (A) adducted because of breath-holding with glottis closed. **B** Scan 9 mm cephalad to **A** shows air in the right laryngeal ventricle as a low-density area (vertical marker) anterior to the arytenoid cartilages (A). (Scans are 1.5 mm thick.) (Courtesy of Dr. Robert L. Stern, Concord, Calif.)

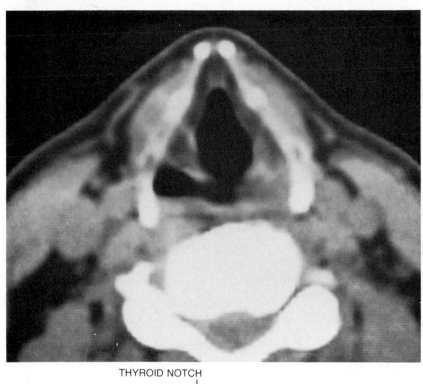

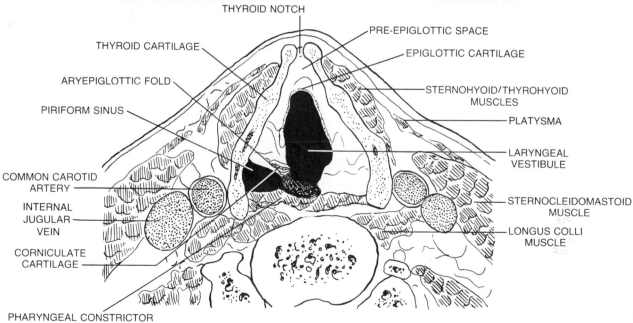

Figure 3–13. Normal supraglottic larynx. CT scan (top) at the level of the thyroid notch accompanied by a labeled schema (bottom).

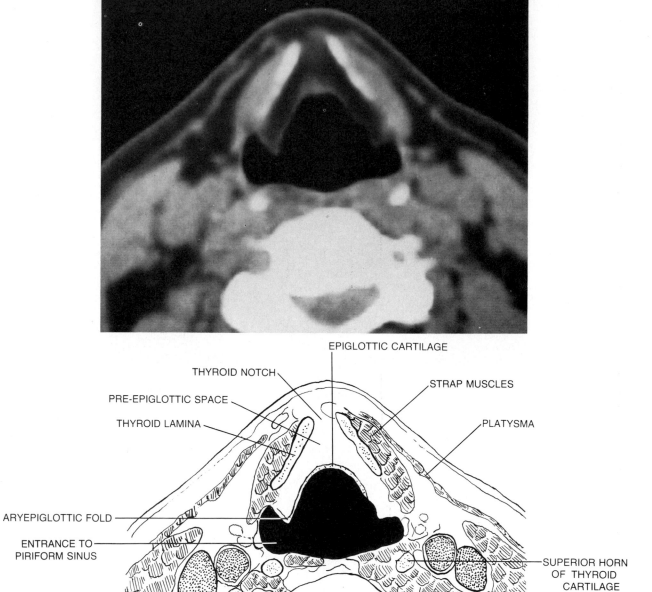

Figure 3–14. Normal supraglottic larynx. CT scan (top) at the level of the top of the thyroid cartilage accompanied by a labeled schema (bottom).

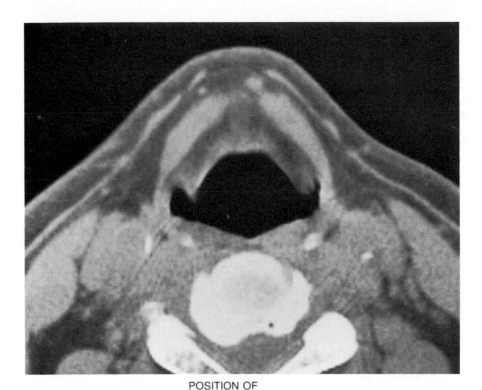

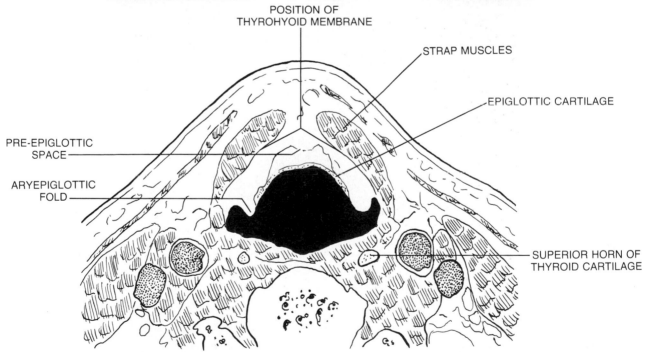

Figure 3–15. Normal supraglottic larynx. CT scan (top) at the level of the thyrohyoid membrane accompanied by a labeled schema (bottom).

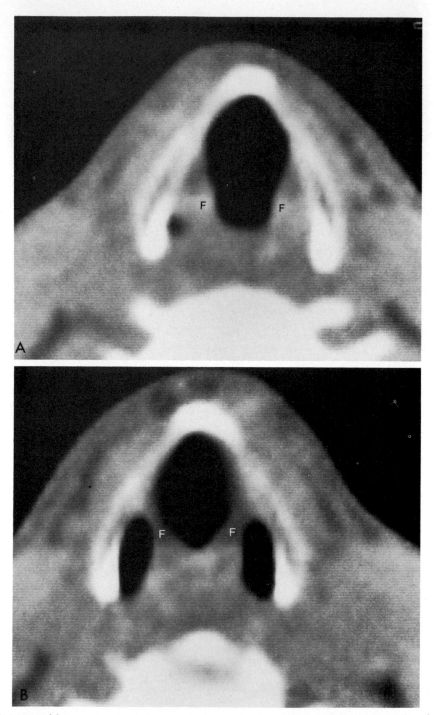

Figure 3–16. Normal low supraglottic larynx during quiet breathing and phonation. **A** CT scan during quiet breathing shows piriform sinuses collapsed and aryepiglottic folds (F) poorly displayed. **B** In scan obtained at the same level during phonation, the piriform sinuses are distended and the aryepiglottic folds (F) are thrown into relief.

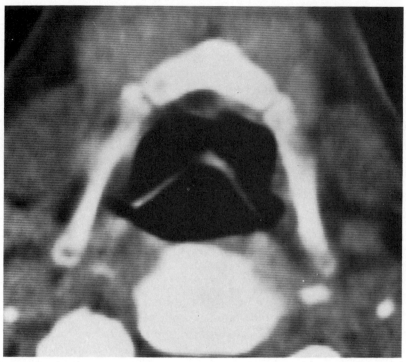

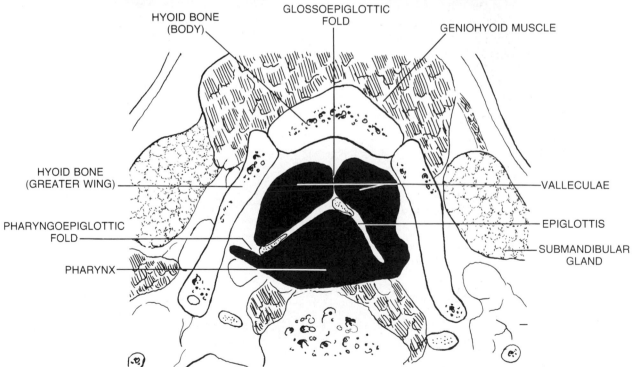

Figure 3–17. Normal hyoid bone and epiglottis. CT scan (top) accompanied by a labeled schema (bottom).

between the two sides and between patients. During quiet breathing, the sinuses are partially collapsed, and the most inferior level at which they are visible is from 5 to 25 mm above the true vocal cords.[14] During phonation, the sinuses distend and project downward to the level of the true vocal cords or within 5 mm of them (Fig. 3–11).

TECHNIQUES OF EXAMINATION

To obtain optimal CT scans of a small organ such as the larynx, meticulous attention must be given to the technical details of the examination. Nondiagnostic and even misleading images can be created unless adequate care is taken in such matters as patient positioning or respiratory maneuvers. In general, procedural details for CT of the larynx have not been documented in the literature.

RESPIRATION

The structures of the endolarynx are both motile and mobile, and the potential for distortion of their images on CT scans is considerable. The initial portion of the examination must be performed with the larynx in a state of complete relaxation, i.e., with the true vocal cords abducted. The patient is instructed to breathe quietly through the mouth without holding the breath at end inspiration or end expiration.

Following a series of scans through the larynx obtained during quiet breathing, an additional series should be obtained during a maneuver that will produce adduction of the true vocal cords and distention of the piriform sinuses. Scans during phonation of a low-pitched letter "E" are the easiest to obtain and the most reproducible.[3, 14] During phonation, the arytenoid cartilages adduct toward the midline (Fig. 3–10A,B). The piriform sinuses are distended and the aryepiglottic folds brought into relief. Scans obtained during a Valsalva maneuver will also show adduction of the true cords, but the images from this maneuver are less reproducible because the larynx moves vertically.

POSITION

The patient should be supine, with a pad between the shoulders to straighten the upper thorax. The arms should be pulled down along the side of the body as far as possible to avoid streak artifacts from the shoulder girdle. A useful adjunct is to have the patient grasp a sheet passed under the feet. The long axis of the larynx should be perpendicular to the plane of the image. The head (orbitomeatal line) is extended 35 to 40° to the vertical axis. When feasible, a lateral projection radiograph (computed radiograph, digital radiograph, scout view) should be obtained while the patient phonates the letter "E" (Fig. 3–18). The true vocal cords and laryngeal cartilages can be seen and the scanner gantry tilted or the position of the head altered to correctly align the larynx perpendicular to the plane of the scan. The

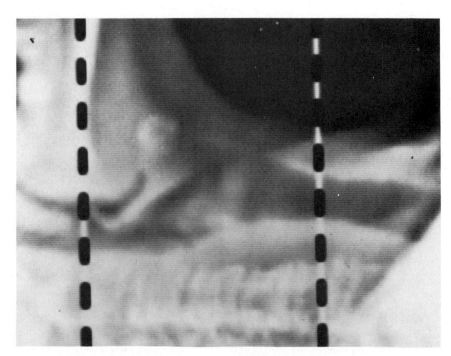

Figure 3–18. Lateral projection radiograph of the larynx. The laryngeal cartilages and vocal cords are visible and show precise levels for scanning. Dashed lines indicate region for scanning; in this case, the proximal trachea was included.

head is then immobilized in this position with either tape or a head holder.

A convenient routine is to start scanning at the lower border of the cricoid cartilage, which is easily palpated or seen on the projection radiograph. Five-millimeter collimation with contiguous scans as far cephalad as the valleculae will assure demonstration of the entire larynx. Twelve to 15 scans are usually required.

Modification to the field-of-interest should be undertaken with supraglottic tumors, for which the field should be extended cephalad to the angle of the mandible. With subglottic tumors the field is extended caudad to include the trachea and upper mediastinum.

CONTRAST MATERIAL

Intravenous contrast medium has not been shown to assist in the diagnosis of lesions within the larynx or piriform sinuses. Detection of cervical lymph node enlargement, however, is important in the evaluation of laryngeal carcinoma. Because the neck around the larynx contains numerous arteries and veins, opacification of these vessels is necessary to differentiate them from lymph nodes. Sixty or 76 per cent contrast medium should be administered by rapid-drip infusion or bolus injection to a total of 125 to 150 ml (35.25 to 42.3 grams of organically bound iodine). The timing of contrast medium infusion in relationship to scanning should maximize intravascular contrast. We have found that a bolus of 50 to 75 ml of 76 per cent contrast medium injected during rapid, sequential scanning with advancement of the scanner table is usually successful in demonstrating the vascular structures of the neck.

TECHNICAL CONSIDERATIONS

Recent improvements in scanner capabilities have facilitated imaging of the larynx. Many of the original studies of the larynx were obtained with scan times of 18 seconds or longer and relatively poor spatial resolution.[1, 2, 16, 17] Diagnostic examinations are possible with this equipment, but fine detail of the larynx is frequently not shown. Several of the newer scanners allow primary magnification of an area the size of the larynx with better temporal and spatial resolution; the highest resolution possible should be employed.[18] Balanced against this desirable feature is a need to maintain rapid scan times, in the range of under 5 seconds.

Special computer software allowing reconstruction of the scans with enhanced bone detail is available with some scanners. These scans produce excellent visualization of the laryngeal cartilages (Fig. 3–19).

Rapid sequential scanning with incrementation of the scanner table improves registration of the scans, with less likelihood of the patient moving during the imaging sequence.[18a] Images reformat-

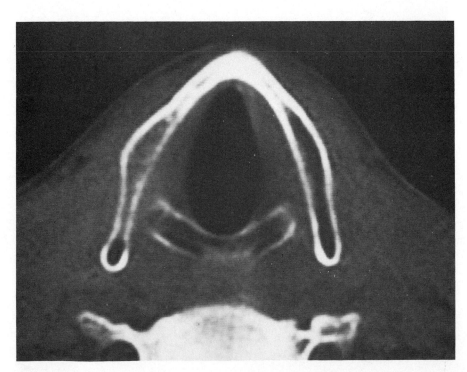

Figure 3–19. Laryngeal cartilages with enhanced bone detail. CT scan shows detail of inner and outer cortex of thyroid and cricoid cartilages.

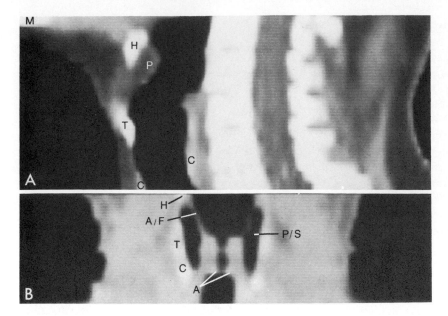

Figure 3–20. Multiplanar images of the normal larynx after reformation. **A** Image in the midsagittal plane of the larynx shows mandible (M), hyoid bone (H), thyroid cartilage (T), and cricoid cartilage (C). A low-density pre-epiglottic space (P) is visible anterior to epiglottic cartilage. **B** Image in coronal plane through the posterior half of the larynx during phonation shows hyoid bone (H), thyroid cartilage (T), cricoid cartilage (C), and distended piriform sinuses (P/S) lateral to the aryepiglottic folds (A/F). The arytenoid cartilages (A) are at the inferior extent of the true and false cords.

ted in the coronal or sagittal planes can be generated from multiple transverse scans, although they have not assisted in the diagnosis of laryngeal disease (Fig. 3–20A,B).[3, 19] Direct coronal CT scans of the neck and upper mediastinum can be made using scanners with a large aperture in their gantry (Fig. 21A,B).[20, 21] Reported experience with this last technique is limited, but the technique does have advantages compared with multiplanar reformatted images: Examination time is reduced and image quality improved.

CT images of the larynx are viewed at monitor settings appropriate for both calcified cartilage and soft tissue. A window level of 65 to 80 Hounsfield Units (H) and window width of 500 H are suitable. Additional images at the level of the

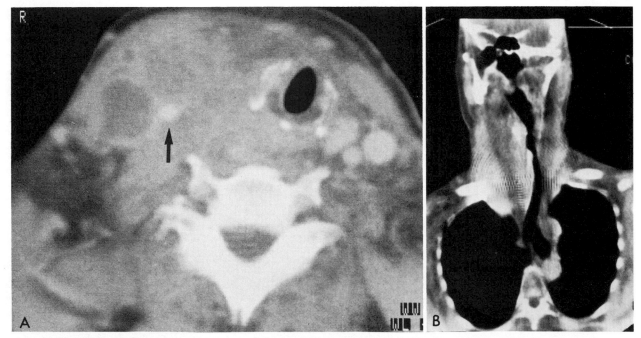

Figure 3–21. Direct coronal CT scan of the neck and upper mediastinum. Patient with infiltrating carcinoma of the thyroid gland. **A** Transverse CT scan of the larynx shows a mass displacing the larynx to the left and encasing the right common carotid artery (arrow). **B** Direct coronal CT scan demonstrates the extent of the mass in the right neck and superior mediastinum and narrowing of the displaced trachea. (From van Waes PFGM, Zonneveld FW: Direct coronal body computed tomography. J Comput Assist Tomogr 6: 58, 1982. Reprinted by permission.)

vocal cords are viewed at a window level of about −300 H and width of 1000 H, to show detail of the soft tissue–air interfaces of the endolarynx.

PATHOLOGY

NON-NEOPLASTIC LESIONS

The larynx can be affected by a variety of congenital, inflammatory, connective tissue, and idiopathic diseases. CT scans can show the size and extent of the disease process and detail the cross-sectional area and adequacy of the airway. Laryngeal CT is usually not capable of tissue characterization and cannot differentiate edema, inflammation, and neoplasia.

Granulomatous Diseases

The larynx is affected by both infectious granulomatous and noninfectious granulomatous diseases. In general, biopsy is required for diagnosis because the gross appearances are nonspecific.

Sarcoidosis is a systemic inflammatory disorder characterized by a granulomatous lesion containing noncaseating epitheloid tubercles. The incidence of laryngeal involvement is only 1.3 per cent of patients with sarcoidosis and rarely is the larynx the only site of disease.[22–24] Patients with laryngeal sarcoid present with hoarseness, cough, dysphasia, and dyspnea. Upper-airway obstruction can occur.[25] The larynx is diffusely edematous, often with the epiglottis and supraglottic larynx most severely affected. The true vocal cords are less frequently involved, but neuritis of the recurrent laryngeal nerve can occur and result in unilateral vocal cord paralysis.[22] Laryngoscopy reveals mucosal changes consisting of edema, erythema, nodules, and masslike lesions. We have seen one case of sarcoidosis in which CT scans showed marked thickening of the epiglottis and aryepiglottic folds. The glottis in this case showed diffuse thickening (Fig. 3–22A,B). Treatment of laryngeal sarcoidosis consists of systemic steroids with local steroid injections and, in selected cases, surgical excision.

Tuberculosis of the larynx virtually occurs only in patients with active pulmonary tuberculosis. Symptoms are hoarseness, cough, and pain that frequently radiates to one ear. Constitutional symptoms and dysphasia are evident in less than 50 per cent of patients.[25] Most commonly involved are the epiglottis and posterior laryngeal structures—areas that are readily visible with indirect laryngoscopy.[26, 27] The diagnosis is usually made by direct laryngoscopy and biopsy. In some cases, the vocal cords are predominantly involved and may have the appearance of an exophytic carcinoma. The CT findings have not been described but should show a diffuse thickening and increasing density of the paralaryngeal and preepiglottic tissues. The epiglottis and aryepiglottic folds should likewise be thickened. Encroachment on the laryngeal airway may be evident, although severe compromise of the airway seldom occurs. The CT appearance should be nonspecific and cannot differentiate laryngeal tuberculosis from other diffuse granulomatous processes or a diffusely infiltrating circumglottic carcinoma. Involvement of the cervical lymph nodes is common.

Other chronic granulomatous diseases due to specific infectious agents can also involve the larynx. With most of them, additional areas of the upper airway are affected simultaneously or prior to laryngeal involvement. *Scleroma of the larynx* (rhinoscleroma) is caused by the bacillus *Klebsiella rhinoscleromatis* (von Frisch bacillus).[25] It is a chronic granulomatous disease of central and southern Europe and South America. The incidence of scleroma is increasing both in other countries and in the United States. The nose is the most commonly involved site, but the larynx, pharynx, trachea, and bronchi can also be affected without nasal involvement. Acute laryngeal obstruction can occur in the initial, exudative stage. Untreated, the disease progresses to proliferative and cicatricial stages, resulting in stenosis throughout the upper respiratory tract.

Leprosy of the larynx usually occurs after involvement of the skin, oral cavity, and nose. The mucous membrane shows a diffuse nodular infiltration. Late respiratory obstruction due to vocal cord involvement may necessitate tracheostomy or surgery for laryngeal stenosis.

Tertiary or congenital *syphilis of the larynx* can produce punched-out ulcers or nodular infiltration. Healing is accompanied by deforming scar formation and, as with leprosy, may necessitate surgical intervention.

Mycotic infections of the larynx are rare and usually are associated with disease at other sites.[28] Symptoms include hoarseness, hemoptysis, and cough. Laryngeal histoplasmosis is mostly seen with the mucocutaneous form of the disease. Endoscopy reveals a nodular granulomatous mass, or ulceration. Laryngeal blastomycosis can also show nodular granulations and ulcerations. Pulmonary disease is usually evident as well as skin lesions. Coccidioidomycosis rarely involves the supraglottic larynx and its appearance is similar to those of the other mycotic infections. Candidiasis

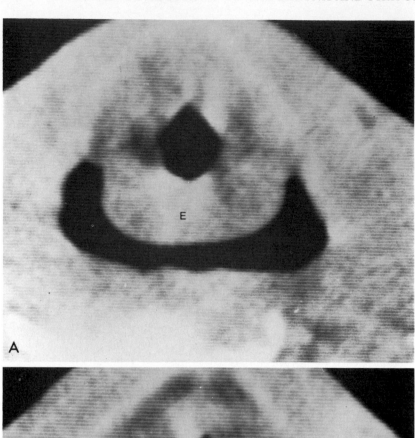

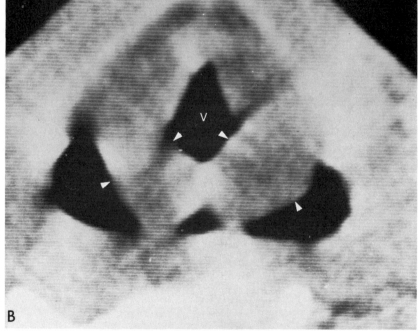

Figure 3–22. Supraglottic larynx in patient with sarcoidosis. **A** CT scan shows that the epiglottis (E) is markedly thickened and the pre-epiglottic space is diffusely increased in CT density. **B** Scan 1 cm caudad to **A,** the aryepiglottic folds are symmetrically thickened (arrowheads) and the laryngeal vestibule (V) is reduced in area. (Courtesy of Drs. J. P. Smith and J. Livoni, Sacramento, Calif.)

of the larynx is usually seen in immunocompromised patients or as a superinfection in patients receiving systemic antibiotics. Pain and dysphasia are the common symptoms, although respiratory obstruction can occur from sloughing of the thick membranous exudate, which can be observed at endoscopy.

Nonspecific, post-traumatic granulomas of the larynx are common; they are caused by endotracheal intubation and are bilateral in 50 per cent of cases.[29]

Their typical location is along the free margins of the true vocal cords in their posterior third adjacent to the vocal processes of the arytenoid cartilages. They may also occur along the lower borders of the aryepiglottic folds. The CT findings of these granulomas is a focal thickening of the involved region, often with increased CT density of the adjacent tissues. This appearance is nonspecific and should not be mistaken for tumor infiltration.[30]

Collagen Vascular Diseases

The collagen vascular diseases form an overlapping group of conditions in which fibrinoid necrosis of the walls of small vessels is a constant finding. They are multisystem disorders, and the larynx is frequently involved. Symptoms can include hoarseness, dyspnea, dysphasia, odynophagia, and respiratory obstruction.

Rheumatoid lesions affect the larynx in up to 26 per cent of patients who have generalized rheumatoid disease.[31] Arthritis of the cricoarytenoid joints is the most common cause of symptoms and can lead to ankylosis and subluxation. Indirect or direct laryngoscopy will show decreased vocal cord motion. Neuritis of the recurrent laryngeal nerve can also cause decreased vocal cord movement and must be differentiated from cricoarytenoid arthritis. CT scans during quiet breathing may reveal anterior displacement of the arytenoid cartilage.[32] During phonation, decreased adduction of the arytenoid will be seen. Rheumatoid nodules and polyps have been described on the vocal cords but are rare. Computed tomography will show localized masses in addition to the other features of rheumatoid disease.

Cricoarytenoid arthritis, mucosal ulcerations, scarring, and laryngeal stenosis can also be found in systemic lupus erythematosus, progressive systemic sclerosis, polyarteritis, and Wegener granulomatosis. In all of these conditions, laryngeal involvement is part of the systemic disease.

Polyps and Cysts

Laryngeal polyps and cysts are frequently traumatic and possibly infectious lesions that can produce endolaryngeal masses. Their appearance on CT scans can be confused with laryngeal carcinomas, but an understanding of their typical sites and appearances can lead to the correct diagnosis.

Fibrous or fibroangiomatous polyps are among the most common lesions encountered in the larynx.[33] They are a form of traumatic laryngitis and seen most often in singers and professional speakers. These nodular masses characteristically occur on the free margin of the true vocal cords at the junction of the anterior and middle thirds (Fig. 3–23) and are frequently bilateral. Occasionally, vocal polyps, also caused by abuse of the voice, are diffusely situated on the vocal cords. Surgical removal may be indicated in patients unresponsive to voice therapy.

Saccular (congenital) cysts of the larynx constitute only 2 to 3 per cent of all congenital anomalies of the larynx[34] and can develop in infancy or in later life. The most common saccular cyst is the cyst of the aryepiglottic fold; it is presumed to result from maldevelopment of the appendix of the laryngeal ventricle.[35] When distended with mucus, these cysts can be up to 6 to 7 cm in diameter. They originate in the paralaryngeal tissue at the level of the false cords and enlarge along planes of least resistance. They are particularly well demonstrated on CT scans of the larynx. If the

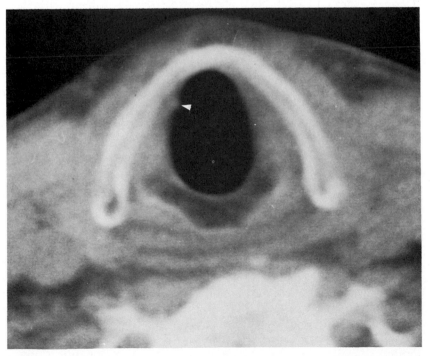

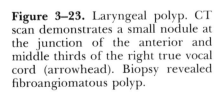

Figure 3–23. Laryngeal polyp. CT scan demonstrates a small nodule at the junction of the anterior and middle thirds of the right true vocal cord (arrowhead). Biopsy revealed fibroangiomatous polyp.

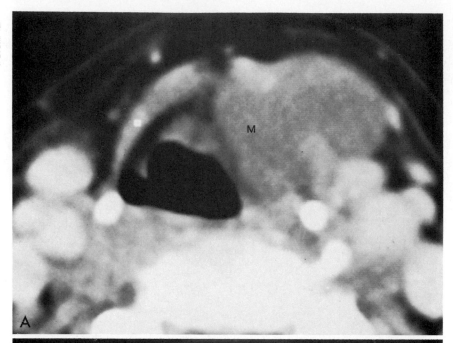

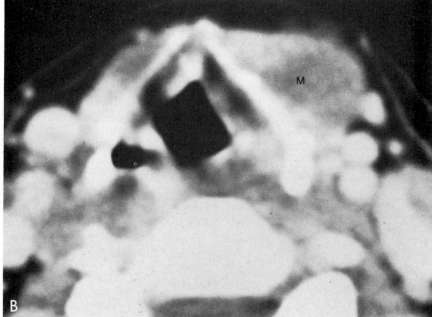

Figure 3–24. Saccular (congenital) cyst of the larynx. **A** CT scan at the level of the thyrohyoid membrane shows low density cystic mass (M) in the left pre-epiglottic space extending into the neck. **B** Scan 1 cm caudad to **A,** the external component of the cyst is still visible, and the left piriform sinus is obliterated. (Courtesy of Dr. W. J. Kilman, Dallas, Tex.)

cyst extends upward, it will thicken the anterior aryepiglottic fold or bulge into the anterior wall of the laryngeal vestibule. If it is directed anteromedially, it can reach through the pre-epiglottic space and present as a mass in the ipsilateral vallecula. Occasionally, these cysts will project laterally through the thyrohyoid membrane and will appear as a mass in the side of the neck (Fig. 3–24A,B). On CT scans, the cyst wall and cyst contents are readily apparent. With the aid of adjacent scans, the position of the cyst within the larynx can be determined and a correct diagnosis made.

Congenital cysts also occur along the tracts of the primitive second, third, and fourth branchial clefts. Although they do not involve the endolarynx, cysts arising from the third and fourth clefts can pierce the thyrohyoid membrane and communicate with a piriform sinus (see Chapter 2).

Thyroglossal duct cysts, like branchial cleft cysts, are not intrinsic to the larynx but can impinge on laryngeal structures. The thyroglossal duct extends downward in the midline from the base of the tongue, in front of the hyoid bone and thyroid cartilage, as far as the isthmus of the thyroid gland. Cysts can occur anywhere along the course of the duct tract but are most common around the hyoid bone. Those arising below the hyoid bone bulge into the pre-epiglottic space to displace the epiglottic cartilage posteriorly. On CT scans, the cystic nature of these lesions is readily apparent. A midline position of a cyst strongly favors the diagnosis of a thyroglossal duct cyst.

Laryngocele

In adults, the normal appendix, or saccule, of the laryngeal ventricle measures only 5 to 15 mm in length. In some apes, such as the orangutan, the laryngeal appendix is much larger than in humans and can even extend into the axilla. It is normally visible on CT scans obtained during phonation in about 10 per cent of adults as a round air-density structure immediately medial to the cartilage of the thyroid lamina at the junction of its anterior and middle thirds.

A laryngocele, or laryngeal aerocele, is an enlargement and elongation of the normal ventricular appendix. Over 90 per cent of laryngoceles present in adult life when the ventricular appendix becomes swollen or occasionally infected.[36] They are bilateral in almost 25 per cent of cases. Occupations that are associated with increased in-

tralaryngeal pressure, such as the blowing of wind instruments, probably predisposes to the development of laryngoceles.

Laryngoceles are classified into three types: internal, external, and mixed.[37] *Internal laryngoceles* are confined to the soft tissues of the larynx. Similar to saccular cysts of the larynx, they can extend anterosuperiorly into the pre-epiglottic space and even as far cephalad as the valleculae. They can also project posterosuperiorly into an aryepiglottic fold.

External laryngoceles expand laterally through the thyrohyoid membrane posterior to the thyrohyoid muscles. This is a relatively weak area, in which the superior laryngeal vessels and internal laryngeal nerve penetrate the membrane.

Laryngoceles are called *mixed* when cystic spaces are present both medial to the thyroid cartilage and external to it. The mixed type is the most common laryngocele, followed by the internal, and then the external type. In almost 20 per cent of cases, a laryngeal tumor, most commonly a carcinoma, is found in conjunction with a laryngocele.

With few exceptions, the clinical and radiographic diagnosis of an uncomplicated laryngocele is straightforward. Conventional radiographs

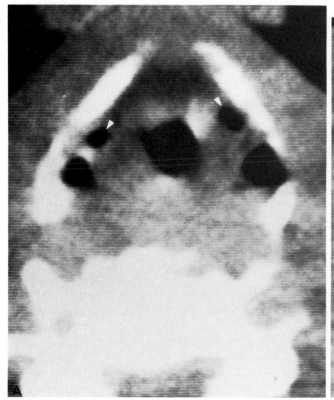
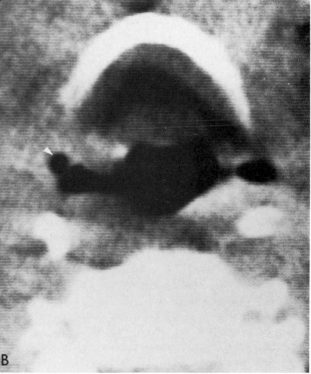

Figure 3–25. Bilateral laryngoceles. **A** CT scan at the level of the thyroid notch shows bilateral air-containing laryngoceles (arrowheads). **B** Scan 15 mm cephalad to **A,** at the level of the thyrohyoid membrane and hyoid bone, the right laryngocele is still evident deep to the piriform sinus (arrowhead). (Courtesy of Dr. M. Reid, Sacramento, Calif.)

and tomograms reveal an air-containing space within the paralaryngeal tissue, pre-epiglottic space or aryepiglottic fold or lateral to the thyrohyoid membrane. If the laryngocele contains liquid and air, one or two air-fluid levels are visible. CT scans will show the exact location of both internal and external laryngoceles (Fig. 3–25A,B).[37a, 37b] Occasionally, a large excavating laryngeal carcinoma can superficially resemble a laryngocele.[35]

If the neck of the laryngocele is obstructed by chronic inflammation or by a tumor and the laryngocele becomes filled with mucus, CT scans will show a circumscribed fluid-density mass arising above the level of the false cord and extending superiorly.[38] The CT appearance of the laryngocele is then indistinguishable from that of a lateral saccular cyst to which laryngoceles are embryologically related.[39] Direct laryngoscopy is indicated in all patients with a laryngocele to exclude a ventricular tumor.

TRAUMA

Trauma to the larynx is uncommon but increasing in frequency, and recent interest in this injury has stimulated improved methods of diagnosis and treatment. A complete understanding of the types of injury that can affect the larynx, their significance, and their management is essential for the interpretation of the CT scans.

Trauma to the larynx may be internal or external. Internal trauma from intubation rarely results in severe damage to the larynx. Inhalation of noxious gases and liquids (e.g., smoke, steam, acids, caustics, and corrosives) causes various degrees of mucosal damage, edema, and granulation-tissue formation.[40] CT can be a useful adjunct to endoscopy for internal trauma to the larynx if marked supraglottic swelling and stenosis are present.

External trauma is either penetrating or blunt injury. Penetrating injuries are usually evaluated clinically, and exploratory surgery is frequently indicated.

Blunt Laryngeal Injury

Blunt injury to the larynx is caused by compression of the neck against the spine by an object that does not penetrate the soft tissues. The cause frequently depends on the age of the patient. In children and adolescents, swinging bats and sticks or collision with a stretched wire while riding a two-wheeled vehicle are the most common causes of blunt injury. In adults, dashboard or steering wheel injuries are the most common.

Symptoms can be marked or subtle. The voice will usually change, varying from hoarseness to aphonia. Cough is evidence of laryngeal irritation. Hemoptysis and pain are nonspecific findings. Dyspnea and symptoms of airway compromise usually indicate serious structural damage.

Physical examination of the neck may reveal the type of laryngeal injury, or it may be limited by the presence of severe edema or hematoma. Extensive subcutaneous emphysema may be present, indicating a mucosal tear. There may be palpable distortion of the laryngeal cartilages or an appreciably displaced fracture of the thyroid cartilage.[41] Loss of the normal prominence of the cricoid cartilage strongly suggests a fracture at the subglottic level.

It is frequently difficult clinically to assess the extent of laryngeal injury. Other more apparent injuries of the head and neck or of other parts of the body may distract the physician. Nevertheless, to avoid poor functional results, every effort should be made to determine the extent of laryngeal injury and initiate early therapy.[42, 43]

Endoscopy should be undertaken early and radiographic studies obtained as soon as an adequate airway has been secured. The usual radiographic examinations include frontal and lateral views of the soft tissues of the neck and radiographs of the cervical spine.[40] Concomitant injuries to the cervical esophagus should also be considered.

Computed Tomography of the Injured Larynx

Although conventional radiographs can provide considerable information about the injured larynx, CT has greatly extended the noninvasive assessment of the damage and is capable of great precision in demonstrating disruption of the laryngeal cartilages and soft tissues. Reported experience with this technique in laryngeal injuries is limited, and the indications for CT scanning have not been detailed.[44] The indications for exploratory surgery have been established[45, 46] and are presented next. These are the clinical circumstances in which CT scanning is most likely to assist in the evaluation of the patient.

AIRWAY OBSTRUCTION. Sufficient trauma to cause compromise of the airway will usually result in secondary stenosis. A prompt surgical approach is indicated.

SUBCUTANEOUS EMPHYSEMA. Extensive subcutaneous emphysema is indicative of a mucosal tear large enough to warrant surgical closure.

EXPOSED CARTILAGE. Endoscopic visualization of exposed fragments of cartilage usually indicates severe disruption of the laryngeal skeleton and a need for surgical repair of the larynx.

FRACTURED CRICOID CARTILAGE. Cricoid fractures are frequently associated with acute airway obstruction and necessitate tracheostomy. Inadequate treatment of subglottic injuries frequently leads to chronic stenosis.[47]

FISTULOUS TRACTS. Endoscopic or radiographic evidence of a false passage or fistulous tract from the larynx is not common but does necessitate surgical repair.

ARYTENOID DISRUPTION. Avulsion or dislocation of the arytenoid cartilages requires repositioning in the acute phase of the injury. Arytenoid dislocations are frequently associated with damage to the true or false cords, and restoration of vocal function may not be achieved even with surgical repair.[47]

Classification of Injuries and CT Findings

LARYNGEAL EDEMA, HEMATOMA, MINOR LACERATIONS. Extensive swelling of the endolaryngeal soft tissues can occur without skeletal damage. At the supraglottic level, blood and edema fluid can distend the fibrofatty tissues of the pre-epiglottic space and aryepiglottic folds (Figs. 3–26A–D and 3–27A–C). The CT density of these structures will be increased. CT scans can also show swelling of the true and false cords.

Careful attention should be directed to the positions of the arytenoid cartilages. Scans obtained both during quiet breathing and phonation are important. Motion of the arytenoids and function of the true vocal cords can be limited by the mass effect of a hematoma or by dislocation at the cricoarytenoid joint.

At the subglottic level, blood or edema tends to spread around the airway beneath the vocal cords within the cricoid cartilage. This spread is readily shown on CT scans as soft-tissue density within the cricoid cartilage.

Computed tomography is an excellent method for demonstrating gas within the soft tissues of the larynx and neck (Fig. 3–28). This finding of gas is an indication for careful endoscopy to exclude significant mucosal lacerations and skeletal exposure.

In general, the role of CT scanning is to extend the clinical examination by providing information about the cartilaginous structures, soft tissues, and airway. When conservative management is being considered for soft tissue injury of the lar-

ynx, CT scans can confirm that the cartilages are not damaged and the airway is adequate.

SKELETAL INJURIES AND EXTENSIVE SOFT-TISSUE LACERATION. With severe laryngeal injuries, CT scans are the most precise noninvasive method for determining the sites of soft-tissue swelling and skeletal disruption. Skeletal injuries of the larynx are classified regionally into supraglottic, glottic, subglottic, and transglottic. Although two or more regions are frequently involved, this classification serves for descriptive purposes.

Supraglottic Injury. Patients with supraglottic injuries typically have the early onset of airway obstruction and difficulty in swallowing. Skeletal injuries to the supraglottic larynx involve the thyroid and epiglottic cartilages. A vertical paramedian fracture of the thyroid cartilage is the most common type of injury, although transverse, oblique, or comminuted fractures can all occur.[46] Vertical fractures tend to occur in young patients, who have compliant, partially calcified thyroid cartilages. With transverse fractures, the upper fragment tends to displace superiorly and posteriorly (Fig. 3–29). Extensive soft-tissue damage and lacerations of the true and false cords and of the aryepiglottic folds are frequently associated with transverse fractures. CT scans will demonstrate marked swelling of the involved soft tissues. Mucosal lacerations should be suspected if gas is shown in the soft tissues.

A common supraglottic injury is avulsion of the epiglottic cartilage from the thyroid cartilage. The thyroepiglottic ligament is ruptured with marked bleeding around the base of the epiglottis, which is displaced posteriorly and superiorly. This injury is suspected from CT scans by an increase in the depth and CT density of the inferior pre-epiglottic space. With high resolution images, the displaced epiglottic cartilage itself can be seen. However, CT cannot reliably differentiate avulsion of the epiglottis from hematoma and edema of the pre-epiglottic space when there is no rupture of the thyroepiglottic ligament. With a transverse or vertical fracture of the thyroid cartilage, avulsion of the epiglottic cartilage should be considered.

When damage to the lower aryepiglottic folds is extensive, the capsule of the cricoarytenoid joint may also be damaged. An arytenoid cartilage may then dislocate, usually in a posterosuperior direction. Careful attention should be given to the position and mobility of the arytenoid cartilages and true vocal cords.

Glottic Injury. As with injury at other sites in the larynx, glottic injuries are usually from

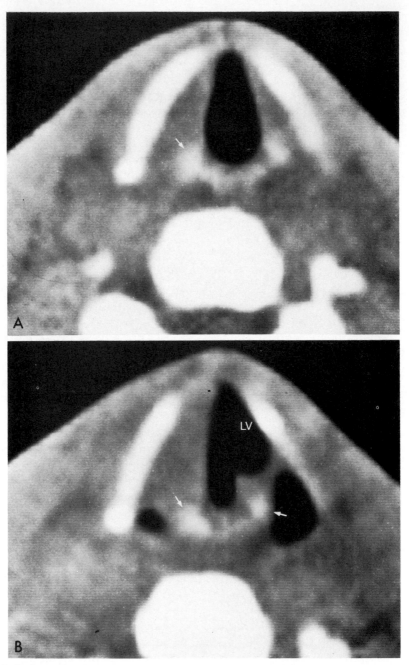

Figure 3–26. Soft-tissue hematoma and edema. **A** CT scan at the level of the vocal cords during quiet breathing shows thickening of the right vocal cord and slight medial displacement of the right arytenoid cartilage (arrow). **B**   Scan at about the same level during phonation; both arytenoid cartilages are adducted (arrows), the right piriform sinus is compressed, and the left laryngeal ventricle (LV) is normally prominent.

Illustration continued on opposite page

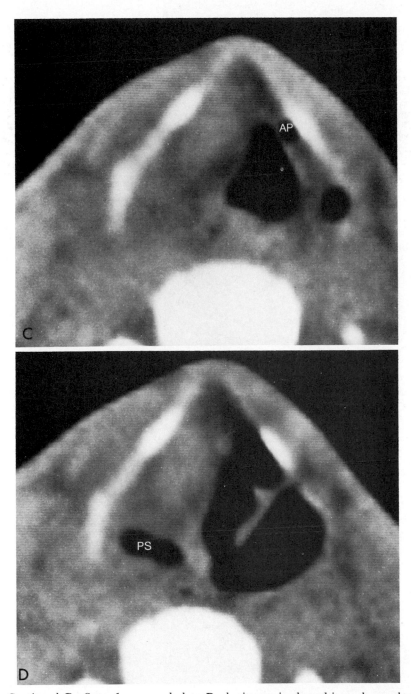

Figure 3–26. *Continued* **C**   Scan 1 cm caudad to **B,** during quiet breathing, shows that the right supraglottic larynx is swollen. The normal appendix (Ap) of the left ventricle is evident. **D**   CT scan
during phonation, at same level as **C** shows posterior displacement of the right piriform sinus (PS)
with soft tissue between the sinus and the thyroid cartilage. The right aryepiglottic fold is thickened.
No cartilage injury was seen.

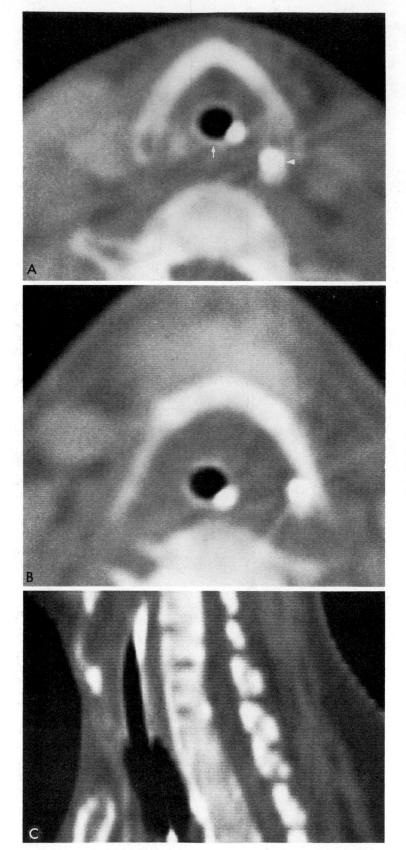

Figure 3–27. Marked laryngeal edema. **A** CT scan at the level of the middle of the thyroid cartilage shows marked edema obscuring endolaryngeal landmarks. Patient is intubated (arrow) and has nasogastric tube (arrowhead) in place. **B** Scan 2 cm cephalad to **A**, soft tissue fills the supraglottic larynx. **C** Multiplanar image after reformation shows extent of the supraglottic, glottic, and subglottic edema. There were no injuries to the laryngeal skeleton.

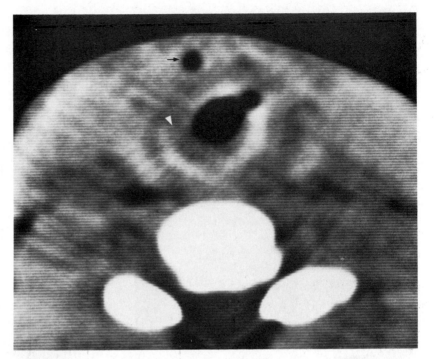

Figure 3–28. Gas in the soft tissues of the neck. CT scan at the level of the cricoid cartilage shows gas in the neck (arrow), cricoid cartilage fracture (arrowhead), and subglottic edema. At surgery, a mucosal tear was found. (Courtesy of Dr. Pierre A. Schnyder, Lausanne, Switzerland.)

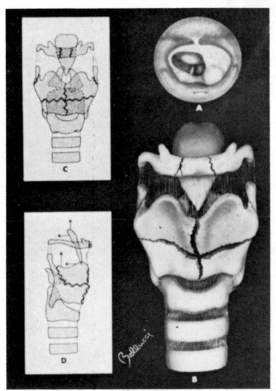

Figure 3–29. Schema of transverse and vertical fractures of the thyroid cartilage. **A** Endoscopy shows marked soft-tissue swelling of the supraglottic region. **B** Schema shows thyroid cartilage and hyoid bone fractures in multiple directions. **C, D** Schemata demonstrate superior fragments of the thyroid cartilage and epiglottis displaced posteriorly and superiorly. (From Ogura JH, Heeneman H, Spector GJ: Laryngotracheal trauma: Diagnosis and treatment. Can J Otolaryngol 2:112, 1973. Reprinted by permission.)

compression of the larynx against the cervical spine. Parasagittal, transverse, oblique, and comminuted fractures of the thyroid cartilage are frequently associated with damage to the true and false cords and the anterior commissure (Fig. 3–30). Posterior displacement of fragments of the thyroid cartilage may be evident on CT scans at the glottic level (Figs. 3–31A–C). The thyroarytenoid muscles within the true cords can rupture or be avulsed, with lacerations of the cords and aryepiglottic folds.

CT scans will show marked soft-tissue swelling at the level of the glottis. Encroachment on the airway will be evident as a reduction in the cross-sectional area of the lumen. One or both arytenoid cartilages are frequently subluxated or dislocated in an anterior or anterosuperior direction (Figs. 3–32A–C). Careful observation of the cartilaginous fragments seen on CT scans will usually reveal the displaced arytenoid cartilage. Detection of air in the swollen soft tissues of the larynx or neck is highly suspicious of a mucosal laceration.

Loss of function and immobility of the true vocal cords can be from one or more of several causes and CT scans may assist in determining which of these is present:

1. Dislocation of one or both arytenoid cartilages.
2. Avulsion of a true vocal cord.
3. Edema of the true vocal cords.
4. Injury to the recurrent laryngeal nerve.

Dislocation of an arytenoid may be detected by

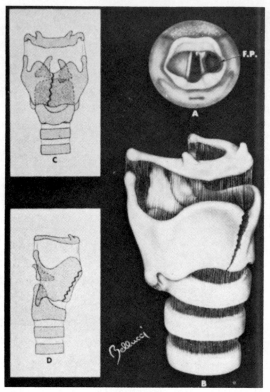

Figure 3–30. Glottic injury. **A** Endoscopy reveals a mucosal tear, or false passage (F.P.), and exposed cartilage. **B** Schema shows that vertical paramedian fractures of the thyroid cartilage are most common. **C, D** Schemata demonstrate that the alignment of the larynx is usually normal. (From Ogura JH, Heeneman H, Spector GJ: Laryngotracheal trauma: Diagnosis and treatment. Can J Otolaryngol 2:112, 1973. Reprinted by permission.)

means of endoscopy or suspected from an abnormal position on CT scans. The contralateral ary-epiglottic fold will be thickened, and the piriform sinus will be prominent.[44] There are no reliable findings on CT scans of an avulsed true vocal cord, but marked soft-tissue swelling will be manifest.

Subglottic Injury. The hallmark of subglottic injury to the laryngeal skeleton is a fracture or fractures of the cricoid cartilage. Airway obstruction is common and is usually severe and immediate. Detection of cricoid fractures is most important. Morgenstern[48] showed that subglottic injuries, unless repaired, frequently result in instability, chronic scarring, and stenosis of the larynx. The cricoid cartilage is the only complete cartilaginous ring in the airway and fractures from compression tend to occur in two places. Direct frontal force will fracture the cricoid cartilage anteriorly and posteriorly. Oblique force will produce ipsilateral and contralateral fractures.

Fractures of the anterior arch of the cricoid ring can usually be suspected clinically from a loss of the normal prominence of the cricoid (Fig. 3–33); however, soft-tissue swelling and subcutaneous emphysema can obscure this finding. CT can readily demonstrate fragments of the cricoid cartilage and their encroachment on the airway (Fig. 3–34A,B). Reduction in the anteroposterior diameter of the cricoid cartilage with distortion of its normal round shape is strong evidence of a comminuted cricoid fracture. With severe blunt trauma, multiple fragments may be evident. The cricopharyngeal muscles attach to the lateral margins of the cricoid cartilage. With anterior and posterior fractures, the cricoid cartilage can appear to be sprung open. The fragments are retracted posterolaterally, contributing to the decrease in the anteroposterior diameter of the airway.

Fractures of the cricoid cartilage are frequently found in conjunction with fractures of the thyroid cartilage, disruption of the cricoarytenoid joint, and separation of the cricothyroid joint. Careful scrutiny of all of the CT scans can reveal these various components of the injury. Frequently, concomitant damage to the recurrent laryngeal nerves and paralysis of the vocal cords are present. Demonstration of a fracture involving the posterior half of the cricoid cartilage should raise suspicion of injury to the recurrent laryngeal nerve.

When the force of the injury is directed to the cricothyroid membrane, the major component of the injury is stenosis in the upper subglottic region.[41] Obstruction to the airway will be from posterior displacement of the thyroid cartilage and its contents, while the cricoid cartilage remains in normal position. Careful examination of serial scans through the larynx will show narrowing and loss of alignment of the larynx in the subglottic region.

Complete avulsion of the trachea from the larynx is a rare type of severe subglottic injury. Most patients die immediately; early diagnosis is essential in those who survive long enough to reach a hospital. Airway obstruction is progressive, and vocal cord paralysis due to injury of the recurrent laryngeal nerves is frequent. The patient is usually aphonic, and prominent features in the neck are contusion, swelling, and subcutaneous emphysema. The avulsed trachea will retract downward toward the sternum, and the larynx will retract upward, and in many cases rotate around its axis.

Radiographic procedures that have been sug-

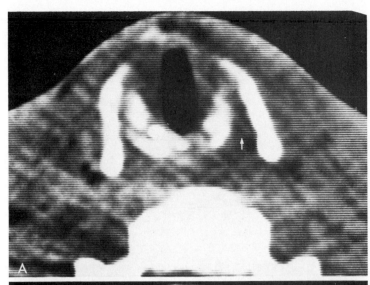

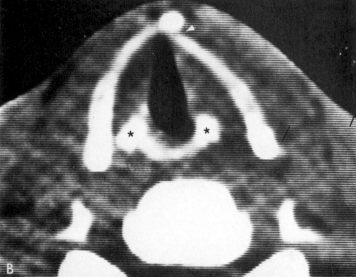

Figure 3–31. Neck injury with fracture of the thyroid cartilage. **A** CT scan at the level of the upper cricoid cartilage shows widening of the left cricothyroid space (arrow), indicating separation at the cricothyroid joint. **B** Scan 1 cm cephalad to **A,** an anterior left paramedian fracture of the thyroid cartilage is visible (arrowhead). The arytenoid cartilages (asterisks) are in normal position. Cricothyroid separation is confirmed. **C** At the supraglottic level, a comminuted fracture of the left lamina of the thyroid cartilage is visible.

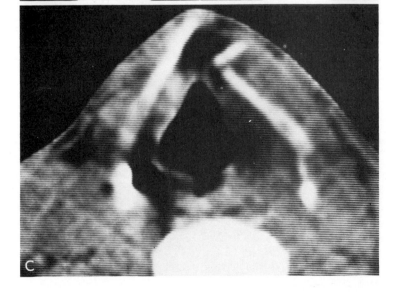

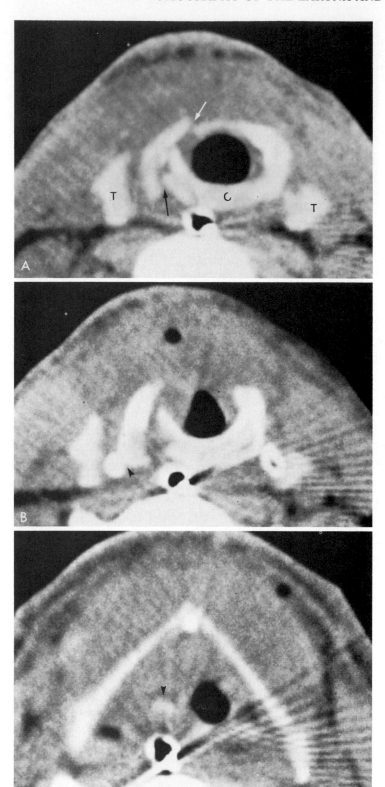

Figure 3–32. Comminuted fracture of the cricoid cartilage with marked edema, hemorrhage, and dislocated arytenoid. **A** CT scan at the subglottic level shows comminuted fractures (arrows) of the right side of cricoid ring (C). The dense lateral structures are the thyroid gland (T). Edema is visible within the cricoid cartilage. **B** Scan 1 cm cephalad to **A,** the fractured right inferior horn (arrowhead) of the thyroid cartilage is seen. Gas is visible in the edematous neck. **C** Scan 1.5 cm cephalad to **B,** marked edema of the endolarynx and an anteriorly dislocated arytenoid cartilage (arrowhead) are visible.

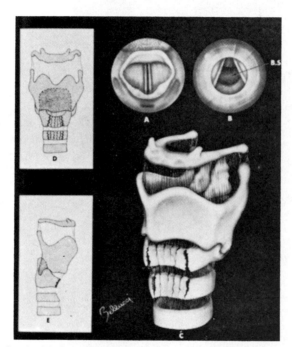

Figure 3–33. Schema of cricoid fracture from subglottic injury. **A, B** Endoscopy shows bilateral vocal-cord paralysis with a blind sac (B.S.) visible if the vocal cords are wedged apart. **C** Schema shows presence of fractures of the anterior arch of the cricoid cartilage and first tracheal ring. **D, E** Schemata show that the cricoid cartilage is displaced posteriorly, leading to loss of cricoid prominence. (From Ogura JH, Heeneman H, Spector, GJ: Laryngotracheal trauma: Diagnosis and treatment. Can J Otolaryngol 2:112, 1973. Reprinted by permission.)

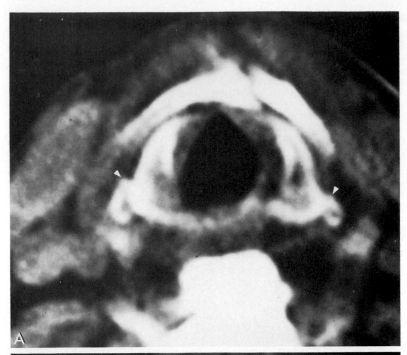

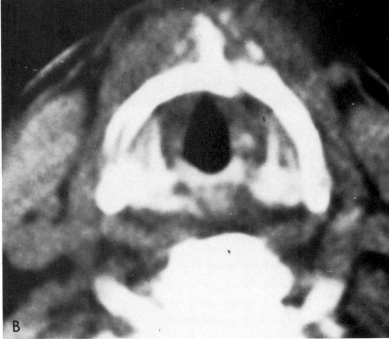

Figure 3–34. Fractures of the cricoid and thyroid cartilages. **A** CT scan at subglottic level shows anterior and posterior fractures of the cricoid cartilage, which is reduced in size in the antero-posterior direction. Fractures of the anterior thyroid cartilage and of inferior horns (arrowheads) are shown. **B** Scan 1 cm cephalad to **A,** fragments from the thyroid cartilage are visible. (Courtesy of Dr. A. A. Mancuso, Salt Lake City, Utah.)

gested[49, 50] for the assessment of laryngotracheal disruption include radiography of the soft tissues of the neck, laryngography, and esophagography. The displaced, obliquely situated cricoid cartilage will produce a confusing appearance on CT scans. Associated cricoid fractures and disruption of the cricothyroid joints will further distort laryngeal structures. A high index of suspicion for this injury is necessary to suggest the diagnosis from CT scans and to enable the radiologist to advocate immediate further investigation.

NEOPLASMS

Benign Neoplasms

True benign neoplasms of the larynx, except for squamous cell papillomas, are uncommon. Benign masses are more frequently non-neoplastic than neoplastic and include cysts, nodules, polyps, granulomas, and hematomas. Without biopsy and histologic examination, many of these non-neoplastic lesions are indistinguishable from neoplasms. Most benign tumors of the larynx are of

Table 3–1. CLASSIFICATION OF BENIGN
NEOPLASMS OF THE LARYNX*

Epithelial
  Epithelial polyp
  Squamous cell papilloma
  Adenoma
  Oncocytoma (oxyphil adenoma)
  Benign mixed tumor (R)†
Connective tissue
  Fibroma
  Chondroma
  Hemangioma
  Leiomyoma
  Lipoma (R)†
  Rhabdomyoma (R)†
Neurogenic
  Neurilemoma
  Neurofibroma
  Chemodectoma (glomus) (R)†
  Granular cell tumor (myoblastoma)
Hematopoietic
  Plasmacytoma
Miscellaneous
  Hamartoma (R)†
  Adenolipoma (R)†
  Lymphangioma (cystic hygroma, secondary (R)†
  Branchiogenic cyst

*Adapted from Barney PL: Histopathologic problems and
frozen section diagnosis in diseases of the larynx. Otolaryngol
Clin North Am 3:493, 1970.
  †(R) = rare.

epithelial, connective tissue, or neurogenic origin
(Table 3–1). They are usually slow growing and
tend to recur if incompletely excised.

The CT findings of benign neoplasms have not
been extensively described. A benign neoplasm
may, however, be encountered in a patient suspected clinically of having laryngeal carcinoma.
Alternatively, CT scans may be obtained to determine the extent of a known benign neoplasm.

PAPILLOMAS. Squamous cell papillomas can be
single or multiple. They are the most common
laryngeal tumor in children and tend to be multiple. In adults, they are usually solitary.[51]

Papillomas usually arise in the anterior half of
the larynx at the level of the true vocal cords or
anterior commissure, and large lesions can cause
airway obstructions.[52] Because papillomas do not
penetrate deeply into the paralaryngeal tissues,
destruction by microelectrocautery, cryotherapy,
or laser beam therapy produces good results.[53]

Juvenile papillomatosis is an aggressive form of
squamous cell papilloma (Fig. 3–35A,B). The papillomas tend to be multiple and the recurrence
rate is high.[52] They have a propensity for spreading to the trachea and bronchi. If repeated exci-

sion does not control the laryngeal lesions,
treacheostomy becomes necessary.

CHONDROMAS. Of the cartilaginous tumors of
the larynx, 80 per cent are benign chondromas.[54, 55]
Most arise from the inner surface of the posterolateral portion of the cricoid cartilage.[56] Less commonly, they originate from the thyroid, arytenoid, or epiglottic cartilages. Symptoms are often
insidious, consisting of dyspnea, hoarseness, a
sense of fullness in the throat, or a lump in the
neck.

Conventional radiographs or xeroradiographs
typically show granular or punctate calcifications.[54]
CT scans can demonstrate the lesion's site of origin, its cartilaginous component, distortion of the
laryngeal skeleton, and the severity of airway obstruction (Fig. 3–36A,B).

HEMANGIOMAS. Hemangioma of the larynx occurs in infants, children, and adults. The adult
form is the most common and usually arises on
the true vocal cords, but it may be supraglottic or
subglottic.[57] Hemangiomas in infants and children are predominantly subglottic and of the cavernous type. Approximately 50 per cent of children with laryngeal hemangioma have similar
lesions on the skin, especially on the head and
neck. Symptoms are usually of dysnea, cough,
and hoarseness. When large, these lesions can
cause airway obstruction that necessitates tracheostomy. As with other benign tumors, CT scans
can probably assist in determining the origin and
extent of laryngeal hemangiomas. The CT findings have not been reported, but in one case that
we studied, calcifications within the lesion suggested the correct diagnosis (Figs. 3–37A–D).

NEUROGENIC TUMORS. Neurofibromas and
schwannomas of the larynx are rare tumors that
can occur at any age. They are slow growing and
symptoms are often insidious. Symptoms relate to
the site of origin, which is most commonly an aryepiglottic fold. Malignant neurogenic tumors do
not occur in the larynx. The CT findings have not
been described but should be of a nonspecific
mass in an aryepiglottic fold or on a vocal cord.
In a patient with neurofibromatosis, demonstration of a laryngeal mass on CT scans should suggest the diagnosis of a neurofibroma. Multiplicity
of the lesions is also suggestive of neurogenic
tumors.

Malignant Neoplasms

An understanding of the role of radiology, and
specifically computed tomography in the diagnosis and management of laryngeal cancer, requires

Text continued on page 112

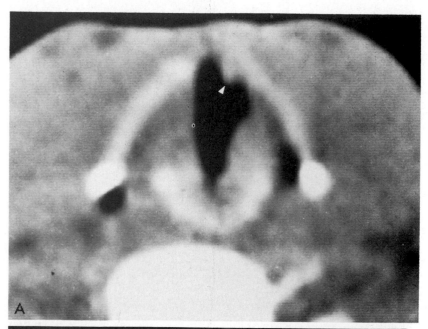

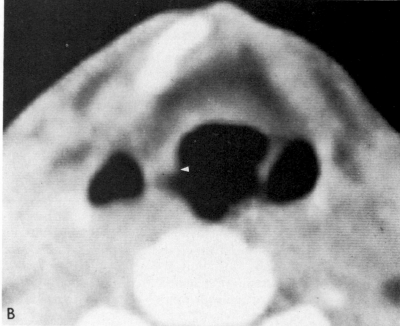

Figure 3–35. Juvenile papillomatosis. **A** CT scan at the level of the true vocal cords shows a papilloma (arrowhead) at the left side of the anterior commisure. **B** Scan 15 cm cephalad to **A,** during phonation, shows thickening of the right aryepiglottic fold from an additional papilloma (arrowhead).

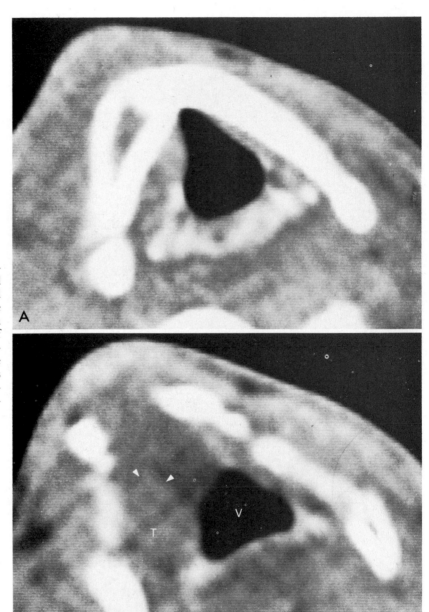

Figure 3–36. Chondroma of the thyroid cartilage. **A** CT scan at the level of the true vocal cord shows marked distortion of the right lamina of the thyroid cartilage. **B** Scan 15 mm cephalad to **A,** at about the level of the thyroid notch, the thyroid cartilage is still markedly distorted and the larynx is rotated. Tumor (T) extends into the pre-epiglottic space (arrowheads), displacing the laryngeal vestibule (V).

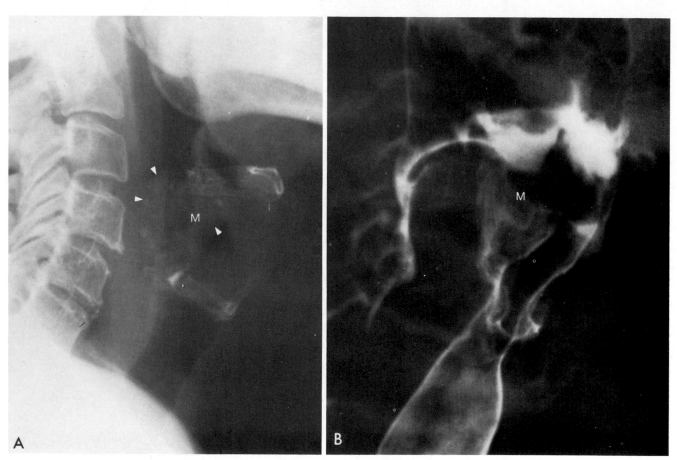

Figure 3–37. Hemangioma of the larynx. **A** Lateral radiograph of the neck shows a mass (M) in the posterior supraglottic region (arrowheads). Round calcifications are visible within the mass. **B** Oblique view from laryngogram confirms the pressure of the mass (M).

Illustration continued on opposite page

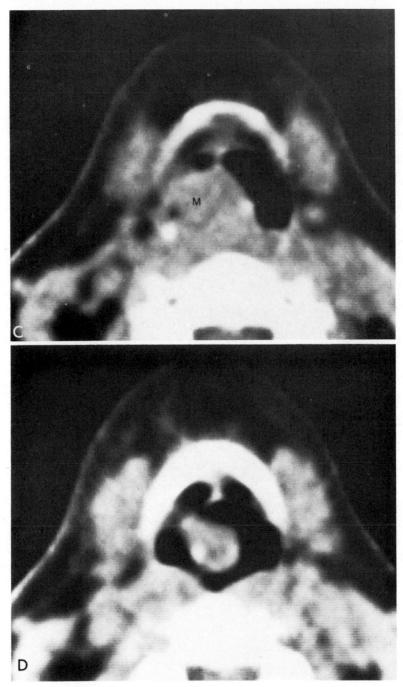

Figure 3–37. *Continued* **C** CT scan at level of the thyrohyoid membrane shows the mass (M) thickening the right aryepiglottic fold and distorting the right piriform sinus. **D** Scan 5 mm cephalad to **C,** the epiglottis and right pharyngoepiglottic fold are thickened. (Abnormal round calcifications are visible in **C** and **D**. The biopsy diagnosis was hemangioma.)

detailed knowledge of the site or origin, routes of spread, staging, and treatment options. Laryngeal cancer comprises 2 to 5 per cent of all malignant neoplasms. The disease is more common in males than in females by a ratio of 10 to 1, and its peak incidence is in the fifth, sixth, and seventh decades.[58] The incidence varies geographically, occurring more in Asia and India than in the United States or Europe. The cause of laryngeal cancer remains obscure, although strong associations with alcohol consumption, smoking, and airborne irritants have been demonstrated.[59, 60] Postcricoid cancer in women is associated with the Plummer-Vinson syndrome. A higher incidence of laryngeal cancer has also been demonstrated in patients with laryngeal tuberculosis and syphilis.

PREMALIGNANT LESIONS. The term refers to a lesion that is reversible or can develop into frank malignancy. Several epithelial lesions of the larynx can, with time, become the site of laryngeal carcinomas. Keratotic papillomas are warty lesions that probably have malignant potential. Both squamous cell carcinoma and verrucose carcinoma may arise from them. Both acanthosis and pseudoepitheliomatous hyperplasias cause thick-

Table 3–2.   CLASSIFICATION OF MALIGNANT NEOPLASMS OF THE LARYNX*

Epithelial
   Squamous cell carcinoma
   Verrucous carcinoma
   Malignant mixed tumor
   "Spindle cell" carcinoma (R)†
   Adenosquamous carcinoma (R)†
   Basal cell carcinoma (R)†
   Malignant melanoma (R)†
   Adenoid cystic adenocarcinoma (R)†
   Squamous carcinoma with pseudosarcomatous change (R)
   Adenocarcinoma (R)†
   Malignant mixed tumor
   Oat cell carcinoma (R)†
Connective tissue
   Fibrosarcoma (R)†
   Chondrosarcoma
   Liposarcoma (R)†
   Angiosarcoma (R)†
   Rhabdomyosarcoma (R)†
Hematopoietic
   Reticulosarcoma
   Acute leukemia
   Lymphosarcoma
Miscellaneous
   Metastatic carcinoma (R)†

*Adapted from Barney PL: Histopathologic problems and frozen section diagnosis in diseases of the larynx. Otolaryngol Clin North Am 3:493, 1970.
†(R) = rare.

Table 3–3.   ANATOMIC CLASSIFICATION OF CANCER OF THE LARYNX

Region	Site
Supraglottis	Epilarynx
	Posterior surface of suprahyoid epiglottis (including the tip)
	Aryepiglottic fold
	Arytenoid
	Vestibulum
	Infrahyoid epiglottis
	Ventricular bands (false vocal cords)
	Ventricular cavities
Glottis	Vocal cords
	Anterior commissure
	Posterior commissure
Subglottis	

ening of the laryngeal mucosa but are not known to be associated with malignancy. Leukoplakia, bowenoid dyskeratosis, and chronic laryngeal dyskeratosis are all forms of abnormal laryngeal mucosa. The incidence of malignancy developing from these three conditions is controversial and varies from 3 to 40 per cent.[58, 61] Compounding the problem is that these conditions can be mistaken for carcinoma in situ, which almost certainly progresses to invasive cancer.

PATHOLOGY. More than 95 per cent of all laryngeal malignancies are squamous cell carcinomas (Table 3–2). They tend to be well differentiated and remain localized for a relatively long time; but once deep infiltration has occurred, they can spread rapidly. The direction and rapidity of spread of a laryngeal tumor are dependent primarily on its site of origin.

Adenocarcinoma of the larynx is much less common than squamous cell carcinoma. Subgroups of adenocarcinoma are cylindromas and mucoepidermoid carcinomas.[62] Mixed adenosquamous cell carcinoma, oat cell carcinoma, and "spindle cell" carcinoma are all uncommon. Other malignant tumors of the larynx are rare.

SITE OF ORIGIN AND CLASSIFICATION. The site of origin of laryngeal cancer has direct bearing on its direction and rapidity of spread. Carcinoma of the larynx is classified by its anatomic region of origin and by its site within that region (Table 3–3). The incidence of laryngeal cancer varies for each region. The general range of frequency of laryngeal cancer according to region is glottic—50 to 60 per cent, supraglottic—20 to 30 per cent, piriform sinus—10 to 20 per cent, and subglottic—2 to 5 per cent.[63–66] Extension of tumor to secondarily involve the subglottic space, however, can occur in up to 25 per cent of cases of glottic cancer.[67]

STAGING. With appropriate treatment, laryngeal cancer has one of the highest rates of cure of any malignancy arising from an internal organ of the body. Therapy for malignant laryngeal tumors is dependent on the precision of the initial staging of the disease. The therapy of these neoplasms presents special problems because preservation of speech has a high priority but must not be allowed to jeopardize eradication of the tumor.

The staging of laryngeal cancer proposed by the American Joint Committee for Cancer Staging and End-Stage Results Reporting[12] is now widely accepted and used. This system employs the TNM-staging classification for each of the three anatomic regions of the larynx (Table 3–3) as follows: T defines the degree of extension of the tumor based on clinical examination, endoscopy, and radiologic imaging modalities; N defines the status of the regional lymph nodes, usually assessed clinically but *with computed tomography* able to extend the clinical examination; and M denotes the presence or absence of distant metastases, assessed by *all available examining modalities.*

The initial examination before surgical confirmation or treatment is called the "clinical-diagnostic" staging and is the situation in which radiology is most extensively used. Because no account is taken of the histopathologic character of the tumor, this essentially macroscopic extent of the tumor often does not reflect the microscopic extent.

A primary tumor (T) in each anatomic region is considered in terms of its extent (Table 3–4). In the clinical diagnostic staging of regional lymph nodes (N), the actual size of the nodal masses are measured, with allowance made for the intervening soft tissue. There are three stages of positive nodes (Table 3–5). Midline nodes are considered ipsilateral. Distant metastases (M) are either present or absent.

Glottic cancer is defined as a malignant tumor originating on the true vocal cords. About 75 per cent of glottic carcinomas arise on the anterior half of the true cord near the anterior commissure, 15 per cent arise near the middle of the cord, and only 10 per cent arise on the posterior half.

Subglottic cancer originates below the true cords and above a plane through the inferior border of the cricoid cartilage.

Table 3–4. CLASSIFICATION OF PRIMARY TUMOR (T)

Primary tumor	TX	Tumor that cannot be assessed
	T0	No evidence of primary tumor
Supraglottis	T1S	Carcinoma in situ
	T1	Tumor confined to site of origin with normal mobility
	T2	Tumor involves adjacent supraglottic site(s) or glottis without fixation
	T3	Tumor limited to larynx with fixation and/or extension to involve postcricoid area, medial wall of piriform sinus, or pre-epiglottic space
	T4	Massive tumor extending beyond the larynx to involve oropharynx, soft tissues of neck, or thyroid cartilage
Glottis	T1S	Carcinoma in situ
	T1	Tumor confined to vocal cord(s) with normal mobility (includes involvement of anterior or posterior commissures)
	T2	Supraglottic and/or subglottic extension of tumor with normal or impaired cord mobility
	T3	Tumor confined to the larynx with cord fixation
	T4	Massive tumor with thyroid cartilage destruction and/or extension beyond the confines of the larynx
Subglottis	T1S	Carcinoma in situ
	T1	Tumor confined to the subglottic region
	T2	Tumor extension to vocal cords with normal or impaired cord mobility
	T3	Tumor confined to larynx with cord fixation
	T4	Massive tumor with cartilage destruction or extension beyond the confines of the larynx, or both

Supraglottic cancer arises between the tip of the lingular surface of the epiglottis and the laryngeal ventricles. Of the 20 to 30 per cent of laryngeal cancers that arise in the supraglottic region, 10 per cent originate from the false cords, 8.5 per cent from the epiglottis, 5 per cent from the aryepiglottic folds, 2.5 per cent from the laryngeal ventricles, and 2 per cent from the area of the arytenoid cartilages.[64, 66]

Transglottic cancer is defined as a tumor extending vertically across the laryngeal ventricle to involve the supraglottic and glottic regions.[68, 69]

Table 3–5.   CLASSIFICATION OF REGIONAL
NODES (N)

NX	Nodes cannot be assessed
N0	No clinically positive node
N1	Single, clinically positive, homolateral node 3 cm or less in diameter
N2	Single, clinically positive, homolateral node more than 3 cm but not more than 6 cm in diameter; or multiple, clinically positive, homolateral nodes, none more than 6 cm in diameter.
N2a	Single, clinically positive, homolateral node more than 3 cm but not more than 6 cm in diameter
N2b	Multiple, clinically positive, homolateral nodes, none more than 6 cm in diameter
N3	Massive homolateral node(s), bilateral nodes, or contralateral node(s)
N3a	Clinically positive, homolateral node(s), one more than 6 cm in diameter
N3b	Bilateral, clinically positive nodes (in this situation, each side of the neck should be staged separately, e.g., N3b: right N2a, left N1)
N3c	Contralateral, clinically positive node only

Most arise from the true vocal cords and invade the laryngeal ventricle. Spread of this tumor may be mucosal or by deep penetration of the paralaryngeal tissues.[68]

DISSEMINATION.   Essential to the interpretation of CT scans of laryngeal cancers is an understanding of their growth potential and their mode of spread. In general, they have defined predilections for their growth patterns and directions of local invasion. Their sites of origin and the normal structural barriers to tumor growth are the main determinants of dissemination. The frequency of nodal metastasis is likewise dependent on the site at which the tumor arises.

Glottic Region.   As stated previously, 50 to 60 per cent of laryngeal carcinomas arise from the true vocal cords. They are frequently well differentiated and slow growing. Early tumors (Stage T1) are localized, with mobility of the true cords being maintained. The free margins of the true cords do not contain lymphatics; therefore, nodal metastases are rare.

CT scans obtained of early vocal cord lesions usually show no abnormality, but they may show minimal cordal thickening that is indistinguishable from normal variations in cord thickness. The density resolution of present CT scanners does not allow for differentiation between tumor tissue and the vocalis muscle; thus detection of tumor depends on the recognition of abnormal thickening or irregularity of the true cord (Fig. 3–38). New, high-resolution CT scanners may be able to reveal tumor extension within the cord. In our experience, for early (Stage T1) glottic tumors, CT scans have not provided information additional to that obtained from direct laryngoscopy.

Glottic cancer spreads anteriorly, posteriorly, inferiorly, or laterally into the paraglottic space. Anterior extension is to the anterior commissure, and CT scans are extremely accurate in demonstrating tumor involvement at this site. In the normal larynx having a wide angle to the thyroid cartilage, the airway is directly behind the thyroid

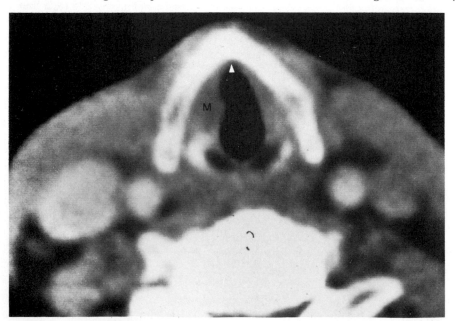

Figure 3–38. Early (Stage T1) squamous cell carcinoma of the right true vocal cord. CT scan at the level of the true vocal cords shows slight asymmetry, with thickening of the midportion of the right true vocal cord (M). The small amount of tissue (arrowhead) at the anterior commissure is normal.

cartilage.[14, 18] The anterior-commissure tendon, the point at which the two vocal ligaments attach to the thyroid cartilage, is not normally visible. However, with a narrow thyroid angle, 1 to 2 mm of soft tissue can be visible (Fig. 3–8). Any additional soft tissue at the anterior commissure is abnormal and indicative of tumor extension (Figs. 3–39A–C). Cancer that has reached the anterior commissure can grow in several directions. It can extend inferiorly to the subglottic space and cricothyroid membrane; contralaterally to the opposite true vocal cord; superiorly to the pre-epiglottic space; and anteriorly into the thyroid cartilage.

Subglottic extension of the tumor is of great importance because it directly affects staging and therapy. Computed tomography is as accurate as direct laryngoscopy in the demonstration of subglottic tumor and is particularly useful for showing inferior extension from bulky cordal masses.[3, 4, 19] The CT diagnosis of subglottic tumor is made by determining the relationship of the tumor mass to the level of the true vocal cords. With the larynx in a relaxed state during quiet breathing, the true vocal cords are identified by the vocal processes of the arytenoid cartilages, or, the most inferior image through the arytenoid cartilages. During phonation, the adducted true vocal cords are normally visible. We allow 5 mm caudad to the level of the arytenoid cartilages to encompass the undersurface of the true cords. Any soft tissue within the cricoid cartilage extending further inferiorly is indicative of subglottic tumor (Figs. 3–39C and 3–40A–C).[3] If the patient's head is not adequately extended, the anterior portions of the vocal cords can project below the arytenoid cartilages and mimic a thickened anterior commissure.

The thyroid cartilage at the anterior commissure is devoid of perichondrium, which resists tumor spread[70]; therefore, tumor at this site can readily invade the thyroid cartilage and cricothyroid membrane (Fig. 3–41). Dissemination in this direction is not easily detected clinically or endoscopically. The CT scan finding of thyroid cartilage invasion has a decisive effect on staging because the tumor is then classified as an advanced (Stage T4) lesion.[12]

Superior extension of tumor from the anterior commissure into the pre-epiglottic space (T2) is difficult to detect endoscopically. CT scanning is the only method for finding subtle tumor spread in this direction.[3, 71] At this site, tumor mass contrasts markedly with the normal low CT density of the pre-epiglottic fibroadipose tissue (Fig. 3–42A–D). Once the tumor has gained access to the pre-epiglottic space, it may remain on the ipsilateral side, cross the midline to the contralateral side of the pre-epiglottic space, or extend posteriorly into an anterior aryepiglottic fold.

Glottic cancer commonly spreads to the opposite true vocal cord once the anterior commissure has been infiltrated. This route of spread can usually be detected at endoscopy and confirmed by biopsy of the abnormal-appearing contralateral cord. CT scans can frequently demonstrate contralateral spread (Fig. 3–43), but when both cords are symmetrically thickened, the lack of asymmetry makes detection more difficult (Fig. 3–41).[72] The abnormal depth of tissue at the anterior commissure must be recognized to suspect contralateral tumor growth. Advanced, bilateral disease may be overlooked unless the abnormal tissue at the anterior commissure is appreciated.

Posterior extension of glottic cancer is to the arytenoid cartilage, posterior commissure, and cricoarytenoid joint. Spread around the arytenoid cartilage can displace the cartilage medially and the cartilage will appear adducted on CT scans during quiet breathing. Alternatively, the tumor can fix the arytenoid cartilage in the abducted position, making it immobile during phonation (Fig. 44A,B). Both of these findings indicate an advanced (Stage T3) tumor. Once the tumor has gained access to the posterior commissure, it can cross to the contralateral vocal cord or escape laterally into the tissues of the neck (Fig. 3–45A,B). Widening or asymmetry of more than 1 to 2 mm of the distance between thyroid and cricoid cartilages indicates tumor extension into the lateral cricothyroid space (Fig. 3–46A–C).

Direct lateral extension of glottic cancer is into the paralaryngeal tissues between the conus elasticus and thyroid cartilage. The paraglottic portion of the paralaryngeal space is an important route for tumor infiltration. It communicates with the pre-epiglottic space anterosuperiorly and with the soft tissue of the neck, between the thyroid and cricoid cartilages; glottic tumors can spread in either of these directions. The piriform sinus limits the paraglottic space posteriorly. Encroachment on the anterior wall of the piriform sinus is most easily detected from CT scans obtained during phonation. Tumor in the paraglottic space can directly penetrate the thyroid cartilage; its ossified portions offer the least resistance to tumor invasion. The difficulties with detection of cartilage invasion are dealt with below.

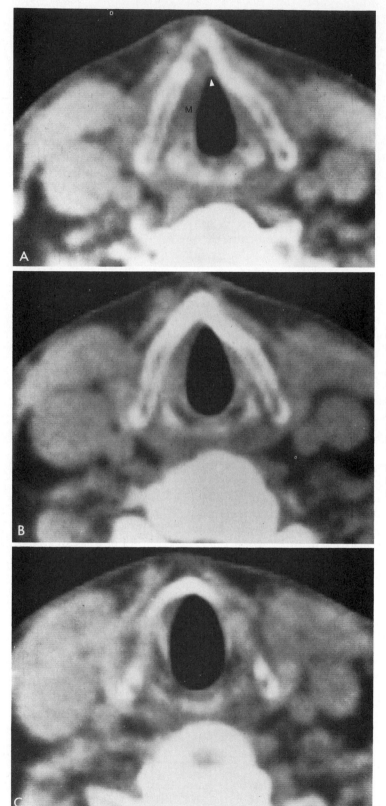

Figure 3–39. Cordal tumor with extension to anterior commissure and subglottic region. **A** CT scan through the base of the arytenoid cartilages shows thickening of the right true vocal cord (M) and asymmetric soft tissue (arrowhead) at the anterior commissure. **B** Scan 5 mm caudad to **A,** the undersurface of the right true vocal cord is thick. Tumor persists at the low anterior commissure. **C** Scan 10 mm caudad to **B,** the tumor present anteriorly on the right represents a subtle extension to the subglottic region. Endoscopy confirmed these CT findings.

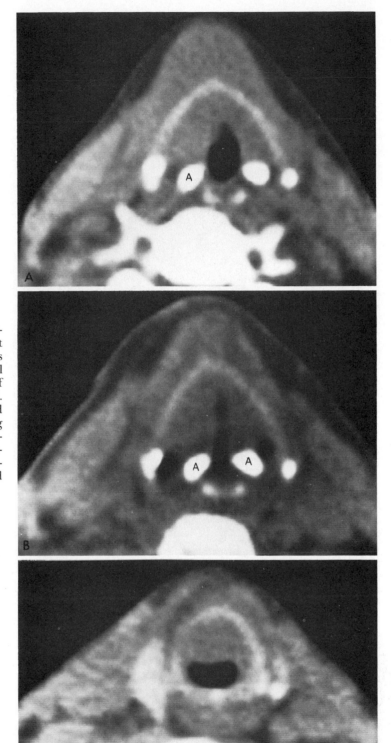

Figure 3–40. Anterior commissure and subglottic extension of tumor. **A** CT scan at about the level of the true vocal cords shows tumor markedly thickening the right vocal cord and anterior commissure. The degree of extension to the left cannot be determined. The right arytenoid cartilage (A) is displaced medially. **B** Scan at the same level, during phonation; both arytenoid cartilages (A) adduct, indicating that cordal fixation is not present. **C** Scan 15 mm caudad to **B** shows extensive tumor within the arch of the cricoid cartilage.

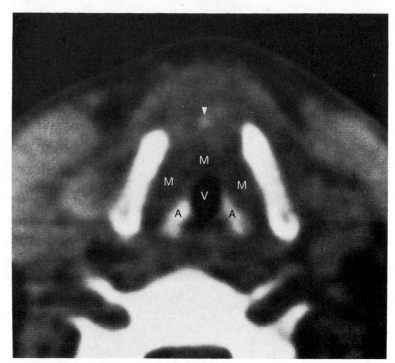

Figure 3–41. Cartilage destruction from glottic tumor. CT scan through the arytenoid cartilages (A) shows narrowing of the laryngeal vestibule (V) from a circumglottic tumor (M). The thyroid cartilage is destroyed anteriorly. A small amount of residual cartilage is seen (arrowhead). The soft-tissue mass seen anteriorly should raise the suspicion of extralaryngeal spread of the tumor.

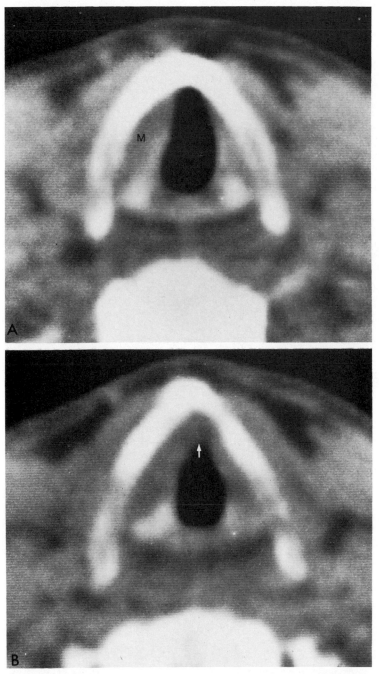

Figure 3–42. Infiltration of glottic cancer into the pre-epiglottic space. **A**   CT scan through the glottis demonstrates slight tumor thickening of the right true vocal cord (M). **B**   Scan 5 mm cephalad to **A** shows tumor at the junction (arrow) of the inferior pre-epiglottic space and the anterior commissure.

Illustration continued on following page

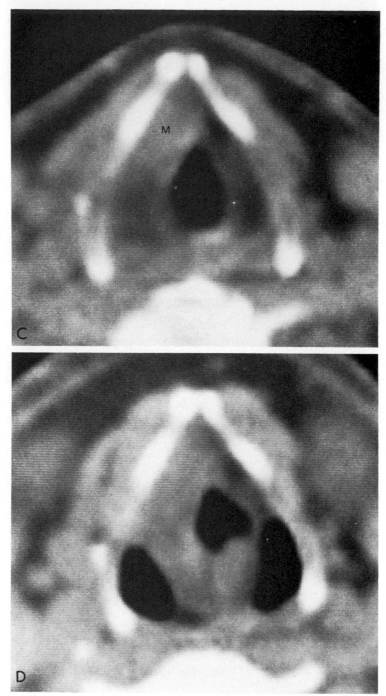

Figure 3–42. *Continued* **C**   Scan 10 mm cephalad to **B,** increased CT density from tumor (M) is seen on the right side of the pre-epiglottic space. The piriform sinuses are collapsed. **D**   At same level as **C,** during phonation; the piriform sinuses are distended, showing tumor infiltration into the right ary-epiglottic fold.

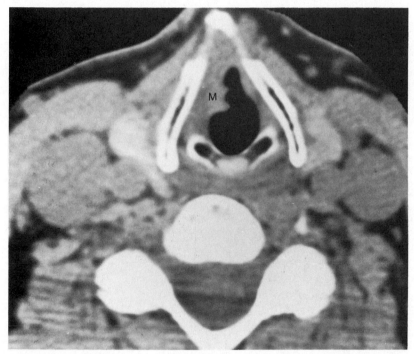

Figure 3–43. Right true vocal cord tumor with contralateral extension. CT scan through the right glottic tumor mass (M) shows extension to the anterior commissure and the contralateral anterior third of the left true vocal cord. The difference in CT density between the tumor and the vocal cords is visible (GE 9800 scan). (Courtesy of Dr. Lincoln L. Berland, Milwaukee, Wis.)

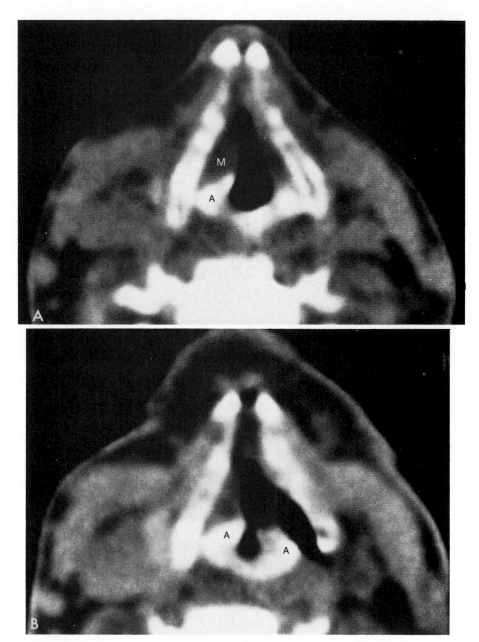

Figure 3–44. Right glottic tumor with fixation of true vocal cord. **A**   CT scan during quiet breathing shows cordal mass (M) displacing the vocal process of the right arytenoid cartilage (A) medially. **B**   Scan at same level, during phonation; the left arytenoid (A) moves normally; right arytenoid (A) remains immobile in abducted position. (From Gamsu G, Webb WR, Shallit JB, Moss AA: CT in carcinoma of the larynx and pyriform sinus: Value of phonation scans. AJR 136:577, 1981. © 1981, American Roentgen Ray Society. Reprinted by permission.)

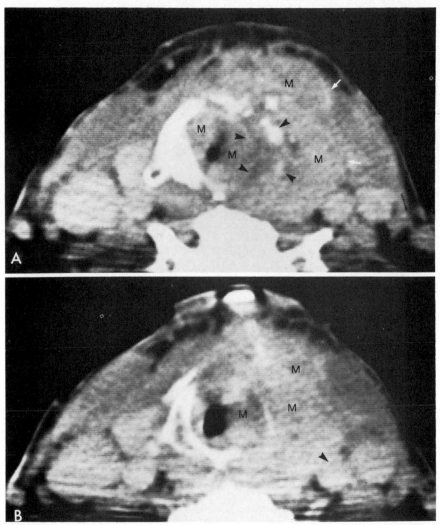

Figure 3–45. Extensive laryngeal tumor with lateral extension into the neck. **A**   CT scan immediately below the glottis shows extensive endolaryngeal tumor mass (M). The tumor infiltrates the left side between the destroyed cricoid (medial arrowheads) and thyroid (lateral arrowheads) cartilages and extends into left side of the neck (arrows). **B**   Scan 5 mm caudad to **A;** additional subglottic tumor is evident. The tumor (M) displaces and contacts the left common carotid artery (arrowhead). The top of a tracheostomy tube is visible anteriorly.

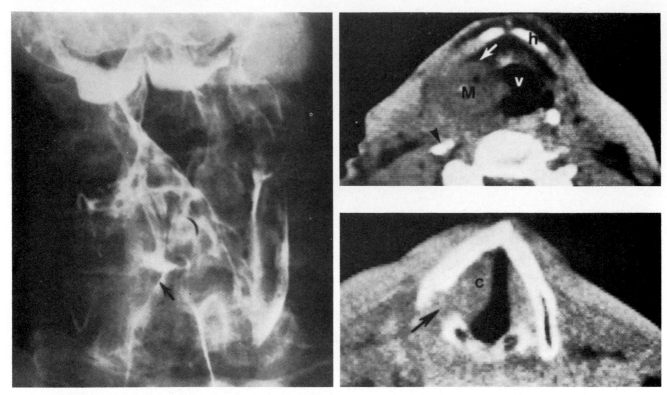

Figure 3–46. Transglottic carcinoma with invasion into cricothyroid space. **A** Laryngogram shows an extensive mass in the supraglottic region obliterating the right piriform sinus and causing deviation of aryepiglottic fold. The right true vocal cord (arrow) is fixed in the adducted position. **B** CT scan at the level of the hyoid bone (h) demonstrates a mass (M) obliterating the right piriform sinus and extending to the lateral and posterior pharyngeal wall. The right side of the pre-epiglottic space (arrow) is infiltrated by tumor, which encroaches on the laryngeal vestibule (V). The right superior thyroid horn (arrowhead) is displaced posteriorly. **C** CT scan through the true vocal cords shows tumor extension with widening of the right cricothyroid space (arrow). The right vocal cord (C) is adducted. (From Archer CR, Sagel SS, Yeager VL, Martin S, Friedman WH: Staging of the carcinoma of the larynx: Comparative accuracy of CT and laryngography. AJR 136: 571, 1981. © 1981, American Roentgen Ray Society. Reprinted by permission.)

Supraglottic Region. Twenty to 30 per cent of laryngeal carcinomas arise in the supraglottic region. The supraglottic region of the larynx develops from the pharyngeal anlage, whereas the glottic and subglottic regions are derived from the lung and tracheal anlage. The lymphatics of the supraglottic region are abundant and separate from the two inferior regions. They drain laterally and superiorly through the thyrohyoid membrane to the jugulodigastric and jugulocarotid nodes (see Chapter 2). Nodal metastases from supraglottic tumors are thus frequent and tend to be high in the neck.

The biologic behavior and surgical treatment of supraglottic cancer have led to the division of this region into two subregions.[73] The *superior subregion* is the epilarynx and consists of the posterior surface of the epiglottis (including the tip), the mucosa over the arytenoid cartilages, and the aryepiglottic folds. Some investigators have used the terms "marginal" or "transitional" for epila-

ryngeal tumors and consider them hypopharyngeal.[66, 74, 75] In the American system of classification, these tumors are included within the larynx. The *inferior subregion* is the vestibulum and consists of the infrahyoid epiglottis, the false vocal cords, and the laryngeal ventricles.

When first diagnosed, supraglottic cancers are usually more advanced than glottic cancers. They frequently metastasize to regional lymph nodes and invade surrounding structures.[58] Epilaryngeal tumors infiltrate the valleculae, base of the tongue, walls of the pharynx, infrahyoid epiglottis, pre-epiglottic space, and aryepiglottic folds. Vestibulum tumors infiltrate especially into the lateral paralaryngeal tissues, pre-epiglottic space, and thyroid cartilage. The epiglottic cartilage is fenestrated and offers little resistance to tumor spread. Once the pre-epiglottic space and lower vestibulum have been invaded, the tumor can spread caudally to the anterior commissure and even to the subglottic region. Tumors that extend caudally have a propensity for invading the thyroid cartilage.

Supraglottic cancers frequently are more extensive than clinically suspected.[58] CT scans can demonstrate deep penetration of these tumors and thereby help to avoid excessively limited surgery that would not eradicate the tumor. The pre-epiglottic space is well shown on CT scans and an increase in its CT density indicates tumor infiltration or edema associated with the tumor (Fig. 3–47A–C). Edema cannot be differentiated from tumor by clinical or radiologic means, including CT scans, and will be resected or included in the radiation field along with the tumor. The extent of penetration of the pre-epiglottic space and contralateral spread can be established from CT scans, both of which are of special importance (Fig. 3–48A–C).[3, 76, 77] The normal midline CT density of the hyoepiglottic ligament should not be mistaken for that of tumor (Fig. 3–15).

Superior extension of cancer into the valleculae can be difficult to detect with CT unless it is extensive. Because the valleculae are normally asymmetric and because their base is in the plane of the scan, they are not well demonstrated on CT scans. Fortunately, tumor in this area is easily assessed by endoscopy. Thickening of the median glossoepiglottic and lateral pharyngoepiglottic folds, however, should be recognizable on CT scans (Fig. 3–48C).

Extension of tumor into the aryepiglottic folds and caudad to the region of the arytenoid cartilages is well demonstrated on CT scans. The normal variation in thickness of the aryepiglottic folds should be remembered. During quiet breathing, the piriform sinuses are usually collapsed, and the thickness of the aryepiglottic folds cannot be determined. On CT scans during quiet breathing, an aryepiglottic fold tumor frequently cannot be differentiated from a piriform sinus tumor. CT scans obtained during phonation will show distention of the piriform sinuses and thinning of the normal aryepiglottic fold. Phonation thus allows for easier CT demonstration and localization of the tumor (Fig. 3–49A–C). Tumor extension into an aryepiglottic fold is recognizable by thickening of the fold (Fig. 3–50). In the anterior quarter of the fold, tumor will show replacement of fibroadipose tissue by a high CT density mass.

Lateral extension of supraglottic tumors is into the paralaryngeal soft tissues (Fig. 3–51). Paralaryngeal tumor is recognizable as a mass that frequently displaces the piriform sinus posteriorly. Distortion of a piriform sinus is more easily evaluated when the sinus is distended during phonation.[3] Deep lateral penetration by tumor can occasionally manifest as destruction of a lateral lamina of the thyroid cartilage.

Subglottic Region. Tumors arising in the subglottic region are rare, whereas subglottic extension of cordal or even supraglottic tumors are common.[64–67] True subglottic tumors disseminate early and widely.[78] Lymphatic spread is through the cricothyroid membrane to the prelaryngeal, pretracheal, and cervical nodes bilaterally. Subglottic tumors frequently disseminate to the hypopharynx, trachea, and thyroid gland. When subglottic tumors are being scanned, the CT examination should be extended inferiorly to include the lower neck and upper mediastinum. The subglottic region is particularly well demonstrated with CT because of the absence of normal soft tissue between the cricoid cartilage and airway below the level of the true cords. Any soft tissue in this region is abnormal (Fig. 3–52A,B). Inferior extension of subglottic tumor to the trachea can be difficult to assess by laryngoscopy, but is well seen on CT scans as a mass between the airway and the tracheal wall. Extension through the cricothyroid membrane into the soft tissues of the neck is seen on CT scans as an abnormal soft-tissue mass. Contrast medium by intravenous infusion can assist in determining the margins of the mass. Superior extension of tumor to the undersurface of the true vocal cords can be difficult to detect with CT. Thin sections and high-resolution images can sometimes demonstrate a plane between the tumor and true vocal cords. When CT scans obtained during quiet breathing and during phonation reveal immobility of an arytenoid cartilage, cordal fixation is present and tumor extension to the vocal cord can be assumed. Destruction of the cricoid cartilage is common,[79] but CT scans should not be overinterpreted. A normal, thin anterior cricoid arch or tilting of the cricoid cartilage may be misinterpreted as cartilage destruction.

Transglottic Tumors. Laryngeal tumors that span the laryngeal ventricle to involve both the true and false cords are called transglottic.[68, 69, 79] They are advanced tumors, and vocal cord fixation is frequently present. The tumor can originate in the laryngeal ventricle, as do about 2.5 per cent of squamous cell carcinomas of the larynx. Alternatively, transglottic tumors can represent advanced disease that has spread from the glottic or supraglottic region. Dissemination may be superficial and obvious at endoscopy or deep by way of

Text continued on page 132

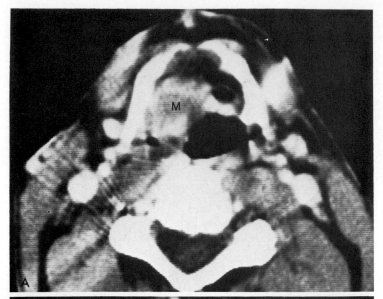

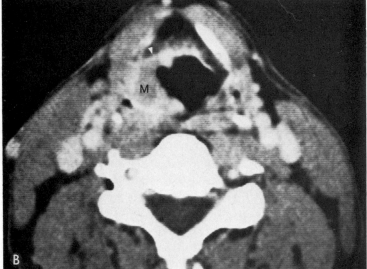

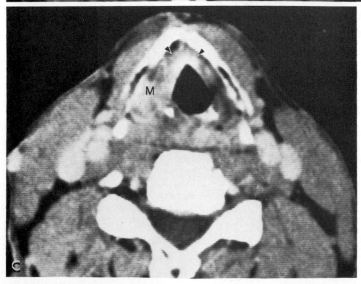

Figure 3–47. Epiglottic carcinoma with endoscopically undetected invasion into pre-epiglottic space. **A** CT scan at the level of the hyoid bone shows a large tumor mass (M) in the right pre-epiglottic space. The entrance to the right piriform sinus is stenosed. **B** Scan 15 mm caudad to **A** through the superior border of the thyroid cartilage; the right aryepiglottic fold is thickened and the right lateral pre-epiglottic space demonstrates increased CT density due to tumor (arrowhead). **C** Scan 5 mm caudad to **B,** through the false vocal cords; the right paralaryngeal tissues contain tumor mass (M) that extends anteriorly into the low pre-epiglottic space (arrowheads).

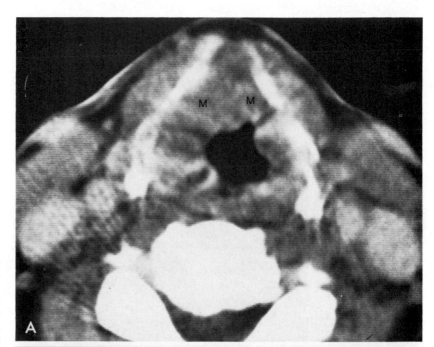

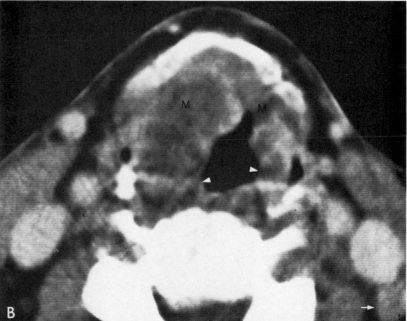

Figure 3–48. Supraglottic tumor with extension to pre-epiglottic space, valleculae, and pharyngoepiglottic folds. **A** CT scan through the thyroid notch shows extensive bilateral tumor mass (M) in the pre-epiglottic space. **B** Scan 15 mm cephalad to **A,** the tumor mass (M) surrounds the anterior endolarynx, filling the pre-epiglottic space and thickening both aryepiglottic folds (arrowheads). An enlarged lymph node is present on the left (arrow).

Illustration continued on following page

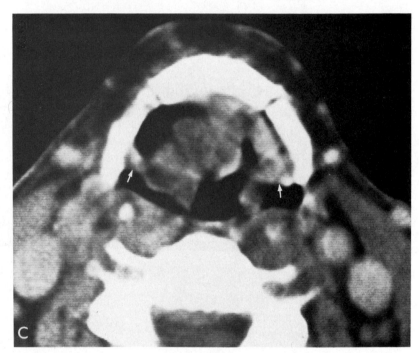

Figure 3–48. *Continued* **C** Scan 10 mm caudad to **B,** the tumor invades both valleculae and pharyngoepiglottic folds (arrows).

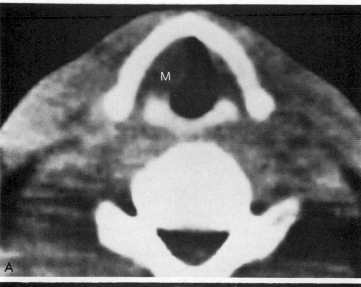

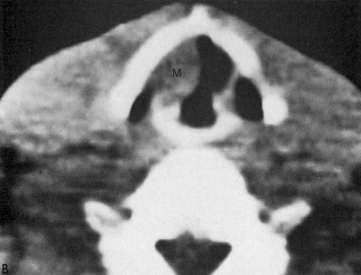

Figure 3–49. Tumor invading the low aryepiglottic fold. **A** CT scan during quiet breathing at about the level of the false vocal cords shows the tumor mass (M) on the right side. **B** Scan at the same level, during phonation; the mass (M) is evident on the right, impinging on the anterior wall of the piriform sinus. **C** Scan 10 cm cephalad to **B**, also obtained during phonation; the tumor mass (M) is visible extending into the right aryepiglottic fold.

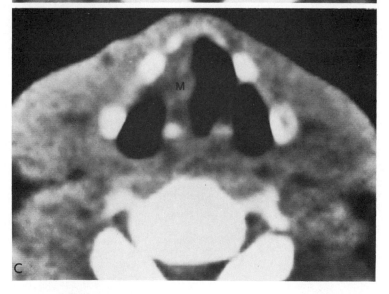

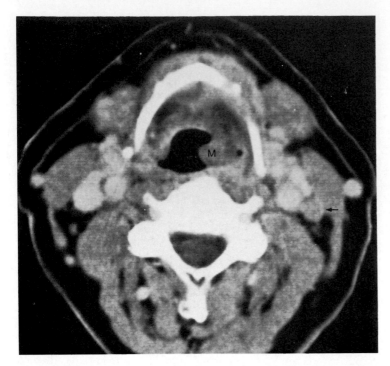

Figure 3–50. Left transglottic tumor thickening the upper aryepiglottic fold. CT scan demonstrates tumor mass (M) causing thickening of the upper aryepiglottic fold. The tumor surrounds the piriform sinus and extends into the pre-epiglottic space. An enlarged lymph node (arrow) is visible on the left.

Figure 3–51. Right supraglottic tumor extending into the neck. CT scan shows tumor from the right aryepiglottic fold extending directly into the right side of the neck. A low-density tumor mass (M) compresses the vessels and is delineated by intravenous contrast medium.

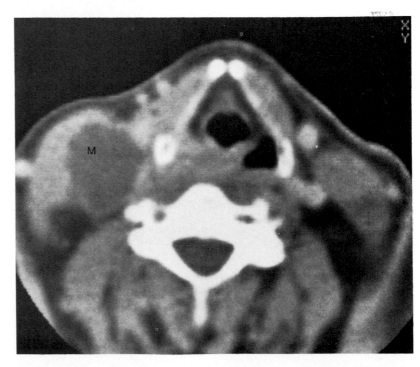

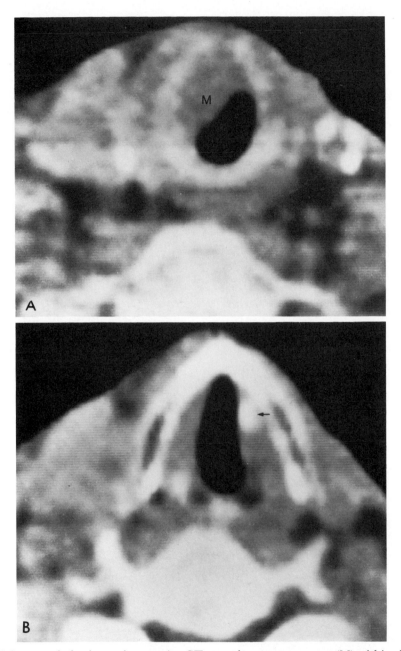

Figure 3–52. Primary subglottic carcinoma. **A**   CT scan shows tumor mass (M) within the cricoid ring. **B**   Scan 15 mm cephalad to **A,** showing that the right true vocal cord is normal. The left true vocal cord contains high-density Teflon (arrow), which had been injected previously. Intermediate scans and endoscopy demonstrated a plane of separation between the tumor and the glottis.

the paralaryngeal soft tissues. CT scans of the thyroid cartilage and cricothyroid area should be carefully examined because these tumors have a propensity for lateral invasion into cartilage and beyond the confines of the larynx (Fig. 3–46A–C).

Piriform Sinus Tumors. These are usually classified as being within the inferior hypopharynx and not the larynx.[12] They are included because of their intimate contact with the larynx. Tumors arising in the piriform sinus have a high incidence of nodal metastases when first seen because lymphatic channels course around their anterior wall and, therefore, early lymphatic invasion is common. Piriform sinus cancers also disseminate early by direct infiltration.[76, 79] Spread is inferior into the paralaryngeal tissue lateral to the true and false vocal cords, supramedially to the aryepiglottic folds and pre-epiglottic space, and laterally through or around the thyroid cartilage.

Endoscopic observation of piriform sinus cancer is difficult and frequently underestimates the extent of the lesion.[80] CT can appreciably assist the clinical and endoscopic examinations in localizing and staging of the tumor.[1, 3, 76] Any soft tissue between air in the piriform sinus and the inner margin of the thyroid cartilage indicates tumor (Fig. 3–53). Inferior extension of the tumor is to the level of the false and true vocal cords. Asymmetry of the paralaryngeal soft tissues in this region is most easily evaluated from CT scans obtained during quiet breathing. The cricothyroid space lateral to the conus elasticus is a potential path for extralaryngeal spread. Superoanterior infiltration of an aryepiglottic fold is assessed from CT scans obtained during phonation. Abnormal asymmetry in thickness or increased CT density of an aryepiglottic fold is indicative of tumor spread (Fig. 3–54A,B). Tumor in the pre-epiglottic space means advanced disease (Stage T2). Direct lateral extension of the tumor is common and indicated by destruction of the lateral lamina of the thyroid cartilage or asymmetry of the soft tissues adjacent to the thyroid cartilage and thyrohyoid membrane (Fig. 3–53). Direct extension of tumor into the soft tissue of the neck often cannot be differentiated on CT scans from matted lymph nodes adjacent to the larynx.

SKELETAL DESTRUCTION AND DISTORTION.   Demonstration of cartilage invasion or destruction is important in laryngeal and piriform sinus cancer because this finding indicates advanced (stage T4) disease[12] and profoundly affects treatment. Endoscopy cannot demonstrate destruction of cartilage, and radiographs are relatively insensitive. The high-density resolution and transverse display of CT make it the most accurate method of detecting tumor disruption of the laryngeal skeleton.

The incidence of tumor invasion of the laryngeal skeleton depends on the site of origin of the tumor. Kirscher[79] studied serial sections of 200

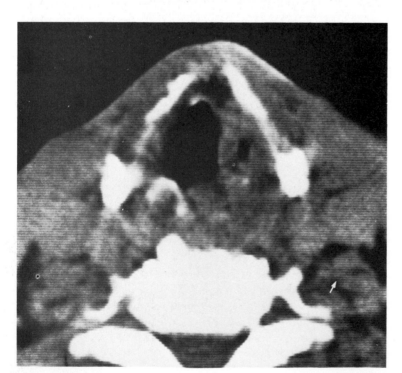

Figure 3–53. Left piriform sinus carcinoma. CT scan demonstrates tumor surrounding the left piriform sinus and separating it from the inner margin of the thyroid lamina. Slight pre-epiglottic space invasion is visible. The carotid sheath lymph nodes (arrow) are enlarged.

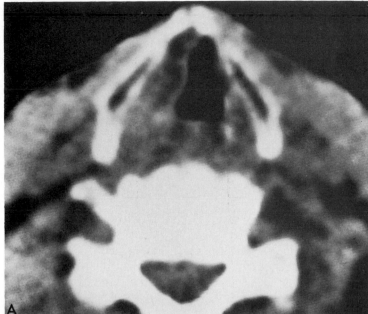

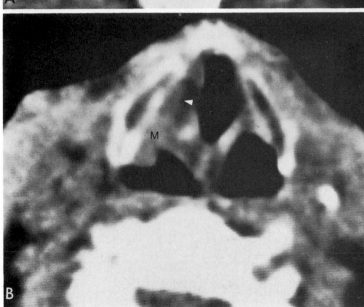

Figure 3–54. Right piriform sinus tumor. **A** CT scan immediately below thyroid notch shows asymmetry of paralaryngeal tissues, which are thickened on the right. **B** Scan at about the same level, during phonation; tumor mass (M) is evident on the anterior wall of the piriform sinus, extending anteriorly (arrowhead) and into the aryepiglottic fold.

surgically resected larynges and found a marked variation in the incidence of invasion of the laryngeal skeleton. He found that 60 per cent of transglottic, 50 per cent of subglottic, 45 per cent of piriform sinus, and 0 per cent of supraglottic tumors had cartilage invasion. Glottic cancer invaded the thyroid lamina in only 10 per cent of cases, usually when subglottic extension of tumor had occurred. These incidences have been confirmed by several investigators in patients studied by CT scanning.[19, 76, 81, 82] One study[82] reported that chondrosclerosis, with increased CT density as well as chondrolysis, with decreased CT density, could be seen in laryngeal cartilages contain-

ing tumor. This potentially important observation has not been confirmed.

Marked destruction of the thyroid and cricoid cartilages is readily demonstrated on CT scans (Figs. 3–41, 3–45A,B, 3–55, 3–56, and 3–57A–C). Demonstration of small areas of cartilage infiltration is one of the most difficult aspects of computed laryngeal tomography. The upper and lower margins of the thyroid cartilage are curved and normally appear ill defined and irregular on CT scans. The degree and symmetry of cartilage calcification or ossification vary.[17, 83, 84] Most CT studies have used scanners with insufficient spatial resolution to detect subtle cartilage invasion.

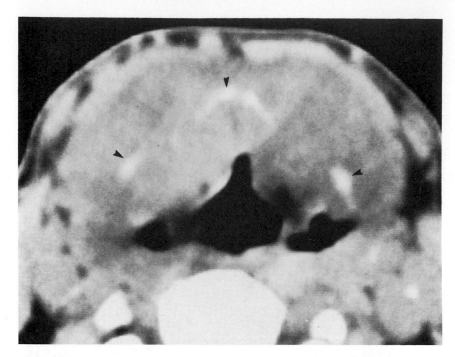

Figure 3–55. Exploded thyroid cartilage. CT scan shows a large tumor extending directly from the larynx into the anterior neck, destroying thyroid cartilage. Fragments of cartilage (arrowheads) are visible within the tumor.

Figure 3–56. Transglottic tumor extending into the neck, destroying the outer wall of thyroid cartilage. CT scan shows endolaryngeal tumor mass (M) with neck tumor on the left. Thyroid cartilage is distorted and tilted, and its left outer wall is destroyed.

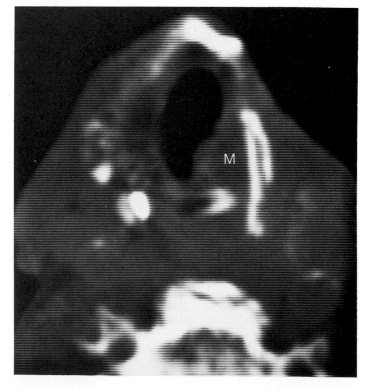

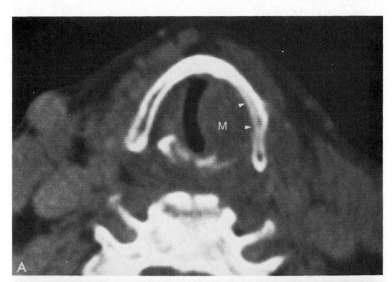

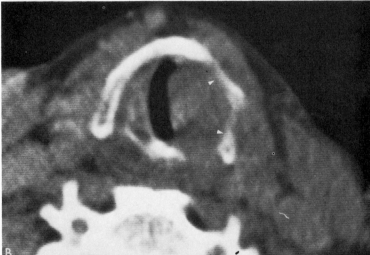

Figure 3–57. Destruction of arytenoid and cricoid cartilages and subglottic extension of tumor. **A** CT scan through the true vocal cords shows a left tumor mass (M) destroying the left arytenoid cartilage. The inner margin of the thyroid cartilage (arrowheads) is irregular but not definitely invaded. **B** On CT scan 0.5 cm caudad to **A,** the bulky mass is still present. The thyroid cartilage (arrowheads) is distorted. The cricoid cartilage not visible. **C** CT scan 1 cm caudad to **B** demonstrates marked destruction of the left side of the cricoid cartilage (C). Subglottic extension of tumor (T) is present. The lateral mass (M) represents tumor infiltration into the neck through the cricothyroid membrane.

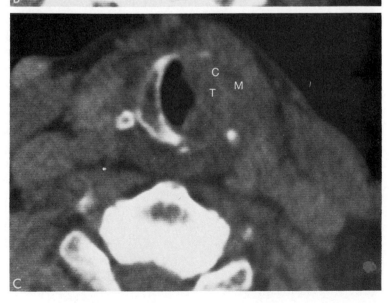

The small size and mobility of the laryngeal cartilages are drawbacks in obtaining detailed scans. New, high-resolution fast scanners should improve the demonstration of the laryngeal skeleton. We consider interruption of the cortex of the cartilage a necessary finding for a definite diagnosis of tumor invasion (Fig. 3–56). Irregularity of the cortex of a laryngeal cartilage is nonspecific and can be misleading.

Mancuso and Hanafee[85] have been the only investigators to have dealt in detail with distortions of the laryngeal skeleton by laryngeal cancer. They found two types of distortions: deformation of the shape of the thyroid cartilage, and disturbance of the normal relationships of the laryngeal cartilages to one another. Both of these abnormalities are not specific for tumor because they can also occur with trauma, inflammatory lesions, benign masses, and radiation chondronecrosis, as well as after surgery.

The thyroid laminae are relatively weak, and their shape can be deformed by bulky masses or abnormal stresses. They can buckle inward or bow outward. In our experience, these distortions do not signify tumor invasion of the cartilage (Fig. 3–58A,B), and their importance must still be demonstrated.

Disturbances in alignment of the cricoid, thyroid, and arytenoid cartilages and of the hyoid bone are common with but not specific for laryngeal tumors. The alignment of these cartilages can vary normally with change in patient position and with respiratory maneuvers. Before a diagnosis of abnormal tilting or rotation of the thyroid cartilage or hyoid bone is considered, correct alignment of the head and neck must be assured. Bulky masses or cricothyroid joint disruption can cause the thyroid cartilage to tilt forward on the cricoid or to rotate about the long axis of the larynx. These distortions do not directly assist in determining tumor extent but may draw the observer's attention to specific regions of the larynx. Frequently, minor buckling or bowing of the thyroid cartilage is due to previous trauma, which may not be remembered by the patient.

An increase in the normal 2- to 3-mm transverse distance between the lateral cricoid and posteromedial thyroid surfaces is a strong indication of tumor invasion into this region. The normal vertical distance between the thyroid cartilage and hyoid bone can be increased by a large mass in the pre-epiglottic space. The thyroid cartilage and hyoid bone normally overlap each other during a Valsalva maneuver or during phonation so that both will be demonstrated on the same CT scan.

Failure of the thyroid cartilage to overlap the hyoid bone is a radiographic sign of infiltration of pre-epiglottic space by tumor.[86] Because the tumor itself can be demonstrated on CT scans, this indirect evidence of pre-epiglottic space invasion is not necessary for diagnosis. In general, a diagnosis of tumor distortion or invasion of the laryngeal skeleton should not be considered from CT scans unless an adjacent mass is visible.

CORDAL FIXATION.   Endoscopically determined immobility of a true vocal cord is defined as cordal fixation. The significance of this finding was first recognized in 1959 by Lenz and colleagues.[87] Patients with laryngeal tumors that cause cordal fixation generally have a lower survival rate than those with laryngeal tumors and vocal cord mobility.[88, 89] The failure rate for radiation therapy when there is cordal fixation is high, and in most situations hemilaryngectomy is inadequate for eradication of the tumor. Total laryngectomy is the usual surgical procedure for removal of a tumor with cordal fixation.

The American Joint Committee Staging System classifies tumors with cordal fixation as advanced (Stage T3) lesions.[12] Five mechanisms[90] can cause cordal fixation from laryngeal tumor:

1. Complete replacement of the thyroarytenoid muscle by tumor can immobilize the true vocal cord.

2. Lateral extension of the tumor to the thyroid cartilage can bind and immobilize the vocal cord, although the thyroarytenoid muscle is not completely replaced by tumor.

3. A bulky tumor of the true cord can prevent motion of the vocal cord without either the first or second mechanism being present.

4. Subglottic extension of the tumor, particularily posteriorly, can fix the vocal cord to the cricoid cartilage.

5. Finally, cricoarytenoid joint invasion by tumor can freeze the joint and immobilize the true vocal cord.

Immobility of the vocal cord is readily confirmed by CT performed during quiet breathing and during phonation.[3] Two patterns of abnormality can be seen. The arytenoid cartilage can be in an abducted position during quiet breathing and not adduct during phonation (Fig. 3–44A,B). Alternatively, the arytenoid cartilage can be in an adducted position both during quiet breathing and phonation. However, these findings alone are not specific because vocal cord paralysis from damage to the recurrent laryngeal nerve can have the same CT scan patterns of abnormality.

Computed tomography can accurately demon-

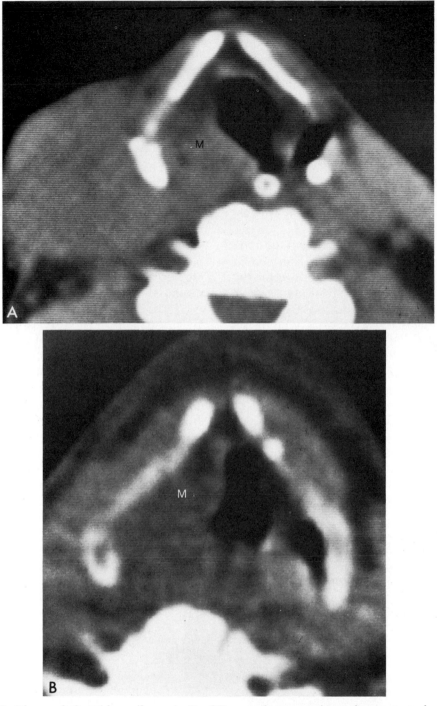

Figure 3–58. Distorted thyroid cartilage. **A, B** CT scans in two patients demonstrate large endolaryngeal masses (M) distorting the shape of the thyroid lamina on the right. The lamina was not invaded in either case.

strate the mechanism of cordal fixation from a tumor.[91] Tumor mass infiltrating both the arytenoid cartilage and the cricoarytenoid joint is the most common finding. In this circumstance, CT scans can demonstrate lateral penetration of tumor beyond the larynx that has not been seen at endoscopy. CT scans are also extremely accurate in showing posterior subglottic extension of the tumor within the cricoid cartilage; this extension is seen as a soft-tissue mass below the level of the true vocal cords. Occasionally, old laryngeal trauma is revealed by the CT scans and can explain a clinical diagnosis of cordal fixation. We have seen several patients in whom the CT scans indicated cordal fixation that had not been detected at indirect laryngoscopy; repeat endoscopy confirmed the CT scan findings.

REGIONAL LYMPH NODE METASTASES. The most important determinant of the survival of patients with laryngeal cancer is the presence of tumor in the cervical lymph nodes. Survival decreases approximately 40 per cent when cervical lymph nodes contain tumor and are palpable. The incidence of nodal metastases varies with the degree of histologic differentiation and the growth pattern of the tumor as well as with the tumor's location and size. The highest correlation of the metastatic rate is with the location of the tumor.[92, 93]

Small glottic tumors have an incidence of nodal metastases of only 0 to 2 per cent. When the tumor has spread locally to the anterior commissure, subglottic region, or posterior commissure, the incidence of regional metastases increases to 5 to 16 per cent. Occult metastases occur in approximately 5 per cent of patients. When tumor extends to the subglottic region, lymph nodes around the thyroid gland and upper trachea can contain metastatic deposits.

Supraglottic cancers are often larger than glottic cancers when first discovered, and the supraglottic region has a more abundant lymphatic supply than the glottis. The incidence of nodal metastases is 20 to 50 per cent (Fig. 3–59), half of which are not clinically palpable.

Primary subglottic tumors are rare but do tend to metastasize to regional nodes, and the incidence is approximately 25 per cent. As with subglottic extension of glottic tumors, primary subglottic tumors can metastasize to the upper mediastinal nodes.

Transglottic cancer is advanced disease, and this is reflected in its high incidence of metastasis. Regional tumor metastases are found at neck exploration in 40 to 50 per cent of patients with transglottic cancer; 30 per cent of the time the metastases are occult and not palpable (Fig. 3–50).

Piriform sinus tumors are also usually advanced when first diagnosed, and this region has abundant lymphatics. The incidence of regional metastases is 50 to 75 per cent (Fig. 3–53); with up to 40 per cent of them being occult. Supraglottic and piriform sinus tumors metastasize upward to the jugulodiagastric lymph nodes; therefore, this area should always be included in the CT examination.

CT scanning is the first imaging modality to allow assessment of the cervical lymph nodes. Mancuso and colleagues[94] found that CT is sensitive in detecting cervical lymph node enlargement from laryngeal carcinoma. In several instances in their study, CT was able to show nonpalpable lymph nodes. Cervical lymph nodes must be distinguished from blood vessels. If rapid sequential scanning with incrementation of the scanner table is available, high concentrations of intravascular contrast medium (Fig. 3–47A–C) can be obtained. A slow bolus injection of 50 to 75 ml of contrast medium is started and scanning begun after 20

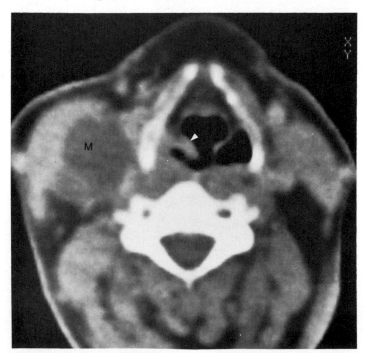

Figure 3–59. Large mass of matted lymph nodes in the neck. CT scan shows aryepiglottic tumor on the right (arrowhead) invading laterally. Large, low-density mass (M) is matted lymph nodes containing tumor.

ml has been injected. The injection is continued throughout the scanning sequence.

In the patient with laryngeal cancer, enlarged lymph nodes may not necessarily contain cancer; in one group of patients with supraglottic cancer, 45 per cent of the palpable nodes were found histologically to be benign.[95] Mancuso and colleagues[94] have described the sites of cervical lymph nodes and proposed diagnostic criteria for separating malignant involvement of nodes from reactive hyperplasia (see Chapter 2). Future studies are needed to confirm these proposals.

TREATMENT AND PROGNOSIS. The treatment of laryngeal cancer is by radiotherapy, surgery, or both.[58, 66, 96–104] Any of several surgical procedures can be employed for laryngeal cancer (Table 3–6), and the choice varies with the tumor and the preference of the physician. If cervical lymph nodes are palpable, some form of neck dissection is usually indicated. The approach in an individual patient requires determination of the precise site and extent of tumor. Therapy differs for each anatomic region of the larynx.

Glottic Region. The cure rate for Stage T1 tumors of the glottis is 85 to 95 per cent using either irradiation or surgery. In most instances, irradiation is preferred because vocal function is better preserved. Stage T2 glottic cancers have a 60 to 80 per cent cure rate with irradiation, and surgery can salvage most of the failures of radiotherapy. In some instances of more advanced lesions, such as subglottic extension of the tumor or invasion of the vocal process of the arytenoid cartilage, hemilaryngectomy is an alternative to irradiation.

The choice of treatment for Stage T3 glottic lesions with cordal fixation remains controversial. The surgical approach can be hemilaryngectomy or total laryngectomy.[102, 104] Alternatively, radiotherapy has been used with early assessment of

the response of the tumor.[66] If CT scans demonstrate deep infiltration of a Stage T3 tumor with cartilage destruction or subglottic extension, an aggressive surgical approach is usually indicated. The cure rate for Stage T3 lesions is about 70 per cent when there are no palpable neck nodes. The larger and the more profuse the cervical lymphadenopathy, the worse the prognosis. Stage T4 glottic cancer is treated by initial total laryngectomy or by irradiation followed by total laryngectomy. The cure rate is about 50 per cent if there are no nodal metastases, and considerably worse if palpable nodes are present.

Supraglottic Region. Early Stage T1 and T2 tumors are not commonly found in the supraglottic larynx but are amenable to treatment by irradiation.[66] The cure rate is 75 to 85 per cent when surgery is used to salvage the failures from irradiation.

Larger Stage T2 and T3 lesions are treated by irradiation, surgery, or radiotherapy followed by supraglottic laryngectomy or total laryngectomy. The cure rate is 60 to 70 per cent, decreasing with the presence of palpable cervical lymph nodes. The CT scan demonstration of tumor invasion of the thyroid cartilage, of the pre-epiglottic space, or through the thyrohyoid membrane indicates the need for an aggressive surgical approach.

Subglottic Region. Because subglottic cancers can be difficult to evaluate by endoscopy, CT scanning can appreciably assist in defining their inferior extent. In general, subglottic cancer that is small and that does not extend inferiorly more than 1 cm below the vocal cord can be treated by hemilaryngectomy. More extensive tumors require total laryngectomy.

Transglottic Tumors. Transglottic cancer can be treated by hemilaryngectomy in selected instances of smaller tumors. Tumors that are bilateral, impair vocal cord mobility, extend to the subglottic region for more than 5 mm, or invade cartilage require total laryngectomy. CT can demonstrate clinically undetected cartilage invasion as well as extension to the contralateral pre-epiglottic space or to the subglottic region. Under these circumstances, total laryngectomy will be indicated to try to avoid possible recurrence of tumor. Clinically undetected nodal enlargement can also be demonstrated by CT and indicates the need for a neck dissection.

COMPARISON OF IMAGING MODALITIES. Several reports have compared computed tomography with conventional tomography and laryngogra-

Table 3–6. SURGICAL PROCEDURES FOR CANCER OF THE LARYNX*

Partial laryngectomy by laryngofissure
    Partial lateral laryngectomy
    Partial frontal-lateral laryngectomy
    Lateral hemilaryngectomy
Partial laryngectomy by pharyngotomy
    Epiglottidectomy
    Partial horizontal laryngectomy
Total laryngectomy

*Adapted from English GM: Malignant neoplasms of the larynx. In English GM (ed): Otaryngology. Hagerstown, Md, Harper & Row, 1976, p 542.

phy in the evaluation of patients with laryngeal cancer.[2, 4, 19, 70, 77, 81] These reports highlight both the advantages and drawbacks of CT. In general, CT has proved to be superior to laryngography in 90 to 95 per cent of cases. CT scans show deep penetration of laryngeal tumors better than laryngography or conventional tomography. Yaeger and colleagues[84] emphasized the difficulties of CT demonstration of cartilage invasion and the potential for overinterpretation of the CT images. High-resolution fast scanners are capable of greatly improving detection of cartilage invasion and destruction.

The inability of CT to routinely demonstrate the laryngeal ventricles is initially disturbing to radiologists who are accustomed to interpreting laryngograms. In the interpretation of CT images of the larynx, the reference points are the laryngeal skeleton, joints, spaces, the true vocal cords, and the aryepiglottic folds. Instead of indirectly indicating the presence of tumor lateral to the laryngeal ventricle, CT can show the mass directly. Subtle tumor infiltration of the ventricle, however, requires endoscopic observation, and CT scans should not be expected to demonstrate this. In many institutions that have adopted CT of the larynx, laryngography and conventional tomography have become uncommon procedures.

INDICATIONS FOR COMPUTED TOMOGRAPHY OF THE LARYNX

The indications for laryngeal CT have not been established. In 1979, the Society for Computed Body Tomography, in a special report[105] offered limited recommendations for the neck. The larynx is included in the general statement, "determination of the extent of primary and secondary neoplasms of the neck" and "localization of foreign bodies."

Our knowledge of laryngeal CT has progressed considerably since 1979, and more specific detailed indications can now be proposed. Patients with laryngeal disorders will virtually always have endoscopy. The additional information that CT scanning can provide should be the prime consideration. Most non-neoplastic lesions of the larynx can be satisfactorily evaluated by clinical examination and laryngoscopy. With bulky masses, CT can determine the extent of the lesion and the degree of distortion of the laryngeal skeleton. The adequacy of the airway can also be ascertained using CT. CT is indicated whenever laryngoscopy is

considered not to have adequately demonstrated the lesion.

Reported experience with CT of the traumatized larynx has been limited. The clinical circumstances in which CT would be indicated are still to be clarified. Reasonable situations for CT include airway obstruction, subcutaneous gas in the neck, vocal disturbances, suspected foreign body, and any patient being considered for neck exploration.

Cancer of the larynx is the primary condition for which CT has been used. Improvements in direct laryngoscopy have made this a precise method for observing the surface of the endolarynx. Small glottic and small supraglottic tumors that can be treated by radiotherapy will proably not benefit by further evaluation using CT. Larger glottic tumors with extension to the commissures or with cordal fixation are indications for laryngeal CT. Most supraglottic, subglottic, and piriform sinus tumors should be examined by CT. CT can show deep infiltration of the tumor, cartilage invasion, and enlarged nonpalpable deep cervical or mediastinal lymph nodes. Unsuspected cordal fixation can be demonstrated by CT. All of these CT findings can have a profound influence on therapy. The role of laryngeal CT in staging of laryngeal and piriform sinus tumors and in modifying therapy is only beginning to be understood. Large, detailed studies with prolonged patient observation and in which fast, high-resolution CT scanners are used are still needed to determine the full efficacy of laryngeal CT.

REFERENCES

1. Mancuso AA, Calcaterra TC, Hanafee WN: Computed tomography of the larynx. Radiol Clin North Am 16:195, 1978.
2. Ward PH, Hanafee W, Mancuso AA, Shallit J, Berci G: Evaluation of computerized tomography, cinelaryngoscopy, and laryngography in determining the extent of laryngeal disease. Ann Otol 88:454, 1979.
3. Gamsu G, Webb WR, Shallit JB, Moss AA: CT in carcinoma of the larynx and piriform sinus: Value of phonation scans. AJR 136:577, 1981.
4. Friedman WH, Archer CR, Yeager VL, Katsantonis GP: Computed tomography vs. laryngography: A comparison of relative diagnostic value. Otolaryngol Head Neck Surg 89:579, 1981.
5. Lockhart RD, Hamilton GF, Fyfe FW: Anatomy of the Human Body. London, Faber & Faber Limited, 1959, pp 535–541.
6. Gray H: The respiratory system. In Goss CM (ed): Anatomy of the Human Body. Philadelphia, Lea & Febiger, 1966, p 1125.
7. Gray H: The respiratory system. In Goss CM (ed): Anatomy of the Human Body. Philadelphia, Lea & Febiger, 1966, p 1127.

8. Pressman JJ, Kelemen G: Physiology of the larynx. Physiol Rev 35:506, 1955.
9. Ardran GM, Kemp FH: The mechanism of the larynx: I: The movements of the arytenoid and cricoid cartilages. Br J Radiol 39:641, 1966.
10. Last RJ: Anatomy Regional and Applied, ed 5. Edinburgh, Churchill Livingston, 1972, p 573.
11. Ardran GM, Kemp FH: The mechanism of the larynx: II: The epiglottis and closure of the larynx. Br J Radiol 40:372, 1967.
12. American Joint Committee for Cancer Staging and End-Results Reporting: Manual for Staging of Cancer. Chicago, Whiting Press, 1978, pp 39–41.
13. Bassett LW, Hanafee WN, Canalis RF: The appendix of the ventricle of the larynx. Radiology 120:571, 1976.
14. Gamsu G, Mark AS, Webb WR: Computed tomography of the normal larynx during quiet breathing and phonation. J Comput Assist Tomogr 5:353, 1981.
15. Mancuso AA, Hanafee WN: Computed Tomography of the Head and Neck. Baltimore, Williams & Wilkins, 1982, pp 5–7.
16. Mancuso AA, Hanafee WN, Juillard GJF, Winter J, Calcaterra TC: The role of computed tomography in the management of cancer of the larynx. Radiology 124:243, 1977.
17. Archer CR, Friedman WH, Yeager VL, Katsantonis GP: Evaluation of laryngeal cancer by computed tomography. J Comput Assist Tomogr 2:618, 1978.
18. Sagel SS, AufderHeide JF, Aronberg DJ, Stanley RJ, Archer CR: High resolution computed tomography in the staging of carcinoma of the larynx. Laryngoscope 91:292, 1981.
18a. Silverman PM, Korobkin M, Thompson WM, Johnson GA, Cole TB, Fisher SR: Work in progress: High-resolution thin-section computed tomography of the larynx. Radiology 145:723, 1982.
19. Scott M, Forsted DH, Rominger CJ, Brennan M: Computed tomographic evaluation of the laryngeal neoplasms. Radiology 140:141, 1981.
20. van Waes PFGM, Zonneveld FW: Patient positioning for direct coronal computed tomography of the entire body. Radiology 142:531, 1982.
21. van Waes PFGM, Zonneveld FW: Direct coronal body computed tomography. J Comput Assist Tomogr 6:58, 1982.
22. Caldarelli DD, Friedberg SA, Harris AA: Medical and surgical aspects of the granulomatous diseases of the larynx. Otolaryngol Clin North Am 12:767, 1979.
23. Mayock RL, Bertrand P, Morrison CE, Scott JH: Manifestations of sarcoidosis: Analysis of 145 patients with a review of nine series selected from the literature. Am J Med 35:67, 1963.
24. Carasso B: Sarcoidosis of the larynx causing airway obstruction. Chest 65:693, 1974.
25. Bower JS, Belen JE, Weg JG, Dantzker DR: Manifestations and treatment of laryngeal sarcoidosis. Am Rev Respir Dis 122:325, 1980.
26. Proctor DF: Laryngeal tuberculosis in the negro. Am Rev Tuberc 47:582, 1943.
27. Travis LW, Hybels RL, Newman MA: Tuberculosis of the larynx. Laryngoscope 86:549, 1976.
28. Friedmann I: Granulomas of the larynx. Paparella MM, Shumrick DA (eds): Otolaryngology, 2nd ed, vol. 3. Philadelphia, WB Saunders Company, 1980, pp 2459–2461.
29. Friedmann I: Granulomas of the larynx. Paparella MM and Shumrick DA (eds): Otolaryngology, 2nd ed, vol. 3. Philadelphia, WB Saunders Company, 1980, p 2449.
30. Proctor DF, Edgerton MT: Chronic complete traumatic occlusion in the larynx secondary to endotracheal anesthesia and its plastic correction. Ann Otol 68:187, 1959.
31. Bridger MWM, Jahn AF, van Nostrand AWP: Laryngeal rheumatoid arthritis. Laryngoscope 90:296, 1980.
32. Mancuso AA, Hanafee WN: Computed Tomography of the Head and Neck. Baltimore, Williams & Wilkins, 1982, p 72.
33. Salmon LFW: Chronic laryngitis. In Ballantyne J, Groves J (eds): Scott-Brown's Diseases of the Ear, Nose and Throat, vol. 4, ed 4. London, Butterworths, 1979, pp 395–401.
34. Holinger PH, Brown WT: Congenital webs, cysts, laryngoceles, and other anomalies of the larynx. Ann Otol Rhinol Laryngol 76:744, 1967.
35. Bachman AL: Benign, non-neoplastic conditions of the larynx and pharynx. Radiol Clin North Am 16:273, 1978.
36. Canalis FF, Maxwell DS, Hemenway WG: Laryngocele—An updated review. J Otolaryngol 6:191, 1977.
37. Landing BH, Dixon LG: Congenital malformations and genetic disorders of the respiratory tract. Am Rev Respir Dis 120:151, 1979.
37a. Silverman PM, Korobkin M: Computed tomographic evaluation of laryngoceles. Radiology 145:104, 1982.
37b. Glazer HS, Mauro MA, Aronberg DJ, Lee JKT, Johnston DE, Sagel SS: Computed tomography of laryngoceles. AJR 140:549, 1983.
38. Mancuso AA, Hanafee WN: Computed Tomography of the Head and Neck. Baltimore, Williams & Wilkins, 1982, pp 72–73.
39. DeSanto LW: Laryngocele, laryngeal mucocele, large saccules, and laryngeal saccular cysts: A developmental spectrum. Laryngoscope 84:1291, 1974.
40. Greene R, Stark P: Trauma of the larynx and trachea. Radiol Clin North Am 16:309, 1978.
41. Templer JW: Trauma to the larynx and cervical trachea. In Otolaryngology, English GM (ed): Hagerstown, Md, Harper & Row, 1976, pp 555–565.
42. Montgomery WW: The surgical management of supraglottic and subglottic stenosis. Ann Otol Rhinol Laryngol 77:534, 1968.
43. Ogura JH, Powers WE: Functional restitution of traumatic stenosis of the larynx and pharynx. Laryngoscope 74:1081, 1964.
44. Mancuso AA, Hanafee WN: Computed tomography of the injured larynx. Radiology 133:139, 1979.
45. Ogura JH, Heeneman H, Spector GJ: Laryngo-tracheal trauma: diagnosis and treatment. Canad J Otolaryngol 2:112, 1973.
46. Brandenburg JH: Management of acute blunt laryngeal injuries. Otolaryngol Clin North Am 12:741, 1979.
47. Cohn AM, Larson DL: Laryngeal injury: A critical review. Arch Otolaryngol 102:166, 1976.
48. Morgenstein KM: Treatment of the fractured larynx: Use of a new grafting technique. Arch Otolaryngol 101:157, 1975.
49. Alonso WA: Surgical management and complications of acute laryngo-tracheal disruption. Otolaryngol Clin North Am 12:753, 1979.

50. Unger JD, Shaffer KA: The radiology of laryngeal and tracheal stenosis. Otolaryngol Clin North Am 12:783, 1979.

51. Shaw H: Tumors of the larynx. In Ballantyne J, Groves J (eds): Scott-Brown's Diseases of the Ear, Nose and Throat, vol 4, ed 4. London, Butterworths, 1979, pp 423–426.

52. Ogura JH, Thawley SE: Cysts and tumors of the larynx. In Paparella MM, Shumrick DA (eds): Otolaryngology, vol 3, ed 2. Philadelphia, WB Saunders Company, 1980, pp 2507–2508.

53. Lyons GD, Lousteau RJ, Mouney DF: CO$_2$ laser laryngoscopy in a variety of lesions. Laryngoscope 86:1658, 1976.

54. Weber AL, Shortsleeve M, Goodman M, Montgomery W, Grillo HC: Cartilaginous tumors of the larynx and trachea. Radiol Clin North Am 16:261, 1978.

55. Barsocchini LM, McCoy G: Tumors of the larynx. Ann Otol Rhinol Laryngol 77:146, 1968.

56. Singh J, Black MJ, Fried I: Cartilaginous tumors of the larynx: A review of literature and two case experiences. Laryngoscope 90:1872, 1980.

57. English GM: Benign neoplasms of the larynx. In English GM (ed): Otolaryngology. Hagerstown, Harper & Row, 1976, pp 528–529.

58. Harrison DFN: Carcinoma of the larynx. Br Med J 2(5657):615, 1969.

59. Kissin B, Kaley MM, Su WH, Lerner R: Head and neck cancer in alcoholics: The relationship to drinking, smoking, and dietary patterns. JAMA 224:1174, 1973.

60. Wynder EL, Bross IJ, Day E: A study of environmental factors in cancer of the larynx. Cancer 9:86, 1956.

61. McGavran MH, Bauter WC, Ogura JH: Isolated laryngeal keratosis. Laryngoscope 70:932, 1960.

62. Whicker JH, Neel HB, Devine KD: Adenocarcinoma of the larynx. Am Laryngol Assoc, Proc 95th Ann Mtg, 1974.

63. Ogura JH, Spector GJ: The larynx. In Nealon TF (ed): Management of the Patient with Cancer. Philadephia, WB Saunders Company, 1976, pp 206–238.

64. Kirchner JA, Cornog JL, Holmes RE: Transglottic cancer: Its growth and spread within the larynx. Arch Otolaryngol 99:247, 1974.

65. Lee JG: Detection of residual carcinoma of the oral cavity, oropharynx, hypopharynx and larynx: A study of surgical margins. Trans Am Acad Ophthalmol Otolaryngol 78:49, 1974.

66. Lederman M: Radiotherapy of cancer of the larynx. J Laryngol Otol 84:867, 1970.

67. Norris CM: Laryngectomy and neck dissection. Otolaryngol Clin North Am 2:667, 1969.

68. Tucker GF Jr: The anatomy of laryngeal cancer. Can J Otolaryngol 3:417, 1974.

69. Kirschner JA: One hundred laryngeal cancers studied by serial section. Ann Otolaryngol 78:689, 1969.

70. Tucker GF, Alonso WA, Tucker JA, Cowan M, Druck N: The anterior commissure revisited. Ann Otol 82:625, 1973.

71. Mancuso AA, Hanafee WN: A comparative evaluation of computed tomography and laryngography. Radiology 133:131, 1979.

72. Mancuso AA, Hanafee WN: Computed Tomography of the Head and Neck. Baltimore, Williams & Wilkins, 1982, pp 28–29.

73. English GM: Malignant neoplasms of the larynx. In English GM (ed): Otolaryngology. Hagerstown, Harper & Row, 1976, p 536.

74. Ducuing J, Ducuing L: Les Tumeurs Malignés des Voies Aerodigestives Supérieures. Paris, 1949.

75. Fletcher GN, Hamberger AD: Cause of failure in irradiation of squamous cell carcinoma of the supraglottic larynx. Radiology 111:697, 1974.

76. Larsson S, Mancuso A, Hoover L, Hanafee W: Differentiation of pyriform sinus cancer from supraglottic laryngeal cancer by computed tomography. Radiology 141:427, 1981.

77. Archer CR, Sagel SS, Yeager VL, Martin S, Friedman WH: Staging of carcinoma of the larynx: Comparative accuracy of CT and laryngography. AJR 136:571, 1981.

78. Stell PM, Tobin KE: The behavior of cancer affecting the subglottic space. Can J Otolaryngol 250:620, 1974.

79. Kirchner JA: Two hundred laryngeal cancers: Patterns of growth and spread as seen in serial section. Laryngoscope 87:474, 1977.

80. Kirchner JA: Pyriform sinus cancer: A clinical and laboratory study. Ann Otol Rhinol Laryngol 84:793, 1975.

81. Parsons CA, Chapman P, Counter RT, Grundy A: The role of computed tomography in tumours of the larynx. Clin Radiol 31:529, 1980.

82. Lloyd GAS, Michaels L, Phelps PD: The demonstration of cartilaginous involvement in laryngeal carcinoma by computerized tomography. Clin Otolaryngol 6:171, 1981.

83. Hately W, Evison G, Samuel E: The pattern of ossification in the laryngeal cartilages: A radiological study. Br J Radiol 38:585, 1965.

84. Yeager VL, Lawson C, Archer CR: Ossification of the laryngeal cartilages as it relates to computed tomography. Invest Radiol 17:11, 1982.

85. Mancuso AA, Hanafee WN: Computed Tomography of the Head and Neck. Baltimore, Williams & Wilkins, 1982, pp 32–34.

86. Jing BS: Roentgen examination of laryngeal cancer: A critical evaluation. Can J Otolaryngol 4:64, 1975.

87. Lenz M, Okraineta C, Berne AS: Radiotherapy of cancer of the larynx. In Pack GT, Ariel IM (eds): Treatment of Cancer and Allied Disease. New York, PB Hoeber, Inc, 1959, p 542.

88. Mårtensson B, Fluur E, Jacobson F: Aspects of treatment of cancer of the larynx. Ann Otolaryngol 76:313, 1967.

89. Vermund H: Role of radiotherapy in cancer of the larynx, as related to the T.N.M. system of staging. Cancer 5:485, 1970.

90. Kirchner JA: Clinical significance of fixed vocal cord. Laryngoscope 81:1029, 1971.

91. Mancuso AA, Tamakawa Y, Hanafee WN: CT of the fixed vocal cord. AJR 135:529, 1980.

92. McGavran MH, Bauer WC, Ogura JH: The incidence of cervical lymph node metastases from epidermoid carcinoma of the larynx and their relationship to certain characteristics of the primary tumor. Cancer 14:55, 1961.

93. Cocke EW: Cancer of the larynx: Surgery. Cancer 26:201, 1976.

94. Mancuso AA, Maceri D, Rice D, Hanafee WN: CT of cervical lymph node cancer. AJR 136:381, 1981.

95. Cummings CW: Incidence of nodal metastasis in T2 supraglottic carcinoma. Arch Otolaryngol 99:268, 1974.

96. Hendrickson FR: Programmed preoperative radiation therapy for carcinoma of the larynx. Otolaryngol Clin North Am 3:589, 1970.

97. Goldman JL, Gunsberg MJ, Friedman WH, Ryan JR, Bloom BS: Combined therapy for cancer of the laryngopharynx. Arch Otolaryngol 92:221, 1970.

98. Bryce DP, Rider WD: Preoperative irradiation in the treatment of advanced laryngeal carcinoma. Laryngoscope 81:1481, 1971.

99. Shumrick DA: Supraglottic laryngectomy: Its plan in the treatment of laryngeal cancer. Arch Otolaryngol 89:629, 1969.

100. Kirchner JA, Som ML: The anterior commissure technique of partial laryngectomy: Clinical and laboratory observations. Laryngoscope 85:1308, 1975.

101. Ogura JH, Sessions DG, Spector GJ: Analysis of surgical therapy for epidermoid carcinoma of the laryngeal glottis. Laryngoscope 85:1522, 1975.

102. Lesinski SG, Bauer WC, Ogura JH: Hemilaryngectomy for T3 (fixed cord) epidermoid carcinoma of larynx. Laryngoscope 86:1563, 1976.

103. Ogura JH: Selection of patients for conservative surgery of the larynx and pharynx. Tran Am Acad Ophthalmol Otol 76:741, 1972.

104. Bryce DP, Ireland PI, Rider WD: Experience in the surgical and radiological treatment of 500 cases of carcinoma of the larynx. Ann Otolaryngol 72:416, 1963.

105. Society for Computed Body Tomography: New indications for computed body tomography. AJR 133:115, 1979.

4 COMPUTED TOMOGRAPHY OF THE TRACHEA AND CENTRAL BRONCHI

Gordon Gamsu

Computed tomography (CT) is an excellent method for visualizing mediastinal structures. However, descriptions of the normal CT anatomy of the trachea and bronchi are limited.[1–4] The use of CT scanning in abnormalities of the trachea and bronchi has been reported only briefly.[5 6] The trachea and major bronchi generally lie in a plane perpendicular to the CT image and are well displayed in cross section. The tracheobronchial tree is visible on CT scans as far peripherally as seg-mental and occasionally subsegmental bronchi.[6] This chapter will deal with these airways.

ANATOMY

The trachea is a fibromuscular and cartilaginous tube 10 to 12 cm long (Fig. 4–1).[7] It extends from the lower border of the cricoid cartilage in the neck to its bifurcation at the tracheal carina in the mediastinum. The trachea is a midline structure until near its termination, where it inclines slightly to the right. Its walls are parallel except for two minor indentations. The impression of the aortic arch on the left anterolateral wall of the trachea can be seen on CT scans in many normal persons. An indentation from the arch of the azygos vein is seen less frequently.

The tracheal wall comprises 20 to 22 horseshoe-shaped cartilages open posteriorly.[8] The cartilages are connected posteriorly by a thick fibromuscular membrane. The diameter of the trachea is normally 11 to 30 mm (mean, 19.5 mm in males; 17.5 mm in females).[9]

Six to 9 cm after entering the thorax, the trachea divides into two main bronchi.[2] The right main bronchus is 2.2 cm long, the left is 5 cm.[10, 11] The diameter of the right main bronchus averages 15.3 mm, the left 13 mm, when measured on chest radiographs at full inspiration.[12]

RIGHT BRANCHING PATTERN. On the right, the short main bronchus divides into an upper lobe bronchus and an intermediate bronchus. The right upper-lobe bronchus passes laterally for 1 to 2 cm before dividing into its three segmental

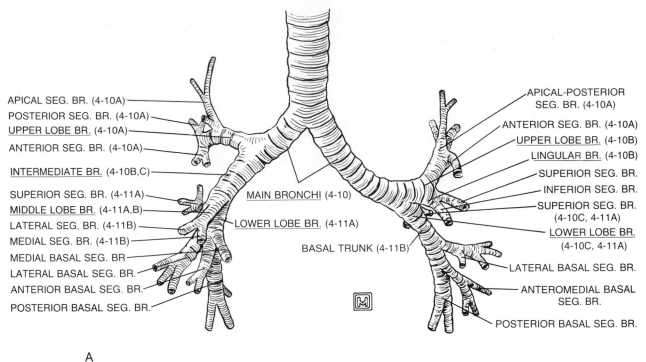

APICAL SEG. BR. (4-10A)
POSTERIOR SEG. BR. (4-10A)
UPPER LOBE BR. (4-10A)
ANTERIOR SEG. BR. (4-10A)

INTERMEDIATE BR. (4-10B,C)

SUPERIOR SEG. BR. (4-11A)
MIDDLE LOBE BR. (4-11A,B)
LATERAL SEG. BR. (4-11B)
MEDIAL SEG. BR. (4-11B)
MEDIAL BASAL SEG. BR
LATERAL BASAL SEG. BR.
ANTERIOR BASAL SEG. BR.
POSTERIOR BASAL SEG. BR.

MAIN BRONCHI (4-10)

LOWER LOBE BR. (4-11A)

BASAL TRUNK (4-11B)

APICAL-POSTERIOR
SEG. BR. (4-10A)
ANTERIOR SEG. BR. (4-10A)
UPPER LOBE BR. (4-10B)
LINGULAR BR. (4-10B)
SUPERIOR SEG. BR.
INFERIOR SEG. BR.
SUPERIOR SEG. BR.
(4-10C, 4-11A)
LOWER LOBE BR.
(4-10C, 4-11A)
LATERAL BASAL SEG. BR.
ANTEROMEDIAL BASAL
SEG. BR.
POSTERIOR BASAL SEG. BR.

A

FRONTAL PROJECTION

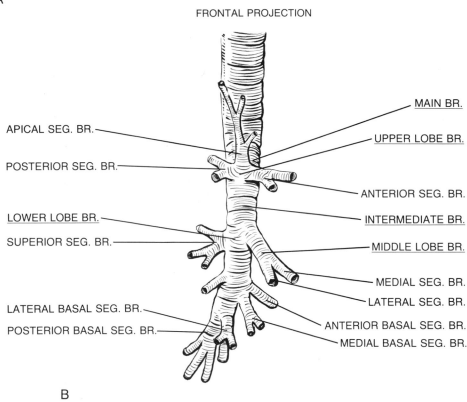

APICAL SEG. BR.

POSTERIOR SEG. BR.

LOWER LOBE BR.
SUPERIOR SEG. BR.

LATERAL BASAL SEG. BR.
POSTERIOR BASAL SEG. BR.

MAIN BR.

UPPER LOBE BR.

ANTERIOR SEG. BR.

INTERMEDIATE BR.

MIDDLE LOBE BR.

MEDIAL SEG. BR.
LATERAL SEG. BR.
ANTERIOR BASAL SEG. BR.
MEDIAL BASAL SEG. BR.

B

RIGHT LATERAL PROJECTION

Figure 4–1. Schema of lower trachea and central bronchi. The bronchial tree is shown in frontal projection (**A**) and right lateral projection (**B**).

Illustration continued on opposite page

bronchi.[3, 4] The branching pattern is moderately variable, but on CT scans, all three segmental bronchi are usually visible. The intermediate bronchus is 3 to 4 cm long and courses in a su-

perior-inferior direction. The middle lobe bronchus arises from the anterolateral wall of the intermediate bronchus and passes inferiorly, laterally, and anteriorly in an oblique direction for 1 to 2

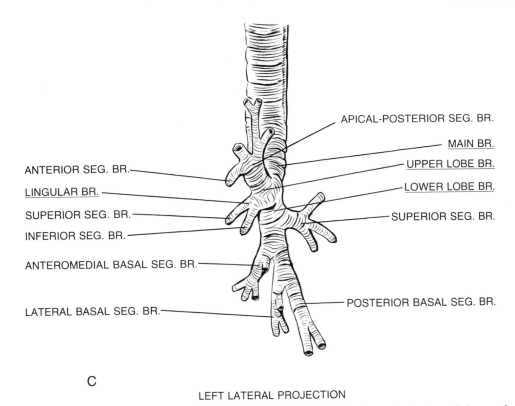

APICAL-POSTERIOR SEG. BR.

MAIN BR.

UPPER LOBE BR.

LOWER LOBE BR.

SUPERIOR SEG. BR.

POSTERIOR BASAL SEG. BR.

ANTERIOR SEG. BR.

LINGULAR BR.

SUPERIOR SEG. BR.

INFERIOR SEG. BR.

ANTEROMEDIAL BASAL SEG. BR.

LATERAL BASAL SEG. BR.

C

LEFT LATERAL PROJECTION

Figure 4–1. *Continued* **C** Bronchial tree, shown in left lateral projection. In **A, B,** and **C,** numbers in parentheses refer to figures showing the relevant anatomic features. (See also Chapter 6, Figs. 6–1 through 6–9.)

cm before dividing into its medial and lateral segmental bronchi. After giving off the middle lobe bronchus, the intermediate bronchus continues as the right lower lobe bronchus. The first segmental branch of the right lower lobe is the superior segmental bronchus. It arises from the posterior wall of the lower lobe bronchus at a slightly lower level than the middle lobe bronchus. One to 2 cm beyond the origin of the superior segmental bronchus, the right lower lobe bronchus divides into its four basal segments (medial, anterior, lateral, and posterior).

LEFT BRANCHING PATTERN. The branching pattern of the left bronchial tree is different from that of the right. The long left main bronchus divides directly into upper and lower lobe bronchi. The upper lobe bronchus gives off a lingular branch from its anterior-inferior surface and most commonly continues as a common trunk, which divides into anterior and apical-posterior branches.[13] Less commonly, the left upper lobe bronchus trifurcates into anterior, lingular, and apical-posterior bronchi. The lingular bronchus, which is the least frequently visualized major airway on CT scans, is directed anteroinferiorly for 2 to 3 cm and then bifurcates into superior and inferior segmental bronchi. The absence of an in-

termediate bronchus, combined with a longer main bronchus, results in a left lower lobe bronchus that arises 1 to 2 cm cephalad to the right lower lobe bronchus. As on the right, the first branch of the lower lobe is the posteriorly directed superior segmental bronchus. The three basal segmental bronchi (anteromedial, lateral, and posterior) arise 1 to 2 cm distal to the origin of the superior segmental bronchus.

TRACHEA

The extrathoracic trachea begins at the lower border of the cricoid cartilage and ends at the thoracic inlet, a distance of 2 to 4 cm.[2] The subglottic larynx, within the cricoid cartilage, is always circular on CT scans and the airway is close to the underlying perichondrium. Immediately below the cricoid cartilage, the extrathoracic trachea assumes a horseshoe, elliptical, or circular configuration (Fig. 4–2). In about 50 per cent of normal people, the posterior tracheal membrane protrudes slightly into the tracheal air column.[2]

The thyroid gland encases the anterior and lateral walls of the extrathoracic trachea (Fig. 4–3). It is always visible on CT scans and extends vertically for 2 to 4 cm. The thyroid gland is usually denser than the surrounding soft tissues because

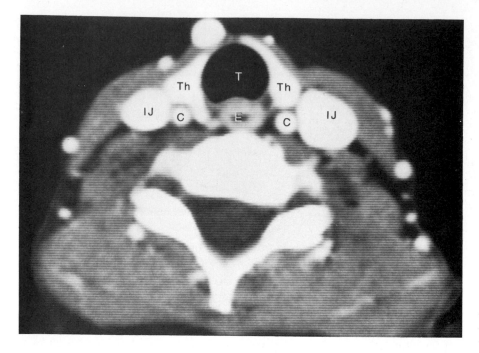

Figure 4–2. Normal extrathoracic trachea. CT scan shows trachea (T) with the esophagus (E) protruding at the posterior tracheal membrane. The thyroid gland (Th) is lateral and anterior to the trachea. The common carotid arteries (C) and internal jugular veins (IJ) are posterolateral to the trachea. Multiple superficial cervical veins are opacified by intravenous contrast material.

of its iodine content. The sternohyoid and sternothyroid muscles, together with a variable quantity of fat, also border the anterior wall of the extrathoracic trachea.

The common carotid arteries and jugular veins are lateral to the middle and posterior thirds of the extrathoracic trachea (Fig. 4–3). Occasionally, they are slightly behind the coronal plane through the trachea. The right common carotid artery is usually more anterior than the left. The right internal jugular vein lies lateral to the right common carotid artery and is usually larger than the left internal jugular vein, which is anterolateral to the left common carotid artery.

The thoracic inlet is a sloping plane at the junction of the thorax and neck. It extends from the

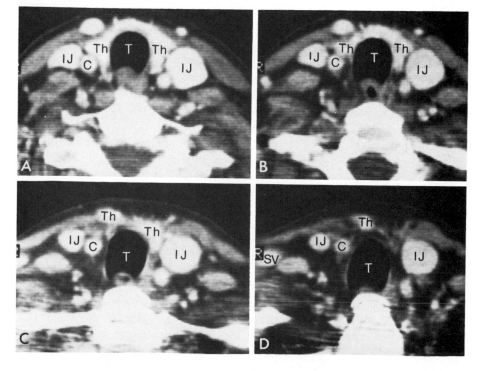

Figure 4–3. Normal extrathoracic trachea. **A–D** Sequential CT scans 1 cm thick through the lower neck. The middle and lower poles of the thyroid gland (Th) are anterior and lateral to the horseshoe-shaped trachea (T). The right carotid artery (C) courses from anterior to posterior. The internal jugular veins (IJ) and right subclavian vein (SV) are anterolateral to the trachea.

suprasternal (jugular) notch anteriorly to the first thoracic vertebral body posteriorly. Below this level the trachea is intrathoracic and makes its first contact with the right lung 1 to 3 cm above the suprasternal notch. The relationship of the great arteries and veins to the trachea changes rapidly at the thoracic inlet (Fig. 4–4) (see also Chapter 5, Fig. 5–12). The innominate artery is visible on CT scans opposite the right anterior third of the trachea, where it divides to form the right subclavian and common carotid arteries. The right internal jugular and subclavian veins join to form the right brachiocephalic vein lateral to the innominate artery. The left common carotid artery is next to the middle or posterior third of the left tracheal wall. The left subclavian artery is initially posterior to the trachea and then courses anterolaterally towards the left first rib. The esophagus at the level of the thoracic inlet is always directly behind the trachea in or slightly to the left of the midline. The inferior extent of the strap muscles is directly anterior to the trachea.

The apices of the lungs are evident on CT scans at the level at which the trachea becomes intrathoracic. The intrathoracic trachea is 6 to 9 cm long (mean 7.5 ± 0.8 cm).[2] The shape of the normal intrathoracic trachea on CT scans varies from person to person and at different levels in the same person. The usual shape is circular or slightly oval (Fig. 4–5). It is also frequently horseshoe-shaped, with a flat posterior wall. Less commonly, it has the shape of an inverted pear or it can be almost square.

The tracheal wall is usually visible on CT scans as a distinct thin line against a background of low CT density mediastinal fat, except where lung parenchyma or vessels contact the trachea. Distinct calcification of the tracheal cartilages is usually seen only in people over the age of 40 (Fig. 4–5). It is visible as small, discontinuous high CT densities within the tracheal wall. Soft-tissue density is not normally present within the outline of the tracheal wall. Occasionally, a glob of mucus can be seen in the trachea or major bronchi (Fig. 4–6).

The relationship of the intrathoracic trachea to the vessels around it and to the esophagus depends on the level of the scan. The great vessels are in front and to the left of the upper 2 to 4 cm of the intrathoracic trachea. The innominate artery is directly anterior to the trachea in about 40 per cent of normal people. In the remainder, it is either slightly to the left or the right of the midline (Fig. 4–7). The left common carotid artery is to the left of and anterior to the trachea in its lower portion and to the left of and lateral to the trachea in its upper portion. The left subclavian artery has a variable anteroposterior relationship to the upper intrathoracic trachea. In about half of normal people, it is directly lateral to the middle third of the trachea. In most of the remainder, it is lateral to the anterior third, while in a small minority, it is lateral to the posterior third. Mediastinal fat usually separates the upper trachea from the left lung and surrounds the left subclavian artery to a variable degree.

On the right side of the upper mediastinum, the right lung first makes contact with the posterolateral surface of the trachea. One to 2 cm caudad, contact is with the posterior half to two thirds of the right tracheal wall. The superior vena cava is always anterior and to the right of the trachea; only near the thoracic inlet does the right brachiocephalic vein assume a position lateral to the trachea. In the supine position, one third to two thirds of the posterior wall of the trachea is in contact with the right lung (Fig. 4–7).[14–16] In most subjects, the rest of the posterior wall of the trachea is bordered by the esophagus or by mediastinal fat. In about 15 per cent of subjects, the retrotracheal space is small, and the trachea is in direct contact with the spine. Under these conditions, the esophagus is entirely to the left of the trachea.

Below the level of the great vessels, the aortic arch is visible over a vertical distance of 1 to 2 cm, anterior and to the left of the trachea. On CT scans, the aortic arch frequently produces a slight flattening of the left anterolateral wall of the trachea but does not otherwise distort the normal trachea (Fig. 4–8). Inferior to the thoracic inlet, the only vascular structure bordering the right tracheal wall is the azygos arch, which is usually visible on CT scans at a level immediately above the tracheal carina.

The trachea assumes a horizontal oval shape in its most inferior 1 to 2 cm (Fig. 4–9). The arch of the azygos vein is visible to the right of the inferior trachea, and the fat-containing pretracheal space separates the lower trachea from the ascending aorta.[17] The left side of the lower trachea forms the base of the aortic-pulmonic window. However, on CT scans obtained with the scanner gantry in the vertical position, a distinctive aortic-pulmonic window is seen in only a third of subjects. In the remainder, the inferior surface of

Text continued on page 154

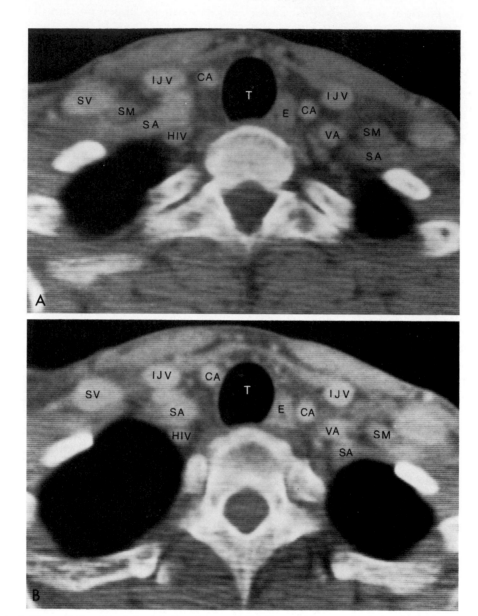

Figure 4–4. Normal thoracic inlet. **A–D**   Sequential CT scans 5 mm thick through the thoracic inlet from above down. The trachea (T) is midline and the esophagus (E) is to the left. On the right side the subclavian artery (SA) is behind the anterior scalene muscle (SM) in **A,** and the right subclavian vein (SV) and internal jugular vein (IJV) in **A** through **D**. The right common carotid artery (CA) stays close to the trachea. **A–D**   The right highest intercostal vein (HIV) is behind the subclavian artery. On the left, the common carotid artery (CA) is lateral to the esophagus. The left subclavian artery courses from posterior to anterior. The internal jugular vein (IJV) and subclavian join anterior and lateral to the common carotid artery. **A–C**   The left vertebral artery (VA) is posterior and lateral to the common carotid artery.

Illustration continued on opposite page

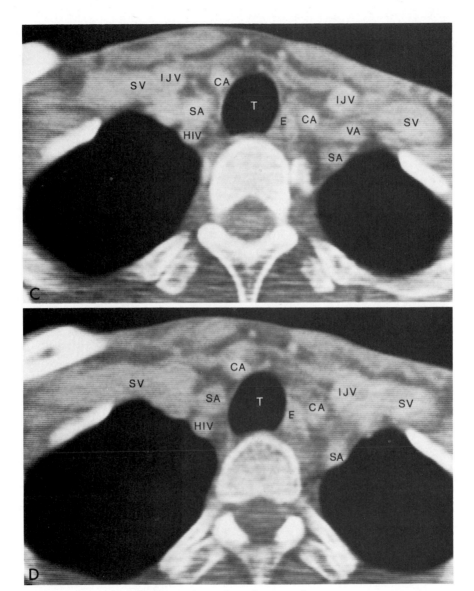

Figure 4–4. *See legend on opposite page*

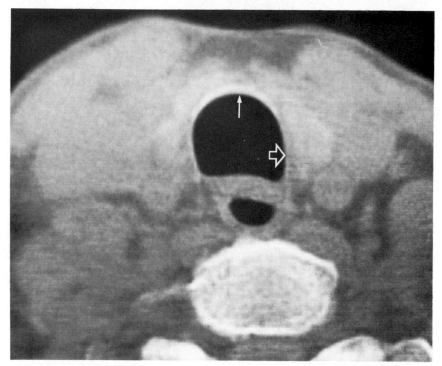

Figure 4–5. Normal tracheal cartilage calcification. High-resolution CT scan shows a calcified tracheal cartilage (arrow). The tracheal wall is demonstrated on the left side (open arrow).

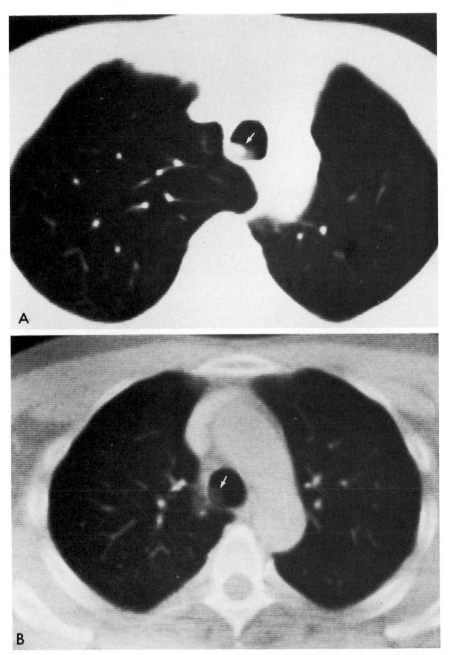

Figure 4–6. Mucus in the tracheal lumen. **A** CT scan at "lung" window settings (level −259 H; width 1000 H) shows a glob of mucus in the trachea (arrow). **B** In a second patient, CT scan at extended window settings (level −360 H; width 1664 H) shows the relationship of a glob of mucus (arrow) to the tracheal wall.

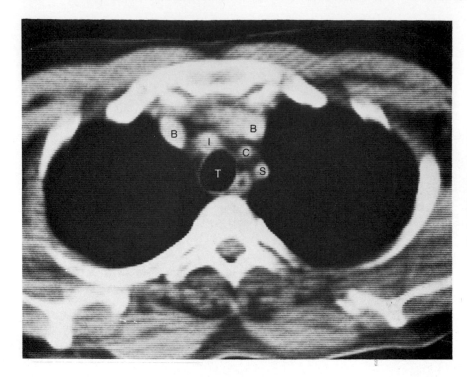

Figure 4–7. Normal upper intrathoracic trachea. CT scan shows a circular trachea (T). The innominate artery (I), left common carotid artery (C), and left subclavian artery (S) are anterior or to the left. The brachiocephalic veins (B) are well forward of the trachea.

the aortic arch or the superior surface of the left pulmonary artery obscures the aortic-pulmonic window.

CENTRAL BRONCHI

The frequency with which a central bronchus is seen on CT scans depends on the size of the bronchus, its orientation relative to the plane of the scan, and the scan thickness.[3, 4] The main bronchi, intermediate bronchus, and lobar bronchi are normally all visible. Segmental bronchi that are in cross section or image along their axis, are also usually demonstrated. The middle lobe, lingular, and basal bronchi course obliquely and are well seen on CT scans 1 cm thick only 60 to 80 per cent of the time. On thinner sections, these

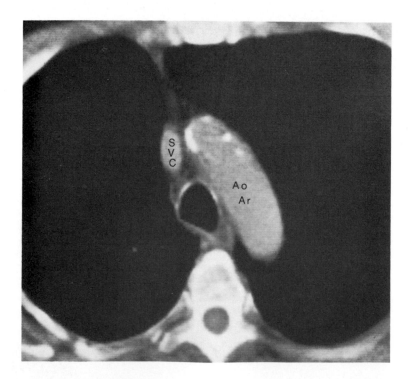

Figure 4–8. Normal trachea at the aortic arch. CT scan shows aortic arch (AoAr) that slightly flattens the left anterolateral wall of the trachea. The superior vena cava (SVC) is anterior and to the right.

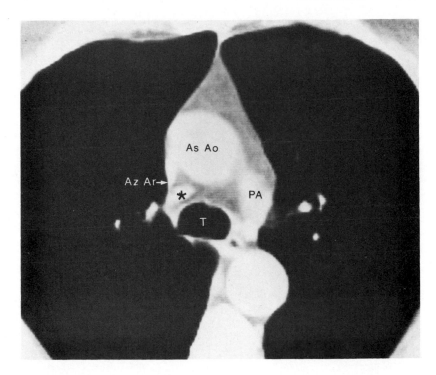

Figure 4–9. Normal trachea immediately above carina. CT scan shows the trachea (T) having an oval shape. The pretracheal space containing a normal azygos lymph node (asterisk) separates the trachea from the ascending aorta (AsAo). A short segment of azygos arch (AzAr) and the pulmonary artery (PA) are also visible.

bronchi are seen more frequently. Bronchi beyond segmental branches are not routinely seen with CT. (The relationships of the bronchi to the pulmonary arteries and veins are discussed in Chapter 6.)

The short right main bronchus can be seen coursing inferiorly and laterally on one or two adjacent scans. It then divides into a right upper lobe bronchus and an intermediate bronchus. The upper lobe bronchus normally courses laterally for 1 to 2 cm and can be seen on one or two contiguous scans (Fig. 4–10A). The anterior and posterior segmental bronchi are demonstrated on the same scan as the lobar bronchus. They are oriented in a near-horizontal plane and pass forward and backward, respectively. The anterior segmental bronchus is more horizontal than the posterior segmental bronchus and visible over a greater length. The apical bronchus is almost always seen in cross section, at levels 1 to 2 cm cephalad to the lobar bronchus.

The intermediate bronchus is visible in almost perfect cross section as it courses vertically from the origin of the right upper lobe bronchus to the origin of the middle lobe bronchus. On three to four contiguous images, it appears as a ring bordered by lung posteriorly and the interlobar branch of the right pulmonary artery anterolaterally (Figs. 4–10B,C).

The origin and entire length of the middle lobe bronchus are seen on one to two contiguous

scans, arising from the anterolateral surface of the intermediate bronchus (Figs. 4–11A,B). It courses anteriorly, laterally, and inferiorly for 1 to 3 cm before dividing into its medial and lateral segmental bronchi. In about 60 per cent of normal subjects, the segmental bronchi are of equal size. In the remainder, the medial segmental bronchus predominates and can be recognized on CT scans as the larger of the two.[3] The lateral segmental bronchus is in a more horizontal plane and frequently demonstrated over a greater length than the medial segmental bronchus.

At about the level of the origin of the middle lobe bronchus, the bronchus to the superior segment of the right lower lobe is directed posteriorly and slightly laterally (Fig. 4–11A). Its proximal 1 to 3 cm is always seen, frequently accompanied by a branch of the pulmonary artery on its lateral side. The superior segmental bronchus originates at the level of the right middle lobe bronchus, 1 cm caudad to it, or because of the orientation of the lung in the chest, can even appear to be 1 cm cephalad. Lung borders the posterior hilum at this level and is in contact with the posterior and often medial walls of the intermediate bronchus as well as the medial wall of the superior segmental bronchus.

The short right lower lobe bronchus distal to the superior segmental bronchus courses in a vertical plane and is usually visible on only one CT scan. The right pulmonary artery is lateral to the bronchus; the inferior pulmonary vein, posterior; and parenchyma of the lung, anterior. The basal segmental bronchi originate approximately 1 cm distal to the right middle lobe bronchus and course in oblique directions. Frequently, only two to three of the basal bronchi are demonstrated on CT scans. The inferior pulmonary vein courses from lateral to medial, behind the dividing basal segmental bronchi, and is always visible on CT scans.

The left main bronchus is considerably longer than the right main bronchus and is visible on three to four contiguous CT scans 1 cm thick (Fig. 4–10). Its orifice and proximal segment, immediately distal to the tracheal carina, are directly medial to the left pulmonary artery, anterior to the descending aorta, and posterior to the left superior pulmonary vein (Fig. 4–10A). The distal left main bronchus and the left upper lobe bronchus are visible at two contiguous levels, 2 to 4 cm be-

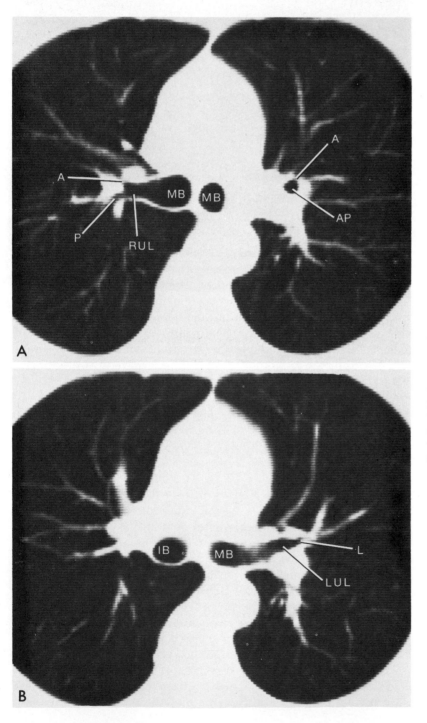

Figure 4–10. Normal proximal bronchi. Sequential CT scans 1 cm thick. **A** Scan through the tracheal carina shows both main bronchi (MB). The right upper lobe bronchus (RUL) gives origin to anterior (A) and posterior (P) segmental bronchi. The apical-posterior (A-P) and orifice of the anterior (A) segmental bronchi are demonstrated on the left. **B** Scan shows the intermediate bronchus (IB) on the right, and on the left the horizontal segment of the main bronchus (MB), the left upper lobe bronchus (LUL), and the proximal lingular bronchus (L).

Illustration continued on opposite page

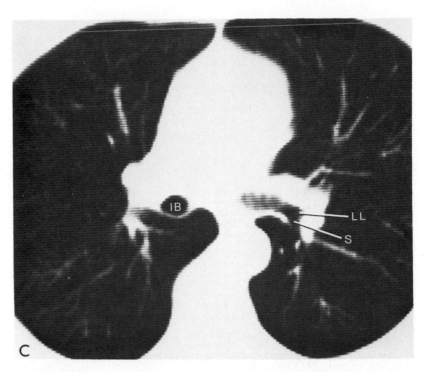

Figure 4–10. *Continued* **C** Scan still shows the intermediate bronchus (IB) on the right. On the left, the lower lobe (LL) bronchus gives origin to the superior segmental (S) bronchus.

low the tracheal carina. On the cephalad of these two scans, the posterior wall of the left upper lobe bronchus appears slightly concave where it is in contact with the descending left pulmonary artery (Fig. 4–10B). In almost 90 per cent of people, the left lung extends medial to the descending left pulmonary artery and anterior and lateral to the descending aorta.[18] This tongue of lung contacts the posterior wall of the distal left main bronchus and proximal left upper lobe bronchus and is visible on one to three successive CT scans. In the remaining patients, lung is precluded from this retrobronchial recess by a tortuous aorta or narrow anteroposterior diameter of the chest.

On the upper of the two scans through the left upper lobe bronchus, the bronchus terminates in one of two branching patterns. In 75 per cent of subjects, a single bronchus is visible coursing in a cephalad direction. This bronchus is the common trunk for the anterior segmental and apical-posterior segmental bronchi (Fig. 4–10A). In the remaining 25 per cent, the left upper lobe bronchus trifurcates into anterior, apical-posterior, and lingular bronchi.

The origin of the left lower lobe bronchus is demonstrated on the lower of the two scans through the distal left main bronchus and proximal left upper lobe bronchus (Fig. 4–10C). Frequently, a spur indicates the orifices of the left lower lobe and left upper lobe bronchi.

The anterior segmental bronchus of the left upper lobe courses in an anterior and slightly lateral direction. In most people, it has a horizontal course and is visible for 1 to 3 cm. The apical-posterior segmental bronchus is seen 1 to 2 cm above the left upper lobe bronchus, at the level of the proximal left main bronchus.

The lingular bronchus is only seen in about 60 per cent of people. It is immediately caudad to the anterior segmental bronchus and courses in an anterior, lateral, and inferior direction, obliquely to the plane of the CT scan (Fig. 4–10C). The superior and inferior segmental bronchi of the lingula are seen only occasionally on CT scans.

The left lower lobe bronchus is usually demonstrated on the same scan as the lingular bronchus. It orifice is anteromedial to the descending left pulmonary artery. The superior segmental bronchus of the left lower lobe arises from the posterior wall of the left lower lobe bronchus within 1 cm of its origin (Figs. 4–10C and 4–11A). It is not always visible on CT scans, but its posterior direction is easily recognized when present. The descending pulmonary artery is lateral and a portion of the parenchyma of the left lower lobe usually medial to the superior segmental bronchus. One to 2 cm below the origin of the superior segmental bronchus, one to three of the three basal bronchi to the left lower lobe are demonstrated in cross section. As on the right, a tributary of the

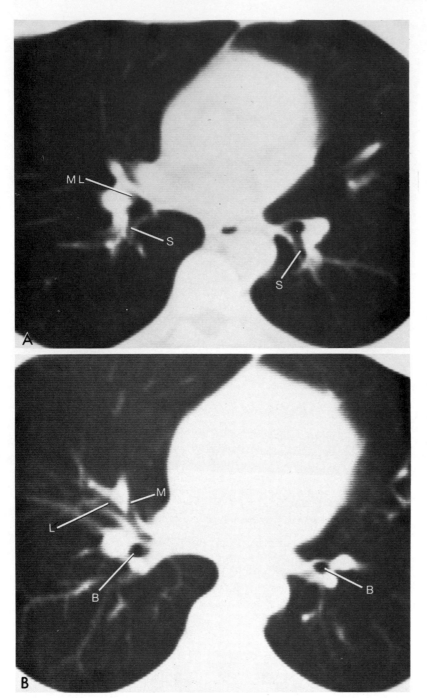

Figure 4–11. Normal middle lobe and left lower lobe bronchi. Two sequential CT scans 1 cm thick. **A** Scan shows on the right the origin of the middle lobe (ML) bronchus arising from the anterolateral wall of the intermediate bronchus. The superior segmental (S) bronchus of the right lower lobe courses posteriorly. On the left, the superior segmental (S) bronchus arises from the posterior wall of the left lower lobe bronchus. **B** Scan 1 cm caudad to scan in **A** demonstrates the lateral (L) and medial (M) segmental bronchi of the middle lobe and the basal trunk (B) of the right lower lobe. The right and left basal trunks (B) are anterior to the inferior pulmonary veins.

inferior pulmonary vein courses from lateral to medial across the back of the hilum at this level.

TECHNIQUES OF EXAMINATION

Computed tomography of the trachea and bronchi is performed in a manner similar to that of the rest of the thorax (see also Chapters 5 through 7). The patient is usually in the supine position. When the region of primary concern is the extrathoracic trachea, the patient's arms are positioned at the side, with the shoulders pulled down as far as possible. If the intrathoracic, mediastinal portion of the trachea, or the central bronchi are the region of interest, the patient's arms are usually positioned above the head to eliminate streak artifacts from the shoulder girdle and arms. A computed projection radiograph (scout view, projection view) can be obtained at the beginning of the examination to localize the area that will be scanned.

In most circumstances, CT scans of the trachea and bronchi are performed while the patient suspends respiration at full inspiration. With modern scanners, patients can suspend respiration for the time required for a single or multiple scans. A few deep breaths before scanning can aid the patient in suspending respiration for the required time. In older patients who are unable to hold their breath, scanning can be undertaken during quiet mouth breathing. Occasionally, scans during a specific respiratory maneuver can assist in the diagnosis of tracheal abnormality. For example, a Valsalva maneuver will increase intratracheal pressure and distend the extrathoracic trachea, allowing segments of abnormal tracheal compliance to be demonstrated. Forced expiratory maneuvers cause a marked reduction in the cross-sectional area of the normal trachea and central bronchi. When fast scanners are available, segments of abnormal tracheal collapse can sometimes be detected during forced expiration.

Intravenous injection or infusion of contrast medium has not been shown to directly assist in the diagnosis or characterization of tracheal or bronchial masses. Contrast medium will, however, detail the mediastinal and cervical vessels. During scanning, 125 to 150 ml of 60 to 76 per cent contrast material can be administered by slow infusion or by a series of bolus injections. A mass impinging on the trachea or a bronchus can be a large-vessel or a soft-tissue tumor. CT scans with high levels of intravascular contrast material will differentiate between the two. High levels of contrast can be achieved by rapid intravascular injection of a 25- to 30-ml bolus of contrast material during a series of rapid sequential scans (dynamic scanning). Scanning may be carried out at a single level or, when the scanner table can be incremented with a short interscan delay, multiple levels through the abnormality can be scanned.

CT scans of the trachea and bronchi are viewed at several window levels and widths on the scanner console. Narrowing of the trachea and bronchi is best detected at a window level of -250 to -500 Hounsfield Units (H) and a window width of 500 or 1000 H. At these settings, normal and abnormal airways will have a smaller caliber than at mediastinal window settings. The most precise monitor settings for measurement of the airways is a window level midway between the air in the airway and the soft tissue around the airway (approximately -600 H), and a narrow window width. The hilar contours are viewed at window settings usually used for the lung fields (level -500 H, width 1000 H). Masses within the trachea or invading the tracheal wall are viewed at window settings normally used for the mediastinum (level 0 to 60 H, width 150 to 300 H).

In most instances, CT scans of the trachea and bronchi are obtained at 1-cm intervals using scans 1 cm thick. These scans are usually sufficient to demonstrate abnormalities of this area of the respiratory system. When uncertainty exists as to the presence of an abnormality, additional scans of 0.5 cm should be obtained through the area. The greater spatial resolution can improve the demonstration, especially of endobronchial masses.

PATHOLOGY

GENERALIZED TRACHEAL ABNORMALITIES

Increased Tracheal Caliber

TRACHEOBRONCHOMEGALY (TRACHIECTASIS, MOU-NIER-KUHN SYNDROME). This is a distinctive condition consisting of marked dilation of the trachea and central bronchi, in association with chronic respiratory tract infections.[19, 20] The clinical features are ineffective chronic cough and recurrent bronchitis or pneumonia. Tracheobronchomegaly probably results from a congenital defect of the elastic and muscle fibers within the tracheal and bronchial walls. Typically, the trachea and central bronchi are involved, but occasionally bronchial involvement alone is found. Studies of pedigrees suggest a genetic disease, and an association with the Ehlers-Danlos syndrome has been described.[21]

Radiographically, the condition is characterized by a greatly increased tracheal caliber, which measures 35 to 50 mm or more in diameter.[20] The tracheal air column has an irregular, corrugated appearance caused by the protrusion of redundant mucosa between the cartilaginous rings. CT scans show the enlarged trachea and central bronchi. Detection of concomitant lung disease is possible. Bronchiectasis, bronchiolectasis, bullous emphysema, diffuse emphysema, chronic bronchitis, and pulmonary fibrosis can all be present and sometimes evident on CT scans of the thorax.

TRACHEOBRONCHOMALACIA. Described by Williams and Campbell,[22] this condition is characterized by a deficiency of cartilage in the tracheobronchial tree. It is a developmental defect and can be associated with other congenital anomalies such as cleft palate and laryngomalacia. As with tracheobronchomegaly, there is excessive flaccidity of the tracheal wall and recurrent pneumonia and bronchietasis. The trachea and central bronchi are dilated on radiographs during inspiration and collapse with expiration. The CT findings should be similar to those of tracheobronchomegaly, although tracheobronchomalacia is a more severe condition and most patients die from respiratory failure in childhood.

Decreased Tracheal Caliber

Diffuse narrowing of the trachea is uncommon and usually due to a specific cause. Symptoms are often nonspecific, consisting of dyspnea, cough, wheezing, and sometimes hoarseness, or stridor. Five entities should be considered when dealing with diffuse tracheal narrowing: saber-sheath trachea, amyloidosis, relapsing polychondritis, tracheobronchopathia osteochondroplastica, and scleroma.

SABER-SHEATH TRACHEA. In some patients with chronic obstructive pulmonary disease, the intrathoracic trachea has a "saber-sheath" configuration.[23, 24] The coronal dimension is narrow and is less than two thirds of the sagittal diameter at the same level (Fig. 4–12A). In one study, 95 per cent of patients with a saber-sheath trachea had clinical evidence of chronic obstructive lung disease, 100 per cent had a history of smoking, and 80 per cent had symptoms of chronic bronchitis.[23] The cause of a saber-sheath trachea is unknown.

Chest radiographs show the abnormal configuration of the trachea, and the tracheal wall may appear thickened. CT scans do not demonstrate abnormal soft tissue within the tracheal lumen or thickening of the tracheal wall.[2] On CT scans, the tracheal cartilages are usually densely calcified. The coronal narrowing of the intrathoracic trachea is due to an abnormal configuration of the tracheal cartilages, which have a narrow anterior arch. CT scans during forced expiration have shown that the intrathoracic trachea narrows abnormally.[2] Instead of the posterior tracheal membrane invaginating to reduce the lumen of the trachea, as in normal subjects, the lateral walls of the trachea collapse inward (Fig. 4–12B).

AMYLOIDOSIS. Deposition of the protein-polysaccharide complex known as amyloid within the respiratory system can occur in both the primary and secondary forms of the disease.[25, 26] Deposition can involve the lungs, resulting in pulmonary nodules, or it can be limited to the trachea and bronchi. In the latter form, amyloid is in the sub-

mucosal and muscular layers of the airway wall. Irregular, lardlike masses encroach on the tracheal lumen and produce focal or diffuse narrowing of the airway. Mediastinal and hilar lymphadenopathy can be present. The airway narrowing can be seen on conventional chest radiographs, conventional tomograms, or CT scans (Fig. 4–13). CT scans will show thickening of the tracheal wall. Diagnosis is usually made by bronchoscopy and biopsy of the tracheal or central bronchial masses.

RELAPSING POLYCHONDRITIS. Relapsing polychondritis is an unusual systemic disease that affects cartilage at many sites throughout the body, including the ears, nose, joints, and tracheobronchial tree.[27, 28] Cartilage is destroyed and replaced by fibrous tissue. Respiratory distress is common and death from respiratory failure can occur.[28] The cause of relapsing polychondritis is unknown. The cartilage destruction appears to be mediated by lysosomal enzymes that destroy connective tissue and release chondroitin sulfate from the cartilage matrix.[29] Anticartilage antibodies have been found in some patients.[28, 29]

The diagnosis can be suspected from recurrent episodes of inflammation of cartilage, most commonly of the nose and ear. Deafness and arthritis are frequently present. Radiographs and CT scans usually show generalized, fixed narrowing of the trachea and bronchi. Flaccidity of the airway has been described in one case.[30]

TRACHEOBRONCHOPATHIA OSTEOCHONDROPLASTICA. Occurring almost exclusively in older men, tracheobronchopathia osteochondroplastica is a degenerative disease characterized by the formation of nodules of bone and cartilage within the submucosa of the trachea and bronchi.[31–33] These nodules produce sessile and polypoid masses that narrow the tracheal and central bronchial lumen irregularly.[31] The airways appear beaded on tomography and on positive contrast studies. On conventional tomograms and CT scans, plaques and calcifications are frequently seen in the anterior and lateral walls of the trachea (Figs. 4–14A,B). The lesions are confined to parts of the trachea and bronchi that normally contain cartilage; the posterior tracheal membrane is spared. More peripheral lesions can cause obstruction of segmental and lobar bronchi, giving rise to atelectasis and obstructive pneumonitis.[32]

The condition may not be suspected during life and the diagnosis may only be made at necropsy.[34] The beaded appearance seen at bronchoscopy is typical and the diagnosis readily confirmed.[33]

SCLEROMA. Scleroma is a specific chronic granulomatous condition caused by a strain of the

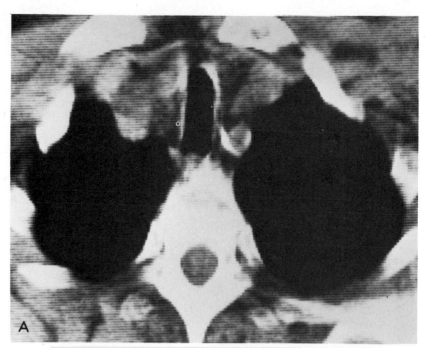

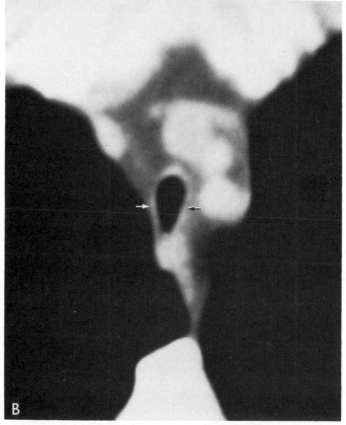

Figure 4–12. Saber-sheath trachea. **A** CT scan shows the typical configuration of a saber-sheath trachea. The anteroposterior dimension is increased and the lateral dimension decreased. The anterior arch is excessively narrow. **B** Scan during forced expiration in a different patient with a saber-sheath trachea shows abnormal inward collapse of the lateral walls of the trachea (arrows).

Friedlander's bacillus *(Bacillus rhinoscleromatis)*.[35] It is endemic in parts of Eastern Europe, Russia, South America, and Asia and is being seen with increasing frequency in North America. The nose is the main site of infection, but the larynx, trachea, and bronchi can be involved. Continuity be-

tween the nasal granulomas and the airway may or may not be evident. The age distribution is from childhood to old age. Symptoms include nasal obstruction, hoarseness, dyspnea, and cough.

The trachea is not involved unless laryngoscleroma is present.[35] Subglottic stenosis is the most

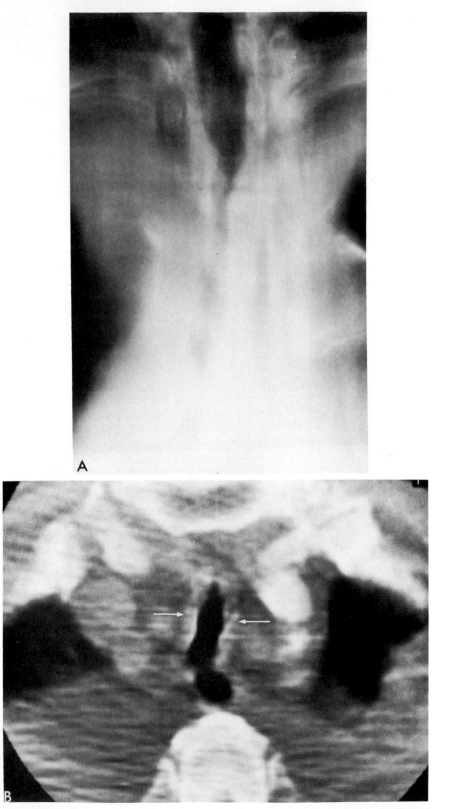

Figure 4–13. Amyloid of the trachea. **A**   Conventional tomogram demonstrates diffuse, irregular narrowing of the trachea air column. **B**   CT scan through the upper intrathoracic trachea shows irregular thickening of the tracheal wall.

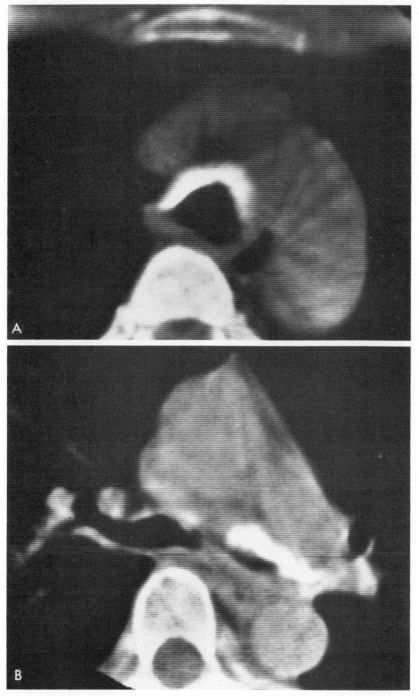

Figure 4–14. Tracheobronchopathia osteochondroplastica. **A**   CT scan through the midtrachea shows dense calcification of the tracheal cartilage. The tracheal lumen is near normal in caliber. **B**   CT scan at the level of the tracheal carina demonstrates dense, irregular calcification of the main bronchi. The left main bronchus is distorted and narrowed.

common tracheal abnormality. Diffuse, uniform tracheal narrowing from mucosal thickening or multiple masses can also be seen.

LOCALIZED TRACHEAL ABNORMALITIES

Neoplasms

Localized lesions of the trachea can be primary benign or malignant neoplasms, inflammatory masses, pseudotumors caused by a variety of conditions, secondary invasion from malignant neoplasms arising in adjacent organs, or metastatic deposits (Table 4–1). Extrinsic compression of the trachea can also present clinically and radiographically as a tracheal mass. Tracheal stenosis and granulomas after intubation, instrumentation, or tracheal injury can also appear to be masslike lesions of the trachea.

The symptoms of focal tracheal lesions are frequently nonspecific and mimic a variety of pulmonary diseases. Most symptoms related to airway obstruction. Many patients are treated for asthma or chronic bronchitis before the possibility of a focal tracheal lesion is suspected.

BENIGN NEOPLASMS.   These constitute a minority of benign tracheal masses. Inflammatory, post-traumatic, and infiltrative lesions are all more common. Most benign tracheal neoplasms are found in the pediatric age group; squamous cell papilloma, fibroma, and hemangioma are the most common.[36, 37] In adults, the most common benign tumors are chondroma, papilloma, fibroma, hemangioma, and granular cell myoblastoma.[37]

Chondromas of the trachea are rare neoplasms.[38–41] In one report, three chondromas were found among 84 primary and secondary neoplasms of the trachea.[42] The tumor appears at bronchoscopy as a smooth, well-circumscribed, hard mass covered by normal epithelium. Chondromas tend to recur if inadequately excised.

Squamous cell papillomas are sessile or papillary nodular masses, limited to the tracheal mucosa. They can be single or multiple. Multiple papillomas of the trachea can be from the spread of laryngeal papillomatosis. Recurrence is frequent, and repeated surgical excisions may be necessary.

Fibromas of the trachea occur as a mixture of fibrous tissue with other tissue elements to produce fibroadenomas, neurofibromas, myxofibromas, and chondrofibromas. None of these shows specific characteristics.

Table 4–1.   CAUSES OF A TRACHEAL MASS

Inflammatory granuloma	Post-traumatic Tuberculosis Fungus Wegener's granulomatosis Scleroma Laryngeal papillomatosis
Benign neoplasms	Chondroma, hamartoma Squamous cell papilloma Fibroma Hemangioma Granular cell myoblastoma Leiomyoma Others (neurilemoma, lipoma, fibrous histiocytoma, benign mixed tumors)
Malignant neoplasms	Squamous cell carcinoma Adenoid cystic carcinoma (cylindroma) Adenocarcinoma Sarcoma Carcinoid Other (pseudosarcoma, oat cell carcinoma, lymphoma, plasmacytoma, melanoma, hemangioendothelioma)
Invasion from adjacent neoplasm	Thyroid Lung Esophagus
Metastasis from distant site	Breast Colon Genitourinary Melanoma
Extrinsic compression	Neoplasm Aneurysm Vascular ring
Idiopathic	Goiter Amyloid Tracheopathia osteochondroplastica

Other benign neoplasms and non-neoplastic masses can occur in the trachea (Table 4–1). They are usually well defined and sessile or pedunculated. They do not invade deeply into the tracheal wall. Their diagnosis is based on histologic characteristics from biopsy specimens or from the excised tumor.

Most benign neoplasms are evident on well-penetrated chest radiographs or conventional tomograms at the time they are suspected clinically. Benign lesions are usually less than 2 cm in size and are well circumscribed.[42] They will invariably project into the lumen of the trachea. Malignant tracheal neoplasms can have similar radiographic features and be indistinguishable from benign tumors. Calcification is frequently visible in cartilaginous tumors, such as chondroma and hamartoma. CT scans may be obtained in patients with suspected tracheal neoplasms to detect invasion of the tumor through the tracheal wall.[2] CT scans demonstrate the superficial intratracheal site of a benign tracheal neoplasm and can accurately localize the position and extent of the lesion. The tracheal wall is visible on CT scans and the tumor should be clearly seen limited by the tracheal cartilages. CT scans are more sensitive than conventional tomograms in detecting calcification within lung and mediastinal masses. Calcification within benign tracheal tumors, such as chondromas, should be readily visible on CT scans. CT scans can also assess the severity of airway narrowing by a mass and the cross-sectional area of the airway can be measured.

PRIMARY MALIGNANT NEOPLASMS. These are uncommon, accounting for less than 0.1 per cent of malignancies.[43, 44] Malignant tumors of laryngeal and bronchial origin are, respectively, at least 75 and 180 times more common.[42] In adults, primary malignant tumors of the trachea are slightly more common than benign tumors. Carcinomas account for 80 to 90 per cent of tracheal malignancies.[37, 43] Squamous cell carcinoma derived from tracheal epithelium is the most frequent, and adenoid cystic carcinoma (cylindroma) arising from mucous glands in the tracheal wall is next in frequency. In a study by Houston and colleagues,[43] 51 per cent of malignant tracheal neoplasms were squamous cell carcinoma and 40 per cent adenoid cystic carcinoma. Sarcoma, lymphoma, plasmacytoma, adenocarcinoma, chondrosarcoma, malignant carcinoid, and oat cell carcinoma have all been reported but are rare tumors.

The most common location for tracheal neoplasms is the lower third of the trachea, 35 to 44 per cent arising in this location.[37, 43, 45, 46] Squamous cell carcinoma is particularly common in the distal trachea, over half arising within 3 to 4 cm of the tracheal carina. The extrathoracic, proximal trachea is the next most frequent site for squamous cell carcinoma and the most common site for other malignant tumors.

The symptoms of tracheal malignancies are frequently nonspecific, leading to a delay in diagnosis that averages 10 months.[46] Up to 75 per cent of the area of the trachea must be obstructed before symptoms of obstruction occur. Cough occurs in 33 to 85 per cent of patients, hemoptysis in 27 to 66 per cent and dyspnea in 20 to 75 per cent.[43, 45, 46] Weight loss and dysphagia are late symptoms. Proximal tracheal tumors can interfere with vocal cord function or cause recurrent laryngeal nerve paralysis, both resulting in hoarseness. Distal tracheal tumors can prolapse into a main bronchus and produce symptoms of bronchial obstruction.[37]

Pulmonary function studies are useful in localizing airway obstruction above the tracheal carina.[47] In particular, the shape of the flow:volume loop can show the presence of tracheal narrowing from a tracheal neoplasm (Fig. 4–15). In the absence of peripheral obstruction from emphysema or chronic bronchitis, the flow:volume loop is sensitive in detecting tracheal stenosis when the airway is reduced to less than 6 to 8 mm in diameter.

Chest radiographs are of limited value in detecting tracheal tumors.[46, 48, 49] Karlan and colleagues[46] found that in only 4 of 11 patients with tracheal tumors was the chest radiograph prospectively interpreted as abnormal. Penetration of the mediastinum on most chest radiographs is insufficient to allow adequate visualization of the tracheal lumen. Oblique views of the chest wall project the tracheal air column away from the spine and are often helpful in visualizing suspected endotracheal masses (Fig. 4–15B). Coned-down radiographs of the thoracic inlet and of the soft tissues of the neck can also assist in demonstrating a tracheal tumor.

Conventional tomography in anteroposterior or lateral projection is the most valuable standard radiographic technique for detecting and localizing tracheal masses (Fig. 4–15C).[46, 49, 50] In a series by Houston and co-workers,[43] conventional tracheal tomography was of diagnostic assistance in 16 of 18 cases of tracheal neoplasms. In 13 of 16 patients with an abnormal tracheogram, the chest radiograph had been considered normal.

Tracheograms using iodinated oil, barium suspension, or tantalum as the contrast medium can demonstrate an endotracheal mass and its site of origin.[51–53] The dynamic relationship of the mass to the airway can aid in explaining the symptoms of tracheal stenosis. The configuration of the area of narrowing will usually differentiate neoplasms from benign structures. Tracheography, however, cannot define extratracheal extension of a tumor.[2] Tracheography is also potentially hazardous and deaths have been reported from this procedure.[49]

Malignant tracheal tumors appear on CT scans as a mass of soft-tissue CT density within the tracheal wall. The posterior and lateral walls of the

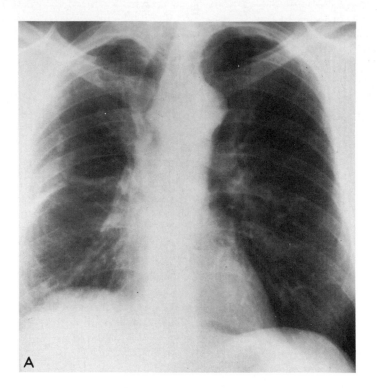

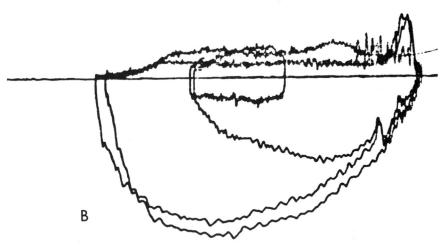

Figure 4–15. Primary adenocarcinoma of the trachea. **A**   Frontal chest radiograph shows a mass projection into the intrathoracic tracheal air column. **B**   Flow:volume loop with flow on the vertical axis and volume of the horizontal axis demonstrates marked limitation of expiratory flow with a plateau on the expiratory curve.

Illustration continued on opposite page

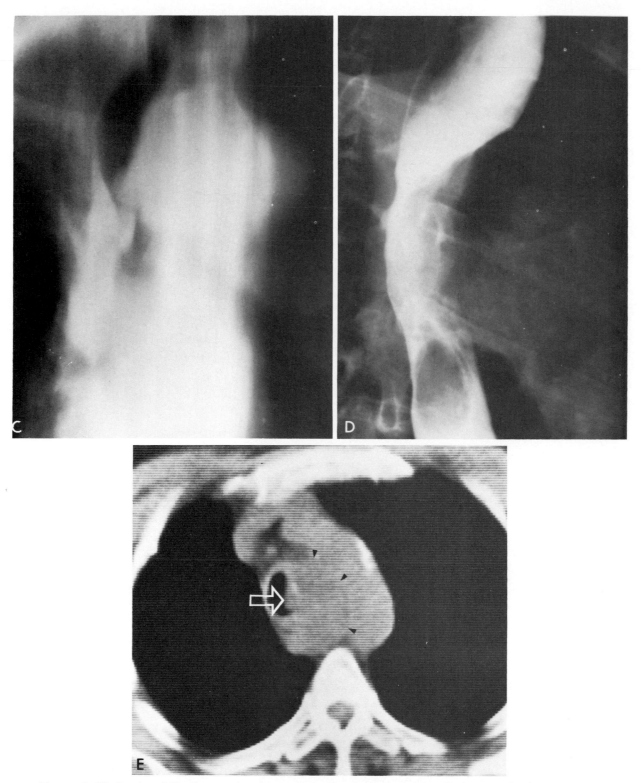

Figure 4–15. *Continued* **C**   Conventional tomogram clearly demonstrates the intratracheal tumor. The mediastinal contour suggests an extratracheal component to the mass. **D**   Esophagram shows extrinsic compression of the esophagus, confirming an extratracheal mass. **E**   CT scan most accurately demonstrates the mass (open arrow) within a tracheal cartilage and the mediastinal extension (arrowheads) of the carcinoma.

trachea are the most frequent sites for tracheal tumors to arise. Tumors are most often sessile and eccentric, producing an asymmetric narrowing of the tracheal lumen (Figs. 4–16A–C). They can, however, be polypoid and entirely intraluminal.[43, 47, 49] Approximately 10 per cent of malignant tracheal neoplasms are circumferential, a finding that is not seen with benign tumors.[43] Malignant tracheal tumors extend directly into the mediastinum in 30 to 40 per cent of patients.[45, 46] In some patients, a mediastinal mass can be seen on chest radiographs or conventional tomograms. CT is, however, more accurate than other imaging modalities in demonstrating the extent of mediastinal invasion of tracheal neoplasms.[2, 53a] CT scans can show extension through the tracheal wall as well as encasement of mediastinal structures. Benign tumors rarely show extension through the tracheal wall into the mediastinum.

SECONDARY MALIGNANT NEOPLASMS. Mediastinal masses commonly compress the trachea without invading the tracheal wall. These masses

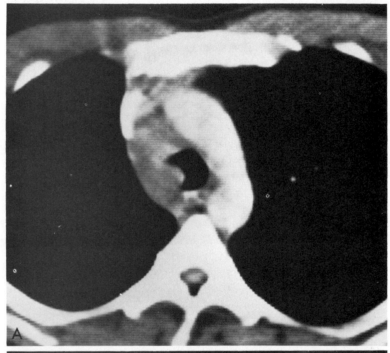

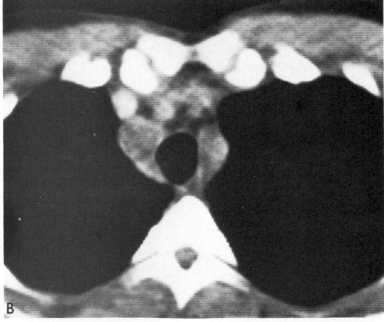

Figure 4–16. Carcinoid of the trachea. **A** CT scan shows an intratracheal tumor on the right with mediastinal extension causing widening of the right paratracheal stripe. **B** CT scan, 2 cm cephalad to the scan in **A,** demonstrates superior extratracheal extension of tumor.

Illustration continued on opposite page

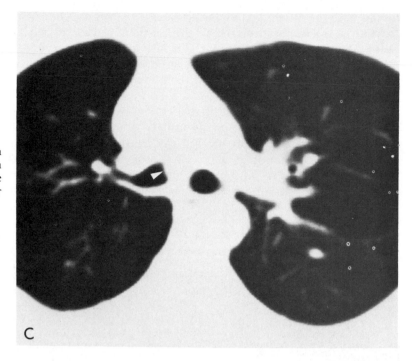

Figure 4–16. *Continued* **C**   CT scan through the tracheal carina shows an impression (arrowhead) on the medial wall of the right main bronchus, indicating inferior extension of the carcinoid tumor.

produce a smooth, concentric, impression on the tracheal lumen and frequently displace the trachea toward the contralateral side. CT scans can usually demonstrate the cause of tracheal compression. The most common cause is a dilated innominate artery or aortic arch. A goiter in the neck or superior mediastinum is also a frequent cause (Fig. 4–17). CT scans after infusion of contrast material will show enhancement of a dilated vessel. Most goiters demonstrate marked and pro-

longed enhancement after infusion of contrast material.[54]

Malignant neoplasms can either directly invade the trachea or, less commonly, metastasize to the tracheal mucosa. Carcinoma arising in the thyroid gland, esophagus, larynx, and lung is responsible for most cases of invasion of the trachea.[2, 42, 55, 56] CT scans show asymmetric tracheal narrowing and a soft-tissue mass within the tracheal cartilages. An adjacent mediastinal mass is usually

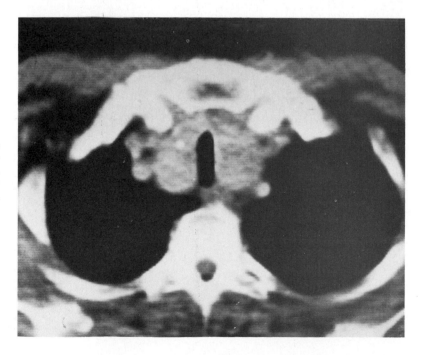

Figure 4–17. Tracheal compression by a goiter. CT scan through the upper mediastinum shows mediastinal extension of a goiter encasing and compressing the trachea. Calcification is demonstrated on the right in the goiter.

demonstrated. When a mediastinal mass is not apparent, a secondary tumor of the trachea can mimic a primary tracheal tumor. The CT appearance of an intraluminal mass is not specific for tumor invasion, and endoscopy with biopsy is required for diagnosis.

Subglottic extension of laryngeal carcinoma to the proximal trachea is most accurately demonstrated on CT scans.[57] The level of the true vocal cords is readily identified and a soft-tissue mass extending below the inferior margin of the cricoid cartilage indicates proximal tracheal extension of the neoplasm (Fig. 4–18). Carcinoma of

the larynx can also involve the tracheal stoma and adjacent tracheal wall in patients who have had a laryngectomy.[58] CT can assist in defining stoma recurrence of a laryngeal carcinoma by demonstrating the extent of the tumor within the tracheal wall and of the mass around the trachea. The severity of tracheal narrowing can also be assessed from CT scans.

Esophageal neoplasms that arise in the upper third of the esophagus can encase and invade the trachea. CT scans can show encasement of the trachea and direct extension of the tumor through the tracheal wall (Fig. 4–19).[56, 59] Esophageal car-

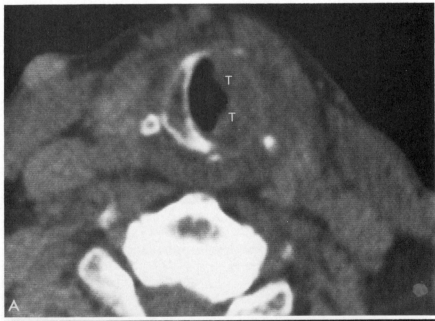

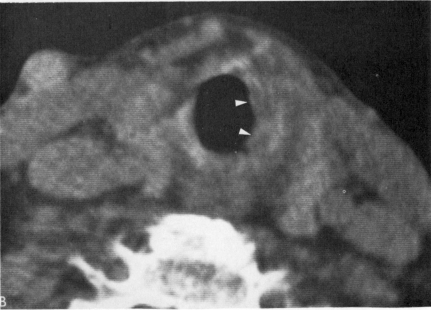

Figure 4–18. Tracheal extension of laryngeal carcinoma. **A** CT scan through the subglottic larynx shows extensive tumor (T) destroying the left half of the cricoid cartilage. **B** CT scan, 15 mm caudad to the scan in **A** demonstrates tumor on the right growing into the proximal trachea (arrowheads) (confirmed at laryngectomy).

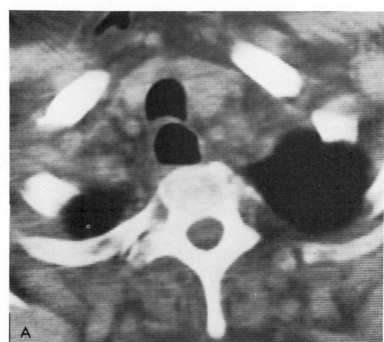

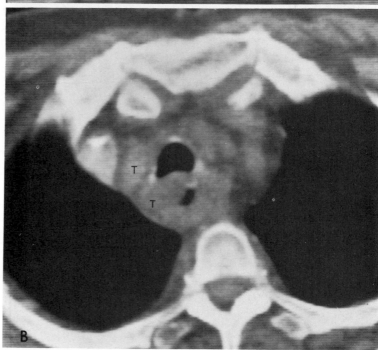

Figure 4–19. Esophageal carcinoma extending around trachea. **A** CT scan at the thoracic inlet shows a normal trachea and an air-filled, distended esophagus. **B** CT scans, 3 cm caudad to scan in **A,** shows esophageal tumor (T) extending around the right side of the trachea.

cinoma can, however, invaginate the unsupported posterior tracheal membrane without extending through the tracheal wall (Fig. 4–20). Blurring of the margins between the esophagus and trachea has been described as a sensitive and easily apparent CT finding, indicating tracheal invasion by esophageal carcinoma.[56, 59] A plane of separation between the esophagus and trachea, however, is not always visible on CT scans, and invasion of tumor into the outer layers of the tracheal wall probably cannot be determined with CT.

Hematogenous metastases to the tracheal mucosa are rare. They are most commonly from breast carcinoma, melanoma, and genitourinary tract malignancies. CT scans will show a polypoid mass within the tracheal wall (Fig. 4–21). Extensive metastasis can simulate a primary tracheal tumor (Fig. 4–22).

Strictures

Intubation or tracheostomy for assisted ventilation is being used with increasing frequency but

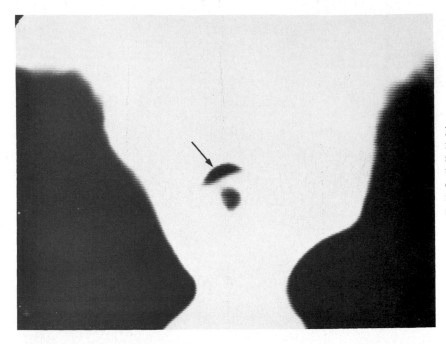

Figure 4–20. Esophageal cancer mimicking tracheal stenosis. CT scan shows marked narrowing of the trachea (arrow). The esophageal cancer is invaginating the posterior tracheal membrane. (Bronchoscopy showed no tumor in the trachea.)

can result in damage to the tracheal wall.[60–62] Neck trauma is also a common cause of tracheal injury. The trachea can become scarred, resulting in a segment of fixed stenosis. Alternatively, a tracheal segment can become flaccid (tracheomalacia). Advances in tracheal surgery have made resection of long tracheal segments possible.[63–65] Imaging studies of the injured trachea not only must detect the site of abnormality, but also must precisely determine the severity and length of the stenosis and the compliance of the airway. CT scans can demonstrate the site of narrowing in most patients with fixed tracheal stenosis.[2] It can also differentiate granulation and scar tissue within the tracheal cartilages (Fig. 4–23) from collapse of the tracheal cartilages (Figs. 4–24 and 4–25).

In patients with tracheal webs or short segments of stenosis, CT scans may not show the airway narrowing. Presumably, the soft tissue of the stenosis is obscured by volume averaging with air in the tracheal lumen. CT scans obtained in recumbent patients tend to overestimate the severity of stenosis when compared with tracheograms.

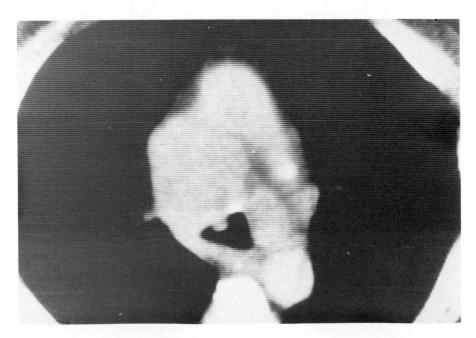

Figure 4–21. Unsuspected tracheal metastasis from bronchogenic carcinoma. CT scan immediately above the tracheal carina shows an unsuspected endotracheal metastasis. Nodal tumor masses are also present anterior and to the left of the trachea.

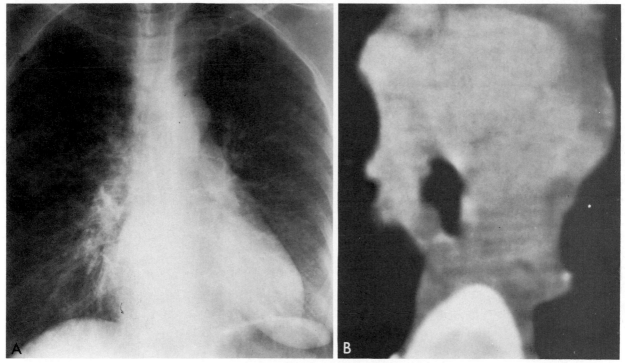

Figure 4–22. Metastasis to the trachea from breast carcinoma. **A** Frontal chest radiograph shows thickening of the walls of the mediastinal trachea. A right mastectomy is evident. **B** CT scan demonstrates irregular circumferential narrowing of the trachea by tumor. The right wall of the trachea is thickened. (Tumor confirmed by bronchoscopy and biopsy.)

CT scans cannot evaluate the tracheal mucosa, and the length of trachea resected is usually longer than the abnormality detected on CT scans. CT scans obtained during suspended respiration cannot demonstrate segments of tracheomalacia. CT scans obtained during forced expiration using high-spatial-resolution, fast scanners may, in the future, be capable of detecting tracheomalacia. At present, conventional tomography and tracheography appear to be better than CT scanning for assessing tracheal stenosis from tracheal injury.

LOCALIZED BRONCHIAL ABNORMALITIES

Focal lesions of the central bronchi (tracheal carina to segmental bronchi) cover a broad spectrum of diseases. Tumors, however, are far more common in the central bronchi than in the trachea. Bronchogenic carcinoma accounts for more than 90 per cent of neoplasms, and benign tumors of the central bronchi are uncommon.[66, 67] In one series, covering a 10-year period, 11,626 bronchoscopies were performed and 2000 bronchogenic carcinomas discovered, whereas only 11 benign neoplasms were found.[68] Nonneoplastic

benign masses in the central bronchi are equally uncommon.

Inflammatory Strictures and Granulomas

Bronchial disease is common in both primary and reinfection tuberculosis. In primary tuberculosis, bronchial narrowing is usually the result of compression of bronchi by enlarged lymph nodes.[69, 70] Tuberculous granulation tissue of the bronchial mucosa is uncommon.

Occasionally, infection in a lymph node will erode the bronchial wall, causing stenosis or occlusion of the bronchus.[69, 71] The bronchi of the anterior segment of an upper lobe or the medial segment of the middle lobe are most commonly involved. In reinfection tuberculosis, endobronchial involvement results in mucosal ulcerations, scarring, and bronchostenosis. Bronchial disease is frequent within the bronchi subtending a tuberculous cavity or focal area of caseation. The diagnosis of endobronchial tuberculosis is usually made by bronchoscopy and biopsy of the abnormal mucosa. CT scans can localize areas of bronchial wall thickening and stenosis before bronchoscopy.

Bronchostenosis is rare or absent in most

Text continued on page 178

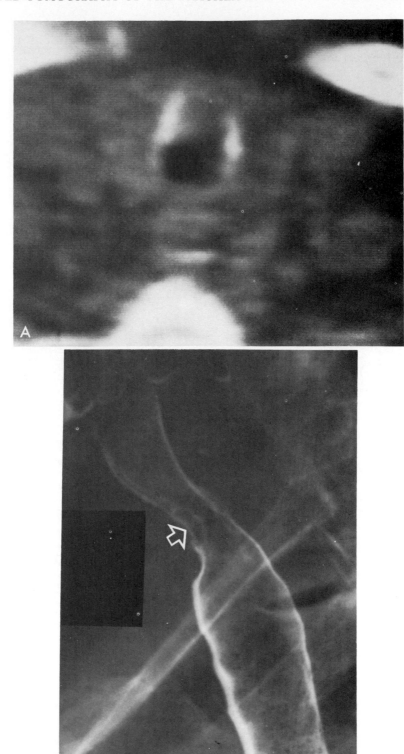

Figure 4–23. Tracheal stenosis from previous tracheostomy. **A**   CT scan through the stenotic segment shows soft tissue anteriorly within the tracheal cartilage. The tracheal lumen at the stenosis is 4.9×6.0 mm in diameter. The length of stenosis as determined from sequential CT scans, was 2 cm. **B**   Oblique view from tracheogram shows tracheal stenosis with heaped-up granulation tissue anteriorly (arrow). The minimum diameter of the stenosis is 4.5×5.5 mm. The abnormal segment is 3.5 to 4.0 cm long. (At surgery, 4 cm of trachea was resected.) (From Gamsu G, Webb WR: Computed tomography of the trachea: Normal and abnormal. AJR 139:321–326, 1982. © American Roentgen Ray Society. Used with permission.)

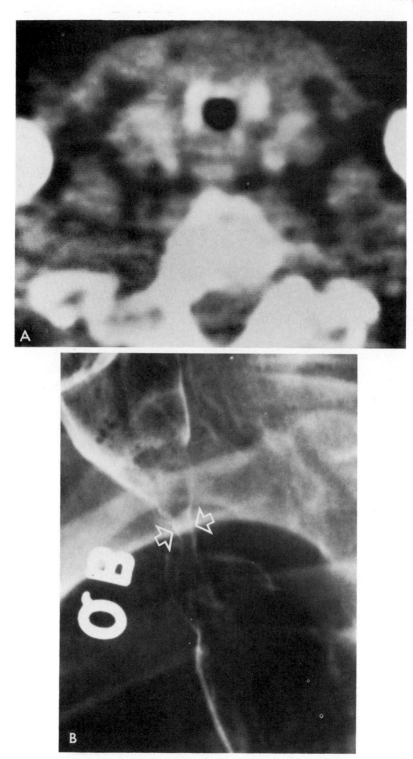

Figure 4–24. Tracheal stenosis from previous tracheostomy. **A** CT scan through site of stenosis demonstrates collapse of the tracheal cartilage around the stenosis. The stenosis is 2.8 mm in diameter. (From Gamsu G, Webb WR: Computed tomography of the trachea: Normal and abnormal. AJR 139:321–326, 1982. © American Roentgen Ray Society. Used with permission.) **B** Oblique view from tracheogram shows the severe circumferential stenosis. The narrowest diameter of the stenosis (arrows) is 4.5 mm.

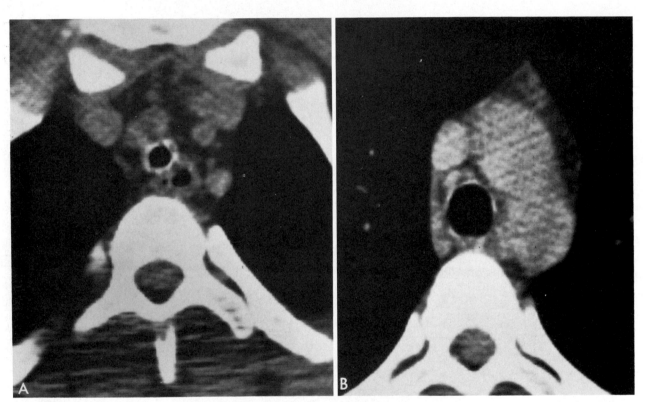

Figure 4–25. Tracheal stenosis after prolonged intubation. **A** CT scan through the stenosis shows collapse of a tracheal cartilage around the stenosed trachea. (Significance of tracheal cartilage extending circumferentially is unknown.) **B** CT scan, 4 cm caudad to the scan in **A,** shows the normal tracheal size for comparison.

Illustration continued on opposite page

Figure 4–25. *Continued* **C** CT scan is a magnified view of the scan in **A** and demonstrates the cursor method for measuring tracheal diameter. The lumen measures 6.9 mm (at this window level, −16 H, the luminal diameter is overestimated). **D** Reformatted sagittal image shows the site and length of stenosis but does not augment the transverse axial scans. (Courtesy of Dr. Edward Baker, San Francisco, Cal.)

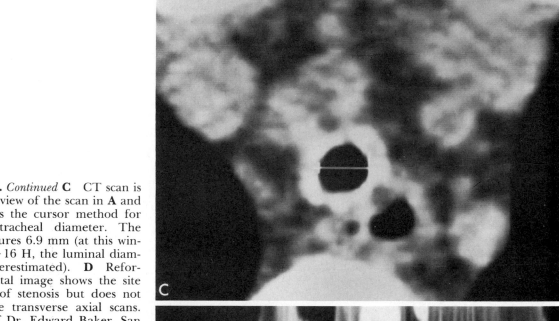
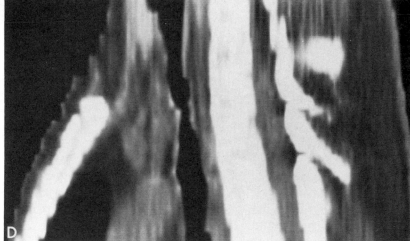

mycotic granulomatous diseases such as histoplasmosis, coccidioidiomycosis, or blastomycosis. Central bronchial obstruction occurs uncommonly in cryptococcosis. When present, the radiographic appearances are frequently mistaken for bronchogenic carcinoma.[72, 73] The CT findings have not been described but presumably will also mimic those of a lung carcinoma. Sarcoidosis does cause bronchostenosis in the advanced stages of the disease.[74–76] One or more segmental or lobar bronchi can be involved. CT can be used in these circumstances to localize areas of narrowing before bronchoscopy and biopsy.

The CT findings of inflammatory strictures of the bronchi have not been described. In our experience, sites of airway narrowing as far distal as the segmental bronchi can be detected as easily with CT as with conventional tomography. However, bronchial wall thickening, mediastinal and hilar adenopathy, and unsuspected parenchymal disease that are not apparent from conventional tomograms can all be seen on CT scans.

Bronchiectasis

Bronchiectasis is a permanent abnormal dilatation of bronchi resulting from destruction of the elastic and muscular components of the bronchial wall. The most common form of bronchiectasis results from necrotizing bacterial infections in childhood.[77] Antibiotics and vaccines have markedly decreased the incidence of bronchiectasis in the developed countries. The condition, however, does remain a major problem in less developed regions of the world. Congenital forms of bronchiectasis exist, although they are uncommon.

Congenital anomalies of the bronchi, such as bronchomalacia, are frequently associated with bronchiectasis. About 20 per cent of patients with dextrocardia have associated bronchiectasis (Kartagener's syndrome). This syndrome is one variety of a genetically determined group of disorders known as the immotile-cilia syndrome.[78] Other hereditary or familial conditions such as cystic fibrosis have a breakdown in local defense mechanisms of the lung.[79] Deficiency in systemic defense mechanisms such as immunodeficiency states and allergic conditions such as bronchopulmonary aspergillosis can also be complicated by bronchiectasis.

The majority of patients with bronchiectasis have an abnormal chest radiograph.[80, 81] The usual radiographic findings reflect the pathologic changes. Bronchi are increased in size and their walls more prominent than normal. The vessels in the involved areas of the lung appear ill-defined and are crowded together, reflecting volume loss of the affected lung segments. Cystic spaces, sometimes containing fluid levels, are indicative of advanced disease.

Bronchography is the only commonly used method for establishing the diagnosis and determining the extent of bronchiectasis. Bronchography is now performed only before surgery to determine the distribution of lung segments involved with bronchiectasis.

Naidich and colleagues[82] described the CT findings in six cases of bronchiectasis. In all patients, CT scans revealed abnormalities indicative of the disease. In patients with cylindrical or varicose bronchiectasis, the normally invisible intraparenchymal bronchi are thick-walled and dilated. In patients with cystic bronchiectasis, the characteristic CT findings are thick-walled cystic spaces, which are either grouped together in a cluster or strung together in a linear fashion (Fig. 4–26). Fluid levels within the cysts are readily demonstrated on CT scans. When segmental or lobar collapse accompanies bronchiectasis, the crowded dilated bronchi are seen against a background of increased CT density.

The dilated bronchi of bronchiectasis are easily differentiated from bullae and blebs.[82] Bullae and blebs are thin-walled and peripheral and are not accompanied by branches of the pulmonary artery.

Bronchial Adenoma and Benign Tumors

The most frequent benign tumors of the large central bronchi are bronchial adenomas, lipomas, fibromas, and hamartomas.[36, 83] Granular cell myoblastoma, leiomyoma, chondroma, neurogenic tumors, papilloma, and bronchogenic cysts also can occur within or adjacent to the central bronchi.[36, 68, 83, 84]

BRONCHIAL ADENOMAS. These are uncommon, constituting only 0.6 to 1.2 per cent of tracheobronchial neoplasms.[85–87] Over 85 per cent of adenomas arising within the bronchial tree are of the carcinoid variety of adenoma.[86–88] Cylindromas (adenoid cystic carcinomas) make up only 6 to 12 per cent of bronchial adenomas, but account for 95 per cent of tracheal adenomas.[86–89] Carcinoid tumors are low-grade carcinomas and frequently locally invasive. They can metastasize to regional lymph nodes and to distant sites. Most arise in the central bronchi and are visible on CT scans (Fig. 4–27). Bronchial obstruction is the most common presentation and CT scans will reveal atelectasis and consolidation in the subtended segment or lobe. Recurrent episodes of infection can lead to bronchietasis or lung abscess. The obstructing mass as well as the commonly present extension of the tumor beyond the bronchial wall can be visible on CT scans.[53a] Enlargement of regional lymph nodes can be from metastatic tumor or reactive hyperplasia of the nodes from concomitant infection (Fig. 4–27D,E). Partial bronchial obstruction can result in obstructed emphysema, which will be evident on CT scans as an area of decreased CT density peripheral to the tumor.

CHONDROMATOUS HAMARTOMAS.   These are the most common true benign neoplasms of the lung. Despite their bronchial origin, they usually present as a solitary pulmonary nodule and are rarely endobronchial masses.[90] Calcification occurs in about 30 percent of all chondromatous hamartomas and the frequency of calcification increases with tumor size. The pattern of

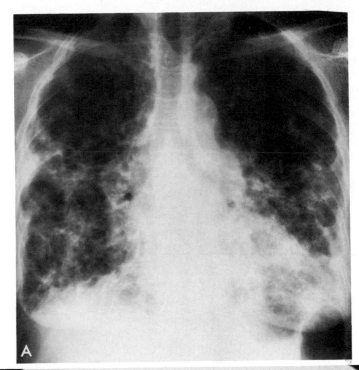

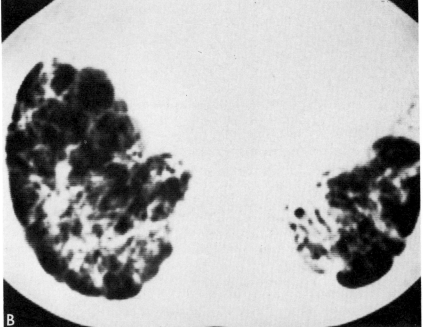

Figure 4–26. Bronchiectasis in a patient with acquired immunodeficiency. **A** Frontal chest radiograph shows extensive bronchiectasis, bands of scarring, and peripheral bullae. **B** CT scan through the lower lobes demonstrates thick-walled bronchi, clusters of cystic bronchial dilatation, and extensive subpleural bullae.

Illustration continued on following page

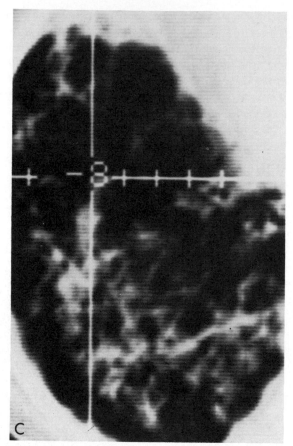

Figure 4–26. *Continued* **C** CT scan with a 1-cm scale overlay shows the cystic bronchial spaces to be 0.5 to 2.0 cm in diameter.

calcification is stippled or conglomerate; conglomerate or "popcorn" calcification is rarely seen with other lesions.[91] Endobronchial hamartomas can be resected bronchoscopically and do not tend to recur.[83]

SQUAMOUS PAPILLOMAS. These are an abnormal proliferation of airway mucosal cells and are thought to be of viral origin. Most lesions arise in the larynx. Distal spread to the trachea, bronchi, and lung parenchyma occurs in only a small minority of patients. Bronchography and CT scans can show the endobronchial masses. Bronchoscopic excision of the lesions is the preferred treatment, but the lesions recur in over 90 per cent of patients.[36, 83]

OTHER TUMORS. Other benign tumors of the bronchi are all rare and their demonstration on CT scans has not been reported. Granular cell myoblastomas and lipomas tend to occur in the major bronchi and cause airway obstruction. About 50 per cent of leiomyomas arise within the central bronchi and the remainder occur in the lung parenchyma. Bronchial fibromas are only

rarely endobronchial. Tumors of neurogenic origin also rarely arise within the bronchi and most present as a solitary pulmonary nodule. The most common presentation when these tumors are endobronchial is with segmental or lobar collapse. CT scans should localize the site of the tumor and will demonstrate the distal collapsed lung. The CT appearance of these tumors, although not described, should be nonspecific and will not differentiate these lesions from other masses causing bronchial obstruction. The focal appearance of the tumor without extrabronchial extension may suggest a benign tumor. Bronchoscopy and biopsy are usually required for diagnosis.

Central Bronchogenic Carcinoma

Over the past 50 years in the western hemisphere, bronchogenic carcinoma has established itself as the most common fatal malignancy in men, and in women the incidence continues to increase alarmingly.[92] The prevalence, however, varies widely among countries and racial groups.[93, 94]

The frequency with which bronchogenic carcinoma arises in a central location varies with the histologic type of tumor.[95, 96] Squamous cell carcinoma most commonly arises centrally, predominantly in segmental bronchi; it is less common in lobar or main bronchi. Atelectasis or a hilar mass is therefore the most common presentation. Small-cell undifferentiated carcinoma also usually arises centrally as a hilar mass, or an area of lung atelectasis or pneumonitis. Large-cell undifferentiated carcinoma infrequently has a central origin, and adenocarcinoma arises predominantly in the lung parenchyma away from the central bronchi.

The radiographic and CT features of bronchogenic carcinoma are determined by the site of origin of the tumor, its size, and its growth pattern and dissemination. At the time of presentation, most bronchogenic carcinomas are no longer amenable to surgical cure.[97]

The appearance on CT scans of bronchogenic carcinoma arising in a central location has not been described in detail.[5, 6, 98] The following description is based largely on our own observations. The most common radiographic[99–101] and CT[98] findings are the result of bronchial obstruction. Atelectasis, obstructive fluid retention, and obstructive pneumonitis all result from bronchial obstruction.[95]

Narrowing or obstruction of bronchi can be demonstrated when bronchi that are routinely seen on CT scans are involved. These are the main bronchi, intermediate bronchus, lobar bronchi, segmental bronchi of the upper lobes, and the superior segmental bronchi of the lower lobes. The segmental bronchi to the lingular, middle lobe, and basal bronchi of both lower lobes are not always visible in normal adults, and narrowing of these bronchi is less easily seen on CT scans.

Complete bronchial obstruction is most often seen with segmental bronchial tumors (Fig. 4–28).[98] The degree of volume loss of the lung distal to an obstruction is variable. The lung can collapse and be reduced to its minimal volume. Alternatively, the obstructed lung can become filled with desquamated material, mucus, and fluid and lose little of its volume. In both instances, CT scans will show an absence of air bronchograms in

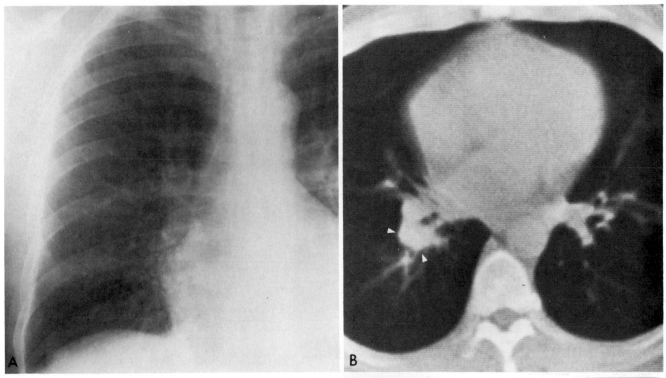

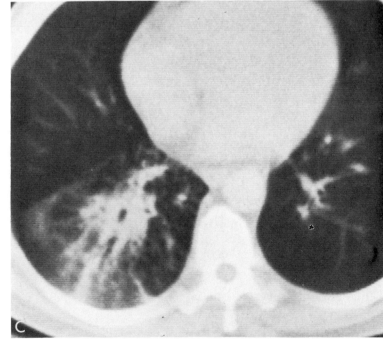

Figure 4–27. Bronchial carcinoid in a patient with obstructive pneumonia. **A** Frontal radiograph shows fullness of the right inferior hilum and patchy consolidation in the right lower lobe. **B** CT scan through the lower lobe basal segmental bronchi demonstrates a lobulated mass (arrowheads) compressing the bronchi. **C** CT scan, 2 cm caudal to the scan in **B,** shows consolidation and loss of volume in the posterior and lateral basal segments of the right lower lobe.

Illustration continued on following page

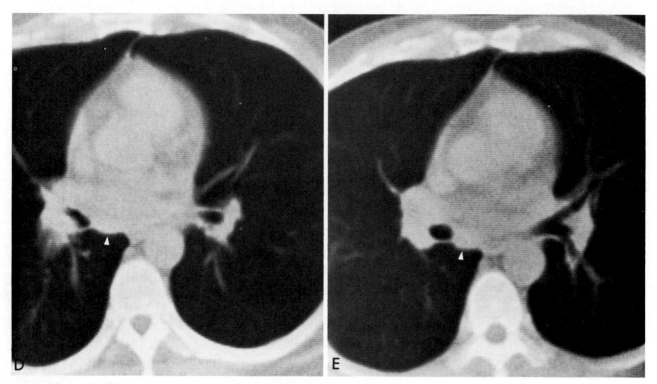

Figure 4–27. *Continued* **D**   CT scan through the basal trunk of the right lower lobe shows narrowing of the bronchus and a lymph node medially (arrowhead). **E**   CT scan, 1 cm cephalad to the scan in **D,** confirms the presence of the azygoesophageal lymph node (arrowhead). (At thoracotomy, a 1.3 × 2.0 cm carcinoid compressed the posterior and lateral basal segmental bronchi. Lymphadenopathy showed reactive hyperplasia without tumor.)

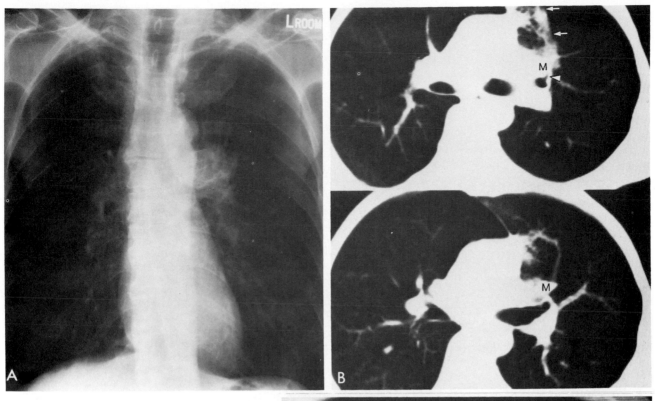

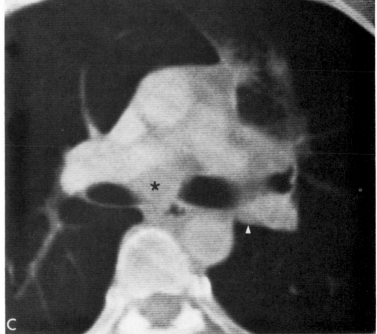

Figure 4–28. Bronchogenic carcinoma with segmental atelectasis. **A** Frontal radiograph shows a left upper hilar mass. **B** Adjacent CT scans through the left main and upper lobe bronchi demonstrate a left anterior hilar mass (M), narrowing of the anterior segmental bronchus (arrowhead), and atelectasis of the anterior segment (arrows). **C** CT scan, (scan **B** upper panel) at extended window settings confirms the mass and bronchial obstruction. A retrobronchial lymph node medial to the left pulmonary artery (arrowhead) and subcarinal adenopathy (asterisk) are also present.

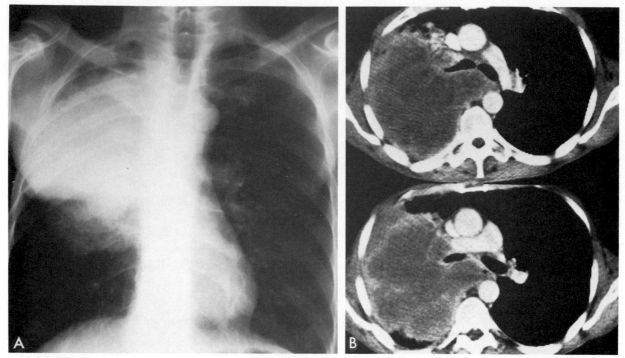

Figure 4–29. Bronchogenic carcinoma producing bronchial obstruction and a fluid-filled lobe. **A** Frontal radiograph shows dense opacification of the right upper lobe without loss of volume or air bronchograms. **B** Adjacent CT scans demonstrate inhomogeneous opacification of the right upper lobe. The right upper lobe bronchus narrows and terminates (upper panel). The bronchi are displaced anteriorly. The intermediate bronchus is compressed (lower panel). The proximal tumor cannot be differentiated from the fluid-filled upper lobe on these scans. (After radiation therapy to the right hilum, the right upper lobe reaerated.)

the area, which suggests obstruction of the proximal bronchus (Fig. 4–29).

Atelectasis of the lung subtended by the obstructing tumor is readily demonstrated on CT scans (Fig. 4–30). Occasionally, the lung distal to a segmental or lobar obstruction remains inflated, presumably due to collateral ventilation (Fig. 4–31). Low window levels on the CT console (−500 to −600 H) can give a false appearance of bronchial obstruction. Patency of the bronchus can be demonstrated if higher window levels (20 to 50 H) are used.

The main bronchi, intermediate bronchus, and lobar bronchi frequently show tumor narrowing, and less commonly obstructing, the airway lumen. A mass representing the tumor is usually seen around the narrow bronchus on CT scans. In general, it is not possible on CT scans to differentiate intrinsic tumor producing narrowing of a bronchus from extrinsic compression of a bronchus by the tumor. Displacement of bronchi from an adjacent mass is frequent and can help in confirming the presence of a tumor (Figs. 4–29 and 4–30).

Thickening of the wall of a bronchus can be seen on CT scans at the sites where lung normally makes contact with the bronchial tree. The posterior walls of the right main bronchus, right upper lobe bronchus, intermediate bronchus, distal left main bronchus, and left lower lobe bronchus are such sites. Tumor infiltration of these bronchial walls and lymphadenopathy can both cause thickening of the bronchial wall.[98] Irregularity of a thickened wall usually indicates tumor infiltration and correlates with the bronchoscopic finding of endobronchial tumor (Fig. 4–32).

Of bronchogenic carcinomas, 12 to 35 per cent present as an enlargement of one hilum on chest radiographs.[99, 100] The hilar enlargement can be from a central tumor arising in a hilar bronchus or from hilar adenopathy from a peripheral tumor. In most instances of a centrally arising tumor or hilar adenopathy, CT scans show abnormal enlargement and an abnormal contour to the hilum. Contour abnormalities can occur anywhere within the hilum, but are most easily appreciated when they are lateral and posterior to the hilar vessels. If interpretation of the CT scans is equivocal, a bolus injection of intravenous contrast material during rapid sequential (dynamic) scanning can separate the tumor mass from the hilar vessels (Fig. 4–33). A consolidated or collapsed lung in continuity with the hilum obscures the hilar contours on CT scans, and the abnormal hilum cannot be demonstrated. Similarly, a large pleural effusion can prevent assessment of hilar contours.

Bronchial obstruction predisposes to infection in the subtended lung segment. Obstructive pneumonitis or abscess formation can result. Generally, the proximal tumor mass cannot be separated from the distal obstructive pneumonitis or abscess on CT scans (Fig. 4–34). The endobronchial obstruction, however, is usually evident.

Bronchogenic carcinoma rarely produces hyperinflation and air trapping of the lung subtended by a partially obstructed bronchus. We have not seen CT scans in such a case; however, hyperlucency is readily demonstrated on CT scans at appropriate window settings. In addition, the proximal bronchial tumor should be demonstrated.

Sputum cytologic screening of people at high risk for development of bronchogenic carcinoma and in patients with respiratory symptoms have shown some cases with malignant cells in their sputum, although their chest radiographs are normal.[102, 103] In most of these patients, the tumor arises from a central bronchus. Before fibrobronchoscopy and CT scanning, bronchography was advocated for the localization of the occult neoplasm,[104] but this procedure is no longer recommended. Painstaking fibrobronchoscopy can reveal the neoplasm in more than half of the patients.[105] CT scanning can localize the tumor in some cases and direct bronchoscopy to areas of special concern (Fig. 4–35).

Of major importance in CT scanning of the thorax in patients with bronchogenic carcinoma is the demonstration of intrathoracic metastases and local spread of the tumor. Lymphatic spread is usually to the hilar, mediastinal, or supraclavicular lymph nodes. Central bronchogenic carcinoma also frequently invades the mediastinum by direct growth of the tumor (see Chapters 5 and 6).

Spread of bronchogenic carcinoma by way of the lymphatic system and the blood stream can be to the lung on the side of the primary tumor or to the contralateral lung. In our experience, the spatial resolution of present CT scanners does not permit the demonstration of lymphangitic carcinomatosis. CT scans are, however, more sensitive than chest radiographs or conventional tomograms in detection of pulmonary nodules. In pa-

tients with bronchogenic carcinoma, the frequency with which nodules demonstrated only on CT scans are metastases has not been established.

Pleural effusion is present at the time of diagnosis in 2 to 5 per cent of patients with bronchogenic carcinoma.[99, 104] Most patients with pleural effusion have nonresectable tumor. Serous effusion usually indicates hilar lymph node involvement and lymphatic blockage. Pleural deposits from bronchogenic carcinoma causing pleural effusion are usually not visible on CT scans.

INDICATIONS FOR COMPUTED TOMOGRAPHY OF THE TRACHEA AND BRONCHI

The indications for CT scanning in imaging abnormalities of the trachea and bronchi have not been determined.[106, 107] The normal contrast provided by air within the airway lumen allows detection of most focal masses in the trachea and central bronchi. Oblique radiographs, coned-down views, and conventional tomograms demonstrate most lesions protruding into the trachea and bronchi.

CT scanning has replaced conventional tomography for the investigation of most mediastinal and hilar masses. When the patient's symptoms, pulmonary function studies, or chest radiographs suggest compression or displacement of the trachea by an extrinsic mass, CT scans are likely to demonstrate the cause. A dilated or aberrant vessel, or mediastinal extension of a goiter are the most common causes and both are readily diagnosed from CT scans. Extrinsic compression of the bronchi within a hilum is usually due to lymphadenopathy or a bronchogenic carcinoma.

CT scanning is probably indicated in all patients with masses that appear to be arising from the tracheal wall. Most of these will have nonspecific findings on CT scans, but the position and extent of the abnormality can be precisely demonstrated. If the mass contains calcium deposits, a benign tumor of cartilaginous origin should be considered. Rarely, a chondrosarcoma will show this finding. Extension of the mass beyond the confines of the tracheal wall is very suggestive of a malignant neoplasm. Unless disease in other organs or parts of the respiratory tract make the diagnosis obvious, endoscopy and biopsy will be invariably necessary for diagnosis.

The use of CT scanning for tracheal stenosis

Text continued on page 192

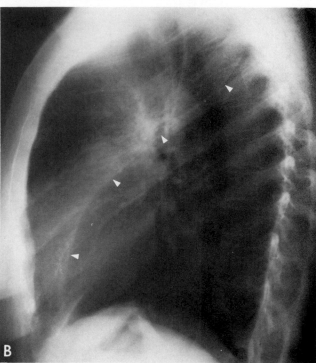

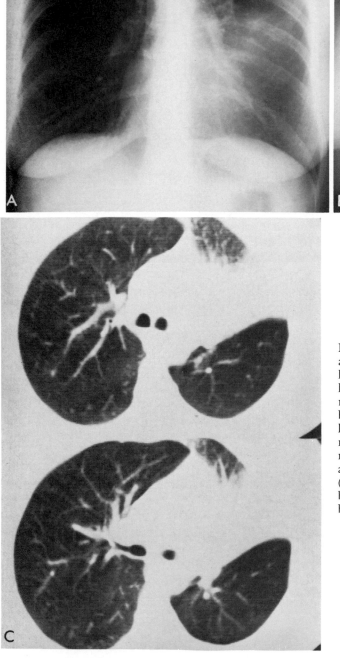

Figure 4–30. Bronchogenic carcinoma causing partial atelectasis of the left upper lobe. **A, B** Frontal (**A**) and lateral (**B**) radiographs show partial left upper lobe atelectasis. The major fissure (arrows) is displaced anteriorly. **C, D** Sequential CT scans through the left main bronchus and proximal left lower lobe bronchus show no left upper lobe bronchus. Anterior displacement of the major fissure is confirmed. The anterior segment remains partially aerated. **E** CT scan, (same as scan **D** but at mediastinal window settings) shows the tumor mass (M) in the anticipated position of the left upper lobe. (At bronchoscopy, tumor occluded the left upper lobe bronchus.)

Illustration continued on opposite page

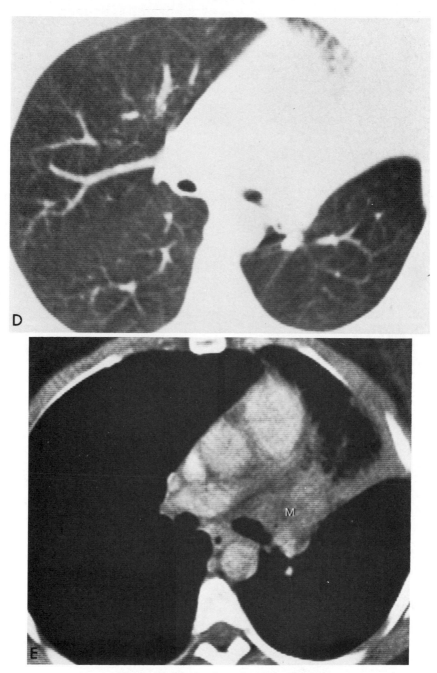

Figure 4–30. *See legend on opposite page*

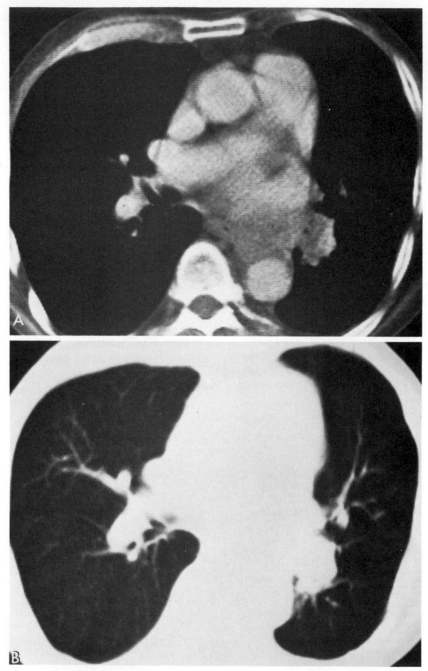

Figure 4–31. Bronchogenic carcinoma causing marked bronchial narrowing without atelectasis. CT scans at the same level: **A** at mediastinal window settings and **B** at lung window settings. **A**   CT scan shows tumor mass surrounding and narrowing the left basal bronchus and directly invading the mediastinum between the descending aorta and left atrium. **B**   CT scan shows the lobular mass. At these window settings the basal trunk is not seen. The left lung is small and hyperlucent (decreased CT density). (Marked bronchial narrowing was confirmed at bronchoscopy.)

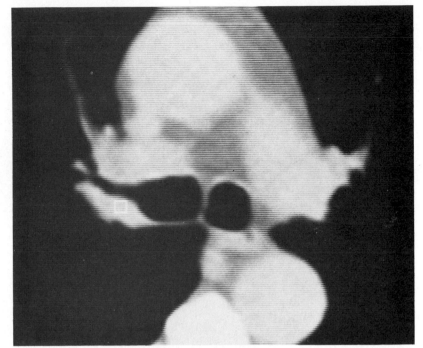

Figure 4–32. Endobronchial bronchogenic carcinoma causing irregular narrowing of the right upper lobe bronchus. CT scan shows narrowing of the right upper lobe bronchus. The bronchial wall is thickened and irregular (cursor). (Tumor confirmed by bronchoscopy and biopsy.)

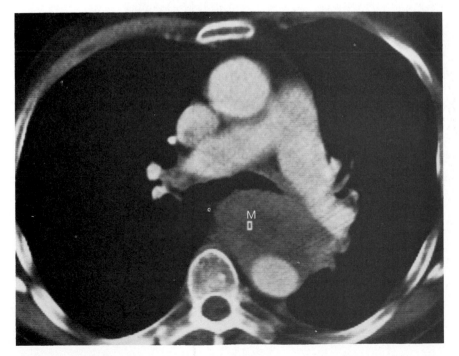

Figure 4–33. Intravenous bolus injection of contrast material in discriminating mass from vessels. CT scan after injection of contrast material separates the retrobronchial tumor mass (M) from the left pulmonary artery and descending aorta.

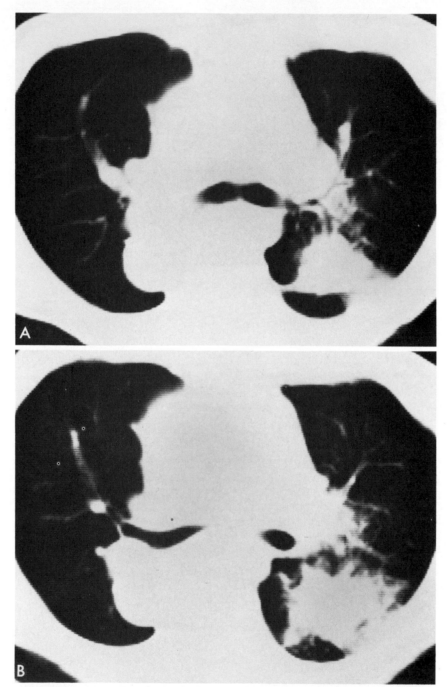

Figure 4–34. Bronchial narrowing from bronchogenic carcinoma causing persistent pneumonia. **A** CT scan through the left upper lobe and anterior and posterior segmental bronchi shows diffuse bronchial narrowing. Consolidation is demonstrated in the posterior segmental of the left upper lobe. Adenopathy is present behind the left upper lobe bronchus. **B** CT scan, 1 cm caudad to the scan in **A,** shows thickening of the posterior wall of the left intermediate bronchus. The left hilum is enlarged and excessively lobulated. (The patient has situs inversus.)

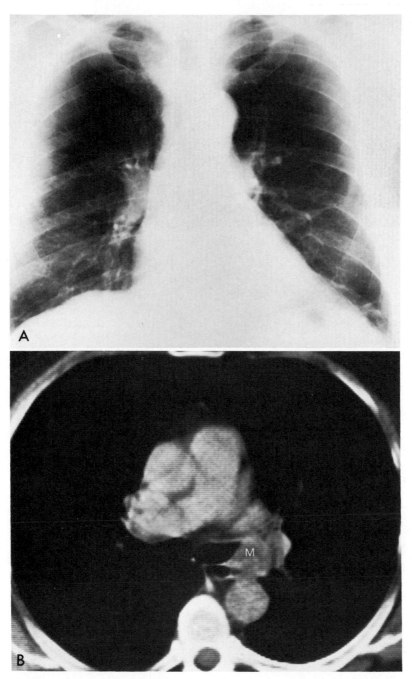

Figure 4–35. Bronchogenic carcinoma in a patient with malignant cells in the sputum. **A**   Frontal radiograph shows mild dilatation of central pulmonary arteries and scarring at left base. **B**   CT scan through the left main bronchus shows an endobronchial mass (M) almost completely occluding the distal left main bronchus.

Illustration continued on following page

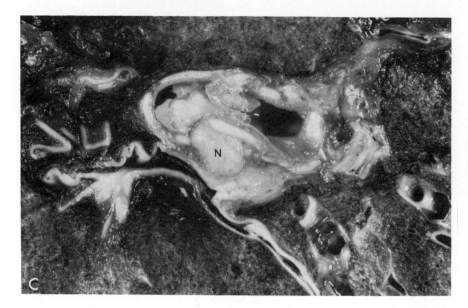

Figure 4–35. *Continued* **C**   A left lung section from the pneumonectomy specimen, demonstrates the endobronchial carcinoma. Node (N) posterior to the bronchus showed reactive hyperplasia.

from tracheal injury requires further clarification. In our experience, CT scans do not offer advantages over conventional tomography and tracheography.

CT scanning of the entire thorax and upper abdomen is indicated in patients with endobronchial lesions suspected of being malignant neoplasms. CT scans can demonstrate sites suspicious for spread of bronchogenic carcinoma to the mediastinum, bony thorax, lung parenchyma, adrenal glands, and liver. In several instances, we have guided the bronchoscopist to perform a biopsy of or to brush abnormal bronchial sites beyond the range of direct endoscopic visibility. CT scans are also excellent for demonstrating suspected areas of atelectasis and obstructive pneumonitis.

The relative sensitivity of conventional tomography and CT scanning for detecting areas of bronchial narrowing has not been established.[108] However, CT scans provide more information than tomograms about the mediastinum and remainder of the thorax and should be the favored modality for investigating endobronchial lesions. Several aspects of CT scanning of the trachea and bronchi are still controversial, and the challenge of determining the precise indications remains.

REFERENCES

1. Kittredge RD: Computed tomography of the trachea: A review. Comput Tomogr 5:44, 1981.
2. Gamsu G, Webb WR: Computed tomography of the trachea: Normal and abnormal. AJR 139:321, 1982.
3. Naidich DP, Terry PB, Stitik FP, Siegelman SS: Computed tomography of the bronchi: 1. Normal anatomy. J Comput Assist Tomogr 4:746, 1980.
4. Webb WR, Glazer G, Gamsu G: Computed tomography of the normal pulmonary hilum. J Comput Assist Tomogr 5:476, 1981.
5. Naidich DP, Stitik FP, Khouri NF, Terry PB, Siegelman SS: Computed tomography of the bronchi: 2. Pathology. J Comput Assist Tomogr 4:754, 1980.
6. Webb WR, Gamsu G, Glazer G: Computed tomography of the abnormal pulmonary hilum. J Comput Assist Tomogr 5:485, 1981.
7. Gray H: Trachea. In Goss CM (ed): Anatomy of the Human Body, 28th American edition. Philadelphia, Lea & Febiger, 1966, pp 1137–1139.
8. Fraser RG, Paré JAP: Diagnosis of Diseases of the Chest, 2nd ed., vol 1. Philadelphia, WB Saunders Company, 1977, p 56.
9. Merendino KA, Kiriluk LB: Human measurements involved in tracheobronchial resection and reconstruction procedures: Report of case of bronchial adenoma. Surgery 35:590, 1954.
10. Jesseph JE, Merendino KA: The dimensional interrelationships of the major components of the human tracheobronchial tree. Surg Gynecol Obstet 105:210, 1957.
11. Fraser RG: Measurements of the caliber of human bronchi in three phases of respiration by cinebronchography. J Can Assoc Radiol 12:102, 1961.
12. Boyden EA, Hartmann JF: An analysis of variations in the bronchopulmonary segments of the left upper lobes of fifty lungs. Am J Anat 79:321, 1946.
13. Landing BH: Congenital malformations and genetic disorders of the respiratory tract (larynx, trachea, bronchi, and lungs). Am Rev Respir Dis 120:151, 1979.
14. Kormano M, Yrjana J: The posterior tracheal band: Correlation between computed tomography and chest radiography. Radiology 136:689, 1980.
15. Cimmino CV: The esophageal-pleural stripe: An update. Radiology 140:609, 1981.
16. Speckman JM, Gamsu G, Webb WR: Alterations in CT mediastinal anatomy produced by an azygos lobe. AJR 137:47, 1981.
17. Schnyder PA, Gamsu G: CT of the pretracheal retrocaval space. AJR 136:303, 1981.
18. Webb WR, Gamsu G: Computed tomography of the left

retrobronchial stripe. J Comput Assist Tomogr 7:65, 1983.

19. Himalstein MR, Gallagher JC: Tracheobronchiomegaly. Ann Otol Rhinol Laryngol 82:223, 1973.

20. Bateson EM, Woo-Ming M: Tracheobronchiomegaly. Clin Radiol 24:354, 1978.

21. Aaby GV, Blake HA: Tracheobronchiomegaly. Ann Thorac Surg 2:64, 1966.

22. Williams H, Campbell P: Generalized bronchiectasis associated with deficiency of cartilage in the bronchial tree. Arch Dis Child 35:182, 1960.

23. Greene R: Saber-sheath trachea: Relation to chronic obstructive pulmonary disease. AJR 130:441, 1978.

24. Rubenstein J, Weisbrod G, Steinhardt MI: Atypical appearances of saber-sheath trachea. Radiology 127:41, 1978.

25. Wilson SR, Sanders DE, Delarue NC: Intrathoracic manifestations of amyloid disease. Radiology 120:283, 1976.

26. Cook AJ, Weinstein M, Powell RD: Diffuse amyloidosis of the tracheobronchial tree: Bronchographic manifestations. Radiology 107:303, 1973.

27. Kilman WJ: Narrowing of the airway in relapsing polychondritis. Radiology 126:373, 1978.

28. Hughes RAC, Berry CL, Seifert M, Lessof MH: Relapsing polychondritis. QJ Med 41:363, 1972.

29. Dolan DL, Lemmon GB Jr, Teitelbaum SL: Relapsing polychondritis. Analytical literature review and studies on pathogenesis. Am J Med 41:285, 1966.

30. Gibson GJ, Davis P: Respiratory complications of relapsing polychondritis. Thorax 29:726, 1974.

31. Howland WJ Jr, Good CA: The radiographic features of tracheopathia osteoplastica. Radiology 71:847, 1958.

32. Secrest PG, Kendig TA, Beland AJ: Tracheobronchopathia osteochondroplastica. Am J Med 36:815, 1964.

33. Bergeron D, Cormier Y, Desmeules M: Tracheobronchopathia osteochondroplastica. Am Rev Respir Dis 114:803, 1976.

34. Baird RB, McCartney JN: Tracheopathia osteoplastica. Thorax 21:321, 1966.

35. Massoud GE, Awwad HK: Scleroma of the upper airpassages. J Faculty Radiol 10:44, 1959.

36. Caldarola VT, Harrison EG Jr, Clagett OT, Schmidt HW: Benign tumors and tumorlike conditions of the trachea and bronchi. Ann Otol Rhinol Laryngol 73:1042, 1964.

37. Gilbert JG, Mazzarella LA, Feit LJ: Primary tracheal tumors in the infant and adult. Arch Otolaryngol 58:1, 1953.

38. Weber AL, Shortsleeve M, Goodman M, Montgomery W, Grillo HC: Cartilaginous tumors of the larynx and trachea. Radiol Clin North Am 16:261, 1978.

39. Piaget F: Benign tumors of the trachea. Ann Otolaryngol (Paris) 53:182, 1966.

40. Renault P: Tracheal chondroma. J Fr Med Chir Thorac 25:481, 1971.

41. Rishovits G: Tracheobronchial chondroma. Tuberkulozis 14:182, 1961.

42. Weber AL, Grillo HC: Tracheal tumors. A radiological, clinical, and pathological evaluation of 84 cases. Radiol Clin North Am 16:227, 1978.

43. Houston HE, Payne WS, Harrison EG Jr, Olsen AM: Primary cancers of the trachea. Arch Surg 99:132, 1969.

44. Ranke EJ, Presley SS, Holinger PH: Tracheogenic carcinoma. JAMA 182:519, 1962.

45. Hajdu SI, Huvos AG, Goodner JT, Foote FW Jr, Beattie EJ Jr: Carcinoma of the trachea. Clinicopathologic study of 41 cases. Cancer 25:1448, 1970.

46. Karlan MS, Livingston PA, Baker DC Jr: Diagnosis of tracheal tumors. Ann Otol Rhinol Laryngol 82:790, 1973.

47. Gamsu G, Borson DB, Webb WR: Structure and function in tracheal stenosis. Am Rev Respir Dis 121:519, 1980.

48. Fleming RJ, Medina J, Seaman WB: Roentgenographic aspects of tracheal tumors. Radiology 79:628, 1962.

49. Janower ML, Grillo HC, MacMillan AS Jr, James AE Jr: The radiological appearance of carcinoma of the trachea. Radiology 96:39, 1970.

50. Muhm JR, Crowe JK: The evaluation of tracheal abnormalities by tomography. Radiol Clin North Am 14:95, 1976.

51. Dunbar JS, Skinner GB, Wortzman G, Stuart JR: An investigation of effects of opaque media on the lungs with comparison of barium sulfate, lipiodol and dionosil. AJR 82:902, 1959.

52. Gamsu G, Nadel JA: New technique for roentgenographic study of airways and lungs using powdered tantalum. Cancer 30:1353, 1972.

53. Momose KJ, MacMillan AS Jr: Roentgenologic investigations of the larynx and trachea. Radiol Clin North Am 16:321, 1978.

53a. Naidich DP, McCauley DI, Siegelman SS: Computed tomography of bronchial adenomas. J Comput Assist Tomogr 6:725, 1982.

54. Glazer GM, Axel L, Moss AA: CT diagnosis of mediastinal thyroid. AJR 138:495, 1982.

55. Djalilian M, Beahrs OH, Devine KD, Weiland LH, DeSanto LW; Intraluminal involvement of the larynx and trachea by thyroid cancer. Am J Surg 128:500, 1974.

56. Daffner RH, Halber MD, Postlethwait RW, Korobkin M, Thompson WM: CT of the esophagus: II. Carcinoma. AJR 133:1051, 1979.

57. Gamsu G, Webb WR, Shallit JB, Moss AA: CT in carcinoma of the larynx and pyriform sinus: Value of phonation scans. AJR 136:577, 1981.

58. Calem WS, Freund HR: Subglottic carcinoma with extensive tracheal involvement. Surgery 50:894, 1961.

59. Moss AA, Schnyder P, Thoeni RF, Margulis AR: Esophageal carcinoma: Pretherapy staging by computed tomography. AJR 136:1051, 1981.

60. MacMillan AS, James AE Jr, Stitik FP, Grillo HC: Radiological evaluation of post-tracheostomy lesions. Thorax 26:696, 1971.

61. Harley HRS: Laryngotracheal obstruction complicating tracheostomy or endotracheal intubation with assisted respiration. Thorax 26:493, 1971.

62. Dunn CR, Dunn DL, Moser KM: Determinants of tracheal injury by cuffed tracheostomy tubes. Chest 65:128, 1974.

63. Gillo HC: Reconstruction of the trachea: Experience in 100 cases. Thorax 28:667, 1973.

64. Bergstrom B, Ollman B, Lindholm CE: Endotracheal excision of fibrous tracheal stenosis and subsequent prolonged stenting. Chest 71:1, 1977.

65. Ross JAT: Techniques in the surgical repair of tracheal stenosis. Otolaryngol Clin North Am 12:893, 1979.

66. Atetras A, Bjork VO, Fors B: Benign broncho-pulmonary neoplasms. Dis Chest 44:498, 1963.

67. Rinker CT, Garrotto LJ, Lee KR, Templeton AW: Bronchography: Diagnostic signs and accuracy in pulmonary carcinoma. Am J Roentgenol Rad Ther Nucl Med 104:802, 1968.

68. Donoghue FE, Andersen HA, McDonald JR: Unusual bronchial tumors. Ann Otol Rhinol Laryngol 65:820, 1956.

69. Weber AL, Bird TK, Janower ML: Primary tuberculosis in childhood with particular emphasis on changes affecting the tracheobronchial tree. AJR 103:123, 1968.

70. Singh D, Richards WF: Obstructive emphysema in primary pulmonary tuberculosis. Tubercle 38:397, 1957.

71. Daly JF: Endoscopic aspects of primary tuberculosis in children. Ann Otol Rhinol Laryngol 67:1089, 1958.

72. Long RF, Berens SV, Shambhag GR: An unusual manifestation of pulmonary eryptococcosis (case report). Br J Radiol 45:757, 1972.

73. Meighan JW; Pulmonary cryptococcosis mimicking carcinoma of the lung. Radiology 103:61, 1972.

74. Citron KM, Scadding JG: Stenosing non-caseating tuberculosis (sarcoidosis) of the bronchi. Thorax 12:10, 1957.

75. Goldenberg GJ, Greenspan RH: Middle-lobe atelectasis due to endobronchial sarcoidosis, with hypercalcemia and renal impairment. N Engl J Med 262:1112, 1960.

76. Olsson T, Bjornstad-Pettersen H, Stjernberg NL: Bronchostenosis due to sarcoidosis: A cause of atelectasis and airway obstruction simulating pulmonary neoplasm and chronic obstructive pulmonary disease. Chest 75:663, 1979.

77. Crofton J: Diagnosis and treatment of bronchiectasis: I. Diagnosis. II. Treatment and prevention. Br Med J 1:721, 1966.

78. Eliasson R, Mossberg B, Camner P, Afzelius BA: The immotile-cilia syndrome: A congenital ciliary abnormality as an etiologic factor in chronic airway infections and male sterility. N Engl J Med 297:1, 1977.

79. Wood RF, Boat TF, Doershuk CF: Cystic fibrosis. Am Rev Respir Dis 113:833, 1976.

80. Gudbjerg CE: Roentgenologic diagnosis of bronchiectasis: An analysis of 112 cases. Acta Radiol 43:209, 1955.

81. Gudbjerg CE: Bronchiectasis; radiological diagnosis and prognosis after operative treatment. Acta Radiol (Suppl) 143, 1957.

82. Naidich DP, McCauley DI, Khouri NF, Stitik FP, Siegelman SS: Computed tomography of bronchiectasis. J Comput Assist Tomogr 6:437, 1982.

83. Miller DR: Benign tumors of lung and tracheobronchial tree. Ann Thorac Surg 8:542, 1969.

84. Peleg H, Pauzner Y: Benign tumors of the lung. Dis Chest 47:179, 1965.

85. Burcharth F, Axelsson C: Bronchial adenomas. Thorax 27:442, 1972.

86. Donahue JK, Weichert RF, Ochsner JL: Bronchial adenoma. Ann Surg 167:873, 1968.

87. Marks C, Marks M: Bronchial adenoma: A clinicopathologic study. Chest 71:376, 1977.

88. Bower G: Bronchial adenoma: A review of twenty-eight cases. Am Rev Respir Dis 92:558, 1965.

89. Giustra PE, Stassa G: The multiple presentations of bronchial adenomas. Radiology 93:1013, 1969.

90. Bateson EM, Abbott EK: Mixed tumors of the lung, or hamartochondromas: A review of the radiological appearances of cases published in the literature and a report of fifteen new cases. Clin Radiol 11:232, 1960.

91. O'Keefe ME, Good CA, McDonald JR: Calcification in solitary nodules of the lung. Am J Roentgenol Rad Ther Nucl Med 77:1023, 1957.

92. Silverberg E, Holleb AI: Cancer statistics, 1974-worldwide epidemiology. Cancer 24:2, 1974.

93. Hammond EC: Lung cancer death rates in England and Wales compared with those in the U.S.A. Br Med J 2:649, 1958.

94. Korpela A, Magnus K: The incidence of lung cancer in Finland and Norway. Br J Cancer 15:393, 1961.

95. Cohen S, Hossain MS: Primary carcinoma of the lung: A review of 417 histologically proved cases. Dis Chest 49:67, 1966.

96. Kreyberg L, Liebow AA, Uehlinger EA: Histological Typing of Lung Tumours. Geneva, World Health Organization, 1967.

97. Moutain CF: Surgical prospects and priorities for clinical research. Cancer Chemother Rep 4:19, 1973.

98. Webb WR, Gamsu G, Speckman JM: Computed tomography of the pulmonary hilum in patients with bronchogenic carcinoma. J Comput Assist Tomogr 7:219, 1983.

99. Byrd RB, Carr DT, Miller WE, Payne WS, Woolner LB: Radiographic abnormalities in carcinoma of the lung as related to histological cell type. Thorax 24:573, 1969.

100. Lehar TJ, Carr DT, Miller WE, Payne WS, Woolner LB: Roentgenographic appearance of bronchogenic adenocarcinoma. Am Rev Respir Dis 96:245, 1967.

101. Rigler LG: The earliest roentgenographic signs of carcinoma of the lung. JAMA 195:655, 1966.

102. Pearson FG, Thompson DW, Delarue NC: Experience with the cytologic detection, localization, and treatment of radiographically undemonstrable bronchial carcinoma. J Thorac Cardiovasc Surg 54:371, 1967.

103. Grzybowski S, Coy P: Early diagnosis of carcinoma of the lung. Cancer 25:113, 1970.

104. Lerner MA, Rosebash H, Frank HA, Fleischner FG: Radiologic localization and management of cytologically discovered bronchial carcinoma. N Engl J Med 264:480, 1961.

105. Marsh BR, Frost JK, Erozan YS, Carter D: Occult bronchogenic carcinoma: Endoscopic localization and television documentation. Cancer 30:1348, 1972.

106. Society for Computed Body Tomography: New indications for computed body tomography. AJR 133:115, 1979.

107. Heitzman ER: Computed tomography of the thorax: Current perspectives. AJR 136:2, 1981.

108. Hughes RL, Mintzer RA, Shields TW, Jensik RJ, Cugell DW: Management of the hilar mass. Chest 79:1, 1981.

5 COMPUTED TOMOGRAPHY OF THE MEDIASTINUM

Gordon Gamsu

ANATOMY

Cross-sectional imaging allows evaluation of the mediastinum from a perspective totally different from that obtained with conventional radiography or tomography. Individual mediastinal structures and their relationships can be visualized. Interpretation of computed mediastinal tomograms requires thorough knowledge of both conventional and cross-sectional anatomy of the mediastinum.[1] The newer cross-sectional anatomic texts are useful aids.[2-4] To distinguish between normal and abnormal mediastinal structures requires an appreciation of the anatomic variations in individuals of different ages and physiques. Familiarity with the variations in density of mediastinal tissue, especially of mediastinal fat, and in the caliber of the mediastinal vessels is also important. Distortions of the mediastinal structures produced by musculoskeletal, pleural, and pulmonary diseases must also be understood.

In this chapter, unless otherwise stated, we will assume that the computed tomographic (CT) scans are transverse and that the patient is supine. Anatomic orientation will be conventional with

195

"anterior," "ventral," "in front of" meaning toward the patient's front; "posterior," "dorsal," "behind" meaning toward the patient's back; "superior," "cephalad," "above" meaning toward the patient's head; and "inferior," "caudad," "below" meaning toward the patient's feet.

The mediastinum extends from the sternum anteriorly to the vertebral bodies posteriorly. It is bounded laterally by the parietal mediastinal pleura of each lung. Below the thoracic inlet, the mediastinum is dominated by its vascular structures, the trachea, and the esophagus. The heart and pericardium will be dealt with in Chapter 9.

VASCULAR STRUCTURES

Upper Mediastinum

Above the aortic arch and below the thoracic inlet, a distance of 2 to 4 cm, the great arteries (arch vessels) and veins are uniformly positioned within the mediastinum (Figs. 5–1 through 5–4).[5–8] They are always visible on CT scans in the transverse plane. Intravenous administration of contrast material renders them more easily visible.

The innominate artery varies slightly in its position within the mediastinum. In about half of normal individuals, it is directly anterior to the trachea. In the remainder, it is either slightly to the right or left of the midline but still anterior to the trachea. The left common carotid artery is to the left of the intrathoracic trachea. At its origin, it is distinctly anterior to the trachea. Toward the thoracic inlet it is to the left of the anterior half of the trachea. The left common carotid artery is usually surrounded by mediastinal fat and only rarely is in contact with the left lung. The left subclavian artery lies to the left of the middle or anterior third of the trachea in most individuals. About 10 per cent of the time, it is lateral to the posterior third of the trachea. The amount of mediastinal fat surrounding the left subclavian artery varies among people, and in most the artery is separated from the left lung.

The venous structures in the upper mediastinum are the right and left brachiocephalic veins, both of which are in front of the arch vessels (Figs. 5–1 through 5–4). The left brachiocephalic vein courses anterior to the root of the arch vessels, or aortic arch, and joins the right brachiocephalic vein to form the superior vena cava (SVC) (Figs. 5–5 and 5–6). The inferior portion of the right brachiocephalic vein is well forward and to the right of the trachea. Only near the thoracic inlet does it assume a position lateral to the trachea.

Below the great vessels, the aortic arch is visible for a vertical distance of 1 to 2 cm (Fig. 5–5). As the arch courses posteriorly and to the left, it sometimes causes slight flattening of the left anterolateral wall of the trachea, with which it is in contact. The anterior aspect of the aortic arch has the SVC on its right side and the left lung on its left side. The midportion of the aortic arch is left of the trachea. The posterior aspect of the arch lies near the left wall of the esophagus.

The SVC is in front of the trachea, separated from it by the pretracheal space (Fig. 5–6). It is elliptical, with its long axis oriented toward the right or, less commonly, directly anteroposterior.[9] The SVC is normally about half the size of the ascending aorta, but at times it is much smaller and may appear as a thin, slit-like structure.

The ascending aorta lies midway between the sternum and spine (Figs. 5–6 through 5–9). It extends vertically for 3 to 4 cm. About two thirds of the time, the ascending aorta directly contacts the left lung. In the remainder, it is separated from the left lung by mediastinal fat. The upper ascending aorta is separated from the lower trachea by fat within the pretracheal space (Figs. 5–6 and 5–8), while the lower portion of the ascending aorta is close to the right pulmonary artery (Figs. 5–7 and 5–9B). The main pulmonary artery is interposed between the lower ascending aorta and the left lung (Fig. 5–9B). To the right of the lower ascending aorta, and slightly posterior, lies the SVC and the top of the right atrium (Figs. 5–7 and 5–9).

The positional relationship of the descending aorta to the spinal column and esophagus varies with age and physique. In most people, the descending aorta is contiguous with the left anterolateral aspect of the spine. It can, however, be in the midline or excessively tortuous and situated directly left of the spine. Except in older patients, the left lung inserts between the descending aorta and the left pulmonary artery, an area well shown by computed tomography. Any soft tissue between the descending aorta, the descending left pulmonary artery, and the left main bronchus is indicative of enlarged lymph nodes or a mass in this region.

The only consistent vascular structure to the right of the intrathoracic trachea is the arch of the azygos vein (Fig. 5–8). The ascending azygos vein is usually in the midline or slightly to the right, along the spinal column (Fig. 5–9A,B). At the level of the tracheal carina, or 1 to 2 cm above it, the azygos vein arches around the right wall of the trachea to enter the posterior wall of the SVC.

Text continued on page 206

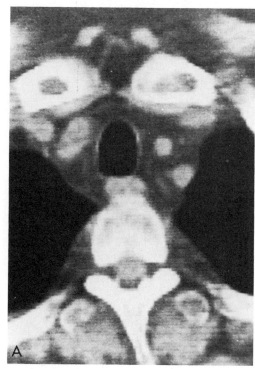

Figure 5–1. Normal upper mediastinal anatomy. **A** CT scan in a 35-year-old obese man, at the level of the proximal clavicles. **B** Schematic representation of the mediastinum at the same level. Contrast medium has not been infused.

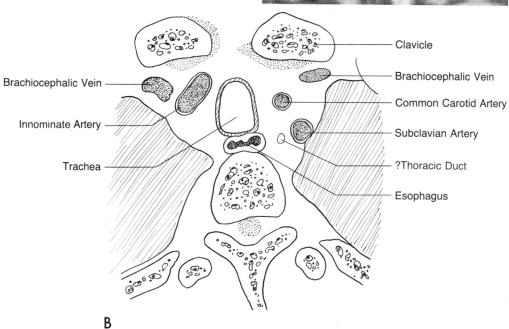

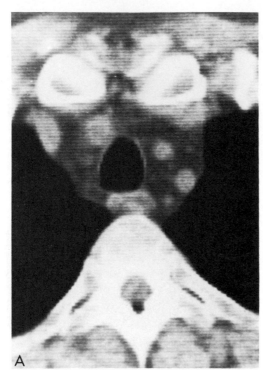

Figure 5–2. Normal upper mediastinal anatomy. **A** CT scan in a 35-year-old obese man, at the level of the suprasternal notch (1 cm caudad to Fig. 5–1). **B** Schematic representation of the mediastinum at the same level. Contrast medium has not been infused.

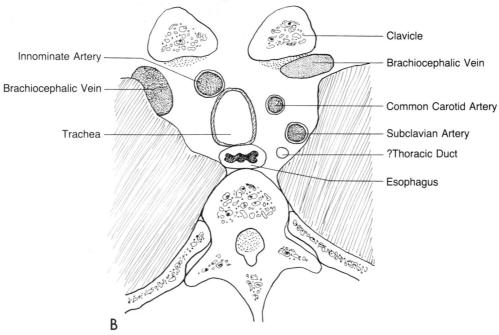

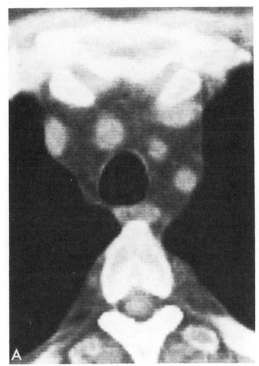

Figure 5–3. Normal upper mediastinal anatomy. **A** CT scan in a 35-year-old obese man, at the level of the manubrium (1 cm caudad to Fig. 5–2). **B** Schematic representation of the mediastinum at the same level. Contrast medium has not been infused.

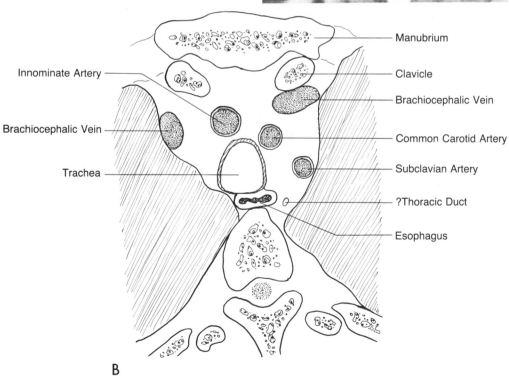

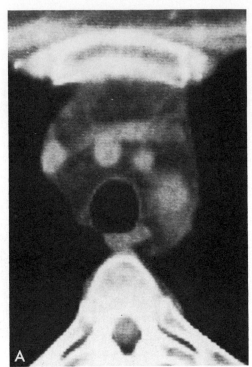

Figure 5–4. Normal upper mediastinal anatomy. **A** CT scan in a 35-year-old obese man, at the level of the origin of the great vessels (1 cm caudad to Fig. 5–3). **B** Schematic representation of the mediastinum at the same level. Contrast medium has not been infused.

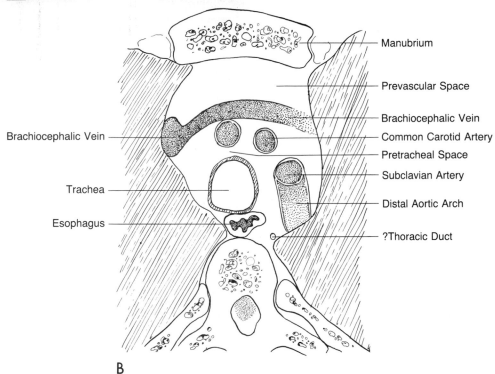

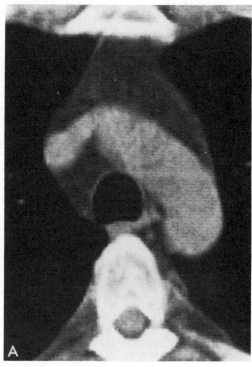

Figure 5–5. Normal upper mediastinal anatomy. **A** CT scan in a 35-year-old obese man, at the level of the aortic arch (1 cm caudad to Fig. 5–4). **B** Schematic representation of the mediastinum at the same level. Contrast medium has not been infused.

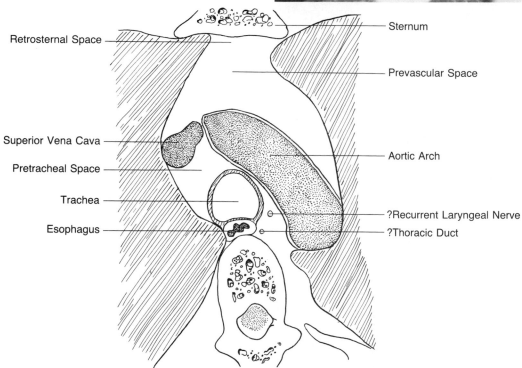

Retrosternal Space

Sternum

Prevascular Space

Superior Vena Cava

Pretracheal Space

Trachea

Esophagus

Aortic Arch

?Recurrent Laryngeal Nerve

?Thoracic Duct

B

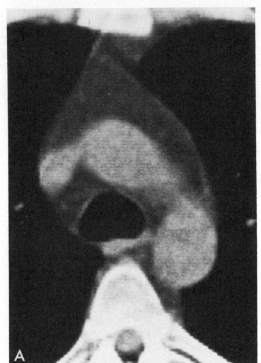

Figure 5–6. Normal upper mediastinal anatomy. **A** CT scan in a 35-year-old obese man, immediately above the tracheal bifurcation (1 cm caudad to Fig. 5–5). **B** Schematic representation of the mediastinum at the same level. Contrast medium has not been infused.

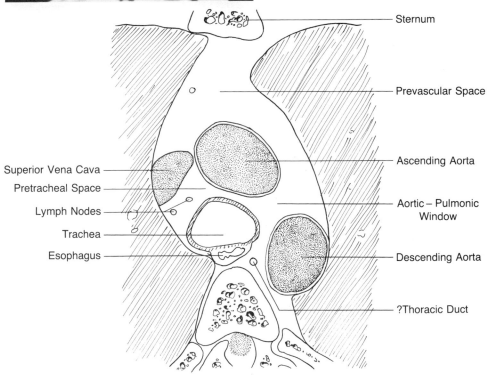

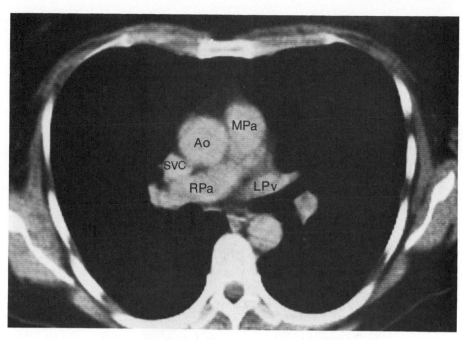

Figure 5–7. Normal mediastinal anatomy at the level of the aortic root (Ao). The main pulmonary artery (MPa) is to the left of the aorta. The right pulmonary artery (RPa) is behind the aorta and superior vena cava (SVC). The left superior pulmonary vein (LPv) is in front of the left main bronchus.

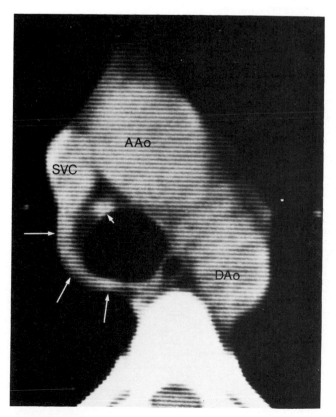

Figure 5–8. Normal mediastinal anatomy at the level of the azygos arch (long arrows), 1 cm below the aortic arch. The azygos vein enters the posterior superior vena cava (SVC). The upper ascending aorta (AAo), descending aorta (DAo), and a single azygos lymph node (short arrow) are demonstrated.

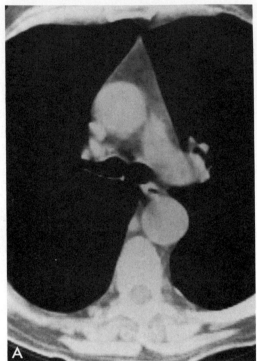

Figure 5–9. Normal anatomy of mediastinal segments of the left and right pulmonary arteries, after intravenous infusion of contrast material. **A**   CT scan *(left)* and schematic drawing *(right)* made at the same level show left pulmonary artery coursing lateral to and over the left main bronchus. A tongue of lung extends between the left pulmonary artery and descending aorta. The anterior trunk lies between the superior vena cava and the right main bronchus.

Illustration continued on opposite page

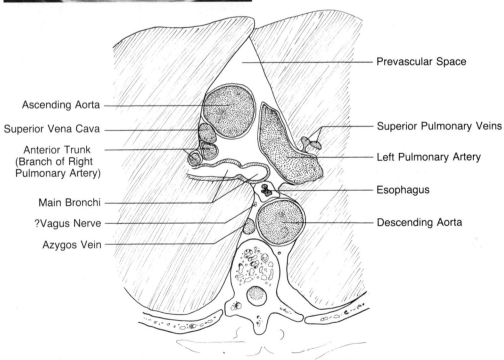

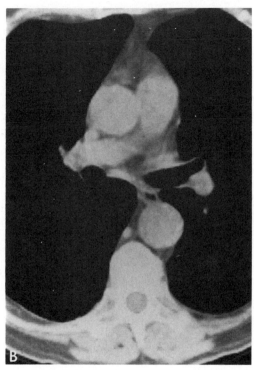

Figure 5–9. *Continued* **B** Two centimeters caudad, the right pulmonary artery is visible between the superior vena cava and the intermediate bronchus. The left descending pulmonary artery is posterior to the left main bronchus and still separated from the descending aorta by lung.

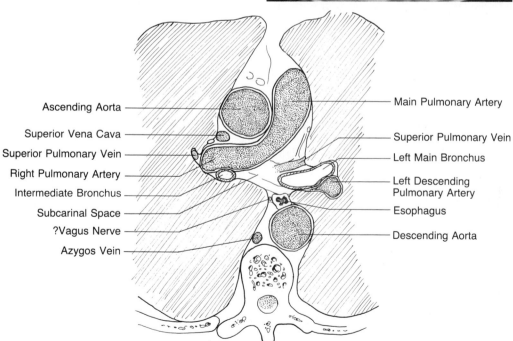

Ascending Aorta

Superior Vena Cava

Superior Pulmonary Vein

Right Pulmonary Artery

Intermediate Bronchus

Subcarinal Space

?Vagus Nerve

Azygos Vein

Main Pulmonary Artery

Superior Pulmonary Vein

Left Main Bronchus

Left Descending Pulmonary Artery

Esophagus

Descending Aorta

Middle Mediastinum

The vascular structures of the middle mediastinum are the pulmonary arteries and veins, the aorta, the azygos and hemiazygos veins, and the SVC (Figs. 5–7 through 5–9).

The main pulmonary artery is visible over a vertical distance of 1 to 2 cm. It lies to the left of the ascending aorta and is flanked by the left lung anteriorly and laterally. The right pulmonary artery courses posterolaterally, to the right. It is situated behind the root of the aorta and the SVC and in front of the right main bronchus and intermediate bronchus. The anteroposterior diameter of the right pulmonary artery is 2.0 ± 0.4 cm, measured at computed tomographic window levels set for the mediastinum—about 20 to 50 Hounsfield Units (H).[10] The left pulmonary artery lies in a transverse plane 1 to 2 cm above the right pulmonary artery and at the level of or 1 cm below the tracheal carina (Fig. 5–9A). It appears as a continuation of the main pulmonary artery as it arches over the left main bronchus to enter the left pulmonary hilum.

Lower Mediastinum

The vascular structures contained in the lower mediastinum are the heart (see Chapter 9), the descending aorta, the azygos vein, and the hemiazygos vein (Fig. 5–10).

Before it enters the abdomen through the diaphragmatic retrocrural space, the descending aorta assumes a near midline position. The cali-

ber and the degree of tortuosity of the descending aorta vary depending on age and physique and on whether vascular disease is present. The normal ascending aorta is about 1.5 times larger in diameter than the descending aorta. It measures 3.0 to 4.0 cm, being wider toward its base.[10] In most people, the azygos vein is to the right and the hemiazygos vein is posterior to the descending aorta.

Thoracic Inlet

At the level of the thoracic inlet, 1 to 3 cm above the suprasternal notch, the vascular structures of the mediastinum undergo an abrupt reorientation (Figs. 5–11 through 5–13). The innominate artery assumes a position to the right of the anterior third of the trachea; it then divides into the right common carotid artery and the right subclavian artery. The right common carotid artery remains close to the right side of the trachea, whereas the right subclavian artery courses laterally toward the first rib (Fig. 5–12). The right brachiocephalic vein assumes a position to the right of the posterior or middle third of the trachea and receives its tributaries, the right internal jugular vein and the right subclavian vein. On the opposite side, the left common carotid artery takes up a position opposite the middle or posterior third of the left side of the trachea (Fig. 5–13). The left subclavian artery, meanwhile, moves anteriorly toward the left first rib. The left brachiocephalic vein maintains its anterolateral posi-

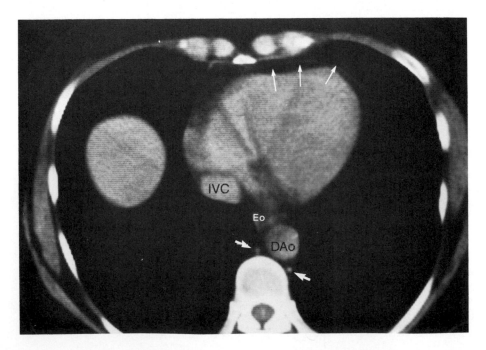

Figure 5–10. Normal anatomy of the lower mediastinum. The descending aorta (DAo) is at the left anterolateral aspect of the spine. The inferior vena cava (IVC) is anterior and to the right of the esophagus (Eo). Normal pericardium (long arrows) surrounds the anterior myocardium. Azygos and hemiazygos veins are to the right and behind the aorta, respectively (short arrows).

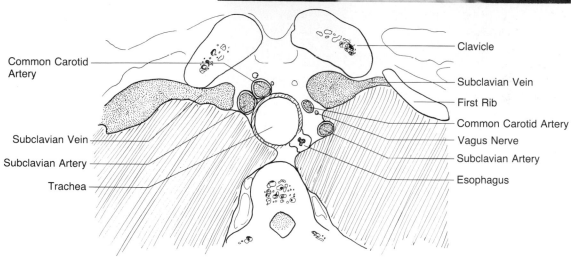

Figure 5–11. Normal anatomy at the level of the thoracic inlet. **A** CT scan after intravenous infusion of contrast medium, in a 50-year-old woman. **B** Schematic representation of the mediastinum at the same level.

Common Carotid Artery

Clavicle

Subclavian Vein

First Rib

Common Carotid Artery

Vagus Nerve

Subclavian Vein

Subclavian Artery

Subclavian Artery

Trachea

Esophagus

B

tion, receiving the left internal jugular and left subclavian veins.

MEDIASTINAL SPACES

The vessels, heart, trachea, mediastinal pleura, and bony structures that border the mediastinum create real or potential spaces.[1, 11] The computed tomographic appearances of these spaces have not been reported in detail, and the following description is based largely on observation of scans of 100 adult patients who had no significant mediastinal disease.

Retrosternal Space

The parietal mediastinal pleura becomes adherent to the inner thoracic cage lateral to the sternum.[12, 13] The retrosternal space is immediately behind and to either side of the sternum for a distance of about the width of the sternum (Figs.

5–4 through 5–6). It is limited anteriorly by transverse thoracic muscle.[14] Posteriorly it is continuous with the prevascular space. This space contains fat and connective tissue and varies markedly in size among individuals. The anterior margins of the two lungs may appose and be separated only by their pleural surfaces (Fig. 5–7). In obese individuals, up to 2 cm of mediastinal tissue can separate the lungs and the sternum then abuts low-density mediastinal fat posteriorly.

The inner margin of the thoracic cage lateral to the sternum has a predictable contour. When viewed at mediastinal window levels, it is slightly concave about half the time. The other half of the time, it appears straight. In about 10 per cent of people, the costochondral junctions cause a slight indentation. At the level of the anterior ends of the first ribs, a prominent indentation into the subapex of the lung is common.

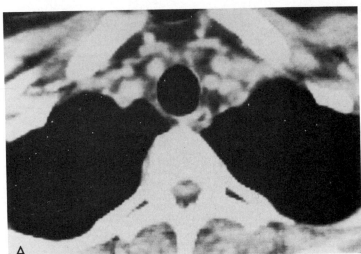

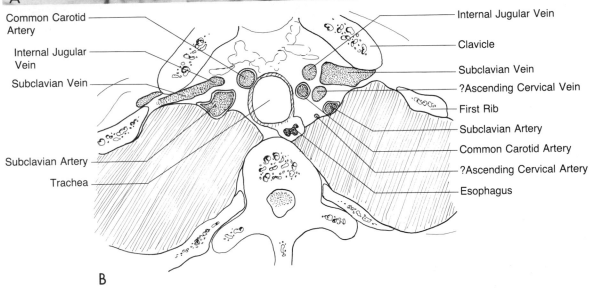

Figure 5–12. Normal anatomy at the level of the thoracic inlet. **A** CT scan 1 cm cephalad to Figure 5–11, after intravenous infusion of contrast medium, in a 50-year-old woman. **B** Schematic representation of the mediastinum at the same level.

Common Carotid Artery

Internal Jugular Vein

Subclavian Vein

Subclavian Artery

Trachea

Internal Jugular Vein

Clavicle

Subclavian Vein

?Ascending Cervical Vein

First Rib

Subclavian Artery

Common Carotid Artery

?Ascending Cervical Artery

Esophagus

Figure 5–13. Normal anatomy at the level of the thoracic inlet. **A** CT scan 1 cm cephalad to Figure 5–2, after intravenous infusion of contrast medium, in a 50-year-old woman. **B** Schematic representation of the mediastinum at the same level.

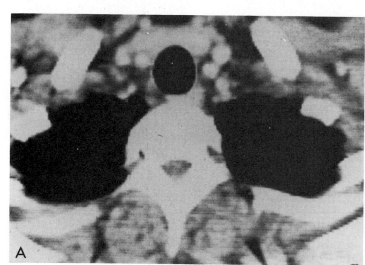

A

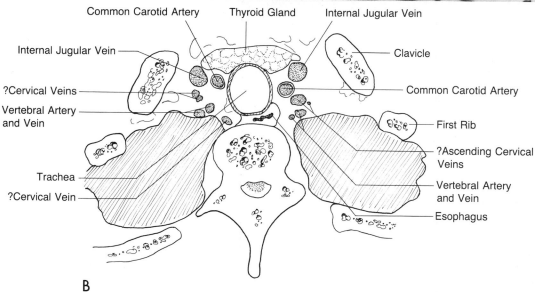

Common Carotid Artery   Thyroid Gland   Internal Jugular Vein

Internal Jugular Vein   Clavicle

?Cervical Veins   Common Carotid Artery

Vertebral Artery and Vein   First Rib

?Ascending Cervical Veins

Trachea   Vertebral Artery and Vein

?Cervical Vein   Esophagus

B

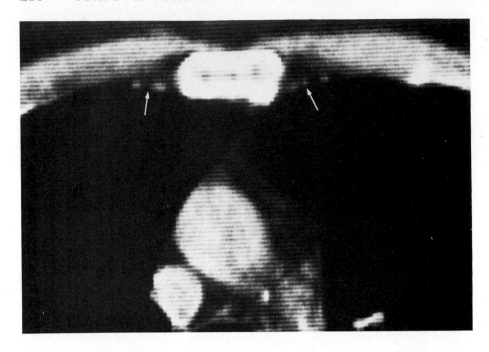

Figure 5–14. Normal internal mammary vessels. CT scan in a 48-year-old man, after contrast material infusion. Three vessels are visible on the left and two on the right (arrows), that were not demonstrated before contrast material infusion.

Small lymph nodes are normally present along the internal mammary vascular bundle, but they are rarely visible on CT scans. The internal mammary vascular bundles are not discernible without intravenously administered contrast material. After contrast infusion, one to three, but usually two, of these vascular structures are visible on each side of the sternum (Fig. 5–14). The internal mammary vessels are immediately subpleural and 2 to 5 cm from the midline (i.e., lateral to the sternum by one third to one half of its width).

Prevascular Space

The mediastinum anterior to the great vessels, ascending aorta, and anterior aortic arch forms the prevascular space (Figs. 5–4 through 5–8). It is continuous with the retrosternal space and is bordered by the lungs laterally. Posteriorly it is limited by the ascending aorta and arch vessels. It is, however, continuous with the aortic-pulmonic window lateral to the aortic arch and ascending aorta on the left side. The size of the prevascular space depends on the patient's adiposity and physique. The density of the fat in the prevascular space also varies considerably in normal people. Less than half of the time is the typical low density of fat found. About one third of the time, the density of the prevascular space is that of soft tissue, and in the remainder the density is irregular and inhomogeneous. Ill-defined bands of higher density are frequently visible crossing the prevascular space.

The normal contents of the prevascular space are the left brachiocephalic vein and the thymus gland. At the level of the origin of the arch vessels, or the upper ascending aorta, the left brachiocephalic vein crosses from upper left to lower right. If unopacified with contrast, the left brachiocephalic vein may be mistaken for an anterior mediastinal mass.[15]

Baron and colleagues[16] described the appearance of the normal thymus and the frequency with which it is seen on CT scans. The thymus is visible in all normal people under age 30, but in only 17 per cent of those over 49 years old. The density of the normal thymus decreases with age from above 30 H to less than −10 H. In one study of patients under age 20,[17] the size, appearance, and density of the normal thymus varied markedly. The gland, however, did tend to conform to the structures of the mediastinum and chest. It also usually had smooth lateral contours, whether convex or concave. A sharp, angular, lateral margin was only occasionally visible with CT. The thymus has an arrowhead, or bilobed, shape and is about 1 to 4 cm wide and 0.4 to 1.5 cm thick (Fig. 5–15A,B). The posterior cleft seen in the normal thymus has been emphasized by Moore and co-workers (Fig. 5–15B).[18] Dixon and colleagues[19] have correlated the mean CT number of the prevascular space with the percentage of residual thymus in this area assessed histologically. They confirm that this area is frequently inhomogeneous, at least partially because of variations in thymic involution and in fatty replacement.

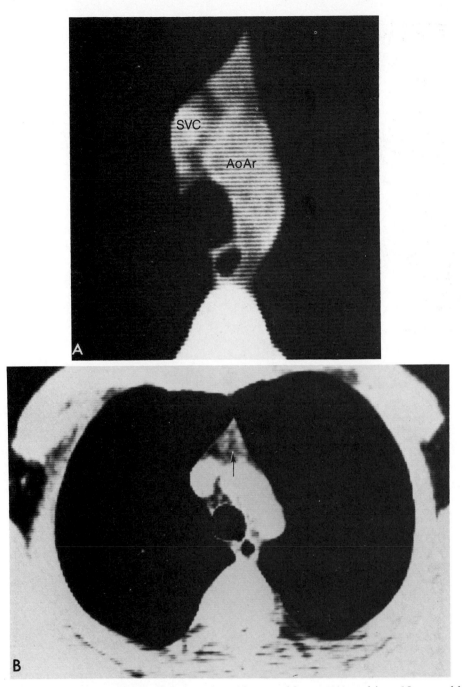

Figure 5–15. Normal thymus. **A, B** CT scans in a 22-year-old man **(A)** and in a 13-year-old boy **(B)**. A pyramidal structure lies in front of the aortic arch (AoAr) and superior vena cava (SVC). It does not bulge the anterior mediastinal pleura. A posterior cleft (arrow) is visible in the boy.

Lymph nodes are not normally visible in the prevascular space. However, in patients who have had granulomatous disease, small noncalcified nodes are commonly shown. In about 5 per cent of people, a tubular structure is visible lateral to the aortic arch (Fig. 5–16). This structure is probably either a mediastinal vein or the phrenic nerve, but its nature is not certain at this time.

Pretracheal Space

The pretracheal space has particular significance in computed mediastinal tomography. It contains many lymph nodes draining both lungs and the mediastinal organs. In addition, it is the space through which transcervical mediastinoscopy is performed. The pretracheal space does

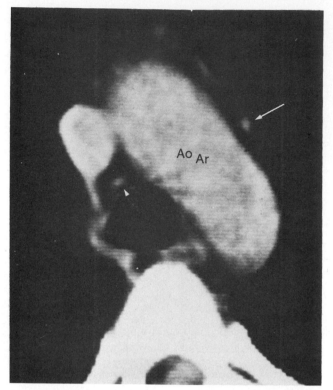

Figure 5–16. Normal mediastinal anatomy. CT scan in an adult man. Lateral to the aortic arch (AoAr) is a small tubular structure, probably the phrenic nerve or a mediastinal vein (arrow). A single normal azygos node is visible (arrowhead).

not border the lungs. On conventional radiographs, masses or lymph nodes must be of considerable size before becoming visible, but CT scans can demonstrate subtle enlargement of lymph nodes.

The pretracheal space extends vertically from the thoracic inlet to the tracheal carina (Figs. 5–1 to 5–6, 5–16, 5–17). The structures bordering the space depend on the level in the mediastinum. At lower levels, the space is bounded by the anterior convexity of the trachea, the medial wall of the azygos arch, the posteromedial wall of the superior vena cava, and the posterior wall of the ascending aorta (Fig. 5–8).[20] On the left side it is limited by the aortic arch or, in about 10 per cent of patients, it is continuous with the aortic-pulmonic window (Fig. 5–17). At upper levels, above the aortic arch, the pretracheal space is between the anterior arch of the trachea and the great vessels. The space contains the innominate artery in front of the trachea and the left common carotid and left subclavian arteries to the left. The superior vena cava and right brachiocephalic vein bound the pretracheal space on the right. Above the thoracic inlet the space continues into the deep fascial spaces of the neck.

The surface area of the pretracheal spaces varies widely among people. It increases with increasing mediastinal fat, age, and aortic unfolding. The CT density of the space is usually uniform and less than 0 H. As with mediastinal "fat" in general, the density varies among individuals. In one study[20] the mean density of inferior pretracheal space in normal individuals was found to range from -107 H to $+48$ H.

The pretracheal space contains fat and fibrous connective tissue and, around the trachea, numerous lymph nodes. However, the only lymph nodes regularly visible on CT scans of the mediastinum are the azygos nodes. In 50 to 90 per cent of normal individuals, one node is visible medial to the azygos arch (Figs. 5–8, 5–16, and 5–17). In 10 to 30 per cent, two nodes can be seen, and occasionally a third node is present. Normal azygos nodes are 5.5 ± 2.8 mm in diameter, measured at window settings suitable for viewing the mediastinum.[20] These nodes can, however, meas-

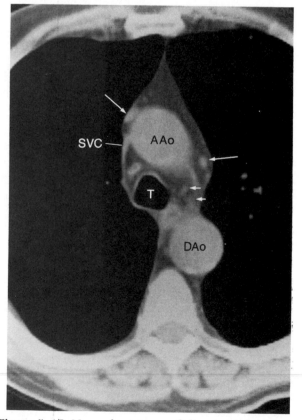

Figure 5–17. Normal anatomy of the pretracheal space and aortic-pulmonic window. Patient is a 76-year-old man who had had granulomatous disease. The pretracheal space lies between the trachea (T), the ascending aorta (AAo), and the superior vena cava (SVC). The aortic pulmonic window is between the ascending and descending aorta (DAo). Small lymph nodes (long arrows) are demonstrated in the prevascular space and in the aortic pulmonic window (short arrows).

ure up to 10 or 12 mm in diameter. We have sometimes seen additional small nodes 1 to 5 cm above the tracheal carina.

Aortic-Pulmonic Window

The aortic-pulmonic window is situated beneath the aortic arch and above the left pulmonary artery.[21] This space is bounded medially by the lower trachea and esophagus, and laterally by the left lung. It may be continuous with the inferior pretracheal space medially and the prevascular space lateral to the ascending aorta (Fig. 5–17).

On chest radiographs, the aortic-pulmonic window has a height of 2 to 3 cm. On CT scans obtained with the patient supine, the window frequently spans less than a single 1-cm scan. In more than 75 per cent of individuals, the window is obscured by volume-averaging from the undersurface of the aortic arch and the superior surface of the left pulmonary artery. The left lung rarely appears to penetrate this space, when viewed on CT scans, although it does appear to do so on chest radiographs.

The aortic-pulmonic window usually shows markedly inhomogeneous CT density; high-density bands frequently course through it. Lying between two pulsatile vascular structures, it is also frequently distorted by streak artifacts.

The aortic-pulmonic window contains lymph nodes (including the ductus node), the ligamentum arteriosum, and the recurrent laryngeal nerve. In our experience, normal lymph nodes are rarely visible within the window. Occasionally, a tubular structure appears to course across it, which may be the ligamentum arteriosum, but this has not been proved.

Subcarinal Space

Extending inferiorly from the pretracheal space is the subcarinal space. This is one of the more difficult areas of the mediastinum to assess using conventional radiographs. The height of the subcarinal space is approximately 2 cm. Its upper portion is bounded anteriorly by the right pulmonary artery, and on the left side by the mediastinal portion of the left superior pulmonary vein (Figs. 5–7 and 5–9B). The right and left main bronchi flank the space on either side. Posterior in the space is the esophagus, which is usually to the left of the midline, and the azygos vein, which is anterior to the spine. The right lung contacts the mediastinum behind the right main bronchus and bounds the subcarinal space posterolaterally. In its lower portion, the space is limited

on the right by the intermediate bronchus and inferiorly by the left atrium. In asthenic individuals, and in patients with emphysema, the aorta may be in the midline and form the posterior border of the subcarinal space.

The space normally contains mediastinal fat and connective tissue, and its CT density is moderately inhomogeneous. Three to five lymph nodes normally occupy the subcarinal space.[22, 23] In our experience, we have observed a single small lymph node immediately beneath the tracheal carina in about 10 per cent of people. Lymph nodes are not otherwise visible on CT scans of this region.

Retrotracheal Space and Posterior Mediastinum

The mediastinum posterior to the trachea and heart is elegantly displayed by computed tomography.[24, 25] Between the thoracic inlet and the azygos arch, the appearance of the retrotracheal region is determined by the relative positions of the esophagus and aorta and by the degree of contact of the right lung with the mediastinum. In about 50 per cent of individuals, the right lung contacts one quarter to one half of the posterior wall of the trachea (Fig. 5–11).[9] In the other 50 per cent, the right lung penetrates the retrotracheal mediastinum to a lesser extent, and the retrotracheal space is filled with mediastinal fat and connective tissue. Occasionally, if the trachea lies close to the spinal column, the space is small, and lung is precluded from entering it. In the supine patient, the midesophagus is often to the left of the midline. About one third of the time, the center of the esophagus is completely to the left of the lower trachea.

Variations in size, shape, and configuration of the posterior mediastinum are evident in the retrocardiac region. The position of the descending aorta varies with age, physique, and degree of lung inflation. It may be distinctly to the left of the spinal column, or it may approach the midline (Fig. 5–10). Toward the diaphragmatic crura, the descending aorta is in the midline. The esophagus likewise varies in position until it approaches the diaphragm. The ascending azygos vein maintains a fairly constant position in the midline or slightly to the right of midline anterior to the spinal column.

The lower posterior mediastinum is in direct continuity with the subcarinal space (Fig. 5–7). The right lung always contacts the posterior wall of the right main bronchus and intermediate bronchus. Posteromedial to the bronchial tree,

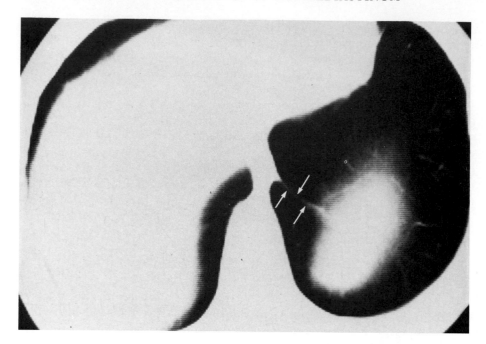

Figure 5–18. Normal anatomy of the lower mediastinum. A linear structure (arrows), representing the inferior pulmonary ligament, extends laterally from the mediastinum near the esophagus.

the right lung may intrude deeply into the posterior mediastinum and contact the esophagus, aorta, and azygos vein. Alternatively, the lower posterior mediastinum may be filled with mediastinal fat, preventing the lung from contact with these structures. In the latter instance, the right border of the posterior mediastinum is a straight line from the intermediate bronchus, pulmonary vein, or left atrium to the spine. In about 20 per cent of individuals, the anteroposterior dimension of the posterior mediastinum is small. The bronchial tree, right pulmonary vein, and heart are all close to the spine. In normal adults, the contour of the right posteroinferior mediastinum is almost always concave or straight. Occasionally, the esophagus bulges to the right in this area and can be mistaken for a mass or adenopathy. In children and infants, the mediastinum itself may bulge to the right, producing a right posterior mediastinal convexity.

In our experience, normal lymph nodes are not visible on CT scans of the posterior mediastinum. The azygos vein is seen in most people after infusion of contrast material; and in 25 to 50 per cent of people, the hemiazygos vein is also visible ascending on the left side immediately behind the descending aorta.

In about 10 per cent of people, a structure is seen that probably represents the inferior pulmonary ligament, although this has not been described or proved. It appears as a thin line immediately above the diaphragm, extending laterally from the lower mediastinum for 2 to 3 cm (Fig. 5–18).

Retrocrural Space

The retrocrural space is a distinctive and well-defined inferior extension of the posterior mediastinum.[8, 26] Before the development of computed tomography, this area received little recognition. The diaphragmatic crura originate as tendons that blend with the anterior longitudinal ligament of the lumbar vertebrae (Fig. 5–19). The muscular fibers of the two crura intermingle to form the aortic hiatus. The right crus is noticeably larger and longer than the left. Each crus passes from one side of the vertebral body to the anterior wall of the aorta. Several structures, in addition to the aorta, traverse this space. The thoracic duct and azygos vein lie to the right of the aorta; the hemiazygos vein is to the left. Intercostal arteries and splanchnic nerves also course through the retrocrural space. The CT density of this space has not been measured but usually appears uniform and low, equivalent to that of retroperitoneal fat. Except for the aorta, the normal structures within the retrocrural space do not measure more than 6 mm in diameter when viewed at a window width of 200 H and a level of 10 to 30 H. Some of the structures seen on CT scans opacify with intravenous contrast material, and normal lymph nodes either are small or are not seen.

MEDIASTINAL LINES

Mediastinal lines observed on chest radiographs are either interfaces between the lung and mediastinum or sites where the two lungs approach

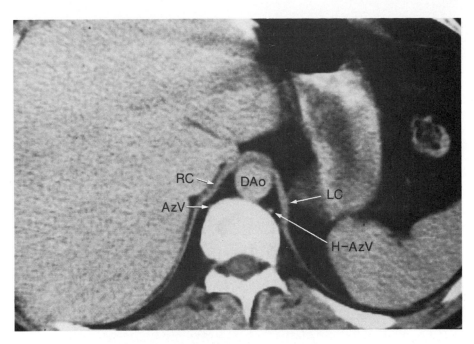

Figure 5–19. Normal anatomy of the retrocrural space. The right diaphragmatic crus (RC) meets the left crus (LC) anterior to the descending aorta (DAo). The azygos vein (AzV) (better seen at other levels in this patient) and hemiazygos vein (H-AzV) are visible.

each other. Computed mediastinal tomography permits observation of mediastinal lines in a transverse plane and allows for insight as to their nature.

Anterior Junction Line

The anterior junction line lies anterior to the aorta and heart, where the anteromedial portion of each lung approaches the midline. It is seen on 20 to 25 per cent of anteroposterior radiographs of normal chests, commencing at the manubrium and extending inferiorly and slightly to the left for several centimeters.[27, 28] The line represents the visceral and parietal pleurae and a small quantity of mediastinal fat between them. This region of the mediastinum is well demonstrated on CT scans, and the reason for the anterior junction line being visible on chest radiographs in only 20 to 25 per cent of individuals is evident (Fig. 5–20). In the other 75 to 80 per cent, the lungs are separated by enough mediastinal fat as not to approach each other. If the anterior junc-

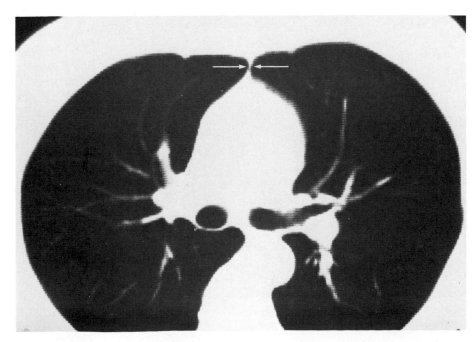

Figure 5–20. Normal anatomy of the anterior junction line. The two lungs approach the midline anterior to the ascending aorta. The line (arrows) is composed of four layers of pleura and a varying amount of mediastinal fat and fibrous tissue.

tion line is obliterated by disease, CT scans can demonstrate the cause, which may be ascending aorta prominence or an aneurysm, lymphadenopathy, tumor, or mediastinal infiltration.[29]

Posterior Junction Line

The two lungs approach each other behind the esophagus and in front of the spine above the aortic arch. On chest radiographs of the erect patient, the posterior junction line projects vertically as a somewhat thick stripe through the tracheal air column. It invariably extends above the suprasternal notch, which distinguishes it from the anterior junction line. Variations in the normal thickness of the posterior junction line limit its use in defining mediastinal disease. On CT scans of the supine patient, mediastinal structures tend to lie against the spine, so it is unusual for the lungs to appose posteriorly (Fig. 5–21A). On CT scans of the prone patient, the posterior junction line is seen more frequently.

When air is present in the esophagus, a soft tissue stripe may appear on frontal radiographs and on CT scans separating air in the lungs from air within the esophagus (Fig. 5–21B). This is the esophageal-pleural stripe and may be present on

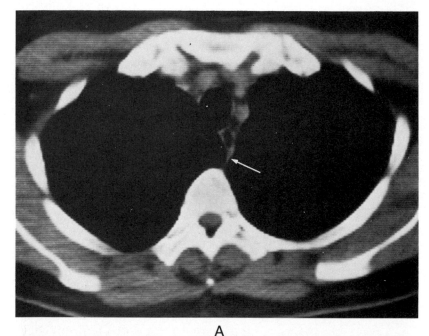

A

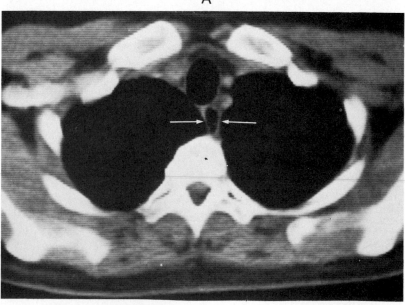

B

Figure 5–21. Normal anatomy of the posterior junction line. Patient is a 39-year-old man. **A** The two lungs appose behind the esophagus to produce a single line (arrow). **B** Two centimeters cephalad, air in the esophagus produces right and left esophageal-pleural stripes (arrows).

either or both sides of the esophagus.[30–32] The stripe comprises visceral and parietal pleurae, mediastinal fat, and the esophageal wall. Thickening of the esophageal-pleural stripe may be due to diseases affecting pleura, mediastinal contents, or the esophageal wall, and computed tomography can elegantly display the cause.

Right Paratracheal Stripe

The right paratracheal stripe is an important and sensitive indicator of disease on chest radiographs. In most adults, this stripe or line is up to 4 mm thick when measured between air in the right lung and air in the trachea.[29, 33] The stripe comprises pleura, mediastinal fat, connective tissue, and the wall of the trachea. On computed tomograms, the right wall of the trachea is well shown in all individuals (Figs. 5–1 to 5–6, 5–11, 5–12). The extent of contact of the right lung with the right wall of the trachea varies, but in most instances, the posterior one half to two thirds of the trachea contacts the right lung. Absence of the right paratracheal stripe on radiographs may be due not to disease but to excessive mediastinal fat separating the trachea from the right lung. Abnormal thickening of the stripe can be caused by tracheal, mediastinal, or pleural disease. The most common cause is enlarged pretracheal lymph nodes extending to the right of the trachea. Computed tomography can usually show the cause of an abnormally wide right paratracheal stripe.

Posterior Tracheal Band or Stripe

On about 80 per cent of well-penetrated lateral chest radiographs, a line up to 5 mm wide can be seen posterior to the tracheal air column.[24, 25, 34] The posterior tracheal stripe consists of tracheal wall, mediastinal tissue, and pleura, separating air in the trachea from air in the right lung (Fig. 5–15B). This stripe is in fact the posterior continuation of the right paratracheal stripe. It may not be visible, however, on chest radiographs when the right lung does not enter the retrotracheal mediastinum sufficiently to produce a tangential interface. On computed tomograms of the supine patient, the right lung normally contacts less than 50 per cent of the posterior tracheal wall. Presumably, on CT scans of prone patients and chest radiographs of erect patients, contact will be greater. This stripe is absent on chest radiographs when there is a very small tracheoesophageal recess or a fat-filled retrotracheal space (visible on CT scans). The width of the posterior tracheal stripe can vary over its length with differing amounts of retrotracheal tissue.

The posterior stripe may appear thickened on chest radiographs when the esophagus contains air and is in midline because the anterior esophageal wall then contributes to the thickness of the stripe (Fig. 5–15A). Computed tomograms can distinguish between thickening of the stripe due to disease and thickening due to variation in the position of the esophagus.

Abnormal thickening of the stripe is most commonly caused by primary or recurrent carcinoma of the esophagus.[35] Thickening may also result from esophageal dilatation, an aberrant subclavian artery, tracheal tumors, and mediastinal lymphadenopathy.

TECHNIQUES OF EXAMINATION

The technique for performing computed tomography of the thorax and mediastinum differs markedly among institutions.[36] In most hospitals, the study is limited by constraints of time, the technical capabilities of the equipment, and the availability of clinical information. A routine format becomes established and, in our opinion, insufficient consideration is given to the potential for extending the examination. An eclectic approach should be adopted for each patient, and the technique modified to obtain the scans most appropriate to the problem being investigated. The literature is deficient in describing how varying lung volumes and patient positions as well as different respiratory maneuvers can increase the diagnostic information from mediastinal CT. The optimum dose of contrast material and timing of contrast infusion have been studied,[37–40] but the results of these studies are often not fully exploited.

RESPIRATION

Most patients are able to suspend respiration long enough to complete at least one scan or, with modern equipment, multiple scans. If possible, CT scans should always be obtained with the patient holding the breath. If breath-holding is not possible, the patient should breathe quietly through the mouth to minimize motion artifacts.

The optimum lung volume for mediastinal scanning is maximum deep inspiration (total lung capacity), which is reproducible and provides the best demonstration of the lungs and mediastinum. Most patients achieve full inspiration more comfortably and are able to sustain this lung volume after taking a few deep breaths. This may be a useful routine to adopt, especially for older patients. The effects of respiratory maneuvers, such as a Valsalva maneuver, on CT images of normal mediastinal structures and on mediastinal masses of different types have not been reported.

POSITION

Most computed tomograms of the thorax are obtained with the patient supine. In adults, the patient's arms are placed above the head to reduce scan artifacts. Little is known about the appearance of the mediastinum on scans obtained with the patient prone, in which position the heart and mediastinum tend to fall forward toward the sternum (Fig. 5–22A,B).[41]

For the evaluation of posterior mediastinal masses or structures such as the esophagus, prone scans may be more appropriate, although this has not been investigated. Scans can also be obtained with the patient in the decubitus position, although this position does not seem to offer advantages in the mediastinum. Scanners with a wide aperture allow the examination to be performed with the patient seated; direct coronal scans are then possible.[42] This position may improve the imaging of posterior mediastinal lesions and lesion near the diaphragm, but such imaging awaits further evaluation.

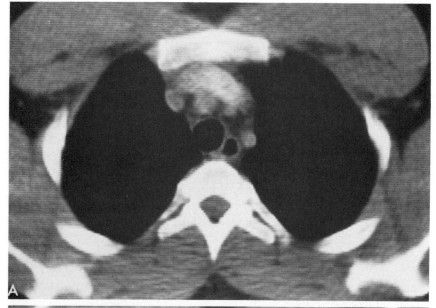

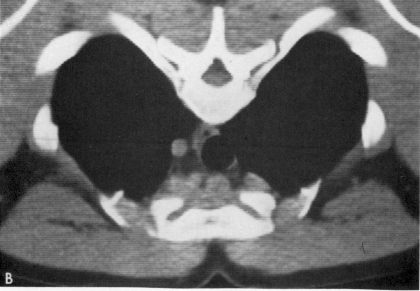

Figure 5–22. Normal upper mediastinal anatomy. **A, B** Differences between supine (**A**) and prone (**B**) images. On the prone scan, the arch vessels are displaced forward against the sternum. The left brachiocephalic vein is compressed and no longer seen. The esophagus assumes a near midline position.

CONTRAST MATERIAL

Use of intravenous contrast material greatly facilitates the interpretation of CT scans of the mediastinum. Intravenous contrast medium details vascular landmarks, facilitates the detection of vessel enlargement and abnormal vessels, and by enhancement can show highly vascular masses.

In most institutions, computed mediastinal tomography is performed only after intravenous infusion of contrast material.[36] The accepted precautions with intravenous iodinated contrast agents must be observed. The usual adult dose is 125 to 150 ml of 60 per cent contrast (35.25 to 42.3 g of organically bound iodine) administered by rapid intravenous drip.[37] Two thirds of the contrast medium should be infused in the first 5 minutes. After the infusion of contrast medium, the intravascular iodine concentration rapidly reaches a peak, then steeply declines.[38, 39] The examination should therefore be completed while the contrast material is being infused. A technique should be developed to achieve maximum intravascular iodine concentration. For unusually long examinations, administration of repeated boluses of contrast material may be a suitable alternative to the drip technique.

Several commercial scanners are capable of performing rapid sequential scanning with an interscan delay of seconds. This modification allows an intravenous bolus of contrast material to be followed throughout the vascular bed (Fig. 5–23). A bolus of 25 to 30 ml of 76 or 90 per cent is injected in less than 10 seconds. An extremely high intravascular concentration of contrast medium is achieved, providing several advantages.[40] Masses can be more easily separated from vessels, and veins can be differentiated from arteries (Fig. 5–23). Intravascular thrombi and emboli can be demonstrated. Aortic dissections can be more easily defined. Small vascular structures, such as coronary artery bypass grafts, may also be shown.

TECHNICAL CONSIDERATIONS

The major cause of degradation of images of the mediastinum is the presence of streak artifacts from the edges of pulsatile vascular structures.[43] These artifacts can be diminished by technique manipulations. For the mediastinum, the shortest possible scan time should be used.[43] Streak artifacts occur less toward the center of the field, and meticulous attention should be given to patient positioning. In general, the finer the resolution of the scans, the greater the number of scan artifacts. A large scan-file should therefore be used. For example, with the GE 8800 scanner we employ a 42-cm file.

Projection radiographs (e.g., scout views) are useful in planning computed mediastinal tomography. For evaluation of focal lesions, the projection radiograph can be correlated with the conventional chest radiographs to determine the number of CT scans needed to demonstrate the area of interest. A projection radiograph is especially useful in planning CT investigation of vascular lesions, including anomalies of the great vessels and aortic dissections, where specific levels are to be studied with rapid sequential scans.

The most appropriate window levels and win-

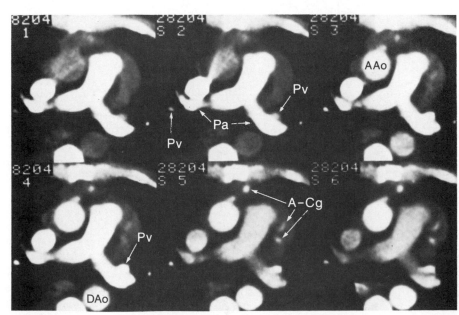

Figure 5–23. Anatomy demonstrated by six rapid sequential scans. Scans were obtained at intervals of approximately 3 sec. The pulmonary arteries (Pa) can be separated from pulmonary veins (Pv). The ascending aorta (AAo) and descending aorta (DAo) opacify in sequence. Incidentally visible are three aortocoronary bypass grafts (A-Cg).

dow widths for viewing the mediastinum are determined by the equipment and the eye of the beholder. Generally, for the mediastinum, a window width between 100 and 250 H and a window level between 10 and 60 H are used.

PATHOLOGY

VASCULAR LESIONS

Arterial Anomalies of the Mediastinum

The embryonically paired aortic arches may develop anomalously and result in specific malformations of the thoracic aorta and arch vessels (Fig. 5–24 and Table 5–1). The majority of patients with aortic arch anomalies are asymptomatic. When a complete vascular ring is present, symptoms may result from airway or esophageal compression. Most patients with arch malformations will have a chest radiograph suggestive of the anomaly. In patients with aortic arch anoma-

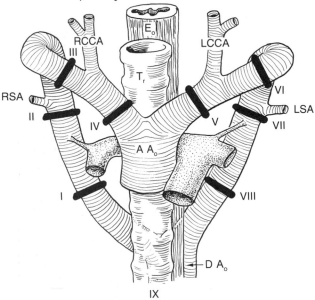

Figure 5–24. Schematic representation of the embryonic development of the paired aortic arches with sites of potential interruption. The ascending aorta (AAo) divides into a right and left arch. The right arch gives rise to the common carotid artery (RCCA) and right subclavian artery (RSA), whereas the left arch gives off the left common carotid artery (LCCA) and left subclavian artery (LSA). The aortic arches unite behind the trachea (Tr) and esophagus (Eo) to form the descending aorta (DAo)   I = Normal. II = Left aortic arch with aortic diverticulum. III = Left aortic arch with an aberrant right subclavian artery. IV = Left aortic arch with an aberrant right innominate artery. V = Right aortic arch with an aberrant left innominate artery. VI = Right aortic arch with an aberrant left subclavian artery. VII = Right aortic arch with mirror image branching (rare). VIII = Right aortic arch with mirror image branching (common). IX = Double aortic arch (no interruption).

Table 5–1.   AORTIC ARCH ANOMALIES

Left aortic arch with aberrant right subclavian artery
Left aortic arch with aberrant right innominate artery
Left aortic arch with right descending aorta
Right aortic arch with mirror-image branching
Right aortic arch with aberrant left subclavian artery
Right aortic arch with aberrant left innominate artery
Right aortic arch with isolation of the left subclavian artery
Double aortic arch with both arches patent
Double aortic arch with partial atresia of one
Cervical aortic arch
Atresia of the aortic arch
Coarctation of the aorta
Aortic valve atresia
Supravalvular aortic stenosis

lies, CT scans are often obtained to investigate a mediastinal mass or mediastinal widening. Baron and co-workers[44] found five of 71 mediastinal masses evaluated with CT to be arch anomalies. Arch anomalies can also be incidental and can present potentially confusing findings in a patient undergoing CT scanning for other reasons. Webb[45] and McLaughlin[46] and their colleagues showed that if an aortic anomaly is suspected, computed tomography is a simple, noninvasive method for accurately determining the abnormality. Only the more common arterial anomalies and those that have been noted on CT scans will be discussed.

COARCTATION OF THE AORTA. This is a localized deformity of the media resulting in an infolding of the aortic wall.[47] An eccentric narrowing of the aortic lumen results. Coarctation most often occurs distal to the left subclavian artery. Usually the segments of aorta between the left subclavian artery and the coarctation are also hypoplastic and slightly narrowed.

The CT findings in two patients with coarctation of the aorta and one patient after repair of a coarctation have been reported.[48] Images reformatted in the plane of the aortic arch showed a narrow, deformed aortic isthmus—the segment of aorta between the left subclavian artery and the ligamentum arteriosum. The coarctation itself was probably not seen. The relatively poor spatial resolution of presently available scanners and the reformatted images derived from them probably do not allow for accurate imaging of the degree of stenosis of most aortic coarctations. At present, CT cannot image webs or short strictures in such vessels as the aorta.

The CT findings in one case of pseudocoarctation of the aorta have also been described.[49] The high, anteriorly situated distal arch and the buckled proximal descending aorta could be demonstrated. Also, a portion of the left lung was seen indenting the mediastinum between the redundant aortic arch and the spine. The latter finding is occasionally seen in normal individuals and may not be specific for pseudocoarctation. It is unlikely that these computed tomographic features can allow the diagnosis of pseudocoarctation of the aorta to be made with any accuracy.

ABERRANT SUBCLAVIAN ARTERY. An aberrant right subclavian artery in the presence of an otherwise normal aorta is the most common anomaly of aortic arch development, occurring in approximately one in 200 people.[50] The anomalous subclavian artery arises from the distal aortic arch as its last major vessel. The aberrant artery crosses the posterior mediastinum obliquely upward from left to right. Symptoms are uncommon, but widening of the superior mediastinum and bowing of the trachea anteriorly are not infrequently seen on chest radiographs (Fig. 5–25A). Several CT findings reflect the aortic maldevelopment. The aortic arch is higher than normal with a more directly anteroposterior orientation.[45] The aberrant right subclavian artery arises from the most su-

perior portion of the arch or from the beginning of the descending aorta (Fig. 5–25B). Dilatation of the origin of the aberrant right subclavian artery is common, and if excessive, is called a diverticulum of the aorta (Fig. 5–25C). Unless recognized as the dilated segment of an anomalous artery, it can be misdiagnosed as an aortic aneurysm.[45, 46]

An aberrant left subclavian artery arises from a right aortic arch and is less common than an aberrant right subclavian artery, occurring in approximately one in 1000 people.[51, 52] About 10 per cent of patients with this anomaly will also have congenital heart disease. The CT appearances of the malformed aorta and aberrant left subclavian artery are similar to those seen with an aberrant right subclavian artery, although the posterior portion of the aortic arch is often more midline than normal, assuming a position behind the trachea and displacing the esophagus to the left.

RIGHT AORTIC ARCH MALFORMATIONS. By definition, a right aortic arch is to the right of the trachea and esophagus. The normal arrangement of the arch vessels is determined by the site at

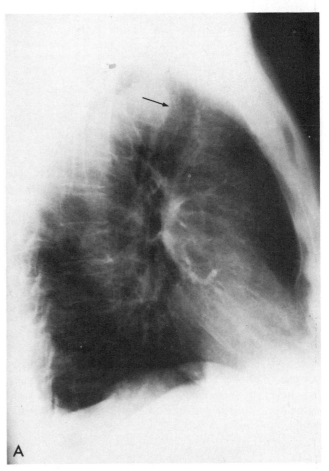

Figure 5–25. Aberrant right subclavian artery. Patient is an asymptomatic 71-year-old man. **A** A retrotracheal mass displaces the trachea (arrow) anteriorly.

Illustration continued on following page

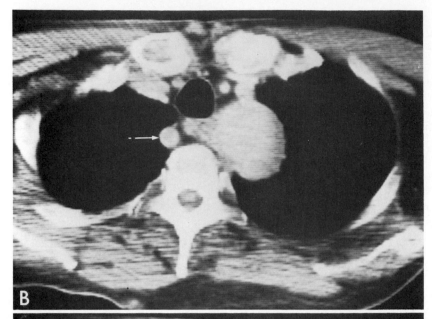

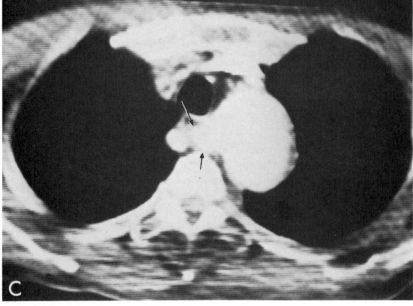

Figure 5–25. *Continued* **B** At the level of the mass, an abnormally situated right subclavian artery (arrow), as well as the retrotracheal mass, is visible. The aortic arch is abnormally high. **C** After a bolus of contrast material has been injected, the retrotracheal mass is shown to be the dilated proximal portion of the anomalous right subclavian artery (arrows).

which the left aortic arch is embryonically interrupted.

With a right aortic arch and aberrant left subclavian artery, embryonic interruption is between the left common carotid artery and the left subclavian artery (Fig. 5–24). This form of arch malformation has been detailed earlier in this chapter.

Two kinds of aberrant left subclavian artery can occur. In one, the descending aorta descends on the left of the spine. In the other, it descends on the right (Fig. 5–26A,B). With both variations, a vascular ring is present, although tracheoesophageal compression is rare.

An additional very rare anomaly of the right aortic arch, which can be diagnosed from computed tomograms, is the aberrant left innominate artery. With computed tomography, the branching order of the arch vessels can usually be ascertained. In the case of an aberrant left innominate artery, the origin of the right common carotid artery is before the right subclavian artery. The anomalous aberrant left innominate artery will arise from the medial aspect of the distal right arch and will produce a symptomatic vascular ring.

When aortic interruption is distal to the left subclavian artery, mirror-image branching is produced.[53] Two types are found; the commoner oc-

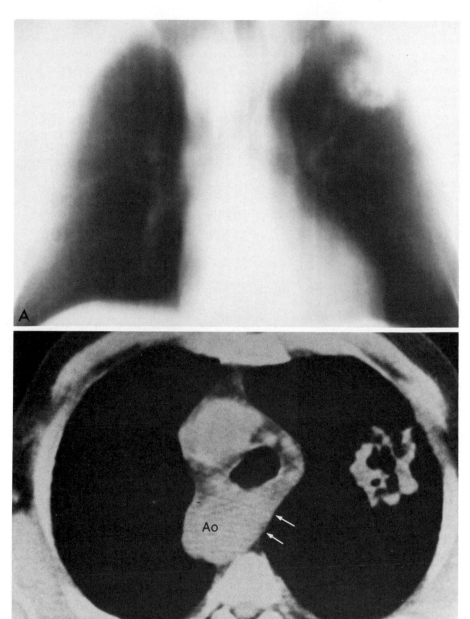

Figure 5–26. Right aortic arch with aberrant left subclavian artery. Patient is a 68-year-old man. **A** A conventional tomogram shows a left upper lobe bronchogenic carcinoma and right mediastinal mass. **B** CT scan shows that the right mediastinal mass is a right aortic arch (Ao). The dilated proximal portion (arrows) of an anomalous left subclavian artery is also demonstrated.

curs when interruption is distal to the left ductus arteriosus and a vascular ring is not produced. Virtually all patients with this type of branching will have congenital heart disease, usually tetralogy of Fallot or truncus arteriosus. A rare form of mirror-image right aortic arch occurs when the left arch is interrupted proximal to the left ductus arteriosus.[54]

The CT findings in most of the rare forms of right aortic arch malformations have not been described. However, the diagnoses can readily be made using computed tomography. For example, if a right aortic arch with mirror-image branching

of the arch vessels is shown and if a dilated retrotracheal aorta is seen, the rarer form of mirror-image branching should be suggested.

DOUBLE AORTIC ARCH. Double aortic arch is the most important of the arch anomalies producing a vascular ring.[55] It is rarely associated with congenital heart disease, but symptoms of tracheoesophageal compression are common. Two broad groups of double aortic arch are found. In the first, both arches are patent and functional; in the second group, a portion of the left arch is atretic.

The CT findings in double aortic arch have

been described in a few cases.[45, 46] They accurately reflect the anatomic position of the aortic arches and arch vessels. The right arch is usually the larger and higher, and it courses behind the esophagus to join the left arch (Fig. 5–27A–D). The aorta usually descends on the left. The images near the thoracic inlet will demonstrate the four arch vessels, situated symmetrically around the trachea and each arising independently from the two aortas (Fig. 5–27A).

RARE ARTERIAL ANOMALIES. The CT findings in one or two cases of uncommon anomalies of the aorta and pulmonary artery have been reported. Among these anomalies are an aneurysm of the ductus arteriosus, a left aortic arch with right descending aorta, an anomalous left pulmonary artery, transposition of the great vessels, and a hypoplastic right pulmonary artery.[45, 56–58a] As with the more common vascular anomalies, CT scanning using intravenous infusion of contrast material enables the diagnosis to be made with a high degree of accuracy.

Venous Anomalies of the Mediastinum

Anomalies of the great thoracic veins rarely result in symptoms but can cause confusing mediastinal contours on chest radiographs that call for further evaluation using CT. They may also produce unusual vascular structures that can be seen incidentally on computed tomograms obtained

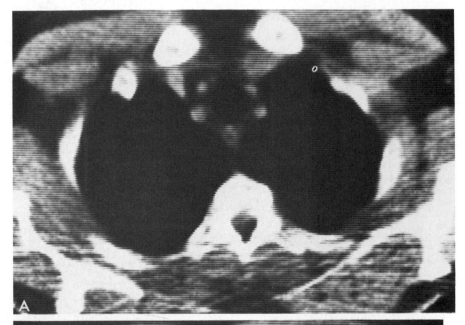

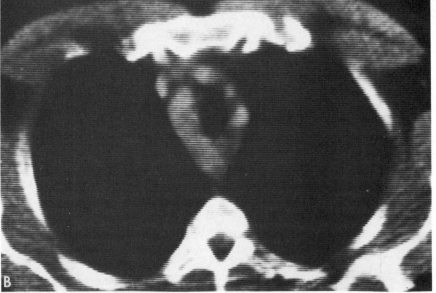

Figure 5–27. Double aortic arch. Patient is an asymptomatic young man with a superior mediastinal mass. **A** Above the aortic arches, four vessels are positioned symmetrically around the trachea. **B** Two centimeters caudad, a right arch becomes visible.

Illustration continued on opposite page

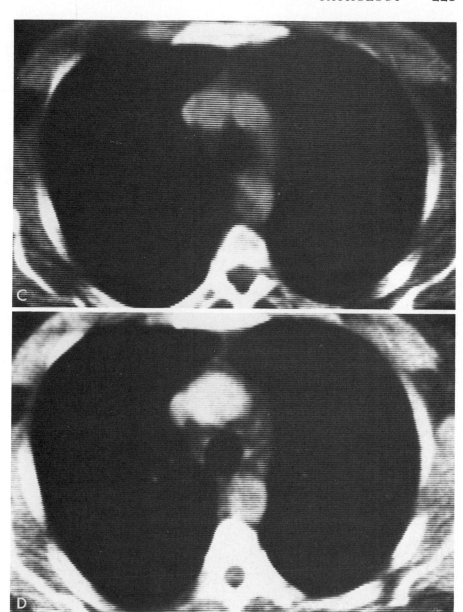

Figure 5–27. *Continued* **C** Two centimeters further caudad, the left aortic arch is now visible. **D** An additional one centimeter caudad, a single ascending and descending aorta appears.

for other reasons. It is important, therefore, to recognize them and to know their appearance.

Anomalous development may involve the vena caval systems or the azygos systems. Only the more common anomalies, for which the CT findings have been reported, are discussed here. The principles apply to other venous anomalies, and computed tomography should be able to define them accurately.

AZYGOS LOBE. The most common maldevelopment of the thoracic veins is lateral displacement of the arch of the azygos vein. This anomaly occurs in 0.4 to 1.0 per cent of the population and is referred to as the azygos lobe because the medial portion of the right upper lobe is trapped by the azygos fissure and vein. The embryonic

derivation of the malposition of the azygos vein is from premature descent of the right posterior cardinal vein. A portion of the right upper lobe lung bud becomes trapped between it and the mediastinum.

Computed tomography has been instrumental in defining the spectrum of alterations in mediastinal anatomy associated with an azygos lobe.[9] The azygos vein is displaced cephalad and joins the SVC in an abnormal position close to the junction of the left and right brachiocephalic veins. The superior 2 to 3 cm of the ascending azygos vein lies to the right of the spine and, as it leaves the spine, may resemble a lung nodule when viewed on a single scan. Frequently the axis of the SVC is abnormally oriented toward the left.

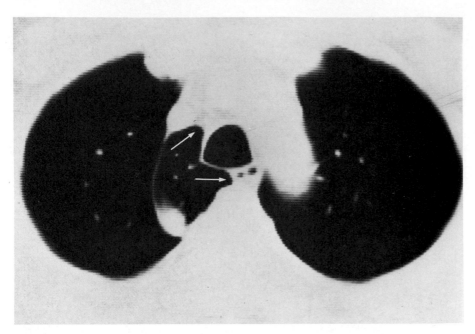

Figure 5–28. Azygos lobe. Lung within the azygos lobe protrudes into the mediastinum behind the superior vena cava (upper arrow) and the trachea (lower arrow).

The contact between the right upper lobe and the mediastinum also differs from normal when an azygos lobe is present. The lung often intrudes between the SVC and the trachea to an excessive degree and contacts their medioposterior and anterior walls, respectively (Fig. 5–28). This intrusion can often be seen on lateral chest radiographs as a lucency behind the SVC. The lung within the azygos lobe also often intrudes into the retrotracheal space, displacing the esophagus to the left and outlining the posterior wall of the trachea.

LEFT SUPERIOR VENA CAVA.   Persistence of the embryonic left anterior cardinal vein results in a left SVC. This is a relatively common anomaly, present in 0.3 per cent of normal individuals and about 5 per cent of patients with congenital heart disease.[59–61] Most people with a left SVC also have the right SVC. In two thirds of these, the left brachiocephalic vein is small or absent. The left SVC may be smaller than its counterpart on the right or the two may be equal in size. Communication of the left SVC with the hemiazygos system may be present. In patients with a left SVC, an additional contour to the left superior mediastinum is frequently visible on frontal radiographs. CT scans may be obtained to investigate this abnormal contour, or, alternatively, a left SVC may be an incidental finding on scans obtained for other reasons.

The CT findings of a left SVC are readily apparent.[62, 63] Within the upper mediastinum, the left SVC is positioned lateral to the left common carotid artery and anterior to the left subclavian artery (Fig. 5–29A). As it descends, the vein is visible left of the aortic arch and main pulmonary artery (Fig. 29B). It then passes in front of the left hilum and enters the oblique coronary vein and coronary sinus posterior to the left atrium and ventricle. In the upper mediastinum, the position of the left SVC resembles that of its counterpart on the right, whereas at lower levels it is more posterior. When there is a left SVC, the left brachiocephalic vein is seen on CT scans in a minority of patients.

AZYGOS AND HEMIAZYGOS CONTINUATION OF THE INFERIOR VENA CAVA.   The inferior vena cava (IVC) is derived from three sets of paired veins: supracardinal, subcardinal, and postcardinal.[64] If the infrahepatic segment of the IVC, derived from subcardinal veins, fails to achieve patency, the intermediate segments of the supracardinal veins will join the IVC to the azygos or hemiazygos systems.

Berdon and Baker[65] have shown that azygos continuation of the IVC may be suspected from the radiographic appearances of an enlarged azygos system. However, an enlarged azygos system has frequently been mistaken for a mediastinal mass or for posterior mediastinal lymphadenopathy. With hemiazygos continuation of the IVC, the dilated hemiazygos vein may not communicate with the azygos system and will course up the left side of the mediastinum to produce a retroaortic mass. The suprahepatic portion of the IVC is derived from hepatic sinusoids and the in-

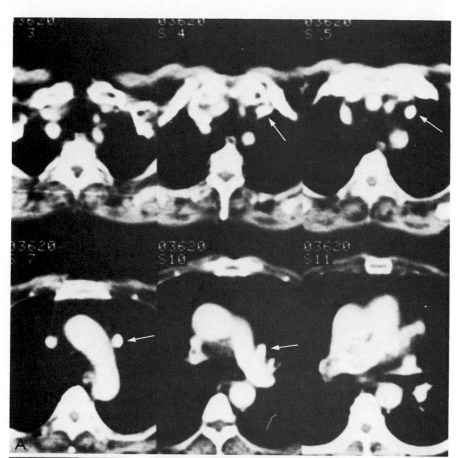

Figure 5–29. Persistent left superior vena cava. **A** Serial contiguous 1-cm images show the left superior vena cava (arrows) descending on the left side of the mediastinum. A normal right superior vena cava is present. The left brachiocephalic vein is not visible. **B** CT scans reformatted in the coronal plane, in another patients, demonstrate a persistent left superior vena cava descending lateral to the aorta and main pulmonary artery.

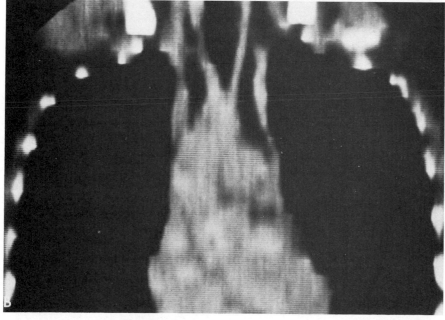

trathoracic IVC is usually present with azygos continuation. Therefore, the finding of an IVC on chest radiographs does not preclude the diagnosis of azygos or hemiazygos continuation.

The CT findings of azygos continuation of the IVC, or of hemiazygos continuation of the IVC with connection to the azygos system, are definitive enough to exclude the use of venography for diagnosis.[66–68a] In patients with azygos continuation of the IVC or with hemiazygos continuation of the IVC with connection to the azygos vein, findings in the upper thorax are the same. The

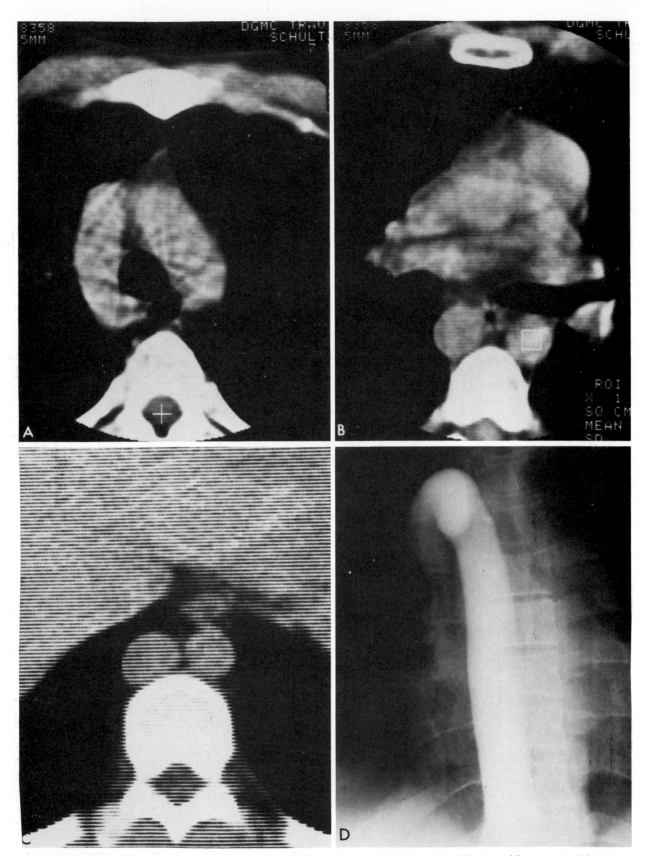

Figure 5–30. Azygos continuation of the inferior vena cava. Patient is a 29-year-old woman with a mass in the right upper mediastinum. **A** CT scan at the level of the aortic arch shows an enlarged azygos arch to the right of the trachea. **B, C** At the level of the tracheal carina and diaphragm, the ascending azygos vein is equal in size to the descending aorta. **D** The thoracic portion of an inferior venacavogram shows the dilated azygos vein. The cephalic portion of the inferior vena cava was absent.

ascending azygos vein, the azygos arch, and the distal SVC are dilated from increased blood flow. In azygos continuation, the dilated azygos vein exits the abdomen through the retrocrural space. Without infusion of contrast medium, the dilated azygos vein can be mistaken for a retrocrural mass. The vein ascends in a normal position in front of the spine along or slightly right of the midline (Fig. 5–30A–D). The dilated azygos is often equal to the aorta in diameter. With hemiazygos continuation of the IVC, having an azygos connection, the dilated hemiazygos vein lies posterior to the aorta and to the left of the spine (Fig. 5–31).[69] It then crosses the posterior mediastinum to join the azygos system. In hemiazygos continuation of the IVC, without azygos connection, the dilated hemiazygos vein stays on the left and drains into a dilated left superior intercostal vein or persistent left SVC.[70]

Several anomalies associated with azygos and hemiazygos continuation of the IVC can occur and should be sought on CT scans. Among these are a left IVC, duplication of the IVC, polysplenia, and congenital heart disease.

RARE VENOUS ANOMALIES. The CT findings for many less common malformations of the thoracic veins have not been reported. However, CT should be able to detail any venous malformation of the chest. Bolus injections of contrast medium with rapid sequential scanning will usually assist in defining these anomalies.

DISEASES OF THE THORACIC AORTA

Aortic Aneurysms

The demonstration and characterization of thoracic aortic aneurysms by CT scans have been described in several reports.[71–76] By definition, an aneurysm of the thoracic aorta is a dilatation of all components of the vessel wall. The morphologic types of aortic aneurysms are saccular, fusiform, dissecting, false, and sinus of Valsalva. This section deals only with saccular and fusiform aneurysms. Acquired aortic aneurysms are arteriosclerotic, luetic, mycotic, traumatic, or from medial necrosis; both saccular and fusiform aneurysms are most commonly arteriosclerotic. The diameter of a fusiform aneurysm is by definition greater than 4 cm.[77] A saccular aneurysm can be smaller than 4 cm and still be considered an aneurysm. Fomon and colleagues[78] have shown that the potential for rupture of an aortic aneurysm is directly related to its wall tension and thus to the size of the aneurysm. Aneurysms less than 5 cm in diameter have a negligible incidence of rupture. Those that are 5 to 10 cm in diameter, if untreated, have an approximately 10 per cent chance of rupturing. Aneurysms more than 10 cm have a 50 per cent chance of rupturing.

The majority of thoracic aortic aneurysms can be suspected from chest radiographs.[79, 80] The most common radiographic findings are a mediastinal mass or an enlarged segment of the aorta that often contains wall calcification. Displacement and, less frequently, compression of the esophagus or of the trachea and bronchi may be visible on radiographs. Erosion of thoracic vertebrae and posterior ribs can also occur but is uncommon.

Computed tomography can delineate a mediastinal mass as an aneurysm, characterize it, and show its exact location. Fusiform thoracic aortic aneurysms have characteristic computed tomographic appearances and, in most patients, the diagnosis is readily apparent (Fig. 5–32A,B).[74–76] The findings show the following: dilatation of the aorta, usually greater than 4 cm in diameter; cur-

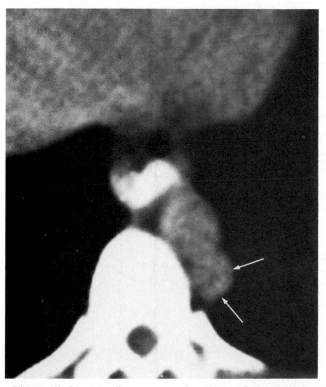

Figure 5–31. Hemiazygos continuation of the inferior vena cava. Patient is a 36-year-old woman who had carcinoma of the cervix and demonstrated a posterior mediastinal mass on chest radiographs. A dilated hemiazygos vein (arrows) is demonstrated behind the aorta at the level of the diaphragm. The vessel opacified with contrast material to the same degree as the aorta. Contrast material is present in the esophagus. (Courtesy of Dr. J. Mall, San Francisco, Cal.)

vilinear or plaquelike calcification; intraluminal thrombus; contrast enhancement of the patent portion of the lumen; displacement of mediastinal structures; and bone erosion.

Thrombus within thoracic aortic aneurysms is seen on CT scans in 86 to 100 per cent of patients (Fig. 5–33).[74, 75] These figures apply to arteriosclerotic aneurysms but are probably similar to those for aneurysms from other causes. Machida and Tasaka[75] have shown that the most common configuration is a complete ring of thrombus surrounding the aortic lumen. In our experience, rings of thrombus occur mainly in large fusiform aneurysms. Smaller thrombi tend to form crescents involving from one quarter to more than two thirds the circumference of the aneurysm.[74]

Calcification in the wall of aortic aneurysms is visible on CT scans in 83 to 100 per cent of patients (Fig. 5–32A and 5–33).[74 75] It tends to be in discontinuous plaques and curvilinear segments. Machida and Tasaka[75] reported calcification within the mural thrombus of aortic aneurysms in 17 per cent of patients, a finding that has not been confirmed. This important observation should be substantiated because it may confuse the interpretation of the images.

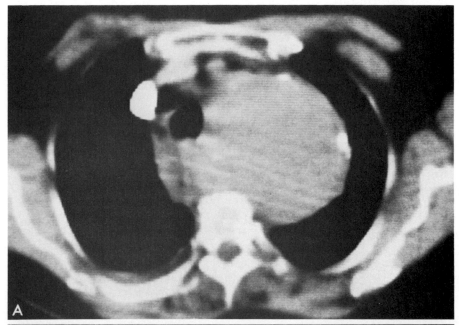

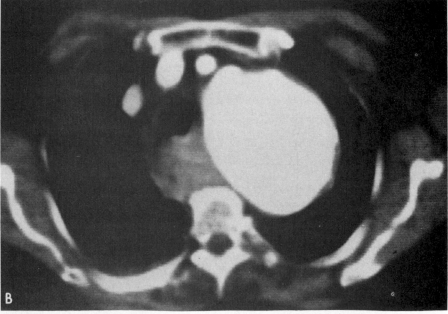

Figure 5–32. Ruptured aortic aneurysm. Patient is a 68-year-old woman with clinical suspicion of aortic rupture. **A** CT scan shortly after contrast material injection shows a large aortic aneurysm with a rim of calcification. The superior vena cava is opacified. **B** CT scan from later in the scan sequence reveals almost complete opacification of the aneurysm. A retrotracheal mass is from a mediastinal hematoma.

Illustration continued on opposite page

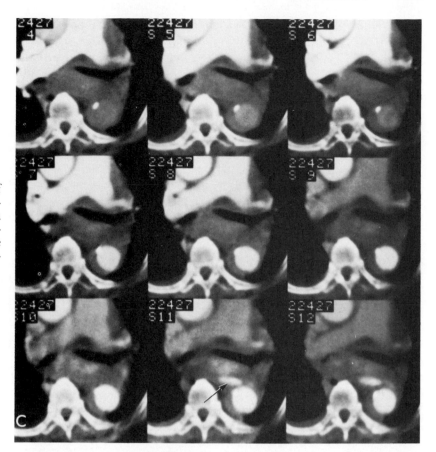

Figure 5–32. *Continued* **C** A series of CT scans, at a lower level, shows opacification of a normal-caliber aorta and escape of contrast material (arrow) into the mediastinum. Extensive mediastinal hematoma is demonstrated.

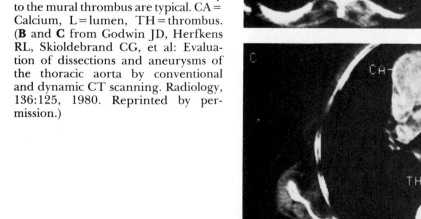

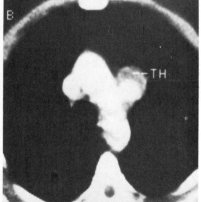

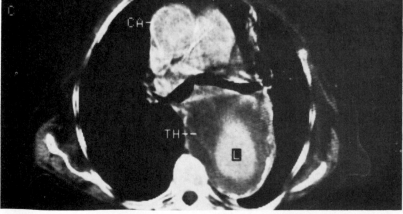

Figure 5–33. Aortic aneurysm in three patients. The configuration of the aortic lumen and its relationship to the mural thrombus are typical. CA = Calcium, L = lumen, TH = thrombus. (**B** and **C** from Godwin JD, Herfkens RL, Skioldebrand CG, et al: Evaluation of dissections and aneurysms of the thoracic aorta by conventional and dynamic CT scanning. Radiology, 136:125, 1980. Reprinted by permission.)

The most common site of thoracic aneurysms is in the descending aorta.[80] The esophagus is displaced to the right, whereas the trachea and bronchi are displaced anteriorly. The arch of the aorta is the next most common site; the ascending aorta is the least common. Aneurysms of the arch and ascending aorta will produce the anticipated displacement and compression of mediastinal structures. Fusiform aneurysms rarely involve the entire aorta.

The CT findings of a leaking or ruptured thoracic aortic aneurysm have been referred to,[81] but they have not been reported in detail. We have observed one such case. The mediastinum showed extensive soft tissue density from mediastinal hematoma. A left pleural effusion was evident. With a bolus injection of contrast medium, the material could be seen to escape beyond the confines of the aorta (Fig. 5–32C). Unfortunately, the patient died shortly after the examination.

Thoracic aortic aneurysms can undoubtedly be diagnosed with a high degree of accuracy using good quality CT scans and infused contrast material (Fig. 5–33 and 5–34A–C). Bolus injections of contrast with rapid sequential scans can assist in detailing the aneurysm. However, for computed tomography to replace aortography in the preoperative assessment of patients with aortic aneurysms, it must provide all the information required to determine the surgical approach to the disease because excision of the aneurysm is the only definitive therapy.[82, 83] The site of the aneurysm and whether the arch vessels are affected must be apparent. Whether the aneurysm is sac-cular or fusiform and whether the remainder of the aorta is normal must also be shown. Because CT scanning can provide this information, it should replace aortography in the preoperative evaluation of most patients with aortic aneurysms.

Aortic Dissections

Aortic dissection is the most common acute emergency involving the aorta.[84] In fact, 10 to 25 per cent of aortic "dilatations" seen on chest radiographs are due to chronic, undiagnosed dissection. Dissection results from a tear in the vessel wall with penetration of blood into the media to create a false channel, or false lumen. The false channel is usually between the inner one third and outer two thirds of the media. Predisposing weakness of the media in the form of Erdheim's cystic medial necrosis, Marfan syndrome, Ehlers-Danlos syndrome, or arteritis is present in most cases.[85] Arteriosclerosis and syphilis account for less than 5 per cent of cases.

The classification of aortic dissection into three types by DeBakey and colleagues[86] has become generally accepted. Each type of dissection is directly related to prognosis and therapy. Type 1 affects the ascending and descending aorta and accounts for 60 to 70 per cent of aortic dissections. Type 2 affects only the ascending aorta and does not extend beyond the left subclavian artery; this is the rarest type of dissection. Type 3 extends distally from the aortic isthmus, which is near the aortic insertion of the ligamentum arteriosus.

The chest radiograph in aortic dissection fre-

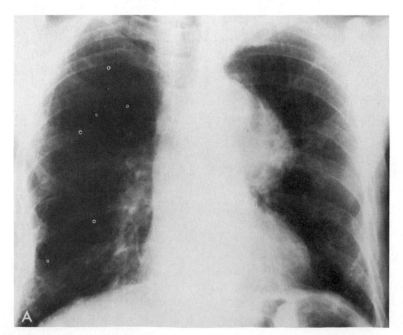

Figure 5–34. Bronchogenic carcinoma simulating aortic aneurysm. Patient is a 79-year-old man. **A** Chest radiograph shows a left para-aortic mass thought to be an aortic aneurysm.

Illustration continued on opposite page

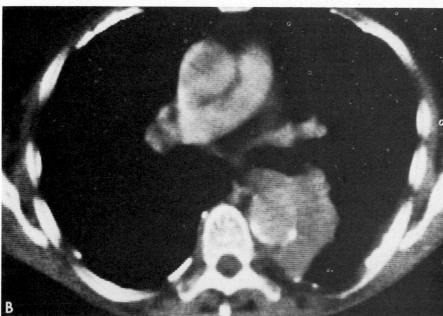

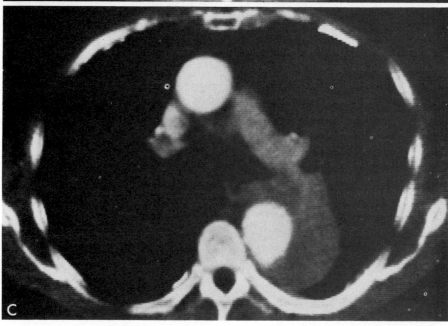

Figure 5–34. *Continued* **B** CT scan shows the large mass surrounding the calcified aortic lumen. The pleural plaques and calcification are indicative of asbestos pleural disease. **C** CT scan after injection of a bolus of contrast material demonstrates a normal aorta surrounded by the mass.

quently shows abnormality, but the findings are not always specific.[87, 88] Widening of the aorta or a progressive change in its configuration on sequential radiographs is highly suspicious, and the site of mediastinal widening may suggest the type of dissection. An unexplained discrepancy between the sizes of the ascending and descending aorta also suggests dissection. The esophagus and trachea may be displaced, but this can also be seen with aortic aneurysms. A left pleural effusion, an apical pleural cap, or paraspinous widening may each indicate leakage from an aorta dissection. Enlargement of the cardiac silhouette,

or evidence of acute left heart failure, may be due to aortic insufficiency or hemopericardium. The most specific radiographic sign of aortic dissection is displacement of intimal calcification away from the outer margin of the aorta by at least 4 to 5 mm, although this sign is found in only a small minority of patients.

The CT findings of aortic dissection, as described by various investigators[74, 76, 89–91] are similar. Two studies[91, 92] in which computed tomograms were obtained before, or without, infusion of contrast material showed that a difference in CT density between the true and false lumens of the dissection could be seen in about half the patients. Displacement of intimal calcification away from the apparent wall of the aorta was also demonstrated and was more apparent before than after contrast material infusion.

Computed tomograms obtained after infusion of contrast material are generally more revealing than those obtained before. In the patient undergoing CT scanning for a suspected aortic dissection, the examination should probably be performed only after administration of intravenous contrast material. High concentrations of intravascular contrast material are desirable. Rapid sequential scanning after a manual injection of 20 to 30 ml of 76 or 90 per cent contrast material in about 3 seconds is most helpful in diagnosis.

A series of five to seven rapid sequential scans is obtained initially at each of three levels: through the aortic arch, at the tracheal bifurcation, and immediately above the diaphragm.[74] A frontal

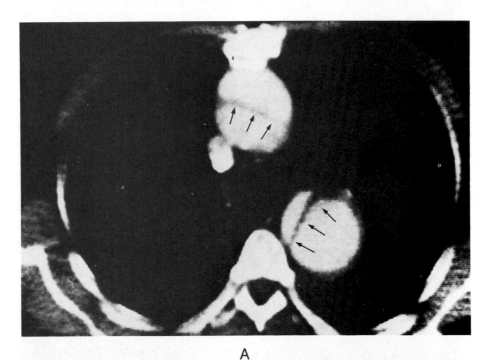

A

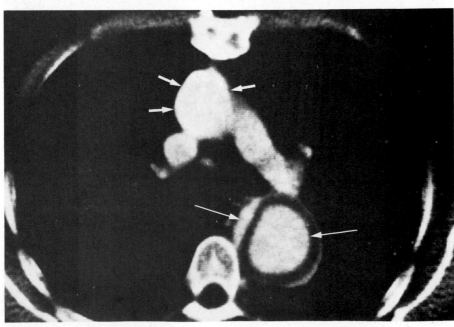

B

Figure 5–35. Type 1 aortic dissection. Patient is an elderly man with recurrent aortic dissection. **A** CT scan at the level of the proximal ascending and descending aorta demonstrate distinct flaps (arrows) with opacification of two lumens. **B** CT scan two centimeters caudad, at the level of the pulmonary artery, the two channels (long arrows) are still evident, although unequal in size. The larger channel has a circumferential lining of mural thrombus and, therefore, probably represents the true lumen. A graft (short arrows) is visible in the ascending aorta. (From Lipton MJ, Boyd DP: Contrast media in dynamic computed tomography of the heart and great vessels. *In* Felix R, Kazner E., Wegener OH [eds.]: Contrast Media in Computed Tomography. Amsterdam, Excerpta Medica, 1981, pp. 204–213. Reprinted by permission.)

projection radiograph assists in determining the correct levels for the sequential scans. If a Type 1 or Type 3 dissection is shown on the initial computed tomograms, the scanning should be continued to determine the inferior extent of the dissection and the status of the abdominal arteries. After this series of sequential scans, the entire thoracic aorta and arch vessels should be scanned during infusion of contrast material.

When a dissection is present, the outer diameter of the aorta is invariably larger than 5 cm but usually less than 10 cm.[89] The diameter of the opacified true lumen is usually smaller than normal and often appears flattened or distorted. The space between the opacified true lumen and the outer aortic margin contains the opacified or unopacified false lumen. A discrepancy in the size of the ascending and descending aorta is only a confirmatory sign of aortic dissection.

The definitive CT finding for acute aortic dissection is the presence of two opacified channels with an intimal flap between them (Fig. 5–35A,B).[74, 89–91] The two channels are visible in about 75 per cent of symptomatic patients with acute aortic dissection. In the thoracic aorta, the false lumen is usually posterolateral. The CT density of contrast within the true lumen is often different from that of the false lumen, reflecting a difference in the flow rate of contrast material in each channel. The slower flow is usually in the false lumen, and this can be demonstrated with the use of rapid sequential scanning. Alternatively, serial field-of-interest measurements of CT density can be obtained from the true and false lumens and can be plotted as time-density curves (Fig. 5–36). Computed tomography is more sensitive than angiography in demonstrating any difference in opacification between the two channels.

Calcified, atheromatous plaques occur in the intima of the aortic wall and are particularly well displayed on CT scans. In 25 to 56 per cent of patients with aortic dissection, these plaques become displaced along with the intima, away from the rest of the aortic wall (Fig. 5–37).[74, 89–91] Several investigators[89–91] assume that intimal calcification displaced inward from the aortic contour is pathognomonic of aortic dissection. This assumption is probably incorrect because there are some conditions in which a soft-tissue density between the plaque and the apparent aortic contour can

Figure 5–36. Type 3 aortic dissection as seen on a CT scan with time-density plot from multiple sequential scans. Fields-of-interest are plotted from the ascending aorta (ASC AO), true lumen (TRUE), and false lumen (FALSE). The relative increase in attenuation values (vertical axis) reflects the passage of a bolus of contrast material through the areas of interest. "Flow" through the false lumen is slower than through the true lumen or through the ascending aorta.

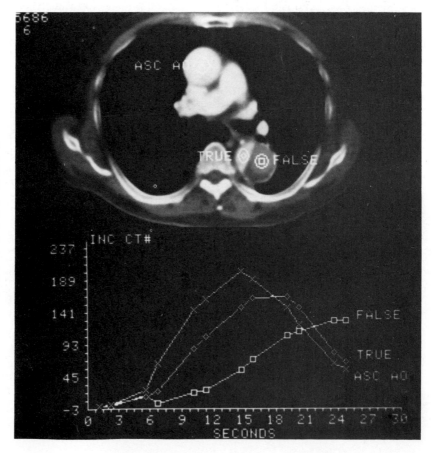

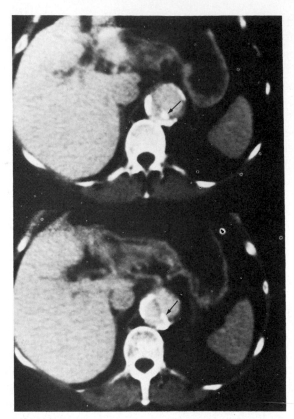

Figure 5–37. Aortic dissection with displaced intimal calcification. Adjacent CT scans show an intimal flap with calcium (arrows) within the flap. Both channels of the dissection have opacified with contrast material.

produce the same appearance.[92a] For example, calcification within a mural thrombus of an aortic aneurysm can appear displaced from the aortic wall. A periaortic hematoma or incidental soft-tissue mass surrounding the aorta (Fig. 5–34A–C) likewise can separate a calcified plaque from the apparent outer contour of the aorta. If two lumina are opacified with contrast material, the diagnosis of aortic dissection can be made. Occasionally, a saccular aneurysm contiguous with the calcified aortic wall gives the appearance of displaced calcification. Therefore, aortic dissection should not be diagnosed from the appearance of "displaced" calcification alone. The CT findings of dissection are visible over numerous levels, and all the scans should be examined before the final diagnosis is considered.

In about 25 per cent of patients with acute aortic dissections, the false channel is thrombosed and does not opacify. The false channel is thrombosed more frequently with subacute and chronic aortic dissection. If seen on only a few scans, a thrombosed false lumen without displaced intimal calcification may be confused with a fusiform aortic aneurysm containing a crescentic thrombus. The site and length of an aortic dissection, together with its other features, should make the differentiation possible in most cases.

The role of CT in evaluating patients with suspected aortic dissection varies for different institutions. The merits of surgical relative to intensive medical therapy for some aortic dissections are still controversial.[93–97] The use of computed tomography will thus be determined by the way in which patients with suspected aortic dissection are managed in each hospital.

In general, patients with Types 1 and 2 dissections are surgical candidates, whereas those with Type 3 are treated medically. Irrespective of therapy, the diagnosis of the presence and type of dissection should be made promptly, once the patient's condition has stabilized. Emergency CT scans should be performed within hours of the patient's admission to the hospital. Definitive therapy is based on the site of intimal tear, the extent of dissecting hematoma, the degree of involvement of aortic branches, the presence of an associated aneurysm or pseudoaneurysm, and whether the false channel is patent.[98]

As in the case of aortic aneurysm, if computed tomography provides all this information, aortography can be precluded. Patients in whom the false channel is thrombosed are usually excluded for surgical therapy and further angiographic studies are not warranted. Also, if a definite diagnosis of a Type 3 dissection can be made, surgery is usually not indicated and aortography is unnecessary.

Computed tomography should be used as the initial examination for patients suspected of having subacute or chronic aortic dissection. The majority of these patients are treated medically, and computed tomography is a relatively noninvasive method of confirming the diagnosis and the type of dissection.

Patients treated either surgically or medically for aortic dissection are prone to serious immediate and long-term complications.[99, 100] Complications consist of extension of the dissecting hematoma; aneurysm formation, which occurs in 15 to 25 per cent of patients; aortic valvular insufficiency; and aortic rupture. Turley and colleagues[101] showed a remarkably high incidence of persistent patency of the false channel after surgery. Radiographic and angiographic monitoring of patients with a persistent false channel has been advocated,[102] but computed tomography is a convenient and rapid method of repeatedly evaluating the aorta.[101, 103] After surgery, CT scans should be performed in a manner similar to that previously described. The examination should be directed toward the detection of potential complications. Teflon grafts, often inserted at the site of the intimal tear, are radiodense and visible on CT scans (Fig. 5–35*B*).[103] Dacron grafts, however, are usually not dense enough to be visible with computed tomography. After many years, Dacron grafts may calcify and can be seen radiographically and with computed tomography.

OBSTRUCTION OF THE SUPERIOR VENA CAVA

Obstruction of the superior vena cava is not as rare as formerly thought.[104, 105] Most patients with superior vena cava syndrome have a malignant tumor involving the mediastinum. In over 80 per cent of cases, the responsible tumor is a bronchogenic carcinoma, commonly arising in the right upper lobe.[106, 107] Other responsible malignancies originate in the thymus or thyroid or are lymphomas or metastases to the mediastinal lymph nodes. Benign causes of the syndrome are fibrosing mediastinitis, granulomatous mediastinitis (especially histoplasmosis), multinodular goiter, aortic aneurysm, trauma, irradiation, and primary thrombosis of the SVC. In a minority of patients, no cause can be found.[108] One cause has been reported to be thrombosis resulting from indwelling catheters.[109]

SVC obstruction produces a distinct constellation of clinical findings.[109] Suffusion and cyanosis of the face may be accompanied by edema of the head, neck, and arms. The veins of the head and neck are prominently distended. Dilated collateral veins of the chest wall are often visible. Venous pressure in the upper extremities is elevated above 25 cm of saline.

Radiographs of the chest frequently reveal a mediastinal mass.[108, 109] The mass may be the compressing tumor, but it may also be composed of dilated mediastinal azygos veins.[110] CT scanning can usually confirm the diagnosis and define the site of venous obstruction (Fig. 5–38*A*).[111] Occasionally, the SVC is intact and bilateral occlusion of brachiocephalic veins will be found with computed tomography. Dilated collateral venous channels involving the azygos system and passing through the chest wall are also often visible on CT scans.[112] With neoplasms, computed tomography can determine the extent of the tumor mass and the presence of additional mediastinal

disease. Brown and colleagues[113] reported three cases of SVC obstruction, two due to bronchogenic carcinoma and one to lymphoma. In each case, a mediastinal mass could be seen compressing the SVC.

The thoracic veins are well defined on CT scans.[114, 115] After contrast material infusion, venous thrombosis can be readily demonstrated.[116, 117] In most patients undergoing mediastinal computed tomography, contrast material is infused into an upper extremity or neck vein and contrast material–related flow patterns, especially with a bolus injection, can simulate venous thrombosis (Fig. 5–38*B*). Therefore, care should be taken in interpreting these examinations.[118] As a general rule, contrast material should be infused simultaneously into both upper extremities in patients with suspected venous thrombosis.

MEDIASTINAL LYMPHADENOPATHY

The detection of mediastinal lymph node enlargement is an important function of pulmonary radiology. Computed tomography has been advocated for the detection of mediastinal lymphadenopathy not apparent with conventional radiographic modalities. However, the frequency with which normal mediastinal lymph nodes are seen on CT scans and their range in size has not been established. The significance of enlarged lymph nodes in diseases of the mediastinum also remains controversial. In general, enlarged mediastinal lymph nodes appear as discrete, nonenhanced, round or slightly irregular densities of various sizes. The mediastinal lymph nodes demonstrate soft-tissue density, which usually distinguishes them easily from the background of mediastinal fat and connective tissue.

The main lymph node groups of the mediastinum are the internal mammary, prevascular, pretracheal, aortic-pulmonic, subcarinal, posterior mediastinal, and circumcardiac nodes. The literature is deficient in the description of normal mediastinal nodes. Presented next are CT findings, based mainly on our own observations.

INTERNAL MAMMARY LYMPH NODES. Normal internal mammary lymph nodes are not demonstrated on CT scans. After infusion of contrast medium, one to three small structures are usually visible, representing internal mammary vessels (Fig. 5–14). Enlarged internal mammary nodes exhibit a characteristic focal soft-tissue convexity protruding into the lung lateral to the sternum (Fig. 5–39). Ege[119] and Rose and colleagues[120] have shown that the position of the internal mam-

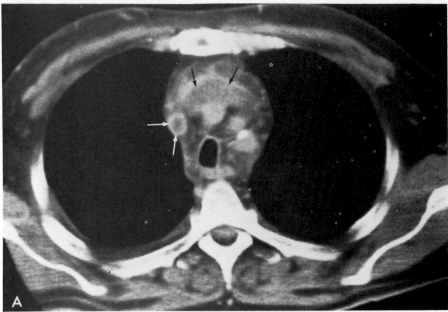

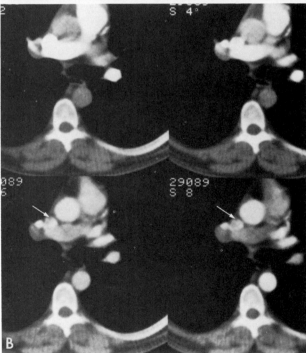

Figure 5–38. Venous thrombosis and pseudothrombosis. **A** CT scan at the level of the arch vessels in a man with right upper lobe squamous cell carcinoma and superior vena cava syndrome. Thrombus outlined by contrast material is visible within the right (white arrows) and left (black arrows) brachiocephalic veins. Opacified collateral veins are evident in the anterior chest wall and behind the spinous process of the vertebra. At levels more caudad, the superior vena cava was occluded by tumor. (Courtesy of Dr. S. London, Oakland, Cal.) **B** Sequential CT scans show pseudothrombosis in a patient with coronary artery bypass grafts. The trailing end of the bolus of contrast material passing through the superior vena cava produces a false appearance of thrombosis (arrows.)

mary nodes varies from midline to 5.3 cm from the midline. Costal cartilages can also produce a convexity lateral to the sternum; by observation of contiguous scans, this potential pitfall in diagnosis can usually be eliminated. Internal mammary lymph nodes are infrequently seen in patients who have had granulomatous disease. In our experience, these nodes are also rarely affected by metastatic bronchogenic carcinoma. Internal mammary lymph node enlargement has been reported in patients with metastatic breast carcinoma.[121–123]

Computed tomography, in conjunction with other imaging studies, can assist in the staging of breast cancer and in the detection of nodal recurrence. In our institution, CT scans showed internal mammary lymph node enlargement in a patient with lymphosarcoma, which was the first indication of recurrence. Internal mammary lymph node enlargement may be suspected from lateral chest radiographs, but the enlargement must be relatively massive. Computed tomography is considerably more sensitive for detection of nodes in this area.

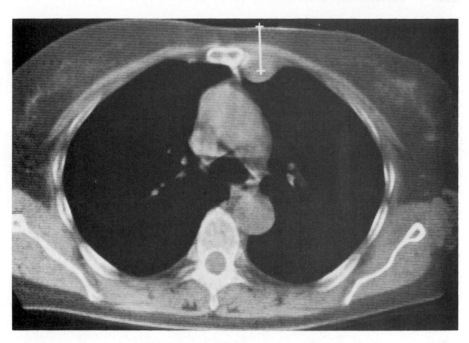

Figure 5–39. Enlarged internal mammary lymph node. Patient is a 64-year-old asymptomatic woman who showed a retrosternal density on a routine lateral chest radiograph. CT scan shows normal internal mammary vessels are present on the right. The mass on the left (bottom of marker) represents an enlarged internal mammary lymph node. Other scans showed a breast mass on the left that had not been palpable but was subsequently found to be carcinoma. (Courtesy of Dr. J. A. Kaiser, San Francisco, Cal.)

PREVASCULAR LYMPH NODES. These are seen on CT scans in about 10 per cent of patients. They appear as discrete, round densities less than about 5 mm in diameter. These nodes may represent the residue of prior granulomatous disease or they may be normal nodes. Enlarged prevascular lymph nodes are commonly due to bronchogenic carcinoma, lymphoma, sarcoidosis, metastasis, and many other conditions that can affect thoracic lymph nodes.[5, 124–131] The CT appearance of prevascular adenopathy varies from discrete, round or slightly irregular densities to large lobulated masses (Fig. 5–40A,B). Lymphoma characteristically produces lobulated masses of matted nodes. Computed tomography is more sensitive than chest radiographs or conventional tomograms in the detection and identification of prevascular lymphadenopathy.

PRETRACHEAL LYMPH NODES. The pretracheal space, between the anterior trachea and the ascending aorta and arch vessels, contains numerous lymph nodes.[132] The azygos lymph nodes are the only normal mediastinal nodes seen frequently on CT scans.[20] They are present in 50 to 90 per cent of normal people and are 5.5 ± 2.8 mm in diameter. An occasional azygos node can be up to 10 or 11 mm in transverse diameter (Figs. 5–8 and 5–17). Lymph nodes at other sites in the pretracheal space are smaller and infrequently visible. When present on CT scans, they probably reflect minimal enlargement due to prior granulomatous or inflammatory disease. The azygos and other pretracheal lymph nodes

are the mediastinal nodes most commonly enlarged. They are usually discrete and because of their position may be detected only from CT scans (Fig. 5–41). Only when these lymph nodes are sufficiently enlarged to protrude to the right of the mediastinum will they be visible on chest radiographs and conventional tomograms, producing a widening of the right paratracheal stripe.[33]

AORTIC-PULMONIC LYMPH NODES. The aortic-pulmonic window is not well demonstrated on CT scans because it is usually less than 1 cm in height and often suffers from partial superimposition of the superior surface of the left pulmonary artery or the undersurface of the aortic arch. Small round densities less than 5 mm in diameter, probably representing lymph nodes, are visible in the aortic-pulmonic window in less than 10 per cent of individuals. The aortic pulmonic window occasionally contains an irregular tubular density, presumably the ligamentum arteriosum, that should not be mistaken for an enlarged lymph node. Enlarged lymph nodes in the aortic-pulmonic window typically appear as round or slightly irregular, nonenhanced densities (Figs. 5–40B and 5–41). Chest radiographs are sensitive in detecting aortic-pulmonic window adenopathy. With CT, we have not found lymphadenopathy in the aortic-pulmonic window that was not first seen with chest radiographs.

SUBCARINAL LYMPH NODES. In patients who have had granulomatous disease, a few small calcified or noncalcified lymph nodes are often visi-

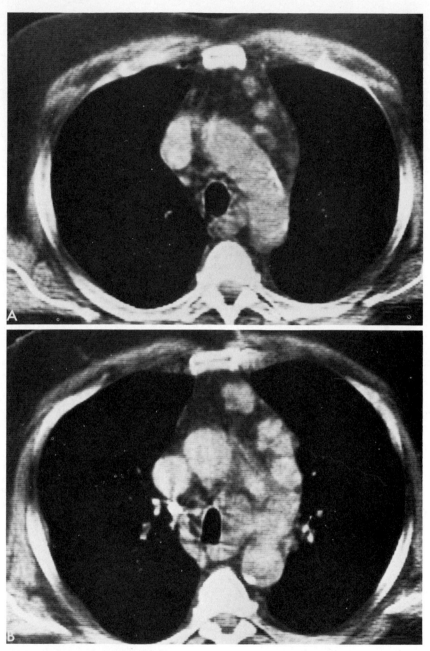

Figure 5–40. Enlarged lymph nodes in the prevascular space and aortic pulmonic window. Patient is elderly, with poorly differentiated carcinoma of the left lung. **A**   CT scan shows enlarged nodes in the prevascular space anterior to the aortic arch. **B**   CT scan two centimeters caudad to A, demonstrates massively enlarged nodes in front of the ascending aorta, in the aortic pulmonic window, and to the left of the trachea. (Nodes of this size in a patient with bronchogenic carcinoma have a high probability of being malignant. Only the paratracheal node could be reached by cervical mediastinoscopy. The calcified azygos node behind the superior vena cava is due to previous granulomatous disease.)

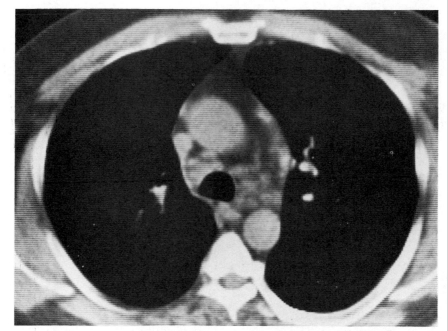

Figure 5–41. Enlarged lymph nodes in the pretracheal space and aortic-pulmonic window. Patient is a man with melanoma and previous histoplasmosis. CT scan shows multiple discrete nodes less than 1 cm in diameter; their profusion is abnormal. Biopsy showed the nodes to be due to the histoplasmosis.

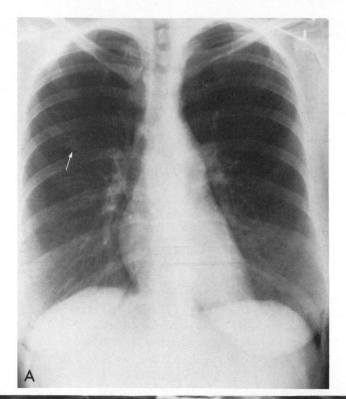

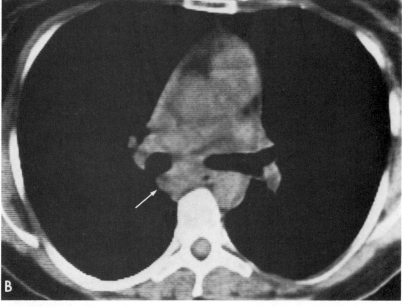

Figure 5–42. Enlarged subcarinal lymph nodes. Patient is a 31-year-old woman with choriocarcinoma and a right lung nodule. **A** The chest radiograph shows a lung nodule (arrow), but a normal mediastinum. **B** CT scan demonstrates a large subcarinal mass of nodes (arrow) behind the intermediate bronchus and to the right of the trachea. Biopsy of a skin lesion showed the patient had coccidioidomycosis. Metastatic disease was not present in the chest.

ble on CT scans in the subcarinal area. Subcarinal lymph nodes can be markedly enlarged without being visible on the chest radiographs (Fig. 5–42A,B). Computed tomography is considerably more sensitive than conventional chest radiographs or tomograms in detecting subcarinal lymphadenopathy.

POSTERIOR MEDIASTINAL LYMPH NODES. Focal displacement or widening of one or both paraspinal interfaces, detected from chest radio-

graphs, is a common diagnostic problem.[133, 134] Inflammatory, traumatic, or neoplastic disease extending from the spine may cause widening of the paraspinous line. Changes in the vertebral column are usually recognized from chest or bone radiographs. In the absence of vertebral body abnormalities, lymph node enlargement becomes a common cause of paraspinal displacement. Enlarged lymph nodes may be due to lymphoma, metastasis, or inflammation. Efremidis and co-

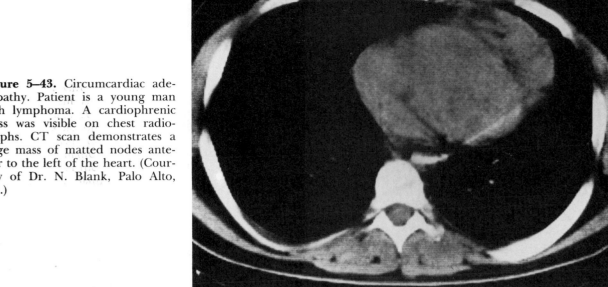

Figure 5–43. Circumcardiac adenopathy. Patient is a young man with lymphoma. A cardiophrenic mass was visible on chest radiographs. CT scan demonstrates a large mass of matted nodes anterior to the left of the heart. (Courtesy of Dr. N. Blank, Palo Alto, Cal.)

workers[133] showed that computed tomography is an excellent method of investigating paraspinous widening; they were able to confirm radiographic findings and determine the extent of disease in 11 patients with paraspinal widening. Enlarged paravertebral lymph nodes appear as discrete, nonenhanced densities, often displacing normal mediastinal structures. Computed tomography is more sensitive than lymphangiography in detecting and identifying posterior mediastinal adenopathy.[133] Occasionally, steroid-induced lipomatosis causes paraspinal widening. CT scanning can readily demonstrate this finding.[134a]

CIRCUMCARDIAC LYMPH NODES. These lymph nodes form a chain around the pericardial attachment to the diaphragm. Normal circumcardiac nodes cannot be shown on CT scans. In our experience, circumcardiac nodes have not been commonly involved in most diseases affecting the thorax or in disease metastatic to the mediastinum. Lymphoma, however, classically affects the circumcardiac nodes (Fig. 5–43).[135a] On CT scans, circumcardiac lymph node enlargement can be distinguished from masses in this area, especially an epicardic fat pad or a pleuropericardial cyst.[136]

BENIGN LESIONS

Computed tomography is widely advocated and rapidly becoming the procedure of choice for investigating suspected diseases within the mediastinum. It is used to detect mediastinal abnormalities not visible on chest radiographs and to characterize and determine the precise location of lesions initially detected by other imaging modalities. Interpretation of the CT scans often profoundly influences patient management; this is especially true when lesions are diagnosed as benign. Information gained from CT scans usually

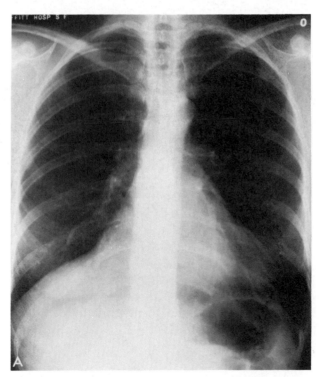

Figure 5–44. Mediastinal thymolipoma. Patient is a 52-year-old asymptomatic woman whose chest radiographs showed an anterior mediastinal density unchanged over three years. **A** Chest radiograph shows the low density mass extending to the left and to the right of the mediastinum.

Illustration continued on following page

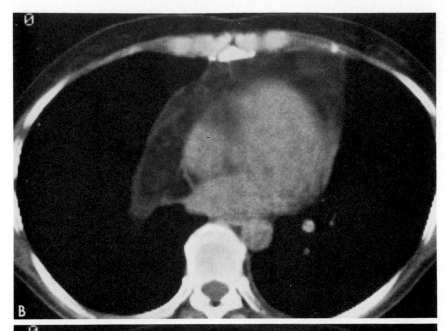

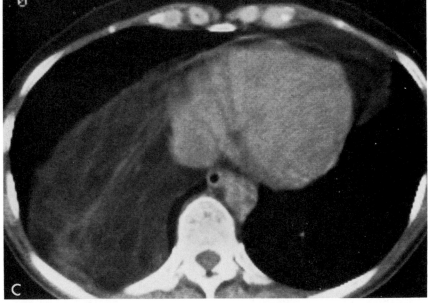

Figure 5–44. *Continued* **B, C** CT scans at the base of the heart **(B)** and immediately above the diaphragm **(C)** show the mass enveloping the anterior aspect of the heart and extending to the right posterior chest wall. Strands of fibrous tissue course through the mass. A thoracotomy, a large thymolipoma was removed.

obviates further investigation. When CT is able to identify a mediastinal mass as a vessel, fatty mass, or thin-walled cyst, benignity is usually assumed. However, the findings indicating benignity of solid, soft-tissue masses have not been established,[44] and further investigation is necessary in this area.

Fatty Lesions

With the advent of CT, the frequent deposition of fat within the mediastinum has become apparent.[137, 138] Fat is easily identified by its low density (−20 H to −100 H). In the study by Pugatch and colleagues,[139] almost half of 39 benign mediastinal abnormalities investigated with CT were composed of fat. Fatty lesions occurred in the superior, anterior, and posterior mediastinum, although the superior mediastinum was the most common site of mediastinal adiposity or lipomatosis. In two other studies, fat-containing lesions constituted 3 to 10 per cent of all mediastinal lesions evaluated using CT.[127, 140] The usual clinical circumstances leading to investigation with CT occurs when a superior mediastinal mass or diffuse mediastinal widening is seen on chest radiographs.[138] The patient is often obese or may be receiving steroids. On CT scans, mediastinal fat in obese patients usually appears low in CT density and of uniform consistency.

Localized fatty masses visible on CT scans can

have a number of causes. A prominent epicardial fat pad is the most common fatty mass in the thorax and is easily recognized on CT scans. Lipomas are usually in the anterior mediastinum, but they also occur in the middle and posterior mediastinum and adjacent to the diaphragm.[141] Thymolipomas are anterior mediastinal masses and indistinguishable on CT scans from lipomas (Fig. 5–44A–C). Extraperitoneal or omental fat can herniate through the foramen of Morgagni or of Bochdalek or through the esophageal hiatus.

Specific Hounsfield units that can categorically define mediastinal fat as benign have not been reported. Therefore, the diagnosis of benignity of a fatty mass is presumptive. Liposarcoma is a rare mediastinal tumor, occurring most commonly in the posterior mediastinum and occasionally in the anterior mediastinum. Liposarcoma should have a higher density than benign fat, should be inhomogeneous, and should show features of mediastinal invasion.

Cystic Lesions

Cystic lesions constitute approximately 15 to 20 per cent of mediastinal masses.[142, 143] The most common are bronchogenic, enterogenous, pleuropericardial, and thymic cysts. Most benign mediastinal cysts do not produce symptoms and can become large before they are discovered. They are usually found incidentally on chest radiographs.

Cystic masses that are shown by CT scans to be thin-walled with a distinctive, defined margin are usually benign.[125] Most mediastinal cysts will have a density of 0 H to 20 H, which is less than that of soft tissue. However, considerable care should be taken in diagnosing mediastinal cysts. Some benign cystic lesions have viscous fluid with a density in the range of 20 H to 50 H, equivalent to that of solid tumors.[5, 144] In addition, a variety of solid mediastinal masses, whether benign or malignant, can undergo cystic degeneration and the cystic components can be easily misinterpreted as benign cysts.[145]

Bronchogenic and enterogenous cysts arise from the airway and esophagus respectively, most commonly at the level of the tracheal carina. They frequently protrude into the posterior mediastinum and may be extremely large when first discovered.[146, 147] An abrupt increase in size can be caused by hemorrhage into the cyst. On CT scans, bronchogenic cysts appear unilocular with uniform density (Fig. 5–45A,B). Their attenuation value depends on the contents of the cyst, and can vary from 0 to over 100 H.[147a, 147b] The wall of the cyst is usually thin and the inner margin smooth. Although bronchogenic cysts can displace adjacent structures, they are usually clearly demarked from the surrounding mediastinum.

Pleuropericardial cysts are congenital, smooth, round-to-oval lesions that are invariably in contact with the pericardium. In about two-thirds of instances, they arise from the right cardiophrenic angle. Other sites of origin are the left cardiophrenic angle, the anterior and superior mediastinum, and, rarely, the pericardium posterior to the heart.[148] Occasionally, pleuropericardial cysts are pedunculated, and on CT scans the connection of the cyst to the pericardium is not evident. They appear smooth and thin-walled,[149] and their contents are homogeneous with a density usually ranging from 0 H to 20 H, but sometimes higher. These lesions are maleable, and as Pugatch and colleagues[143] showed, they can change shape on CT scans when the patient is in the prone or decubitus position.

True congenital thymic cysts are rare and originate from the thymopharyngeal duct.[150] They can occur anywhere along the course of the embryonic thymus gland from the angle of the mandible to the manubrium. Most do not cause symptoms, but if large, they can produce tracheal or cardiac compression.[151, 152] Mediastinal thymic cysts are usually round and are frequently multiloculated. Hemorrhage into the cyst is common and the cyst cavity often contains old blood, necrotic material, and cholesterol crystals. It can thus be anticipated that the CT attenuation values of the cyst fluid may vary considerably from those of water.

Thymomas often undergo cystic degeneration. If the degeneration is extensive, the computed tomographic and gross appearance of the lesion is indistinguishable from that of a thymic cyst.[150] Cystic degeneration can also occur in Hodgkin's disease and germinoma of the thymus and produce a similar appearance. An anterior or superior mediastinal cyst is seldom a congenital thymic cyst, and the commoner, more ominous alternative lesions should be considered first in the diagnosis.

Pancreatic pseudocysts rarely present as masses in the posterior or inferior mediastinum. If they do, CT can demonstrate their cystic nature and their extension through the retrocrural portion of the diaphragm[153, 154] (Fig. 5–46). We have seen one pancreatic pseudocyst in which the cyst wall appeared thick on CT scans. Computed tomography is probably the most precise method of de-

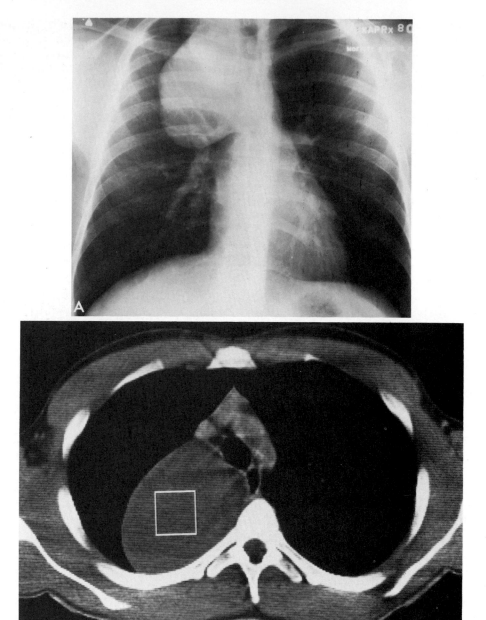

Figure 5–45. Bronchogenic cyst. Patient is a young man with an incidental upper respiratory infection. **A** The chest radiograph reveals a huge right upper mediastinal mass. **B** CT scan shows the mass extending from the right of the trachea to the posterior chest wall. It has a uniform appearance and a measured density of 13.25 H. The cyst extended vertically from the lower pole of the thyroid gland to the tracheal carina.

termining the thoracic and abdominal extent of a pancreatic pseudocyst.

Dermoid cysts and cystic teratomas can be benign or malignant, cystic or solid; the cystic lesions tend to be benign. One reported benign cystic teratoma[155] demonstrated CT findings of a well-circumscribed, anterior mediastinal mass composed of fat and soft-tissue density. Subsequent studies have shown marked variability in the thickness of the wall and the CT density of

the contents of benign cystic teratomas.[155a, 155b] Whether CT can differentiate benign from malignant dermoids or teratomas is not known.

Vascular Lesions

As mentioned, CT will commonly show a mediastinal mass to be an abnormally dilated or aberrant vessel. In general, a mass that enhances with intravenous contrast material to the same degree as the aorta or arch vessels is a dilated or

lung appears on CT scans as a homogeneous or inhomogeneous mass continuous with the mediastinum, and it is not possible to determine whether tumor has invaded the mediastinum.

Computed tomography is the most sensitive radiologic method of detecting mediastinal lymph node enlargement. The frequency of mediastinal nodal involvement at the time of initial presentation of lung carcinoma depends on the histologic type and the site of the tumor. In one representative series reported by Whitcomb and colleagues,[193] mediastinal lymph node metastases were present in 68 per cent of patients having small cell carcinoma, in 52 per cent of patients having large cell carcinoma, 29 per cent of patients having adenocarcinoma, and 11 per cent of

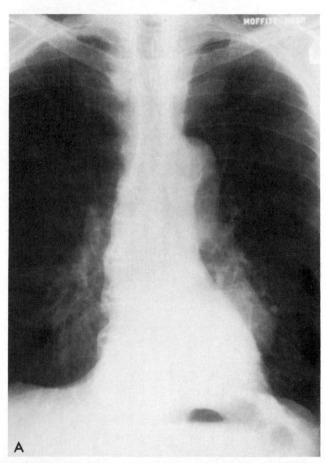

Figure 5–52. Bronchogenic carcinoma appearing to invade the mediastinum. Patient is a 72-year-old man. **A** Chest radiograph shows left lower lobe atelectasis from a squamous cell carcinoma occluding the left lower lobe bronchus. **B** CT scan shows the left lower lobe atelectasis and a mass effect between the pulmonary artery and descending aorta. The mass also appears to be between the esophagus and left atrium (arrows). Thoracotomy disclosed that the aorta was not encased and that the collapsed lung had no mediastinal attachments. A 2-cm lymph node beneath the left pulmonary artery showed reactive hyperplasia.

Illustration continued on following page

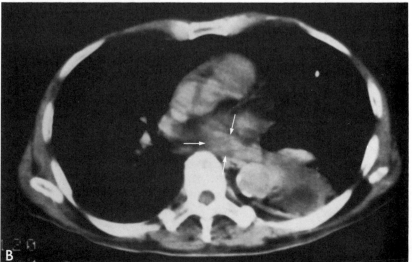

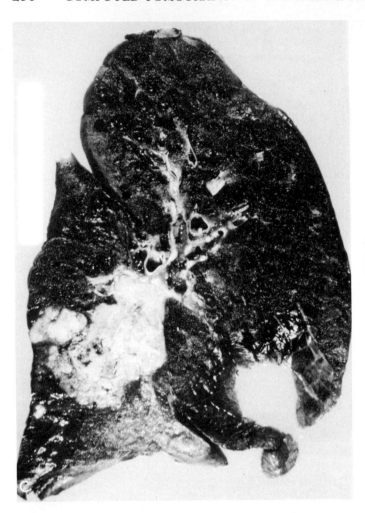

Figure 5–52. *Continued* **C** A section from the pneumonectomy specimen, shows the tumor extending to the pleura but not crossing it.

patients having squamous cell carcinoma. In fact, the incidence of mediastinal lymph node metastases is 20 to 40 per cent in patients considered clinically to have resectable lung carcinoma.[194–198]

Chest radiographs and conventional tomograms have a sensitivity of only about 50 per cent in detecting mediastinal lymph node metastases. However, false-positive radiographic interpretations of mediastinal lymph node metastases are uncommon. Central tumors and tumors with associated lung collapse have about a 50 per cent incidence of mediastinal lymph node metastases. Peripheral lesions are less likely to have mediastinal metastases; when the metastases are present, they are often visible on chest radiographs.

The ability of CT scans to demonstrate mediastinal lymph node involvement by bronchogenic carcinoma has been studied by numerous investigators (Table 5–2).[125, 126, 128–130, 199–202] Many of these did not compare their CT scan results with those for conventional imaging modalities. In addition, the criteria for abnormal nodes varied considerably between studies. It is also not possi-

ble to ascertain the accuracy of CT scans for patients whose chest radiographs or conventional tomograms showed no abnormality. The overall CT accuracy rate of 0.81 (Table 5–2) is high, considering the known incidence of small mediastinal nodes containing metastatic tumor. The relatively high predictive value of 0.86 for a negative test indicates that if CT scans show no evidence of mediastinal adenopathy, invasive diagnostic procedures will usually be unrewarding. The false-positive and false-negative rates in these studies (Table 5–2) were not explained.

It is well known that reactive hyperplasia or pre-existing granulomatous disease also causes mediastinal lymph node enlargement.[36, 129] White and co-workers[203] have shown that the probability of mediastinal lymph nodes containing tumor metastatic from bronchogenic carcinoma is related to the size of the nodes. Nodes larger than 1.7 cm in diameter usually contain tumor, whereas smaller nodes are indeterminate. The significance of small nodes detected only by CT thus remains problematic.

Table 5–2. COMPUTED TOMOGRAPHY IN MEDIASTINAL LYMPH NODE STAGING OF BRONCHOGENIC CARCINOMA*†

Author Year	Crowe et al.[124] 1978	Shevland et al.[126] 1978	Underwood et al.[199] 1979	Mintzer et al.[128] 1979	Eckolm et al.[129] 1980	Hirlman et al.[130] 1980	Faling et al.[201] 1981	Rea et al.[200] 1981	Osborne et al.[202] 1982	
Scanner	EMI 5000, 5005	EMI 1010	EMI 5005	EMI 5005	Tomoscan 300	EMI 5000	Delta 2010	Delta 2020	—	
Scan time (sec)	19.0	19.0	19.0	19.0	4.2	19.0	2.0	2.0	5.0	
Image thickness (mm)	15.0	15.0	13.0	13.0	12.0	13.0	10.0	15.0	8 or 10	
No. patients	44	37	18	49	35	50	51	22	42	348
TP	21.0	16.0	4.0	12.0	2.0	23.0	15.0	4.0	17.0	114.0
FN	1.0	2.0	5.0	4.0	5.0	7.0	2.0	1.0	1.0	28.0
FP	0	1.0	1.0	4.0	15.0	1.0	2.0	4.0	9.0	37.0
TN	22.0	18.0	8.0	29.0	13.0	19.0	32.0	13.0	15.0	169.0
Sensitivity	0.95	0.89	0.44	0.75	0.29	0.77	0.88	0.80	0.94	0.80
Specificity	1.0	0.95	0.89	0.88	0.46	0.95	0.94	0.76	0.63	0.82
Overall accuracy	0.98	0.92	0.67	0.84	0.43	0.84	0.92	0.77	0.76	0.81
PV of + test	1.0	0.94	0.80	0.75	0.12	0.96	0.88	0.50	0.65	0.75
PV of − test	0.96	0.90	0.62	0.88	0.72	0.73	0.94	0.93	0.94	0.86

*Confirmed by mediastinoscopy and/or thoracotomy.

†Criteria for abnormal lymph nodes varied widely among studies.

Abbreviations: TP=true-positive results, FN=false-negative results, FP=false-positive results, TN=true-negative results, PV=predictive value.

Definitions: Sensitivity $= \dfrac{TP}{TP+FN}$; specificity $= \dfrac{TN}{FP+TN}$; overall accuracy $= \dfrac{TP+TN}{TP+FN+FP+TN}$; PV of + test $= \dfrac{TP}{TP+FP}$; PV of − test $= \dfrac{TN}{TN+FN}$.

The staging of bronchogenic carcinoma cannot be directly translated into surgical resectability. For the individual patient with bronchogenic carcinoma, the physician's decision as to whether resection should be attempted is complex.[204] The aggressiveness of surgeons varies widely and, in some hospitals, the presence of mediastinal tumor is not a contraindication to resection.[195, 196] Concomitant disease, age, symptoms, and the presence of distant metastases must all be taken into consideration. An excellent review of the problem by Mittman and Bruderman[204] is available. Recommendations based solely on CT findings would, therefore, be inadequate. Computed tomography does have a role in the evaluation of bronchogenic carcinoma, although its limitations and pitfalls in interpretation have been sparsely documented.[204a]

If nodal enlargement or widening of the mediastinum is unequivocally shown on chest radiographs, CT will not give additional information. The overwhelming probability is that the tumor involves the mediastinum, although confirmation of the mediastinal tumor by a surgical procedure may sometimes be warranted. CT scans should probably be performed for all central lesions and for peripheral lesions known to be large cell or undifferentiated carcinoma if chest radiographs show the mediastinum to be normal. If CT scans show direct mediastinal spread of a central tumor, the tumor is probably not resectable.

Because large cell and undifferentiated tumors have a high incidence of mediastinal metastases, they should be fully assessed using CT. The CT interpretation that there are no enlarged mediastinal lymph nodes probably obviates the need for a preliminary staging procedure such as mediastinoscopy or parasternal mediastinotomy. Enlarged mediastinal nodes that are seen only on CT scans should be biopsied by the most appropriate route. The decision as to resectability will then be based on the histologic type of the tumor, the nature and site of the metastatic nodes and other factors just detailed.

Squamous cell carcinomas and adenocarcinomas that are peripheral and well differentiated are the most controversial. When the chest radiograph shows a normal mediastinum, the incidence of mediastinal node spread of these tumors is low. The probability that small mediastinal lymph nodes, detected only by CT, contain tumor is also low. Nevertheless, many surgeons will consider regional resection of nodes in these patients. Computed mediastinal tomography does not seem to provide information that can assist in the management of this group of patients.

The recommendations just made are provisional and highlight a lack of sufficient information regarding CT assessment of bronchogenic carcinoma. They also reflect the diverse and changing attitude of clinicians to the handling of patients with bronchogenic carcinoma. The definitive studies of the efficacy of CT in the management and staging of bronchogenic carcinoma will be difficult to accomplish and are still to be performed.

MALIGNANT LYMPHOMA

The malignant lymphomas form part of a spectrum of lymphoproliferative disorders, all of which may affect the mediastinum and lungs. There is no universally accepted classification of malignant lymphomas. The descriptive, histologic classification in Table 5–3 is widely used, but may be replaced when concepts of lymphoid physiology have become better understood.[205] The major determinants of prognosis in malignant lymphoma are the histologic type and the stage of disease at presentation.[206] The staging of malignant lymphoma has a more profound influence on prognosis of Hodgkin's disease than of non-Hodgkin's lymphoma.

Survival, especially in Hodgkin's disease, is related to early, adequate, and appropriate therapy.[207] Precise determination of the site and extent of disease is important in selecting the optimum type of therapy. The staging of malignant lymphomas proposed by the Rye Conference, or modifications of this staging, are generally accepted[208] (Table 5–4).

New methods for diagnosing and treating patients with malignant lymphomas are continually being developed. For therapy to be appropriate, extensive evaluation of the lymph nodes and affected organs is undertaken. Among the nonra-

Table 5–3. CLASSIFICATION OF MALIGNANT LYMPHOMAS

Hodgkin's disease
  Lymphocyte predominance
  Nodular sclerosis
  Mixed cellularity
  Lymphocyte depletion
Non-Hodgkin's lymphoma
  Lymphocytic, well differentiated
  Lymphocytic, poorly differentiated
  Mixed, lymphocytic and histiocytic
  Histiocytic
  Undifferentiated

Table 5–4. THE STAGES OF HODGKIN'S DISEASE*

Stage	Characteristics
I	Involvement of a single lymph node region or of a single extralymphatic organ or site
II	Involvement limited to one side of the diaphragm, to either two or more lymph node regions, or to localized involvement of an extralymphatic site and one or more lymph node regions
III	Involvement of lymph node regions on both sides of the diaphragm, which may include localized involvement of an extralymphatic site or spleen
IV	Diffuse or disseminated involvement of one or more extralymphatic organs or any liver involvement, with or without associated lymph node involvement

Each case is further classified as
A—If the patient is asymptomatic
B—If any of the following is present
  • Unexplained weight loss of more than 10 per cent of body weight in the preceding 6 months
  • Unexplained fever, with temperatures above 38°C
  • Night sweats

*Adapted from Desforges JF, Rutherford CJ, Piro A: Hodgkin's disease. N Engl J Med 30:1212, 1979. Used with permission.

diologic investigations are hematologic and bone marrow studies and sampling of tissues from abdominal organs, lymph nodes at multiple sites, and the spleen. Radiologic studies include chest radiography, isotope studies, lung and mediastinal tomography, and lymphangiography.

Hodgkin's disease has a more predictable behavior than non-Hodgkin's lymphoma because it tends to spread to contiguous nodal chains.[209] This pattern is reflected in the chest radiographs. The most common finding in intrathoracic lymphoma is mediastinal lymph node enlargement. Filly, Blank, and Castellino,[210] in a study of 300 patients with untreated malignant lymphoma, found radiographically demonstrated intrathoracic disease in 67 per cent of the patients having Hodgkin's disease and 43 per cent of the patients having non-Hodgkin's lymphoma. Involved lymph nodes in the prevascular and pretracheal compartments were found alone, or in combination with other nodal groups, in 90 per cent of those with Hodgkin's disease and in only 46 per cent of those with non-Hodgkin's lymphoma. Internal mammary lymph node enlargement was much more frequent in Hodgkin's disease, whereas isolated posterior mediastinal and paracardiac nodal enlargement was found only in non-Hodgkin's lymphoma. Hilar lymphadenopathy was found in about 20 per cent of patients with mediastinal

Hodgkin's disease and correlated closely with lung involvement. Conventional whole-lung tomography demonstrated additional information in 21.4 per cent of the patients in whom it was performed.[211] However, in only 4.5 per cent did whole-lung tomography lead to changes in the initial staging of the disease or in the treatment plan.

CT could potentially have more influence than conventional tomography on the staging of malignant lymphoma. Computed tomography has made a major impact on the staging of the malignant lymphomas in the abdomen,[212–214] but its role in staging thoracic disease has not received the same intense interest, both because gross mediastinal and lung involvement is readily recognized using conventional techniques and because the advantages of thoracic CT have not been appreciated. These advantages were seen in two studies of the role of thoracic CT in the management of patients with Hodgkin's disease and with non-Hodgkin's lymphoma.[215, 216] Both studies emphasized the ability of CT to detect and show the precise location of mediastinal, hilar, lung, and pleural disease. In many cases, unsuspected disease was found that altered the staging of the malignant lymphoma and the subsequent therapy.

Three patterns of mediastinal tumor distribution are found in both Hodgkin's disease and non-Hodgkin's lymphoma.[216] The first is a mass-

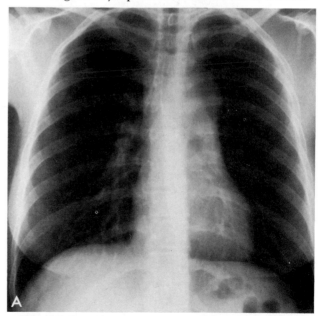

Figure 5–53. Lymphoma with extrapleural spread. Patient is a 25-year-old woman with lymphoma of the left axial and supraclavicular region. **A** Chest radiograph reveals an anterior mediastinal mass extending to the left.

Illustration continued on following page

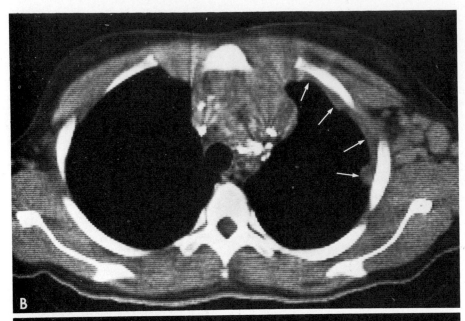

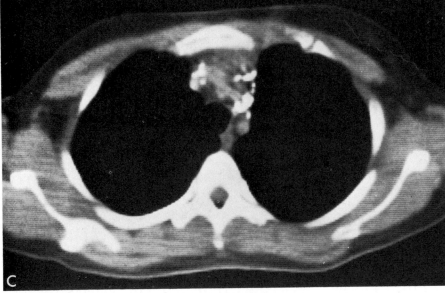

Figure 5–53. *Continued* **B** CT scan at the level of the arch vessels, demonstrates a mediastinal mass composed of enlarged nodes. Anterior extrapleural spread on the left side (arrows) was not evident on the conventional radiographs. Contrast material within the nodes is a result of previously lymphangiography. Left axillary nodal enlargement is visible. **C** CT scan obtained after treatment shows that the mediastinal mass, extrapleural lymphoma, and axillary nodes have regressed.

like expansion of the medastinal lymph nodes, which is confined to the mediastinum. The mediastinal mass may be either symmetric or asymmetric. The second pattern is an extension of tumor from the mediastinum along the lymphoid tissue around the bronchi. CT scans demonstrate this form of continuous spread into the lung with greater sensitivity than do chest radiographs or conventional tomograms. The third pattern is extrapleural extension of tumor from mediastinal tumor either anteriorly or posteriorly (Fig. 5–53A–C). Pilepich and colleagues[216] found the third form of spread in over 50 per cent of patients having mediastinal lymphoma. In 9 of 15 patients, the portals for radiation therapy would

not have included the entire tumor without the additional information provided by CT. In four patients, CT demonstrated invasion of tumor into the chest wall from the extrapleural spread, which caused the proposed therapy to be altered (Fig. 5–54).

A possible advantage of CT is its ability to detect subtle enlargement of mediastinal lymph nodes.[125, 215] Ellert and Kreel[215] studied the distribution of lymph node enlargement in both Hodgkin's disease and non-Hodgkin's lymphoma using CT. Mediastinal lymphadenopathy was found in 57 per cent of patients with Hodgkin's disease and 46 per cent of patients with non-Hodgkin's lymphoma. Enlarged posterior mediastinal nodes

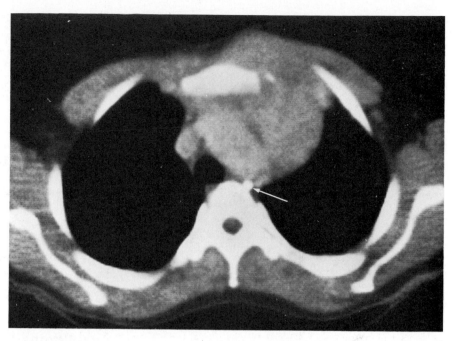

Figure 5–54. Lymphoma invading the chest wall. Patient is a 24-year-old woman with nodular, sclerosing Hodgkin disease of the anterior mediastinum. CT scan shows a large mass of matted nodes in front of the aortic arch, extending into the chest wall on the left. The extension was not suspected or apparent on conventional radiographs. The thoracic duct (arrow) is opacified.

were seen with equal frequency in the two groups. Enlarged retrocrural nodes were more common in non-Hodgkin's lymphoma. However, in only one patient did CT detect mediastinal adenopathy when all other imaging modalities failed to demonstrate any intrathoracic disease. Unsuspected findings in the chest, seen only with CT, included chest wall invasion, subpleural parenchymal nodules, pleural effusion, and thymic enlargement.[215, 216]

Computed tomography is also beneficial in detecting recurrent lymphoma after therapy. The clinical indications for CT in suspected recurrence of thoracic malignant lymphoma have not been established. In 72 patients who were either clinically suspected of having recurrent lymphoma or clinically thought to be free of disease, the most common CT finding was mediastinal lymphadenopathy, present in 41 per cent of the patients with Hodgkin's disease and 33 per cent of the patients with non-Hodgkin's lymphoma.[215] Additional CT findings were pulmonary nodules, pleural effusions, and pulmonary infiltrates.

Effective use of CT scans in the radiologic approach to the initial and subsequent evaluations of the patient with lymphoma requires close cooperation between clinician and radiologist. Simple algorithms are not applicable and the kind of examination will be determined by the type of malignant lymphoma, the staging of disease based on other investigations, and the proposed treatment plan.

In summary, CT, by virtue of its great sensitivity, can be useful in detecting:

1. Subtle mediastinal nodal enlargement not appreciated on conventional radiographs or enlarged hilar nodes obscured by bulky mediastinal masses.

2. Infiltration of tumor into the lungs from mediastinal disease.

3. Anterior and posterior extrapleural spread from mediastinal adenopathy.

4. Pulmonary nodules, pleural effusion, and chest wall invasion.

North and colleagues[217] showed the detrimental influence of mediastinal involvement seen at initial presentation on the survival of patients with Hodgkin's disease. They recommended routine computed mediastinal tomography in all patients who have low cervical or supraclavicular adenopathy and in those suspected of having mediastinal disease.

INDICATIONS FOR COMPUTED TOMOGRAPHY OF THE MEDIASTINUM

Intense interest in CT has been shown by the radiologic and medical communities. Pleas have been made for the development of firm indications and specific guidelines for using CT. The response has been exceedingly slow, and only now are tentative suggestions possible. The liter-

Table 5–5.   INDICATIONS FOR MEDIASTINAL
CT*

Evaluation of problems presented by chest radiograph
  Mass
    Differentiation among cystic, fatty, or solid nature
    Localization relative to other mediastinal structures
  Mediastinal widening
    Assessment of whether cause is pathologic or an
      anatomic variation
    Distinction among solid mass, vascular anomaly,
      aneurysm, and physiologic fat deposition
  Hilum
    Differentiation of enlarged pulmonary artery from solid
      mass when conventional tomography fails to make or is
      not capable of making this distinction
  Paraspinal-line widening
    Distinction among lymph node enlargement, vascular
      cause, and anatomic variant
Search for occult thymic lesion
    Detection of thymoma or hyperplasia in selected patients
      with myasthenia gravis when plain chest radiography is
      negative or suspicious

*Adapted from the Society for Computed Body Tomography: New indications for computed body tomography. AJR 133:115, 1979. © American Roentgen Ray Society. Used with permission.

ature has consisted largely of anecdotal reports, small series of cases, and inadequately documented information. The national cooperative studies necessary to gather sufficient data of good quality have not been instituted.

General indications for computed tomography of the body were proposed in 1977 by the American College of Radiology and the Institute of Medicine of the National Academy of Science.[218, 219] More specific indications were offered in 1979 by the Society for Computed Tomography[220] and are reproduced in part in Table 5–5. Rapid technical advances in scanners have made these indications too limited. Improvements in such aspects of CT as spatial resolution and rapid sequential scanning have opened new avenues for computed mediastinal tomography, and further advances can be anticipated. For practical purposes, CT of the mediastinum is now used to characterize disease through determination of its attenuation values or enhancement with intravenous contrast material; detect disease not evident using other modalities; and localize the extent of disease within the mediastinum.

CT CHARACTERIZATION OF DISEASE

The attenuation coefficients of biologic tissues as measured by the Hounsfield number (H) have a reasonably linear relationship to the physical density of the tissue.[221] Attenuation values (CT density) in the mediastinum are sufficiently precise to differentiate fat, cyst fluid, and soft tissue in most cases. However, the cystic component of some mediastinal masses can approach soft-tissue density. Infusion of contrast material will usually demonstrate the cystic components of a mediastinal mass.

In most circumstances, CT is the examination of choice for investigating mediastinal or paramediastinal abnormalities detected on or suspected from chest radiographs. In most situations, CT provides more information than does conventional tomography. If CT is indicated, conventional tomography should not be performed. The CT images are usually easier to interpret, and a more definitive statement of abnormality can be made. Computed tomography can show whether the mass is a vessel (such as an aneurysm or an anomalous vessel), a solid tumor, lymphadenopathy, fat accumulation, or a cyst. It can also reveal the extent of the lesion, any distortion of normal structures, and any associated involvement of the chest wall and spine.

Diffuse mediastinal widening is a common problem in chest radiography. In most cases, if the patient is asymptomatic and the chest radiograph shows no other abnormality, the mediastinal widening is due to deposition of normal fat. Although CT can easily demonstrate mediastinal adiposity, it should rarely be needed to confirm a diagnosis that can be made with confidence from chest radiographs.

A second situation in which the potential for the overuse of CT exists is the cardiophrenic angle mass frequently seen on chest radiographs. In the asymptomatic patient, these lesions are invariably benign and do not require treatment. Although CT can differentiate an epicardial fat pad from a pleuropericardial cyst, the differentiation is seldom of any clinical importance. However, in the symptomatic patient, or in the patient with possible mediastinal adenopathy, a cardiophrenic angle mass has entirely different significance. In this case, CT detection of enlarged circumcardiac lymph nodes can be of critical importance in determining patient management.

The role of CT in the diagnosis and follow-up assessment of patients with aortic dissection has not been finalized. Fast scanners, with rapid sequential scanning capabilities, can allow a confident diagnosis of the presence or absence of aortic dissection. They can also define with accuracy the patency of the false channel. Still undocumented is whether CT can provide all the information required for the surgical approach to treatment and obviate aortography in some or all patients.

CT Detection of Disease

The efficacy of CT in detecting disease not suspected from chest radiographs has been difficult to document. CT is more sensitive than conventional tomography in the detection of such lesions as mediastinal adenopathy, small thymomas, and parathyroid adenomas. Adequately determining the sensitivity and specificity of CT in these clinical situations has been difficult.

Computed tomography has shown great sensitivity in the detection of mediastinal adenopathy in patients with bronchogenic carcinoma. However, CT cannot make a histologic diagnosis, and the significance of enlarged mediastinal lymph nodes still requires critical investigation. A substantial percentage of enlarged nodes detected only on CT scans do not contain tumor. Bronchogenic carcinoma should not be considered surgically unresectable solely on the finding of mediastinal adenopathy.

The ability of CT to show mediastinal invasion by central bronchogenic tumors should not be overestimated because this interpretation is at times exceedingly difficult. Tumor masses adjacent to the mediastinum, with or without collapsed lung around them, often do not show a clear-cut plane of separation from the mediastinum.

In patients with myasthenia gravis or hyperparathyroidism, CT can demonstrate small mediastinal tumors not apparent on chest radiographs. The sensitivity and specificity of CT in the detection of tumor in these patients requires further confirmation.

The use of computed mediastinal tomography in staging lymphoma is intimately related to changing forms of therapy and also warrants further investigation. In most patients, the bulky mediastinal lymphadenopathy associated with lymphoma is readily apparent on chest radiographs or on conventional tomograms. CT scans can detect lymphadenopathy not apparent using other imaging modalities, but small, subtle lymphadenopathy is relatively uncommon in cases of lymphoma. The frequency and significance of extrapleural extension has been discussed only once[216] and requires further assessment. Similarly, the CT detection of direct extension of lymphomatous tissue from the mediastinum and hilum into the lung parenchyma is important but has not been fully clarified.

The role of CT in assessing many diseases of the mediastinum is in flux. Most reports to date have been anecdotal and limited in scope. Although the capabilities of this imaging modality have been substantiated, larger and more detailed studies must now be undertaken. We can anticipate a better understanding of the role of computed mediastinal tomography and the indications for its use as, over the next few years, more data become available and technical improvements in equipment stabilize. A list of indications based on the most recent available information is given in Table 5–6.

Table 5–6. INDICATIONS FOR COMPUTED
MEDIASTINAL TOMOGRAPHY

Staging of and planning treatment for bronchogenic
 carcinoma
Staging of and planning treatment for lymphoma
Staging of and planning treatment for esophageal carcinoma
 (see Chapter 12)
Detection of thymoma
Detection of parathyroid adenoma
Detection of aortic dissection
Detection of adenopathy
Characterization of mediastinal mass
Characterization of paramediastinal mass
Characterization of mediastinal goiter
Characterization of mediastinal widening (qualified
 indication)
Characterization of aortic aneurysm
Characterization of paraspinous widening
Characterization of cardiophrenic masses (qualified
 indication)
Localization of mediastinal abscess

REFERENCES

1. Heitzman ER: The Mediastinum: Radiologic Correlations with Anatomy and Pathology. St. Louis, CV Mosby Company, 1977.
2. Carter BL, Morehead J, Wolpert SM, Hammerschlag SB, Griffiths HJ: Cross-Sectional Anatomy. Computed Tomography and Ultrasound Correlation. New York, Appleton-Century-Crofts, 1977.
3. Peterson RR: A Cross-Sectional Approach to Anatomy. Chicago, Year Book Medical Publishers, Inc, 1980.
4. Department of Radiology, SUNY Upstate Medical Center: An Atlas of Cross-Sectional Anatomy: Computed Tomography, Ultrasound, Radiography, Gross Anatomy. In Kieffer SA, Heitzman ER (eds): Hagerstown, Md, Harper & Row, 1979.
5. Heitzman ER, Goldwin RL, Proto AV: Radiologic analysis of the mediastinum utilizing computed tomography. Radiol Clin North Am 15:309, 1977.
6. Jost RG, Sagel SS, Stanley RJ, Levitt RG: Computed tomography of the thorax. Radiology 126:125, 1978.
7. Kolbenstvedt A, Kolmannskog F, Aakhus T: Arterial structures of the chest and abdomen at computer tomography. Acta Radiol (Diagn) 20:703, 1979.

8. Goldwin RL, Heitzman ER, Proto AV: Computed tomography of the mediastinum: Normal anatomy and indications for the use of CT. Radiology 124:235, 1977.

9. Speckman JM, Gamsu G, Webb WR: Alterations in CT mediastinal anatomy produced by an azygos lobe. AJR 137:47, 1981.

10. Guthaner DF, Wexler L, Harell G: CT demonstration of cardiac structures. AJR 133:75, 1979.

11. Hyson EA, Ravin CE: Radiographic features of mediastinal anatomy. Chest 75:609, 1979.

12. Sone S, Higashihara T, Morimoto S, Yokota K, Ikezoe J, Masaoka A, Monden Y, Kagotani T: Normal anatomy of thymus and anterior mediastinum by pneumomediastinography. AJR 134:81, 1980.

13. Mitsuoka A, Kitano M, Ishii S: Gas-contrasted computed tomography of the mediastinum. J Comput Assist Tomogr 5:588, 1981.

14. Warwick R, Williams PR: Gray's Anatomy. Philadelphia, WB Saunders Company, 1973.

15. Taber P, Chang LWM, Campion GM: The left brachiocephalic vein simulating aortic dissection on computed tomography. J Comput Assist Tomogr 3:360, 1979.

16. Baron RL, Lee JKT, Sagel SS, Peterson RR: Computed tomography of the normal thymus. Radiology 142:121, 1982.

17. Heiberg E, Wolverson MK, Sundaram M, Nouri S: Normal thymus: CT characteristics in subjects under age 20. AJR 138:491, 1982.

18. Moore AV, Korobkin M, Olanow W, Breiman RS, Ram PC, Hidalgo H: CT of the normal and abnormal thymus gland: Surgical and pathologic correlation on 40 patients. Presented at the Annual Meeting of the Radiological Society of North America, Chicago, November 15–19, 1981.

19. Dixon AK, Hilton CJ, Williams GT: Computed tomography and histological correlation of the thymic remnant. Clin Radiol 32:225, 1981.

20. Schnyder PA, Gamsu G: CT of the pretracheal retrocaval space. AJR 136:303, 1981.

21. Heitzman ER, Lane EJ, Hammack DB, Rimmler LJ: Radiological evaluation of the aortic-pulmonic window. Radiology 116:513, 1975.

22. Beck E, Beattie EJ Jr: The lymph nodes in the mediastinum. J Int Coll Surg 29:247, 1958.

23. Nohl HC: The Spread of Carcinoma of the Bronchus. Chicago, Year Book Medical Publishers, Inc, 1962.

24. Kormano M, Yrjana J: The posterior tracheal band: Correlation between computed tomography and chest radiography. Radiology 136:689, 1980.

25. Cimmino CV: The esophageal-pleural stripe: An update. Radiology 140:609, 1981.

26. Callen PW, Korobkin M, Isherwood I: Computed tomographic evaluation of the retrocrural prevertebral space. AJR 129:907, 1977.

27. Cimmino CV: The anterior mediastinal line on chest roentgenograms. Radiology 82:459, 1964.

28. Berne AS, Gerle RD, Mitchell GE: The mediastinum: Normal roentgen anatomy and radiologic technics. Semin Roentgenol 4:3, 1969.

29. Figley MM: Mediastinal minutiae. Semin Roentgenol 4:22, 1969.

30. Proto AV, Lane EJ: Air in the esophagus: A frequent radiographic finding. AJR 129:433, 1977.

31. Heitzman ER, Scrivani JV, Martino J, Moro J: The azygous vein and its pleural reflections: I. Normal anatomy. Radiology 101:249, 1971.

32. DeGinder WL: Pleuro-esophageal line in normal chest roentgenograms. JAMA 167:437, 1958.

33. Savoca CJ, Austin JHM, Goldberg HI: The right paratracheal stripe. Radiology 122:295, 1977.

34. Putman CE, Curtis AM, Westfriend M, McLoud TC: Thickening of the posterior tracheal stripe: A sign of squamous cell carcinoma of the esophagus. Radiology 121:533, 1976.

35. Yrjana J: The posterior tracheal band and recurrent esophageal carcinoma. Radiology 136:615, 1980.

36. Heitzman ER: Computed tomography of the thorax: Current perspectives. AJR 136:2, 1981.

37. Carter BL, Ignatow SB: Neck and mediastinal angiography by computed tomography scan. Radiology 122:515, 1977.

38. Newhouse JH, Murphy RX Jr: Tissue distribution of soluble contrast: Effect of dose variation and changes with time. AJR 136:463, 1981.

39. Burgener FA, Hamlin DJ: Contrast enhancement in abdominal CT: Bolus vs. infusion. AJR 137:351, 1981.

40. Young SW, Noon MA, Nassi M, Castellino RA: Dynamic computed tomography body scanning. J Comput Assist Tomogr 4:168, 1980.

41. Ball WS, Wicks JD, Mettler FA Jr: Prone-supine change in organ position: CT demonstration. AJR 135:815, 1980.

42. van Waes PFGM, Zonneveld FW: Patient positioning for direct coronal computed tomography of the entire body. Radiology 142:531, 1982.

43. Brown LR, Muhm JR, Sheedy PF II: Computed tomography of the chest. In Putman CE (ed): Pulmonary Diagnosis Imaging and Other Techniques. New York, Appleton-Century-Crofts, 1981, p 83.

44. Baron RL, Levitt RG, Sagel SS, Stanley RJ: Computed tomography in the evaluation of mediastinal widening. Radiology 138:107, 1981.

45. Webb WR, Gamsu G, Speckman JM, Kaiser JA, Federle MP, Lipton MJ: CT demonstration of mediastinal aortic arch anomalies. J Comput Assist Tomogr 6:445, 1982.

46. McLoughlin MJ, Weisbrod G, Wise DJ, Yeung HPH: Computed tomography in congenital anomalies of the aortic arch and great vessels. Radiology 138:399, 1981.

47. Shuford WH, Sybers RG: The Aortic Arch and Its Malformations: With Emphasis on the Angiographic Features. Springfield, Ill, Charles C Thomas, 1974, pp 215–244.

48. Godwin JD, Herfkens RJ, Brundage BH, Lipton MJ: Evaluation of coarctation of the aorta by computed tomography. J Comput Assist Tomogr 5:153, 1981.

49. Gaupp RJ, Fagan CJ, Davis M, Epstein NE: Pseudocoarctation of the aorta. J Comput Assist Tomogr 5:571, 1981.

50. Klinkhamer AC: Aberrant right subclavian artery. Clinical and roentgenologic aspects. AJR 97:438, 1966.

51. Steward JR, Owings WK, Titus JL: Right aortic arch: Plain film diagnosis and significance. AJR 97:377, 1966.

52. Baron MG: Right aortic arch. Circulation 44:1137, 1971.

53. Shuford WH, Sybers RG, Edwards FK: The three types of right aortic arch. AJR 109:67, 1970.

54. Taber P, Chang LWM, Campion GM: Diagnosis of

retro-esophageal right aortic arch by computed tomography. J Comput Assist Tomogr 3:684, 1979.

55. Shuford WH, Sybers RG, Weens HS: The angiographic features of double aortic arch. AJR 116:125, 1972.

56. Cohen BA, Efremidis SC, Dan SJ, Robinson B, Rabinowitz JG: Aneurysm of the ductus arteriosus in an adult: J Comput Assist Tomogr 5:421, 1981.

57. Stone DN, Bein ME, Garris JB: Anomalous left pulmonary artery: Two new adult cases. AJR 135:1259, 1980.

58. Baron RL, Gutierrez FR, Sagel SS, Levitt RG, McKnight RC: CT of anomalies of the mediastinal vessels. AJR 137:571, 1981.

58a. Gilman MJ, Somogyi J, Taber M: Hypoplastic right pulmonary artery in the hypogenetic lung syndrome. J Comput Assist Tomogr 6:1015, 1982.

59. Cha EM, Khoury GH: Persistent left superior vena cava: Radiologic and clinical significance. Radiology 103:375, 1972.

60. Winter FS: Persistent left superior vena cava: Survey of world literature and report of thirty additional cases. Angiology 5:90, 1954.

61. Campbell M, Deuchar DC: The left-sided superior vena cava. Br Heart J 16:423, 1954.

62. Huggins TJ, Lesar ML, Friedman AC, Pyatt RS, Thane TT: CT appearance of persistent left superior vena cava. J Comput Assist Tomogr 6:294, 1982.

63. Webb WR, Gamsu G, Speckman JM, Kaiser JA, Federle MP, Lipton MJ: Computed tomographic demonstration of mediastinal venous anomalies. AJR 139:157, 1982.

64. Chuang VP, Mena CE, Hoskins PA: Congenital anomalies of the inferior vena cava. Review of embryogenesis and presentation of a simplified classification. Br J Radiol 47:206, 1974.

65. Berdon WE, Baker DH: Plain film findings in azygos continuation of the inferior vena cava. AJR 104:452, 1968.

66. Ginaldi S, Chuang VP, Wallace S: Absence of the hepatic segment of the inferior vena cava with azygos continuation. J Comput Assist Tomogr 4:112, 1980.

67. Breckenridge JW, Kinlaw WB: Azygos continuation of inferior vena cava: CT appearance. J Comput Assist Tomogr 4:392, 1980.

68. Churchill RJ, Wesby G III, Marsan RE, Moncada R, Reynes CJ, Love L: Computed tomographic demonstration of anomalous inferior vena cava with azygos continuation. J Comput Assist Tomogr 4:398, 1980.

68a. Smathers RL, Buschi AJ, Pope TL Jr, Brenbridge AN, Williamson BR: The azygous arch: Normal and pathologic CT appearance. AJR 139:477, 1982.

69. Floyd GD, Nelson WP: Developmental interruption of the inferior vena cava with azygos and hemiazygos substitution. Unusual radiographic features. Radiology 119:55, 1976.

70. Haswell DM, Berrigan TJ Jr: Anomalous inferior vena cava with accessory hemiazygos continuation. Radiology 119:51, 1976.

71. Axelbaum SP, Schellinger D, Gomes MN, Ferris RA, Hakkal HG. Computed tomographic evaluation of aortic aneurysms. AJR 127:75, 1976.

72. Kazui T, Takeda H, Yamacishi M, et al: The application of computerized tomography for diagnosis of thoracic and abdominal aneurysm. Jpn J Thorac Surg 31:904, 1978.

73. Korobkin M, Kressel HY, Moss AA, Koehler RE: Com-

puted tomographic angiography of the body. Radiology 126:807, 1978.

74. Godwin JD, Herfkens RL, Skiöldebrand CG, Federle MP, Lipton MJ: Evaluation of dissections and aneurysms of the thoracic aorta by conventional and dynamic CT scanning. Radiology 136:125, 1980.

75. Machida K, Tasaka A: CT patterns of mural thrombus in aortic aneurysms. J Comput Assist Tomogr 4:840, 1980.

76. Egan TJ, Neiman HL, Herman RJ, Malave SR, Sanders JH: Computed tomography in the diagnosis of aortic aneurysm dissection of traumatic injury. Radiology 136:141, 1980.

77. Cooley RN, Schreiber MH: Radiology of the heart and great vessels. Golden's Diagnostic Radiology, 3rd ed. Baltimore, Williams & Wilkins, 1978, p 603–604.

78. Fomon JJ, Kurzweg FT, Broadaway RK: Aneurysms of the aorta: A review. Ann Surg 165:557, 1967.

79. Higgins CB, Silverman NR, Harris RD, Albertson KW: Localized aneurysms of the descending thoracic aorta. Clin Radiol 26:475, 1975.

80. Joyce JW, Fairbairn JF II, Kincaid OW, Juergens JL: Aneurysms of the thoracic aorta: A clinical study with special reference to prognosis. Circulation 29:176, 1964.

81. Brown LR, Muhm JR, Sheedy PF II: Computed tomography of the chest. Pulmonary Diagnosis Imaging and Other Techniques. In Putman CE (ed): New York, Appleton-Century-Crofts, 1981, pp 83–90.

82. Bahnson HT: Definitive treatment of saccular aneurysms of the aorta with excision of sac and aortic suture. Surg Gynecol Obstet 96:382, 1953.

83. Cooley DA, DeBakey ME: Surgical considerations of intrathoracic aneurysms of the aorta and great vessels. Ann Surg 135:660, 1952.

84. Sorensen HR, Olsen H: Ruptured and dissection aneurysms of the aorta. Acta Chir Scand 128:644, 1964.

85. Hirst AE, Johns VJ, Kime SW: Dissecting aneurysms of the aorta: A review of 505 cases. Medicine 37:217, 1958.

86. DeBakey ME, Henley WS, Cooley DA, Morris GC, Crawford ES, Beall AC Jr: Surgical management of dissecting aneurysm involving ascending aorta. J Cardiovasc Surg 5:200, 1964.

87. Itzchak Y, Rosenthal T, Adar R, Rubinstein ZJ, Lieberman V, Deutsch V: Dissecting aneurysm of the thoracic aorta: Reappraisal of radiologic diagnosis. AJR 125:559, 1975.

88. Eyler WR, Clark MD: Dissecting aneurysms of the aorta: Roentgen manifestations including a comparison with other types of aneurysms. Radiology 85:1047, 1965.

89. Gross SC, Barr I, Eyler WR, Khaja F, Goldstein S: Computed tomography in dissection of the thoracic aorta. Radiology 136:135, 1980.

90. Larde D, Belloir C, Vasile N, Frija J, Ferrane J: Computed tomography of aortic dissection. Radiology 136:147, 1980.

91. Heiberg E, Wolverson M, Sundaram M, Connors J, Susman N: CT findings in thoracic aortic dissection. AJR 136:13, 1981.

92. Suchato C, Pekanan P, Singjaroen T, Sereerat P: Indication of dissecting aortic aneurysm on noncontrast computed tomography. J Comput Assist Tomogr 4:115, 1980.

92a. Godwin JD, Breiman RS, Speckman JM: Problems and

pitfalls in the evaluation of thoracic aortic dissection by computed tomography. J Comput Assist Tomogr 6:750, 1982

93. Attar S, Fardin R, Ayella R, McLaughlin JS: Medical vs. surgical treatment of acute dissecting aneurysms. Arch Surg 103:568, 1971.

94. Daily PO, Trueblood HW, Stinson EB, Wuerflein RD, Shumway NE: Management of acute aortic dissections. Ann Thorac Surg 10:237, 1970.

95. Dalen JE, Alpert JS, Cohn LH, Black H, Collins JJ: Dissection of the thoracic aorta—Medical or surgical therapy? Am J Cardiol 34:803, 1974.

96. McFarland J, Willerson JT, Dinsmore RE, Austen WG, Buckley MJ, Sanders CA, DeSanctis RW: The medical treatment of dissecting aortic aneurysms. N Engl J Med 286:115, 1972.

97. Strong WW, Moggio RA, Stansel HC Jr: Acute aortic dissection—Twelve-year medical and surgical experience. J Thorac Cardiovasc Surg 68:815, 1974.

98. Wheat MW Jr: Dissecting aneurysms of the aorta. In Sabiston DC Jr (ed): Textbook of Surgery, 11th ed. Philadelphia, WB Saunders Company, 1977, p 1886–1891.

99. Miller DC, Stinson EB, Oyer PE, Rossiter SJ, Reitz BA, Griepp RB, Shumway NE: The operative treatment of aortic dissections: Experience with 111 patients over a 14 year period. J Thorac Cardiovasc Surg 78:365, 1979.

100. Thomas CS Jr, Alford WC Jr, Burrus GR, Frist RA, Stoney WS: The effectiveness of surgical treatment of acute aortic dissection. Ann Thorac Surg 26:42, 1978.

101. Turley K, Ullyot DJ, Godwin JD, et al: Repair of thoracic aortic dissection. Evaluation of false lumen utilizing computed tomography. J Thorac Cardiovasc Surg 81:61, 1981.

102. Guthaner DF, Miller DC, Silverman JF, et al: Fate of the false lumen following surgical repair of aortic dissections: An angiographic study. Radiology 133:1, 1979.

103. Godwin JD, Turley K, Herfkens RJ, Lipton MJ: Computed tomography for follow-up of chronic aortic dissections. Radiology 139:655, 1981.

104. Bruckner WJ: Significance of superior vena caval syndrome. Arch Intern Med 102:88, 1958.

105. Failor JH, Edwards JE, Hodgson CH: Etiologic factors in obstruction of the superior vena cava: A pathologic study. Proc Staff Meet Mayo Clin 33:671, 1958.

106. Ghosh BC, Cliffton EE: Malignant tumors with superior vena cava obstruction. NY State J Med 73:283, 1973.

107. Nogeire C, Mincer F, Botstein C: Long survival in patients with bronchogenic carcinoma complicated by superior vena caval obstruction. Chest 75:325, 1979.

108. Steinberg I: Dilatation of the hemiazygos veins in superior vena caval occlusion simulating mediastinal tumor. AJR 87:248, 1962.

109. Parish JM, Marschke RF Jr, Dines DE, Lee RE: Etiologic considerations in superior vena cava syndrome. Mayo Clin Proc 56:407, 1981.

110. Berk RN: Dilatation of the left superior intercostal vein in the plain-film diagnosis of chronic superior vena caval obstruction. Radiology 83:419, 1964.

111. Mori KW: Dynamic scanning in the evaluation of superior vena cava syndrome. CT/T Clinical Symposium 4:81, 1981.

112. Hidalgo H, Korobkin M, Breiman RS, Heaston DK, Moore AV, Ram PC: CT demonstration of subcuta-neous venous collaterals. J Comput Assist Tomogr 6:514, 1982.

113. Brown LR, Muhm JR, Sheedy PF II: Computed tomography of the chest. In Pulmonary Diagnosis Imaging and Other Techniques. In Putman CE (ed): New York, Appleton-Century-Crofts, 1981, p 81.

114. Kolbenstvedt A, Kolmannskog F, Aakhus T: Venous structures of the chest and abdomen at computer tomography. Acta Radiol (Diagn) 20:513, 1979.

115. Kormano MJ, Dean PB, Hamlin DJ: Upper extremity contrast medium infusion in computed tomography of upper mediastinal masses. J Comput Assist Tomogr 4:617, 1980.

116. Zerhouni EA, Barth KH, Siegelman SS: Demonstration of venous thrombosis by computed tomography. AJR 134:753, 1980.

117. Vujic I, Stanley J, Tyminski LJ: Computed tomography of suspected caval thrombosis secondary to proximal extension of phlebitis from the leg. Radiology 140:437, 1981.

118. Godwin JD, Webb WR: Contrast-related flow phenomena mimicking pathology on thoracic computed tomography. J Comput Assist Tomogr 6:460, 1982.

119. Ege G: Internal mammary lymphoscintigraphy. Radiology 118:101, 1976.

120. Rose CM, Kaplan WD, Marck A: Lymphoscintigraphy of the internal mammary lymph nodes. Int J Radiat Oncol Biol Phys (Suppl 2) 2:102, 1977.

121. Munzenrider JE, Tchakarova I, Castro M, Carter B: Computerized body tomography in breast cancer. Cancer 43:137, 1979.

122. Gouliamos AD, Carter BL, Emani B: Computed tomography of the chest wall. Radiology 134:433, 1980.

123. Meyer JE, Munzenrider JE: Computed tomographic demonstration of internal mammary lymph-node metastasis in patients with locally recurrent breast carcinoma. Radiology 139:661, 1981.

124. Kreel L: Computed tomography of the thorax. Radiol Clin North Am 16:575, 1978.

125. Crowe JK, Brown LR, Muhm JR: Computed tomography of the mediastinum. Radiology 128:75, 1978.

126. Shevland JE, Chiu LC, Schapiro RL, Young JA, Rossi NP: The role of conventional tomography and computed tomography in assessing the resectability of primary lung cancer: A preliminary report. Comput Tomogr 2:1, 1978.

127. McLoud TC, Wittenberg J, Ferruci JT Jr: Computed tomography of the thorax and standard radiographic evaluation of the chest: A comparative study. J Comput Assist Tomogr 3:170, 1979.

128. Mintzer RA, Malave SR, Neiman HL, Michaelis LL, Vanecko RM, Sanders JH: Computed vs. conventional tomography in evaluation of primary and secondary pulmonary neoplasms. Radiology 132:653, 1979.

129. Ekholm S, Albrechtsson U, Kugelberg J, Tylen U: Computed tomography in preoperative staging of bronchogenic carcinoma. J Comput Assist Tomogr 4:763, 1980.

130. Hirleman MT, Yiu-Chiu VS, Chiu LC, Schapiro RL: The resectability of primary lung carcinoma: A diagnostic staging review. Comput Tomogr 4:146, 1980.

131. Putman CE, Rothman SL, Littner MR, Allen WE, Schachter EN, McLoud TC, Bein ME, Gee JB: Computerized tomography in pulmonary sarcoid. Comput Tomogr 1:197, 1977.

132. Heitzman ER: The Mediastinum: Radiologic Correlations with Anatomy and Pathology. St. Louis, CV Mosby Company, 1977, p 257–263.

133. Efremidis SC, Dan SJ, Cohen BA, Mitty HA, Rabinowitz JG: Displaced paraspinal line: Role of CT and lymphography. AJR 136:505, 1981.

134. Cohen WN, Seidelmann FE, Bryan PJ: Computed tomography of localized adipose deposits presenting as tumor masses. AJR 128:1007, 1977.

134a. Streiter ML, Schneider HJ, Proto AV: Steroid-induced thoracic lipomatosis: Paraspinal involvement. AJR 139:679, 1982.

135. Castellino RA, Blank N: Adenopathy of the cardiophrenic angle (diaphragmatic) lymph nodes. Radiology 114:509, 1972.

135a. Jochelson MS, Balikian JP, Mauch P, Liebman H: Peri- and paracardial involvement in lymphoma: A radiographic study of 11 cases. AJR 40:483, 1983.

136. Bledin A, Bernardino ME, Libshitz HI: Cardiophrenic angle nodes: An unusual CT finding of advanced metastatic disease. Comput Tomogr 4:193, 1980.

137. Rohlfing BM, Korobkin M, Hall AD: Computed tomography of intrathoracic omental herniation and other mediastinal fatty masses. J Comput Assist Tomogr 1:181, 1977.

138. Bein ME, Mancuso AA, Mink JH, Hansen GC: Computed tomography in the evaluation of mediastinal lipomatosis. J Comput Assist Tomogr 2:379, 1978.

139. Pugatch RD, Faling LJ, Robbins AH, Spira R: CT diagnosis of benign mediastinal abnormalities. AJR 134:685, 1980.

140. Mendez G Jr, Isikoff MB, Isikoff SK, Sinner WN: Fatty tumors of the thorax demonstrated by CT. AJR 133:207, 1979.

141. Rothman SLG, Simeone JF, Allen WE, Putman CE, Redman HC: Computerized tomography in the assessment of diseases of the thorax. Comput Tomogr 1:181, 1977.

142. Oldham HN Jr, Sabiston DC Jr: Primary tumors and cysts of the mediastinum. Monogr Surg Sci 4:243, 1967.

143. Oldham HN Jr: Mediastinal tumors and cysts (collective review). Ann Thorac Surg 11:246, 1971.

144. Marvasti MA, Mitchell GE, Burke WA, Meyer JA: Misleading density of mediastinal cysts on computerized tomography. Ann Thorac Surg 31:167, 1981.

145. Federle MP, Callen PW: Cystic Hodgkin's lymphoma of the thymus: Computed tomography appearance. J Comput Assist Tomogr 3:542, 1979.

146. Wychulis AR, Payne WS, Clagett OT, Woolner LB: Surgical treatment of mediastinal tumors. A 40-year experience. J Thorac Cardiovasc Surg 62:379, 1971.

147. Benjamin SP, McCormack LJ, Effler DB, Groves LK: Critical review—"Primary tumours of the mediastinum." Chest 62:297, 1972.

147a. Nakata H, Nakayama C, Kimoto T, Nakayama T, Tsukamoto Y, Nobe T, Suzuki H: Computed tomography of mediastinal bronchogenic cysts. J Comput Assist Tomogr 6:733, 1982.

147b. Mendelson DS, Rose JS, Efremidis SC, Kirschner PA, Cohen BA: Bronchogenic cysts with high CT numbers. AJR 140: 463, 1983.

148. Rogers CI, Seymour EQ, Brock JG: Atypical pericardial cyst location: The value of computed tomography. J Comput Assist Tomogr 4:683, 1980.

149. Pugatch RD, Braver JH, Robbins AH, Faling LJ: CT diagnosis of pericardial cysts. AJR 131:515, 1978.

150. Rosai J, Levine GD: Tumors of the Thymus. Washington, DC, Armed Forces Institute of Pathology, 1976, pp 207–211.

151. Gouliamos A, Striggaris K, Lolas C, Deligeorgi-Politi H, Vlahos L: Thymic cyst. J Comput Assist Tomogr 6:172, 1982.

152. Alee G, Logue B, Mansour K: Thymic cyts simulating multiple cardiovascular abnormalities and presenting with pericarditis and pericardial tamponade. Am J Cardiol 31:377, 1973.

153. Weinfeld A, Kaplan JO: Mediastinal pancreatic pseudocyst. Gastrointest Radiol 4:343, 1979.

154. Ovens GR, Arger PH, Mulhern CB Jr, Coleman BG, Gohel V: CT evaluation of mediastinal pseudocyst. J Comput Assist Tomogr 4:256, 1980.

155. Scully RE, Galdabini JJ, McNeely U: Weekly clinicopathological exercises. Case Records of the Massachusetts General Hospital 296:1467, 1977.

155a. Friedman AC, Pyatt RS, Hartman DS, Downey EF Jr, Olson WB: CT of benign cystic teratomas. AJR 138:659, 1982.

155b. Suzuki M, Takashima T, Itoh H, Choutoh S, Kawamura I, Watanabe Y: Computed tomography of mediastinal teratomas. J Comput Assist Tomogr 7:74, 1983.

156. Komaiko MS, Lee ME, Birnberg FA: The contrast enhanced paravascular neoplasm: A potential CT pitfall. J Comput Assist Tomogr 4:516, 1980.

157. Livesay JJ, Mink JH, Fee HJ, Bein ME, Sample WF, Mulder DG: The use of computed tomography to evaluate suspected mediastinal tumors. Ann Thorac Surg 27:305, 1979.

158. Webb WR, Jeffrey RB, Godwin JD: Thoracic computed tomography in superior sulcus tumors. J Comput Assist Tomogr 5:361, 1981.

159. Brown LR, Muhm JR, Gray JE: Radiographic detection of thymoma. AJR 134:1181, 1980.

160. Fon GT, Bein ME, Mancuso AA, Keesey JC, Lupetin AR, Wong WS: Computed tomography of the anterior mediastinum in myasthenia gravis. Radiology 142:135, 1982.

161. Batata MA, Martini N, Huvos AG, Aguilar RI, Beattie EJ: Thymomas: Clinicopathologic features, therapy, and prognosis. Cancer 34:398, 1974.

162. Goldman AJ, Herrmann C, Keesey JC, Mulder DG, Brown WJ: Myasthenia gravis and invasive thymoma: A 20-year experience. Neurology 25:1021, 1975.

163. Lattes R: Thymoma and other tumors of the thymus: An analysis of 107 cases. Cancer 15:1224, 1962.

164. Sellors TH, Thackray AC, Thomson AD: Tumours of the thymus. A review of 88 operation cases. Thorax 22:193, 1967.

165. Good CA: Roentgenologic findings in myasthenia gravis associated with thymic tumor. AJR 57:305, 1947.

166. Kreel L: Radiology in myasthenia gravis. Proc Soc Med 61:757, 1968.

167. Rosenthal T, Hertz M, Samra Y, Shahin N: Thymoma: Clinical and additional radiologic signs. Chest 65:428, 1974.

168. Mink JH, Bein ME, Sukov R, Herrmann C Jr, Winter J, Sample WF, Mulder D: Computed tomography of the anterior mediastinum in patients with myasthenia gravis and suspected thymoma. AJR 130:239, 1978.

169. Aita JF, Wanamaker WM: Body computerized tomography and the thymus. Arch Neurol 36:20, 1979.

170. Rosai J, Levine GD: Atlas of Tumor Pathology, 2nd Series. Tumors of the Thymus. Washington, DC, Armed Forces Institute of Pathology, 1976, pp 132–140.

171. Moore AV, Korobkin M, Powers B, Olanow W, Ravin CE, Putman CE, Breiman RS: Thymoma detection by mediastinal CT: Patients with myasthenia gravis. AJR 138:217, 1982.

172. Baron RL, Lee JKT, Sagel SS, Levitt RG: Computed tomography of the abnormal thymus. Radiology 142:127, 1982.

173. Zerhouni EA, Scott WW Jr, Baker RR, Wharam MD, Siegelman SS: Invasive thymomas: Diagnosis and evaluation by computed tomography. J Comput Assist Tomogr 6:92, 1982.

174. Wychulis AR, Payne WS, Clagett OT, Woolner LB: Surgical treatment of mediastinal tumors. J Thorac Cardiovasc Surg 62:379, 1971.

175. Benjamin SP, McCormack IJ, Effler DB, Groves LK: Primary tumors of the mediastinum. Chest 62:297, 1972.

176. Binder RE, Pugatch RD, Faling LJ, Kanter RA, Sawin CT: Diagnosis of posterior mediastinal goiter by computed tomography. J Comput Assist Tomogr 4:552, 1980.

177. Irwin RS, Braman SS, Arvanitidis AN, Hamolsky MW: [131]I thyroid scanning in preoperative diagnosis of mediastinal goiter. Ann Intern Med 89:73, 1978.

178. Kaneko T, Matsumoto M, Fukui K, Hori T, Katayama K: Clinical evaluation of thyroid CT values in various thyroid conditions. Comput Tomogr 3:1, 1979.

179. Machida K, Yoshikawa K: Aberrant thyroid gland demonstrated by computed tomography. J Comput Assist Tomogr 35:689, 1979.

179a. Morris UL, Colletti PM, Ralls PW, Boswell WD, Lapin SA, Quinn M, Halls JM: CT demonstration of intrathoracic thyroid tissue. J Comput Assist Tomogr 6:821, 1982.

179b. Bashist B, Ellis K, Gold RP: Computed tomography of intrathoracic goiters. AJR 140:455, 1983.

180. Sekiya T, Tada S, Kawakami K, Kino M, Fukuda K, Watanabe H: Clinical application of computed tomography to thyroid disease. Comput Tomogr 3:185, 1979.

181. Glazer GM, Axel L, Moss AA: CT diagnosis of mediastinal thyroid. AJR 138:495, 1982.

182. Krudy AG, Doppman JL, Brennan MF: The detection of mediastinal parathyroid glands by computed tomography, selective arteriography, and venous sampling. Radiology 140:739, 1981.

183. Brennan MF, Doppman JL, Marx SJ, Spiegel AM, Brown EM, Aurback GD: Reoperative parathyroid surgery for persistent hyperparathyroidism. Surgery 83:669, 1978.

184. Doppman JL, Krudy AG, Brennan MF, Schneider P, Lasker RD, Marx SJ: CT appearance of enlarged parathyroid glands in the posterior superior mediastinum. J Comput Assist Tomogr 6:1099, 1982.

185. Sommer B, Welter HF, Spelsberg F, Scherer U, Lissner J: Computed tomography for localizing enlarged parathyroid glands in primary hyperparathyroidism. J Comput Assist Tomogr 6:521, 1982.

186. Leigh TF, Weens HS: The Mediastinum. Springfield, Ill, Charles C Thomas, 1959.

187. Oldham HN Jr, Sabiston DC Jr: The mediastinum. In Sabiston DC Jr (ed): Textbook of Surgery. The Biological Basis of Modern Surgical Practice, 11th ed. Philadelphia, WB Saunders Company, 1977, pp 2153–2154.

187a. de Graaff CS, Falke Th, Bakker W: Computerized tomography in acute mediastinitis. Europ J Radiol 1:180, 1981.

188. Hammond EC: Lung cancer death rates in England and Wales compared with those in the U.S.A. Br Med J 2:649, 1958.

189. Silverberg E, Holleb AI: Cancer statistics, 1974-world-wide epidemiology. CA 24:2, 1974.

190. Mountain CF, Carr, DT, Anderson WAD: Clinical staging of lung cancer. AJR 120:130, 1974.

191. Carr DT: The staging of lung cancer. Am Rev Respir Dis 117:819, 1978.

192. American Joint Committee: Manual for Staging of Cancer 1978. Chicago, Whiting Press, 1978.

193. Whitcomb ME, Barham E, Goldman AL, Green DC: Indications for mediastinoscopy in bronchogenic carcinoma. Am Rev Respir Dis 113:189, 1976.

194. Acosta JL, Manfredi F: Selective mediastinoscopy. Chest 71:150, 1977.

195. Naruke T, Suemasu K, Ishikawa S: Lymph node mapping and curability at various levels of metastasis in resected lung cancer. J Thorac Cardiovasc Surg 76:832, 1978.

196. Martini N: Identification and prognostic implications of mediastinal lymph node metastases in carcinoma of the lung. Lung Cancer: Progress in Therapeutic Research. In Muggia F, Rozencweig M (eds). New York, Raven Press, 1979, pp 251–255.

197. Ashraf MH, Milsom PL, Walesby RK: Selection by mediastinoscopy and long-term survival in bronchial carcinoma. Ann Thorac Surg 30:208, 1980.

198. Jolly PC, Li W, Anderson RP: Anterior and cervical mediastinoscopy for determining operability and predicting resectability in lung cancer. J Thorac Cardiovasc Surg 79:366, 1980.

199. Underwood GH Jr, Hooper RG, Axelbaum Sp, Goodwin DW: Computed tomographic scanning of the thorax in the staging of bronchogenic carcinoma. N Engl J Med 300:777, 1979.

200. Rea HH, Shevland JE, House AJS: Accuracy of computed tomographic scanning in assessment of the mediastinum in bronchial carcinoma. J Thorac Cardiovasc Surg 81:825, 1981.

201. Faling LJ, Pugatch RD, Jung-Legg Y, Daly BDT Jr, Hong WK: CT scanning of the mediastinum in the staging of bronchogenic carcinoma. Am Rev Respir Dis 124:690, 1981.

202. Osborne DR, Korobkin M, Ravin CE, Putman CE, Wolfe NC, Sealy WC, Young WG, Breiman R, Heaston D, Ram P, Halber M: Comparison of plain radiography, conventional tomography, and computed tomography in detecting intrathoracic lymph node metastases from lung carcinoma. Radiology 142:157, 1982.

203. White MJ, Levitt RG, Baron RL, Sagel SS, Roper CL, Marbarger JP: Role of CT scanning in the evaluation of bronchogenic carcinoma. Presented at the Annual meeting of the Radiological Society of North America, Chicago, November 15–19, 1981.

204. Mittman C, Bruderman I: Lung Cancer: To operate or not? Am Rev Respir Dis 116:477, 1977.

204a. Baron RL, Levitt RG, Sagel SS, White MJ, Roper CL, Marbarger JP: Computed tomography in the preoperative evaluation of bronchogenic carcinoma. Radiology 145:727, 1982.

205. Lukes RJ, Craver LF, Hall TC, Rappaport H, Ruben P: Report of the nomenclature committee. Cancer Res 26:1311, 1966.

206. Korst DR, Meyer OO, Jaeschke WH: Survival in Hodgkin's disease: A study of patients with at least ten-year survival. Arch Intern Med 134:1043, 1974.

207. Henry L: Long survival in Hodgkin's disease. Clin Radiol 21:203, 1970.

208. Bragg DG: The clinical, pathologic and radiographic spectrum of the intrathoracic lymphomas. Invest Radiol 13:2, 1978.

209. Rosenberg SA, Kaplan HS: Evidence for an orderly progression in the spread of Hodgkin's disease. Cancer Res 26:1225, 1966.

210. Filly R, Blank N, Castellino RA: Radiographic distribution of intrathoracic disease in previously untreated patients with Hodgkin's disease and non-Hodgkin's lymphoma. Radiology 120:277, 1976.

211. Castellino RA, Filly R, Blank N: Routine full-lung tomography in the initial staging and treatment planning of patients with Hodgkin's disease and non-Hodgkin's lymphoma. Cancer 38:1130, 1976.

212. Alcorn FS, Mategrano VC, Pelasnick JP, Clark JW: Contributions of computed tomography in the staging and management of malignant lymphoma. Radiology 125:717, 1977.

213. Jones SE, Tobias DA, Waldman RS: Computed tomographic scanning in patients with lymphoma. Cancer 41:480, 1978.

214. Breiman RS, Castellino RA, Harell GS, Marshall WH, Glatstein E, Kaplan HS: CT-pathologic correlations in Hodgkin's disease and non-Hodgkin's lymphoma. Radiology 126:159, 1978.

215. Ellert J, Kreel L: The role of computed tomography in the initial staging and subsequent management of the lymphomas. J Comput Assist Tomogr 4:368, 1980.

216. Pilepich MV, Rene JB, Munzenrider JE, Carter BL: Contribution of computed tomography to the treatment of lymphomas. AJR 131:69, 1978.

217. North LB, Fuller LM, Hagemeister FB, Rodgers RW, Butler JJ, Shullenberger CC: Importance of initial mediastinal adenopathy in Hodgkin disease. AJR 138:229, 1982.

218. New policy outlines—Role of CT. Am Coll Radiol Bull 33:2, 1977.

219. Institute of Medicine: Computed Tomographic Scanning: A Policy Statement. Washington, DC, National Academy of Sciences, 1977.

220. Society for Computed Body Tomography: New indications for computed body tomography. AJR 133:115, 1979.

221. Phelps ME, Gado MH, Hoffman EJ: Correlation of effective atomic number and electron density with attenuation coefficients measured with polychromatic x-rays. Radiology 117:585, 1975.

6 COMPUTED TOMOGRAPHY OF THE PULMONARY HILA

Gordon Gamsu

The transverse axial anatomy of the hila is relatively simple when the relationships of the pulmonary arteries and veins to the bronchial tree are understood. The variations in the relative positions of the arteries, veins, and bronchi are small and do not produce major differences among patients in the appearances of the hila. The normal computed tomographic (CT) anatomy of the pulmonary hila has been described only within the past few years.[1, 2]

ANATOMY

The pulmonary hilum cannot be defined anatomically with precision, but it is generally considered to be "the depression on the mediastinal surface of the lung where the bronchus and the blood vessels and nerves enter."[3] More important than a strict definition of the hilum is an understanding of the anatomy of the pulmonary arteries and veins and their relationship to the bronchial tree, from the site in the mediastinum where they approach the lungs to their segmental branches and tributaries. The bronchial anatomy has been detailed in Chapter 4. The branches of the pulmonary artery tend to accompany their respective bronchi as they course from the mediastinum into each lung. In contrast, the pulmonary veins do not follow the bronchi and are more variable in position.

The right pulmonary artery divides within the mediastinum into upper and lower divisional arteries. The upper division of the right pulmonary artery (anterior trunk) is immediately in front of the right main bronchus. It rapidly divides, usually into three branches, each of which accompa-

271

nies a right upper lobe segmental bronchus. The apical arterial branch is anteromedial to its bronchus. The anterior and posterior pulmonary arterial branches tend to be medial to their respective bronchi. The lower division of the right pulmonary artery (interlobar artery) is anterolateral to the intermediate bronchus. The first branches of the interlobar artery are one to three ascending branches arising from its anterolateral surface to supply the right upper lobe. Next are branches accompanying the superior segmental bronchus of the right lower lobe and, at a slightly lower level, the right middle lobe bronchus. The superior segmental artery and right middle lobe

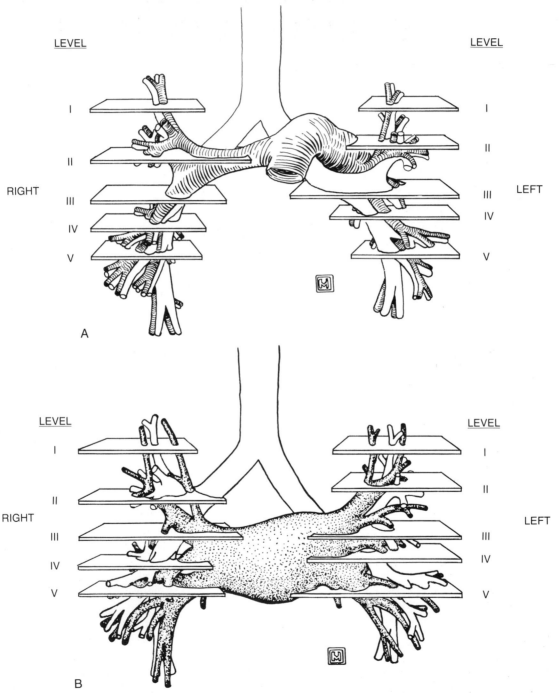

Figure 6–1. Schema of the normal hila. **A, B** The bronchial tree is shown in frontal projection in relationship to the pulmonary arteries **(A)** and pulmonary veins **(B)**. (Designated levels refer to levels in the text and to Figures 6–2 through 6–9.)

artery tend to be lateral to their respective bronchi, but they vary in position. The basal branches of the interlobar artery accompany the basal segmental bronchi but vary slightly in position.

The veins contributing to the hilar contours on the right side are the superior, middle, and inferior pulmonary veins. The right superior pulmonary vein is a relatively constant structure with two major tributaries. In most people the posterior right pulmonary vein lies lateral to the apical bronchus and courses forward in the angle between the anterior and posterior segmental bronchi of the right upper lobe. It joins the apical anterior pulmonary vein in front of the interlobar artery before entering the mediastinum. The middle pulmonary vein (or middle lobe tributary of the superior pulmonary vein) drains primarily the middle lobe and passes medial to the middle lobe bronchus. It then enters the mediastinum and joins with the superior pulmonary vein. The right inferior pulmonary vein drains primarily the lower lobe. It is the only vascular structure that crosses behind the bronchial tree on the right, which it does at about the level of the basal segmental bronchi.

The top of the left hilum is about 2 cm higher than the right, and its vascular structures vary more in position than those on the right. The left pulmonary artery does not divide into distinct upper and lower divisions. Four to eight upper lobe arterial branches arise from the superior and lateral surfaces of the main trunk of the left pulmonary artery. The branch most constantly present is an apical segmental artery coursing medial to the apical posterior segmental bronchus. An anterior branch medial to the anterior segmental bronchus is also frequently present. A posterior subsegmental branch is an inconstant finding. The left pulmonary artery passes over the left main bronchus and turns rapidly caudad as the descending left pulmonary artery. A posterior branch to the superior segment of the left lower lobe and an anterior branch to the lingular segments of the left upper lobe are the first two major branches of the descending left pulmonary artery as it courses lateral to the lower lobe bronchus. The pulmonary artery branches of both the lingular and the superior segments accompany their respective bronchi. Multiple lateral branches supplying portions of the left lower lobe are also often present. The descending left pulmonary artery divides with the basal segmental bronchi to supply the remainder of the left lower lobe.

The left pulmonary veins are similar to those found on the right. The superior pulmonary vein has posterior and apical anterior tributaries that converge and enter the mediastinum anterior to the left main bronchus. The middle pulmonary vein tributary of the superior pulmonary vein tends to drain the lingular segments of the left upper lobe and enters the mediastinum slightly caudad to the superior pulmonary vein. The inferior pulmonary vein is a posterior structure and, as on the right, passes posterior to the dividing lower lobe segmental bronchi.

The most accurate assessment of the normal and abnormal hilum is based on the hilar contours. The description of the hilar contours will be for CT window settings usually used to view the lungs (level -300 to -500 H; width 1000 H). The intramediastinal pulmonary arteries and veins are best seen at monitor settings suitable for viewing the mediastinum (level 10 to 60 H; width 250 to 500 H). The frequency with which CT scans demonstrate the hilar bronchi, arteries, and veins depends on their size and orientation. The largest central structures and those cut either transversely or longitudinally are usually visible. The segmental bronchi and vessels that course obliquely through the plane of the image, such as the middle lobe segmental bronchi, are shown less frequently.

For descriptive purposes, we will deal with CT appearances of the right and left hila separately and sequentially from superior to inferior levels (Fig. 6–1). Figures 6–1 through 6–9 are serial, contiguous 1-cm CT scans through the normal hila from superior to inferior levels. Each CT image is accompanied by a labeled schema of the hilum at that level.

RIGHT HILUM

Right Superior Hilum (Apical Segmental Bronchus, Level 1)

The superior right hilum is always identified at a level close to the tracheal bifurcation (Fig. 6–2). The apical segmental bronchus is seen in cross section lateral to the lower trachea or right main bronchus and is usually flanked on its medial side by the apical segmental pulmonary artery and on its lateral side by the posterior tributary of the superior pulmonary vein. CT scans may show branches of these vessels coursing outward from the right superior hilum, but normally additional tissue or density is not visible at this level.

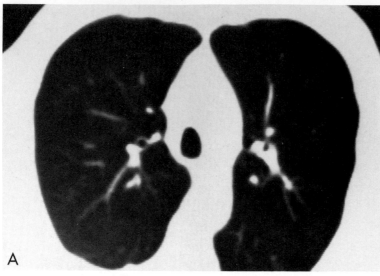

Figure 6–2. Superior hila. **A** CT scan. **B** Line drawing.

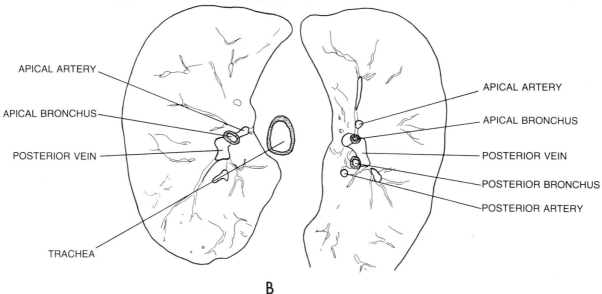

APICAL ARTERY

APICAL BRONCHUS

POSTERIOR VEIN

TRACHEA

APICAL ARTERY

APICAL BRONCHUS

POSTERIOR VEIN

POSTERIOR BRONCHUS

POSTERIOR ARTERY

B

Right Upper Hilum (Right Main Bronchus, Level 2)

The right main bronchus bifurcates into the right upper lobe bronchus and the intermediate bronchus about 1 cm below the tracheal carina (Fig. 6–3). The upper lobe bronchus arises from the lateral aspect of the main bronchus and courses laterally for 1 to 2 cm. It then usually trifurcates into anterior, posterior, and apical segmental bronchi. CT scans show the main bronchus and the anterior and posterior segmental bronchi on one image. The anterior segmental bronchus lies in a more horizontal plane than the posterior bronchus, which is directed obliquely cephalad. The anterior bronchus is thus frequently seen over a greater distance than its posterior counterpart.

The upper division of the right pulmonary artery (anterior trunk) lies anterior to the right main bronchus (Figs. 6–3, 6–4). In the transverse axial plane it is cut obliquely and produces an oval density immediately anterior to the right main bronchus and continuous with the mediastinum. The anteroposterior diameter of the anterior trunk is approximately equal to the diameter of the adjacent right main bronchus. At this level or slightly caudad, the horizontal anterior segmental pulmonary artery is medial to the anterior segmental bronchus. The posterior tributary of the superior pulmonary vein is present relatively constantly; it was found in 82 per cent of 50 lungs studied by Boyden and Scannell.[4] It is distinctive on CT images, situated laterally in the angle between the anterior and posterior segmental bron-

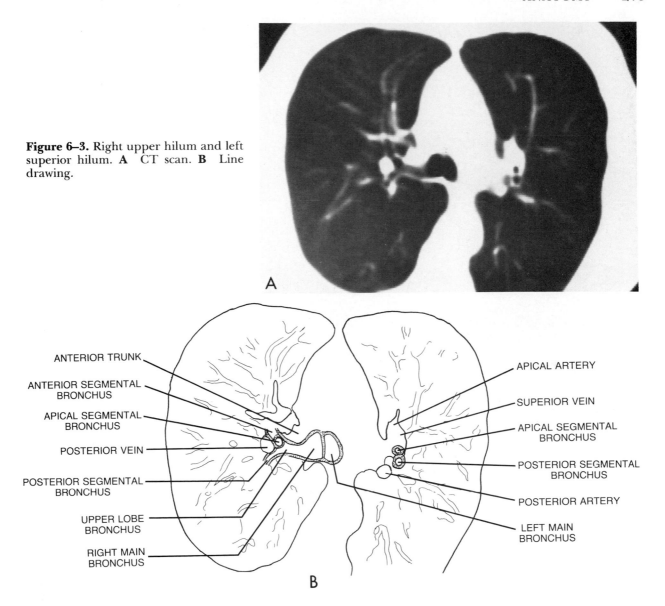

Figure 6–3. Right upper hilum and left superior hilum. **A** CT scan. **B** Line drawing.

ANTERIOR TRUNK

ANTERIOR SEGMENTAL BRONCHUS

APICAL SEGMENTAL BRONCHUS

POSTERIOR VEIN

POSTERIOR SEGMENTAL BRONCHUS

UPPER LOBE BRONCHUS

RIGHT MAIN BRONCHUS

APICAL ARTERY

SUPERIOR VEIN

APICAL SEGMENTAL BRONCHUS

POSTERIOR SEGMENTAL BRONCHUS

POSTERIOR ARTERY

LEFT MAIN BRONCHUS

chi as a round or slightly oval structure (Fig. 6–3). Also visible at this level, but less constant in position, is the apical anterior tributary of the superior pulmonary vein, which forms a subpleural convexity to the anterior hilus between the truncus anterior and the superior vena cava.

The posterior upper right hilum is devoid of vascular structures. The lung is usually close to the posterior wall of the distal right main stem bronchus and right upper lobe bronchus and medial to the posterior segmental bronchus (Figs. 6–3, 6–4).

Right Middle Hilum (Intermediate Bronchus, Level 3)

The intermediate bronchus extends vertically 3 to 4 cm, between the origin of the right upper lobe and the right middle lobe bronchi (Figs. 6–5 and 6–6). It is present in cross section on three or four adjacent images 1 cm thick. The interlobar pulmonary artery courses laterally and inferiorly from the mediastinum to assume a position anterolateral to the intermediate bronchus.

In its upper portion, the interlobar artery gives rise to two to four ascending branches that supply the anterior and lateral regions of the right upper lobe. At this level, the posterior pulmonary vein lies near the apical anterior pulmonary vein in the anterior hilum (Fig. 6–4). The two veins usually produce adjacent convexities on the anterior surface of the interlobar artery, lateral to the superior vena cava and upper right atrium (Fig. 6–4).

One to 2 cm lower, the interlobar artery takes up a more lateral position in relation to the inter-

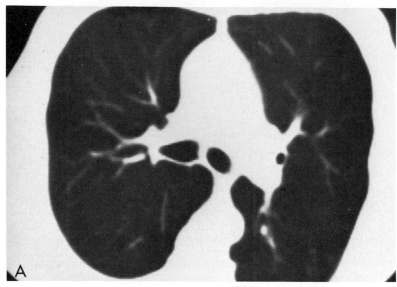

Figure 6–4. Right upper hilum and left upper hilum. **A** CT scan. **B** Line drawing.

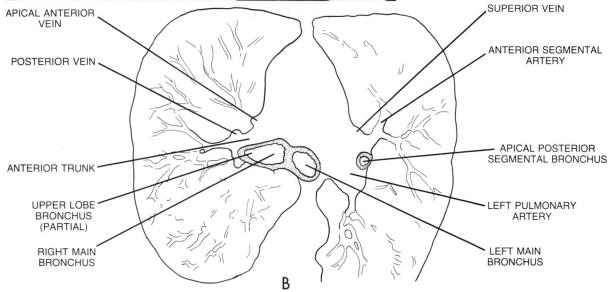

APICAL ANTERIOR VEIN

POSTERIOR VEIN

ANTERIOR TRUNK

UPPER LOBE BRONCHUS (PARTIAL)

RIGHT MAIN BRONCHUS

SUPERIOR VEIN

ANTERIOR SEGMENTAL ARTERY

APICAL POSTERIOR SEGMENTAL BRONCHUS

LEFT PULMONARY ARTERY

LEFT MAIN BRONCHUS

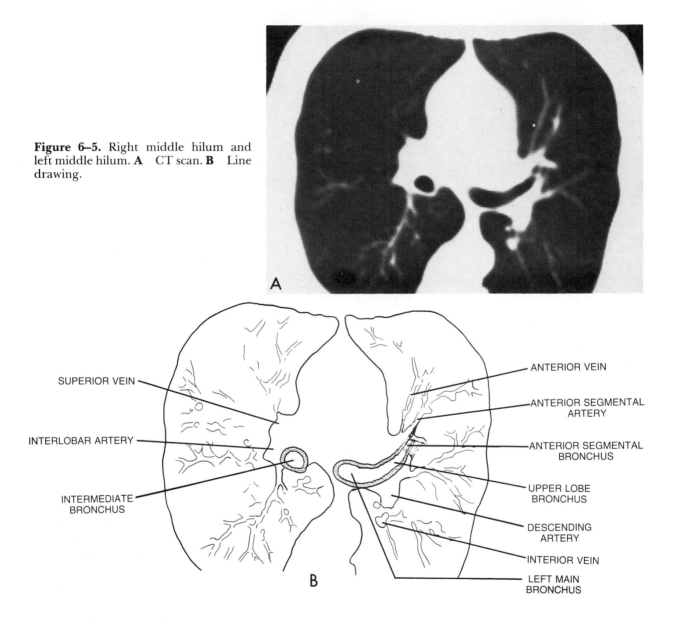

Figure 6–5. Right middle hilum and left middle hilum. **A** CT scan. **B** Line drawing.

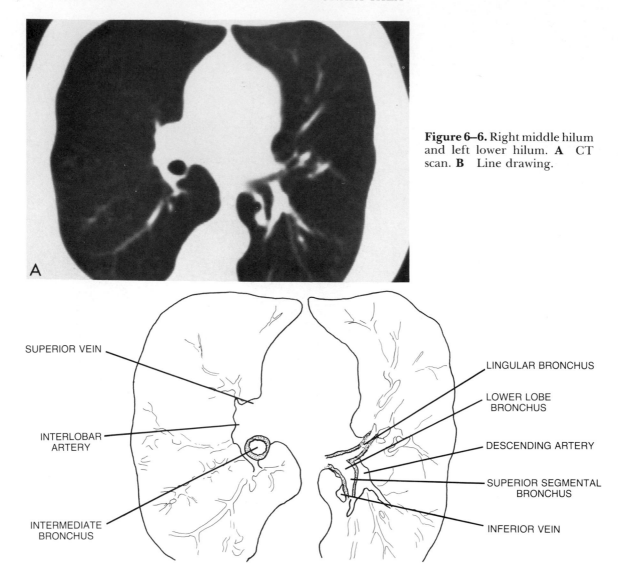

Figure 6–6. Right middle hilum and left lower hilum. **A** CT scan. **B** Line drawing.

mediate bronchus (Fig. 6–6). One to three branches course posteriorly to supply the superior segment of the right lower lobe (Figs. 6–6, 6–7). These branches, together with the interlobar artery, give the hilar contour a reverse comma or elongated S shape at this level. One or more inconstant branches may also arise from the anterior surface of the interlobar artery at this level. These branches supply the anterior segment of the right upper lobe. The two pulmonary veins of the anterior hilum combine at about this level to form the superior pulmonary vein, which then enters the mediastinum.

Right Lower Hilum (Middle Lobe Bronchus, Level 4)

The right middle lobe bronchus arises from the anterolateral surface of the intermediate bron-

chus 4 to 5 cm below the tracheal carina. It courses anteriorly, laterally, and inferiorly for 1 to 3 cm before dividing into its segmental bronchi (Fig. 6–7). The middle lobe bronchus is routinely visible at this level, usually on two adjacent images; the medial and lateral segmental bronchi of the middle lobe, however, cannot always be seen on CT scans. The bronchus to the superior segment of the right lower lobe is usually visible at the level of the orifice of the right middle lobe bronchus, or 1 cm superiorly (Fig. 6–7). It arises from the posterolateral right lower lobe bronchus. CT scans at the level of the right middle lobe and superior segmental bronchi clearly show the descending right pulmonary artery. It now lies lateral to the bronchi between the right middle lobe bronchus anteriorly and the superior segmental bronchus posteriorly, forming a distinct

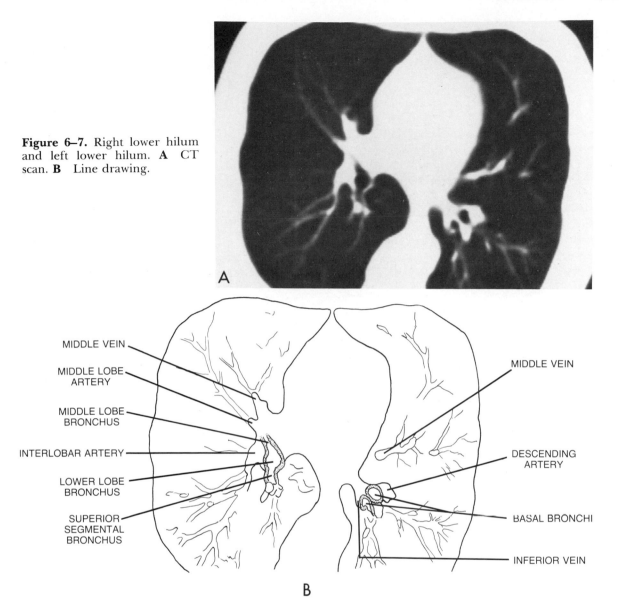

Figure 6–7. Right lower hilum and left lower hilum. **A** CT scan. **B** Line drawing.

MIDDLE VEIN

MIDDLE LOBE ARTERY

MIDDLE LOBE BRONCHUS

INTERLOBAR ARTERY

LOWER LOBE BRONCHUS

SUPERIOR SEGMENTAL BRONCHUS

MIDDLE VEIN

DESCENDING ARTERY

BASAL BRONCHI

INFERIOR VEIN

B

oval density with a smooth lateral contour. As many as three branches, but usually only one, arise from its anterolateral surface, coursing forward to accompany the right middle lobe bronchi (Fig. 6–7).[5] At about the same level, pulmonary artery branches to the superior segment of the lower lobe extend posteriorly to accompany the superior segmental bronchus on its lateral surface. The middle pulmonary vein tributary of the superior pulmonary vein can be seen between the right middle lobe bronchus and the mediastinum approximately 50 per cent of the time.

Lung tissue always outlines the posterior hilum at this level, sharply defining the posterior wall and often part of the medial wall of the intermediate bronchus and adjacent mediastinum. When the superior segmental bronchus is visible, its me-

dial wall contacts the parenchyma of the right lower lobe.

Right Inferior Hilum (Basal Bronchi, Level 5)

The right lower lobe bronchus divides into its four basal segmental bronchi approximately 1 cm below the level of the origin of the right middle lobe bronchus (Fig. 6–8).[6] CT scans always show one or more basal segmental bronchi, but rarely do they show all four (Figs. 6–8, 6–9). At this level, the relationship of the segmental pulmonary artery branches to the bronchial tree varies. The branching pulmonary arteries course in oblique planes. At their branch points, they often have a lobular, round, or oval appearance, usually adjacent to bronchi.

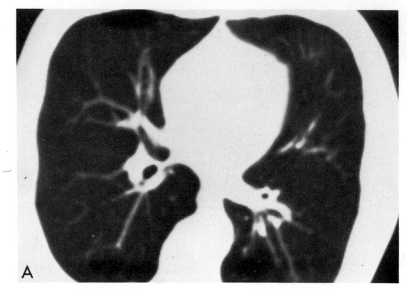

Figure 6–8. Right lower hilum and left inferior hilum. **A** CT scan. **B** Line drawing.

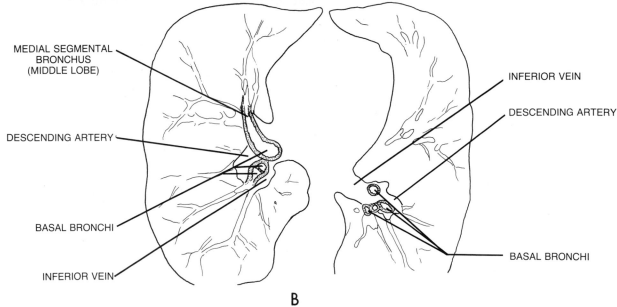

MEDIAL SEGMENTAL BRONCHUS (MIDDLE LOBE)

DESCENDING ARTERY

BASAL BRONCHI

INFERIOR VEIN

INFERIOR VEIN

DESCENDING ARTERY

BASAL BRONCHI

B

CT scans at about the level of the origin of the segmental bronchi always show the right inferior pulmonary vein (Figs. 6–8, 6–9). It passes behind the bronchial tree and courses medially toward the left atrium. Usually, the inferior pulmonary vein is relatively horizontal and can be seen for 2 to 4 cm before entering the posterolateral left atrium. This is the only level below the azygos vein at which lung does not contact the posterior surface of the right bronchial tree.

LEFT HILUM

Left Superior Hilum (Apical Posterior Bronchus, Level 1)

The left superior hilum is similar in appearance to the right superior hilum. At the level of the tracheal carina, or 1 cm cephalad, the apical posterior bronchus is always visible in cross section. Occasionally both the apical and posterior subsegmental bronchi are seen (Figs. 6–2, 6–3). A vein analogous to the right posterior pulmonary vein lies lateral to the bronchus in over half of normal subjects (Fig. 6–2).[7] It is the only normal structure lateral to the bronchus at this level. An additional vein frequently is present anterior to the apical posterior bronchus. One of the upper lobe pulmonary artery branches is usually present medial to the bronchial tree (Fig. 6–3).

At a slightly caudad level, the top of the left pulmonary artery is close to the medial side of the apical posterior bronchus. Four to eight arterial branches to the left upper lobe arise from the superior surface of the left pulmonary artery as it

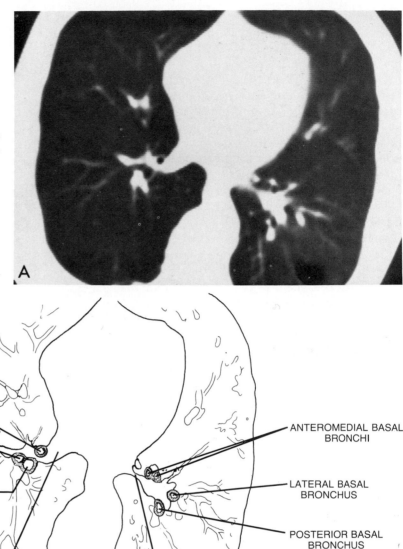

Figure 6–9. Right inferior hilum and left inferior hilum. **A** CT scan. **B** Line drawing.

MEDIAL BASAL BRONCHUS

LATERAL BASAL BRONCHUS

POSTERIOR BASAL BRONCHUS

INFERIOR VEIN

ANTEROMEDIAL BASAL BRONCHI

LATERAL BASAL BRONCHUS

POSTERIOR BASAL BRONCHUS

INFERIOR VEIN

B

arches over the left main bronchus. The contour of the superior surface of the left pulmonary artery is thus variable and irregular.

Left Upper Hilum (Left Pulmonary Artery, Level 2)

The normal hilar contour at this level varies little. CT scans 1 to 2 cm below the tracheal carina pass through the horizontal segment of the left pulmonary artery, above the left main bronchus and proximal left upper lobe bronchus (Fig. 6–4). The artery has an oval appearance and is directly lateral to the proximal left main bronchus. About 75 per cent of the time, the anterior segmental bronchus to the left upper lobe arises with the apical posterior segmental bronchus from a common trunk.[8] At this level, or 1 cm caudad, the an-

terior segmental bronchus is visible about 90 per cent of the time (Fig. 6–5). It usually has a horizontal orientation and can be seen for 1 to 3 cm of its length. The posterior hilum is formed by the pulmonary artery, which is smoothly rounded and gives off one to three arterial branches. The anterior hilum, medial to the anterior segmental bronchus, is variably lobulated. The CT appearance of the anterior hilum is a composite of the superior pulmonary vein and one or more branches of the pulmonary artery to the anterior segment of the left upper lobe (Figs. 6–4, 6–5).

Left Middle Hilum (Left Upper Lobe Bronchus, Level 3)

On the left side, 2 to 4 cm below the tracheal carina, the main bronchus divides into the left upper lobe and left lower lobe bronchi. This is at the level of the midportion of the intermediate bronchus on the right side. The left upper lobe bronchus courses anterolaterally and is visible on one or two adjacent CT images. The left upper lobe rapidly divides into its segmental branches. In 75 per cent of people, the anterior and apical posterior segmental bronchi arise as a common trunk, and the lingular bronchus appears as the continuation of the left upper lobe bronchus, coursing anteriorly, laterally, and inferiorly (Fig. 6–6). In 25 per cent of people, the left upper lobe bronchus trifurcates into anterior, apical-posterior, and lingular bronchi, and the anterior segmental bronchus may be visible at this level. The course of the proximal anterior segmental bronchus parallels the lingular bronchus, and it may be difficult to differentiate the two. The lingular bronchus is visible only about 60 per cent of the time.

The contour of the left hilum at this level is relatively simple. Anterior to the left upper lobe bronchus and medial to the anterior or lingular segmental bronchi, the hilum consists of pulmonary venous structures. The superior pulmonary vein enters the mediastinum at about this level to produce a small but variable anterior convexity (Figs. 6–4, 6–5). Depending on its size and position, the vein may extend inferiorly to lie medial to the lingular bronchus as well. Lateral to the lower lobe bronchus and behind the upper lobe bronchus, the descending left pulmonary artery forms a distinct oval density (Fig. 6–6); this appearance is similar to that of the right hilum at the level of the origin of the right middle lobe bronchus. Both anterior and posterior arterial branches arise from the pulmonary artery at this level, producing a somewhat lobular appearance. An arterial branch to the lingula can be seen in about half of normal persons, and a posterior branch to the superior segment of the lower lobe can be found in about 80 per cent.

A small segment of the posterior wall of the left main bronchus and the medial wall of the left lower lobe bronchus are usually contacted by lung (Figs. 6–5, 6–6). A portion of the superior segment of the left lower lobe invaginates between the descending pulmonary artery and bronchus laterally and the aorta and esophagus medially. When the anteroposterior diameter of the chest is narrow or the aorta is dilated, lung is absent from this area. The proximity of lung to the bronchial tree facilitates the recognition of bronchial abnormalities at this level.

Left Lower Hilum (Left Lower Lobe Bronchus, Level 4)

Three to 5 cm below the tracheal carina and 1 cm distal to the origin of the left lower lobe bronchus, the superior segmental bronchus to the lower lobe is seen along its axis (Fig. 6–6). As on the right, the proximal superior segmental bronchus is usually seen on only one image and only about 50 per cent of the time. It extends directly posteriorly, usually flanked by a branch of the pulmonary artery on its lateral side and a tributary of the inferior pulmonary vein medially. At this level, the pulmonary artery is lateral to the lower lobe bronchus and has a bilobed or oval contour. CT images sometimes show the middle pulmonary tributary of the superior pulmonary vein as it crosses in front of the hilum toward the left atrium (Fig. 6–7).

Left Inferior Hilum (Basal Bronchi, Level 5)

The left inferior hilum is very similar in appearance to the right inferior hilum and is usually seen at about the same level. CT scans show the left inferior pulmonary vein in all subjects as it passes behind the dividing lower lobe segmental bronchi (Figs. 6–8, 6–9). The segmental pulmonary arteries are visible in cross section as oval or elongated segments near the bronchi they accompany.

TECHNIQUES OF EXAMINATION

Computed tomography of the hila is usually performed as part of an examination of the entire thorax. The hilar images should be observed while the patient is still in the scanner, as additional images, with or without further contrast, are frequently used to define any abnormality that is detected. The techniques used for CT of the thorax vary widely among institutions.[9] With modern equipment, the study can be modified to suit the problem under consideration. Rapid sequential scanning (dynamic scanning) after injection of a bolus of contrast material is a useful method of defining the hilar vessels. Dynamic scanning with incrementation of the scanner table, during contrast medium infusion, gives excellent detail of the hilar vessels.[9a]

RESPIRATION AND POSITION

Scanning should be performed during suspended respiration at maximal inspiration. In

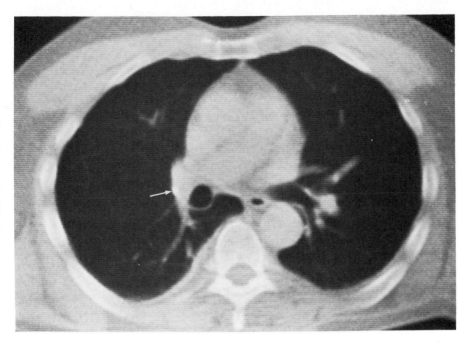

Figure 6–10. Normal hila at extended window settings (level −360 H; width 1664 H). CT scan at the level of the intermediate bronchus on the right. Bronchi, hilar contours, and mediastinal structures are all well displayed. An incidental small calcified node is present lateral to the interlobar pulmonary artery (arrow).

older patients and patients who are dyspneic, a few preliminary deep breaths will make it easier to maintain full inspiration. If breath holding is not possible, quiet breathing will reduce motion artifacts.

The supine position is usually used, with the patient's arms extended above the head. Although the hila have limited mobility, the prone or decubitus position offers no advantage over the supine position.

CONTRAST MEDIUM

Contrast medium will usually have been administered to opacify the mediastinal vessels. The hilar vessels will necessarily be opacified, and masses can be distinguished from enlarged vessels within the hilum. The usual dose of contrast medium is 125 to 150 ml of 60 per cent contrast (35.25 to 42.3 g of organically bound iodine). The most frequent method of administering contrast is by

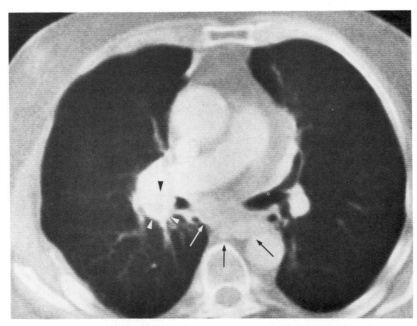

Figure 6–11. Metastatic bronchogenic carcinoma: extended window settings. CT scan, after a bolus of contrast material, shows narrowing of the intermediate bronchus from hilar adenopathy posterior to the right interlobar pulmonary artery (arrowheads), and extensive subcarinal lymphadenopathy (arrows).

rapid-drip infusion. Alternatively, a large bolus of contrast medium (75 ml of 60 per cent contrast) can be given immediately before scanning. When higher concentrations of intravascular iodine are required, a bolus injection of 25 to 30 ml of 76 to 90 per cent contrast should be given, followed by rapid sequential scanning at a specific level. For rapid sequential scanning, scan times must be less than 5 seconds, with an interscan delay of only 1 to 2 seconds.

TECHNICAL CONSIDERATIONS

Evaluating the pulmonary hila requires observation of a wide range of CT densities. The most accurate assessment of hilar contours and normal bronchi is achieved with settings used for the lungs. A window level between -300 and -500 Hounsfield Units (H) and a window width of 1000 H are usually used. These settings, however, obscure detail of adjacent mediastinal structures and tend to yield underestimations of the internal diameter of the bronchi. Abnormal bronchial narrowing is overestimated at lung window settings. The hilar structures, adjacent mediastinum, and bronchi should also be observed at mediastinal window settings. A window level of 10 to 60 H and a window width of 250 to 500 H are normally used. Rapid sequential scans through the hila are also viewed at these mediastinal window settings.

We recently reviewed images of the hila using an extended window of -1000 to 4000 H. At a window level of -350 to -450 H and a window width of 1400 to 1800 H, the hilar contours and structures, as well as the bronchi, can be seen on a single image (Fig. 6–10). Although image contrast is reduced, the lungs can be adequately evaluated from these images. These window settings provide a suitable compromise for observing the lungs, hilar structures, and bronchi. Bronchial narrowing and obstruction are more precisely delineated than at lung window settings. The relationship of hilar abnormalities to adjacent mediastinal structures can be seen more easily at these extended window settings (Fig. 6–11).

PATHOLOGY

CT SIGNS OF HILAR ABNORMALITIES

To identify an abnormal hilum requires detailed knowledge of the normal variations in hilar contours and bronchial appearances at each level. This understanding can only be achieved by careful observation of many normal cases. CT of the hila uses as a basis the bronchial anatomy and the relationship of the vascular hilar structures to the bronchial tree. Normal hila are composed predominantly of bronchi and vessels. At extended window settings, a small quantity of mediastinal fat may extend into the hilum; any other tissue is abnormal. The objective findings of an abnormal hilum are found posteriorly, where lung normally contacts the bronchial tree. The finding of endobronchial abnormalities in conjunction with an adjacent mass also helps to identify an abnormal hilum. Local or generalized alteration or irregularity in hilar contours is at least partially subjective and is more difficult to define precisely. Because hilar abnormalities are frequently focal, involving only one or two levels, a systematic evaluation of each level on both sides is essential.

Abnormal Right Hilum

Abnormalities of the superior right hilum are relatively easy to detect. The apical segmental bronchus is invariably present in cross section, and the vessels accompanying the bronchus are only slightly bigger than the bronchus. Any larger mass or density should raise suspicion of an abnormality (Fig. 6–12A–F). Obliteration or narrowing of the bronchus is invariably accompanied by a mass in this region.

At the level of the right upper lobe bronchus, the presence of a greater amount of tissue in the posterior hilum than the anticipated thickness of the bronchial wall is abnormal (Figs. 6–12E,F and 6–13A–C). Laterally, the posterior pulmonary vein is usually present between the anterior and posterior segmental bronchi. It is about one half to three quarters the size of the right main bronchus. Any additional density lateral to the bronchial bifurcation indicates lymphadenopathy or a mass. Anteriorly, the anterior trunk should not be larger than about one and a half times the size of the adjacent right main bronchus. The anterior trunk has multiple branches that course anteriorly and laterally, but the main artery should not extend lateral to a vertical plane through the posterior pulmonary vein.

At the level of the intermediate bronchus, the posterior right hilum is also relatively easy to evaluate. The right lung routinely contacts the posterior bronchial tree for the full length of the intermediate bronchus. The lateral and anterior surfaces of the hilum at this level are the most difficult areas in which to detect subtle abnormalities. The interlobar pulmonary artery lies partially in front of and partially lateral to the intermediate bronchus. Its branches extend laterally, superiorly, and posteriorly, and they course in oblique planes to the transverse axial image. The CT appearance of the anterior hilar contour is a composite of the superior pulmonary vein and the descending pulmonary artery; the contour normally is lobulated. Bronchial narrowing, posterior hilar density, and a focal bulge laterally or anteriorly are reliable indicators of abnormality. A uniform increase in size of the anterior hilum is difficult to detect, and dynamic scanning is useful in separating vessel from adjacent mass (Fig. 6–14).

At the level of the origin of the right middle lobe bronchus, lung continues to touch the posterior bronchial wall. The interlobar artery lies lateral to the bronchial tree in the angle between the origin of the right middle lobe bronchus and superior segmental bronchus. When viewed at lung window settings, the pulmonary artery fre-

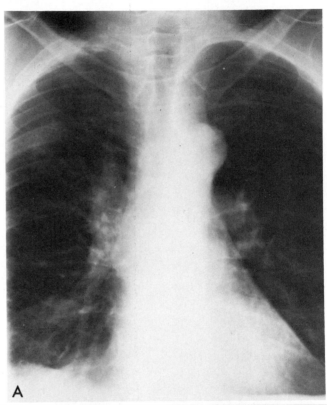

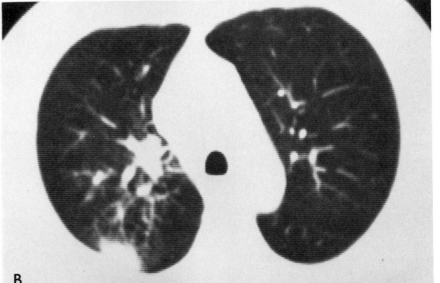

Figure 6–12. Bronchogenic carcinoma with hilar metastases. **A** Frontal radiograph shows a vague right upper lobe mass and enlargement of the superior right hilum. **B** CT scan shows a mass larger than normal vessels, involving the superior right hilum. Posteriorly, the primary tumor is visible.

Illustration continued on following page

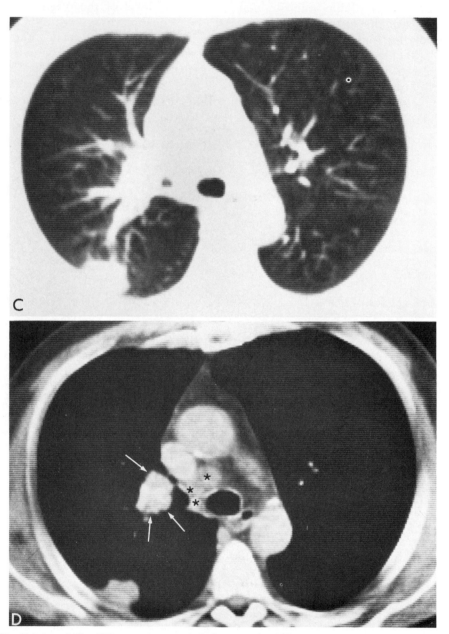

Figure 6–12. *Continued* **C**   CT scan 1 cm caudad to **B;** the hilar mass is still evident, obliterating the apical segmental bronchus. **D**   CT scan at same level as **C,** but at mediastinal window settings, shows multiple metastatic nodes around the apical vessels (arrows). Pretracheal and right paratracheal lymphadenopathy is also present (asterisks).

Illustration continued on opposite page

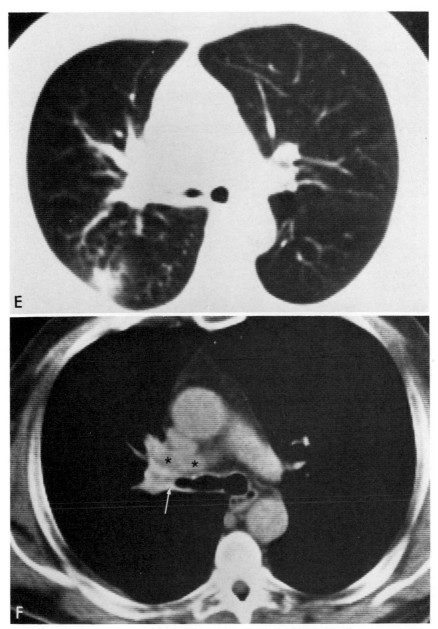

Figure 6–12. *Continued* **E**   CT scan 1 cm caudad to **D** demonstrates narrowing of the right main bronchus and marked stenosis of the right upper lobe bronchus. The posterior walls of these bronchi are thickened by tumor infiltration. **F**   CT scan at same level as **E,** but at mediastinal window settings, confirms stenosis of right upper lobe bronchus (arrow) and adenopathy anterior to it (asterisk). (All endobronchial findings were substantiated at bronchoscopy.)

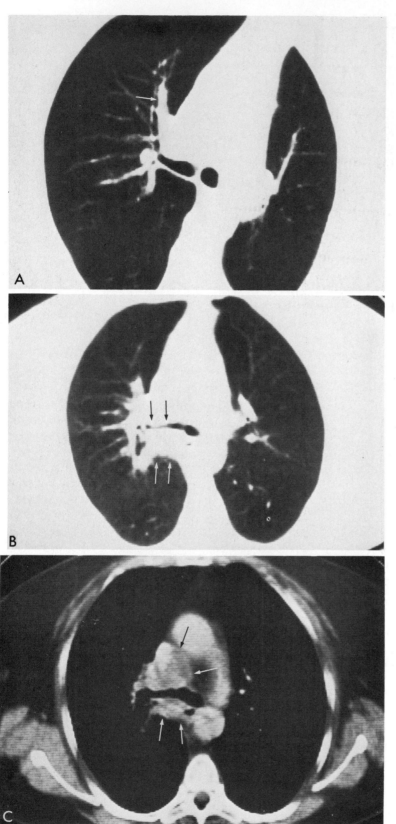

Figure 6–13. Recurrent bronchogenic carcinoma of the right hilum. Squamous cell carcinoma of the left lung previously treated with radiation. **A** CT scan 6 months after irradiation of the mediastinum shows a normal right lateral and posterior hilum. Subsegmental atelectasis is present in the anterior segment of the right upper lobe (arrow). **B** CT scan at the same level as in A, two years later; the right hilum is markedly abnormal. The posterior walls of the main bronchus and right upper lobe bronchus are thickened (arrows). Both bronchi are narrowed, the right posterior pulmonary vein is effaced, and the right hilum is poorly defined. **C** CT scan at the same level as **B,** but at mediastinal window settings, shows metastatic tumor posterior and anterior to the narrow right main and upper lobe bronchi (arrows). The superior vena cava is displaced anteriorly.

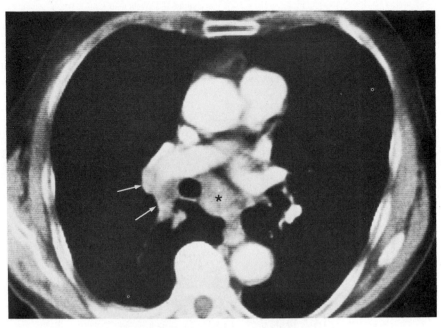

Figure 6–14. Metastatic bronchogenic carcinoma to the right midhilum. CT scan during injection of a 25-ml bolus of contrast material shows a metastatic tumor mass with an irregular contour lateral to the intermediate bronchus and proximal interlobar pulmonary artery (arrows). Extensive subcarinal adenopathy (asterisk) was not seen on conventional radiographs.

quently appears slightly larger than the adjacent lower lobe bronchus. The origins of branching vessels cause the pulmonary artery to appear slightly irregular. As Webb and colleagues[10] demonstrated, lobulation at this level strongly suggests lymphadenopathy or a mass (Fig. 6–15A,B). Bronchial narrowing or an endobronchial mass at this level must be interpreted carefully. The superior segmental bronchus of the lower lobe and the right middle lobe bronchus both course obliquely across the plane of view. Only a short segment of each of these bronchi is present on a single CT scan.

The right pulmonary artery divides into its basal segmental branches about 1 cm below the level of the right middle lobe bronchus. The CT appearance of the pulmonary arterial branches varies as they course through the plane of the image. These branches often appear as small knobs or rounded densities, and they should not be much larger than the adjacent bronchial branches. Abnormal tissue at this level appears as a focal enlargement of the inferior hilum (Fig. 6–16A,B). At about the same level, the right inferior pulmonary vein courses from lateral to medial across the posterior hilum. The anterior hilum, however, is devoid of vascular structures, and lymphadenopathy or a mass will appear as an additional density.

Abnormal Left Hilum

The superior left hilum is analogous to that on the right, with a bronchus and one or two vessels of similar size to the bronchus. The apical-posterior bronchus is seen in cross section. A hilar mass or lymphadenopathy must be of greater extent than the normal vessels in the area to be recognized (Fig. 6–17). Narrowing or obliteration of the bronchus is strong supportive evidence that the hilum is abnormal.

At a slightly lower level, the left pulmonary artery arches over the left main bronchus, producing a laterally convex contour. Arterial branches to the left upper lobe give the hilum an irregular appearance. However, the common trunk that gives rise to the anterior and apical-posterior segmental bronchi and the apical-posterior bronchus forms the lateral boundary of the hilum. A mass present lateral to the bronchus and larger than a normal vessel is abnormal (Fig. 6–18A,B). The anterior left hilum has a distinctive convexity produced by the left superior pulmonary vein before it enters the mediastinum. Absence of this contour indicates an anterior left hilar lesion effacing the normal venous convexity (Fig. 6–18A,B).

At the level of the bifurcation of the left main bronchus into its upper and lower lobe bronchi, the left hilar contour is reasonably simple and similar to the right hilar contour at the level of the right middle lobe bronchus. The origin of the left lower lobe bronchus is visible, as is the descending left pulmonary artery lateral to it. The normal left pulmonary artery at this level should not be more than about one to one and a half times the size of the adjacent bronchus. Extending forward from the bronchial tree is the lingu-

Text continued on page 294

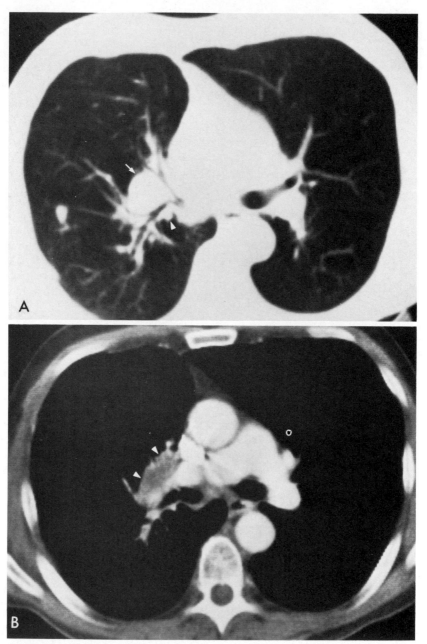

Figure 6–15. Metastatic bronchogenic carcinoma to right lower hilum. **A** CT scan shows a slightly lobulated nodal mass between the right middle lobe and superior segmental bronchi (arrow). The density appears smooth but is too large to be an interlobar artery. A small node is present behind the superior segmental bronchus (arrowhead). **B** CT scan 1 cm cephalad to the one in **A,** during injection of a bolus of contrast medium, shows a mass anterior to the interlobar artery and compressing it (arrowheads).

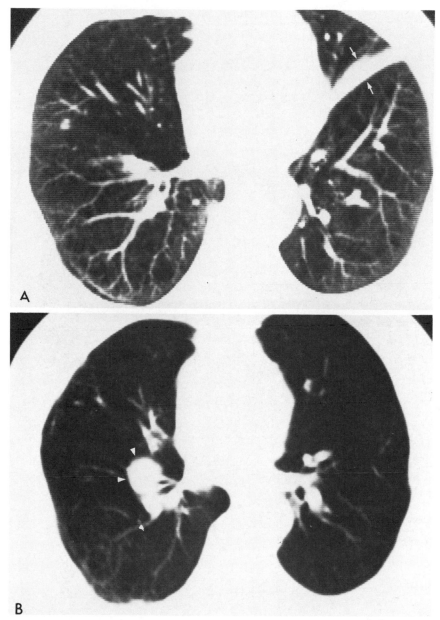

Figure 6–16. Metastatic bronchogenic carcinoma to right inferior hilum. **A** CT scan demonstrates a normal right inferior hilum. Dividing basal bronchi with normal-sized segmental pulmonary artery branches are evident. Incidental segmental atelectasis is present in the lingula (arrows). **B** CT scan 18 months later demonstrates nodal metastases to the right inferior hilum. Lobular lymph nodes are considerably larger than the adjacent bronchi (arrowheads).

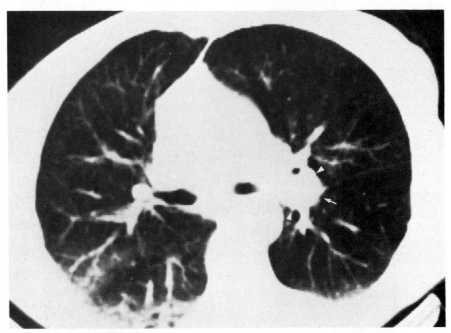

Figure 6–17. Metastatic bronchogenic carcinoma to the left superior hilum. CT scan shows a nodal mass (arrowheads) posterior to the apical-posterior segmental bronchus and displacing it forward. The mass is larger than the normal artery and vein, is lobulated, and has a slightly irregular outline.

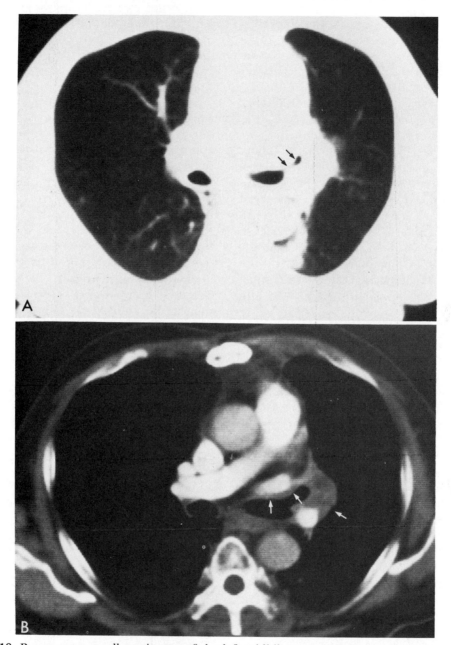

Figure 6–18. Recurrent oat cell carcinoma of the left midhilum. **A** CT scan shows a large mass lateral and posterior to the left upper lobe bronchus, which is narrowed (arrows). Excessive tissue is also present in the anterior hilum. The density posterior to the aorta represents radiation pneumonopathy. **B** CT scan at the same level as **A** during contrast material infusion. The tumor mass (anterior arrows) is demonstrated between the upper lobe bronchus and the superior pulmonary vein. A mass (lateral arrow) is also shown to the left of the descending pulmonary artery.

lar bronchus with the superior pulmonary vein medial to it, joined by its middle pulmonary vein tributary.

Abnormalities of contour at this level appear as masses larger than the expected vessels, or as abnormal lobulation (Fig. 6–19*A–C*). Lymphadenopathy posterior to the left main and left lower lobe bronchi are readily detected between the descending pulmonary artery and the aorta (Figs. 6–19, 6–20).

Below the origin of the lingular bronchus, the left hilum is similar to the inferior right hilum. The left inferior pulmonary vein courses across the posterior hilum and may touch the descending aorta. As on the right, only short segments of the basal pulmonary arteries are present on a single image. They appear as small, lobulated densities near the basal bronchi. Abnormal contours are easily detected in the inferior hilum and appear as focal enlargements greater in size than the anticipated vascular structures (Fig. 6–21*A,B*).

Associated Hilar Abnormalities

Hilar masses, or adenopathy, are frequently accompanied by CT findings that help establish the hilum as abnormal. These findings may also suggest the cause of the abnormality and the most appropriate method of further diagnosis. In the study by Webb and co-workers,[11] more than 50 per cent of patients with an abnormal hilar contour had additional CT findings confirming the abnormality. These included obscuration of normal bronchial walls and vessels, bronchial narrowing, and local abnormalities in the adjacent lung (Figs. 6–12, 6–13, 6–15, 6–18, and 6–21).

The right lung touches the posterior wall of the distal right main bronchus, the right upper lobe bronchus, and the intermediate bronchus in all patients. The left lung touches the posterior wall of the distal left main bronchus and the posteromedial wall of the left lower lobe bronchus in about 90 per cent of patients. Thickening of the bronchial wall or masses in these regions are readily detected with CT.

Schnur and colleagues[12] investigated 36 patients with thickening of the posterior wall of the intermediate bronchus on lateral chest radiographs. The maximal normal thickness of the intermediate bronchus on lateral chest radiographs was 3 mm. Two patterns of abnormal thickening were found: uniform and lobulated. Both patterns were found in patients with metastatic carcinoma or lymphoma. Congestive heart failure,

however, was the most common cause of uniform thickening.

CT scans clearly define the bronchial wall, and although the wall thickness has not been measured by CT, the appearance is uniform. Mediastinal fat and the overlying pleural surfaces do not add to the normal apparent thickness of the bronchial wall.

Both Webb and colleagues[10] and Naidich and associates[13] reported that posterior hilar obscuration is a frequent and sensitive indicator of hilar abnormality. Nonvascular enlargement of a hilum is frequently accompanied by poor definition of the hilar contours. Seven of 25 patients with bronchogenic carcinoma or lymphoma had this finding.[10] Bronchial narrowing was also present in many of these patients, and the poor hilar definition could have been due to obstructive pneumonitis, tumor infiltration of the perihilar lung, or lymphatic obstruction. The significance of this potentially important observation requires further clarification.

CT scans in the transverse axial plane readily demonstrate subtle degrees of bronchial narrowing. Bronchial narrowing may be from intrinsic tumor, extrinsic compression from lymphadenopathy, or compression by vessel enlargement. The apparent diameter of the normal hilar bronchi is critically dependent on the window width and

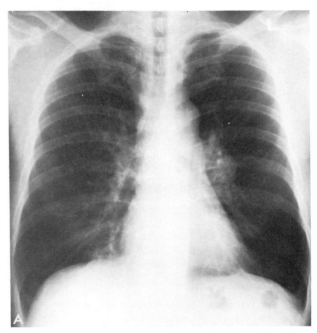

Figure 6–19. Plasmacytoma of the left hilum. **A** Chest radiograph shows that left hilum is enlarged and lobulated.

Illustration continued on opposite page

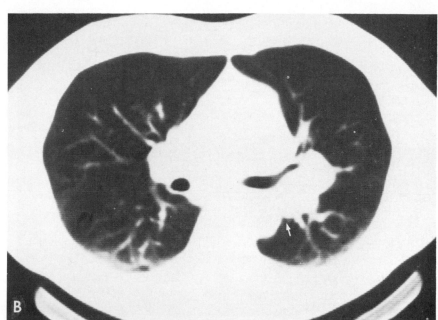

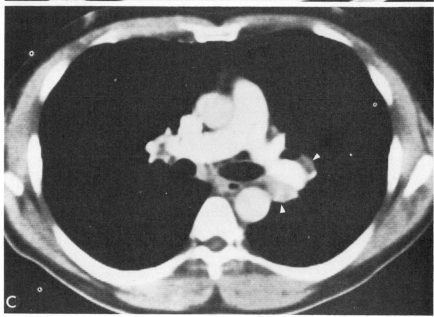

Figure 6–19. *Continued* **B** CT scan at the level of the distal main and left upper lobe bronchi shows a lobulated mass displacing the left upper lobe bronchus anteriorly. The normal space between the descending pulmonary artery and aorta is obliterated (arrow). **C** CT scan during injection of a bolus of contrast material shows the plasmacytoma (arrowheads) medial and lateral to the descending pulmonary artery.

level at which they are viewed. Bronchial narrowing must be evaluated at various settings.

VASCULAR LESIONS OF THE HILA

Development of the Hilar Pulmonary Arteries

The central pulmonary arteries are derived from the paired sixth (pulmonary) primitive aortic arches, which are formed by a ventral bud from the aortic sac and a dorsal bud from the dorsal aorta.[14-16] The pulmonary arch then joins the splanchnic plexus of vessels, which arises with the lung bud off the ventral esophagus. The portion of the splanchnic plexus giving rise to the lung vessels is referred to by Huntington as the "pulmonary postbrachial plexus."[17] The ventral buds, with contributions from the postbrachial plexus, form the pulmonary arteries. The dorsal buds form the left and right ductus arteriosus; normally, only the left ductus persists until birth, after which it becomes the ligamentum arteriosum. Numerous vascular channels form communications between the distal aorta and the postbrachial plexus. Some of these persist as the bronchial arteries, whereas others form potential systemic-pulmonary anastomoses in later life.

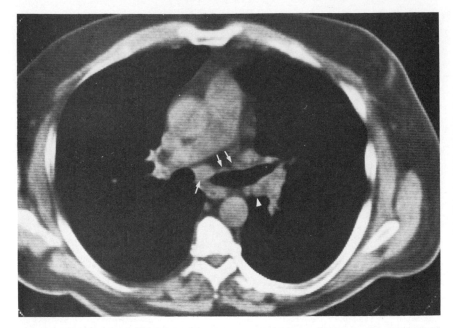

Figure 6–20. Adenopathy posterior to the left main bronchus (prior histoplasmosis). CT scan demonstrates discrete lymph nodes behind the left main bronchus (arrowhead), medial to the descending left pulmonary artery and anterolateral to the descending aorta. Additional lymph nodes are shown in the subcarinal space (medial arrow) and in front of the left main bronchus (anterior arrows).

After absorption of the segments of the aortic arches that do not persist, the primitive truncus arteriosus rotates counterclockwise. The left pulmonary artery is pulled anteriorly, while the right pulmonary artery migrates posteriorly and to the left. Thus, the main pulmonary artery is derived largely from the primitive left pulmonary artery, and the right pulmonary artery appears as a branch vessel of the main and left pulmonary arteries.

Congenital Anomalies of the Hilar Pulmonary Arteries

CONGENITAL UNILATERAL ABSENCE OF A PULMONARY ARTERY. This is a rare anomaly that has been called by many names: "Proximal interruption," "agenesis," "aplasia," "hypoplasia," and "absence of the left or right pulmonary artery" are terms frequently used interchangeably. The embryologic malformation giving rise to absence of a pulmonary artery is probably a failure of the ventral buds of the primitive aortic arch to develop.[18] The intraparenchymal pulmonary vessels derived from the postbrachial plexus are present and patent. Blood is supplied to the lung by the bronchial arteries, or by anomalous vessels from the aorta, or one of the great vessels.

The anomalous pulmonary artery is most frequently located opposite the aorta. When the absent pulmonary artery is on the same side as the aorta, the incidence of cardiac anomalies, particularly tetralogy of Fallot and septal defects, is high. Absence of the right pulmonary artery is frequently associated with a patent ductus arteriosus.

The radiographic features of absence of the pulmonary artery, first described by Danelius,[19] strongly suggest the diagnosis. The affected lung is frequently small, with decreased vascularity and a small hilum. The "lacy" pattern of pulmonary vessels has been attributed to enlarged bronchial arteries. Expiratory radiographs do not reveal delayed expiration on the affected side. Ventilation-perfusion radionuclide scans demonstrating absent pulmonary perfusion with nearly normal ventilation should confirm the diagnosis. Madoff and colleagues[20] first reported the angiographic findings, which are typical.

Naidich and colleagues[13] described the CT appearance in a patient with an absent right pulmonary artery (Fig. 6–22A–D). The right lung was small, and, as anticipated, the mediastinum was displaced. The ipsilateral bronchi appeared intact, but the main and interlobar pulmonary arteries were absent. The contralateral pulmonary arteries and veins were both enlarged, reflecting a long-standing increase in pulmonary flow.

PULMONARY ARTERY DILATATION. The central pulmonary arteries dilate in response to a long-standing increase in intraluminal pressure or blood flow. Segmental dilatation of a pulmonary artery, often called a pulmonary artery aneurysm, usually results from turbulence within the pulmonary artery.[21–23] Both pulmonary valvular stenosis and subvalvular stenosis can produce a jet of turbulent blood directed toward the left pulmo-

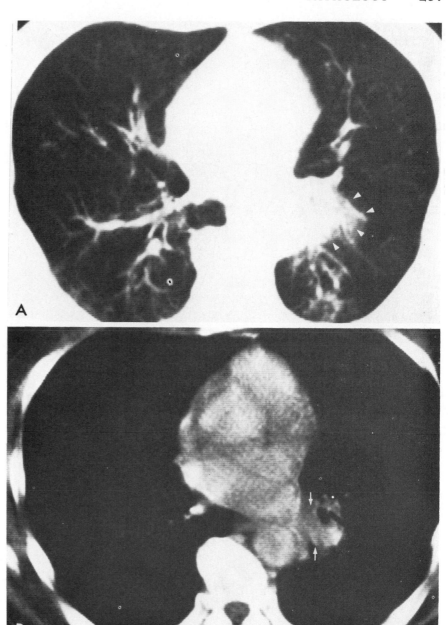

Figure 6–21. Central bronchogenic carcinoma involving left inferior hilum. **A** CT scan shows an ill-defined mass involving the left inferior hilum (arrowheads), posterior to the inferior pulmonary vein and continuous with the aorta. **B** CT scan at mediastinal window settings demonstrates nodes (arrows) medial to the basal bronchi and lateral to the left atrium and aorta. These nodes may be hilar or in the inferior pulmonary ligament and, therefore, mediastinal.

nary artery. Typically, the main and left pulmonary arteries are markedly enlarged, but the right hilar vessels are normal. Congenital pulmonary valvular insufficiency, however, is often associated with dilatation of both central pulmonary arteries and a ventricular septal defect. Segmental dilatation of the central pulmonary arteries may also be seen with mycotic aneurysms, syphilis, trauma, and diseases of defective connective tissue, such as Marfan's syndrome.

True congenital aneurysms of the pulmonary arteries are rare and almost invariably associated with more common malformations of the lung, especially arteriovenous fistula and pulmonary sequestration.[21, 23] Guthaner and co-workers[24] used

CT to measure the normal diameter of the central pulmonary arteries, which fell within a narrow range. The main pulmonary artery measured 2.8 ± 0.3 cm, the left pulmonary artery 2.0 ± 0.2 cm, and the right pulmonary artery 2.0 ± 0.4 cm. O'Callaghan and his colleagues,[25] also using CT, measured the diameter of the right pulmonary artery between the anterior wall of the main bronchus and the posterior wall of the superior vena cava. They found a mean diameter of 1.33 ± 0.15 cm in 25 adult patients without evidence of pulmonary vascular disease. The discrepancy in these measurements has not been explained, and a larger study is necessary.

The CT findings in segmental central pulmo-

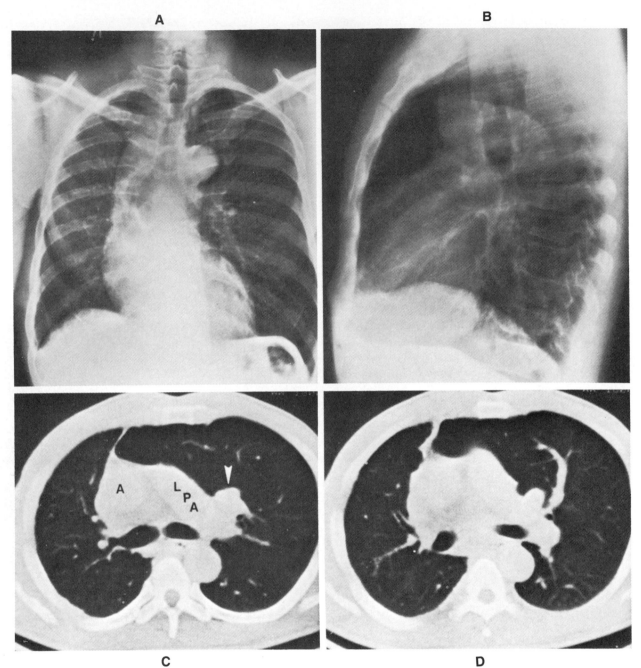

Figure 6–22. Congenital absence of the right pulmonary artery. **A, B** Frontal (**A**) and lateral (**B**) chest radiographs show a small right lung with a small right hilum. **C** CT scan at the level of the tracheal carina confirms the small right lung. The mediastinum is shifted to the right. The bronchi are of normal caliber. The right hilum shows no evidence of a right pulmonary artery, although the right posterior pulmonary vein is in normal position. The left pulmonary artery (LPA) and vein (arrowhead) are prominent. A = Ascending aorta. **D** CT scan at the level of the intermediate bronchus, shows that an interlobar pulmonary artery is also not present. (From Naidich DP, Khouri NF, Stitik FP, McCauley DI, Siegelman SS: Computed tomography of the pulmonary hila. II. Abnormal anatomy. J Comput Assist Tomogr 5:468, 1981. Reprinted by permission.)

nary artery dilatation have not been described. Central pulmonary vascular dilatation should be detected easily with CT scanning after contrast opacification of the vessels.

PULMONARY ARTERY STENOSIS.   Pulmonary artery stenosis without concomitant cardiac disease is a rare anomaly of the pulmonary vascular system. The stenotic segments, or coarctations, can be single or multiple, central or peripheral, short or long, unilateral or bilateral. Poststenotic dilatation is common, and when it is strategically placed, it may be seen as a hilar mass on CT scans.

Coarctations of the pulmonary artery are most frequently associated with congenital cardiac disease. Two major forms of congenital coarctation involve the main pulmonary artery. One is a short web immediately above the pulmonary valve; the other is a longer segment of stenosis, extending to the bifurcation of the main pulmonary artery or even further (Fig. 6–23A,B). Pulmonary valvular stenosis, or tetralogy of Fallot, is commonly present with either form.[21, 26, 27] Stenosis of the pulmonary arteries distal to the bifurcation of the main pulmonary artery is part of several syndromes. In familial pulmonary artery stenosis, supravalvular aortic stenosis is commonly present. When stenosis is from maternal rubella, other stigmata of the syndrome can be found. In the Williams-Beuren syndrome, pulmonary artery stenosis is associated with supravalvular aortic stenosis, mental retardation, and goblin facies.[26] When pulmonary artery stenosis is associated with Takayasu's arteritis or the Ehlers-Danlos syndrome, additional features of these entities will be present.[28]

Chest radiographs may show hilar masses due to poststenotic dilatation of segments of the central pulmonary arteries. In the presence of peripheral stenoses, focal or diffuse regions of lung oligemia may be evident. When pulmonary stenosis is severe, chest radiographs will demonstrate the findings of pulmonary arterial hypertension and cor pulmonale. The CT appearance of pulmonary artery stenosis has not been described, but CT scans should be able to suggest the malformation. CT may be performed in these patients to clarify hilar abnormalities detected on conventional radiographs. In patients in whom surgery is contemplated, detailed pulmonary and cardiac angiography is required to detect multiple lesions.

Anomalous Origin of the Pulmonary Arteries

Anomalous origin of the pulmonary arteries is a complex malformation of the embryonic ventral and dorsal aortic arches and their communication with the postbrachial vascular plexus.[21] Most cases

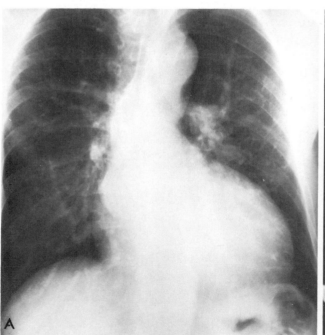
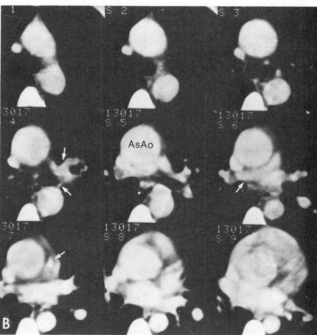

Figure 6–23. Pulmonary artery coarctation in a 23-year-old man. **A** Frontal radiograph shows an enlarged heart with absence of the main pulmonary artery trunk and a narrow cardiac root. The intrapulmonary vessels are increased in size. **B** Serial CT scans through the mediastinum from superior to inferior levels, reveal a dilated ascending aorta (AsAo). The main pulmonary is atretic (S7, arrow). The ductus arteriosus is visible (S4, posterior arrow). Both the left (S4, anterior arrow) and the right (S6, arrow) pulmonary arteries are seen. (At cardiac catheterization, a large ductus arteriosus connected the descending aorta to the left pulmonary artery. Both left and right pulmonary arteries were present and dilated. The main pulmonary artery was atretic.)

Table 6–1. ANOMALOUS ORIGINS OF
PULMONARY ARTERIES

Descending aorta via patent ductus arteriosus
   Ipsilateral to aortic arch
   Contralateral to aortic arch

Innominate or subclavian artery via patent ductus arteriosus
   Contralateral to aortic arch

Ascending aorta
   Right pulmonary artery with left arch
   Left pulmonary artery with right arch (rare)

Left pulmonary artery from right pulmonary artery
Persistent bronchial arteries

---

are associated with congenital heart disease, which usually dominates the clinical picture. The more common varieties are described in Table 6–1.

Stone and associates[29] described the CT findings in two patients with anomalous origin of the left pulmonary artery. The malformed artery arises from the posterior surface of the midportion of the right pulmonary artery and passes from right to left between the lower trachea and esophagus to enter the left hilum. Most patients with this anomaly have airway obstruction before the age of 2 years.[30] Airway obstruction may be from compression by the maldeveloped pulmonary artery sling. In about 50 per cent of patients, however, complete cartilaginous rings are present, causing severe intrinsic tracheal stenosis.

Anomalous origin of the pulmonary arteries in adults is rare, but in the few cases that have been described, an asymptomatic mediastinal or hilar mass was present. Chest radiographs show a right hilar mass that displaces or indents the right main bronchus or lower trachea. CT studies may be obtained to characterize the abnormal hilum. In the patients reported by Stone and colleagues,[29] the abnormal origin and course of the maldeveloped left pulmonary artery was clearly documented by CT scans (Fig. 6–24A–I).

Pulmonary Arterial Hypertension

Radiologists have been intrigued for some time as to whether the caliber of vessels visible on chest radiographs reflects pulmonary hemodynamics. The pulmonary vascular bed is a low-pressure system; the upper limit of normal pressure is close to 30/10 mm Hg, and the mean pressure is 15 to 18 mm Hg.[31] Pressure within the pulmonary circuit is a function of flow and resistance. Flow is determined by cardiac output and resistance by the cross-sectional area of the pulmonary vascular bed. The pulmonary vascular bed contains a large volume of viscous liquid at low pressure that moves in a pulsatile manner.[32] The pulmonary vessels are variably distensible, with active and elastic tension in their walls. They are surrounded by the lungs, which continually change volume and thereby affect the transmural pressure across the pulmonary vessels. The pulmonary circuit can compensate for a two- to threefold increase in flow by decreasing resistance and allowing pressure to remain stable.[33]

A long-standing increase in flow causes adaptive changes in the pulmonary arterial walls, which result in increased pulmonary arterial volume and radiographically visible changes in vessel

---

Figure 6–24. Anomalous origin of the left pulmonary artery. **A** Frontal radiograph shows an abnormal mediastinal density (arrows). The intermediate bronchus (arrowheads) is displaced medially and inferiorly. **B** Lateral radiograph shows airway impression (arrows). Right pulmonary artery and posterior wall of the intermediate bronchus are not visible. **C** Anteroposterior pluridirectional tomogram shows the trachea bifurcating into a hypoplastic right main bronchus and elongated left main bronchus. The proximal left pulmonary artery courses posteriorly between the right main bronchus and the intermediate bronchus. (Arrows and letters at the bottom of Fig. C refer to the planes of the lateral tomograms in **D–G.**) **D** Lateral tomogram at the right hilum shows the right middle and right lower lobe bronchi originate from an anomalous intermediate bronchus. **E** Lateral tomogram shows a posterior impression on the left main bronchus by the left pulmonary artery. **F** Lateral tomogram shows an anomalous vessel continuous with the descending left pulmonary artery. **G** Lateral radiograph shows the left pulmonary artery coursing between the left main bronchus and barium-filled esophagus. **H** CT scan shows a normal right pulmonary artery. **I** CT scan at a level more cephalad than **H** shows that the anomalous left pulmonary artery originates from the posterior right pulmonary artery and continues posteriorly to enter the left hilum (arrow). The esophagus cannot be seen. A = Aorta; AA = ascending aorta; Az = azygous vein; BI = intermediate bronchus; C = carina; DA = descending aorta; LLL = left lower lobe bronchus; LMB = left main bronchus; LPA = left pulmonary artery; dLPA = descending left pulmonary artery; LUL = left upper lobe bronchus; MPA = main pulmonary artery; RLL = right lower lobe bronchus; RML = right middle lobe bronchus; RPA = right pulmonary artery; SVC = superior vena cava; X = air bubble. (From Stone DN, Bein ME, Garris JB: Anomalous left pulmonary artery: two new adult cases. AJR 135:1259, 1980. © 1980, American Roentgen Ray Society. Reprinted by permission.)

caliber. Pulmonary hypertension, a sustained increase in systolic pulmonary arterial pressure above the normal 30 mm Hg,[34] with few exceptions occurs only when the cross-sectional area of the pulmonary vascular bed is reduced and pulmonary vascular resistance is increased. Pulmonary hypertension arises from a primary change in the structure or hemodynamics of the pulmonary vascular system (Table 6–2).

ALTERED STRUCTURE OF THE PULMONARY VASCULATURE. Diseases of the pulmonary artery wall, lungs, pleura, and chest wall may all increase pulmonary arterial pressure irreversibly. Transient pulmonary hypertension may also occur,

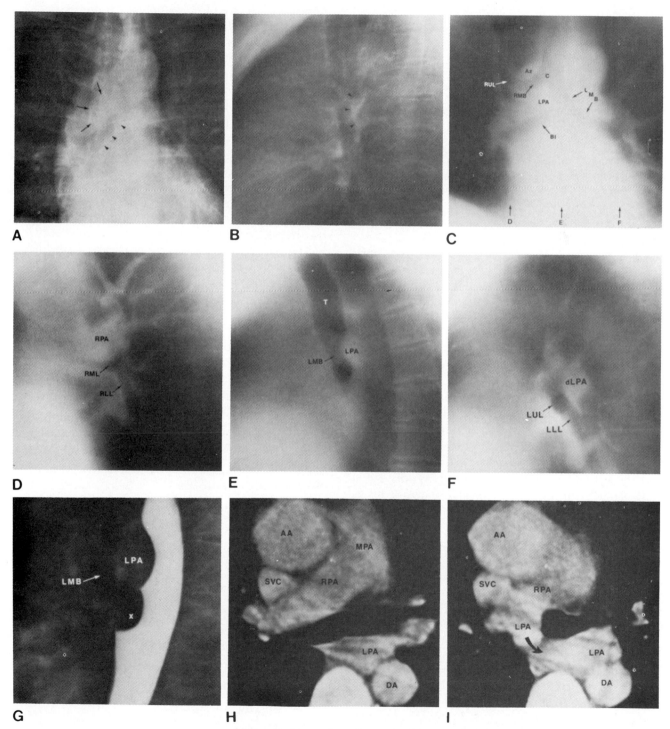

Figure 6–24. *See legend on opposite page*

Table 6–2.   CLASSIFICATION OF PULMONARY
HYPERTENSION

Altered structure
1. Vascular
   a. Primary pulmonary hypertension
   b. Thromboembolic disease
      • Thrombotic emboli
      • Neoplastic emboli
      • Parasitic emboli
      • Foreign body emboli
   c. Pulmonary arteritis
2. Pulmonary
   a. Obstructive lung disease
      • Emphysema
      • Chronic bronchitis
   b. Restrictive and cicatricial lung disease
3. Chest wall deformity
4. Alveolar hypoventilation
Altered hemodynamics
1. Increased flow
   a. Left-to-right shunt
2. Increased venous pressure
   a. Cardiac
      • Left ventricular failure
      • Mitral stenosis
      • Atrial obstruction
   b. Pulmonary venous obstruction

and it can be reversed by supplying 100 per cent oxygen. Focal hypoxia may be a significant stimulus for vasoconstriction. Other contributing factors to pulmonary hypertension include polycythemia, hypervolemia, and systemic-pulmonary arterial anastomoses.

Primary pulmonary hypertension is an uncommon condition, seen predominantly in young females.[35] The prognosis varies, but most patients do not survive longer than one decade from the time of diagnosis. Primary pulmonary hypertension designates a distinctive syndrome resulting from intrinsic, idiopathic obstructive disease of the small pulmonary arteries. The cause of the initial elevation in pulmonary arterial pressure is unknown, but vasoconstriction does play some part. Once hypertension has been present for some time, morphologic changes in the vascular wall lead to fixed, nonreactive pulmonary hypertension. The radiographic features are distinctive: The caliber of the central hilar pulmonary arteries is uniformly increased and the caliber of the peripheral vessels is decreased; right ventricular enlargement may also be evident.

Pulmonary hypertension is a common sequel of both advanced emphysema and chronic bronchitis.[36] The pathophysiology of the elevated pulmonary pressure in these conditions has not been completely clarified. The potential causative factors include hypoxia, destruction of the pulmo-

nary vascular bed, and small pulmonary emboli.[37] Emphysema does not involve the lung uniformly, and in the more affected regions there is a marked decrease in caliber of the vessels subtending them. The more normal areas of the lungs contain normal-appearing vessels, as in lower lobe emphysema caused by alpha-1-antitrypsin deficiency. Patients with chronic bronchitis may have significant airway obstruction and pulmonary hypertension without the radiographic features of the airway disease.

Advanced restrictive and cicatricial lung diseases frequently result in significant pulmonary hypertension. The radiographic features of pulmonary hypertension are often obscured by the concomitant pulmonary disease. Dilated central pulmonary arteries are the only radiographic clue to the developing pulmonary hypertension. Clinically, the diagnosis may not be apparent until right-heart failure supervenes. CT may be able to detect the pulmonary vessel abnormalities at an earlier stage than can chest radiographs, although this has not been determined.

Alveolar hypoventilation exists when alveolar ventilation is insufficient for the metabolic needs of the body. There are several causes of hypoventilation (Table 6–3). The term "alveolar hypoventilation syndrome" is used to designate lesions in which the lungs are normal and ventilatory insufficiency is from neurologic, muscular, or skeletal causes. All of these conditions can result in pulmonary hypertension.

Severe pulmonary hypertension may occur in children with upper airway obstruction,[38–39] in

Table 6–3.   CAUSES OF ALVEOLAR
HYPOVENTILATION

Respiratory center depression
   Anesthesia
   Morphine
   Barbiturates
   Trauma
   Anoxia
Neural conduction defect
   Spinal trauma
   Poliomyelitis
   Curare
   Myasthenia gravis
Respiratory muscle disease
Chest wall restriction
   Arthritis
   Deformity
Pleural restriction
   Fibrothorax
Pulmonary disease
   Restrictive lung disease
   Obstructive lung disease

obese patients with the pickwickian syndrome,[40] and in patients with autonomic dysfunction.[41] The radiographic features are those of pulmonary hypertension; otherwise, the lungs appear normal.

Pulmonary hypertension and cor pulmonale are major but infrequent complications of congenital, paralytic, or idiopathic spinal curvature. Pulmonary hypertension does not usually become clinically manifest until late middle age and should not be given primary consideration in children with kyphoscoliosis. The radiographic manifestations of severe kyphoscoliotic cardiopulmonary disease are extremely difficult to evaluate. The heart and mediastinum are distorted and ro-

tated. The orientation of the main pulmonary arteries is abnormal, and even the intrapulmonary vasculature is difficult to assess.

Approximately 2 per cent of patients with pulmonary emboli have recurrent emboli, which may cause pulmonary hypertension and cor pulmonale.[42–44] A clinical history of repeated, acute attacks is usually available. Recurrent showers of small blood clots that produce pulmonary hypertension without acute clinical attacks are extremely rare. Radiographic manifestations of pulmonary hypertension from recurrent pulmonary emboli are usually different from those seen in other conditions; the central pulmonary arteries are enlarged, whereas the peripheral pulmonary

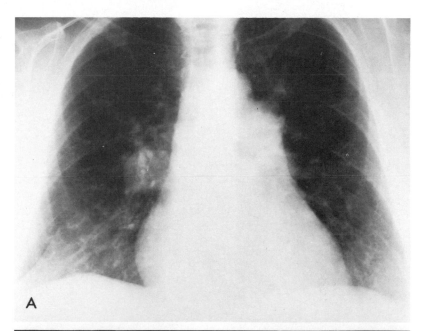

Figure 6–25. Recurrent pulmonary thromboembolism producing pulmonary hypertension in a 57-year-old woman. **A** Frontal radiograph shows cardiomegaly and marked enlargement of the central pulmonary arteries. **B** CT scan reveals massive enlargement of the left pulmonary artery and a large thromboembolus (arrowheads) occluding over 50 per cent of the vessel.

Illustration continued on following page

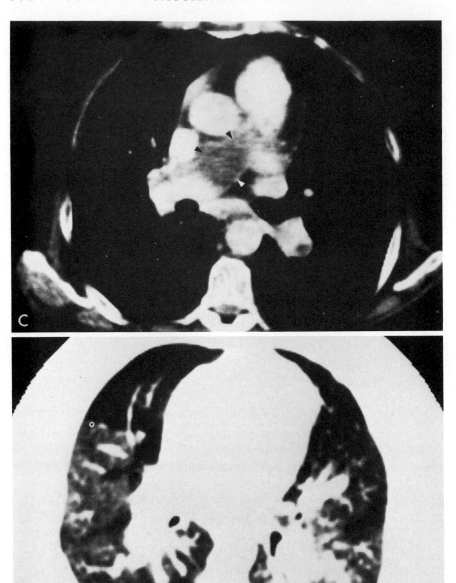

Figure 6–25. *Continued* **C** CT scan 2 cm inferior to B, demonstrates a large thromboembolus (arrowheads) occluding the majority of the right pulmonary artery. **D** CT scan at lung window setting shows that the hila are symmetrically enlarged and the lung CT density is markedly inhomogeneous. (Courtesy of Drs. R. Herfkens and B. H. Brundage, San Francisco, Cal.)

arterial changes are focal and asymmetric (Fig. 6–25A). In affected areas, the lung parenchyma is often markedly oligemic, and the vessels are attenuated; these changes are well demonstrated with CT (Fig. 6–25B–D). The vessels in other areas of the lung maintain a nearly normal appearance and caliber or are increased in diameter.

Neoplastic emboli can affect the lungs in two ways. Large tumor emboli may be swept into the pulmonary arterial bed and produce acute attacks, simulating thrombotic emboli. Large tumor emboli usually originate in the abdominal viscera

that have large direct communications to the inferior vena cava, especially the liver and kidneys. Emboli of tumor cells, mainly from malignant trophoblastic disease and breast carcinoma, can cause insidious pulmonary hypertension without acute attacks.[45] The radiographic features are those of pulmonary hypertension without underlying lung disease.

Rare causes of pulmonary hypertension include parasites, such as those found in schistosomiasis, talc or cotton particles, and even mercury droplets in drug addicts (Fig. 6–26A–C). The radiograph shows symmetric vascular changes without evidence of lung abnormality, unless other diseases coexist.

Conditions that involve the pulmonary arterial walls and cause arterial hypertension may be from morphologic changes in the arterial wall or from vasoconstriction. Pulmonary arteritis from the collagen vascular diseases, including scleroderma, rheumatoid lung disease, systemic lupus erythematosus, and polyarteritis nodosa, can result in pulmonary hypertension without lung parenchymal fibrosis.[46] Drugs and poisons such as aminorex, fumarate, and cobalt have been implicated in the development of pulmonary hypertension, although their mechanisms of action have not been defined.[47]

ALTERED PULMONARY VASCULAR HEMODYNAMICS. Congenital cardiac defects with left-to-right shunts can occur at the level of the pulmonary veins, atria, ventricles, or aorta. Pulmonary blood flow can be substantially increased for a considerable time before pulmonary hypertension develops. The radiographic features of pulmonary hypertension are those associated with increased pulmonary blood flow.[48] In about 10 per cent of patients with atrial septal defects, and rarely in other patients with left-to-right shunts, pulmonary vascular resistance increases and pulmonary hypertension supervenes (the Eisenmenger reaction).

The pathophysiology of the increase in pulmonary vascular resistance is not well understood, but the evidence suggests that reversible vasoconstriction occurs initially and that morphologic changes in the pulmonary vessels develop later.[49] The radiographic manifestations are difficult to see until the condition becomes well established. The central pulmonary vessels dilate, whereas the peripheral pulmonary arteries become narrower. Not until late in the disease do the pulmonary arteries show the severe peripheral attenuation seen in conditions characterized by pulmonary hypertension without increased flow.

Increased pulmonary venous pressure develops from obstruction to flow at the level of the pulmonary veins, left atrium, or mitral valve. Left ventricular failure also increases pulmonary venous pressure. An increase in venous pressure of long duration leads to interstitial pulmonary edema and morphologic changes in the small pulmonary vessels and reduces the cross-sectional area of the pulmonary vascular bed. Reflex pulmonary arterial constriction may also occur. Both factors cause pulmonary arterial hypertension.[50]

The usual radiographic features of pulmonary arterial hypertension coexist with the venous changes. In some cases of mitral stenosis, arterial hypertension is the predominant radiographic feature, and this is accompanied by central artery enlargement, peripheral artery attenuation, and right ventricular prominence. Left atrial enlargement and some radiographic evidence of venous hypertension should be recognizable.

The radiographic features of pulmonary arterial hypertension vary with the cause of the hypertension.[51] Enlargement of the central pulmonary arteries is, however, common to all situations in almost all patients with chronic pulmonary hypertension. Pulmonary hypertension is one of the few conditions in which the caliber of vascular structures can be measured from the chest radiograph. Increase in the diameter of the right descending pulmonary artery is a sensitive indicator of elevation of pulmonary arterial pressure in mitral stenosis, obstructive lung disease, and primary pulmonary hypertension.[36, 41, 52] The diameter of the right interlobar pulmonary artery is usually less than about 16 mm. In patients with chronic pulmonary hypertension, this vessel is usually more than 20 mm in diameter.

The central pulmonary arteries in the medias-

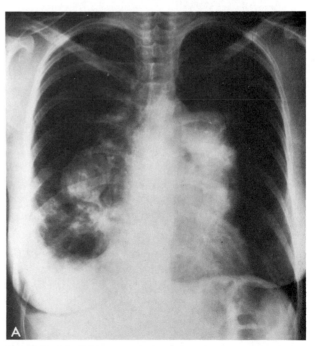

Figure 6–26. Schistosomiasis producing pulmonary hypertension. **A** Frontal radiograph shows massive bilateral hilar enlargement.

Illustration continued on following page

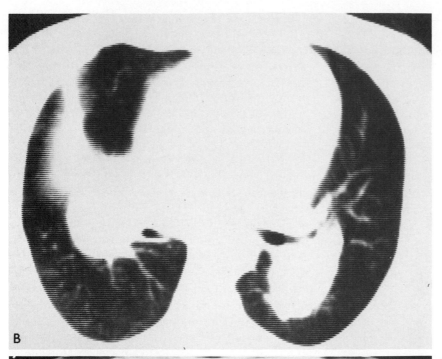

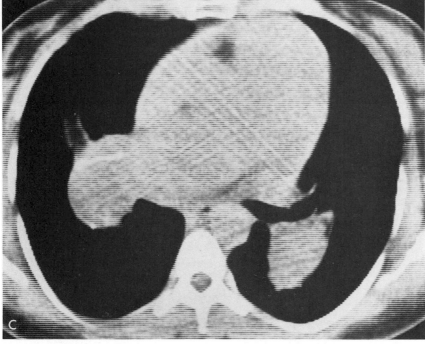

Figure 6–26. *Continued* **B** CT scan shows that the midhila are bilaterally enlarged, with smooth contours and no retrobronchial adenopathy. **C** CT scan at mediastinal window settings (without contrast material infusion) confirms that the hilar enlargement is due to pulmonary artery enlargement. A rim of calcification is visible in the interlobar artery.

tinum and hila can be measured precisely on CT scans. O'Callaghan and co-workers[25] found that the diameter of the right pulmonary artery was 16.6 to 26.6 mm in a small group of patients with pulmonary hypertension. The potential for accurate CT measurement of the interlobar and proximal lung arteries does exist. We have found that the caliber of the main pulmonary artery, measured from CT scans, is an accurate predictor of pulmonary artery pressure. In 32 patients with

cardiopulmonary disease, the calculated cross-sectional area of the main pulmonary artery (normalized for body surface area) predicted mean pulmonary artery pressure with a correlation coefficient (r) of 0.89 (unpublished data).

Occasionally, a patient with pulmonary arterial hypertension has unilateral or bilateral hilar enlargement that cannot be differentiated from hilar lymphadenopathy or a mass. In these circumstances, CT scans can show that the hilar enlargement is due to enlarged pulmonary arteries, and facilitate further evaluation of the patient (Fig. 6–27A–C).

HILAR LYMPHADENOPATHY

The hilar lymph nodes form the major pathway for lymph drainage from the lungs. From the hila, lymph flows through a maze of interconnecting paratracheal, mediastinal, and subdiaphragmatic lymphatic vessels and lymph nodes.[53] The patterns of pulmonary lymph drainage are now recognized as complex and variable. Direct pathways course from the lungs to the aortic pulmonic window and the subcarinal and paraesophageal nodes, bypassing the hila.

CT can provide a topographic display of the hilar nodes that is more precise than conventional tomography. To recognize hilar lymph node enlargement, it is necessary to understand the position of the lymph nodes in the hila. The existing descriptions of hilar lymph nodes are from dissections of specimens in which the anatomy is distorted. In the original anatomic description, Sukiennikow[54] portrayed the hilar lymph nodes as grouped exclusively around the bronchial tree. Although Engel[55] disproved Sukiennikow's observations, this misconception still persists. Descriptions of hilar adenopathy based on radiographic studies frequently emphasize the bronchial relationships of hilar nodes, dismissing the importance of the perivascular nodes, which are also present.

In his detailed description, Engel[55] divided the hilar (bronchopulmonary) lymph nodes into anteromedial and posterolateral groups. The anteromedial nodes are in the bifurcations between the upper and lower lobe bronchi on both sides. On the right side, they are also medial to the intermediate bronchus and lower lobe bronchus; on the left, they are medial to the lower lobe bronchus. The posterolateral nodes are portrayed in his diagrams as situated in the bifurcation between the upper and middle lobe pulmonary artery and posterolateral to the interlobar and lower lobe pulmonary arteries on the right. On the left, the posterolateral nodes are similarly positioned posterior and lateral to the pulmonary arteries. Chang and Zinn[56] described the hilar lymph nodes only in relationship to the bronchial tree. They divided both the left and right hilar lymph nodes into superior, inferior, anterior, and posterior groups. The lymph nodes around the main stem bronchi, lobar bronchi, and segmental bronchi were assigned either an anterior or posterior position.

The transverse axial displays of thoracic anatomy found in various published works do not provide a detailed description of hilar lymph nodes but tend to show them related to both the bronchi and pulmonary arteries.[57] An adequate topographic description of the position and relationships of the hilar nodes is not available. Our observations of small calcified hilar nodes on CT scans indicate that they may be anterior, poste-

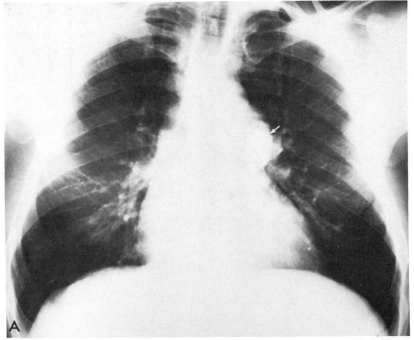

Figure 6–27. Pulmonary hypertension presenting as a left hilar mass. **A** Frontal radiograph reveals a left hilar mass. Curvilinear calcification is present at the edge of the "mass" (arrow).

Illustration continued on following page

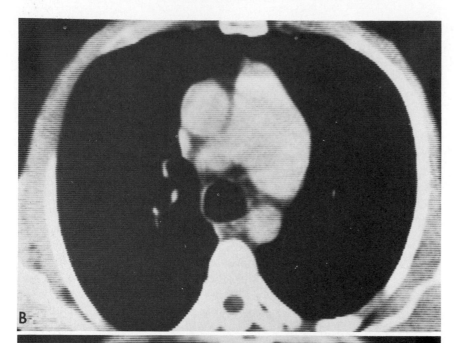

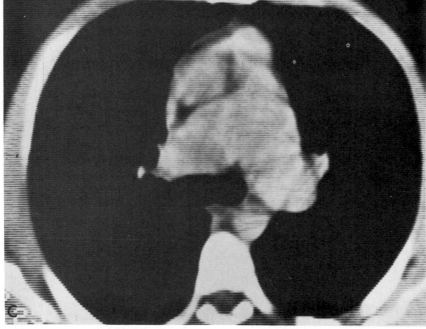

Figure 6–27. *Continued.* **B** CT scan at level of the lower trachea, demonstrates marked enlargement of the main pulmonary artery. **C** CT scan 2 cm caudad to **B** shows enlargement of the right and left pulmonary arteries. (At cardiac catheterization, pulmonary hypertension was found.) (Courtesy of Dr. P. A. Schnyder, Lausanne, Switzerland.)

rior, lateral, or medial to both the bronchi and pulmonary arteries. Those in proximity to the arterial tree may be some distance from the nearest bronchi.

Normal hilar lymph nodes are not visible on conventional radiographs or on CT scans; a hilar node that is visible should be considered abnormal. In patients who have had granulomatous disease, small calcified lymph nodes are frequently present and may be visible on conventional chest radiographs, conventional tomograms, and CT scans.[58]

Of the internal organs, the lungs are in most direct contact with the environment. The hilar lymph nodes form an important part of the lymphoid system, and numerous infectious, inflammatory, and neoplastic diseases involve these lymph nodes.

Hilar lymphadenopathy, which may be marked, is present in almost all patients with primary pulmonary tuberculosis, but it is rare in postprimary disease.[59] The lung on the side of the adenopathy is virtually always abnormal. The distribution of lymph node involvement varies in patients with tuberculosis. Hilar lymph node enlargement is unilateral in approximately 80 per cent of patients and associated with mediastinal adenopathy in about half of these. In the remaining 20 per cent, bilateral, but usually asymmetric, hilar lymph node enlargement is present.

Most of the common bacterial pneumonias are not associated with hilar or mediastinal lymphadenopathy. Patients with unusual bacterial pneumonias may have lymph node enlargement, which can be unilateral or bilateral (Table 6–4). Hilar lymphadenopathy in mycoplasma and viral pneumonia is frequent and usually bilateral.

The fungal infections histoplasmosis and coccidioidomycosis may cause either unilateral or bilateral hilar lymphadenopathy.[60–62] In histoplasmosis, hilar node involvement occurs in the benign form of the disease as well as in the more severe pneumonic form. Occasionally bilateral hilar lymph node enlargement is found without parenchymal disease. In the late healing phase, enlarged lymph nodes may compress the hilar bronchi. Hilar node calcification is a common sequel of histoplasmosis. Enlargement of the hilar nodes is common in the acute phase of coccidioidomycosis. It may be unilateral or bilateral and occurs in conjunction with mediastinal adenopathy in about 50 per cent of patients. Colwell and

Tillman[63] suggested that involvement of mediastinal lymph nodes indicates imminent dissemination of the disease; this suggestion has been questioned.

The neoplasm that most commonly involves the hilar nodes is bronchogenic carcinoma, which is discussed later in this chapter. Metastases to hilar and mediastinal lymph nodes do occur in patients with extrathoracic malignancy and are not rare.

McLoud and co-workers[64] studied the frequency and types of extrathoracic malignancy that produce intrathoracic lymph node metastases. Of 1021 patients with extrathoracic malignant neoplasms, 163 had an abnormal chest radiograph and 25 (15.3 per cent) had hilar or mediastinal metastases or both. The hila were the most frequent site for metastatic adenopathy; seven patients had bilateral and ten patients unilateral lymph node enlargement. The more common sites of the primary malignancy were the head and neck (including the thyroid), the genitourinary tract, and the breast.[64, 65]

Tumors of the stomach and pancreas also tend to metastasize to the hilar lymph nodes. In his study of intrathoracic lymph node metastases from melanoma, Webb emphasized the relative frequency of symmetric bilateral hilar node involvement.[66] Extrathoracic malignancy is, how-

Table 6–4.   CAUSES OF HILAR ADENOPATHY*

	Unilateral	Bilateral
Infectious	Coccidioidomycosis	Anthrax
	Cystic fibrosis	Chicken pox
	Histoplasmosis	Coccidioidomycosis
	Mycoplasma	Cystic fibrosis
	Tuberculosis	Histoplasmosis
	Tularemia	Mononucleosis
	Whooping cough	Mycoplasma
		Plague
		Tropical eosinophilia
		Tuberculosis
Neoplastic	Bronchogenic carcinoma	Extrathoracic metastases
	Extrathoracic metastases	Histiocytic lymphoma
	Histiocytic lymphoma	Hodgkin's disease
	Hodgkin's disease (uncommon)	Immunoblastic lymphadenopathy
		Leukemia
Environmental		Berylliosis
		Extrinsic allergic alveolitis
		Silicosis
Idiopathic	Sarcoidosis (uncommon)	Eosinophilic granulomatosis
		Pulmonary hemosiderosis
		Sarcoidosis

*Modified from Fraser ERG, Pare JAP: Diagnosis of Diseases of the Chest, 2nd ed. Philadelphia, WB Saunders Company, 1979, pp 2300–2305.

ever, an uncommon cause of bilateral hilar adenopathy in unselected patients. Winterbauer and colleagues[67] found that in only 2 of 100 patients was bilateral hilar adenopathy due to extrathoracic malignancy.

Filly and associates[68] described the incidence of hilar lymphadenopathy in patients with untreated lymphoma. Hilar nodal enlargement was demonstrated by conventional chest radiographs or tomograms in approximately 22 per cent of patients with Hodgkin's disease, and approximately 10 per cent of patients with non-Hodgkin's lymphoma. In all but three of their patients, hilar adenopathy was visible on the plain chest radiograph, and conventional tomography seldom detected additional adenopathy.

Winterbauer and colleagues[67] studied 212 patients with lymphoma and an abnormal chest radiograph and found unilateral hilar disease in 7.1 per cent of patients and bilateral adenopathy in 3.8 per cent. An additional 12 patients developed adenopathy during the course of their disease. This incidence was less than that in the study of Filly's.[68] All patients with intrathoracic lymphoma had symptoms when first seen, and physical examination showed extrathoracic disease, which tended to differentiate them from patients with sarcoidosis.

In patients with lymphoma, the low yield of frontal tomography in detecting hilar adenopathy not visible on chest radiographs suggests that CT will provide little additional information. However, the tomographic evaluation of the pulmonary hila in the presence of bulky mediastinal disease is difficult and the finding of hilar lymph node involvement in lymphoma is of prime importance (Figs. 6–28A–C and 6–29A,B). In many institutions, the radiotherapy ports in these patients will be altered to include the ipsilateral lung, and those with Hodgkin's disease may require the addition of chemotherapy.[69] CT examination of the thorax should be strongly considered in patients with lymphoma who have bulky mediastinal disease. A study to determine the frequency of hilar lymphadenopathy in lymphoma not detected by chest radiographs is needed to elucidate this problem.

Sarcoidosis is defined as a disease characterized by the presence in all affected organs or tissues of noncaseating epithelioid cell tubercles (though some fibrinoid necrosis may be present at the centers of a few tubercles); either the condition resolves or the epithelioid cell tubercles are converted into avascular, acellular hyaline fibrous

tissue.[70] This complex definition reflects the obscure etiology and protean manifestations of the disease. Sarcoidosis is a multisystem granulomatous disorder in which mediastinal and hilar adenopathy and pulmonary involvement are frequent. The classic description of the thoracic lymph node distribution in sarcoidosis is one of bilateral hilar and right paratracheal lymphadenopathy.

Kirks and associates[71] found abnormalities on the chest radiograph in 93 per cent of 162 patients in whom sarcoidosis was proved by biopsy. In 84 per cent of those who had abnormal chest radiographs, lymphadenopathy was present, and in 90 per cent involvement included the hilar nodes bilaterally. Paratracheal lymphadenopathy with unilateral hilar node involvement, as in tuberculosis, is unusual with sarcoidosis, but it has been recorded in up to 5 per cent of patients.[72] A more diffuse distribution of the lymphadenopathy has been shown in sarcoidosis, and subcarinal, anterior, and posterior mediastinal lymph node enlargement may be present in up to 20 per cent of patients.[73, 74]

Winterbauer and his associates[67] emphasized that the hilar lymphadenopathy was symmetric in almost all patients. Clinical correlations demonstrated that bilateral hilar adenopathy in the asymptomatic patient with normal results on physical examination could be considered evi-

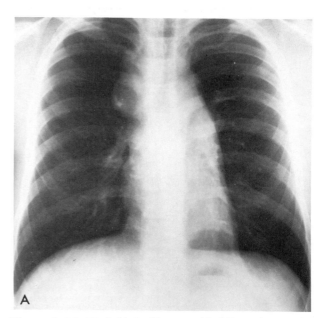

Figure 6–28. Hodgkin's disease with hilar adenopathy in a 23-year-old woman. **A** Frontal radiograph shows a bulky mass projecting to both sides of upper mediastinum. Hilar adenopathy is not visible.

Illustration continued on opposite page

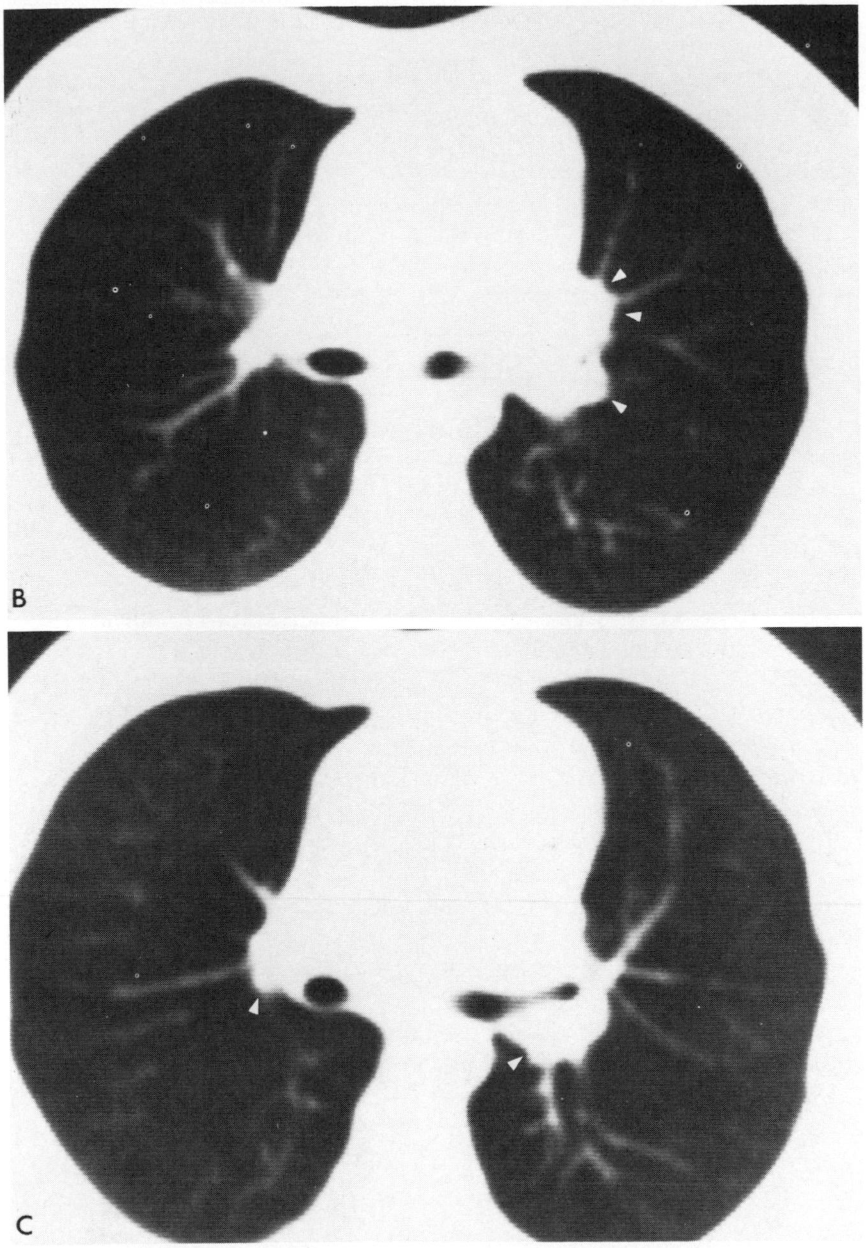

Figure 6–28. *Continued* **B** CT scan at the level of the superior hila shows adenopathy (arrowheads) on the left side, anterior, lateral, and posterior to the apical-posterior bronchus. The bronchus is compressed. **C** CT scan 1 cm caudad to **B** shows that the left hilum is still abnormal, with lobulation laterally and increased size posteriorly (arrowhead). Adenopathy is also present on the right side (arrowhead).

dence of sarcoidosis without the need for further confirmation.

The CT findings of sarcoidosis have mainly supplied information on the pulmonary parenchymal disease.[75, 76] These studies have, however, confirmed the presence of widespread mediastinal lymphadenopathy. The hilar lymph node involvement in patients with sarcoidosis is usually obvious, and CT is not required. In a small percentage of patients, confluent lung disease obscures the hila; in these patients, CT should be considered for detecting hilar disease.

BRONCHOGENIC CARCINOMA

The spread of bronchogenic carcinoma has interested surgeons, internists, pathologists, and ra-

diologists for many years. Lung cancer may spread by direct extension and also by lymphatic and hematogenous metastases. Direct extension occurs into the adjacent pulmonary parenchyma and the adjacent visceral pleura, across interlobar fissures, along the bronchus from which the tumor originates, and also into adjacent structures of the thorax. Lymphatic dissemination of bronchogenic carcinoma is most commonly to hilar lymph nodes, but the carcinoma also spreads directly to mediastinal lymph nodes. The presence of hilar disease not only influences treatment but also may determine prognosis in bronchogenic carcinoma.

Lymphatic metastases occur with marked frequency in patients with lung cancer. The inci-

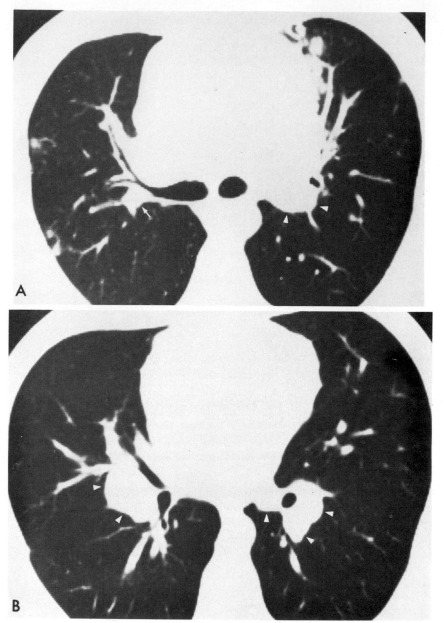

Figure 6–29. Hodgkin's disease with mediastinal, hilar, and parenchymal involvement. **A** CT scan at the level of the right upper lobe bronchus shows that the density in the position of the posterior pulmonary vein is too large for the vein alone (arrow). Extensive bronchial wall thickening is evident, the significance of which is not known. Left posterior hilar adenopathy is also present (arrowheads). **B** CT scan 4 cm caudad to **A,** at the level of the middle lobe bronchus, shows bilateral adenopathy lateral, medial, and posterior to the bronchi (arrowheads). Subpleural nodules are visible in both lungs. (CT scans showed the topographic distribution of the hilar nodes and the extensive lung disease more precisely than did the conventional chest radiographs.)

dence of hilar lymph node involvement is 15 to 40 per cent in patients undergoing pulmonary resection.[77–80] The cell type of the primary tumor affects the incidence of lymphatic spread. In order of increasing frequency, squamous cell carcinoma, adenocarcinoma, large-cell carcinoma, and small-cell carcinoma exhibit lymphatic metastases.[78–80]

The intrapulmonary lymph nodes occur at the bifurcations of the segmental bronchi and their accompanying pulmonary artery branches. Bronchopulmonary lymph nodes are referred to as "hilar" when they are situated along the lower portions of the lobar bronchi and interlobar when situated around the angles formed by the divi-

sions of the right and left main bronchi into their lobar branches.[77] This distinction is usually not necessary, and all central lymph nodes that interface with lung tissue are considered hilar nodes.

Nohl[77] has mapped in detail the hilar and mediastinal lymph nodes involved with bronchogenic carcinoma arising in various locations. On the right side, tumor drainage from all three lobes is into the lymph nodes around the intermediate bronchus, which Borrie[81] called the "lymphatic sump" (Fig. 6–30). These nodes are lateral and medial to the intermediate bronchus; anterior, between the intermediate bronchus and the right interlobar pulmonary artery; and posterior, in the angle between the intermediate bronchus and the

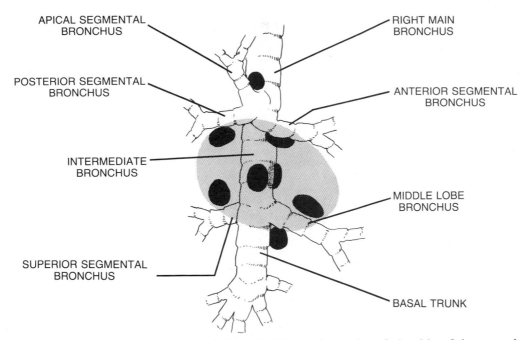

APICAL SEGMENTAL
BRONCHUS

POSTERIOR SEGMENTAL
BRONCHUS

INTERMEDIATE
BRONCHUS

SUPERIOR SEGMENTAL
BRONCHUS

RIGHT MAIN
BRONCHUS

ANTERIOR SEGMENTAL
BRONCHUS

MIDDLE LOBE
BRONCHUS

BASAL TRUNK

Figure 6–30. Right lymphatic sump (shaded area). Schema shows the relationship of the sump lymph nodes to the bronchial tree. (Modified from Shields TW: General Thoracic Surgery. Philadelphia, Lea & Febiger, 1972, p. 76. With permission.)

apical segmental bronchus of the lower lobe (Fig. 6–15*A,B*). Right upper lobe tumors also metastasize to the right superior hilar, azygos, right paratracheal, pretracheal, and post-tracheal lymph nodes (Fig. 6–12*B–F*). Tumors of the right upper lobe rarely involve lymph nodes below the level of the origin of the right middle lobe bronchus or the subcarinal lymph nodes.

Right lower and middle lobe tumors metastasize to the lymph nodes of the lymphatic sump and to the medial side the intermediate bronchus, the subcarinal area, and the paraesophageal nodes at the upper extent of the inferior pulmonary ligament (Figs. 6–11, 6–14, and 6–16). In general, bronchogenic carcinomas arising in the right lower lobe tend to involve the hilar lymph nodes more widely than do upper lobe tumors, and metastases to the right superior hilum are not uncommon.

On the left side, tumors in both the upper and lower lobes drain into the lymphatic sump formed by the lymph nodes between the upper and lower lobe bronchi, those anterior and posterior to the proximal lower lobe bronchus, and also those lateral to the proximal descending left pulmonary artery (Fig. 6–31). The lymph nodes above the superior segmental bronchus of the lower lobe, below the lingular bronchus, and between the lingular and anterior segmental bronchi are also frequently involved by tumors arising in both the left upper and left lower lobes.

Tumors arising in the left lower lobe, in addition to draining upward to involve the sump nodes and other nodes listed previously, have a strong tendency to metastasize to the subcarinal, paraesophageal, and inferior pulmonary ligament lymph nodes. Lower lobe tumors tend not to involve the left superior mediastinum, but when they are advanced, they may cross over to involve the right paratracheal nodes. Tumors arising in the left upper lobe frequently involve the lymph nodes listed earlier, as well as lymph nodes in the left superior hilum and left mediastinum (Fig. 6–17). Unlike tumors in the right upper lobe, left upper lobe tumors do involve the subcarinal lymph nodes. However, involvement of nodes in the inferior left hilum below the infralingular lymph nodes and superior segmental bronchus is rare.

On both the right and left sides, lymph nodes around the main bronchi are frequently involved by tumor. The posterior surfaces of these bronchi are in contact with lung, and lymphadenopathy is readily detected with CT (Figs. 6–12, 6–13, and 6–20). The anterior surfaces of both main bronchi are contiguous with vascular structures. On the right, the pulmonary artery and its anterior trunk are directly in front of the right main bronchus. On the left, the superior pulmonary vein is directly anterior to the left main bronchus. Without intravenous contrast, the vascular structures cannot easily be distinguished from the sur-

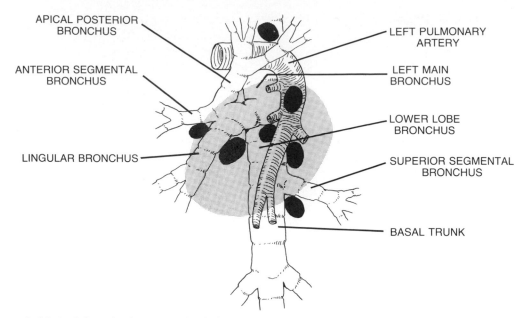

Figure 6–31. Left lymphatic sump (shaded area).   Schema shows the relationship of the sump lymph nodes to the bronchial tree and left pulmonary artery. (Modified from Shields TW: General Thoracic Surgery. Philadelphia, Lea & Febiger, 1972, p. 78. With permission.)

rounding mediastinal tissue, and subtle enlargement of lymph nodes is difficult to detect. Opacification of these vessels with a bolus of contrast medium during rapid sequential scanning is frequently necessary to obtain satisfactory CT images and detect lymph nodes in these regions (Figs. 6–14, 6–18, and 6–19).

The significance of metastases to hilar lymph nodes in patients with bronchogenic carcinoma remains controversial. As a general rule, tumor in the ipsilateral hilar nodes does not preclude resection, if the procedure is technically feasible. Hilar lymphadenopathy frequently necessitates a more extensive resection: either resection of two lobes on the right or a pneumonectomy.

The prognosis for the patient with hilar lymph node tumor is unclear. No consensus has been reached concerning the predictive influence of hilar lymph node metastases found at surgery on long-term survival after resection of primary lung cancer. The reported prognosis for patients with hilar node metastases ranges from extremely poor[82–84] to relatively favorable.[78, 80, 85–88] The prognosis for the patient with hilar adenopathy also varies for different histologic cell types, although again there is no consensus.

Classification of lung cancer according to the definitions and stage grouping rules developed by the American Joint Committee for Cancer Staging and End-Results Reporting contains factors related to the primary tumor (T) and to the pres-

ence of nodal metastases (N). For each more advanced stage of the primary tumor (T), the presence of hilar node metastases worsens the prognosis.[79] In studies showing that hilar node metastases (N_1 lesions) affect prognosis, the 5-year survival rate is intermediate between that associated with absence of nodal metastasis (N_0 tumors) and that associated with metastasis to mediastinal nodes (N_2 tumors).[78] Among patients who undergo resection, those without lymph nodes metastases (N_0) have a 35 to 60 per cent 5-year survival rate, whereas those with hilar node metastases (N_1) have a 15 to 40 per cent 5-year survival rate. The prognosis of patients with adenocarcinoma and hilar metastases is extremely poor, which may be one of the factors explaining the wide discrepancies in the results of different studies.[88]

The use of CT to detect mediastinal lymph node involvement by tumor has been extensively investigated in patients with bronchogenic carcinoma (see Chapter 5). These and other studies clearly show that metastases can exist in normal-sized lymph nodes and that moderately enlarged lymph nodes may not contain metastatic tumor.[77] The same difficulties and reservations are applicable to hilar lymph nodes. The interpretation of lymphadenopathy must always be tempered with the understanding that visibility of the node is not diagnostic of tumor involvement.

The CT appearance of changes in the hilar

Table 6–5. DETECTION OF HILAR LYMPHADENOPATHY IN PATIENTS WITH LUNG CANCER

Author	Mintzer*[89]		Hirleman[90]		Faling[91]		Osborne[92]	
Year	1979		1980		1981		1982	
Scanner	EMI 5005		EMI 5005		Delta 2020			
Scan time (sec)	19.0		19.0		2.0		5.0	
Image thickness (mm)	13.0		13.0		15.0		10.0	
	CVT	CT	CVT	CT	Chest radiol	CT	CVT	CT
No. patients	58	58	47	50	35	35	42	42
TP	15	13	28	25	10	10	12	11
FN	5	7	5	5	5	5	5	6
FP			1	5	3	2	5	3
TN			13	15	17	18	20	22
Sensitivity	0.75	0.65	0.85	0.83	0.67	0.67	0.70	0.65
Specificity			0.93	0.75	0.85	0.90	0.80	0.88
Accuracy			0.87	0.80	0.77	0.80	0.76	0.78
PC of + test			0.97	0.83	0.77	0.83	0.70	0.79
PV of − test			0.72	0.75	0.77	0.78	0.80	0.79

*Incomplete data.

Abbreviations: CVT = conventional tomography; CT = computed tomography; TP = true-positive results; FN = false-negative results; FP = false-positive results; TN = true-negative results; PV = predictive value.

Definitions: Sensitivity = $\dfrac{TP}{TP+FN}$; Specificity = $\dfrac{TN}{FP+TN}$; Accuracy = $\dfrac{TP+FN}{TP+FN+FP+TN}$; PV of + Test = $\dfrac{TP}{TP+FP}$; PV of − Test = $\dfrac{TN}{TN+FN}$

contour due to lymph node enlargement has been described, as have the other CT appearances of lymphadenopathy.[10–12] However, the sensitivity, specificity, and accuracy of CT in detecting hilar lymphadenopathy have only recently been systematically investigated (Table 6–5).[89–92] The combined results from these studies show a sensitivity of 0.70, a specificity of 0.84, and a diagnostic accuracy of 0.81. These results are similar to those for the detection of metastasis in the mediastinum and probably reflect the biologic spread of lung tumors. Normal-sized or slightly enlarged, tumor-containing lymph nodes limit the sensitivity of CT, and, less frequently, reactive hyperplasia and enlargement of hilar lymph nodes decrease the specificity of the examination. Small nodes are also probably more difficult to detect in the hila than in the mediastinum, which further limits the sensitivity of the examination.

INDICATIONS FOR COMPUTED TOMOGRAPHY OF THE HILA

The widespread interest of the medical community in CT has not been matched by a clear understanding of the appropriate use of this imaging modality. The pulmonary hilum is one area in which the efficacy and use of CT have not been reported in adequate detail.

The general indications for computed thoracic tomography proposed in 1977 by the American College of Radiology and the Institute of Medicine of the National Academy of Science were followed in 1979 by more specific indications from the Society for Computed Tomography.[93–95] Technical improvements in scanners and additional information have made these proposals largely obsolete. The single indication for computed tomography listed by the Society for Computed Body Tomography is the "differentiation of enlarged pulmonary artery from solid mass when conventional tomography fails or is not capable of making this distinction".[95]

Generally speaking, CT of the hila is indicated to detect hilar abnormality and to characterize or confirm an abnormality detected by other imaging modalities. Both of these indications must be modified by the clinical circumstances, and careful thought must be given to the potential impact that the information from CT will have on patient management. The sensitivity, specificity, and accuracy of CT relative to other imaging modalities must also be taken into consideration.

CT DETECTION OF HILAR DISEASE

The detection of hilar disease involves finding subtle hilar lymphadenopathy and masses. The accuracy of CT in detecting hilar nodes and masses not suspected from chest radiographs has been difficult to document. The few available studies indicate that CT is at least as sensitive and specific as conventional tomography. Our recent experience has made it clear that with a thorough understanding of hilar anatomy, CT has a greater sensitivity in detecting disease in the medial, pos-

terior, and anterior hilum than does conventional tomography. Lymph nodes lateral to the pulmonary arteries are probably detected with equal sensitivity by the two techniques.

The circumstances in which the detection of hilar nodes or masses affects patient management remain controversial. With most non-neoplastic diseases, subtle hilar adenopathy found by CT but not with conventional radiography is not of value in determining etiology or does not influence patient management. In patients with bron-

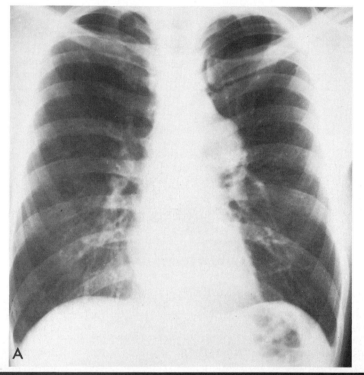

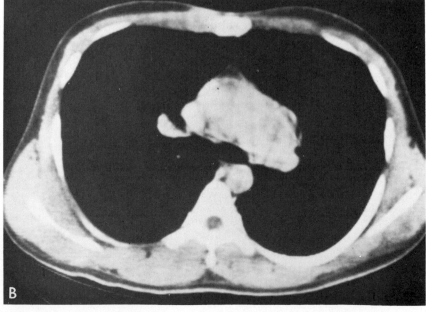

Figure 6–32. Left hilar anaplastic carcinoma showing contrast enhancement. **A** Frontal radiograph shows a left hilar mass. **B** CT scan through the mass and left pulmonary artery, after infusion of contrast material, shows marked contrast enhancement of the mass. A field-of-interest over the mass had a CT density of 86 H, the same as that of the descending aorta. (Courtesy of Dr. D. Klein, San Francisco, Cal.)

chogenic carcinoma, CT is frequently used to determine the stage and resectability of the tumor (also see Chapters 4, 5, and 7). The state of the hila is valuable additional information, even though it may not directly influence the decision to perform surgery. The demonstration of bronchial abnormalities in or adjacent to a hilum may also assist in the bronchoscopic localization of the tumor. In patients with lymphoma, especially Hodgkin's disease with bulky mediastinal nodes, CT may demonstrate hilar lymphadenopathy and affect patient management.

CT CHARACTERIZATION OF HILAR DISEASE

The attenuation values of hilar tissues rarely assist in diagnosis. Abnormalities of hilar contours are caused by nodes, soft tissue masses, or vessels. Fatty or cystic masses of the hila are rare. When unilateral or bilateral hilar enlargement is due to a dilated or anomalous vessel, CT scans clearly show the vascular nature of the mass. Additionally, CT may establish the cause of an abnormally small hilum when absence or atresia of a pulmonary artery is suspected. Very rarely a neoplastic process will show marked enhancement with contrast medium and may be mistaken for a vascular structure in the hilum (Fig. 6–32A,B).[96]

Specific indications for CT of the hila have not been fully established. Additional data and careful studies over the next few years should clarify the clinical circumstances in which CT contributes significantly to diagnosis of hilar disease.

REFERENCES

1. Webb WR, Glazer G, Gamsu G: Computed tomography of the normal pulmonary hilum. J Comput Assist Tomogr 5:476, 1981.
2. Naidich DP, Khouri NF, Scott WW Jr, Wang KP, Siegelman SS: Computed tomography of the pulmonary hila: 1. Normal anatomy. J Comput Assist Tomogr 5:459, 1981.
3. Dorland's Illustrated Medical Dictionary, 26th ed. Philadelphia, WB Saunders Company, 1981, p 609.
4. Boyden EA, Scannell JG: An analysis of variations in the bronchovascular pattern of the right upper lobe of fifty lungs. Am J Anat 82:27, 1948.
5. Boyden EA, Hamre CJ: An analysis of variations in the bronchovascular patterns of the middle lobe in fifty dissected and twenty injected lungs. J Thorac Surg 21:172, 1951.
6. Smith FR, Boyden EA: An analysis of the segmental bronchi of the right lower lobe of fifty injected lungs. J Thorac Surg 18:195, 1949.
7. Boyden EA, Hartmann JF: An analysis of variations in the bronchopulmonary segments of the left upper lobes of fifty lungs. Am J Anat 79:321, 1946.
8. Yamashita H: Roentgenologic Anatomy of the Lung. Tokyo, Igaku-Shoin, 1978, p 8487.
9. Heitzman ER: Computed tomography of the thorax: Current perspectives. AJR 136:2, 1981.
9a. Glazer GM, Francis IR, Gebarski K, Samuels BI, Sorensen KW: Dynamic incremental computed tomography in evaluation of the pulmonary hila. J Comput Assist Tomogr 7:59, 1983.
10. Webb WR, Gamsu G, Glazer G: Computed tomography of the abnormal pulmonary hilum. J Comput Assist Tomogr 5:485, 1981.
11. Webb WR, Gamsu G, Speckman JM: Computed tomography of the pulmonary hilum in patients with bronchogenic carcinoma. J. Comput Assist Tomogr 7:219, 1983.
12. Schnur MJ, Winkler B, Austin JHM: Thickening of the posterior wall of the bronchus intermedius. Radiology 139:551, 1981.
13. Naidich DP, Khouri NF, Stitik FP, McCauley DI, Siegelman SS: Computed tomography of the pulmonary hila: 2. Abnormal anatomy. J Comput Assist Tomogr 5:468, 1981.
14. Bremer JL: On the origin of the pulmonary arteries in mammals. Am J Anat 1:137, 1902.
15. Bremer JL: On the origin of the pulmonary arteries in mammals. II. Anat Rec 3:334, 1909.
16. Bremer JL: An acknowledgment of Federow's work on the pulmonary arteries. Anat Rec 6:491, 1912.
17. Huntington GS: The morphology of the pulmonary artery in the mammalia. Anat Rec 17:165, 1919.
18. Pool PE, Vogel JHK, Blount SG: Congenital unilateral absence of a pulmonary artery: The importance of flow in pulmonary hypertension. Am J Cardiol 10:706, 1962.
19. Danelius G: Absence of the hilar shadow. AJR 47:870, 1942.
20. Madoff IM, Gaensler EA, Strieder JW: Congenital absence of the right pulmonary artery: Diagnosis by angiocardiography with cardiorespiratory studies. N Engl J Med 247:149, 1952.
21. Ellis K, Seaman WB, Griffiths SP, Berdon WE, Baker DH: Some congenital anomalies of the pulmonary arteries. Semin Roentgenol 2:325, 1967.
22. Good CA: Certain vascular abnormalities of the lungs. AJR 65:1009, 1961.
23. Trell E: Pulmonary arterial aneurysm. Thorax 28:644, 1973.
24. Guthaner DF, Wexler L, Harell G: CT demonstration of cardiac structures. AJR 133:75, 1979.
25. O'Callaghan JP, Heitzman ER, Somogyi JW, et al: CT evaluation of pulmonary artery size. J Comput Assist Tomogr 6:101, 1982.
26. Hoeffel JC, Henry M, Jiminez J, Pernot C: Congenital stenosis of the pulmonary artery and its branches. Clin Radiol 25:481, 1974.
27. Baum D, Khoury GH, Ongley PA, Swan HJC, Kincaid OW: Congenital stenosis of the pulmonary artery branches. Circulation 29:680, 1964.
28. Lees MH, Menashe VD, Sunderland CO, Morgan CL, Dawson PJ: Ehlers-Danlos syndrome associated with multiple pulmonary artery stenoses and tortuous systemic arteries. J Pediatr 75:1031, 1969.
29. Stone DN, Bein ME, Garris JB: Anomalous left pulmonary artery: Two new adult cases. AJR 135:1259, 1980.
30. Turner AF, Pacuilli JR, Lau FYK, Mikity VG, Johnson

JL: Partial tracheal obstruction due to anomalous origin of the left pulmonary artery. Calif Med 114:59, 1971.

31. Keele CA, Neil E, Wright S: Applied Physiology, 11th ed. New York, Oxford University Press, 1965.

32. Harris P, Heath D, Apostopoulous A: Extensibility of the pulmonary trunk in heart disease. Br Heart J 27:660, 1965.

33. Caro CG: Physics of blood flow in the lungs. Br Med Bull 19:66, 1963.

34. Fowler NO, Westcott RN, Scott RC: Normal pressure in the right heart and pulmonary artery. Am Heart J 46:264, 1953.

35. Walcott G, Burchell HB, Brown AL: Primary pulmonary hypertension. Am J Med 49:70, 1970.

36. Matthey RA, Schwarz MI, Ellis JH Jr, Steele PP, Siebert PE, Durrance JR, Levin DC: Pulmonary artery hypertension in chronic obstructive pulmonary disease: determination by chest radiography. Invest Radiol 16:95, 1981.

37. Baum GL, Fisher FD: The relationship of fatal pulmonary insufficiency with cor pulmonale, right-sided mural thrombi, and pulmonary embolism. Am J Med Sci 240:609, 1960.

38. Gerald B, Dungan WT: Cor pulmonale edema in children secondary to chronic upper airway obstruction. Radiology 90:679, 1963.

39. Bland JW Jr, Edwards FK: Pulmonary hypertension and congestive heart failure in children with chronic upper airway obstruction. New concepts of etiologic factors. Am J Cardiol 23:830, 1969.

40. Burwell CS, Robin ED, Whaley RD, Bichelmann AS: Extreme obesity associated with alveolar hypoventilation: A Pickwickian syndrome. Am J Med 21:811, 1956.

41. Ravin CE, Greenspan RH, McLoud TC, Lange RC, Langou RA, Putman CE: Redistribution of pulmonary blood flow secondary to pulmonary arterial hypertension. Invest Radiol 15:29, 1980.

42. Paraskos JA, Adelstein SJ, Smith RE, Rickman FD, Grossman N, Dexter L, Dalen JE: Late prognosis of acute pulmonary embolism. N Engl J Med 289:55, 1973.

43. Dalen JE, Alpert JS: Natural history of pulmonary embolism. Prog Cardiovasc Dis 17:257, 1975.

44. Dantzker DR, Bower JS: Partial reversibility of chronic pulmonary hypertension caused by pulmonary thromboembolic disease. Am Rev Resp Dis 124:129, 1981.

45. Evans KT, Cockshott, WP, Hendrickse, P de V: Pulmonary changes in malignant trophoblastic disease. Br J Radiol 38:161, 1965.

46. Steckel RJ, Bein ME, Kelly PM: Pulmonary arterial hypertension in progressive systemic sclerosis. AJR 124:461, 1975.

47. Follath F, Burkart F, Schweizer W: Drug induced pulmonary hypertension? Br Med J 1:265, 1971.

48. Abrams H: Radiologic aspects of increased pulmonary artery pressure and flow. Stanford Med Bull 14:97, 1956.

49. Kimball KG, McIlroy MB: Pulmonary hypertension in patients with congenital heart disease. Am J Med 41:883, 1966.

50. Selzer A, Cohn KE: Natural history of mitral stenosis: Review. Circulation 45:878, 1972.

51. Sidd JJ, Dervan RA, Leland OS, Sasahara AA: Correlation of hemodynamic data and pulmonary angiography in mitral stenosis. Circulation 35:373, 1967.

52. Turner AF, Lau FYK, Jacobson G: A method for the estimation of pulmonary venous and arterial pressures from the routine chest roentgenogram. AJR 116:97, 1972.

53. Dyon JF: Contribution à l'étude du drainage des lymphatiques du poumon. Thesis. Grenoble, Université Scientifique et Médicale de Grenoble, 1973.

54. Sukiennikow W: Dissertation. Berl Klin Wochenschr, 1903 (cited by Engel S: Lung Structure. Springfield, Ill, Charles C Thomas, 1962, pp 74–80).

55. Engel S: Lung Structure. Springfield, Ill, Charles C Thomas, 1962, p 74–80.

56. Chang CHJ, Zinn TW: Roentgen recognition of enlarged hilar lymph nodes: an anatomical review. Radiology 120:291, 1976.

57. Peterson RR: A Cross Sectional Approach to Anatomy. Chicago, Year Book Medical Publishers, Inc, 1980.

58. McLeod RA, Brown LR, Miller WE, DeRemee RA: Evaluation of the pulmonary hila by tomography. Radiol Clin North Am 16:51, 1976.

59. Weber AL, Bird KT, Janower ML: Primary tuberculosis in childhood with particular emphasis on changes affecting the tracheobronchial tree. AJR 103:123, 1968.

60. Curry FJ, Wier JA: Histoplasmosis: A review of one hundred consecutively hospitalized patients. Am Rev Tuberc 77:749, 1958.

61. Murray JF, Howard D: Laboratory acquired histoplasmosis. Am Rev Resp Dis 93:47, 1966.

62. Greendyke WH, Resnick DL, Harvey WC: The varied roentgen manifestations of primary coccidioidomycosis. AJR 109:491, 1970.

63. Colwell JA, Tillman SP: Early recognition and therapy of disseminated coccidioidomycosis. Am J Med 31:676, 1961.

64. McLoud TC, Kalisher L, Stark P, Greene R: Intrathoracic lymph node metastases from extrathoracic neoplasms. AJR 131:403, 1978.

65. Reinke RT, Higgins CB, Niwayama G, Harris RH, Friedman PJ: Bilateral pulmonary hilar lymphadenopathy. Radiology 121:49, 1976.

66. Webb, WR: Hilar and mediastinal lymph node metastases in malignant melanoma. AJR 133:805, 1979.

67. Winterbauer RH, Belic N, Moores KD: Clinical interpretation of bilateral hilar adenopathy. Ann Intern Med 78:65, 1973.

68. Filly R, Blank N, Castellino RA: Radiographic distribution of intrathoracic disease in previously untreated patients with Hodgkin's disease and non-Hodgkin's lymphoma. Radiology 120:277, 1976.

69. Hagemeister FB, Fuller LM, Sullivan JA, North L, Velasquez W, Conrad FG, McLaughlin P, Butler JJ, Shullenberger CC: Treatment of stage I and II mediastinal Hodgkin disease. Radiology 141:783, 1981.

70. Scadding JG: Sarcoidosis. London, Eyre and Spottiswoode, 1967, p 41.

71. Kirks DR, McCormick VD, Greenspan RH: Pulmonary sarcoidosis. Roentgenologic analysis of 150 patients. AJR 117:777, 1973.

72. Rabinowitz JG, Ulreich S, Soriano C: The usual unusual manifestations of sarcoidosis and the "hilar haze" a new diagnostic aid. AJR 120:821, 1974.

73. Bein ME, Putman CE, McLoud TC, Mink JH: A reevaluation of intrathoracic lymphadenopathy in sarcoidosis. AJR 131:409, 1978.

74. Schabel SI, Foote GA, McKee KA: Posterior lymphadenopathy in sarcoidosis. Radiology 129:591, 1978.

75. Putman CE, Rothman SL, Littner MR, Allen WE, Schachter EN, McLoud TC, Bein ME, Gee JBL: Computerized tomography in pulmonary sarcoidosis. Comput Tomogr 1:197, 1977.

76. Solomon A, Kreel L, McNicol M, Johnson N: Computed tomography in pulmonary sarcoidosis. J Comput Assist Tomogr 3:754, 1979.

77. Nohl HC: An investigation into the lymphatic and vascular spread of carcinoma of the bronchus. Thorax 11:172, 1956.

78. Mountain CF: Assessment of the role of surgery for control of lung cancer. Ann Thorac Surg 24:365, 1977.

79. Naruke T, Suemasu K, Ishikawa S: Lymph node mapping and curability at various levels of metastasis in resected lung cancer. J Thorac Cardiovasc Surg 76:832, 1978.

80. Rubinstein I, Baum GL, Kalter Y, Pauzner Y, Lieberman Y, Bubis JJ: The influence of cell type and lymph node metastases on survival of patients with carcinoma of the lung undergoing thoracotomy. Am Rev Resp Dis 119:253, 1979.

81. Borrie J: Primary carcinoma of the bronchus: Prognosis following surgical resection. Ann R Coll Surg Engl 10:165, 1952.

82. Higgins GA, Beebe GW: Bronchogenic carcinoma. Factors in survival. Arch Surg 94:539, 1967.

83. Vincent RG, Takita H, Lane WW, Gutierrez AC, Pickren JW: Surgical therapy of lung cancer. J Thorac Cardiovasc Surg 71:581, 1976.

84. Weiss W, Boucot KR, Cooper DA: The histopathology of bronchogenic carcinoma and its relation to growth rate, metastasis, and prognosis. Cancer 26:965, 1970.

85. Bergh NP, Schersten T: Bronchogenic carcinoma. A followup study of a surgically treated series with special reference to the prognostic significance of lymph node metastasis. Acta Chir Scand (Suppl 347):1, 1965.

86. Shields TW, Yee J, Conn JH, Robinette CD: Relationship of cell type and lymph node metastasis to survival after resction of bronchial carcinoma. Ann Thorac Surg 20:501, 1975.

87. Paulson DL, Reisch JS: Long term survival after resection for bronchogenic carcinoma. Ann Surg 184:324, 1976.

88. Kirsh MM, Rotman H, Argenta L: Bove E, Cimmino V, Tashian J, Ferguson P, Sloan H: Carcinoma of the lung: Results of treatment over ten years. Ann Thorac Surg 21:371, 1976.

89. Mintzer RA, Malave SR, Neiman HL, Michaelis LL, Vanecko RM, Sanders JH: Computed vs. conventional tomography in evaluation of primary and secondary pulmonary neoplasms. Radiology 132:653, 1979.

90. Hirleman MT, YiuChiu VS, Chiu LC, Schapiro RL: The resectability of primary lung carcinoma: A diagnostic staging review. Comput Tomogr 4:146, 1980.

91. Faling LJ, Pugatch RD, JungLegg Y, Daly BDT Jr, Hong WK, Robbins AH, Snider GL: Computed tomographic scanning of the mediastinum in the staging of bronchogenic carcinoma. Am Rev Resp Dis 124:690, 1981.

92. Osborne DR, Korobkin M, Ravin CE, Putman CE, Wolfe WG, Sealy WC, Young WG, Breiman R, Heaston D, Ram P, Halber M: Comparison of plain radiography, conventional tomography, and computed tomography in detecting intrathoracic lymph node metastases from lung carcinoma. Radiology 142:157, 1982.

93. New policy outlines role of CT. Am Coll Radiol Bull 33:2, 1977.

94. Institute of Medicine: Computed Tomographic Scanning: A Policy Statement. Washington, DC, National Academy of Sciences, 1977.

95. Society of Computed Body Tomography: New indications for computed body tomography. AJR 133:115, 1979.

96. Komaiko MS, Lee ME, Birnberg FA: The contrast enhanced paravascular neoplasm: A potential CT pitfall. J Comput Assist Tomogr 4:516, 1980.

7 COMPUTED TOMOGRAPHY OF THE LUNGS

Gordon Gamsu

The conventional chest radiograph is a sensitive, readily available, and relatively inexpensive imaging modality. Air within the lungs provides natural contrast not available in other parts of the body, and the radiographic sensitivity for detection of pulmonary abnormalities is thus considerably greater for the lungs than for other organ systems. The radiographic patterns of pulmonary parenchymal disease are sensitive indicators of the disease processes that involve the lungs. Many lung abnormalities can therefore be diagnosed from the plain chest radiograph. In addition, re-

cent improvements in nonradiologic diagnostic methods and in the treatment of pulmonary disease have decreased the need for complex radiologic imaging studies. For instance, advances in fiberoptic bronchoscopy and percutaneous transthoracic biopsy have led to a direct approach to the diagnosis of many pulmonary abnormalities. For these and other reasons, computed tomography (CT) has had less impact on the imaging of pulmonary parenchymal disease than on imaging of disease elsewhere in the body. CT scanning should be applied only when it can provide reliable diagnostic information unavailable with less sophisticated imaging modalities. Nevertheless, in most medical centers, 15 to 20 per cent of body CT scans are of the thorax, and at least two thirds of these are for imaging of the lungs.

ANATOMY

Computed tomographic anatomy of the lungs, beyond the bronchovascular structures of the hila, has been described only in general terms. The individual lobes of the lung can be localized by their position within each hemithorax. In most people, the entire lengths of the interlobar fissures are not seen on CT scans. With rapid, high-spatial resolution scanners, segments of the major fissures are frequently visible. The positions of the major and minor fissures are, however, apparent in at least 90 per cent of patients.[1, 2] The fissures traverse a 2- to 3-cm wide band of lung characterized by the absence of large vessels (Fig. 7–1A,B).[2a] They course from posterosuperior to inferoanterior for the major fissures and from posterior to anterior in the right mid-lung for the minor fissure. The latter has been referred to as the "right midlung window" and should not be

321

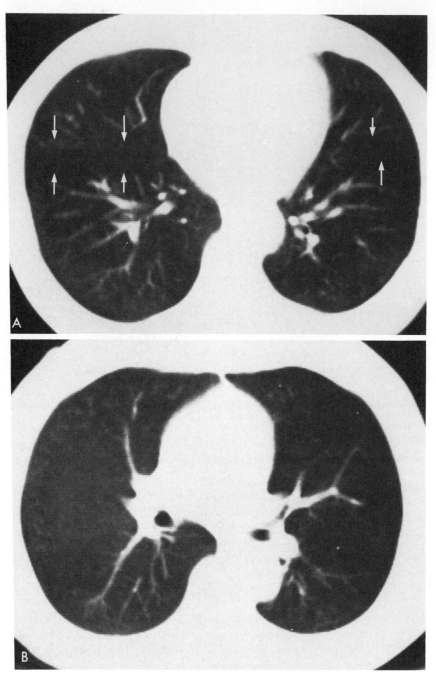

Figure 7–1. Site of interlobar fissures. **A** CT scan through the lower lungs demonstrates the "avascular" planes (arrows) of both major fissures. **B** CT scan shows the avascular plane in the right lung through which the minor fissure courses.

mistaken for an abnormal paucity of vessels in this region.[2b]

The individual bronchopulmonary segments are not separated by boundaries that can be seen on CT scans. Their approximate site within each lobe can be determined from the position and orientation of the segmental bronchus subtending each segment and from their general position within the thorax.

The bronchi divide dichotomously into two daughter branches and are accompanied by branches of the pulmonary artery. Normal bronchi are not demonstrated on CT scans beyond their segmental or subsegmental divisions. They will become visible only if surrounded by consolidation of the lung parenchyma when a bronchus lying in the plane of the CT scan appears as a tubular structure against the increased CT density of the consolidated lung. More often, the bronchus lies in an oblique or vertical plane to the CT scan and appears as a circle, or hole, within the consolidated lung.

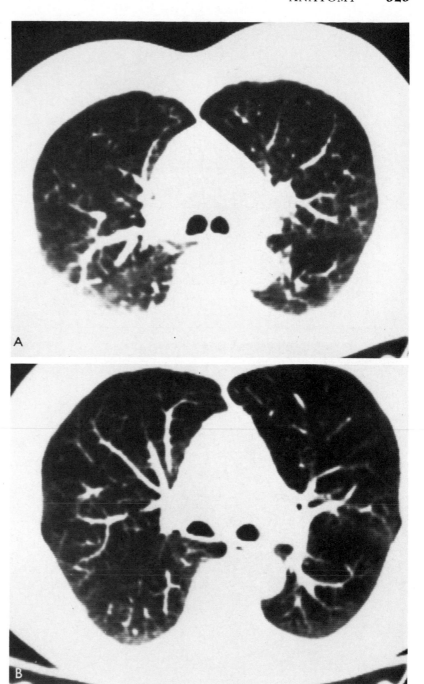

Figure 7–2. Difference in CT appearance with lung volume. **A** CT scan at end-expiration shows prominence of the dependent vessels and an anteroposterior gradient in CT density. The most posterior subsegments of the lungs appear airless. **B** CT scan at approximately the same scan level as in **A,** but at end-inspiration shows less anteroposterior CT density gradient. The dependent lung vessels are nearly equal in caliber to the nondependent vessels.

The blood vessels seen on CT scans of the lung are pulmonary arteries and veins. The general pattern of these vessels is a decrease in caliber from the hila to the periphery of the lungs. In the outer 1 to 2 cm of the lungs, there is a paucity of vessels. The caliber of the vessels seen on CT scans obtained at end-expiration is different from that seen at end-inspiration (Fig. 7–2A,B). At low lung volumes, the normal hydrostatic gradient of the blood volume in the lungs is reflected on CT scans as a prominence of the vessels in the dependent portions of the lung. At high lung volumes, this gradient is less apparent. At very low lung volumes, the most dependent portions of the lung may even appear airless and consolidated. This misleading appearance of abnormality can be corrected by scanning the patient in the prone or decubitus position. The hydrostatic gradient is also seen on CT scans of the lungs in the CT density (attenuation values) of the lung tissue itself. This will be reviewed more extensively in the subsequent section on CT densitometry of the lungs.

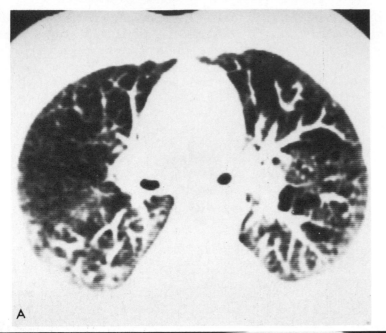

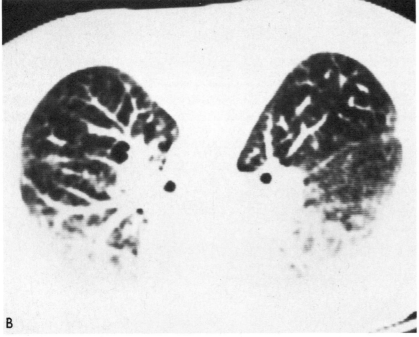

Figure 7–3. Difference in CT appearance on supine and prone CT scans. **A** With the patient in the supine position, CT scan shows prominence of the dependent, lower lobe vessels. **B** With the patient in the prone position, the lower lobes are more expanded and vessel caliber is reduced.

TECHNIQUES OF EXAMINATION

When the lungs are the region of primary concern, patients are usually scanned in the supine position, with their arms above their head to reduce streak artifacts from the shoulder girdle. Occasionally, the addition of CT scans with the patient in the prone position can aid in distinguishing a suspected parenchymal nodule from a vessel in the dependent portion of the lung (Fig. 7–3A,B).[3]

The optimum lung volume for CT scanning of the lungs has been debated at length.[4] In our experience, full inspiration (total lung capacity) is reproducible and easily achieved by most patients. In older or dyspneic patients, a few deep breaths before each scan can help with breath-holding for the required time. With slow scanners, some patients may not be able to suspend respiration for the time required to complete a single scan; in such instances, good quality CT scans can still be obtained during quiet breathing.

Intravenously infused contrast material does not assist in the diagnosis of most focal or diffuse abnormalities of the lungs. Nevertheless, because

CT scanning of the lungs is part of an examination of the entire thorax, intravenous contrast medium is injected or infused to delineate the blood vessels of the mediastinum and hila. When CT scanning is used to evaluate a suspected vascular lesion of the lungs, such as an arteriovenous malformation, high levels of intravascular contrast can be produced by the rapid injection of a bolus of 20 to 40 ml of 76 per cent contrast material. For this type of examination, rapid sequential scanning (dynamic scanning) through the area of abnormality is usually necessary.

A wide range in CT density is present on any CT scan of the thorax. The density differences among chest wall, mediastinum, and lung parenchyma require viewing of the images at several settings on the scanner console. Both the window level and window width must be manipulated to achieve optimum density for evaluation of each structure or area. In general, the lungs are viewed and photographed at a level of −400 to −600 Hounsfield Units (H) and at a window width of 500 to 1000 H. Window settings extended up to 4000 H can be used to demonstrate the mediastinum, lungs, and chest wall on the same scan (Fig. 7–4A). These images are, however, excessively gray, and object contrast is reduced. Narrower window widths decrease the

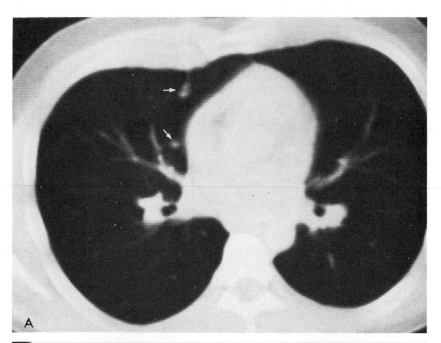

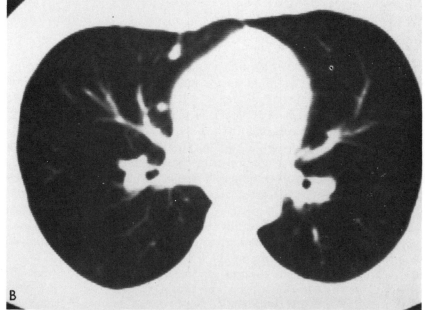

Figure 7–4. Extended window CT image. **A** At a window level of −360 H and a window width of 1664 H, the chest wall, mediastinum, and lungs are shown on one CT scan. The image lacks contrast, and two metastases (arrows) in the middle lobe are not well seen. **B** At a window level of −516 H and a window width of 1000 H, the two metastases are more clearly demonstrated.

gray scale and increase object contrast (Fig. 7–4B). When scan times in the 2- to 5-second range are used, CT images of the lung do not appear degraded by cardiac motion or pulsation of the pulmonary arteries. Scans obtained with longer scan times will show artifacts from the motion of vascular structures.

In most instances, CT scans of the lungs are obtained at 1-cm intervals using 1-cm collimation. These scans are usually sufficient to demonstrate most abnormalities. Scans 0.15 to 0.5 cm thick may be used in special circumstances. For instance, when a pulmonary nodule is suspected from the thicker scans, thinner scans through the area of suspected abnormality should be used. Highly collimated scans can improve resolution for such special procedures as nodule densitometry. A preliminary, projection CT radiograph (scout view) is often used to locate a focal pulmonary abnormality. With many scanners, the levels for scanning can be selected automatically from the projection CT radiograph.

PATHOLOGY

PULMONARY NODULES

Evaluation of pulmonary nodules is by far the most common clinical requirement for CT scanning of the lungs. These involve both the detection of pulmonary nodules and the determination of the nature of a pulmonary nodule detected from conventional radiographs. The value of CT scanning in assessing pulmonary nodules is due mainly to its superior contrast resolution. Whereas the contrast resolution of conventional chest radiographs is 2 to 5 per cent, that of CT scans is about 0.5 per cent. Also, the transverse display of CT images is ideal for separating thoracic structures that overlap on radiographs and decrease the conspicuousness of pulmonary nodules. Nodules that are subpleural, high in the apices of the lungs, in the costophrenic angles, or obscured by mediastinal structures are especially difficult to see on chest radiographs but are readily apparent on CT scans (Fig. 7–5A,B). Many nodules 0.5 to 1 cm in diameter are not apparent on chest radiographs, whereas most pulmonary nodules larger than 2 to 3 mm in diameter are visible on CT scans.

Pulmonary nodules are readily detected on CT scans when they are larger than the pulmonary blood vessels in that portion of the lung. Nodules in the outer third of the lung are therefore more conspicuous than those closer to the hilum. Close observation of contiguous scans is often necessary to distinguish small nodules from vessels. Vessels can usually be seen on adjacent scans as they branch and course through the lungs. The rapid display of serial images on the scanner console can also help in distinguishing vessels from small nodules.[5] The eye integrates the information from serial scans as they demonstrate the course of pulmonary vessels. Small nodules appear as disjointed densities with no vascular connection. The costomanubrial articulation of the first rib can be mistaken for a lung nodule on CT scans (Fig. 7–6 A,B).

The major areas of interest and controversy relate to the evaluation of pulmonary nodules in the patient with potential metastases to the lungs; in the patient who demonstrates a noncalcified, solitary, pulmonary nodule on a chest radiograph; in the patient showing a suspicious but unconfirmed nodule on a chest radiograph; and in the patient with cytologic evidence of malignant cells in the sputum but no apparent abnormalities on the chest radiograph.

Pulmonary Metastasis

CT scans can detect pulmonary nodules with a high degree of sensitivity. Muhm and colleagues[6] found that in 32 of 91 patients, CT scans demonstrated more nodules than were seen on conventional whole lung tomograms. In five of these 32 patients, conventional tomograms failed to show any nodules, whereas CT scans revealed one or more nodules. Shaner and co-workers[7] confirmed these findings in a study of 25 patients with sarcoma or melanoma. Conventional tomograms showed each patient to have one to four pulmonary nodules, whereas CT scans defined additional nodules, usually 3 to 6 mm in diameter, in 12 (48 per cent) of the patients. All 25 patients underwent thoracotomy, and CT scans had correctly demonstrated 78 per cent of all resected nodules greater than 3 mm in diameter.

The clinical significance of pulmonary nodules detected only by CT in a patient with a thoracic or extrathoracic primary neoplasm scanning is controversial. Although the Shaner study[7] found that 60 per cent of these small nodules were benign granulomas or intrapulmonary lymph nodes, Muhm's group[6] found that only 10 to 15 per cent of the nodules in their study were benign. This discrepancy is significant and has not been resolved. For practical purposes, it must be appreciated that nodules detected only on CT scans, even in a patient with a malignant neoplasm, are

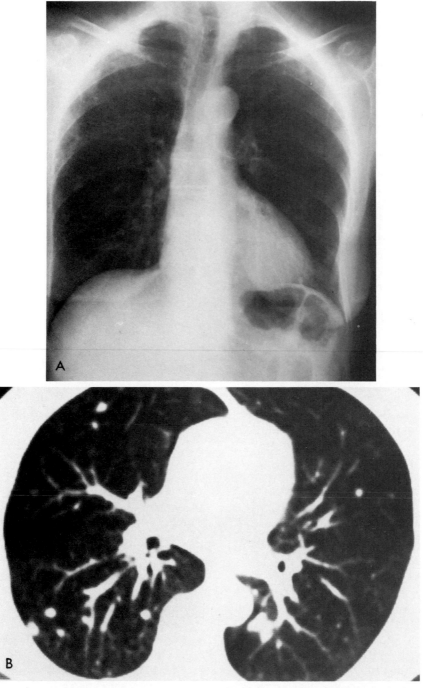

Figure 7–5. Multiple pulmonary nodular metastases. **A**   Frontal chest radiograph shows several suspicious nodules in each lung field. **B**   CT scan through the midthorax reveals numerous small nodules that were not evident on the chest radiograph. CT-guided aspiration biopsy yielded metastatic carcinoma, later found to be from an occult pancreatic tumor.

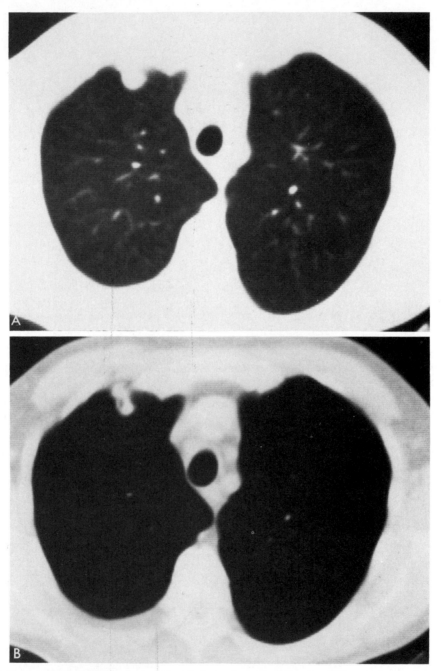

Figure 7–6. Costomanubrial articulation simulating a lung nodule. **A**   CT scan shows the anterior end of the first right rib projecting into the lung and simulating a lung nodule. **B**   CT scan at mediastinal window settings reveals the true nature of this normal variant.

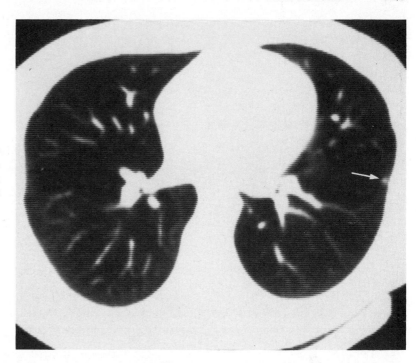

Figure 7–7. Normal intrapulmonary lymph node. CT scan shows a small subpleural nodule (arrow) on the left in a patient with osteogenic sarcoma. This proved to be a normal lymph node.

not necessarily metastases (Fig. 7–7). Depending on the clinical circumstances, additional evaluation is necessary for diagnosis. In some situations, CT-guided percutaneous aspiration biopsy or thoracotomy may be required. Alternatively, repeat CT scanning after 6 to 10 weeks may show enlargement of the nodule or nodules.

In our experience, the high sensitivity of CT scanning should be used in the search for metastatic pulmonary nodules, especially in patients with tumors that have a propensity for metastasizing to the lungs (Table 7–1). In general, CT scanning should replace conventional whole lung tomography for this purpose.

Solitary Pulmonary Nodule

The role of CT scanning in the patient who presents with a solitary pulmonary nodule on a chest radiograph is one of the most controversial issues in thoracic computed tomography. Even without information gained from CT scanning, an integrated plan of management for the patient with a solitary pulmonary nodule, especially when the patient is asymptomatic, has not been formulated.

Table 7–1. SITES LIKELY TO HAVE NODULAR PULMONARY METASTASES

Bone and soft tissue	Colon
Lung	Genitourinary tract
Melanoma	Head and neck

Over the last three decades, extensive studies[8–12] have established the basic facts about the solitary pulmonary nodule. Most of these nodules are granulomas and should not be resected if the correct diagnosis can be established. The surgical mortality rate for resection of a solitary pulmonary nodule, however, is relatively low, particularly when the nodule is benign. A significant proportion (10 to 50 per cent) of *resected* solitary pulmonary nodules are found to be primary or metastatic malignant tumors, and resection does result in a relatively good prognosis for the patient.[13, 14] This indicates that even without the information derived from CT scanning, a significant selection of patients for thoracotomy is possible.

Benignity can be assumed if the nodule shows stability on serial chest radiographs over at least 2 years or if it shows dense or central calcification on chest radiographs or conventional tomograms.[15, 16] In a small proportion of patients, a bronchogenic carcinoma can engulf a calcified nidus; therefore, an eccentric focus of calcification does not exclude malignancy (Fig. 7–8A,B). Bronchogenic carcinomas themselves occasionally calcify, but the calcification is usually very fine and radiographically invisible.

Of 72 patients with a malignant solitary pulmonary nodule studied by O'Keefe and colleagues,[16] ten had calcification visible on radiographs of the resected specimen, but in only one instance was the calcification seen on standard

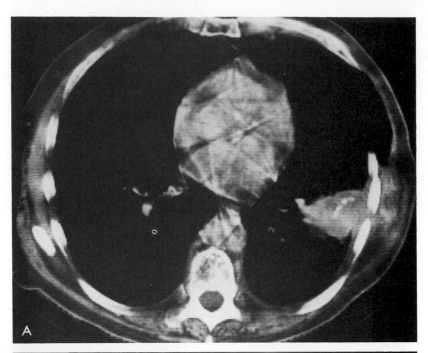

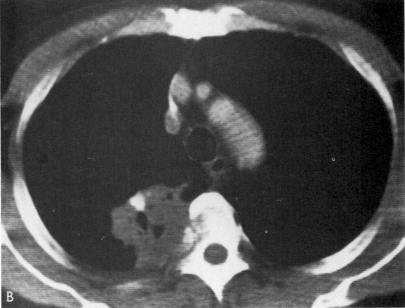

Figure 7–8. Bronchogenic carcinoma containing calcification. **A,B** CT scan shows areas of high CT density within two bronchogenic carcinomas, presumably representing engulfed granulomas.

Figure 7–9. Typical appearance of adenocarcinoma. **A** Frontal radiograph shows an ill-defined mass in the left upper lobe.
Illustration continued on opposite page

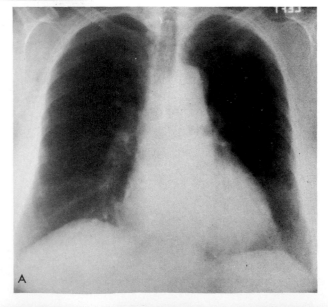

chest radiographs. In the same study, 50 per cent of benign lesions, consisting mainly of granulomas and hematomas, contained calcification. In only 35 per cent of these patients was the calcification visible on chest radiographs. Metastatic malignant tumors, particularly osteogenic sarcoma, chondrosarcoma, and thyroid carcinoma, can show stippled or homogeneous calcification.

Age is also an important factor in deciding the management of the asymptomatic patient with a solitary pulmonary nodule. Pulmonary nodules are rarely malignant in patients under the age of 35 years and resection is seldom indicated.[10]

At present, distinguishing many noncalcified benign from noncalcified malignant pulmonary nodules is not possible using clinical and radiographic criteria. Therefore, a convincing argument can be constructed for resection of all indeterminate solitary pulmonary nodules in patients over the age of 35 years. Equally convincing interpretation of the known facts can be used to argue for all patients to be followed up with periodic chest radiographs. Lillington[17] proposed a widely adopted middle course, in which most patients with indeterminate nodules undergo transbronchial or percutaneous aspiration biopsy of the

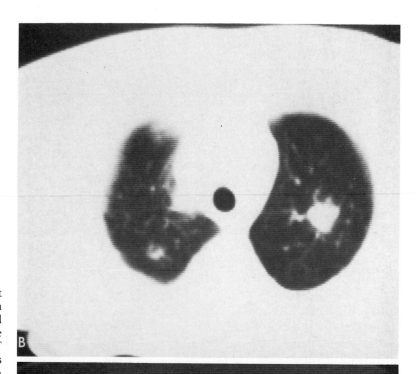

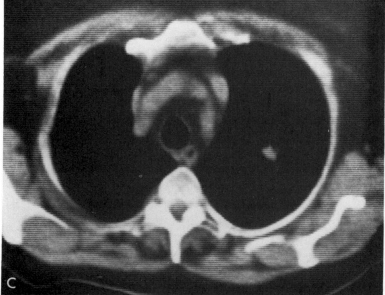

Figure 7–9. *Continued* **B** CT scan at "lung" window settings demonstrates an ill-defined subapical mass on the left and a small granuloma on the right. (These CT appearances are nonspecific.) **C** CT scan at "mediastinal" window settings shows the bronchogenic carcinoma as a smaller nodule. The small granuloma on the right is no longer visible.

nodule to determine whether the lesion is to be observed.

A simple, noninvasive method for distinguishing benign from malignant solitary pulmonary nodules would nevertheless be of great benefit. CT scans do not have the spatial resolution to improve on the radiographic appearance of the gross anatomy of benign and malignant pulmonary nodules. In general, the appearance of a solitary pulmonary nodule on CT scans is similar to that on plain radiographs. Carcinomas can be ill defined, spiculated, lobulated, or well defined (Fig. 7–9A–C).[18] These findings are nonspecific and less well demonstrated on CT scans than they are on chest radiographs. On the other hand, the high-density resolution of CT scans does offer the potential for providing information about the nature of pulmonary nodules.

Phantom studies done by Cann and colleagues[19] have shown that CT scanners are accurate densitometers. In simulated lung nodules, they found that differences of as little as 15 mg/ml^3 of potassium phosphate could be detected using CT densitometry. Using a phantom, Godwin and coworkers[20] studied the relationship of nodule size to the degree of CT scanner collimation and the number of CT voxels free of partial-volume artifacts from surrounding aerated lung. With the resolving element of most scanners, nodules less than 1 cm in diameter require narrow collimation and almost perfect alignment to obtain sufficient voxels from within the nodule for analysis.

Siegelman and associates[21] were the first to describe CT nodule densitometry for distinguishing benign from malignant solitary pulmonary nodules. With careful calibration of the scanner, narrow collimation (2 to 5 mm), and numerical printouts of the CT numbers, an average CT number is obtained from a set of contiguous voxels having the highest CT density. Of 91 noncalcified nodules, 45 were nodular bronchogenic carcinomas and had a representative CT number between 57 and 139 H (mean 92 ± 18 H). Another 13 were nodular metastases, having representative CT numbers ranging from 57 to 147 H (mean 98 H). The remaining 33 nodules were classified as benign and fell into three groups on the basis of CT nodule densitometry. Twenty-seven per cent were indistinguishable from malignant lesions; 60 per cent had a representative CT number above 164 H and were readily distinguishable from the malignant lesions; and 13 per cent had a representative CT number between 147 and 162 H, an intermediate range between benign and malignant.

Overtly calcified nodules all had a representative CT number over 600 H (Fig. 7–10A,B). Thus, about 20 per cent of solitary pulmonary nodules could be classified as benign based on CT densitometry data alone. The high CT numbers are assumed to reflect fine diffuse calcification not visible on radiographs, although high concentrations of collagen (with a CT value of about 400 H) could produce similar findings.

Unfortunately, these results[21] have not been substantiated by at least two other groups.[22, 23] In our experience, only one of 30 noncalcified pulmonary nodules showed high CT numbers in the benign range. The discrepancies in the results of CT nodule densitometry may be due to differences in CT scanner capabilities or in the patient population studied. The difficulties in accurate in vivo CT densitometry in the thorax have been extensively discussed.[19–23] Commercial CT scanners vary in their algorithms and corrections for producing CT numbers.[23a] The CT number for high atomic number materials depends on effective x-ray energy, corrections for filtration and dynamic range, scanner configuration, and other factors.[23b] In the thorax, differing quantities of air, soft tissue, and bone, as well as cardiopulmonary motion, will also influence the resultant CT number. Geographic differences in the causes of pulmonary granulomas (tuberculosis, histoplasmosis, coccidioidomycosis) can also profoundly influence the results of CT nodule densitometry.

Until in vitro studies have quantified the mineral content of various benign pulmonary nodules, the entire basis for CT nodule densitometry remains in question. To summarize, CT nodule densitometry is at present an experimental procedure, requiring further validation. New CT scanners with better hardware and software, as well as such modifications as dual-energy subtraction, promise more precise results for thoracic densitometry.[19]

A second reason for CT scanning in a patient with a solitary pulmonary nodule has been proposed.[24] A solitary pulmonary nodular metastasis may be the only radiographic manifestation of an occult extrathoracic malignancy. Detection of multiple nodules seen only on CT scans could suggest the possibility of metastasis and initiate a search for the primary neoplasm. Nevertheless, the reasoning cannot be considered valid. The frequency of metastasis presenting on chest radiographs as a solitary pulmonary nodule is only 3 to 6 per cent.[10–12] Scanning a large number of patients with solitary pulmonary nodules would un-

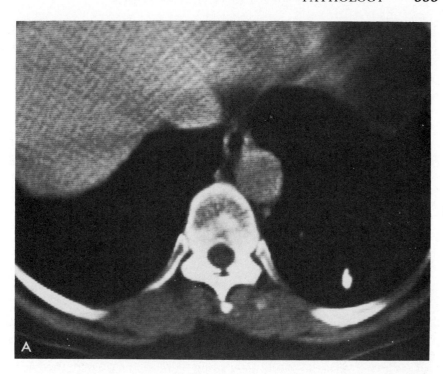

Figure 7–10. Densitometry of overtly mineralized pulmonary nodule. **A** CT scan shows a left lower lobe nodule with a high CT density, equal to that of cortical bone. **B** CT printout shows central voxels in the range of 500 to 700 H.

```
-728-760-722-634-624-616-584-556-546-602-638
-704-740-698-622-516-438-424-432-490-596-644
-682-664-610-494-230 -74-120-290-478-650-670
-604-582-470-254  80 250  74-212-478-642-666
-510-444-304 -96 220 322 114-166-458-590-682
-474-376-222  58 294 240  78-108-328-512-718
-568-448-114 190 344 282 174  38-142-440-734
-664-496 -76 210 436 490 342 162 -66-404-760
-676-426 -54 212 568 678 514 208 -50-420-740
-622-318  -8 278 628 718 554 158-134-496-710
-566-298 -12 262 506 582 410  34-280-582-678
-596-376-108  86 282 368 210 -86-430-622-612
-630-472-266-108  76 130  -6-252-510-600-544
-602-508-368-224 -96 -78-180-368-496-506-458
-570-526-426-314-204-210-328-438-496-494-412
-538-500-402-310-252-310-410-486-498-484-446
-482-444-370-334-364-434-482-512-520-508-444
```

B

doubtedly reveal numerous incidental small granulomas and normal intraparenchymal lymph nodes. The results of the CT studies would be confusing and misleading. Therefore, CT scanning is not indicated for a solitary pulmonary nodule before a diagnosis has been established by other means.

Occult Pulmonary Nodule or Mass

The presence of a small nodule or mass, suspected from chest radiographs, can occasionally be difficult to confirm. The problem can often be resolved with oblique chest radiographs, fluoroscopy with spot-films of the area, or conventional tomograms. Nodules or masses located in the apex of the lung (Fig. 7–11A,B), in the retrocardiac region or subpleurally, can be difficult to demonstrate with these techniques. In a minority of patients, whether a mass is present remains unresolved even after these studies. In our experience, CT scanning is the most sensitive method available for detecting and localizing focal masses

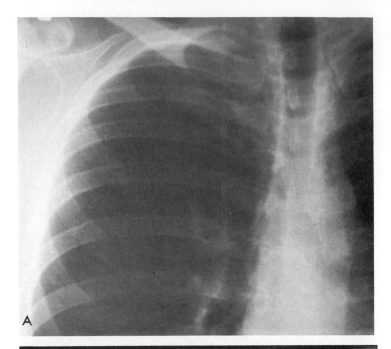

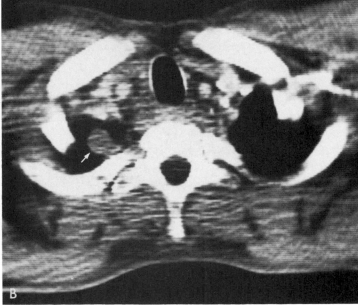

Figure 7–11. Suspicious apical nodule. **A** Frontal chest radiograph shows a possible right apical nodule or focal pleural thickening. **B** CT scan confirms the presence of a lung nodule (arrow) later shown to be a granuloma.

or nodules within the pulmonary parenchyma (Fig. 7–12A,B). We have seen numerous instances of CT scans demonstrating even relatively large nodules that were not visible using more conventional imaging modalities. The frequency of this situation is difficult to determine. In practice, CT scanning should be applied with due consideration of the clinical circumstances. Occasionally, CT scans will demonstrate an occult cavity or a mycetoma within a lung mass which elucidates the cause of hemoptysis.[25, 26]

Sputum cytologic screening of patients with pulmonary symptoms or of people at risk for the development of bronchogenic carcinoma has become widely adopted. Some individuals will have malignant cells in their sputum, although their chest radiograph shows no abnormality.[27, 28] Many such bronchogenic carcinomas are small and centrally located within a bronchus. Detailed fibrobronchoscopy can show more than half of these lesions. In the remainder, CT scanning may demonstrate the occult neoplasm or it may show a suspicious area for subsequent bronchial biopsy, brushing, or washing.

A conceptually related problem occurs in the assessment of a patient who manifests a paraneoplastic syndrome thought to be due to a bronchogenic carcinoma. Bronchogenic carcinoma can cause a variety of paraneoplastic syndromes that are primarily neuromuscular, endocrine, metabolic, skeletal, connective tissue, vascular, and hematologic (Table 7–2).[29, 30] In most patients, the responsible tumor will be seen on chest radiographs. The syndrome, however, can antecede the radiographic appearance of tumor by months or even years. In this instance, CT scanning may disclose the primary tumor or confirm a suspicious radiographic nodule or mass.

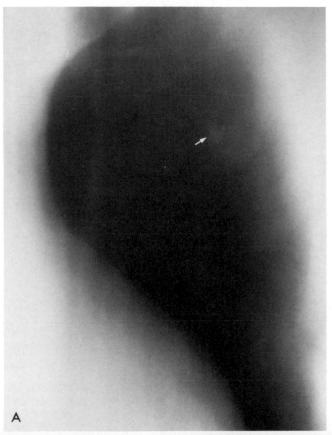

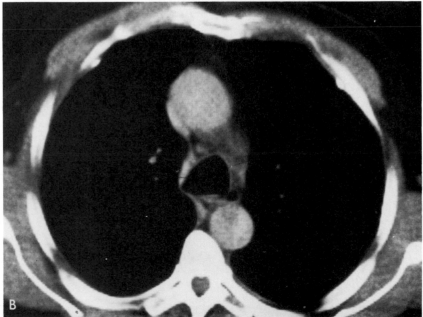

Figure 7–12. Costochondral calcification simulating a lung nodule. **A** Conventional tomogram shows a left upper lung field nodule (arrow), suspicious for being within the lung. **B** CT scan demonstrates that the "nodule" is calcification within the costochondral cartilage of the second rib.

Table 7–2. EXTRATHORACIC MANIFESTATIONS OF BRONCHOGENIC CARCINOMA

Endocrine and metabolic
  Cushing's syndrome
  Hypercalcemia
  Excessive antidiuretic hormone
  Carcinoid syndrome
  Estrogen excretion
Neuromuscular
  Peripheral neuropathy
  Cortical cerebellar degeneration
  Carcinomatous myopathy
  Subacute spinocerebellar degeneration
  Mental aberration
Skeletal and connective tissue
  Clubbing
  Pulmonary hypertrophic osteoarthropathy
  Acanthosis nigricans
  Dermatomyositis
Vascular and hematologic
  Migratory thrombophlebitis
  Nonbacterial verrucous endocarditis
  Anemia
  Fibrinolytic purpura

VASCULAR LESIONS

Rapid, sequential CT scanning (dynamic scanning) after an intravenous bolus injection of contrast material can delineate vascular lesions of the lung.[31] Normal mediastinal and hilar blood vessels will show a predictable increase in CT density from scan to scan following the bolus of contrast material. Similarly, abnormal vessels in the lung will demonstrate enhancement by intravenous contrast material. Many CT scanners can plot the change in CT number with time in order to produce time-density curves for an area-of-interest within the abnormal vessel.[31]

Congenital and acquired abnormalities of the pulmonary vessels are uncommon. Among those that have been diagnosed from CT scans are arteriovenous fistulae,[31, 32] pulmonary vein varices,[31] and pulmonary sequestration.[33] The diagnosis of central pulmonary emboli by CT scanning has been discussed in Chapter 6.

A pulmonary artery–to–pulmonary vein fistula is only one type of abnormal vascular shunt within the lungs. Abnormal communication can also exist between pulmonary arteries and bronchial arteries and between pulmonary veins and bronchial veins.[34, 35] Pulmonary arteriovenous fistulae can be congenital or post-traumatic.[36] The congenital type is much more common. Usually, the abnormal dilated vascular channel is supplied by a single artery and drained by a single vein.[37, 38] Occasionally, many feeding arteries and veins are

present.[39, 40] In about a third of cases, the lesions are multiple, but often only the dominant lesion is seen on chest radiographs. From 40 to 60 per cent of patients have additional lesions outside the thorax, and the condition is then known as hereditary hemorrhagic telangiectasia (Rendu-Osler-Weber syndrome).[40–42]

Pulmonary arteriovenous fistulae can usually be suspected from chest radiographs or conventional tomograms (Fig. 7–13A). The lesion appears as a round or slightly lobular mass, from less than 1 cm to several centimeters in diameter. It is usually in the inner third of the lung. In many patients, the feeding artery emanating from the hilum and the draining vein coursing toward the left atrium are visible. Confirmation of the diagnosis can be obtained by pulmonary angiography or sometimes by radioisotope angiography,[43] but dynamic CT scanning is a more convenient, noninvasive method of confirming the diagnosis and provides a precise anatomic display of the abnormality.[32] When a time-density plot of the lesion shows a contrast peak between the peak of the right side and the peak of the left side of the heart, the pulmonary blood supply to the fistula is confirmed (Fig. 7–13B). In our experience, CT scans obviate the need for angiography unless surgery or embolization of the fistula is being contemplated. Under these circumstances, angiography must be performed to detect any additional lesions because CT has not been shown capable of demonstrating small, radiographically inapparent fistulae. Carefully performed pulmonary angiography of all lung lobes is required.

Pulmonary vein varicosities are uncommon and can be congenital or acquired. They are usually asymptomatic and do not require treatment; they are most often detected from chest radiographs. The tortuous, dilated segment of the pulmonary vein appears as a smooth, round or oval density close to the left atrium.[43–45] It often does not show specific radiographic features, and its nature is suspected from its characteristic position. Dynamic CT scanning is an ideal method for diagnosing pulmonary vein varicosities (Fig. 7–14A,B). After an intravenous bolus of contrast material, the varix will opacify at about the same time as the left atrium. A pulmonary arteriovenous fistula close to the left atrium should have CT scan findings identical to those of a pulmonary vein varicosity.[46] It is doubtful whether CT scans can routinely distinguish a medially situated arteriovenous fistula from a pulmonary vein varicosity.

Abnormal systemic blood supply to a portion of the lung can be due to anomalous vessels that

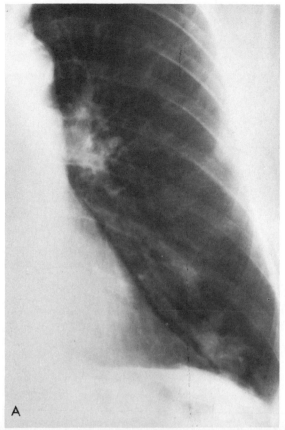

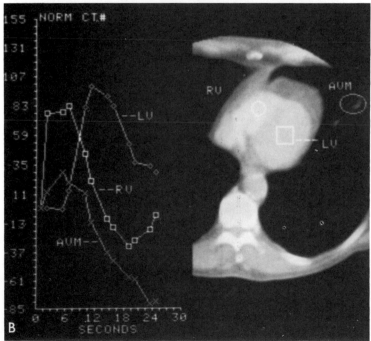

Figure 7–13. Pulmonary arteriovenous fistula. **A**   Frontal radiograph shows a left lower lobe fistula with its feeding artery and draining vein. **B**   Time-density plots derived from areas of interest over the right ventricle (RV), left ventricle (LV), and fistula (AVM) show that the contrast peak from the fistula occurs shortly after the right ventricular peak. (Courtesy of Dr. Robert J. Herfkens, San Francisco)

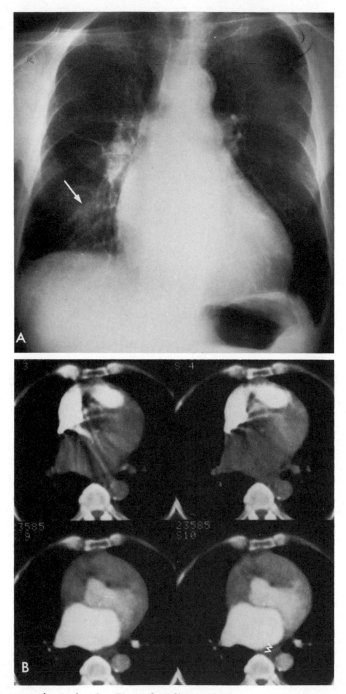

Figure 7–14. Pulmonary vein varix. **A** Frontal radiograph shows a serpiginous mass (arrow) next to the right border of the heart. **B** Serial CT scans through this level demonstrate that the "mass" is a dilated inferior pulmonary vein.

arise from the aorta or its branches, transpleural vessels from the intercostal arteries, or hypertrophied bronchial arteries. The lung itself may otherwise be normal, or it may be dysplastic or damaged (usually from chronic infection). *Pulmonary sequestration* is one of the most common congenital anomalies of the lung. The sequestered portion of lung is characterized by a lack of communication with the tracheobronchial tree and an abnormal systemic blood supply. The abnormal systemic blood supply is from an anomalous vessel arising from the descending aorta in about 70 per cent of cases and from the abdominal aorta, bronchial arteries, intercostal arteries, or aortic arch in the other 30 per cent. When the sequestered lung is clearly within the normal visceral pleura and has its venous drainage to the pulmonary veins, it is referred to as intralobar. When the sequestered lung has its own envelope of pleura and has its venous drainage to systemic veins, it is called extralobar. Many intermediate forms have been described.[47–50]

The radiographic appearance of an intralobar pulmonary sequestration depends on whether or not the sequestered lung is aerated. When the sequestration does not communicate with the rest of the lung, it appears as a sharply circumscribed, homogeneous density, usually in the posterior portion of the lower lobe, almost invariably contiguous with the diaphragm. A sequestration that communicates with the remainder of the lung, usually after being infected, appears cystic. It may exhibit one or more cystic spaces, with or without air-fluid levels.

A definitive diagnosis of pulmonary sequestration usually depends on the demonstration of the anomalous vessels by angiography.[51] In some reported cases,[33, 33a] CT scans showed a large vessel from the left side of the aorta feeding into the sequestration. In one of these cases and in one that we have studied, the septations between the cystic spaces of the sequestration enhanced after a bolus injection of contrast material. In our case, rapid sequential scanning demonstrated this enhancement immediately after the enhancement of the descending thoracic aorta, indicating systemic blood supply to the sequestration. Godwin and Webb[31] described an angioma and an inflammatory mass both with systemic blood supply and showing contrast enhancement immediately after that of the descending thoracic aorta.

Dynamic CT scanning can thus show systemic blood supply to the lung even when the feeding vessels are not demonstrated. Contrast enhancement of the abnormal portion of lung during the arterial phase, after injection of an intravenous bolus of contrast material, should indicate that aortography will show abnormal systemic blood supply.

Pulmonary embolism is the most common acute pulmonary emergency for the hospitalized patient and accounts for an estimated 120,000 deaths per year in the United States. Autopsy studies show that pulmonary embolism is not correctly diagnosed in 60 to 70 per cent of patients who die of it. Pulmonary angiography is the definitive diagnostic modality, but it is not widely available and for the patient can result in complication or even death. An accurate, noninvasive method of diagnosis could improve the diagnostic accuracy for pulmonary embolism. Godwin and co-workers[52] have shown that central pulmonary emboli can be demonstrated on CT scans. After a bolus injection of contrast material, emboli as peripheral as lobar pulmonary arteries can be seen (Fig. 7–15). Ovenfors and colleagues[53] were able to show autologous blood clots in segmental pulmonary arteries in dogs. In our opinion, CT scanning should be used for evaluating suspected chronic pulmonary emboli, as described in Chapter 6. However, further study is necessary before its routine use can be advocated for suspected acute pulmonary embolism.

Indirect evidence of pulmonary emboli might be found in some patients from the CT scan appearance of the lung distal to an occluded artery. Detection of pulmonary infarction distal to sites of pulmonary vascular occlusion has been studied both in patients and in animals. Grossman and colleagues[54] found an increase in CT density in one of six experimentally occluded vessels before infusion of contrast material and in three of six after infusion. In subsequent studies, this group demonstrated decrease in CT density ("oligemia") in areas of lung distal to a balloon occlusion of segmental pulmonary arteries.[55] This finding was consistently demonstrated only in the nondependent portion of the lung. Lourie and co-workers,[56] on the other hand, demonstrated areas of increased density on CT scans of 81 per cent of dogs that had verified infarctions after experimental pulmonary artery occlusion.

In the experiments of Ovenfors and colleagues,[53] infarction was not found distal to the experimental pulmonary emboli. Sinner[57] described various patterns of peripheral wedge-shaped areas of increased CT density in patients with suspected pulmonary emboli. The exact nature of these findings and their specificity, however, was not documented. The increased CT

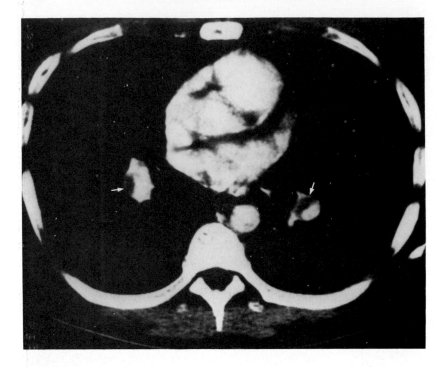

Figure 7–15. Clinically silent chronic pulmonary emboli. After intravenous infusion of contrast material, CT scan demonstrates filling defects (arrows) in the left descending lobar pulmonary artery and interlobar pulmonary artery.

density in an area of lung subtended by a pulmonary embolus can be due to edema, hemorrhage, necrosis of lung tissue, or atelectasis. The clinical significance of this finding in patients with suspected pulmonary embolism awaits further clarification.

DIFFUSE LUNG DISEASE

Description of the CT scan appearances of diffuse lung disease has been limited. In a study of

patients with pulmonary asbestosis,[58] CT scans demonstrated pulmonary parenchymal disease in 33 per cent of the patients, whereas conventional radiographs showed it in only 17 per cent. The major CT finding was a "honeycomb" pattern, mainly at the lung bases. Other features, not readily detected on conventional radiographs, were bullae (small cystic spaces) and transpulmonary bands. On CT scans, bullae appear as areas of low CT density without vessels traversing them.

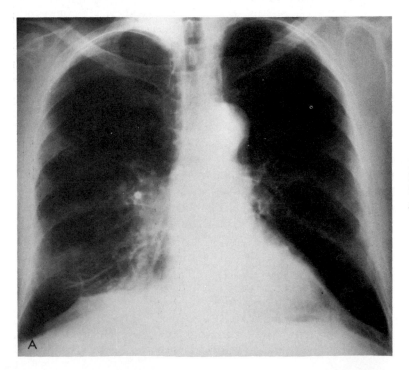

Figure 7–16. Asbestosis with masslike atelectasis. **A**   Frontal chest radiograph shows bilateral ill-defined basal masses.
Illustration continued on opposite page

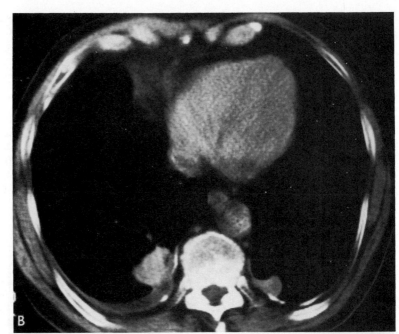

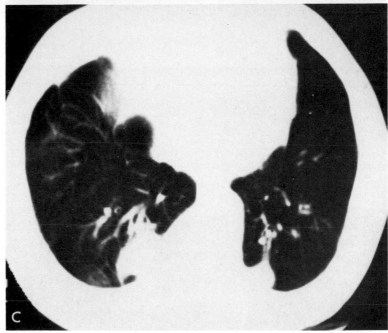

Figure 7–16. *Continued* **B** CT scan at "mediastinal" window settings demonstrates the bilateral lower lobe peripheral masses. Pleural calcification and thickening are evident. **C** The same CT scan at "lung" window settings shows pulmonary vessels and bronchi converging on the masses of atelectatic lung.

They are multiple, often subpleural, and can be from less than 1 to 10 cm in diameter. Transpulmonary bands appear as linear bands of density extending from the cardiophrenic angles and paravertebral recesses into the lungs.

In some patients with asbestosis, a masslike lesion 2 to 6 cm in diameter maybe visible on chest radiographs and CT scans.[59, 60] The lesion is usually located in a lower lobe peripherally, and other pleuroparenchymal CT findings of asbestosis exposure are present (Fig. 7–16A,B). These masses are thought to represent areas of atelectatic lung surrounded by fibrous adhesions ex-

tending from the pleura. CT scans can frequently demonstrate pulmonary vessels and bronchi converging on the mass (Fig. 7–16C). Recognition of the benign nature of these lesions should obviate the need for further evaluation.

In patients without lung disease, the CT density of the lungs as well as the caliber and number of the vessels shows an anteroposterior gradient. In some patients with asbestosis (or other forms of diffuse lung disease), the only CT manifestation of the disease can be loss of the lung vascular gradient. The vessels in the dependent portion of the lung appear similar to those in the nondependent portion. This finding is most apparent on CT scans at low lung volumes and may not be evident when the patient is at full inspiration.

Solomon and colleagues[61] described the CT findings in 34 patients with pulmonary sarcoidosis. As with asbestosis, the most common CT manifestation of pulmonary sarcoidosis was a coarse honeycomb pattern at the lung bases. Because we have seen similar CT appearances in diffuse pulmonary fibrosis from other causes, this finding is probably nonspecific (Figs. 7–17A,B and

7–18A,B). Bullae and nodules can also be seen on the CT scans of patients with sarcoidosis.

Honeycombing seen on chest radiographs as small, thin-wall spaces produce subtle CT scan changes (Fig. 7–19). The honeycomb pattern described on CT scans in patients with asbestosis and sarcoidosis has larger spaces and thicker walls.

In summary, in many patients with diffuse pulmonary fibrosis, CT can show subtle changes not demonstrated on conventional radiographs. How-

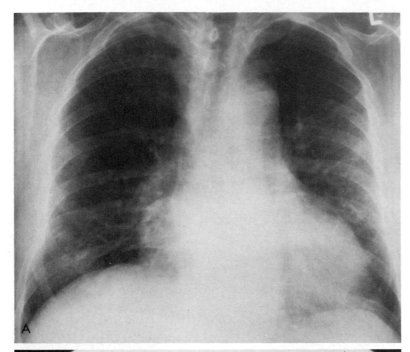

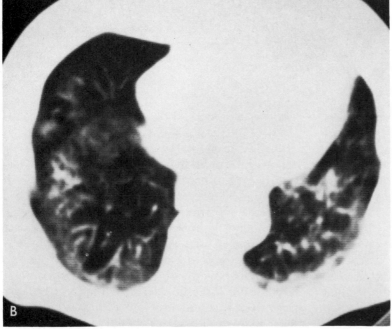

Figure 7–17. Idiopathic pulmonary fibrosis. **A** Frontal chest radiograph shows a diffuse, fine irregular (linear) pattern of disease. **B** CT scan demonstrates many avascular spaces, distortion of the branching pattern of the pulmonary vessels, and posterior bands (probably representing airless lung).

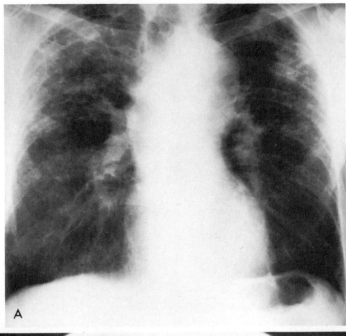

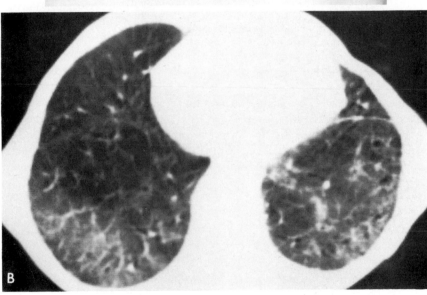

Figure 7–18. Silicosis with pulmonary fibrosis. **A** Frontal radiograph shows fibronodular changes in the upper lobes and a fine irregular pattern at the lung bases. **B** CT scan demonstrates increase in CT density, multiple small bullae, and distortion of the pulmonary vessels.

ever, studies of pulmonary function and gallium radionuclide scans are both recognized methods of detecting subtle diffuse lung disease. Whether CT scans can complement these modalities and provide new information about the stage of activity or nature of the disease processes remains to be defined.

LUNG DENSITOMETRY

The density of the normal lung consists of four main elements: air; blood; walls of bronchi, vessels, and alveoli; and interstitial fluid, in small quantity. The density of the normal lung is neither spatially nor temporally homogeneous. Grav-

itational forces on the lung cause a gradient that results in regional variation in air and blood volume. The dependent portion of the lung contains relatively less air (gas) and more fluid.[62, 63] Temporal changes in lung density occur during the normal respiratory cycle. The density of the lung and the gravitational gradient is greatest on expiration (Fig. 7–2). Robinson and Kreel[63] showed that with subjects supine, the mean CT density (attenuation value) was -766.2 H in the posterior third of the lung and -844.4 H in the anterior third. This anteroposterior gradient in CT density varied from 36 to 188 H at suspended neutral respiration and from 20 to 68 H on deep in-

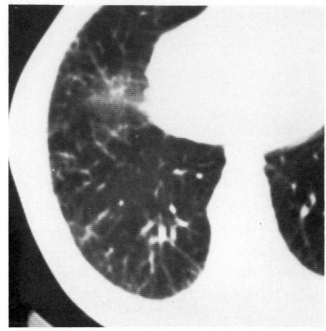

Figure 7–19. Rheumatoid lung disease. CT scan in a patient with a honeycomb pattern on chest radiographs. Subtle, small ring densities are demonstrated throughout the lung, but are most conspicuous at the periphery of the lung.

spiration. These CT findings are similar to those shown by other investigators.[62, 64–66]

Many abnormalities of the lung are reflected in changes in lung density. The noninvasive quantitation of lung disease by the measurement of lung density has interested many investigators. Several methods can be used to measure lung density: fluorodensitometry and videodensitometry, microwave transmission, electrical impedance, Compton scatter, and computed tomography.[67–74] Of these methods, only CT scanning precisely delineates the anatomic localization of the density measurement.[75] A discussion of the basis of quantitative CT and the inherent problems with this method are presented in Chapter 23. The lung is technically the most difficult region of the body for quantitative CT densitometry because density varies greatly within the thorax.

Pulmonary emphysema is characterized pathologically by enlargement of the terminal air spaces of the lung with destruction of alveolar walls. In our experience, the most common CT scan finding is avascular spaces (bullae), measuring up to 10 cm in diameter. These spaces are scattered throughout the lungs, although the number and size vary from one lung zone to another (Fig. 7–20A–C). The walls of the larger of these spaces, or bullae, may be visible. Another prominent feature is distortion of the pulmonary vessels. The normal peripheral decrease in size of the pulmonary vessels is lost and the branching pattern is distorted.[75a] Many vessels appear draped around otherwise invisible bullae. When pulmonary hypertension is present, the central pulmonary arteries, especially the main pulmonary artery, will be enlarged.[75a]

As anticipated, CT densitometry in patients

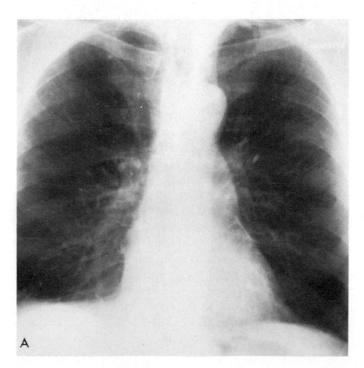

Figure 7–20. Pulmonary emphysema. **A** Frontal chest radiograph shows typical features of emphysema with hyperinflation and peripheral vascular attenuation.

Illustration continued on opposite page

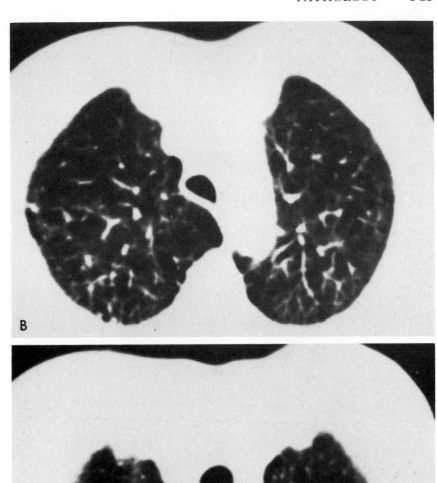

Figure 7–20. *Continued* **B,C** CT scans at two levels demonstrate many avascular spaces, most without visible walls; vascular distortion; and absence of an anteroposterior gradient in vessel caliber.

with advanced emphysema show that the lungs are distinctly less dense than normal.[75a] In one study by Rosenblum and colleagues,[64] the mean CT density of the lungs in patients with emphysema was −860 to −912 H, in contrast to a density of −742 H for normal subjects. Another feature was that the normal anteroposterior gravitational CT density gradient of the lungs was small and inconsistent.

Quantitation of *pulmonary edema* by quantitative CT densitometry has been studied only under experimental conditions in animals. Utell and colleagues[76] detected an increase in lung CT density in pulmonary edema induced by intravenous infusion of air. They found a close correlation be-

tween lung density and postmortem measurements of pulmonary edema. Hedlund and coworkers[77] studied normotensive pulmonary edema induced by oleic acid injury to the lung in dogs. They found that CT density increased from a mean of −802 H to a mean of −757 H. The initial increase in CT density occurred 15 to 30 minutes after oleic acid infusion and was mainly in the periphery and dependent portions of the lung. The increase in lung density presumably reflects accumulation of fluid in the alveolar spaces. The dog lung is poorly lobulated with a small interstitial space and edema fluid will accumulate predominantly in the alveoli. The clinical application of quantitative CT densitometry in detection and assessment of pulmonary edema is not known. At present, the value of CT scanning is insufficiently understood to consider the technique as more than experimental.

A modification of quantitative CT densitometry of the lung was studied by Gur and associates[78] and involved the inhalation of inert xenon gas. They used an 80 per cent concentration of xenon and found CT density typically increased by 50 to 90 H at 2 minutes. Serial CT scans were used to measure the washout of xenon from the lungs over time. Damaged areas of lung demonstrated

decreased CT enhancement and delayed washout. The exciting possibility of obtaining regional ventilation with high spatial resolution[78a] requires further study.

BRONCHOGENIC CARCINOMA

Aspects of CT scanning of bronchogenic carcinoma have been dealt with in Chapters 4, 5, and 6 and in this chapter. Topics that are not covered elsewhere in this book include determination of the extent of bronchogenic carcinoma, CT-guided

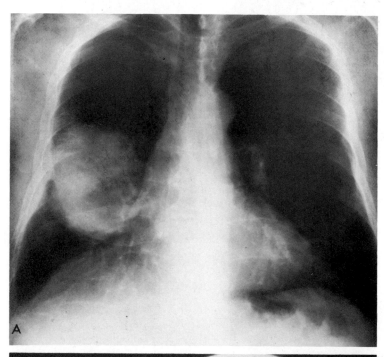

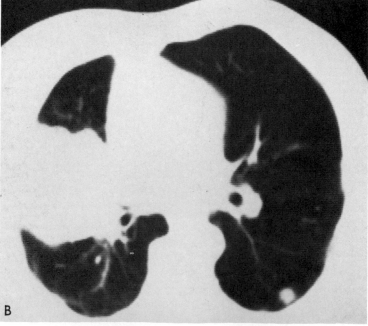

Figure 7–21. Bronchogenic carcinoma with contralateral metastasis. **A** Chest radiograph shows a large, right midlung tumor. **B** CT scan demonstrates a small contralateral nodule not apparent on the chest radiographs. (CT-guided aspiration biopsy of this nodule revealed that it was a metastasis.)

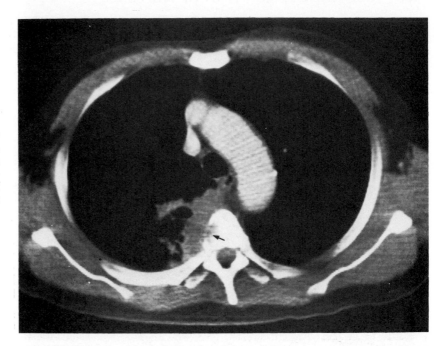

Figure 7–22. Bronchogenic carcinoma with unsuspected destruction of vertebral body. CT scan shows a right posterior bronchogenic carcinoma. Unsuspected destruction of the adjacent vertebral body (arrow) is demonstrated.

aspiration biopsy of thoracic masses, radiotherapy planning, irradiation lung damage, and the CT scan appearance of the thorax after pneumonectomy.

Extent of Bronchogenic Carcinoma

Most articles dealing with CT scanning of bronchogenic carcinoma have discussed the detection of hilar and mediastinal adenopathy and the direct invasion of the mediastinum by bronchogenic carcinoma. These aspects of the staging of bronchogenic carcinoma have been reviewed in previous chapters. Several other findings seen only on CT scans of the thorax and abdomen can assist in determining the extent of bronchogenic carcinoma and profoundly affect management of the patient. These findings may unequivocally demonstrate that the patient is not a candidate for resection, or alternatively they can direct biopsy procedures to areas of metastatic spread of the neoplasm.

Conceptually, the staging of bronchogenic carcinoma is more concerned with describing the disease process than with the individual patient.[79] In clinical practice, the resectability of lung cancer is of greater importance than its staging. Because the aggressiveness of thoracic surgeons varies, criteria for resectability in each medical institution may vary. Therefore, the significance of CT findings regarding resectability must be interpreted in collaboration with the patient's physicians.

CONTRALATERAL TUMOR. In virtually all situations, the presence of metastasis to the contralateral lung is indicative of advanced disease not treatable by surgery. CT scans may show contralateral tumor not seen on chest radiographs (Fig. 7–21A,B). A mass or nodule in the contralateral lung will invariably require biopsy for histologic confirmation of metastasis.

SPINE OR STERNUM DESTRUCTION. Tumor invasion with destruction of the sternum or spine indicates advanced disease and nonresectability. The frequency with which CT scans first detect this finding is difficult to establish. We have seen cases of spine (Fig. 7–22) and sternum destruction that had not been appreciated before the CT scans were obtained.

CHEST WALL INVASION. In most situations, direct tumor invasion of the chest wall is considered nonresectable.[80] Some surgeons, however, will undertake a block-resection of the chest wall. Equivocal CT scans of tumor invasion of the chest wall must be interpreted with caution. Bronchogenic carcinoma tends to respect the pleural surface. We have seen several instances in which tumor against the chest wall produced edema in the adjacent soft tissues that could have been misinterpreted from the CT scans as chest wall invasion.

ADRENAL AND LIVER METASTASES. The incidence of silent liver and adrenal metastases from bronchogenic carcinoma has been studied by several investigators.[81–84b] It varies with the cell type of the tumor. Silent liver metastasis occurs in 10 to 40 per cent of patients, and adrenal metastasis appears in 15 to 40 per cent (Fig. 7–23A,B). Generally, a CT examination of any patient with bronchogenic carcinoma should include the upper abdomen.

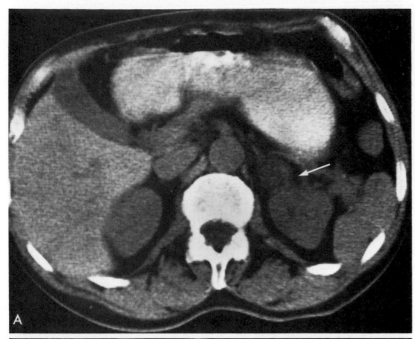

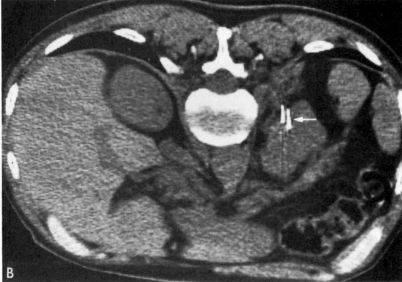

Figure 7–23. Silent adrenal metastasis. **A** CT scan through the upper abdomen in a patient with bronchogenic carcinoma shows a left adrenal mass (arrow). **B** CT scan, with the patient prone, demonstrates the tips of two needles (arrow) for biopsy of the metastasis.

PLEURAL EFFUSION. CT scanning is highly sensitive in demonstrating small pleural effusions. The clinical significance of pleural fluid in the presence of a bronchogenic carcinoma depends on the contents of the fluid and not just its existence.[85, 86] Malignant cells in the fluid indicates nonresectability in over 75 per cent of patients. The CT finding of unsuspected pleural effusion is thus extremely important but does not, by itself, indicate that the tumor is not resectable.

CT-Guided Aspiration Biopsy

Percutaneous needle aspiration has become widely accepted for the biopsy of focal intrathoracic lesions.[87–92] The key to a successful biopsy is precise needle placement within the nodule or mass. In most situations, exact placement of the needle tip can be achieved by using fluoroscopic guidance, preferably in two planes. CT scanning can be used initially to locate a pulmonary mass that is subsequently biopsied using fluoroscopically guided needle placement.[93, 94] The patient should be scanned in the position that will subsequently be used for the biopsy. The depth and distance from surface landmarks of the mass can be precisely measured by means of the CT monitor. This technique works well when the lung lesion is large enough to be demonstrated fluoroscopically in at least one plane. The same technique can also be used for hilar and mediastinal masses.[88]

Certain thoracic masses should be biopsied using computed tomographic rather than fluoroscopic guidance.[95] These are lung lesions that cannot be precisely located fluoroscopically (Fig. 7–24A–C); cavitary lesions in which the wall of the mass must be sampled; and small hilar and central mediastinal masses. Lung nodules as small as 0.8 cm can be successfully aspirated with this technique. The results of CT-guided aspiration biopsy are equal in accuracy to those of fluoroscopic guidance. If a coaxial system[96] is used, the procedure takes 20 to 40 minutes and the incidence of small pneumothoraces is high.[95] A positive diagnosis can often obviate more invasive procedures, and the risks are acceptable.

Radiotherapy Planning

The goal of radiotherapy is to minimize irradiation of normal tissues while adequately treating the tumor. Therapy planning normally uses all available information such as from the physical examination, radiography, bronchoscopy, and surgery. Radiotherapy planning for bronchogenic carcinoma relies heavily on radiographic techniques to determine tumor extent.

The superimposition of thoracic bones, cardiovascular structures, and, occasionally, pleural effusion can make the radiographic assessment of tumor extent difficult. The transverse orientation of CT scans eliminates many of the problems of superimposition. In 40 to 75 per cent of patients, CT scans more clearly delineate tumor extent than do chest radiographs.[97, 98] This information leads to either a decrease or an increase in treatment volume.

It has been found[99, 100] that for the majority of patients in whom treatment volume was altered, CT scans showed tumor that was unsuspected from conventional radiographic studies, resulting in a larger volume of irradiation to include all the tumor. In other patients, CT scans revealed that a smaller volume of irradiation was sufficient to cover the tumor. When the decision is to decrease treatment volume, normal tissue is spared unnecessary irradiation. In some patients, CT scans will show sites of metastasis (such as the mediastinum, adrenals, and liver) that were unsuspected from chest radiographs. In these instances, the stage of the tumor will be altered and the entire therapy protocol may be changed.

In several institutions, the data from CT scans have been incorporated directly into the computers that determine the portals for radiotherapy. In these situations, the accuracy of defining the target volume can approach the precision with which modern radiotherapy machines can deliver irradiation.

Irradiation Injury to the Lung

The severity of irradiation injury to the lung is determined primarily by the total radiation dose, fractionation, and the length of time the radiation is given. Chest radiographs are usually used to follow the course of irradiation lung injury. Radiographic changes are unusual with 3000 rads or less. After a dose of 4000 rads in 4 weeks, some patients demonstrate lung damage, and after 5000 rads in 5 weeks, about 50 per cent of patients show lung damage.[101, 102] Almost all patients receiving 6000 rads exhibit radiographic abnormalities. Symptoms of lung injury are often present when only a third to half of a lung is irradiated.

Ionizing radiation damages cells capable of proliferation by inducing mitotic death. The morphologic changes in lung tissue following irradiation occur on a continuum but can be divided into three phases that occur within the first 6 to 9 months after irradiation.[103] An *exudative phase* is seen during the first 30 days; a *pneumonic phase* lasts through the second and third months; and a *reparative phase* occurs between the third and sixth to ninth month.[104, 105]

In the exudative phase, endothelial and epithelial damage appears with interstitial edema, alveolar proteinosis, and hyaline membranes. In the pneumonic phase, alveolar type II cells and macrophages fill the air spaces.[106] Capillary damage is extensive, and collagen deposition begins. In the reparative phase, many cells proliferate, with profound distortion of lung architecture. Mast cells, among others, predominate and collagen production continues, leading to fibrosis. At 6 to 9 months and beyond, fibrosis of the alveolar walls develops, markedly reducing the number, size, and volume of the alveoli. The number of patent capillaries and small vessels is also greatly reduced.

The radiographic appearance of irradiation lung injury conforms to the morphologic findings.[107, 108] The first abnormalities usually appear 6 to 12 weeks after treatment is completed. The first manifestation is an ill-defined increase in density in the irradiated field that obscures the pulmonary vessels. This may progress to pulmonary consolidation or to a nodular or acinar pat-

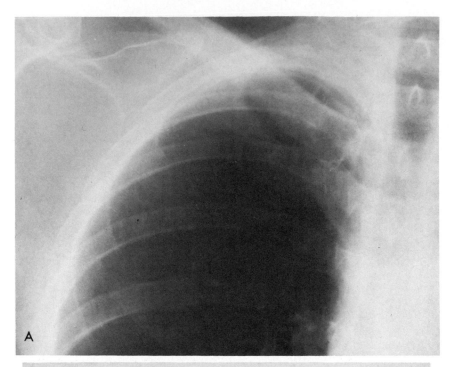

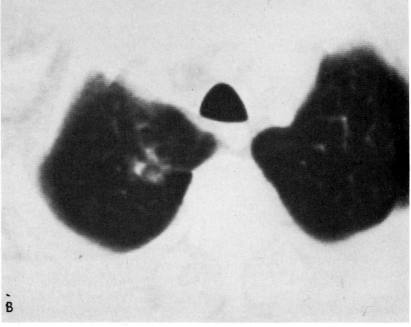

Figure 7–24. CT-guided aspiration biopsy of 1.5-cm lung nodule. **A** Frontal chest radiograph in a patient with probable cerebral metastases shows a small, ill-defined nodule behind the right clavicle. **B** CT scan confirms the 1.5-cm irregular nodule.

Illustration continued on opposite page

tern. The pneumonic changes progress to dense linear streaks, which radiate from the area of involvement. Marked scarring causes volume loss in the irradiated volume of lung. The permanent changes of fibrosis takes 6 to 24 months to evolve.

The CT findings of irradiation lung injury have not been fully described. In our experience, the CT appearances are characteristic, and CT scans seem to be more sensitive than chest radiographs in demonstrating irradiation changes. A single case report[109] described an increase in CT density in the exudative phase. In this case, the pulmonary vessels appeared prominent. In the later fibrotic phase, CT density was markedly increased but limited to the area of irradiation. The involved lung characteristically showed shrinkage. We have found that a nearly straight edge to the region of increased density and prominent bronchi within it are typical of irradiation fibrosis (Fig. 7–25). Whether CT scans will permit early recognition of recurrent tumor in areas of irradiation injury is still to be determined.

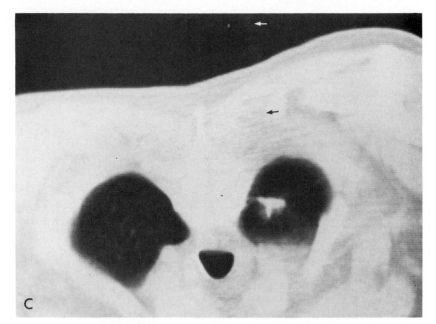

Figure 7–24. *Continued* **C** CT scan, with the patient prone, demonstrates the position of the biopsy needle (arrows). The biopsy specimen showed poorly differentiated adenocarcinoma.

Postpneumonectomy Space

Pneumonectomy results in a large, air-filled space, bounded by parietal pleura. The evacuated hemithorax contains gas and a variable amount of fluid, producing a single, large air-fluid level on chest radiographs. Unless complications occur, the pleural space progressively fills with fluid.[110, 111] Radiographs show filling of the pleural space with fluid in 3 to 24 weeks after pneumonectomy. This filling is usually associated with a gradual decrease in the volume of the hemithorax. The mediastinum shifts toward the side of pneumonec-

tomy, and the ipsilateral hemidiaphragm is elevated.

Biondetti and colleagues,[112] using CT to investigate the postpneumonectomy hemithorax in 22 patients, discovered some interesting and previously undocumented findings. It had been assumed that the fluid in the postpneumonectomy space is resorbed and replaced by connective tissue. In 13 of the 22 patients, fluid was evident on CT scans even years after surgery. They found that generally the postpneumonectomy space was obliterated and the fluid was absent when marked

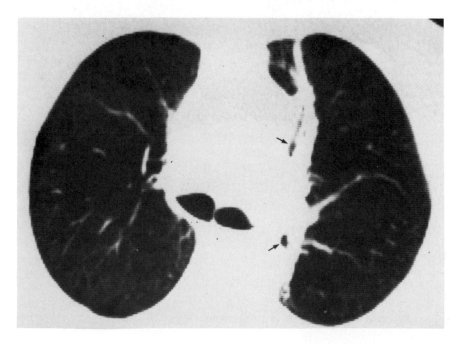

Figure 7–25. Radiation lung injury. CT scan, obtained 5 months after 6500 rads were delivered to the left medial hemithorax and mediastinum, shows a nearly straight edge to the area of irradiation. Dilated bronchi (arrows) are visible within the irradiation fibrosis.

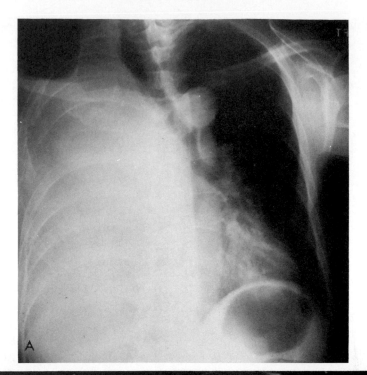

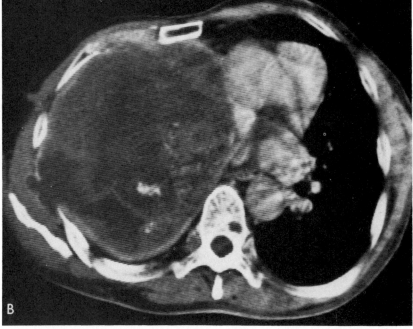

Figure 7–26. Postpneumonectomy tuberculous empyema. **A** Chest radiograph obtained 9 years after right pneumonectomy for tuberculosis shows the heart and mediastinum displaced toward the left. **B** CT scan demonstrates an expanding septated mass filling the right hemithorax, displacing the mediastinum, and invading the chest wall. (At thoracotomy, tuberculous pus was drained.)

mediastinal shift had occurred. Also, after a right pneumonectomy, the mediastinum rotated to the right; after a left pneumonectomy, the mediastinum tended to shift to the left without rotating.

Bronchopleural fistula and empyema are relatively common complications of resectional surgery in patients with bronchogenic neoplasms. Empyema is a dreaded complication with a mortality rate of 16 to 28 per cent.[113, 114] Vigorous therapy with drainage of the pleural space is usu-

ally necessary. An increase in the volume of the fluid-filled hemithorax may be detected from chest radiographs (Fig. 7–26A,B). In our experience, CT scanning has proved accurate in delineating localized empyema following pulmonary resection. The encapsulated fluid can be readily distinguished from free-flowing pleural fluid and from a pleural peel. CT scans obtained with the patient in prone and decubitus positions may help demonstrate the encapsulated fluid collection.

Recurrence of bronchogenic carcinoma after pulmonary resection is common. Between 35 and 70 per cent of patients who die within 1 month after pulmonary resection are found to have had either metastatic spread or persistence of tumor within the thorax.[115, 116] At 1 year after resection, the incidence of tumor rises to 85 per cent. Recurrence of tumor in the ipsilateral hemithorax after pneumonectomy is difficult to detect from radiographs. A shift of the mediastinum toward the contralateral side may indicate a large tumor mass on the side of the pneumonectomy. CT scans can probably demonstrate recurrent tumor at an earlier stage than can chest radiographs.[117] On CT scans, the tumor mass appears denser than the fluid or fibroadipose tissue normally present after pneumonectomy. Further investigation is necessary to determine whether early detection of recurrent bronchogenic carcinoma would appreciably change patient management.

PULMONARY PARENCHYMAL VERSUS PLEURAL DISEASE

Intimate contact of the pleura with the peripheral lung parenchyma can cause difficulty in distinguishing between abnormalities that may be in either place. Oblique radiographs and fluoroscopy can often be of assistance. When the results of these techniques are unhelpful or equivocal, CT scanning is probably indicated. Pugatch and co-workers[118] studied 75 patients with diagnostically problematic disease of the pleura, pulmonary parenchyma, or both. In 28 per cent of the patients, information from the CT scans aided in diagnosis or altered management of the patient. In another 40 per cent, CT scans helped clarify the site and extent of the disease but did not alter therapy.

A peripheral lung nodule seen on chest radiographs can be indistinguishable from a pleural plaque or even from an extrapleural mass indenting the lung. CT scans can readily show this distinction and can accurately locate the abnormality.

In a septic patient with pneumonia, the development of one or more air-fluid levels adjacent to the chest wall is a relatively common and difficult diagnostic problem. The distinction of pyopneumothorax from a peripheral lung abscess is important because each is managed differently. A pyopneumothorax is usually drained by a thoracostomy tube, but a peripheral lung abscess is usually treated with antibiotics and postural drainage.[119] CT scanning can frequently distinguish pyopneumothorax from lung abscess. With pyopneumothorax, the adjacent lung, which is frequently consolidated and demonstrates air bronchograms, is displaced from the chest wall. The air-containing pleural collection is smoothly marginated, usually lentiform in shape, and clearly defined. A lung abscess is irregular in shape, its inner wall is ragged, and its outer edge is poorly defined relative to the surrounding pulmonary parenchymal consolidation (Fig. 7–27A,B).[120] The residua of pulmonary vessels and bronchi often course through a lung abscess and can be seen on CT scans.

Encapsulated (loculated) empyema that does not contain air can be difficult to distinguish from a solid, peripheral lung abscess. Both appear as uniform peripheral densities on chest radiographs. After intravenous infusion of contrast material, the walls of both lesions enhance on CT scans. Their fluid-filled centers show uniform density, or they are septated and do not enhance. Careful inspection of CT scans can sometimes lead to diagnosis of solid empyema. The visceral pleura next to loculated empyema is often thickened and visible between the empyema and the lung. In our experience, CT scans are better than ultrasonograms in localizing empyema for drainage. The CT scan finding of multiple septations within an empyema can indicate that a simple thoracostomy tube will not be successful for drainage. The site of the empyema should be marked on the patient's skin while the patient is still in position on the scanner table. Diagnostic aspiration of an empyema can also be undertaken using CT guidance.

Marked pleural thickening or a large pleural effusion makes conventional radiographs uninterpretable. In these situations, CT scans can often demonstrate any parenchymal, hilar, or mediastinal abnormalities that may be present. Extension of the pleural process to the chest wall may also first be detected from CT scans.

BULLOUS LUNG DISEASE

Large bullae, occur most commonly as an isolated defect in normal lung parenchyma, usually in the upper lobes of lungs in young men.[121] Alternatively, they can be seen as a component of emphysema, chronic bronchitis, or the "end-stage" fibrotic lung. On plain chest radiographs, large bullae appear as focal areas of increased radiolucency. The thin walls of the bullae are usually visible. CT scans can readily show small bullae that are not demonstrated on plain chest radiographs. The avascular areas can be seen on CT

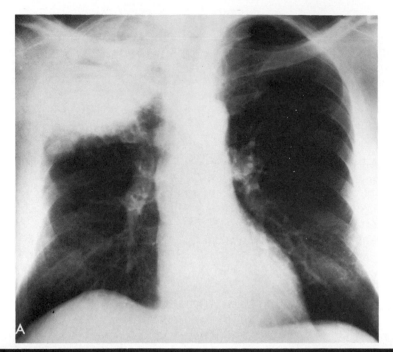

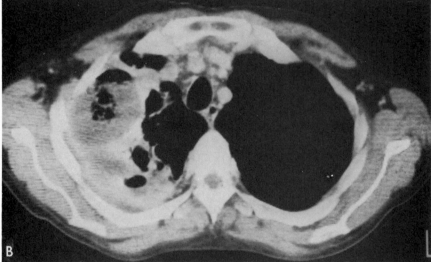

Figure 7–27. Lung abscess. A Frontal chest radiograph demonstrates a right apical density with ill-defined air-fluid levels. B CT scan through the upper lobes shows two air- and fluid-containing spaces with enhanced walls. The residue of the lung tissue is visible within the abscess cavities.

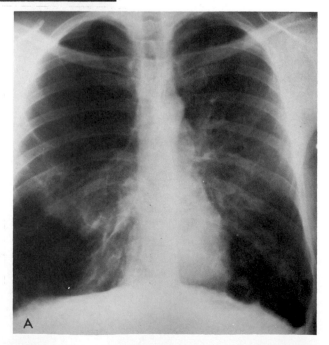

Figure 7–28. Bullous lung disease in a young man. A Frontal radiograph shows a large bulla in the right upper lung field, with small bullae in the right lower and left upper lung fields.
Illustration continued on opposite page

scans even when the walls of the bullae are not visible. Often, the pulmonary vessels appear to be draped around these small avascular areas.

Severe symptoms of airway obstruction are common when large bullae are present.[122, 123] The airway obstruction can be from loss of lung elastic recoil associated with bullae themselves, or they can be due to concomitant lung disease. Resection of large bullae is often considered in an attempt to improve pulmonary function.[124, 125] The best results are obtained when the remainder of the lungs are relatively normal, but when there is diffuse obstructive lung disease, improvement may be marginal and temporary. Specialized pulmonary function studies can aid in determining the functional status of the lungs apart from the bullae.[126] Chest radiographs, radionuclide ventilation and perfusion studies, and pulmonary angiograms have been used to try to detect diffuse bullae within the lungs. CT scans are probably more sensitive than these later techniques for detecting diffuse bullae (Fig. 7–28A–C).[127] The presence of diffuse bullae should mitigate against attempts at surgical resection. CT scans can also demonstrate the size and exact location of localized bullae and assist in the planning of resection.[127]

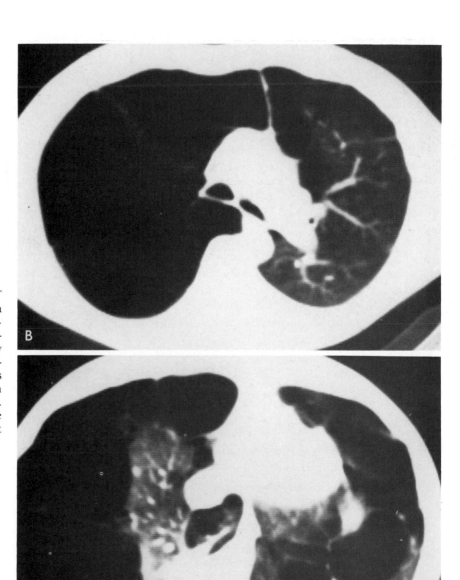

Figure 7–28. *Continued* **B** CT scan through the tracheal carina demonstrates a few septa transversing the right lung bulla. Extensive bullae are present anteriorly on the left. **C** CT scan 5 cm caudad to the one in **B** also shows more extensive changes than can be seen on the chest radiograph. (Resection of the right upper lobe bulla resulted in temporary slight improvement in lung function.)

INDICATIONS FOR COMPUTED TOMOGRAPHY OF THE LUNGS

The indications for CT scanning are less well defined for the lungs than for any other area of the thorax. The number and scope of published articles on CT scanning of the lungs are limited. A 1979 special report by the Society for Computed Body Tomography[128] is generalized and unfortunately incomplete. It emphasizes the detection of occult metastases, bronchogenic carcinoma, and pleural effusion. The approach to defining the extent of intrathoracic spread of bronchogenic carcinoma in selected patients is only mentioned. The search for calcification in indeterminate pulmonary nodules is advocated without introducing the controversy surrounding the issue.

DETECTION OF LUNG DISEASE

The new fast CT scanners have relatively good spatial resolution. This, together with CT's transverse display of images, increases the conspicuity of many pulmonary abnormalities. Occult pulmonary nodules, masses, cavities, and even diffuse lung disease can be detected with greater accuracy from CT scans than from chest radiographs or conventional tomograms. The application of CT scanning in the detection of metastases is still somewhat controversial. Nevertheless, in most situations, CT has replaced conventional tomography in the evaluation of the patient with potential pulmonary metastases. CT scanning is also probably the preferred method for evaluation of the patient with no visible abnormality on the chest radiograph but who exhibits malignant cells in the sputum. A related clinical problem in which CT scanning is valuable is the suspicious mass or nodule seen on chest radiographs that cannot be adequately demonstrated by more conventional imaging techniques.

The application of CT for detecting diffuse lung disease is still to be shown. CT scans can demonstrate abnormalities in such situations as the patient with asbestos exposure and no radiographically visible chest abnormalities. In special circumstances, such as workman's compensation cases, CT scanning may be indicated. Future studies will be necessary to determine which patients with other diffuse fibrotic lung diseases should undergo CT scanning.

The high-contrast resolution of CT scanning, compared with the resolution of other radiographic techniques, does offer the potential for detecting tumor recurrence after pneumonectomy and radiation therapy. These areas have not been fully explored.

LOCALIZATION OF LUNG DISEASE

The combination of contrast resolution, spatial resolution, and transverse anatomic display of CT scans can be used in several situations to precisely locate disease within the thorax and abdomen. Determination of the extent of bronchogenic carcinoma is a prime example. The search for occult lymphogenous and hematogenous dissemination is important in the initial evaluation of the patient with bronchogenic carcinoma. Undoubtedly, CT scanning can facilitate detection of disease spread to the contralateral lung, mediastinum, retroperitoneal lymph nodes, liver, and adrenal glands. Local extension of tumor to pleura, chest wall, spine, and sternum is also often best demonstrated on CT scans.

Separation of pleural from parenchymal lung disease is a second important clinical situation in which CT scanning has proved useful. Precise locating of loculated empyema for surgical drainage or diagnostic aspiration is, in our opinion, best achieved by CT scanning. CT-guided aspiration biopsy of pulmonary, hilar, and even mediastinal nodules and masses has extended the use of biopsy of thoracic lesions without the requirement for thoracotomy.

CHARACTERIZATION OF LUNG DISEASE

Quantitative lung densitometry, in our opinion, has limited clinical application in thoracic CT scanning. Several types of lung abnormalities potentially could be characterized by quantitative lung densitometry. The answer to whether diffuse lung disease can be diagnosed or characterized by the finding of altered CT density awaits refinement in scanner abilities and future studies. Although subtle increases in lung density can be demonstrated in pulmonary edema, the clinical applications are obviously limited. Likewise, a decrease in lung density can be shown in patients with pulmonary emphysema, but again, the probability is that the technique will have limited clinical application.

Densitometry of pulmonary nodules remains an extremely controversial issue. The indeterminate solitary pulmonary nodule is a common clinical problem, and a noninvasive method for determining benignity of at least some solitary pulmonary nodules would be of value. Continued investigation will be necessary to determine whether pulmonary nodule densitometry should be advocated for general clinical use.

Unlike mediastinal and hilar abnormalities, few lung abnormalities are vascular. Therefore, intravenous infusion of contrast material has limited application in lung CT imaging. Suspected arteriovenous malformation, pulmonary vein varix, and, occasionally, pulmonary sequestration can be correctly diagnosed from CT scans, obviating the need for angiography. CT scanning using intravenous contrast infusion or injection should be reserved for selected cases of suspected chronic and acute pulmonary embolism. Whether CT scanning should be used routinely for evaluating patients with hemoptysis and a pulmonary mass is still to be determined.

CT scanning for lung abnormalities has not received the same attention as have other areas. The definitive indications in many clinical situations await future clarification.

REFERENCES

1. Frija J, Schmit P, Katz M, Vadrot D, Laval-Jeantet M: Computed tomography of the pulmonary fissures: Normal anatomy. J Comput Assist Tomogr 6:1069, 1982.
2. Proto AV, Ball JB Jr: Computed tomography of the major and minor fissures. AJR 140:439, 1983.
2a. Marks BW, Kuhns LR: Identification of the pleural fissures with computed tomography. Radiology 143:139, 1982.
2b. Goodman LR, Golkow RS, Steiner RM, Teplick SK, Haskin ME, Himmelstein E, Teplick JG: The right mid-lung window: A potential source of error in computed tomography of the lung. Radiology 143:135, 1982.
3. Spirt BA: Value of the prone position in detecting pulmonary nodules by computed tomography. J Comput Assist Tomogr 4:871, 1980.
4. Heitzman ER: Computed tomography of the thorax: Current perspectives. AJR 136:2, 1981.
5. Kuhns LR, Borlaza GS, Seigel RS: Rapid sequence display of computed tomographic images: An aid in the diagnosis of pulmonary metastases. Radiology 132:747, 1979.
6. Muhm JR, Brown LR, Crowe JK, Sheedy PF II, Hattery RR, Stephens DH: Comparison of whole lung tomography and computed tomography for detecting pulmonary nodules. AJR 131:981, 1978.
7. Shaner EG, Chang AE, Doppman JL, Conkle DM, Flye MW, Rosenberg SA: Comparison of computed and conventional whole lung tomography in detecting pulmonary nodules: A prospective radiologic-pathologic study. AJR 131:51, 1978.
8. Davis EW, Peabody JW Jr, Katz S: The solitary pulmonary nodule. J Thorac Surg 32:728, 1956.
9. McClure CD, Boucot KR, Shipman GA, Gilliam AG, Milmore BK, Lloyd JW: The solitary pulmonary nodule and primary lung malignancy. Arch Environ Health 3:127, 1961.
10. Steele JD: The solitary pulmonary nodule. J Thorac Cardiovasc Surg 46:21, 1963.
11. Vance JW, Good CA, Hodgson CH, Kirklin JW, Gage RP: The solitary circumscribed pulmonary lesion due to bronchogenic carcinoma. Dis Chest 36:231, 1959.
12. Walske BR: The solitary pulmonary nodule. Dis Chest 49:302, 1966.
13. Jackman RJ, Good CA, Clagett OT, Woolner LB: Survival rates in peripheral bronchogenic carcinomas up to 4 centimeters in diameter presenting as solitary nodules. J Thorac Cardiovasc Surg 57:1, 1969.
14. Mountain CF: Surgical management of pulmonary metastases. Postgrad Med 48:128, 1970.
15. Bateson EM: An analysis of 155 solitary lung lesions illustrating the differential diagnosis of mixed tumors of the lung. Clin Radiol 16:51, 1965.
16. O'Keefe ME, Good CA, McDonald JR: Calcification in solitary nodules of the lung. Am J Roentgenol Radium Ther Nucl Med 77:1023, 1957.
17. Lillington GA: The solitary pulmonary nodule—1974. Am Rev Respir Dis 110:699, 1974.
18. Mintzer RA, Malave SR, Neiman HL, Michaelis LL, Vanecko RM, Sanders JH: Computed vs. conventional tomography in evaluation of primary and secondary pulmonary neoplasms. Radiology 132:653, 1979.
19. Cann CE, Gamsu G, Birnberg FA, Webb WR: Quantification of calcium in solitary pulmonary nodules using single- and dual-energy CT. Radiology 145:493, 1982.
20. Godwin JD, Fram EK, Cann CE, Gamsu G: CT densitometry of pulmonary nodules: A phantom study. J Comput Assist Tomogr 6:254, 1982.
21. Siegelman SS, Zerhouni EA, Leo FP, Khouri NF, Stitik FP: CT of the solitary pulmonary nodule. AJR 135:1, 1980.
22. Godwin JD, Speckman JM, Fram EK, Johnson GA, Putman CE, Korobkin M, Breiman RS: Distinguishing benign from malignant pulmonary nodules by computed tomography. Radiology 144:349, 1982.
23. Freundlich IM, Horsley WW, Udall C: Evaluation of pulmonary masses by CT number: A modification of the Siegelman method. Presented at the 67th Annual Meeting of the Radiological Society of North America, Chicago, Nov. 15–19, 1981.
23a. Levi C, Gray JE, McCullough EC, Hattery RR: The unreliability of CT numbers as absolute values. AJR 139:443, 1982.
23b. Zerhouni EA, Spivey JF, Morgan RH, Leo FP, Stitik FP, Siegelman SS: Factors influencing quantitative CT measurements of solitary pulmonary nodules. J Comput Assist Tomogr 6:1075, 1982.
24. Muhm JR, Brown LR, Crowe JK: Detection of pulmonary nodules by computed tomography. AJR 128:267, 1977.
25. Kruglik GD, Wayne KS: Occult lung cavity causing hemoptysis: Recognition by computed tomography. J Comput Assist Tomogr 4:407, 1980.
26. Breuer R, Baigelman W, Pugatch RD: Occult mycetoma. J Comput Assist Tomogr 6:166, 1982.
27. Grzybowski S, Coy P: Early diagnosis of carcinoma of the lung. Cancer 25:113, 1970.
28. Pearson FG, Thompson DW, Delarue NC: Experience with the cytologic detection, localization, and treatment of radiographically undemonstrable bronchial carcinoma. J Thorac Cardiovasc Surg 54:371, 1967.

29. Bower BF, Gordon GS: Hormonal effects of nonendocrine tumors. Ann Rev Med 16:83, 1965.

30. Nathanson L, Hall TC: A spectrum of tumors that produce paraneoplastic syndromes. Lung tumors: 'How they produce their syndromes. Ann NY Acad Sci 230:367, 1974.

31. Godwin JD, Webb WR: Dynamic computed tomography in the evaluation of vascular lung lesions. Radiology 138:629, 1981.

32. Rankin S, Faling LJ, Pugatch RD: CT diagnosis of pulmonary arteriovenous malformations. J Comput Assist Tomogr 6:746, 1982.

33. Paul DJ, Mueller CF: Pulmonary sequestration. J Comput Assist Tomogr 6:163, 1982.

33a. Miller PA, Williamson BRJ, Minor GR, Buschi AJ: Pulmonary sequestration: Visualization of the feeding artery by CT. J Comput Assist Tomogr 6:828, 1982.

34. Kirks DR, Kane PE, Free EA, Taybi H: Systemic arterial supply to normal basilar segments of the left lower lobe. AJR 126:817, 1976.

35. Landing BH: Congenital malformations and genetic disorders of the respiratory tract. Am Rev Respir Dis 120:151, 1979.

36. Gomes MR, Bernatz PE, Dines DE: Pulmonary arteriovenous fistulas. Ann Thorac Surg 7:582, 1969.

37. Hodson CH, Burchell HB, Good CA, Clagett OT: Hereditary hemorrhagic telangiectasia and pulmonary arteriovenous fistula: Survey of a large family. N Engl J Med 261:625, 1959.

38. Stork WJ: Pulmonary arteriovenous fistulas. AJR 74:441, 1955.

39. Abbott OA, Haebich AT, Van Fleit WE: Changing patterns relative to the surgical treatment of pulmonary arteriovenous fistulas. Am Surg 25:674, 1959.

40. Steinberg I, Maisel B, Vogel FS: Pulmonary arteriovenous fistula associated with capillary telangiectasia (Rendu-Osler-Weber disease): Report of a case illustrating use of metal casting for demonstrating the lesion. J Thorac Surg 35:517, 1958.

41. Bjork VO, Intonti F, Aletras H, Madsen R: Varieties of pulmonary arteriovenous aneurysms. Acta Chir Scand 125:69, 1963.

42. Revill D, Matts SGF: Pulmonary arteriovenous aneurysm in heredity telangiectasia. Br J Tuberc 52:222, 1959.

43. Stevenson JS, Maynard CD, Whitley JE: Arteriovenous malformation of the lung: The use of radioisotope angiography. Radiology 99:157, 1971.

44. Bartram C, Strickland B: Pulmonary varices. Br J Radiol 44:927, 1971.

45. Kelvin FM, Boone JA, Peretz D: Pulmonary varix. J Can Assoc Radiol 23:227, 1972.

46. Nelson WP, Hall RJ, Garcia E: Varicosities of the pulmonary veins simulating arteriovenous fistulas. JAMA 195:13, 1966.

47. Blesovsky A: Pulmonary sequestration: A report of an unusual case and a review of the literature. Thorax 22:351, 1967.

48. Halasz NA, Lindskog GE, Liebow AA: Esophago-bronchial fistula and bronchopulmonary sequestration: Report of a case and review of the literature. Ann Surg 155:215, 1962.

49. Iwai K, Shindo G, Hajikano H, Tajima H, Morimoto M, Kosuda T, Yoneuda R: Intralobar pulmonary sequestration, with special reference to developmental pathology. Am Rev Respir Dis 107:911, 1973.

50. Marks C, Wiener SN, Reydman M: Pulmonary sequestration. Chest 61:253, 1972.

51. Savic B, Birtel REJ, Tholen W, Funke HD, Knoche R: Lung sequestration: Report of seven cases and review of 540 published cases. Thorax 34:96, 1979.

52. Godwin JD, Webb WR, Gamsu G, Ovenfors CO: Computed tomography of pulmonary embolism. AJR 135:691, 1980.

53. Ovenfors CO, Godwin JD, Brito AC: Diagnosis of peripheral pulmonary emboli by computed tomography in the living dog. Radiology 141:519, 1981.

54. Grossman ZD, Thomas FD, Gagne G, Mauceri R, Cohen WN, Heitzman ER, Singh A: Transmission computed tomographic diagnosis of experimentally produced acute pulmonary vascular occlusion in the dog. Radiology 131:767, 1979.

55. Grossman ZD, Ritter CA, Tarner RJ, Somogyi JW, Johnson AC, Lyons B, Fernandes P, Thomas FD, Gagne GM, Bassano D, Zens A: Successful identification of oligemic lung by transmission computed tomography after experimentally produced acute pulmonary arterial occlusion in the dog. Invest Radiol 16:275, 1981.

56. Lourie GL, Pizzo SV, Ravin C, Putman C, Thompson WM: Experimental pulmonary infarction in dogs: A comparison of chest radiography and computed tomography. Invest Radiol 17:224, 1982.

57. Sinner WN: Computed tomographic patterns of pulmonary thromboembolism and infarction. J Comput Assist Tomogr 2:395, 1978.

58. Katz D, Kreel L: Computed tomography in pulmonary asbestosis. Clin Radiol 30:207, 1979.

59. Mintzer RA, Gore RM, Vogelzang RL, Holz S: Rounded atelectasis and its association with asbestos-induced pleural disease. Radiology 139:567, 1981.

60. Tylen U, Nilsson U: Computed tomography in pulmonary pseudotumors and their relation to asbestos exposure. J Comput Assist Tomogr 6:229, 1982.

61. Solomon A, Kreel L, McNicol M, Johnson N: Computed tomography in pulmonary sarcoidosis. J Comput Assist Tomogr 3:754, 1979.

62. Wegener OH, Koeppe P, Oeser H: Measurement of lung density by computed tomography. J Comput Assist Tomogr 2:263, 1978.

63. Robinson PJ, Kreel L: Pulmonary tissue attenuation with computed tomography: Comparison of inspiration and expiration scans. J Comput Assist Tomogr 3:740, 1979.

64. Rosenblum LJ, Mauceri RA, Wellenstein DE, Bassano DA, Cohen WN, Heitzman ER: Computed tomography of the lung. Radiology 129:521, 1978.

65. Döhring W: Quantitative analyses of regional pulmonary ventilation using Compton densitometry and computed tomography. Prog Respir Res 11:48, 1979.

66. Rosenblum LJ, Mauceri RA, Wellenstein DE, Thomas FD, Bassano DA, Raasch BN, Chamberlain CC, Heitzman ER: Density patterns in the normal lung as determined by computed tomography. Radiology 137:409, 1980.

67. Kourilsky R, Marchal M, Marchal MT: Recording respiratory function by x-rays: Basic principles. Thorax 20:428, 1965.

68. Silverman NR: Clinical videodensitometry: Pulmonary ventilation analysis. Radiology 103:263, 1972.

69. Zelefsky MN, Schultz RJ, Freeman LM: Assessment of regional lung function and its clinical application by

the combined use of lung scan and gamma densigraphy. Radiology 94:167, 1970.

70. Reiss K, Schuster W: Quantitative measurements of lung function in children by means of Compton backscatter. Radiology 102:613, 1972.

71. Gamsu G, Kaufman L, Swann SJ, Brito AC: Absolute lung density in experimental canine pulmonary edema. Invest Radiol 14:261, 1979.

72. Chevalier PA, Wood EH, Robb Ra, Ritman EL: Synchronous volumetric computed tomography for quantitative studies of structural and functional dynamics of the respiratory system. Prog Respir Res 11:1, 1979.

73. Bragg DG, Durney CH, Johnson CC, Pedersen PC: Monitoring and diagnosis of pulmonary edema by microwaves: A preliminary report. Invest Radiol 12:289, 1977.

74. Weng TR, Spence JA, Polgar G, Nyboer J: Measurement of regional lung function by tetrapolar electrical impedance plethysmography. Chest 76:64, 1979.

75. Hedlung LW, Putman CE: Analysis of lung density by computed tomography. In Putman CE (ed): Pulmonary Diagnosis: Imaging and Other Techniques. New York, Appleton-Century Crofts, 1981, p 107.

75a. Goddard PR, Nicholson EM, Laszlo G, Watt I: Computed tomography in pulmonary emphysema. Clin Radiol 33:379, 1982.

76. Utell MJ, Wandkte JC, Fahey PJ, Baker A, Fischner HW, Hyde RW: Lung weight in normal and edematous dogs by computerized tomography. Fed Proc 38:1326, 1979.

77. Hedlund LW, Effmann EL, Bates WM, Beck JW, Goulding PH, Putman CE: Pulmonary edema: A CT study of regional changes in lung density following oleic acid injury. J Comput Assist Tomogr 6:939, 1982.

78. Gur D, Drayer BP, Borovetz HS, Griffith BP, Hardesty RL, Wolfson SK: Dynamic computed tomography of the lung: Regional ventilation measurements. J Comput Assist Tomogr 3:749, 1979.

78a. Herbert DL, Gur D, Shabason L, Good WF, Rinaldo JE, Snyder JV, Borovetz HS, Mancici MC: Mapping of human local pulmonary ventilation by xenon enhanced computed tomography. J Comput Assist Tomogr 6:1088, 1982.

79. Carr DI: The staging of lung cancer. Am Rev Respir Dis 117:819, 1978.

80. Diagnostic Oncology Case Study: Pulmonary mass in a smoker: Preoperative imaging for staging of lung cancer. AJR 136:739, 1981.

81. Dunnick NR, Ihde DC, Johnston-Early A: Abdominal CT in the evaluation of small cell carcinoma of the lung. AJR 133:1085, 1979.

82. Vas W, Zylak CJ, Mather D, Figueredo A: The value of abdominal computed tomography in the pre-treatment assessment of small cell carcinoma of the lung. Radiology 138:417, 1981.

83. Harper PG, Houang M, Spiro SG, Geddes D, Hodson M, Souhami RL: Computerized axial tomography in the pretreatment assessment of small-cell carcinoma of the bronchus. Cancer 47:1775, 1981.

84. Nielsen ME Jr, Heaston DK, Dunnick NR, Korobkin M: Preoperative CT evaluation of adrenal glands in non-small cell bronchogenic carcinoma. AJR 139:317, 1982.

84a. Poon PY, Feld R, Evans WK, Ege G, Yeoh JL, McLoughlin ML: Computed tomography of the brain, liver, and upper abdomen in the staging of small cell carcinoma of the lung. J Comput Assist Tomogr 6:963, 1982.

84b. Sandler MA, Pearlberg JL, Madrazo BL, Gitschlag KF, Gross SC: Computed tomographic evaluation of the adrenal gland in the preoperative assessment of bronchogenic carcinoma. Radiology 145:733, 1982.

85. Brinkman GL: The significance of pleural effusion complicating otherwise operable bronchogenic carcinoma. Dis Chest 36:152, 1959.

86. Byrd RB, Carr DT, Miller WE, Payne WS, Woolner LB: Radiographic abnormalities in carcinoma of the lung as related to histological cell type. Thorax 24:573, 1969.

87. Dahlgren S, Nordenstrom B: Transthoracic Needle Biopsy. Chicago, Year Book Medical Publishers, 1966, pp 29–41.

88. Fontana RS, Miller WE, Beabout JW, Payne WS, Harrison EG Jr: Transthoracic needle aspiration of discrete pulmonary lesions: Experience in 100 cases. Med Clin North Am 54:961, 1970.

89. Zelch JV, Lalli AF, McCormack LJ, Belovich DM: Aspiration biopsy in diagnosis of pulmonary nodule. Chest 63:149, 1973.

90. Sargent EN, Turner AF, Gordonson J, Schwinn CP, Pashky O: Percutaneous pulmonary needle biopsy: Report of 350 patients. Am J Roentgenol Radium Ther Nucl Med 122:758, 1974.

91. Lalli AF, McCormack LJ, Zelch M, Reich NE, Belovich D: Aspiration biopsies of chest lesions. Radiology 127:35, 1978.

92. Zavala DC, Schoell JE: Ultrathin needle aspiration of the lung in infectious and malignant disease. Am Rev Respir Dis 123:125, 1981.

93. Levy JM, Gordon B, Nykamp PW: Computed tomography-guided percutaneous transthoracic lung biopsy. CT 2:217, 1978.

94. Gobien RP, Skucas J, Paris BS: CT-assisted fluoroscopically guided aspiration biopsy of central hilar and mediastinal masses. Radiology 141:443, 1981.

95. Fink I, Gamsu G, Harter LP: CT-guided aspiration biopsy of the thorax. J Comput Assist Tomogr 6:958, 1982.

96. Greene R: Transthoracic needle aspiration biopsy. In Athanasoulis CA, Pfister RC, Greene RE, Roberson GH (eds): Interventional Radiology. Philadelphia, WB Saunders Company, 1982, pp 587–634.

97. Emami B, Melo A, Carter BL, Munzenrider JE, Prio AJ: Value of computed tomography in radiotherapy of lung cancer. AJR 131:63, 1978.

98. Seydal HG, Kutcher GJ, Steiner RM, Mohiuddin M, Golberg B: Computed tomography in planning radiation therapy for bronchogenic carcinoma. Int J Radiat Oncol Biol Phys 6:601, 1980.

99. Munzenrider JE, Pilepich M, Rene-Ferrero JB, Tchakarova I, Carter BL: Use of body scanner in radiotherapy treatment planning. Cancer 40:170, 1977.

100. Ragan DP, Perez CA: Efficacy of CT-associated two-dimensional treatment planning: Analysis of 45 patients. AJR 131:75, 1978.

101. Libshitz HI, Southard ME: Complications of radiation therapy: The thorax. Semin Roentgenol 9:41, 1974.

102. Salazar OM, Rubin P, Brown JC, Feldstein ML, Keller BE: The assessment of tumor response to irradiation of lung cancer: Continuous versus split-course regimens. Int J Radiat Oncol Biol Phys 1:1107, 1976.

103. Gross NJ: Pulmonary effects of radiation therapy. Ann Intern Med 86:81, 1977.

104. Jennings FL, Arden A: Development of radiation pneumonitis—time and dose factors. Arch Pathol 74:351, 1962.

105. Moosavi H, McDonald S, Rubin P, Cooper R, Stuard ID, Penney D: Early radiation dose-response in lung: An ultrastructural study. Int J Radiat Oncol Biol Phys 2:921, 1977.

106. Phillips TL, Benak S, Ross G: Ultrastructural and cellular effects of ionizing radiation. In Vaeth JM (ed): Frontiers of Radiation Therapy and Oncology, vol 6; Radiation Effect and Tolerance, Normal Tissue. Basel, Karger and Baltimore, University Park Press, 1972, pp. 21–43.

107. Fried JR, Goldberg H: Post-irradiation changes in lungs and thorax: A clinical, roentgenological and pathological study, with emphasis on late and terminal stages. AJR 43:877, 1940.

108. Prato FS, Kurdyak R, Saibil EA, Rider WD, Aspin N: Physiological and radiographic assessment during the development of pulmonary radiation fibrosis. Radiology 122:389, 1977.

109. Nabawi P, Mantravadi R, Breyer D, Capek V: Computed tomography of radiation-induced lung injuries. J Comput Assist Tomogr 5:568, 1981.

110. Andersen JC, Egedorf J, Stougard J: The pleural space succeeding pneumonectomy: A roentgenological and clinical study of 167 cases of bronchogenic carcinoma. Scand J Thorac Cardiovasc Surg 2:70, 1968.

111. Christiansen KH, Morgan SW, Karich AF, Takaro T: Pleural space following pneumonectomy. Ann Thorac Surg 1:298, 1965.

112. Biondette PR, Fiore D, Sartori F, Colognato A, Ravasini R, Romani S: Evaluation of the post-pneumonectomy space by computed tomography. J Comput Assist Tomogr 6:238, 1982.

113. Hood RM, Kirksey TD, Calhoon JH, Arnold HS, Tate RS: The use of automatic stapling devices in pulmonary resection. Ann Thorac Surg 16:85, 1973.

114. Le Roux BT: Empyema thoracis. Br J Surg 52:89, 1965.

115. Spjut JH, Mateo LF: Recurrent and metastatic carcinoma in surgically treated carcinoma of lung: An autopsy survey. Cancer 18:1462, 1955.

116. Weiss W, Gillick JS: The metastatic spread of bronchogenic carcinoma in relation to the interval between resection and death. Chest 71:725, 1977.

117. Crowe JK, Brown LR, Muhm JR: Computed tomography of the mediastinum. Radiology 128:75, 1978.

118. Pugatch RD, Faling LJ, Robbins AH, Snider GL: Differentiation of pleural and pulmonary lesions using computed tomography. J Comput Assist Tomogr 2:601, 1978.

119. Bartlett JG, Gorbach SL, Tally FP, Finegold SM: Bacteriology and treatment of primary lung abscess. Am Rev Respir Dis 109:510, 1974.

120. Baber CE, Hedlund LW, Oddson TA, Putman CE: Differentiating empyemas and peripheral pulmonary abscesses. The value of computed tomography. Radiology 135:755, 1980.

121. Baldwin E de F, Harden KA, Greene DG, Cournand A, Richards DW Jr: Pulmonary insufficiency: IV. A study of 16 cases of large pulmonary air cysts or bullae. Medicine 29:169, 1950.

122. Laurenzi GA, Turino GM, Fishman AP: Bullous disease of the lung. Am J Med 32:361, 1962.

123. Rogers RM, DuBois AB, Blakemore WS: Effect of removal of bullae on airway conductance and conductance volume ratios. J Clin Invest 47:2569, 1968.

124. Wesley JR, Macleod WM, Mullard KS: Evaluation and surgery of bullous emphysema. J Thorac Cardiovasc Surg 63:945, 1972.

125. Harris J: Severe bullous emphysema: Successful surgical management despite poor preoperative blood gas levels and marked pulmonary hypertension. Chest 70:658, 1976.

126. Gelb AF, Gold WM, Nadel JA: Mechanisms limiting airflow in bullous lung disease. Am Rev Respir Dis 107:571, 1973.

127. Fiore D, Biondetti PR, Sartori F, Calabro F: The role of computed tomography in the evaluation of bullous lung disease. J Comput Assist Tomogr 6:105, 1982.

128. Society for Computed Body Tomography: New indications for computed body tomography. AJR 133:115, 1979.

8 COMPUTED TOMOGRAPHY OF THE CHEST WALL, AXILLARY SPACE, PLEURAE, AND DIAPHRAGM

W. Richard Webb

Computed tomography (CT) furnishes considerable information on the chest wall, axillary space, pleurae and diaphragm, although the CT findings in these areas have not been reported in detail. These structures can be involved by contiguous spread of disease from the neighboring lung or mediastinum, or they can be the site of diseases originating from their composite tissues. The cross-sectional format and enhanced density resolution of CT provide information regarding the chest wall that cannot be obtained with conventional radiographic techniques. Furthermore, structures of the chest wall are visible on all CT images of the thorax, and unsuspected chest wall pathology may be detected in patients studied for other reasons.

TECHNIQUES OF EXAMINATION

In general, the chest wall, axillary space, pleurae, and diaphragm are best evaluated using standard techniques for CT of the thorax. Scans are usually obtained at 1-cm intervals with 1-cm collimation during suspended respiration. In most instances, patients are positioned with their arms raised above their head, and the examination is performed from the apex to the base of the lungs. The diaphragm and posterior pleural spaces extend well below the lung bases, and scans inferior to the diaphragmatic cupula must be obtained to evaluate these structures completely. Scanning with the patient in the prone or decubitus position may be of assistance, particu-

larly for evaluating pleural diseases. Free pleural effusions shift to the dependent portion of the pleural space when the patient is moved from the supine position to a prone or decubitus position, whereas loculated effusions or fibrosis show little or no change.[1] The movement of an effusion helps in the diagnosis of a pleural density seen on CT scans and can reveal underlying plumonary parenchymal or pleural lesions that are otherwise obscured.[1] Baber and colleagues[2] have shown that in patients with a loculated collection of air and fluid in the pleural space from a bronchopleural fistula or empyema, movement of the air with a change in patient position enables precise delineation of the size and shape of the cavity.

Mediastinal window settings (mean 20 to 50 Hounsfield Units [H], width 500 to 1000 H) are

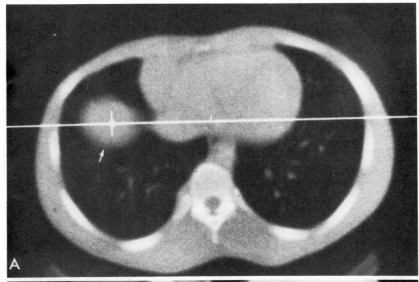

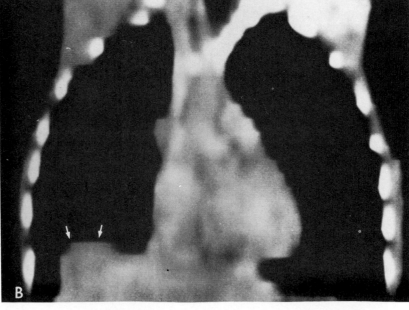

Figure 8–1. Coronal reconstruction. Patient is a 20-year-old man with a thymoma and myasthenia gravis. **A** CT scan shows a density in inferior right hemithorax (arrow). On cross-sectional images it is unclear whether this represents liver or a pleural mass at the diaphragmatic surface. **B** Coronal reconstruction along the plane indicated by the line in **A** shows that the mass (arrows) is less dense than the subjacent liver, and the pleural metastasis can be separated from the normal liver.

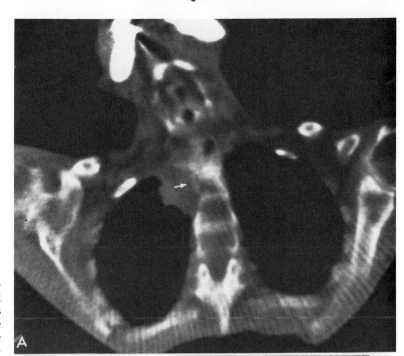

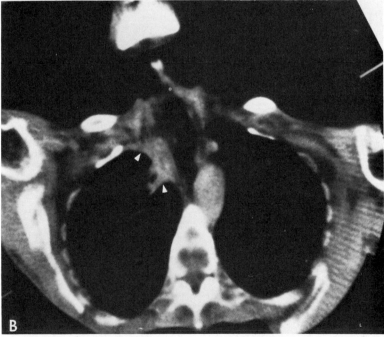

Figure 8–2. Direct coronal computed tomogram. An elderly man with a right superior sulcus (Pancoast) tumor was scanned using direct coronal CT at the levels of the vertebral column (**A**) and the trachea (**B**). **A** The tumor mass is visible medially at the right apex. The right cortical margin of a vertebral body (arrow) has been destroyed by the tumor. **B** Tumor also involves the right paratracheal mediastinum (arrowheads).

most suitable for evaluating the soft tissues of the chest wall, pleurae, and diaphragm. However, lung window settings (level, -500 to -600 H; width, 1000 H) allow more accurate estimation of the size, contour, and appearance of pleural lesions at their interface with adjacent lung. Appropriate window settings must be used to evaluate bony lesions of the chest wall.

Occasionally, multiplanar reconstruction of images can clarify the relationship of chest wall or pleural processes to the lung or mediastinal structures (Fig. 8–1A,B). These reconstructions are particularly helpful to nonradiologists who are more familiar with standard frontal or lateral radiographic projections. Reconstructed images can be valuable in determining the relationship of masses at the lung base to the basal pleura, diaphragm, or upper abdominal organs.

van Waes and Zonneveld[3] demonstrated that direct coronal images can help diagnose intrathoracic disease and provide better resolution than multiplanar reconstructions. With the pa-

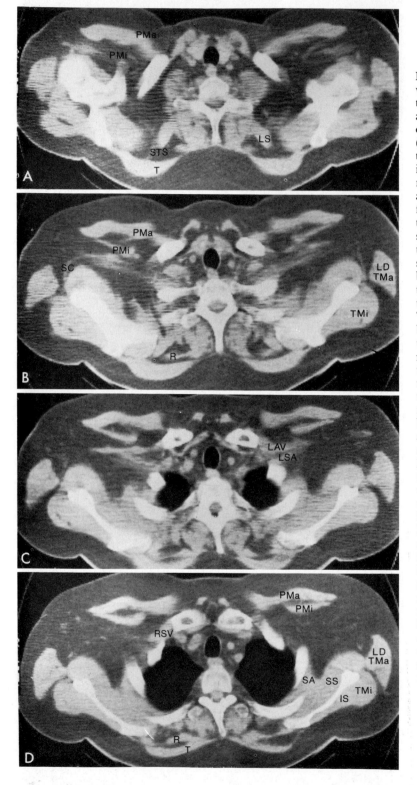

Figure 8–3. Normal anatomy of the chest wall and axilla with arms positioned above the head. **A** CT scan at a level 2 cm above the lung apices shows the clavicular origins of the pectoralis major muscles (PMa) anteriorly. On the right, the insertion of the pectoralis minor muscle (PMi) into the coracoid process of the scapula, marginating the cephalad extent of the axilla, is faintly visible. Posteriorly, the fat-filled subtrapezial space (STS) is ventral to the trapezius muscle (T). The levator scapulae muscle (LS) can be seen clearly in the medial aspect of this space. **B** CT scan 1 cm above the lung apices shows both the pectoralis major (PMa) and pectoralis minor (PMi) muscles, which form the anterior margin of the axillary space. The axillary vessels and branches of the brachial plexus extend laterally within the cephalad portion of the axilla. On the right side, a circumflex scapular (SC) artery or vein is also visible. The first two ribs arise posteriorly; the first is anterior to the second. The subtrapezial space remains visible at this level, with the rhomboideus major (R) muscle in its posterior aspect. **C** CT scan at the level of the lung apices; the first two ribs are again visible. Both the left subclavian (axillary) artery (LSA) and the left axillary vein (LAV) are visible within the axilla. The vein lies anterior to the artery. Both pass between the first rib and clavicle. **D** CT scan 1 cm lower than in **C** clearly shows the right subclavian vein (RSV) passing between the first rib and the clavicular head. The axilla is marginated anteriorly by the pectoralis major (PMa) and pectoralis minor (PMi) muscles; posteriorly by the latissimus dorsi (LD), teres major (TMa), and subscapularis (SS) muscles, and medially by the chest wall and serratus anterior (SA) muscle. Other muscles visible at this level and at lower levels **(E–H)** include the teres minor (TMi) and infraspinatus (IS), trapezius (T), and rhomboideus major (R).

Illustration continued on opposite page

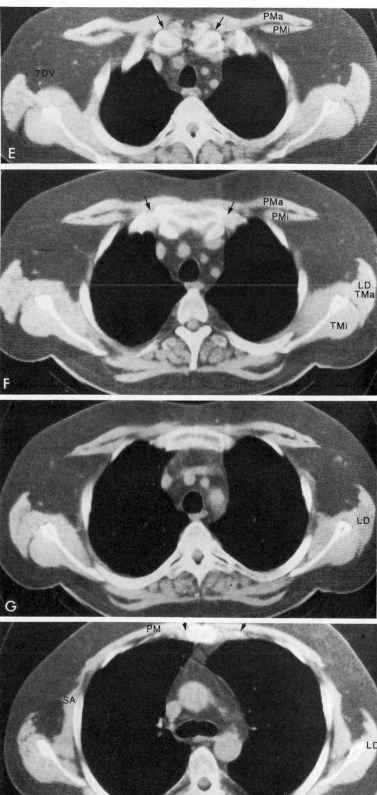

Figure 8–3. *Continued* **E** CT scan at the level of the suprasternal notch. The clavicular heads articulate with the posterolateral aspect of the manubrium (arrows). The joint space, containing a fibrocartilaginous disc, is sharply defined. The thoracodorsal vessels (TDV) are visible at this level and at those above and below and represent large branches of the axillary artery and vein. **F** CT scan 1 cm below **E** shows the first ribs articulating with the lateral margin of the manubrium at its widest point (arrows). The undersurfaces of the clavicular heads are visible as triangular densities posterior to the manubrium. **G** CT scan 1 cm below **F;** at this level, the articulations of the first ribs with the manubrium remain visible. The pectoralis major and pectoralis minor muscles appear thinner than at higher levels, and their sternal and costal origins are visible. The axillary space remains sharply defined. **H** CT scan 3 cm below **G** shows the sternal body in cross section as a much smaller structure than the manubrium. Incompletely calcified costal cartilages (arrows) lie lateral to the manubrium. The pectoral muscles (PM) are now closely applied to the anterior chest wall. The serratus anterior (SA) muscle marginates the medial axilla.

tient seated in the gantry and bending forward, the upper and lower thorax can both be evaluated, but the entire chest cannot be imaged on a single scan. Direct coronal CT can demonstrate the relationships of thoracic lesions to the mediastinum, diaphragm, and chest wall (Fig. 8–2*A,B*). However, few scanners have a sufficiently large aperture to their gantry, and the technique has limited application.

The Chest Wall

ANATOMY

The chest wall consists of the thoracic skeleton and its associated musculature. The axilla and its contents and the breast are discussed in separate sections.

THORACIC SKELETON

The thoracic vertebrae are intermediate in size between the small cervical vertebrae and the larger lumbar vertebrae. When viewed at the level of the neural canals, the vertebral bodies are shaped like an inverted heart and appear as wide in the anteroposterior direction as in the transverse direction (Fig. 8–3*D*). In adults, osteophytes often distort the contour of the thoracic vertebral bodies. Osteophytes usually occur anteriorly and on the right side.[4]

From their articulations with the transverse processes and vertebral bodies, the ribs extend laterally and then obliquely downward and ante-

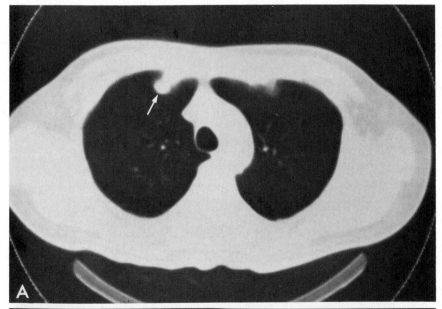

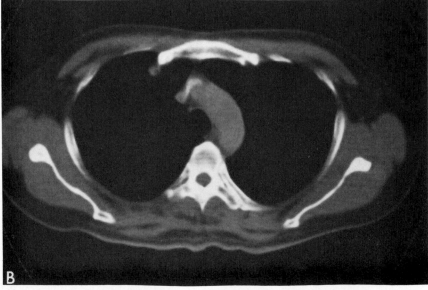

Figure 8–4. Bony spur mimicking a lung nodule. **A** CT scan at the level of the articulation of the first rib and manubrium suggests the presence of a right anterior lung nodule (arrow). **B** On a CT scan at the same level, but at a mediastinal window setting, the "nodule" appears to be of tissue density, rather than bone density, because of volume averaging.

Illustration continued on opposite page

riorly (Fig. 8–3*A–F*). Usually, only a short segment of each rib is visible on a single CT scan; each progressively more anterior rib represents the one arising at a higher thoracic level. Thus, the fifth rib lies anterior to the sixth and the fourth rib anterior to the fifth. At the level of the lung apex, the first rib can be identified by its anterior position and by its articulation with the manubrium immediately below the level of the clavicle.

In some patients, a bony spur projects inferiorly from the undersurface of the first rib at its junction with the manubrium. In cross section, this bony spur can appear to be surrounded by lung and can mimic a lung nodule.[5] This appearance is usually bilateral and symmetrical, providing a clue to its true nature. The "nodule" can

also be seen to be of bone density when viewed at appropriate window settings, and its relationship to the first rib becomes apparent when successively higher images are examined (Fig. 8–4*A–D*).

The manubrium is usually visible over a distance of 3 or 4 cm and is considerably wider than the body of the sternum, which is at lower levels (Fig. 8–3*E–H*). Superiorly, at the level of the suprasternal notch, the heads of the clavicles articulate with the manubrium along its posterolateral margins (Fig. 8–3*E–F*). Destouet and co-workers[6] have shown a clearly defined joint space between the clavicular head and the articular surface of the manubrium. The sternoclavicular joint contains a fibrocartilaginous disk, which can be seen on CT scans when there is gas in the joint space and a normal "vacuum phenomenon" is present.

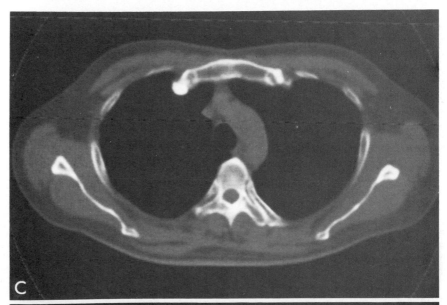

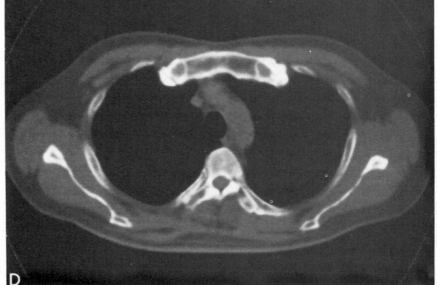

Figure 8–4. *Continued* **C** CT scan at a slightly higher level shows the calcific density of the lesion. Although often symmetric, the bony spur in this patient was present only on the right. **D** CT scan at a higher level shows the relationship of this spur to the articulation of the first rib and manubrium.

At a level 1 cm caudad, the first ribs articulate with the lateral surfaces of the manubrium at its widest point. At this level, the undersurface of the clavicular heads appear triangular and are located medial to the end of the first rib and posterior to the manubrium (Fig. 8–3F).

The junction between the manubrium and sternal body lies in the transverse plane, but it is usually not visible on CT scans. However, this level is defined by the articulations of the second ribs with the sternum. In cross section, the body of the sternum is also narrower and more rectangular than the manubrium (Fig. 8–3F–H). The articulations of the anterior ribs and sternal body are not visible unless their costal cartilages are calcified. Uncalcified costal cartilage can be difficult to distinguish from adjacent intercostal muscle.

Inferiorly, the xiphoid process is seen on CT scans as an extension of the sternal body and is usually ossified in adults. Except for the xiphoid process, the manubrium and sternum have well-defined cortices.

In some patients, deformities of the thoracic skeleton such as pectus excavatum can mimic a mediastinal or hilar mass on plain radiographs. In such patients, CT can help establish the correct diagnosis.[7]

THORACIC MUSCULATURE

The muscles of the chest wall visible on CT scans are those that support and move the shoulder and upper extremity (Fig. 8–3). Anatomically, they also serve to define the boundaries of the axillary space.

The pectoralis major muscle arises from the anterior surface of the sternal half of the clavicle, the anterior surface of the upper sternum, and the cartilages of the upper ribs (Fig. 8–3). From these origins, the muscle fibers converge on a single tendinous insertion at the greater tubercle of the humerus.[8] The pectoralis major varies in size, depending on the patient's muscular development. Inferiorly, the muscle is a thin sheet that is separated from the anterior ribs by only a thin plane of fat. At higher levels, the muscle thickens and is farther from the thoracic cage. Both its sternal and clavicular origins are usually visible.

The pectoralis minor muscle is thinner and lies behind the pectoralis major. It arises from the cranial margins and outer surfaces of the anterior third, fourth, and fifth ribs, and inserts into the coracoid process of the scapula.[8] On CT scans, the pectoralis minor is visible posterior to the upper portion of the pectoralis major (Fig. 8–3). The two muscles are separated only by a layer of fat. The insertion of the pectoralis minor into the coracoid process is also usually visible (Fig. 8–3A).

Posteriorly, several muscles are related to the scapula. These include the subscapularis, infraspinatus, teres major and minor, and latissimus dorsi.[8]

On CT images, the subscapularis lies anterior to the scapula and separates it from the thoracic cage (Fig. 8–3). The subscapularis arises from the axillary portion of the scapula, filling the subscapular fossa, and inserts into the lesser tubercle of the humerus and the capsule of the shoulder joint. Posterior to the scapula, the infraspinatus is visible medial to the much smaller teres minor (Fig. 8–3). Both of these muscles arise from the medial border of the scapula and insert into the greater tubercle of the humerus. CT scans show the teres major and latissimus dorsi lateral to the scapula, but they are difficult to separate at this level. The teres major arises from the inferior angle of the scapula and inserts into the lesser tubercle of the humerus. The latissimus dorsi is a large triangular muscle that covers the lower posterior chest and back (Figs. 8–3B–H). It originates

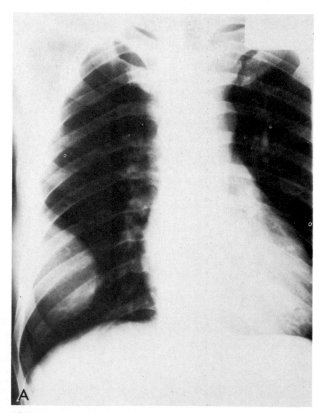

Figure 8–5. Lymphoma with rib destruction. **A** Frontal chest radiograph in a young man shows a well-defined mass in the right hemithorax. The adjacent rib is destroyed.
Illustration continued on opposite page

in a broad aponeurosis, by which it is attached to the spinous processes of the lower thoracic and lumbar vertebrae, and inserts into the humerus.

The serratus anterior is the thin sheet of muscle between the ribs and the scapula. It arises from the superior borders of the first eight or nine ribs and inserts into the ventral surface of the scapula.[8] The serratus anterior is difficult to distinguish from the subscapularis on CT scans (Fig. 8–3).

Within the posterior chest wall, a number of muscles are visible at successive levels. These include the trapezius, rhomboideus major and minor, and the complex group of extensor muscles of the vertebral column (Fig. 8–3). The trapezius is a flat triangular muscle covering the upper pos-

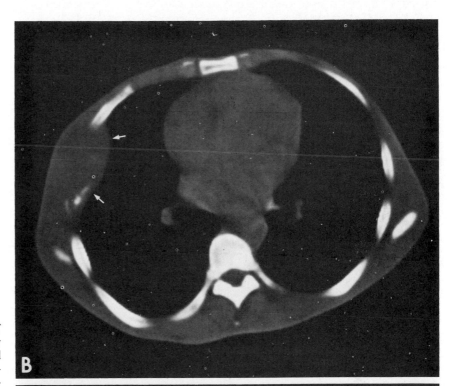

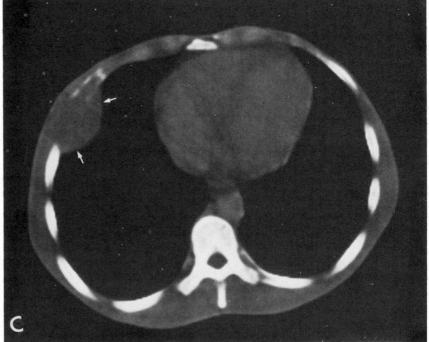

Figure 8–5. *Continued* **B,C** CT scans at two contiguous levels show rib destruction and an extrapleural mass (arrows). The sharp definition of the mass suggests it is limited by the pleura and not invading the lung. Biopsy revealed lymphoma.

terior neck and shoulders. It arises from the spinous processes of the cervical and thoracic vertebrae and inserts into the posterior border of the lateral clavicle, the acromium, and the posterior border of the spine of the scapula. Its insertion into the spine of the scapula can be easily seen on CT scans. The rhomboideus major and minor muscles arise from the spinous processes of the lower cervical and upper thoracic vertebral bodies, pass beneath the trapezius, and descend to attach to the medial margin of the scapula. CT scans below the level of the scapula still show the trapezius, but the rhomboideus muscles are no longer visible.

Deep within the chest wall, the intercostal muscles lie between the visible segments of adjacent ribs.

CHEST WALL ABNORMALITIES

In both adults and children, metastatic tumors involve the thoracic skeleton more commonly than do primary tumors.[9, 10] In adults, adenocarcinomas are the most common; in children, neuroblastoma and leukemia predominate. In adults, the most common primary tumors arising from the thoracic skeleton are chondrosarcoma and myeloma; in children, Ewing's sarcoma is the most common.[9, 10] In both groups, benign tumors occur less commonly than primary malignancies. Osteomyelitis can closely mimic tumor and must be considered in the differential diagnosis of thoracic skeletal lesions.

A majority of patients with malignant tumors of the thoracic skeleton experience chest pain. Other patients first notice a local mass. In most patients, routine radiographs are usually sufficient to establish the diagnosis (Fig. 8–5A–C). In such cases,

CT serves to define the extent of tumor and the degree of involvement of the chest wall and underlying pleura, lung, or mediastinum.[11] Care must be taken to avoid misdiagnosing a partially ossified anterior costal cartilage as a destroyed rib.

Metastatic malignancies to the sternum are common and are more frequent than primary tumors. Primary tumors of the sternum occur slightly more often in the manubrium than in the sternal body, and the xiphoid process is rarely affected. Most primary sternal tumors are chondrosarcomas or myelomas. Benign sternal tumors are very rare, and tumors of the sternum should be considered malignant until proved benign.

Evaluation of the sternoclavicular joints and sternum by conventional tomography is difficult. CT eliminates many of the problems of radiographic tomography, takes less time, is easier for the patient, and provides superior anatomic information.[6] In general, if plain radiographs fail to provide diagnostic information regarding the sternum or sternoclavicular joints, CT rather than conventional tomography is indicated.

Destouet and colleagues[6] reviewed the CT findings in 12 patients with pathologic conditions involving the sternoclavicular joints or sternum. In six patients, sternoclavicular joint dislocations due to trauma were diagnosed. Anterior dislocation of the clavicular head is more common than posterior dislocation, is easier to diagnose clinically, and is easier to treat. Posterior dislocation is more difficult to diagnose clinically, and with conventional radiographic techniques, carries the risk of fatal injury to underlying mediastinal structures. Posterior dislocations are easily detected on cross-sectional images.

Osteomyelitis of the sternum and sternoclavicular joint is uncommon and usually follows surgery or radiotherapy. It also occurs in drug

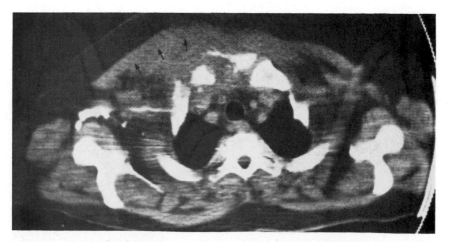

Figure 8–6. Sternoclavicular joint osteomyelitis. Patient is a diabetic man with a staphylococcal infection of the foot and a right chest wall mass. CT scan shows bone destruction and erosion at the right sternoclavicular joint. An associated soft tissue mass displaces the right pectoralis major muscle (arrows) anteriorly.

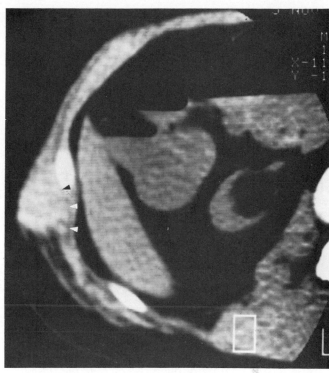

Figure 8–7. Chest wall metastasis. Detail view from CT scan of the lower right chest wall in a 35-year-old man with a pelvic angiosarcoma and a painful right chest wall mass. A soft-tissue mass is visible in the right chest wall. A thin plane of fat (arrowheads) separates the mass from the underlying intercostal muscle. Thus, the mass arises within soft tissues external to the thoracic cage, probably within the serratus anterior muscle. Biopsy revealed metastatic angiosarcoma.

abusers and patients with bacterial endocarditis or mediastinal infections.[6] Osteoporosis, periosteal reaction, and bone erosion are more easily seen with CT than with conventional radiography (Fig. 8–6). Thin sections (5 mm or 1.5 mm) can help demonstrate these subtle abnormalities.

Two of the 12 patients studied by Destouet and co-workers[6] had malignancies (lymphoma and metastatic prostate carcinoma) that caused sternal destruction. CT scans also showed bony sclerosis and the soft tissue extent of the lesions.

Soft-tissue lesions of the chest wall are rare and are usually evident clinically, but CT can be of value in demonstrating involvement of the adjacent bones or intrathoracic structures (Fig. 8–7). Within the superior thorax, soft tissue sarcomas can extend anteriorly under the pectoralis muscles or posteriorly under the subscapularis.[11] Such lesions can be very difficult to palpate, and CT scans often show that their total extent is much greater than is clinically suspected. This information is important to the surgeon.

The most common soft-tissue tumors of the chest wall are lipomas, some of which are dumbbell-shaped, having both an intrathoracic and extrathoracic component.[12] Liposarcomas are the most frequent malignant tumor.[10, 11] Other lesions affecting the chest wall are desmoids, fibrosarcomas, hemangiomas, nerve sheath tumors, rhabdomyosarcomas, and metastases.

RADICAL MASTECTOMY

In patients undergoing radical mastectomy for breast carcinoma, the bulk of the pectoral muscles is surgically removed, along with axillary lymph nodes. Radical mastectomy produces an easily recognizable alteration in axillary anatomy (see Fig. 8–12). Congenital absence of the pectoral muscles has a similar appearance, but the breast tissue is still present. After simple mastectomy, the breast is absent but the pectoral muscles are intact (Fig. 8–8).

INTRATHORACIC LESIONS WITH SECONDARY CHEST WALL INVOLVEMENT

Direct invasion of the chest wall by a peripheral bronchogenic carcinoma is common and was seen in 9 per cent of 110 patients with unresectable tumors studied by Napoli and colleagues.[13] Similarly, Hodgkin's disease can involve structures of the chest wall by direct invasion from the mediastinum or lung in a small percentage of cases.[14] Malignant mesothelioma is a less common tumor that can also invade the chest wall.[15]

Care must be taken in diagnosing chest wall invasion based on the CT appearances. Tumors can abut the visceral pleura without invading the pleura or chest wall. In addition, central bronchogenic carcinoma obstructing a bronchus fre-

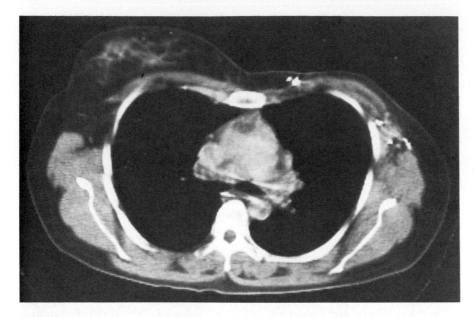

Figure 8–8. Simple mastectomy. CT scan after simple mastectomy; the left breast is absent, but the pectoral muscles are intact.

quently has a peripheral consolidation that mimics a subpleural mass. After thoracotomy or biopsy, edema and hematoma in the chest wall can be mistaken for tumor invasion. Reliable findings of chest wall invasion include bone destruction and a discrete extrapleural mass (Fig. 8–9). Such lesions are readily accessible to biopsy guided by CT.

Several pulmonary infections can involve the chest wall by direct extension.[16] These include actinomycosis, nocardiosis, and tuberculosis (Figs. 8–10A,B). If the chest wall disease is associated with adjacent pulmonary consolidation rather than a mass, differentiation from neoplasm may be possible.

SUPERIOR SULCUS (PANCOAST) TUMORS

Invasive tumors arising in the superior pulmonary sulcus produce the characteristic clinical findings of Horner's syndrome and shoulder and arm pain; this presentation is called Pancoast's

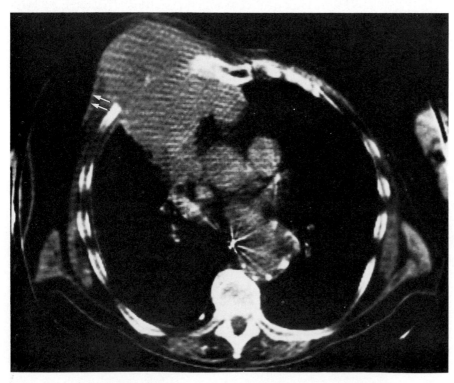

Figure 8–9. Chest wall invasion by bronchogenic carcinoma. Patient is an elderly man scanned because of a right chest wall mass. CT scan shows a large mass elevating the muscle layers of the right chest wall (arrows). The mass also involves the anterior right lung and adjacent anterior mediastinum. This mass represented a squamous cell bronchogenic carcinoma with direct chest wall invasion.

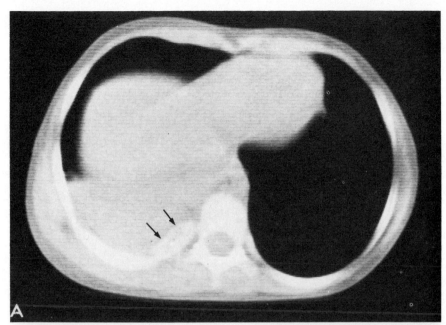

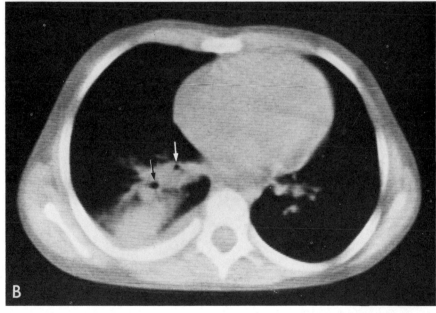

Figure 8–10. Actinomycosis involving lung and chest wall. Patient is a young girl with a low-grade fever and a right posterior chest wall mass. **A** CT scan shows thickening of soft tissues of the posterior chest wall associated with destruction and periostitis of a medial rib (arrows) and dense lower lobe consolidation. **B** CT scan at a higher level; air in bronchi (arrows) and a small pleural effusion are visible. Surgery revealed a large lung abscess, and actinomycosis was cultured. (From Webb WR, Sagel SS: Actinomycosis involving the chest wall: CT findings. AJR 139:1008, 1982. © 1982, American Roentgen Ray Society. Reprinted by permission.)

syndrome.[17] In the past, tumors of the superior sulcus carried a very poor prognosis, but combined therapy with radiation followed by resection of the upper lobe, chest wall, and adjacent structures has resulted in 5-year survival rates of 30 per cent.[18, 19] In patients being considered for this combined therapy, CT scans can provide information on the anatomic extent of tumor spread that is useful in planning both the radiation therapy and the surgical approach to the tumor.[20]

Extension of tumor posteriorly or laterally at the lung apex primarily involves the chest wall and nerves. Although chest wall invasion does not prevent resection, extensive chest wall and bone involvement by tumor makes surgical treatment difficult, and the prognosis of patients with extensive chest wall disease is poor. Invasion of the ribs or vertebral bodies occurs in one third to one half of cases and can usually be seen on CT scans (Fig. 8–11A,B).[20] Anterior and medial extension of tumor can involve the esophagus, trachea, and brachiocephalic vessels. Invasion of these structures usually precludes resection, as does metastasis to mediastinal lymph nodes. In patients with superior sulcus tumors, as with other bronchogenic carcinomas, the detection by CT of mediastinal

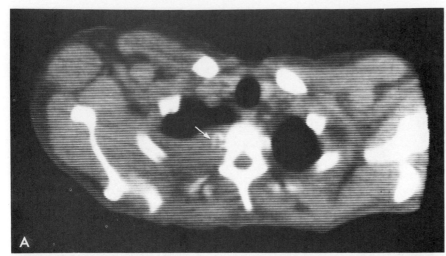

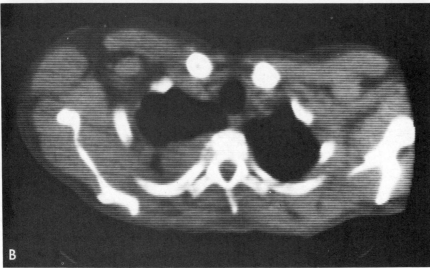

Figure 8–11. Pancoast's tumor. Patient is a 37-year-old man with right shoulder pain and right apical pleural thickening. **A** CT scan 1 cm above the sternal notch shows a posterior tumor mass and partial destruction of the medial third rib (arrow). **B** CT scan at a level 1 cm higher than in **A** again shows destruction of the rib. Biopsy revealed adenocarcinoma; after radiation, en bloc resection was performed. (From Webb WR, Jeffrey RB, Godwin JD: Thoracic computed tomography in superior sulcus tumors. J Comput Assist Tomogr 5:361, 1981. Reprinted by permission.)

invasion can be difficult and has diagnostic limitations. Mediastinal lymphadenopathy in patients with bronchogenic carcinoma must be interpreted with the understanding that enlarged nodes do not necessarily contain tumor (see Chapter 5).

The Axillary Space

ANATOMY

As usually defined, the axilla is bordered by the fascial coverings of the following muscles: anteriorly, the pectoralis major and minor; posteriorly, the latissimus dorsi, teres major, and subscapularis; medially, the chest wall and serratus anterior; and laterally, the coracobrachialis and biceps.[8] These boundaries refer to subjects with their arms at their sides (Fig. 8–12A–C). However, patients are usually scanned with their arms

above their heads so that the arm and its musculature no longer form the lateral margin of the axillary space, and the axilla is open laterally (Fig. 12D–F). On CT scans, the apex, or cephalad extent, of the axilla is best defined by the level at which the pectoralis minor crosses from anterior to posterior above the axillary space and inserts into the coracoid process of the scapula (Fig. 8–3A).

The axilla contains the axillary artery and vein, branches of the brachial plexus, some branches of the intercostal nerves, and a large number of lymph nodes, all surrounded by fat.[8] The axillary vessels and the brachial plexus extend laterally, near the apex of the axilla, close to the pectoralis minor. They are contained within the fibrous axillary sheath, which is continuous with the deep cervical fascia above the first rib. In general, the axillary vein lies below and anterior to the axillary artery, whereas the brachial plexus is largely above and posterior to the artery.[20a] Although each vessel can sometimes be seen on CT images (Fig. 8–3B–D), in many normal persons it is impossible to distinguish artery, vein, and brachial plexus within the axilla (Fig. 8–12D).

The subscapular artery and vein are the largest vascular branches of the axillary vessels.[8] They divide, after a short course, into the thoracodorsal artery and vein medially and the circumflex scapular vessels, branches of which descend along the lateral border of the scapula between the teres major and minor. These vessels are usually visible on high-quality CT scans (Figs. 8–3B–C and 8–12D–F).

The axillary lymph nodes, of which there are 20 to 30,[8] are larger and belong to several groups. A *lateral group* of four to six nodes lies near the undersurface of the axillary vein and drains the arm. An *anterior* or *pectoral group* of four or five nodes lies along the lateral border of the pectoralis minor. Their afferent lymph vessels drain the skin and muscles of the anterior and lateral chest walls and the central and lateral breast. A *posterior* or *subscapular* group of six or seven lymph nodes is situated along the lower margin of the posterior axillary wall, close to a branch of the subscapular artery. They drain the upper back and dorsal part of the neck. A *medial* or *subclavicular group* of six to 12 nodes is posterior to the cranial portion of the pectoralis minor. This group drains a portion of the arm and breast. Last, an *intermediate* or *central group* of three or four large nodes lies deep within the axilla and communicates with all the other node groups. Normal lymph nodes are not usually recognized as such on CT scans of the axilla.

AXILLARY ABNORMALITIES

LYMPHADENOPATHY

Axillary lymph nodes 1 to 1.5 cm in diameter can sometimes be seen in normal patients.[21] Lymph nodes greater than 2 cm in diameter are generally considered pathologic. Axillary lymphadenopathy is most frequently seen in patients with lymphoma or metastatic carcinoma (Figs. 8–13A,B and 8–14A,B). Lymph node masses are most easily detected by observing both axillae for

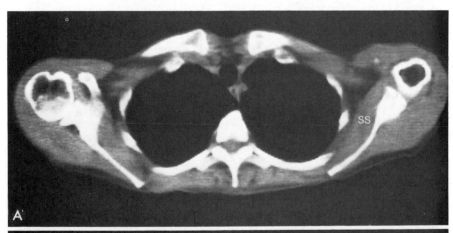

Figure 8–12. Normal axillary anatomy. Patient is a woman who underwent a left radical mastectomy.

Illustration continued on following page

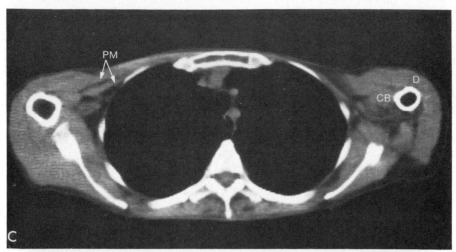

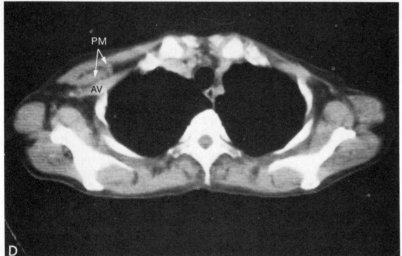

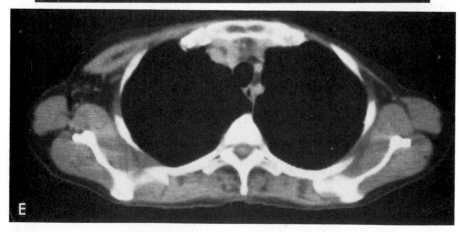

Figure 8–12. *Continued* CT scans were obtained with her arms at her sides (**A–C**) and raised above her head (**D–F**). **A–C** With the arms positioned at the sides, the axilla is marginated anteriorly by the pectoralis major and pectoralis minor (PM) muscles, posteriorly by the subscapularis (SS) and teres major (TM) muscles, and laterally by the coracobrachialis and biceps (CB) muscles. On the left, the great bulk of the pectoral muscles has been removed surgically. The large deltoid muscle (D) is visible laterally. Axillary vessels are clearly visible. **D–F** With the patient's arms positioned above her head, the appearance of the axilla is somewhat altered. Scan levels in **D** through **F** correspond respectively to **A** through **C**. The pectoral muscles (PM) appear thicker, and the clavicle is elevated. The axillary vessels (AV) have a more horizontal course and are more easily seen. The axilla is open laterally. On the left side, the axilla is now open anteriorly because the pectoralis muscle is absent.

Illustration continued on opposite page

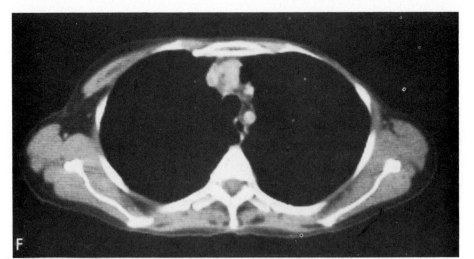

Figure 8–12. *Continued*

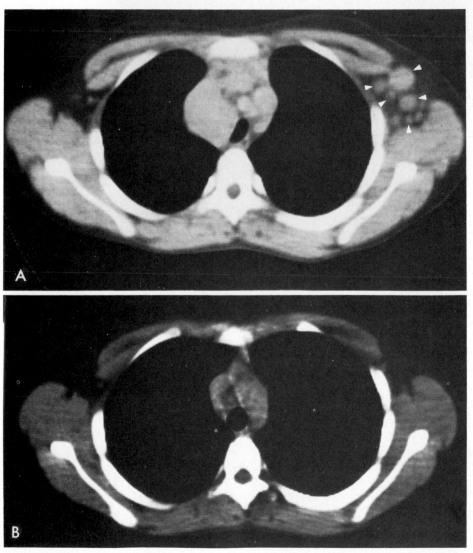

Figure 8–13. Lymphoma with mediastinal and axillary adenopathy. Patient is a young man with Hodgkin's disease. **A**   Initial CT scan shows right mediastinal lymph node enlargement and multiple enlarged left axillary lymph nodes (arrowheads). The right axilla is normal. **B**   CT scan after chemotherapy; the enlargement of both the mediastinal and axillary lymph nodes has resolved.

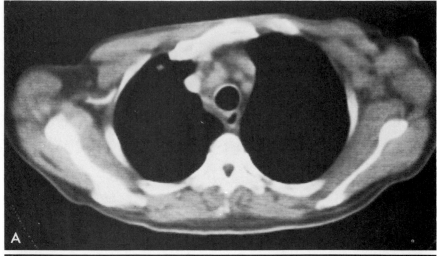

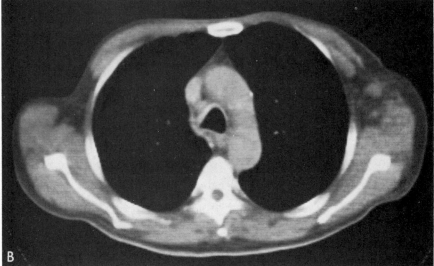

Figure 8–14. Nasopharyngeal carcinoma with axillary metastases. **A** CT scan shows several large clinically palpable lymph nodes within the left axilla. **B** CT scan at a lower level; a smaller minimally enlarged node is present.

asymmetry. Enlarged lymph nodes high within the axilla lie beneath the pectoral muscles and may not be palpable (Fig. 8–15A–C). These nodes, can be detected by CT, although the sensitivity and accuracy of diagnosis have not been determined.[11]

BRACHIAL PLEXUS TUMORS

Although the brachial plexus is not often visible on CT scans as a discrete structure, brachial plexus tumors can be demonstrated.[11, 20a] Tumor involving the brachial plexus is diagnosed when there is a mass in the region of the axillary sheath, and the clinical picture is compatible with brachial plexus involvement (Fig. 8–16A–C).

AXILLARY VEIN OCCLUSION

Occlusion of the axillary vein most frequently occurs as a result of thrombosis or compression by tumor. The condition can be recognized on CT scans after contrast material is injected into an ipsilateral arm vein. Findings include nonopacification of the vein or partial vein opacification with contrast outlining a thrombus (Fig. 8–17A–C). Venous collaterals that are not seen normally become visible in the axilla and chest wall. However, the axillary vein can fail to opacify with contrast material when a more central venous obstruction is present, with stasis of blood in the axillary vein. Small veins in the chest wall sometimes do opacify without venous obstruction being present, especially when the injection is made into a small arm vein or during a Valsalva maneuver.

SUBTRAPEZIAL SPACE

When a patient's arms are raised above the head, an artifactual space becomes visible beneath the trapezius muscle at the level of the upper tho-

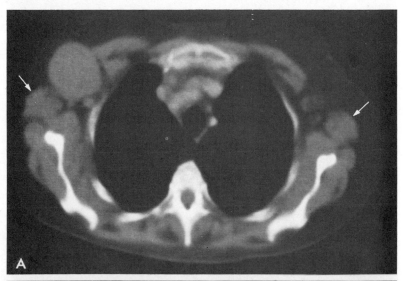

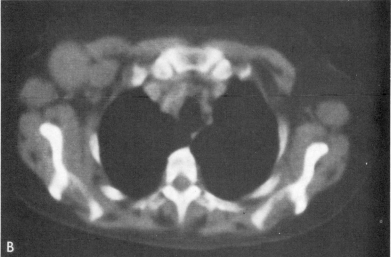

Figure 8–15. Metastatic cervical carcinoma with palpable and nonpalpable lymphadenopathy. **A, B** On CT scans, large lymph nodes involved by tumor are easily visible in the inferior right axilla. The rounded muscle mass of the teres major and latissimus dorsi (arrows) muscles mimics a lymph node mass but is bilateral and symmetric. **C** On CT scan, enlarged lymph node in the apex of the right axilla (arrow), deep below the pectoralis major muscle, displaces an axillary vein posteriorly (arrowhead). The node was not palpable.

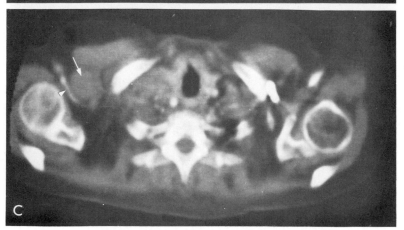

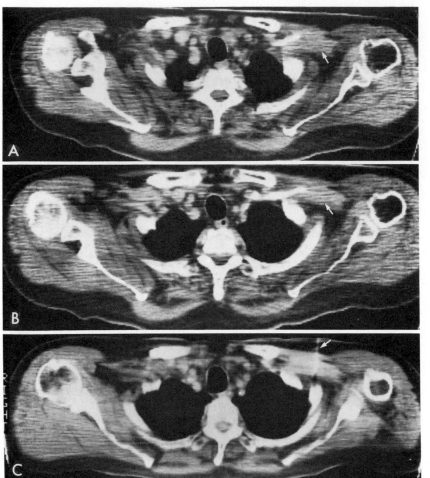

Figure 8–16. Metastatic tumor involving the brachial plexus. Ten years after a left radical mastectomy for breast carcinoma, this woman noticed a tender mass in her left supraclavicular fossa associated with symptoms of left brachial plexitis. **A, B** CT scans show a mass (arrows) posterior to the opacified axillary vein, in the position of the brachial plexus. **C** CT-guided needle biopsy revealed metastatic carcinoma. Arrow indicates needle tip in the mass.

racic and lower cervical vertebrae (Fig. 8–3A,B). This compartment has been termed the *subtrapezial space.*[22] Anteriorly and superiorly it is continuous with the posterior triangle of the neck, and anteriorly and inferiorly with the apex of the axilla. The subtrapezial space contains lymph nodes belonging to the deep cervical chain; when enlarged, these nodes can be seen on CT scans.[22] The levator scapulae and anterior serratus muscles, however, do traverse the subtrapezial space and can cause confusion in the interpretation of CT scans by mimicking lymphadenopathy. The levator scapulae originates from the transverse processes of the upper four cervical vertebrae and inserts into the medial border of the scapula. If the muscle is traced on serial CT scans, it crosses the subtrapezial space from superomedial to inferolateral. A portion of the anterior serratus muscle can also be seen in the subtrapezial space, and has a somewhat triangular outline. Usually, symmetry of these muscles allows differentiation from adenopathy.

THE BREAST

Soft tissues of the breast can be seen easily on CT scans of women in the supine position. Localized breast masses are occasionally visible, but their CT appearance is usually nonspecific.[23] Breast masses detected incidentally on CT images should generally be evaluated by physical examination and conventional mammography (Fig. 8–18A,B).

BREAST MASSES

Special CT scanners can detect and localize some breast carcinomas.[23, 24] In general, it is not possible to distinguish between benign and malignant breast masses on the basis of CT morphology alone.[23] However, breast cancers can show a greater increase in density after intravenous injection of contrast material than do benign tumors, probably as a result of concentration of iodine in the malignant tissue.[24] Thus, particularly in women with dense breasts, a discrete breast mass

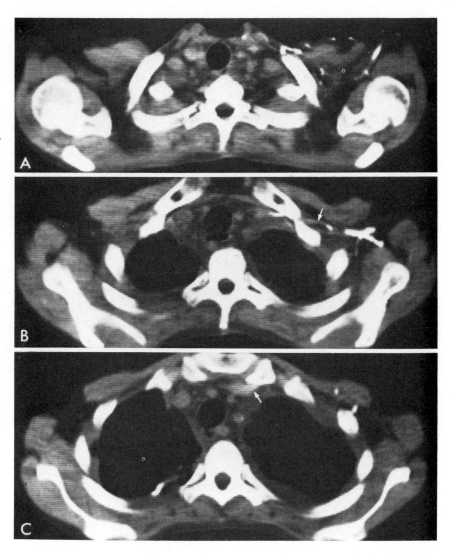

Figure 8–17. Axillary vein occlusion. CT scans at three successive levels after a bolus injection of contrast material into a left arm vein show evidence of axillary vein occlusion. **A** On CT scan numerous small collateral veins are visible within the axilla and anterior chest wall and neck. **B** On a scan at a lower level, the axillary vein is densely opacified laterally, but its caliber is small and it is incompletely seen medially, as it passes between the first rib and the clavicle. The thin line of contrast medially (arrow) may be outlining an intraluminal clot. **C** On scan, the left brachiocephalic vein (arrow) is only faintly opacified by contrast medium. With normal flow, this vein would be more densely opacified after a bolus injection of contrast medium.

may not be visible on mammograms, but CT scans after injection of contrast material can show a localized area of contrast enhancement that indicates the presence of a tumor.[24] Despite this benefit, dedicated breast scanners have not proved cost effective for screening the general population.

Chang and associates[25] reported their experience with breast scanning using a conventional body scanner and obtained results similar to those found with the special scanners.[24] In a group of 67 women with abnormal mammograms or a high risk of breast cancer, CT scans detected 16 of 17 cancers, whereas film mammography detected 12 and physical examination only eight. One cancer detected by CT measured only 4 mm. In general, CT was most useful in patients with dense breasts. In this study, scans 1 cm thick were performed before and after a rapid intravenous drip infusion of 300 ml of contrast agent. The carcinomas

detected by CT showed an increase in density of 46 to 106 H. In three patients with epithelial hyperplasia of the terminal mammary ducts, considered by many to be a precancerous condition, CT showed contrast enhancement of 46 to 100 H.

Ten benign breast lesions were also studied. Five patients with fibrocystic disease had density increases of less than 30 H on postcontrast scans, but three fibroadenomas showed an increase of 44 to 66 H. One breast abscess and one reactive lymph node showed density increases of 66 H and 72 H, respectively. Thus, although postcontrast CT scans cannot always distinguish cancer from benign lesions, CT can be used to localize masses that are potentially malignant and that should be biopsied or excised.

CT cannot replace conventional mammography in the screening or routine evaluation of a breast mass, but it can be indicated in the presence of

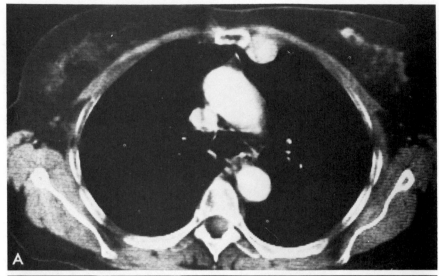

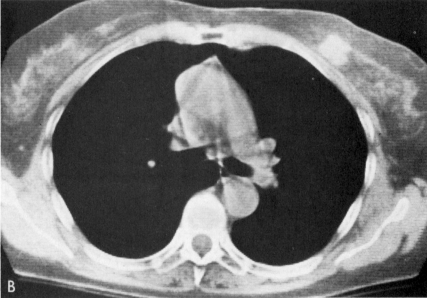

Figure 8–18. Breast carcinoma. CT was performed to evaluate a small retrosternal mass detected on a routine chest radiograph. **A** CT scan shows enlargement of a left internal mammary lymph node and a breast mass. **B** CT scan at a lower level also shows a left breast mass. Needle biopsies of the large internal mammary lymph node and the left breast mass both revealed adenocarcinoma.

dense breasts; a strong clinical suspicion of breast cancer, particularly when the mammogram shows no evidence of tumor; questionable mammographic findings of tumor; and prior biopsy or lumpectomy of breast cancer, when primary radiation therapy is contemplated.[24]

BREAST CARCINOMA

In patients with breast carcinoma, CT can aid the planning of radiation therapy by providing an accurate measurement of chest wall thickness and by detecting internal mammary lymph node metastases.[11, 26, 27]

Metastases to the internal mammary lymph node chain have been found in one third of clinically resectable patients undergoing extended radical mastectomy. Internal mammary node metastases are more frequent in patients with tumors in the central or medial portion of the breast.[26] Because internal mammary metastases are common, irradiating the internal mammary chain significantly improves local control of tumor and survival in patients also treated by radical mastectomy.[26]

Accurate knowledge of the location of the internal mammary lymph nodes is important in planning radiotherapy because these nodes should be irradiated and normal tissues spared. The internal mammary nodes lie in the upper intercostal spaces, lateral to the sternum, and are separated from the pleura only by the endothoracic fascia. Their depth depends on chest wall thickness and is therefore variable. However, CT allows direct measurement of chest wall thickness from the skin to pleura[26]; thus CT guides the therapist in choosing a treatment volume appropriate for irradiating the internal mammary nodes but sparing the lung. Munzenrider and associates[26] recommended that a CT determination of chest wall thickness be made in breast cancer patients considered for electron beam therapy, with which dose distribution varies significantly with depth; in patients treated with tangential radiation; and in patients who are obese or have intact breasts.

CT can show evidence of internal mammary lymph node metastasis not detected with other radiographic modalities.[11, 26, 27] Generally, normal internal mammary lymph nodes are not visible on CT scans, and a visible node is considered abnormal (Fig. 8–18A). Gouliamos and associates[11] found CT evidence of internal mammary node metastases in nine of 64 patients with breast carcinoma. Meyer and Munzenrider[27] used CT to detect internal mammary lymphadenopathy in 18 patients with locally recurrent breast carcinoma. In 12, lymph node enlargement occurred only on

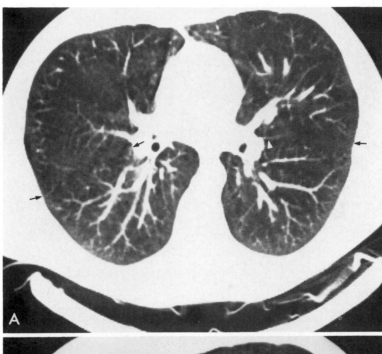

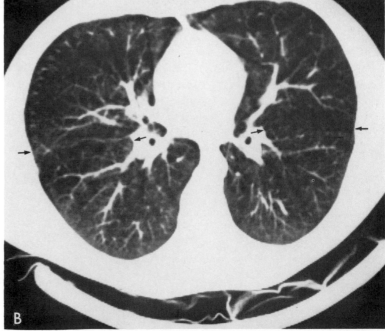

Figure 8–19. Normal fissures. **A** CT scan at the level of midhila shows the plane of the major fissures on both sides (arrows). A medial segment of the left major fissure is visible (arrowhead). **B** CT scan 2 cm caudad to **A** shows the right major fissure (right arrows), and the plane of the left major fissure (left arrows).

the side of the previously treated carcinoma, and in six, it was bilateral. Visible lymph nodes were 7 mm to 2.6 cm in diameter. In only five of the 18 patients were plain radiographic abnormalities visible prospectively. In seven patients, abnormal nodes would have been inadequately treated by routine radiotherapeutic portals. In four patients, CT showed sternal destruction by tumor that was not suspected from the radiographs.

In addition to detecting internal mammary node metastases in patients with breast carcinoma, CT can be used to diagnose axillary lymph node enlargement and metastases to the chest wall or sternum. Gouliamos and colleagues[11] found axillary lymph node enlargement in 21 of 64 patients with breast carcinoma, chest wall involvement in five, and sternal destruction in one.

The CT appearances of augmentation mammoplasty implants have not been described, but they are quite characteristic. The homogeneous water-density implants are normally situated immediately beneath the skin and are distinctly demarcated from the surrounding breast. Higher-density strands may traverse the implant.

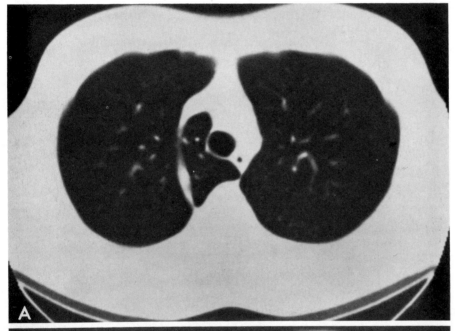

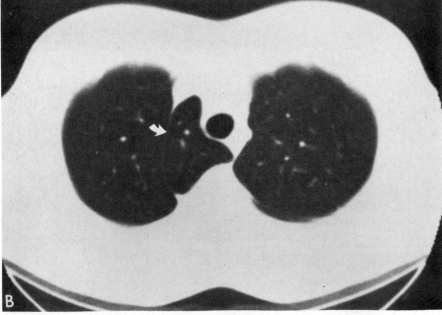

Figure 8–20. Azygos lobe and fissure. **A** CT scan in a patient with an azygos lobe shows the anomalous arch of the azygos vein passing through the right lung. **B** On a scan at a higher level, the azygos fissure (arrow) has a "C" shape. (From Speckman JM, Gamsu G, Webb WR: Alterations in CT mediastinal anatomy produced by an azygos lobe. AJR 137:47, 1981. © 1981, American Roentgen Ray Society. Reprinted by permission.)

The Pleurae
ANATOMY

In general, the visceral and parietal pleural layers cannot be seen on CT scans. However, a knowledge of their anatomy and relationships often allows a reliable diagnosis of pleural disease.

INTRAPULMONARY FISSURES

Because they are thin and oblique relative to the plane of the scan, the normal major fissures are not always seen on CT images. However, the position of each major fissure can be inferred from the position of the avascular plane of lung 2 to 3 cm wide accompanying and paralleling the fissure (Fig. 8–19A,B). CT demonstrated at least part of the avascular plane of the major fissure in 75 to 100 per cent of patients.[28–29b] In our experience, an avascular plane is visible on virtually 100 per cent of CT scans of the chest. In 10 to 20 per cent of patients the major fissures are demonstrated on CT scans as a thin line, although low window levels and narrow window widths can be required to see them. In some patients, a ground-glass band of density is seen in the avascular area, probably reflecting volume averaging of the fissure itself.[28] The minor fissure is invisible, but its plane can also be inferred from the position of the avascular area between the right upper lobe vessels above and the middle lobe vessels below. The avascular plane of lucency, reflecting the position of the minor fissure, is visible in 52 to 100 per cent of patients.[28–29b]

In patients with an azygos lobe, the four layers of the mesoazygos, or azygos fissure, are invariably

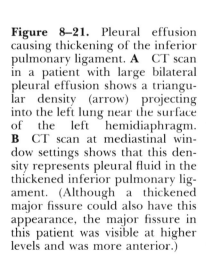

Figure 8–21. Pleural effusion causing thickening of the inferior pulmonary ligament. **A** CT scan in a patient with large bilateral pleural effusion shows a triangular density (arrow) projecting into the left lung near the surface of the left hemidiaphragm. **B** CT scan at mediastinal window settings shows that this density represents pleural fluid in the thickened inferior pulmonary ligament. (Although a thickened major fissure could also have this appearance, the major fissure in this patient was visible at higher levels and was more anterior.)

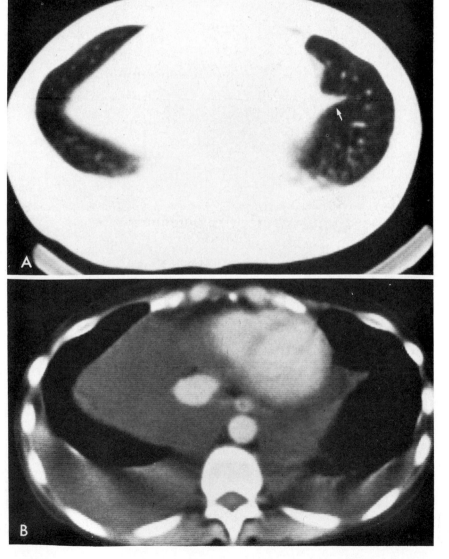

visible above the level of the anomalous azygos vein.[30] The azygos fissure is C-shaped and convex laterally, beginning anteriorly at the right brachiocephalic vein and ending posteriorly at the right anterolateral surface of the vertebral body (Fig. 8–20).

INFERIOR PULMONARY LIGAMENT

On each side, below the level of the pulmonary hilum, the parietal and visceral pleural layers join, forming a fold that extends inferiorly along the mediastinal surface of the lung and ends at the level of the diaphragm. This fold, the inferior pulmonary ligament, anchors the lower lobe.[31] In cross section on CT images viewed at lung windows, it appears as a small triangular density 1 to 2 cm long with its apex pointing laterally into the lung and its base at against the mediastinum (see Chapter 5, Fig. 5–18). On the left, it usually lies adjacent to the esophagus; on the right, it is lateral to the inferior vena cava or esophagus. The caudal portion of the inferior pulmonary ligament extends laterally for several centimeters along the surface of the diaphragm and is visible as a thin linear density. It can become thickened in the presence of a pleural effusion (Fig. 8–21).

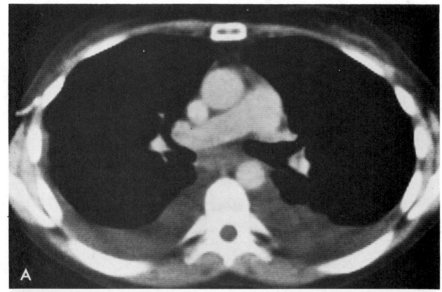

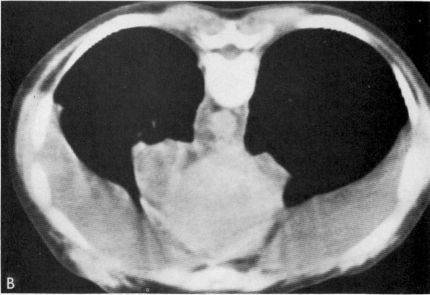

Figure 8–22. Positional shift of pleural fluid in a patient with lymphoma. **A** CT scan with the patient supine shows large bilateral pleural effusions posteriorly. **B** When the patient is scanned prone, the fluid gravitates anteriorly.

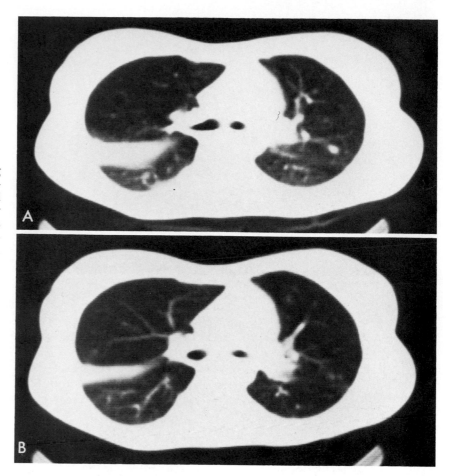

Figure 8–23. Pleural fluid causing thickening of the right major fissure. **A,B** On CT scans, pleural fluid localized to the right major fissure is visible at two contiguous levels. In this patient, the fluid appears as a triangular density, based peripherally, with its apex directed toward the hilum. The lower lobe is displaced posteriorly and medially.

PLEURAL ABNORMALITIES

PLEURAL FLUID COLLECTIONS

In general, collections of pleural fluid are readily recognized on CT scans of the thorax as arcuate areas of homogeneous density paralleling the chest wall.[1] The diagnosis of free pleural fluid requires a change in patient position from supine to decubitus or prone[32] (Figs. 8–22A,B). Large effusions often extend into the major fissures, displacing the lower lobes medially and posteriorly (Figs. 8–23A,B and 8–24A–D).

The visceral pleura covers the surface of the lung, and its inferior extent is defined by the inferior extent of lung in the costophrenic angles. The parietal pleura is contiguous with the chest wall and diaphragm and in the costophrenic angles extends well below the level of the lung base.

Thus, pleural fluid collections in the costophrenic angles can be seen below the lung base and may mimic collections of fluid in the peritoneal cavity. The parallel curvilinear configuration

of the pleural and peritoneal cavities at the level of the perihepatic and perisplenic recesses allows fluid in either cavity to appear as an arcuate or semilunar density displacing liver or spleen away from the adjacent chest wall. The relationship of the fluid collection to the ipsilateral diaphragmatic crus helps to determine its location.[33] Pleural fluid collections in the posterior costophrenic angle lie medial and posterior to the diaphragm and cause lateral displacement of the crus (Fig. 8–25). Peritoneal fluid collections are anterior and lateral to the diaphragm; lateral displacement of the crus is not visible. In patients with both pleural and peritoneal fluid, the diaphragm often can be seen as a curvilinear muscle-density structure with relatively low-density fluid both anteriorly and posteriorly.

To some degree, the specific gravity (density) of pleural fluid obtained at thoracocentesis correlates with the cause of the effusion. Thus, high-density or exudative fluid collections are often associated with infection (empyema) or neoplasm,

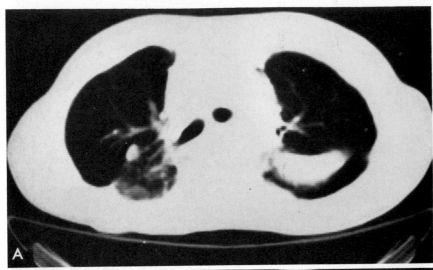

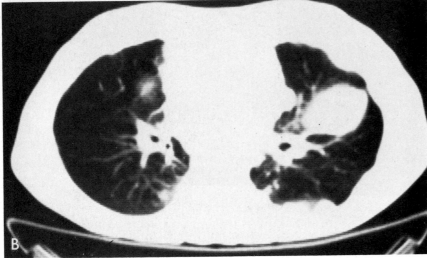

Figure 8–24. Pleural fluid causing thickening of the left major fissure. Patient has lymphoma. **A, B** CT scans show lenticular collections of pleural fluid in the superior **(A)** and inferior **(B)** portions of the left major fissure.

Illustration continued on opposite page

whereas low-density or transudative effusions often are the result of congestive heart failure or other diseases that cause a loss of fluid, but not protein, from the pleural capillaries. Although it might be expected that the CT numbers of pleural fluid collections would correlate well with their specific gravity, CT numbers cannot be reliably used to predict the specific gravity of the fluid or its cause.[32]

EMPYEMA

The term "empyema" is used to describe a purulent pleural effusion due to infection of the pleural space. Empyema is usually diagnosed by thoracocentesis. Culture of material aspirated from the pleural space generally reveals the causative organisms. Most empyemas are caused by *Staphylococcus aureus*, gram-negative enteric bacilli, or mixed anaerobic and aerobic infections.

With conventional radiographic techniques,

empyemas can be difficult or impossible to differentiate from peripheral lung abscesses abutting the chest wall. This distinction is important because empyemas are usually treated by tube thoracostomy and systemic antibiotics, whereas most lung abscesses require appropriate systemic antibiotics and postural drainage.[2]

Baber and co-workers[2] reported the differences between empyemas and peripheral lung abscesses as shown by CT. Typically, an empyema has a regular shape and is round or elliptical in cross section (Fig. 8–26A–C). The outer edge of the lesion is sharply demarcated from adjacent lung. When a bronchopleural fistula is present or when air is introduced into the empyema at thoracocentesis, its inner margin usually appears smooth and its wall is of uniform thickness. Lung abscesses, on the other hand, are irregularly shaped and often contain multiple loculated collections of air and fluid. Their inner surfaces are often irregular

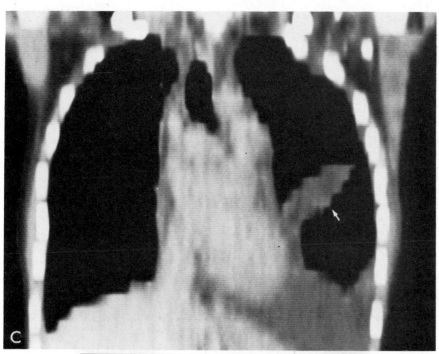

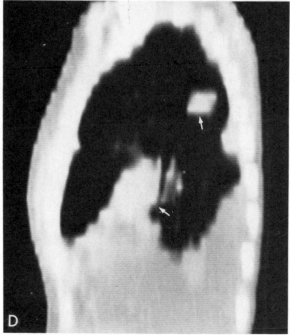

Figure 8–24. *Continued* **C, D** Images in the coronal (**C**) and sagittal (**D**) planes show fluid in the posterior costophrenic angle and in the left major fissure (arrows).

and ragged, and their outer edges are ill defined because of adjacent pulmonary parenchymal consolidation. In some cases, empyema cavities, unlike lung abscess cavities, can change shape when the patient moves from the supine to the prone or decubitus position.

When an abscess or empyema does not contain air and appears solid on plain radiographs, contrast-enhanced CT scans can demonstrate the wall of the lesion and provide a clue as to its fluid-

filled nature (Fig. 8–27A,B).[2] The walls of both empyemas and abscesses enhance with contrast infusion, whereas their fluid-filled centers do not.

The differentiation of pleural and parenchymal processes may not be possible with conventional radiography. Thus, CT provides important information in the majority of patients with pleuroparenchymal disease. Pugatch and colleagues[32] studied 75 patients who had complex pleural processes or combinations of pleural and parenchymal dis-

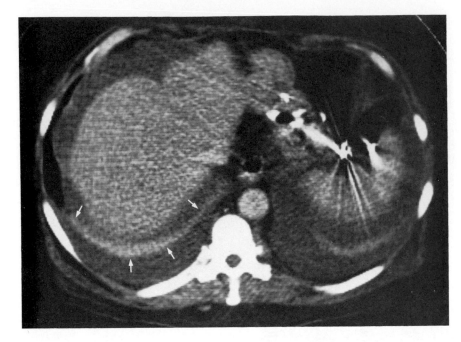

Figure 8–25. Pleural fluid and ascites. CT scan shows the diaphragm (arrows) outlined by fluid on both sides. Pleural fluid is visible posterior to the diaphragm, displacing the diaphragm and crura anteriorly; ascites is visible anterior to the diaphragm, separating it from the liver.

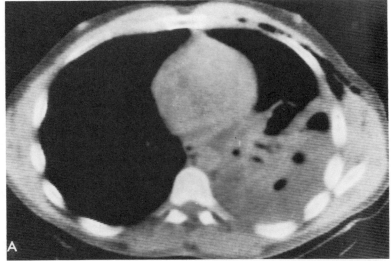

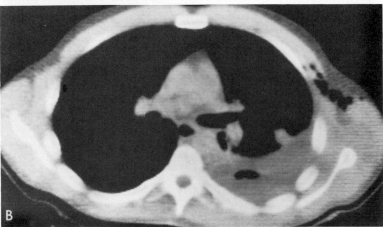

Figure 8–26. Empyema. **A,B** CT scans with the patient supine show a smooth, elliptic or crescentic density containing several collections of air within the posterior left chest. This density is sharply defined from adjacent lung, and, where visible, its wall is of uniform thickness. Subcutaneous empyema reflects the recent placement of a chest tube.

Illustration continued on opposite page

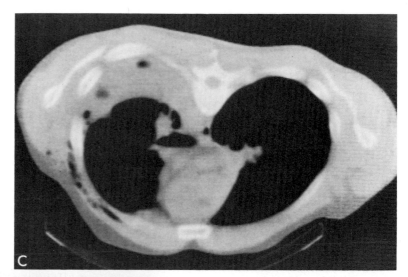

Figure 8–26. *Continued* **C** CT scan at the same level as **B** but with the patient prone shows very little change in the appearance or location of the fluid, which indicates loculation.

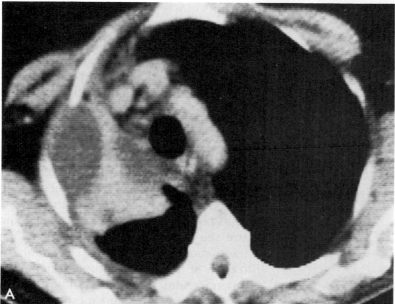

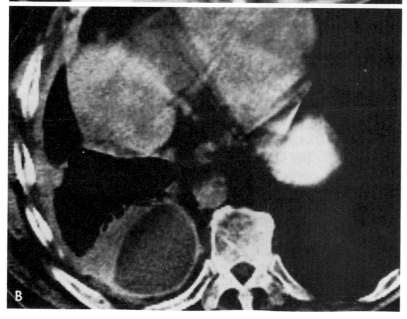

Figure 8–27. Empyema localization in two patients. CT scans show typical features of empyemas without bronchial communication. **A** After right upper lobe lobectomy, scan demonstrates a right upper lentiform empyema with contrast enhancement of the wall. Pleural fluid is present posteriorly. The lung parenchyma around the empyema shows consolidation. **B** Scan shows a right lower empyema with a uniform, low CT density center and a wall of uniform thickness.

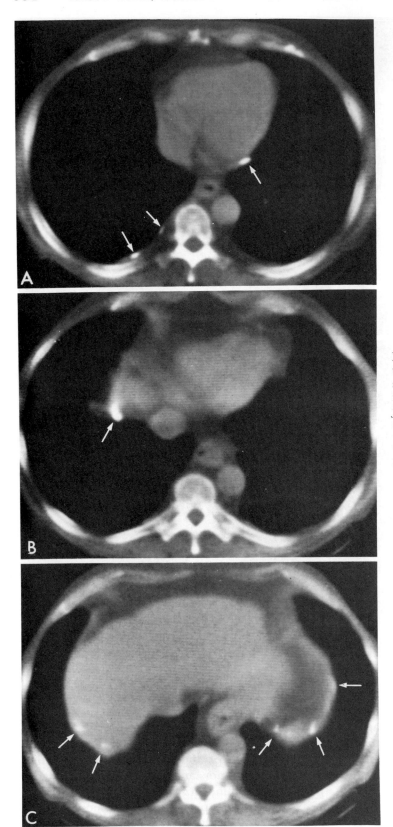

Figure 8–29. Calcified pleural plaques in a patient with asbestos exposure. **A** CT scan shows calcified pleural plaques (arrows) involving the mediastinal pleura and the pleura adjacent to a rib and vertebral body. **B, C** CT scans at lower levels show calcified plaques involving the diaphragmatic pleura (arrows). These calcifications identify the position of the diaphragm adjacent to lung in the posterior costophrenic angles.

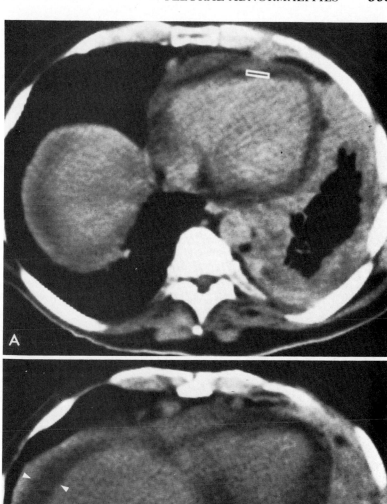
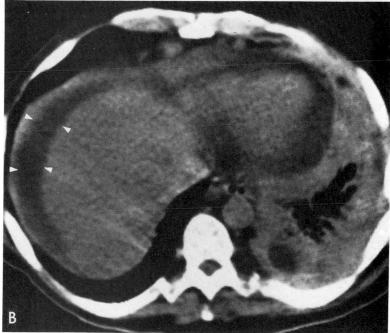

Figure 8–30. Malignant mesothelioma. **A, B** CT scans show encasement of the left lower lobe by a thick, irregular pleural rind that represents tumor. (Tumor also extended into the upper abdomen.) The fluid density separating the right hemidiaphragm from the liver represents ascites (arrowheads).

vanced asbestos-related pleural disease, large and irregular pleural plaques can resemble malignant mesothelioma.

Although pleural thickening is most frequently visible along the lateral chest wall, mediastinal pleural thickening, sometimes with adjacent mediastinal adenopathy, can also be present. The abnormal hemithorax can appear contracted and fixed, with little change in size during inspiration.[35] Pulmonary nodules are frequently hematogenous metastases. Diaphragmatic involvement by tumor can, however, be difficult to demonstrate on CT scans.[36a]

METASTASES

In patients with intrathoracic or extrathoracic tumors, metastases to the pleura can cause nodular pleural thickening and pleural effusions.[1, 37] Usually, pleural effusion masks the underlying pleural lesion, but occasionally the lesion can be seen on CT images. For example, in patients with a malignant thymoma that has metastasized to the pleura, pleural effusion is often lacking and the pleural metastases are visible (Fig. 8–1A,B).[1, 37, 38] They are usually discrete and have obtuse angles at their junction with the chest wall. Flat subpleural masses can occur in patients with lymphoma, and CT is particularly valuable in their detection.[14, 35]

The Diaphragm

ANATOMY

The diaphragm is a dome-shaped muscular sheet that separates the thoracic cavity from the abdomen. Its peripheral part consists of muscle fibers that originate from the circumference of the thoracic cage, converge, and insert into a fibrous central tendon. The muscle fibers can be grouped according to their origin: lumbar, sternal, and costal.

The lumbar fibers arise from the diaphragmatic crura and two aponeurotic arches on each side, called the medial and lateral lumbocostal arches.[8] The right and left diaphragmatic crura (Fig. 8–31A–C) are tendinous structures that arise inferiorly from the anterior surfaces of the upper lumbar vertebral bodies and intervening disks and are continuous with the anterior longitudinal ligament of the spine.[39] The crura ascend along the anterior aspect of the spine, on each side of the aorta, and then pass medially and anteriorly, joining the muscular diaphragm anterior to the aorta, to form the aortic hiatus. The right crus, which is larger and longer than the left, arises from the first three lumbar vertebral levels; the left crus arises from the first two lumbar segments.[39]

The aortic hiatus and the anterior crura are invariably demonstrated by CT. CT scans at caudal levels show the individual crura as discrete oval or round structures posterolateral to the aorta and anterior to the vertebral column. Because the right crus is larger and longer than the left, it has a greater cross-sectional diameter and is visible at lower levels (Chapter 5, Fig. 5–19).

The diaphragmatic crura can be mistaken for enlarged lymph nodes or masses because of their

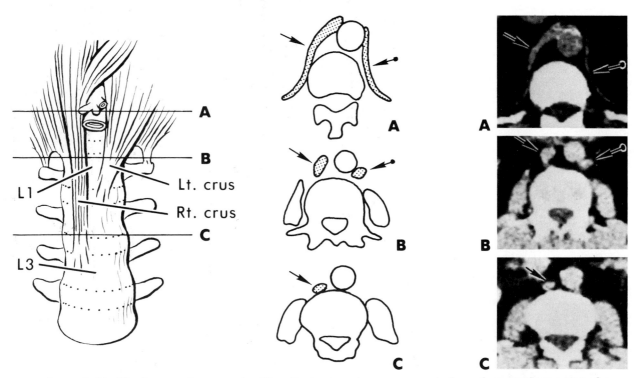

Figure 8–31. Diaphragmatic crura. **A** The diaphragmatic crura ascend along the anterior aspect of the spine, on each side of the aorta, joining anterior to the aorta to form the aortic hiatus. **B, C** The right crus is longer and larger than the left crus and extends to a lower level. The characteristic position of the crura on each side of the aorta allows them to be distinguished from enlarged lymph nodes. (From Callen PW, Filly RA, Korobkin M: Computed tomographic evaluation of the diaphragmatic crura. Radiology 126:413, 1978. Reprinted by permission.)

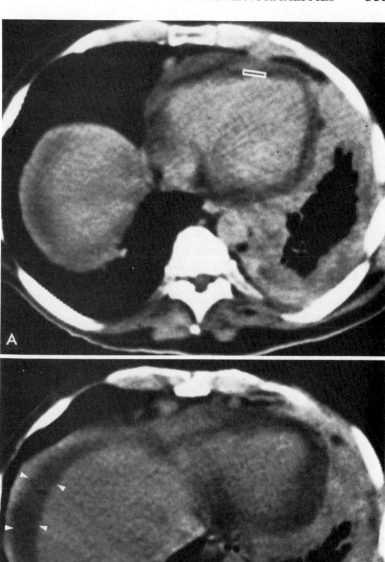

Figure 8–30. Malignant mesothelioma. **A, B** CT scans show encasement of the left lower lobe by a thick, irregular pleural rind that represents tumor. (Tumor also extended into the upper abdomen.) The fluid density separating the right hemidiaphragm from the liver represents ascites (arrowheads).

vanced asbestos-related pleural disease, large and irregular pleural plaques can resemble malignant mesothelioma.

Although pleural thickening is most frequently visible along the lateral chest wall, mediastinal pleural thickening, sometimes with adjacent mediastinal adenopathy, can also be present. The abnormal hemithorax can appear contracted and fixed, with little change in size during inspiration.[35] Pulmonary nodules are frequently hematogenous metastases. Diaphragmatic involvement by tumor can, however, be difficult to demonstrate on CT scans.[36a]

METASTASES

In patients with intrathoracic or extrathoracic tumors, metastases to the pleura can cause nodular pleural thickening and pleural effusions.[1, 37] Usually, pleural effusion masks the underlying pleural lesion, but occasionally the lesion can be seen on CT images. For example, in patients with a malignant thymoma that has metastasized to the pleura, pleural effusion is often lacking and the pleural metastases are visible (Fig. 8–1A,B).[1, 37, 38] They are usually discrete and have obtuse angles at their junction with the chest wall. Flat subpleural masses can occur in patients with lymphoma, and CT is particularly valuable in their detection.[14, 35]

The Diaphragm

ANATOMY

The diaphragm is a dome-shaped muscular sheet that separates the thoracic cavity from the abdomen. Its peripheral part consists of muscle fibers that originate from the circumference of the thoracic cage, converge, and insert into a fibrous central tendon. The muscle fibers can be grouped according to their origin: lumbar, sternal, and costal.

The lumbar fibers arise from the diaphragmatic crura and two aponeurotic arches on each side, called the medial and lateral lumbocostal arches.[8] The right and left diaphragmatic crura (Fig. 8–31A–C) are tendinous structures that arise inferiorly from the anterior surfaces of the upper lumbar vertebral bodies and intervening disks and are continuous with the anterior longitudinal ligament of the spine.[39] The crura ascend along the anterior aspect of the spine, on each side of the aorta, and then pass medially and anteriorly, joining the muscular diaphragm anterior to the aorta, to form the aortic hiatus. The right crus, which is larger and longer than the left, arises from the first three lumbar vertebral levels; the left crus arises from the first two lumbar segments.[39]

The aortic hiatus and the anterior crura are invariably demonstrated by CT. CT scans at caudal levels show the individual crura as discrete oval or round structures posterolateral to the aorta and anterior to the vertebral column. Because the right crus is larger and longer than the left, it has a greater cross-sectional diameter and is visible at lower levels (Chapter 5, Fig. 5–19).

The diaphragmatic crura can be mistaken for enlarged lymph nodes or masses because of their

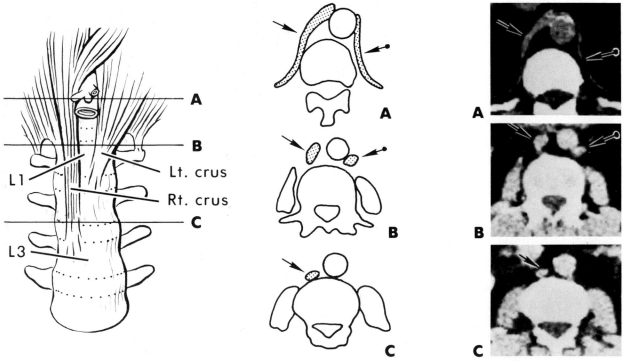

Figure 8–31. Diaphragmatic crura. **A** The diaphragmatic crura ascend along the anterior aspect of the spine, on each side of the aorta, joining anterior to the aorta to form the aortic hiatus. **B, C** The right crus is longer and larger than the left crus and extends to a lower level. The characteristic position of the crura on each side of the aorta allows them to be distinguished from enlarged lymph nodes. (From Callen PW, Filly RA, Korobkin M: Computed tomographic evaluation of the diaphragmatic crura. Radiology 126:413, 1978. Reprinted by permission.)

rounded appearance; para-aortic lymph nodes can indeed be seen in a similar position.[39] However, on contiguous CT scans, the crura merge gradually with the diaphragm at more cephalad levels, which differentiates them from para-aortic lymph nodes.

The medial lumbocostal arch is a tendinous arch that arises medially from the ipsilateral crus and the side of the first or second lumbar vertebral body.[8] It crosses the anterior aspect of the psoas muscle and is attached laterally to the transverse process of the first or second lumbar vertebra. On CT scans, the position of the medial lumbocostal arch can be inferred from the position of the psoas muscle. At this level, the diaphragm is discontinuous and the psoas muscle separates the diaphragmatic crus medially and the posterior leaf of the diaphragm laterally. The lateral lumbocostal arch crosses the anterior surface of the quadratus lumborum and is attached medially to the transverse process of the first lumbar vertebra and laterally to the twelfth rib.

The sternal portion of the diaphragm arises from the dorsum of the xiphoid process, whereas the costal part arises from the inner surfaces of the cartilage and bony surfaces of the inferior six ribs.[8]

Because of the transverse axial plane of the image, the central portion of the diaphragm is not a distinct structure and its position can be inferred only by the position of the lung base and upper abdominal organs. As the more peripheral portions of the diaphragm descend toward their sternal and costal origins, the posterior and lateral portions of the diaphragm become visible adjacent to retroperitoneal fat. Where the diaphragm is contiguous with the liver or spleen, it cannot be delineated by CT.

OPENINGS IN THE DIAPHRAGM

The diaphragm is perforated by several openings that allow structures to pass from the thorax to the abdomen.[8] The aortic hiatus is posterior and lies at the level of the twelfth thoracic vertebra. It is bounded posteriorly by the vertebral body and anteriorly by the crura. Through it pass the aorta, the azygos and hemiazygos veins, the thoracic duct, the intercostal arteries, and the splanchnic nerves. The esophageal hiatus is situated more anteriorly, in the muscular portion of the diaphragm at the level of the tenth thoracic vertebra. Through it pass the esophagus, the vagus nerves, and small blood vessels.[8] The foramen of the inferior vena cava pierces the fibrous central tendon of the diaphragm anterior and to the right of the esophageal hiatus.

Of these three structures, the aortic hiatus is most readily defined. On CT scans, the esophageal foramen is sometimes visible as an opening at the junction of the esophagus and stomach. The foramen of the inferior vena cava must be inferred from the position of the inferior vena cava. The foramina of Morgagni and Bochdalek are not visible on CT scans in normal people.

DIAPHRAGMATIC ABNORMALITIES

HERNIAS

Abdominal or retroperitoneal contents can herniate into the chest through congenital or acquired areas of weakness in the diaphragm or through traumatic diaphragmatic ruptures. Hernias of the stomach through the esophageal hiatus are the most common.

Hernias through the foramen of Bochdalek are uncommon in adults, but are the most common diaphragmatic hernias in infants.[40] Most are left-sided, and although often located in the posterolateral diaphragm, they can occur anywhere along the posterior diaphragm. Bochdalek hernias in adults usually contain retroperitoneal fat or kidney.

Parasternal hernias through Morgagni's foramina are rare, constituting less than 10 per cent of all diaphragmatic hernias.[40, 41] Morgagni's foramina are bounded by sternal slips of the diaphragm medially and by fibers arising from the seventh costal cartilage laterally. Normally, they contain the internal mammary vessels. Most Morgagni hernias occur on the right and, in contrast to Bochdalek hernias, usually contain an extension of the peritoneal sac. Their contents usually include omentum, liver, or bowel.[41]

Diaphragmatic rupture can result from penetrating or nonpenetrating trauma to the abdomen or thorax.[42] Traumatic hernias, however, account for only a small percentage of all diaphragmatic hernias. In nearly all cases, the left hemidiaphragm is affected, with ruptures of the central or posterior diaphragm being most frequent.[42] Omentum, stomach, small or large intestine, spleen, or kidney may all herniate through the diaphragmatic rent.

CT scans sometimes show herniation of abdominal contents into the chest through one of the diaphragmatic foramina. However, the anatomic boundaries of these foramina are often difficult to recognize, and it may not be possible to diagnose a hernia with certainty.[43] Knowledge of the normal positions of the foramina is essential in making the correct diagnosis. A mediastinal hiatal hernia can be diagnosed when the hernia opacifies with oral contrast material or contains both air and liquid and has an air-fluid level on the supine image (Fig. 8–32A,B). Contiguity of a hiatal hernia, with the esophagus above and the stomach below, and its relationship to the esophageal hiatus also assist in diagnosis. Paraesophageal hernias of omental or extraperitoneal fat often cannot be distinguished from a mediastinal lipoma (Fig. 8–33).

In at least one instance, CT has assisted in the diagnosis of traumatic rupture of the diaphragm.[42] In this case, CT scans showed an interruption in the cross-sectional image of the diaphragm that could only indicate a congenital or acquired traumatic defect. However, traumatic rupture of the diaphragm is usually diagnosed from conventional radiographs.[44, 45]

DIAPHRAGMATIC EVENTRATION

Local eventration of the right hemidiaphragm and superior displacement of the liver can be confused radiographically with a peripheral pulmo-

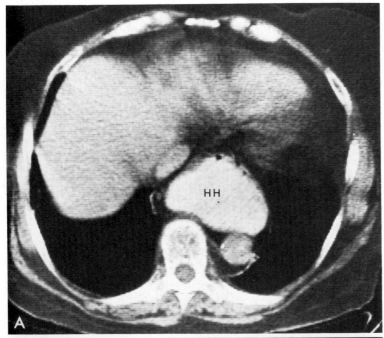

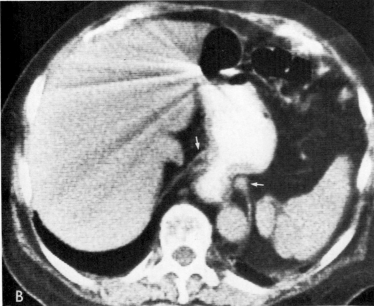

Figure 8–32. Hiatal hernia. **A** CT scan after oral administration of contrast material shows a large opacified hiatal hernia (HH) in the lower mediastinum. **B** At a lower level, the mediastinal hernia communicates anteriorly and laterally through the esophageal hiatus (arrows) with the subdiaphragmatic portion of the stomach.

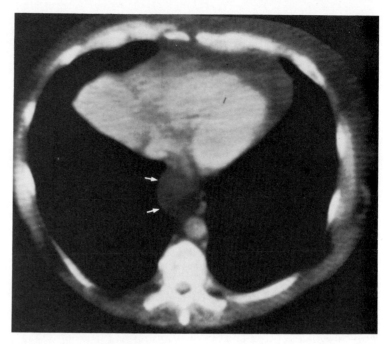

Figure 8–33. Paraesophageal hernia. CT scan near the level of the diaphragm shows a fatty mass in the mediastinum (arrows) compressing the esophagus to the left. (At surgery, a paraesophageal hernia of omentum was found.)

nary or pleural mass. CT scans after infusion of contrast medium can demonstrate opacification of normal intrahepatic vessels in the apparent mass, which identifies it as normal liver.[46] In addition, scans reformatted in the coronal plane can show that the "mass" has the same density as liver.

TUMORS OF THE DIAPHRAGM

Tumors of the diaphragm are rare.[47] Primary benign tumors and primary malignant tumors occur with nearly equal frequency. The most common benign lesions include lipomas, fibromas, neurogenic tumors, and mesothelial or bronchogenic cysts. Primary malignant tumors are generally of fibrous origin, such as fibrosarcoma. Both benign and malignant primary tumors appear radiographically as extrapleural masses.

Most metastatic neoplasms involve the diaphragm by direct extension. Examples of such tumors are carcinomas of the lung, stomach, pancreas, kidney, adrenal gland, and colon, and primary or secondary liver tumors. An invasive tumor can be a well-defined extrapleural mass or it can produce pleural effusion or pulmonary invasion. Radiographically visible hematogenous metastases to the diaphragm are very rare.

The radiographic appearance of a diaphragmatic tumor is nonspecific; most patients with an apparent diaphragmatic mass have a local eventration, a diaphragmatic hernia, or a pleural or pulmonary parenchymal lesion abutting the diaphragm. These conditions can be diagnosed by CT and thus exclude the possibility of a diaphragmatic tumor.

REFERENCES

1. Kreel L: Computed tomography of the lung and pleura. Semin Roentgenol 13:213, 1978.
2. Baber CE, Hedlund LW, Oddson TA, Putman CE: Differentiating empyemas and peripheral pulmonary abscesses. The value of computed tomography. Radiology 135:755, 1980.
3. van Waes PFGM, Zonneveld FW: Direct coronal body computed tomography. J Comput Assist Tomogr 6:58, 1982.
4. Goldberg RP, Carter BL: Absence of thoracic osteophytosis in the area adjacent to the aorta: Computed tomography demonstration. J Comput Assist Tomogr 2:173, 1978.
5. Paling MR, Dwyer A: The first rib as the cause of a "pulmonary nodule" on chest computed tomography. J Comput Assist Tomogr 4:847, 1980.
6. Destouet JM, Gilula LA, Murphy WA, Sagel SS: Computed tomography of the sternoclavicular joint and sternum. Radiology 138:123, 1981.
7. Soteropoulos GC, Cigtay OS, Schellinger D: Pectus excavatum deformities simulating mediastinal masses. J Comput Assist Tomogr 3:596, 1979.
8. Gray H: Anatomy of the Human Body, 28th American ed. In Goss CM (ed): Philadelphia, Lea & Febiger, 1966, pp 416–418, 448–461, 455–456, 614–618, 752–754.
9. Omell GH, Anderson LS, Bramson RJ: Chest wall tumors. Radiol Clin North Am 11:197, 1973.
10. Franken EA Jr, Smith JA, Smith WL: Tumors of the chest wall in infants and children. Pediatr Radiol 6:13, 1977.
11. Gouliamos AD, Carter BL, Emami B: Computed tomography of the chest wall. Radiology 134:433, 1980.
12. Faer MJ, Burnam RE, Beck CL: Transmural thoracic lipoma: Demonstration by computed tomography. AJR 130:161, 1978.
13. Napoli LD, Hansen HH, Muggia FM, Twigg HL: The incidence of osseous involvement in lung cancer, with special reference to the development of osteoblastic changes. Radiology 108:17, 1977.

14. Ellert J, Kreel L: The role of computed tomography in the initial staging and subsequent management of the lymphomas. J Comput Assist Tomogr 4:368, 1980.

15. Alexander E, Clark RA, Colley DP, Mitchell SE: CT of malignant pleural mesothelioma. AJR 137:287, 1981.

16. Webb WR, Sagel SS: Actinomycosis involving the chest wall: CT findings. AJR 139:1007, 1982.

17. Hepper NGG, Herskovic T, Witten DM, Mulder DW, Woolner LB: Thoracic inlet tumors. Ann Intern Med 64:979, 1966.

18. Paulsen DL: Carcinomas in the superior pulmonary sulcus. J Thorac Cardiovasc Surg 70:1095, 1975.

19. Miller JI, Mansour KA, Hatcher CR Jr: Carcinoma of the superior pulmonary sulcus. Ann Thorac Surg 28:44, 1979.

20. Webb WR, Jeffrey RB, Godwin JD: Thoracic computed tomography in superior sulcus tumors. J Comput Assist Tomogr 5:361, 1981.

20a. Gebarski KS, Glazer GM, Gebarski SS: Brachial plexus: Anatomic, radiologic, and pathologic correlation using computed tomography. J Comput Assist Tomogr 6:1058, 1982.

21. Kalisher L: Xeroradiography of axillary lymph node disease. Radiology 115:67, 1975.

22. Thompson JS, Kreel L: The subtrapezial space. J Comput Assist Tomogr 3:355, 1979.

23. McLeod RA, Grisvold JJ, Stephens DH, Beabout JW, Sheedy PF: Computed tomography of soft tissues and breast. Semin Roentgenol 13:267, 1978.

24. Grisvold JJ, Reese DF, Karsell PR: Computed tomographic mammography (CTM). AJR 133:1143, 1979.

25. Chang CHJ, Nesbit DE, Fisher DR, Fritz SL, Dwyer SJ III, Templeton AW, Lin F, Jewell WR: Computed tomographic mammography using a conventional body scanner. AJR 138:553, 1982.

26. Munzenrider JE, Tchakarova I, Castro M, Carter B: Computerized body tomography in breast cancer: I. Internal mammary nodes and radiation treatment planning. Cancer 43:137, 1979.

27. Meyer JE, Munzenrider JE: Computed tomographic demonstration of internal mammary lymph node metastasis in patients with locally recurrent breast carcinoma. Radiology 139:661, 1981.

28. Marks BW, Kuhns LR: Identification of the pleural fissures with computed tomography. Radiology 143:139, 1982.

28a. Frija J, Schmit P, Katz M, Vadrot D, Laval-Jeantet M: Computed tomography of the pulmonary fissures: Normal anatomy. J Comput Assist Tomogr 6:1069, 1982.

28b. Proto AV, Ball JB Jr: Computed tomography of the major and minor fissures. AJR 140:439, 1983.

29. Goodman LR, Golkow RS, Steiner RM, Teplick SK, Haskin ME, Himmelstein E, Teplick JG: The right mid-lung window: A potential source of error in computed tomography of the lung. Radiology 143:135, 1982.

30. Speckman JM, Gamsu G, Webb WR: Alterations in CT mediastinal anatomy produced by an azygos lobe. AJR 137:47, 1981.

31. Rabinowitz JG, Wolf BS: Roentgen significance of the pulmonary ligament. Radiology 87:1013, 1966.

32. Pugatch RD, Faling LJ, Robbins AH, Snider GL: Differentiation of pleural and pulmonary lesions using computed tomography. J Comput Assist Tomogr 2:601, 1978.

33. Dwyer A: The displaced crus: A sign for distinguishing between pleural fluid and ascites on computed tomography. J Comput Assist Tomogr 2:598, 1978.

34. Katz D, Kreel L: Computed tomography in pulmonary asbestosis. Clin Radiol 30:207, 1979.

34a. Webb WR, Cooper C, Gamsu G: Interlobar pleural plaque mimicking a lung nodule in a patient with asbestos exposure. J Comput Assist Tomogr 7:135, 1983.

35. Kreel L: Computed tomography in mesothelioma. Semin Oncol 8:302, 1981.

36. Rabinowitz JG, Efremidis SC, Cohen B, Dan S, Efremidis A, Chahinian AP, Teirstein ASA: A comparative study of mesothelioma and asbestosis using computed tomography and conventional chest radiography. Radiology 144:453, 1982.

36a. Law MR, Gregor A, Husband JE, Kerr IH: Computed tomography in the assessment of malignant mesothelioma of the pleura. Clin Radiol 33:67, 1982.

37. Brown LR, Muhm JR, Gray JE: Radiographic detection of thymoma. AJR 134:1181, 1980.

38. Baron RL, Lee JKT, Sagel SS, Levitt RG: Computed tomography of the abnormal thymus. Radiology 142:127, 1982.

39. Callen PW, Filly RA, Korobkin M: Computed tomographic evaluation of the diaphragmatic crura. Radiology 126:413, 1978.

40. Reed JO, Lang EF: Diaphragmatic hernia in infancy. AJR 82:437, 1959.

41. Betts RA: Subcostosternal diaphragmatic hernia with report of five cases. AJR 75:269, 1956.

42. Heiberg E, Wolverson MK, Hurd RN, Jagannadharao B, Sundaram M: CT recognition of traumatic rupture of the diaphragm. AJR 135:369, 1980.

43. Rohlfing BM, Korobkin M, Hall AD: Computed tomography of intrathoracic omental herniation and other mediastinal fatty masses. J Comput Assist Tomogr 1:181, 1977.

44. Schulman A, Fataar S: CT in diaphragmatic rupture? (letter). AJR 136:1256, 1981.

45. Heiberg E, Sundaram M, Wolverson MK: CT in diaphragmatic rupture? (letter). AJR 136:1256, 1981.

46. Rubinstein ZJ, Solomon A: CT findings in partial eventration of the right diaphragm. J Comput Assist Tomogr 5:719, 1981.

47. Anderson LS, Forrest JV: Tumors of the diaphragm. AJR 119:259, 1973.

9 COMPUTED TOMOGRAPHY OF THE HEART AND PERICARDIUM

Martin J. Lipton

Robert J. Herfkens

Gordon Gamsu

The development of commercial CT scanners[1] has created great interest in applying this type of imaging modality to the diagnosis of cardiac diseases. The excellent spatial and density resolution of a CT scan favors its application in the noninvasive evaluation of heart disease. This chapter deals with advantages and limitations of CT scanning for cardiac and pericardial abnormalities. Although the uses for CT scanning are still being developed, clinical applications have been established and new developments are progressing rapidly.

Heart

CT scanning has several unique advantages over the other modalities currently used for the diagnosis and evaluation of heart disease. Images are displayed in cross-sectional digital form and are stored in the scanner's computer, providing the opportunity for image manipulation, analysis, and direct quantitation. CT scans also have greater density resolution (0.5 to 1.0 per cent) than conventional x-ray film/screen systems (5 to 10 per cent). Calcifications, for example, can be identified with great precision on CT scans (Fig. 9–1). The spatial resolution of CT scans is superior to that of nuclear medicine scintiphotos; and, unlike echocardiography, CT scanning is not impeded by air in the lungs or by the bones of the thoracic cage. The application of CT for cardiac imaging requires special considerations because both cardiac structure and function must be evaluated. Because commercial CT scanners are primarily designed to examine the head and body (where motion is minimal and relatively long exposure times are well tolerated), investigators initially assumed that motion artifacts would preclude imaging of the beating heart.[2, 3]

Cardiac CT studies were at first limited to feasibility studies in postmortem hearts and models.[4–6] The development of CT scanners with scan times of less than 5 seconds, in conjunction with the in-

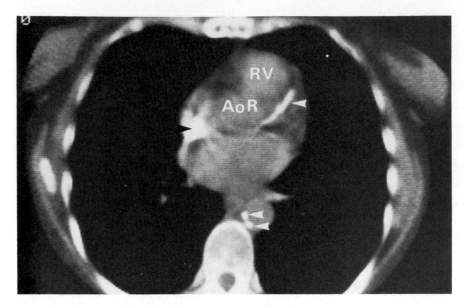

Figure 9–1. Normal anatomy at the level of the aortic root. CT scan shows calcification in the left main coronary artery, left anterior descending coronary artery (anterior white arrowhead), and descending aorta (posterior arrowheads). The aortic root (AoR) is posteromedial to the outflow tract of the right ventricle (RV). Contrast medium has been injected into a peripheral vein and the bolus has reached the superior vena cava (black arrowhead).

intravenous injection of contrast medium, has made in vivo CT cardiac imaging feasible.[7-9]

ANATOMY

The heart begins its embryologic life as a simple tube that subsequently becomes folded and coiled upon itself, so that eventually it has the shape of a blunt cone with an apex and a base. The apex of the heart lies in a caudal and ventral position, pointing to the left.[10] Although its position changes continually during life, the apex in the adult remains close to the left fifth intercostal space approximately 8 cm from the midsternal line.

The heart is overlapped by an extension of the pleura and lungs and the anterior thoracic wall. The base of the heart forms the base of the blunt cone, facing to the right, cranially and also in a dorsal direction. The base comprises primarily the left atrium but also part of the right atrium and a little of the proximal portion of the great vessels. The right atrial border forms the right aspect of the heart on the chest radiograph (Fig. 9–2).[11] The diaphragmatic surface of the heart lies against the diaphragm and comprises the two ventricles. The coronary sulcus marks the plane of the atrioventricular groove.

The left ventricle and a small part of the left atrial appendage form the left border of the heart (Fig. 9–2). The right atrium is larger than the left atrium and has a capacity of approximately 60 ml in the adult; its walls are about 2 mm thick. The right atrial cavity comprises two parts: a principal cavity and an appendage or auricle. The right atrial appendage is shaped like the ear of a dog and is a blind pouch extending cranially between the superior vena cava and the right ventricle. Muscular bundles, termed musculi pectinati because they resemble the teeth of a comb, comprise the internal surface of the atrium.

The superior vena cava opens into the cranial and posterior part of the right atrium. Its orifice directs blood toward the atrioventricular opening. The inferior vena cava opens into the most caudal part of the right atrium near the interatrial septum and its orifice is larger than the superior vena caval opening. The coronary sinus enters the right atrium between the inferior vena cava and the atrioventricular opening. It is responsible for returning blood from the muscle of the heart itself.

The left ventricular chamber is an ellipsoid sphere surrounded by muscular walls 8 to 11 mm thick, which are three times thicker than those of the right ventricle (Fig. 9–3). The left ventricle has two walls: a medial wall (the ventricular septum) which is shared with the right ventricle, and a lateral wall. Both walls are concave toward the cavity. The septum is triangular in shape, with its base located at the level of the aortic valve. It is entirely muscular except for the small membranous septum located just below the right and posterior aortic cusps. The upper third of the septum has a smooth endocardial surface. The other two thirds of the septum and the remainder of the ventricular walls are ridged by interlacing muscles, the trabeculae carnae.[12] The ventricular wall, exclusive of the septum, is often referred to as the free wall of the left ventricle. A line drawn

Figure 9–2. Cardiac chambers and great vessels superimposed on a normal frontal and lateral chest radiographs. **A** Frontal view of the right-sided structures. **B** Frontal view of the left-sided structures. **C** Lateral view of the right-sided structures. **D** Lateral view of the left-sided structures. (Abbreviations: IV = innominate *(brachiocephalic)* vein, SVC = superior vena cava, RA = right atrium, RV = right ventricle, I = right ventricular infundibulum, PT = pulmonary trunk, LMPA = left main pulmonary artery, RMPA = right main pulmonary artery *(interlobar pulmonary artery)*, AA = ascending aorta, AK = aortic knob, LV = left ventricle, LAA = left atrial appendage, LUPV = left upper *(superior)* pulmonary vein, RUPV = right upper *(superior)* pulmonary vein, LA = left atrium, DA = descending aorta.) (Reproduced, with permission, from Elliott LP, Schiebler GL: The X-ray Diagnosis of Congenital Heart Disease in Infants, Children, and Adults, 2nd ed. Springfield, Ill., Charles C Thomas, 1979, pp 28–34.)

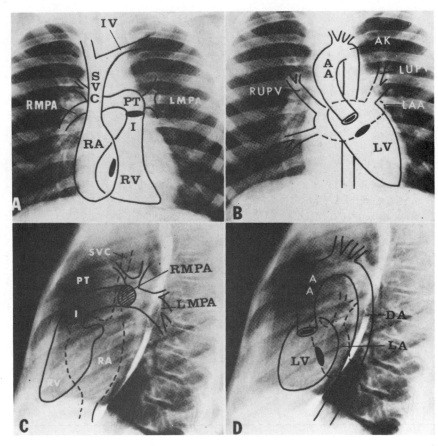

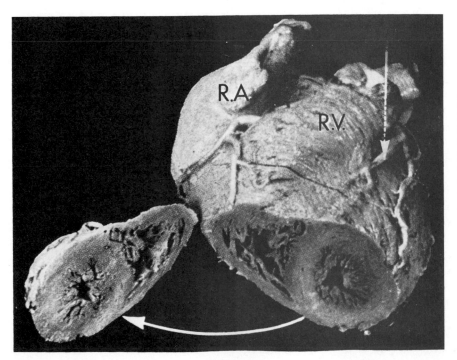

Figure 9–3. Normal heart. Human heart cut in cross section showing the thick-walled left ventricle and thinner-walled right ventricle. The coronary arteries can be seen coursing across the epicardial surface. The left anterior descending coronary artery (arrow) is seen lying along the interventricular groove. Note the markedly irregular trabeculated left ventricular cavity. R.V. = right ventricle; R.A. = right atrium.

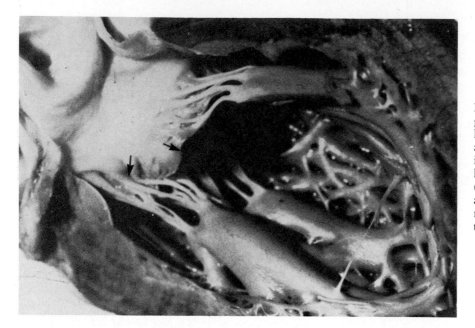

Figure 9–4. Normal heart. Longitudinal section through the left side of the heart, in a right anterior oblique position, showing the anteroseptal mitral valve leaflet and the chordae tendinae (arrows). The papillary muscles and trabeculation result in marked irregularity of the internal architecture of the heart.

from the midpoint of the aortic valve to the cardiac apex can be regarded as the long axis of the chamber. This axis is directed anteriorly, inferiorly and to the left. Although the left ventricle comprises the lower left lateral cardiac border in the frontal chest radiograph, the major portion of its external surface is actually posterolateral.

The right ventricle occupies most of the ventral or sternocostal surface of the heart, anteriorly and to the right of the midline. The right ventricular chamber is triangular and located anteriorly and toward the right of the heart. The right ventricular wall is thinner than the left ventricular wall and, unless thickened, is often poorly defined on CT scans. The pulmonary conus, which is the outflow tract of the right ventricle, swings to the left of the midline and is readily demonstrated on CT scans (Fig. 9–1).

The aortic valve is located at the apex of the outflow tract of the left ventricle. It is a tricuspid valve with the posterior leaflet contiguous with the anterior leaflet of the mitral valve. The aortic valve leaflets cannot be seen routinely on CT scans unless calcified, but their location can be identified. The outflow tract of the left ventricle is irregular but changes to a roughly triangular shape at the sinus of Valsalva. The aortic valve is situated at the triangular sinus of Valsalva and immediately caudal to the circular aortic root (Fig. 9–1). The valve lies in a plane anterior to the left atrium, with the right atrium on the right and the right ventricle and infundibulum on the left.

The mitral valve is located alongside the aortic valve and has two leaflets. The anteroseptal leaflet, the larger and more mobile of the mitral leaf-

lets, is suspended like a curtain diagonally from the top of the posteromedial septum across the ventricular cavity to the anterolateral ventricular wall, separating the left ventricular cavity into an inflow and an outflow tract (Fig. 9–4). The inflow tract, which is funnel-shaped, is formed by the mitral annulus and by both mitral leaflets and their chordae tendinae. It directs blood from the left atrium inferiorly, anteriorly, and to the left. The outflow tract is formed by the inferior surface of the anteroseptal mitral valve leaflet, the ventricular septum, and the free left ventricular wall. It lies at right angles to the inflow tract and directs blood from the apex, superiorly and to the right.[13] The anteromedial mitral leaflet is continuous with supporting tissues of the noncoronary aortic cusps that lie above it. The posterior leaflet, although much shallower in depth than the anterior leaflet, is attached over two thirds of the mitral annulus.

The papillary muscles, located below the anterolateral and posteromedial commissures, arise from the junction of the apical and middle thirds of the ventricular wall (Fig. 9–4). Chordae tendinae are strong chords of fibrous tissue that pass from the papillary muscles to both leaflets of the mitral valve.

The tricuspid valve is oriented vertically, separating the right atrium from the right ventricle. The tricuspid valve cannot be seen on CT scans.

Various anatomic structures on the surface of the heart can be demonstrated on CT scans. The atrioventricular grooves on both the right and left form indentations along the heart borders. The right coronary artery and circumflex coronary artery lie in the right and left atrioventricular grooves, respectively. The left anterior descending coronary artery arises from the left coronary artery and courses along the left anterior surface of the heart over the ventricular septum. The left descending coronary artery is commonly surrounded by fat and its proximal segment is frequently demonstrated on CT scans.

TECHNIQUES OF EXAMINATION

CT scanners allow the operator to select the thickness of each slice of tissue to be scanned. This is accomplished by changing the width of the x-ray fan beam. Scans 1 cm thick are usually used for cardiac purposes, but 5-mm and even 1.5-mm slices can be obtained. Correct selection of the appropriate anatomic level is important, particularly because present instruments can only image one slice level at a time. A digital radiograph (scout view, projection radiograph) is now available on most scanners for improved localization. As the patient is transported on the CT table through the stationary x-ray fan beam, a slit-digital radiograph is taken (Fig. 9–5). This computed radiograph facilitates localization and has two practical applications. First, the scan level can be precisely and automatically reproduced using the scale in Figure 9–5. Second, sequential contiguous scans at multiple levels can be taken. This procedure is

usually performed in conjunction with intravenous infusion of contrast medium and permits the collection of a cubic matrix of CT data (Fig. 9–6). The cube, which is stored in the computer, permits the reconstruction of any axial projection from a plane selected by the operator and defined in a transverse image.

Cardiovascular CT scanning is of limited value without contrast enhancement of the intravascular compartment because the differences in the x-ray attenuation coefficients of blood and muscle are small. Initially, difficulties were encountered in timing the CT scan exposure to coincide with the arrival of a peripherally injected bolus of intravenous contrast medium. The problem was subsequently overcome by modifying CT scanners to perform rapid sequential scanning. The development has become known as dynamic CT and has greatly facilitated the application of CT imaging to the evaluation of cardiovascular disorders.

Intravenous contrast medium can be administered in several ways for cardiac CT scanning. The usual method is a rapid intravenous infusion of 100 to 150 ml of 76 to 90 per cent contrast medium. For dynamic scanning, the rapid injection of a bolus of 25 to 30 ml of contrast medium through an 18-gauge catheter in a medial antecubital vein is suitable (Fig. 9–7). Contrast medium has been injected directly into a coronary artery, providing an excellent demonstration of

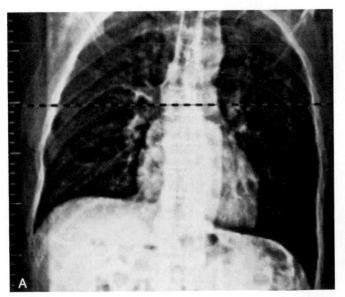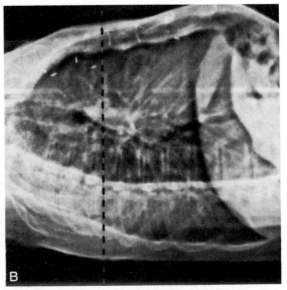

Figure 9–5. Computed radiographs. Anteroposterior (**A**) and lateral (**B**) computed radiographs obtained by transporting the patient through the pulsed x-ray fan beam while the tube is kept stationary. The scanner is being used as a slit-digital radiographic system, and the resulting image has a wide dynamic range; it allows precise slice registration. Three radiopaque surgical clips placed on the ascending aorta can be seen. The dotted line illustrates a suitable scan-level for scanning coronary artery bypass grafts.

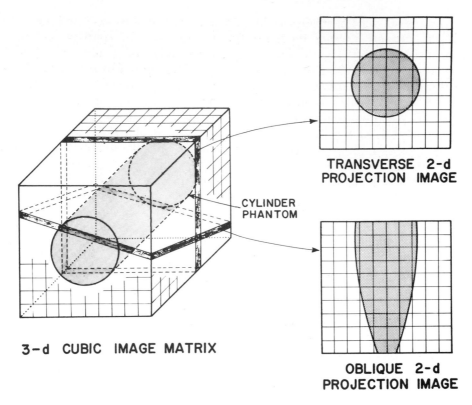

Figure 9–6. Image reformatting from multiplanar scanning. Multiple contiguous scanning provides a three-dimensional cubic matrix of image data stored in the CT computer. The operator can then select any chosen plane in a transverse scan from which the computer reconstructs the appropriate oblique, sagittal or coronal image. This provides projection images resembling angiographic projections, and has diagnostic flexibility and versatility. The oblique plane through the cylinder depicted results in a projection image which may not always be intuitively anticipated.

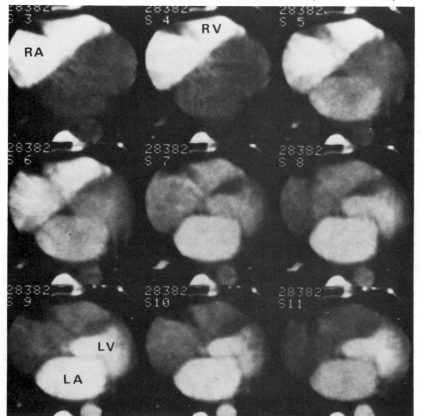

Figure 9–7. Dynamic CT scan through the atrioventricular valves. A dynamic CT scan sequence following a 25-ml peripheral intravenous bolus of Renografin 76. The first scan displayed in this capsule is No. 3 from the series and shows the right atrium (RA) and ventricle (RV). Subsequently the left atrium (LA) and ventricle (LV) are demonstrated. The respective planes of the atrioventricular valves are well seen in scans 6 and 8 through 11.

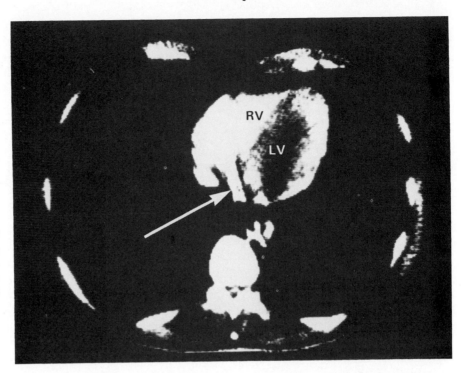

Figure 9–8. Coronary artery injection of contrast medium. A 1-cm thick nongated CT scan obtained with a 4.8-second scan time through the heart at the level of the ventricles following a bolus injection of Renografin 76 into the patient's left main coronary artery. The left ventricular wall is seen to enhance, dramatically outlining the nonenhanced left ventricular (LV) cavity. The venous drainage of the LV myocardium into the coronary sinus (arrow) and subsequently into the right ventricle (RV)—hence enhancement of that cavity—is shown.

cardiac anatomy, but it should not be used routinely (Fig. 9–8).[8]

Rapid incrementation of the scanner table allows multilevel sequential scanning. The whole heart, and, when necessary, the whole thorax, can be scanned by obtaining contiguous slices either 5 or 10 mm thick. Intravenous infusion of contrast medium (1 to 3 ml/kg body weight) is started, and contiguous CT scanning is performed during suspended inspiration. Sagittal, coronal, or oblique images can be reformatted from the multiple CT scans. Rapid dynamic acquisition of these adjacent slices during as few breath-holds as possible improves the quality of the reformatted images.

A further modification of dynamic CT scanning is electrocardiographic-gating (ECG-gating).

This technique allows examination of changes in the heart during the cardiac cycle using present CT scanners with relatively long exposure times (Fig. 9–9).[14–20] The CT programs for ECG-gating are not available on all CT scanners, and the clinical utility of the method is still being defined. Global as well as regional changes in the shape of the ventricular cavities can be demonstrated. Abnormalities in myocardial wall dynamics have also been described in experimental studies.[15, 19] ECG-gated CT scanning permits the measurement of ventricular wall contractility and thickness, which is a sensitive indicator of myocardial ischemia.[18] The tomographic display of CT scans overcomes many of the problems of limited views inherent in the projection images of angiography. Presently

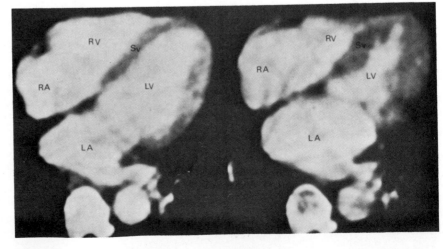

Figure 9–9. ECG-gated cardiac CT scans. CT scan through the ventricles during diastole (left) and systole (right) demonstrate normal contractility of the left ventricle. (Abbreviations: RA = right atrium, RV = right ventricle, SV = interventricular septum, LV = left ventricle, LA = left atrium.) (Reproduced with permission from Lackner K, Thurn P: Computed tomography of the heart: ECG-gated and continuous scans. Radiology 140:414, 1981.)

available whole body scanners allow retrospective or prospective ECG-gating of a single anatomic level at a time. Prospective ECG-gating in which the x-ray tube exposes only during preselected phases of the cardiac cycle (e.g., end-systole and end-diastole), reduces radiation exposure. When intermediate phases of the cardiac cycle are required, either retrospective or continuous prospective gating is necessary. The development of millisecond CT scanners in the near future should enable ECG-gating to reach its full potential (see Chapter 1).

PATHOLOGY

ISCHEMIC HEART DISEASE

Ischemic heart disease, also known as coronary artery disease, is the prime killer of men over the age of 35 and of all adults over the age of 40 in the United States. Each year 1.2 million Americans sustain their first heart attack and at least one third die within a month. Only 50 per cent of surviving patients can be completely rehabilitated. Thus, coronary artery disease is perhaps the most urgent medical problem of our time.[21]

More than 100 million electrocardiograms are performed annually, but a heart attack is often the first confirmation of advanced disease. The sequence of events leading to heart attack is usually gradual, occurring over a number of years. Thus, with a sufficiently sensitive diagnostic procedure, there should be ample opportunity for early diagnosis. The introduction of such a procedure could have a major impact on the success of currently available therapeutic methods.

Stenosis or obstruction of one or more coronary arteries jeopardizes the blood supply to regions of the myocardial wall. The process ultimately results in progressive ischemic damage and replacement of viable heart muscle by connective tissue. This may follow an acute episode of myocardial infarction or it may develop insidiously. The patient's prognosis is related to the size of the myocardial damage, which may be as large as a third of the entire heart.

The tissue changes caused by ischemia are poorly detected by presently available diagnostic techniques. Perhaps the best available procedure for determining myocardial blood flow is the thallium scan. Unfortunately, this procedure gives low-resolution images of the distribution of the radioactive tracer in the heart wall and can only estimate relative myocardial perfusion.

Despite remarkable advances in the development of noninvasive imaging techniques, the diagnostic "gold standard" remains traditional cardiac catheterization with hemodynamic recordings and angiocardiography. Invasive procedures, however, are costly, require patient hospitalization, and carry the risk of major complications. These disadvantages preclude their use for widespread patient screening. Angiocardiography, because it is not three-dimensional and because it is primarily an anatomic study that cannot directly quantitate regional myocardial perfusion, is also limited. Angiography cannot measure myocardial wall thickening or precisely determine the mass of the left ventricle.

The established noninvasive modalities of echocardiography and isotope imaging have contributed greatly to the routine management of patients with ischemic heart disease but have not yet significantly reduced the need for cardiac catheterization. The main reason for this failure is that these techniques, at least at the present time, are unable to provide the necessary structural and functional information obtained by angiocardiography. It is for these reasons that it is worth pursuing computed tomography, which can provide most of this structural and functional information, and may, in the future, be able to measure myocardial blood flow.

Acute Myocardial Infarction

One of the most exciting prospects for CT imaging of the heart is the recognition and quantification of myocardial infarction. CT scans in dogs have shown that infarcted myocardium demonstrates abnormal opacification after intravenous injection or infusion of contrast medium.[3, 4, 6] The density change seen in acute infarcts can involve two phases. An initial low-density region within the area of the infarct relative to normal myocardium, which is probably explained on the basis of inadequate blood supply to this zone, so that the contrast cannot initially reach it. A second, more delayed phase can be seen approximately 5 to 10 minutes following contrast medium infusion. During this phase, the zone of infarction takes up relatively more contrast agent than the surrounding myocardium from which the contrast material has washed out.[8, 9] The increase in density of the infarcted region is probably due to delayed uptake of contrast agent, primarily in the peripheral zone of the infarct, whereas the central zone may not show an increased CT density. The mechanism is not understood but may be due to a breakdown in membrane integrity and intracellular admission of contrast material or to the pooling of contrast material in dilated vessels.

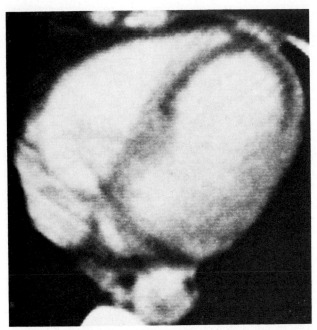

Figure 9–10. Acute myocardial infarction. Nongated CT scan through the ventricles following an intravenous infusion of Conray 400 (1.5 ml/kg body weight) in a patient with an acute (3-day-old) anteroseptal myocardial infarction. The infarcted region is depicted as the dark horseshoe-shaped area of myocardium. The remaining normal myocardium is contrast enhanced, some of which can be seen bordering the infarct. (Reproduced with permission from Boyd DP, Lipton MJ: Cardiac computed tomography. In Harmon GH (ed): IEEE Proceedings on Computed Tomography [in press].)

Multiple CT scans at either 0.5-cm or 1-cm intervals from the apex to the base of the heart encompass the entire ventricular myocardium. The area of infarction can be determined on each CT scan. Thus, from contiguous scans throughout the heart, the total volume of infarcted myocardium can be measured.

CT studies in patients, in whom less contrast material has been injected than in dogs, also demonstrate the initial decreased density or perfusion deficit phase (Fig. 9–10). These findings are being explored for the assessment of the size of myocardial infarction. In patients, however, validation has been limited. In preliminary studies, enzyme indicators of muscle necrosis (e.g., serum creatine phosphokinase levels) that are correlated well with infarct extent, also correlate with CT estimates of infarct size.[22] The delayed enhancement phase has been seen less frequently and less dramatically than in dogs. Further experience with CT scanning of patients after acute infarction will be necessary before the efficacy of this technique for sizing myocardial infarction can be ascertained.

An additional critical need is to find a method of identifying and quantitating areas of jeopardized ischemic myocardium that are viable but at risk of becoming necrotic, as opposed to areas of frankly necrotic myocardium.[23] Such a method, particularly one that is noninvasive, could be repeated easily at short intervals. It would enable the effectiveness of therapeutic measures on infarct size to be evaluated. Although early animal studies indicated that CT scans may have difficulty in demonstrating subendocardial myocardial infarction, later studies did not confirm these findings.[15, 24] The potential ability of CT scanning for these purposes remains to be determined.

Electrocardiographic-gated CT scans can already demonstrate the regional wall motion abnormalities associated with acute infarction (Fig. 9–11). Future developments in CT scanners may allow more extensive evaluation of acute myocardial infarction. Faster cardiac CT scanners with simultaneous multislice capability could well be more accurate than echocardiography or gated

Figure 9–11. Myocardial infarction with akinesia. ECG-gated cardiac CT scans show thinning of the infarcted wall of the left ventricle (LV). The left ventricular cavity is dilated. Scans during diastole *(left)* and systole *(right)* demonstrate akinesia (arrowheads) of the infarcted myocardium. (Reproduced with permission from Lackner K, Thurn P: Computed tomography of the heart: ECG-gated and continuous scans. Radiology 140: 417, 1981.)

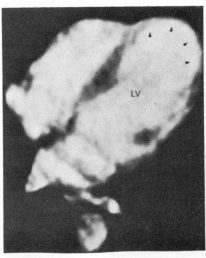
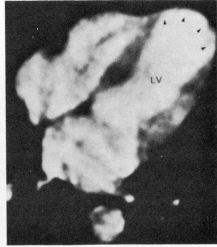

radioisotope methods in demonstrating regional myocardial abnormalities.

Left Ventricular Aneurysm

Left ventricular aneurysm formation is an important complication of acute myocardial infarction and occurs in 12 to 15 per cent of cases.[25, 26] Most aneurysms are chronic and form slowly. The patient becomes symptomatic weeks or months after the acute infarction, exhibiting chronic congestive heart failure or episodes of peripheral emboli.

The anterolateral wall of the left ventricle and interventricular septum are usually involved. The affected myocardium initially demonstrates akinesis but later loses support, becomes dilated, and will show paradoxical motion.[27] During ventricular systole, the aneurysm expands because blood is forced into it from the functional part of the ventricle. The ejection fraction falls, and cardiac output diminishes. During ventricular diastole, the blood in the aneurysm is added to the atrial blood entering the ventricle and results in an increase in resting ventricular volume. The benefits from excision of a ventricular aneurysm are controversial. Systemic embolism, chronic heart failure, and persistent arrhythmia are generally considered indications for surgery.[27] Detection of chronic aneurysm is thus of importance. CT scanning is a simple noninvasive method for detecting and studying ventricular aneurysm.[16, 28] Dynamic CT scanning during bolus injections or drip infusion of contrast medium can demonstrate the marked thinning of the ventricular wall that is usually seen with a ventricular aneurysm. This marked thinning is a well-recognized finding at surgery and could be a useful criterion for defining a left ventricular aneurysm. In addition, distortion of the cardiac contour typically present in left ventricular aneurysms is well demonstrated on CT scans (Fig. 9–12). ECG-gated CT scans can show areas of abnormal contractility of the left ventricular wall.[16] Multiplanar CT scans may assist in selecting patients suitable for aneurysm resection.

Intracardiac Thrombus

The ability to define the internal and external margins of the myocardium is a significant advantage of CT scanning, compared with angiography. After myocardial infarction and open heart surgery, mural thrombi develop within the left ventricular cavity in 20 to 60 per cent of patients.[29, 30] After intravenous contrast medium infusion, the ventricular cavity and the myocardial wall opacify with contrast material. Mural throm-

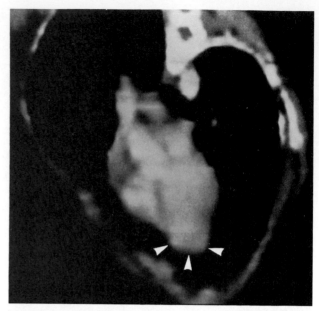

Figure 9–12. Left ventricular aneurysm. Reformatted CT image in an oblique plane shows an apical aneurysm (arrowheads) of the left ventricle.

bus does not change its CT density after contrast medium infusion and is readily seen as a nonenhancing mass within the heart chamber (Fig. 9–13).[31, 32]

In a small series of patients with recent acute infarction or ventricular aneurysm, CT scanning showed at least equivalent accuracy to echocardiography for detecting intraventricular thrombus.[32] Additional studies will be necessary to define the specificity and sensitivity of CT scanning for this purpose.

CT scanning of the heart can detect thrombi in the atria as well as in the ventricles. Tomada and colleagues[33] accurately demonstrated left atrial thrombus in three of 24 patients undergoing mitral valve surgery.

Coronary Artery Bypass Grafts

Approximately 100,000 patients undergo coronary artery bypass graft surgery annually in the United States.[34] The operation bypasses sites of proximal coronary artery stenosis and restores blood flow to the myocardium. Recurrence of symptoms after surgery is common and can result from progressive stenosis of the coronary arteries or from closure of the bypass grafts. Before dynamic CT scanning became available, angiography by selective catheterization of the bypass graft was the only reliable method for demonstrating graft patency.

Dynamic CT scanning after peripheral intravenous injections of 20 to 30 ml of contrast medium is an alternative method of determining graft pat-

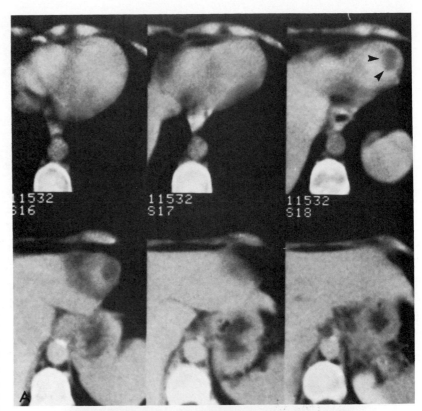

Figure 9–13. Left ventricular thrombus. **A** Six contiguous 1-cm thick CT scans through the ventricles (upper panel) and upper abdomen (lower panel) during contrast material infusion. The filling defect (arrowheads) in the apex of the contrast-enhanced left ventricular cavity is a thrombus (the patient had previous myocardial infarction). **B** A sagittal plane has been selected (vertical line, lower panel) through the thrombus (arrowhead) seen in **A**. The sagittal projection (upper panel) has been reformatted from multiple contiguous scans, showing the thrombus (arrowhead) in relationship to the ventricular cavity.

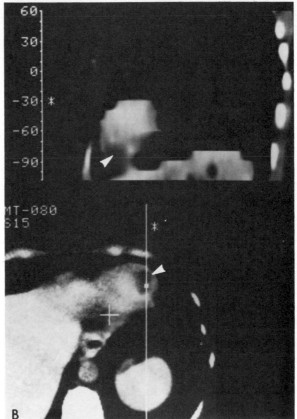

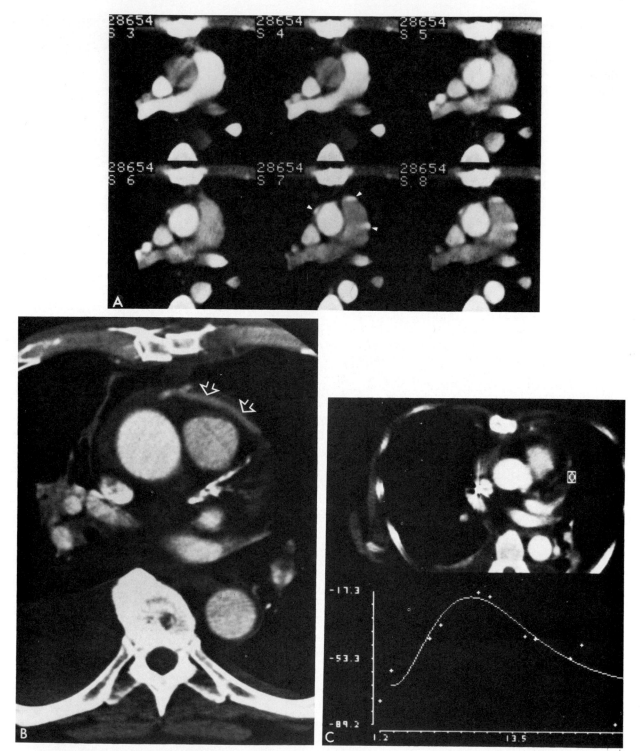

Figure 9–14. Saphenous vein aortocoronary artery bypass grafts. **A** Dynamic CT scan sequence at the level of the aortic root. All three grafts (arrowheads) are seen in cross section, coincident with contrast material reaching the aorta. (Reproduced with permission from Boyd DP, Lipton MJ: Cardiac computed tomography. In Harmon GH (ed): IEEE Proceedings on Computed Tomography [in press].) **B** CT scan in a different patient shortly after aortocoronary artery bypass graft shows the graft (arrows) in longitudinal section anterior to the outflow tract of the right ventricle. The left main and left anterior descending coronary arteries are extensively calcified (GE 9800, 2-second scan). **C** Representative CT scan from a dynamic scan sequence. An area-of-interest cursor is present over a graft on the left. On the lower panel, the CT density measurements have been fitted to a gamma variate curve. Time is on the horizontal axis (seconds) and CT density on the vertical axis (H).

ency.[16, 35–38] Depending on the number and position of the grafts, two to five series of up to 12 rapid sequential scans are obtained through the aortic root. A computed radiograph is useful for selecting the optimum level for scanning. On CT scans, the patent graft will show opacification at about the same time as the passage of the contrast medium through the aorta (Fig. 9–14A,B). Absence of opacification of a graft with a good aortic bolus of contrast medium indicates its occlusion. Both internal mammary artery to coronary artery and saphenous vein aortocoronary bypass grafts can be demonstrated with a diagnostic accuracy between 85 and 95 per cent.[16, 36, 38]

Unfortunately, the technique is limited because significant stenosis in an unoccluded graft cannot be demonstrated on CT scans. Some studies suggest that a semiquantitative estimate of blood flow through grafts can be obtained from the contrast material washout on sequential CT scans.[39] Time-density curves are computed from the change in CT density in an area-of-interest within the graft (Fig. 9–14C). The CT density in the graft rises as the bolus of contrast medium arrives and then slowly falls during the washout phase.

Typically, the rise in CT density takes 2 to 3 seconds and the fall, approximately 10 seconds. Bolus widths of 5 to 10 seconds are typical, and only a small amount of diffusion occurs from the vascular space on the first pass of a bolus.[40] The shape of this time-density curve is best examined by fitting the data to a standard theoretical curve known as a gamma variate.[41] One advantage of this method is that a secondary peak due to rapid recirculation can be eliminated from the analysis by basing the fit on only the first 10 to 15 seconds of data. In a limited number of patients, failure of the data points from an apparently patent graft to fit the gamma variate curve suggested that the flow in the graft was below 50 ml/min. Blood flow through the graft in these patients was determined by electromagnetic flow probes at surgery and by measuring graft diameter and contrast flow velocity from selective angiograms.[39] Despite the problems of heart motion, effects of ionic contrast medium, and delayed mixing (which can produce errors in CT density measurements), the technique is promising as a method of determining blood flow in aortocoronary bypass grafts.

CARDIOMYOPATHY

Cardiomyopathy can be defined as a disease of the myocardium not caused by abnormality of the coronary arteries.[42] Cardiomyopathies are classified both functionally and etiologically (Table 9–1), and both classifications are of practical

Table 9–1. CLASSIFICATION OF CARDIOMYOPATHY

Functional
  Obstructive
  Congestive
  Restrictive
Etiologic
  Primary: Enzyme deficiencies, genetic influences
  Secondary
    Viral infection
    Neurogenic: e.g., Friedreich's ataxia
    Infiltration: e.g., amyloid
    Toxic: e.g., alcohol
    Metabolic: e.g., diabetes mellitus
    Connective tissue disease: e.g., lupus, scleroderma

value. The disease can be difficult to diagnose clinically, and conventional radiographic studies will frequently not assist in diagnosis.

CT scanning in patients with cardiomyopathy has been limited. However, in the obstructive type of cardiomyopathy, some abnormal CT findings can be demonstrated. Obstructive cardiomyopathy is characterized by an asymmetric increase in the muscle mass of the ventricles. The left ventricular cavity is small and heavily trabeculated. CT scans typically show thickening of the myocardial wall and asymmetry of the interventricular septum.[16] Cardiac contractility can be vigorous, so that the left ventricular cavity moves more than usual. CT scans, particularly near the apex of the heart, will demonstrate excessive amounts of motion artifacts. In most patients with obstructive cardiomyopathy, the aortic root is normal in size; this is readily shown on CT scans.

Aortic valve stenosis can also cause hypertrophy of the left ventricle. This is, however, usually symmetrical and invariably associated with enlargement of the aortic root. Both of these findings can be demonstrated on CT scans.

NEOPLASMS

Cardiac neoplasms can be primary or metastatic. Primary neoplasms are rare, occurring in less than 1 in 1000 autopsies.[43] Atrial myxomas account for about 50 per cent of primary neoplasms[44, 45] and can be difficult to diagnose because they can simulate a variety of other cardiac or noncardiac diseases. The other primary cardiac neoplasms are rhabdomyoma, fibroma, lipoma, angioma, papilloma, teratoma, and sarcoma.[46, 47] Cardiac myxomas arise in the left atrium 75 per cent of the time and in the right atrium 20 per cent of the time.

Metastatic tumor to the heart is 10 to 20 times more common than primary tumor, although less than 10 per cent are diagnosed while the patient

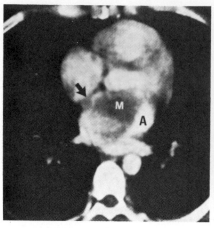
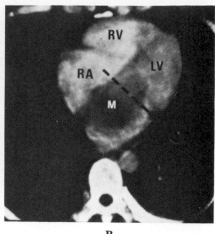

A   **B**

Figure 9–15. Left atrial myxoma. **A** CT scan through the left atrium after an intravenous bolus of contrast material. A large mass (M) in the left atrium (A) is attached to the interatrial septum (arrow). **B** CT scan through the mitral valve (dashed line) shows the mass (M) protruding into the left ventricle (LV). The right atrium (RA) and right ventricle (RV) are normal. (Reproduced with permission from Norlindh T, Lilja B, Nyman U, Hellekant C: Left atrial myxoma demonstrated with CT. AJR 137: 154, 1981. © 1981, American Roentgen Ray Society.)

is still alive.[47–49] The most common tumors to spread hematogenously to the heart are melanoma, breast carcinoma, and lung carcinoma.[48–50] Alternative modes of spread to the heart are direct invasion through the pericardium and tumor growth along the great veins into the heart.

Echocardiography and angiocardiography are the accepted methods of diagnosing both primary and metastatic cardiac tumors.[51, 52] Echocardiography is risk-free and has excellent temporal resolution. Angiocardiography provides excellent spatial and temporal resolution but does entail the risks of cardiac catheterization. CT scans have a high degree of tissue discrimination and can demonstrate abnormalities in the pericardium, mediastinum, and lung around the heart. Several case reports have described the CT scan findings in cardiac myxomas[16, 53, 54] and metastases to the heart.[55–57] In all cases, CT scans after infusion of contrast material showed an intracardiac filling defect representing the tumor mass (Fig. 9–15). The location and extent of the tumor can be demonstrated as well as any additional tumor masses. In one case of a metastatic osteogenic sarcoma, an area of high CT density was found.[55]

Until confirmation of the utility of CT scanning for cardiac tumor is available, this imaging modality must be considered an adjunct. Echocardiography and angiocardiography should remain the primary imaging techniques.

Pericardium

The structure and function of the pericardium has interested physicians for centuries. Hippocrates described the pericardium as a "smooth mantle surrounding the heart and containing a small amount of fluid resembling urine."[58] How-

ever, its role in health and disease is poorly understood and still stimulates active investigation. Investigators have suggested that the pericardium prevents overdilation of the heart,[59–61] reduces friction with surrounding structures,[61] facilitates atrial filling,[59] and moderates the pressure-volume relationships of the cardiac chambers.[61–64] Congenital, neoplastic, infectious, metabolic, traumatic, drug-induced, and primary myocardial diseases can all affect the pericardium.

CT scanning is a sensitive noninvasive method for evaluation of the pericardium in health and disease. It can demonstrate the normal pericardium and adjacent cardiac and extracardiac anatomy. Intravenous contrast material delineates vascular structures but is not always necessary for evaluation of pericardial diseases.

ANATOMY

The pericardium is a two-layered stiff membrane that envelops all four cardiac chambers as well as the origins of the great vessels. The two layers are separated by a small amount of fluid. The pericardium is divided into two distinct layers: the visceral and parietal pericardium. These two become continuous at the attachment to the great vessels and form a closed sac surrounding the heart. The pericardium extends to include the proximal ascending aorta, main pulmonary artery, proximal pulmonary veins, and proximal vena cavae.[65]

The base of the pericardium is attached to the central tendon of the diaphragm. Anteriorly, ligaments attach the pericardium to the sternum from the manubrium to the xyphoid. Posteriorly, additional ligaments extend to the dorsal spine.

The visceral pericardium is a serous layer of mesothelial cells closely applied to the surface of the heart and epicardial fat. The membrane is thin, and its close apposition to cardiac structures prevents visualization of the visceral pericardium on CT scans.

The parietal pericardium is a fibrous layer of tissue composed of serosa, fibrosa, and an outer layer of connective tissue containing blood vessels, nerves, and lymphatics. The normal thickness of the parietal pericardium is 1 to 5 mm. The visceral pericardium is separated from the parietal pericardium by a thin layer of pericardial fluid.

Portions of the normal pericardium can be demonstrated on CT scan in almost all patients (Fig. 9–16A,B).[66–68] The inferior, ventral pericar-

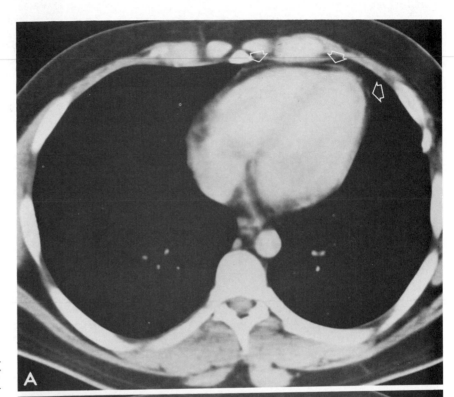

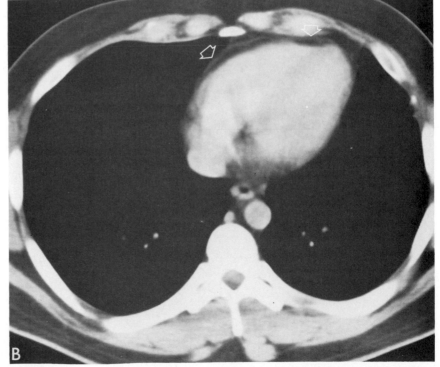

Figure 9–16. Normal pericardium. **A, B** Two adjacent CT scans show the normal pericardium anteriorly and to the left, over the left ventricle (arrows) (GE 9800, 2-second scans).

dium lies between mediastinal and epicardial fat and is the area usually seen on CT scans, especially where epicardial fat surrounds the coronary vessels. This part of the pericardium can have slightly thicker areas than the rest of the pericardium; these areas can be up to 7 mm in thickness, and may be responsible for the pericardium appearing patchy on CT scans.[66]

PATHOLOGY

CONGENITAL ANOMALIES

Congenital malformations of the pericardium are uncommon. These include defects or absence of portions of the pericardium, cysts, diverticula, and benign teratomas.[69] Defects of the pericardium have been recognized since the 16th century. Their cause is obscure but may be secondary to embryologic abnormalities in the vascular supply to the pericardium. Most pericardial defects are partial, and absence of the pericardium occurs in only 9 per cent of cases. Approximately 70 per cent of defects are on the left side. In about half of these, the entire left side of the pericardium is absent and in the other half, the pericardium is partially deficient.[69, 70] Partial defects on the right represent only 4 per cent of cases, whereas diaphragmatic pericardial defects account for 17 per cent.[70]

Approximately a third of patients with pericardial defects have other congenital abnormalities, including atrial septal defect,[71] patent ductus arteriosus,[72] bronchogenic cyst,[73] pulmonary sequestration,[74] mitral stenosis, and tetralogy of Fallot.[70] Patients with cardiac abnormalities can experience atypical chest pain, syncope, and dyspnea. Patients without other congenital abnormalities are usually asymptomatic, and the pericardial defect is found on a routine chest radiograph. Complications include herniation and entrapment of a cardiac chamber, especially an atrial appendage, or compression of a coronary artery.[70, 75]

CT scans readily demonstrate a pericardial defect and may be able to suggest an associated cardiac abnormality. On CT scans, absence of the fibrous parietal pericardium can be noted, as well as the direct contact between lung and cardiac chambers (Fig. 9–17).[66, 76] When absence of the diaphragmatic pericardium is part of a pericardioperitoneal communication, CT scans can show herniation of abdominal organs or fat into the pericardium.[77]

Pericardial cysts and diverticula are uncommon lesions. The majority of pericardial cysts contain clear fluid, with a CT density of 0 to 20 Houns-

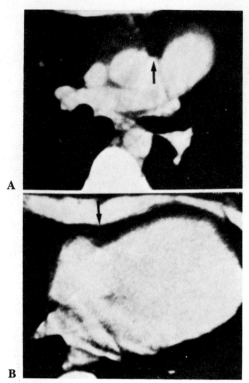

Figure 9–17. Absent left pericardium. **A** CT scan shows aerated lung interposed between the aorta and a prominent main pulmonary artery (arrow). **B** At a caudad level, CT scan demonstrates abrupt termination of the pericardium at an indentation on the anterior cardiac contour (arrow). The heart bulges into the left hemithorax. (Reproduced with permission from Baim RS, MacDonald IL, Wise DJ, Lenkei SC: Computed tomography of absent left pericardium. Radiology 135:128, 1980.)

field Units (H). They are usually located at the right cardiophrenic angle. True pericardial cysts contain all layers of the pericardium and do not communicate with the pericardial space.[78] CT scans provide an excellent method for differentiating pericardial cysts from other masses occurring in this region. On CT scans, pericardial cysts are homogeneous and have a thin smooth wall (Fig. 9–18). Rarely, calcification may occur in the wall of a pericardial cyst.[66, 79, 80]

Congenital diverticula of the pericardium are similar to pericardial cysts but communicate with the pericardium. Their CT appearance should be similar. In our opinion, CT scanning is not warranted in the investigation of an asymptomatic patient with a cardiophrenic angle mass detected on chest radiographs.

EFFUSION

The normal pericardial space contains approximately 20 to 30 ml of fluid. This serouslike fluid is an ultrafiltrate of serum, containing 1.7 to 3.5

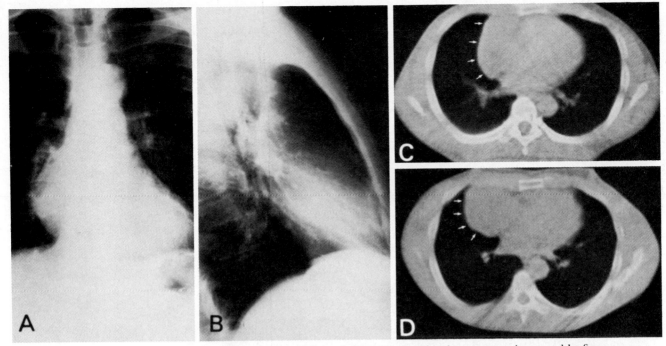

Figure 9–18. Pericardial cyst. Frontal **(A)** and lateral **(B)** radiographs show a mass inseparable from the right heart border. Supine **(C)** and prone **(D)** CT scans demonstrate the mass contiguous with the right side of the heart. The CT density of the mass was that of a cyst. The mass clearly changes shape with change in position of the patient. (Reproduced with permission from Pugatch RD, Braver JH, Robbins AH, Faling LJ: CT diagnosis of pericardial cysts. AJR 131:515, 1978. © 1978, American Roentgen Ray Society.)

per cent protein.[59] Venous or lymphatic obstruction of the drainage from the heart will lead to a pericardial effusion that comes from the visceral pericardium.[81]

The CT density of effusions varies, depending on the protein, cellular, and fat content of the fluid. Common causes of serous effusions are congestive heart failure, hypoalbuminemia, and thoracic irradiation. Serosanguinous effusions usually arise from trauma (including surgery), neoplasm, acute myocardial infarction, and disorders of coagulation. Chylous effusions are rare but can be seen after injury to the thoracic duct. Exusudative effusions are caused by an inflammatory response to infection or neoplasm within the pericardium. Some causes of pleural effusion are cited in Table 9–2.

In the supine patient, a small effusion tends to accumulate posteriorly. A larger effusion forms a layer of fluid that surrounds the heart, displacing the parietal pericardium away from the heart. Pericardial effusion is recognized on CT scans as a layer of fluid density between the heart and mediastinal fat, parietal pleura, mediastinal organs, or the lungs (Fig. 9–19). Pericardial effusion as small as 50 ml of fluid can be detected on CT scans, which is as sensitive as echocardiography.[82, 83] Effusions of 200 ml are required to surround the heart completely.

Table 9–2. CAUSES OF PERICARDITIS AND PERICARDIAL EFFUSION

Infective
  Bacterial
  Tuberculous
  Fungal: Histoplasmosis, actinomycosis
  Viral: Coxsackie B, influenza, ECHO
  Parasitic: Amebiasis, toxoplasmosis, echinococcosis
Postinjury
  Postmyocardial infarction syndrome: Acute myocardial
    infarction
  Postpericardiotomy
  Post-traumatic: Penetrating and non-penetrating wounds
  Physical: Burns, ionizing radiation
Neoplasm
  Lymphoma, leukemia, sarcoma
  Carcinoma: Breast, lung
  Mesothelioma
Connective Tissue Disease
  Lupus erythematosus
  Rheumatic fever
  Rheumatoid arthritis
  Scleroderma
Metabolic
  Uremia
  Hypothyroidism
Drugs
  Procainamide
  Hydrazaline
  Psicofuranine
Dissecting Aortic Aneurysm
Chylopericardium
Idiopathic

THICKENING

Today, pericarditis is most commonly viral and specifically due to coxsackie viruses.[84] Nontuberculous bacterial pericarditis has become uncommon and usually has a predisposing factor such as trauma, surgery, immunosuppression, or infective endocarditis. Tuberculosis and irradiation both cause pericardial thickening that can lead to constriction. Pericarditis and thickening can also be associated with systemic disease such as renal failure, rheumatoid arthritis, scleroderma, and systemic lupus erythematosus.

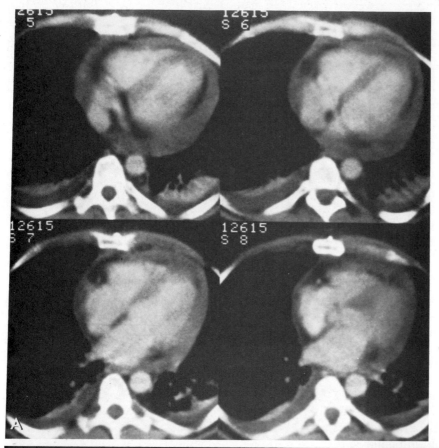

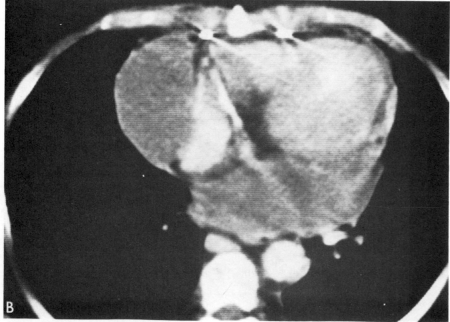

Figure 9–19. Pericardial effusion in three patients. **A** Four sequential CT scans show a moderately large pericardial effusion surrounding the heart. The CT attenuation of the fluid was 6 H. **B** CT scan 6 months after cardiac surgery in a patient with acute chest pain. The scan through the lower heart shows a large pericardial effusion that has accumulated posteriorly and to the right of the heart. Two epicardial pacemaker wires are seen anteriorly. Four hundred milliliters of blood was removed from the pericardium.

Illustration continued on opposite page

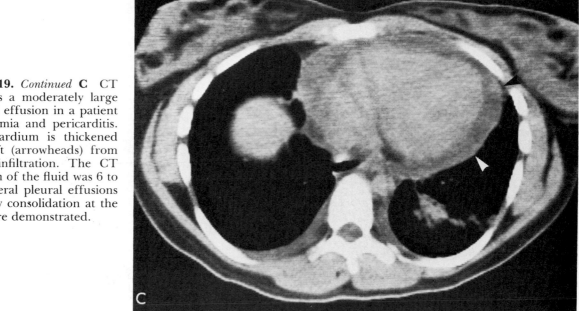

Figure 9–19. *Continued* **C** CT scan shows a moderately large pericardial effusion in a patient with leukemia and pericarditis. The pericardium is thickened on the left (arrowheads) from leukemic infiltration. The CT attenuation of the fluid was 6 to 8 H. Bilateral pleural effusions and patchy consolidation at the left base are demonstrated.

The pericardium responds to many inflammatory stimuli by producing varying amounts of fluid, fibrin deposition, and cellular proliferation. For instance, hemopericardium after surgery can resolve without evidence of pericardial thickening or can result in constrictive pericarditis.[85]

CT scanning offers great promise in solving the difficult clinical problem of separating constrictive pericarditis from restrictive cardiomyopathy. The clinical signs, symptoms and hemodynamic findings of these two conditions are virtually indistinguishable. Echocardiography can be helpful if the constriction is secondary to pericardial effusion. However, echocardiography is relatively insensi-

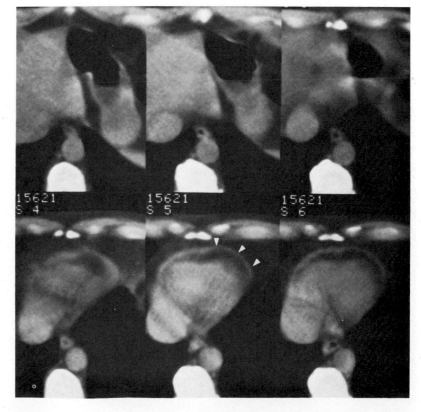

Figure 9–20. Pericardial thickening with constriction. Sequential 1-cm thick CT scans through the heart show a densely thickened pericardium (arrowheads) separated from the myocardium by epicardial fat. The inferior vena cava is dilated. The CT scan appearances combined with the clinical findings led to a diagnosis of constrictive pericarditis.

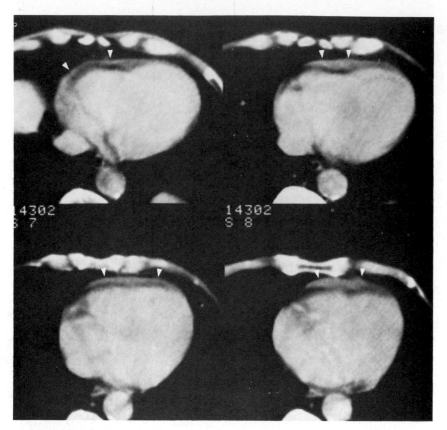

Figure 9–21. Pericardial thickening without constriction. Sequential CT scans through the lower heart show a thickened anterior pericardium (arrowheads). No clinical findings of constriction were present. Patient was being studied for a possible ventricular thrombus.

tive in the detection of pericardial thickening. Several reports have suggested that the CT scan finding of 5 to 20 mm of pericardial thickening can be suggestive of pericardial constriction (Fig. 9–20).[66, 68] A normal pericardium, on the other hand, virtually excludes constriction, leading to the presumptive diagnosis of restrictive cardiomyopathy.

Pericardial thickening, in our experience, does not itself imply constriction unless the clinical signs and hemodynamic changes are present (Fig. 9–21). Prominent thickening without constriction can be seen in several conditions, including the postpericardiotomy and postmyocardial infarction syndromes. These entities occur following cardiac surgery and acute myocardial infarction,

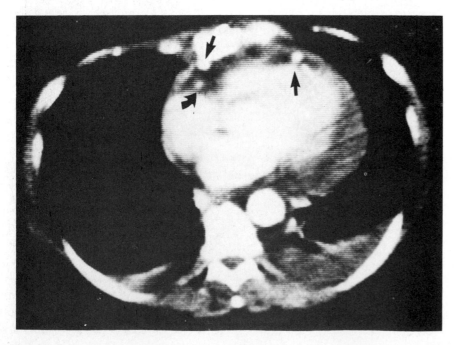

Figure 9–22. Postpericardiotomy syndrome. CT scan after aortocoronary artery bypass surgery. Scan is from a rapid sequential series after intravenous contrast medium injection. Two patent grafts (straight arrows) as well as a large right coronary artery (curved arrow) are demonstrated. Pericardial thickening and effusion and bilateral pleural effusions are evident. (Reproduced with permission from Lipton MJ, Brundage BH, Doherty PW, Herfkens RJ, Berninger WH, Redington RW, Chatterjee K, Carlsson E: Contrast medium-enhanced computed tomography for evaluating ischemic heart disease. Cardiovasc Med 4:1224, 1979.)

respectively, and are most likely immune related. The clinical syndrome includes fever, myalgia, and chest pain, and typically occurs 1 week to 1 year following the initial insult.[86] CT scans of the chest demonstrate prominent pericardial thickening and effusion (Fig. 9–22). Intravenous infusion of contrast material can show enhancement of the thickened pericardium and improve the delineation of pericardial effusion.

CALCIFICATION

Calcification of the pericardium represents the end stage of many inflammatory processes. The most common causes are prior tuberculosis, viral infections, rheumatic fever, and trauma. However, in many instances, no etiology can be found. Histologic study of the pericardium rarely provides a specific diagnosis.[87] Calcification can be microscopic or macroscopic and can encircle the entire heart.[88] The presence of pericardial calcification does not indicate impending constriction.

CT scanning with its high density resolution is the most sensitive method available for detection of calcification. The cross-sectional tomographic format can localize the site of pericardial calcifications (Fig. 9–23A,B). The significance of peri-

Figure 9–23. Tuberculous pericardial calcification with constriction. **A** CT scan shows pericardial calcification on the right (arrowhead) and pericardial thickening on the left (arrows). Right pleural thickening and calcification is also demonstrated. **B** CT scan, 4 cm caudal to scan **A,** shows extensive calcification of the diaphragmatic surface of the pericardium (arrows).

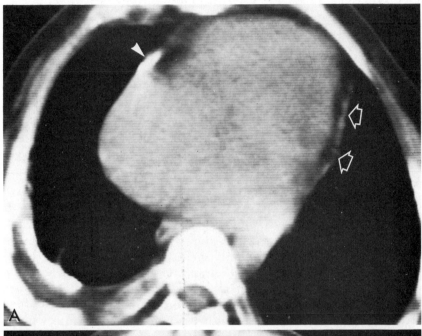

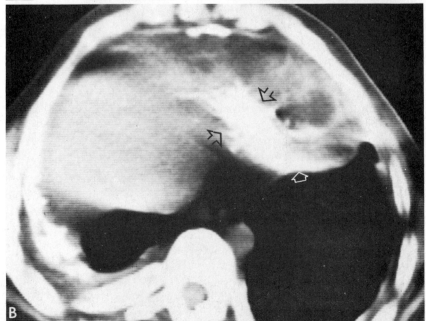

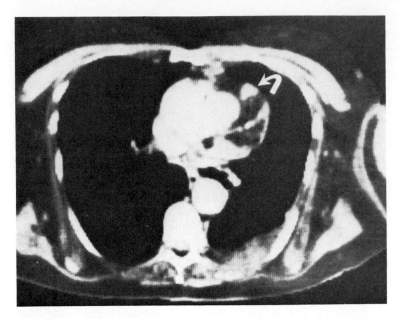

Figure 9–24. Pericardial mesothelioma. CT scan shows a nodular mass arising from the pericardium (arrow). (Reproduced with permission from Moncada R, Baker M, Salinas M, Demos TC, Churchill R, Love L, Reynes C, Hale D, Cardoso M, Pifarr R, Gunnar RM: Diagnostic role of computed tomography in pericardial heart disease: Congenital defects, thickening, neoplasms and effusions. Am Heart J 103:272, 1982.)

cardial calcification, however, should be determined from the patient's symptoms and physical examination.

NEOPLASMS

Primary neoplasms of the pericardium are exceedingly rare. The differentiation of primary malignant myocardial from pericardial tumors can be extremely difficult, if not impossible, even at autopsy. The most common benign tumors are teratoma, lipoma, fibroma, and angioma. Malignant primary pericardial tumors include mesothelioma and both differentiated and undifferentiated sarcoma. The combination of the excellent density resolution and the tomographic format of CT scans provides the most sensitive noninvasive imaging method to localize and characterize neoplasms of the pericardium (Fig. 9–24).

The CT density of malignant pericardial effusion can vary widely, depending on the response of the pericardium. Chylous or pseudochylous effusions, with relatively low attenuation values, can be secondary to neoplastic involvement. Transudative effusions will have intermediate attenuation values. Exudative or hemorrhagic effusions can have higher values, depending on their protein and cellular contents. Unless pericardial masses are evident, the differentiation of malignant effusion from other etiologies, such as radiation-induced pericarditis or idiopathic pericarditis, is not possible with CT scanning. In most cases, pericardiocentesis or thoracotomy and biopsy are necessary for definitive diagnosis of pericardial neoplasms.

Metastasis to the pericardium is much more common than primary pericardial neoplasm. Autopsy series have shown that 5 to 10 per cent of patients with cancer have metastases to the pericardium.[49, 89, 90] In many, however, the pericardial deposits are asymptomatic and not detected before death. Metastasis to the pericardium can occur with almost any neoplasm. Lymphoma, leukemia, breast cancer, and lung carcinoma are the most frequent. Melanoma, although an uncommon tumor, has a high frequency of dissemination to the pericardium.

The principal clinical complication of primary or metastatic neoplasm of the pericardium is pericardial effusion and tamponade.[91] Both can develop insidiously or catastrophically. The clinical features of pericardial tamponade are similar to tumor obstruction of the vena cavae. CT scans after intravenous contrast material infusion frequently separate the two. Although venous obstruction is well demonstrated on CT scans (see Chapter 5), a large pericardial effusion can also be readily shown. The clinical syndrome of cardiac tamponade can also be caused when cardiac restriction results from encasement of the pericardium by tumor. CT scanning is helpful for identifying this type of pericardial involvement.

INDICATIONS FOR COMPUTED TOMOGRAPHY OF THE HEART AND PERICARDIUM

The practical clinical applications of CT scanning of the heart and pericardium are only beginning to be appreciated. In fact, the Special Report of the Society for Computed Body Tomography stated in 1979 that "examinations of intracardiac anatomy are not indicated at this time".[92] Several factors, in fact, do limit the application of cardiac CT scanning:

1. Physiologically, the heart is poorly suited for study by the available, relatively slow CT scanners. The dynamics of myocardial contraction require an instrument with a frequency response in excess of 10 Hz.[93]

2. Many of the studies that have been reported have used specialized fast CT scanners or ECG-gated software, which is not generally available.

3. Computed tomographic scanning of the heart is competing against alternative imaging modalities with excellent spatial or temporal resolution. Sector scan echocardiography, nuclear scalar and tomographic cardiac imaging, digital video subtraction cardiovascular imaging, and angiocardiography all provide detailed images of the heart.[94]

CT scanning has been shown to be of definite value in assessing the patency of coronary artery bypass grafts, cardiac tumors, and intracardiac thrombus. Surprisingly, ungated CT scans taken after contrast material infusion have demonstrated cardiac structures. The detail of cardiac anatomy is nevertheless enhanced by physiologic (ECG) gating of the CT images. In the field of ischemic heart disease, CT can be used to quantitate left ventricular internal measurements and wall thickness. Global and regional assessment of myocardial contractility is possible with ECG-gated images. Limited usefulness has been shown in the diagnosis or evaluation of cardiomyopathy and the effects of coronary artery disease, including myocardial infarction and ventricular aneurysm.

CT scanning for pericardial disease is not severely limited by cardiac motion. The normal pericardium, although only a few millimeters thick, can be demonstrated. CT scans can readily demonstrate pericardial effusion, thickening, tumor, and calcification. The areas in which CT scanning can complement or even provide more information than sector scan echocardiography are pericardial thickening and pericardial tumor.

Many indications and applications of CT scanning of the heart and pericardium require further study and validation. As technologic developments improve CT scanner speed and image manipulation, the goal of functional cardiac imaging should be realized.

REFERENCES

1. Hounsfield GN: Computerized transverse axial scanning (tomography): Part 1: Description of system. Br J Radiol 46:1016, 1973.
2. Ter-Pogossian MM, Weiss ES, Coleman RE: Computed tomography of the heart. AJR 127:79, 1976.
3. Powell WR Jr, Wittenberg J, Maturi RA, Kinsmore RE, Miller SW: Detection of edema associated with myocardial ischemia by computerized tomography in isolated, arrested canine hearts. Circulation 55:99, 1977.
4. Adams DF, Hessel SJ, Judy PF, Stein JA, Abrams HL: Computed tomography of the normal and infarcted myocardium. AJR 126:786, 1976.
5. Lipton MJ, Hayashi TT, Boyd DP, Carlsson E: Ventricular cast volume measurements by computed tomography. Radiology 127:419, 1978.
6. Higgins CB, Sovak M, Schmidt W: Uptake of contrast materials by experimental acute myocardial infarction: A preliminary report. Invest Radiol 13:337, 1978.
7. Gray WR Jr, Parkey RW, Buja LM, Stokely EM, McAllister RE, Bone FJ, Willerson JT: Computed tomography: In vitro evaluation of myocardial infarction. Radiology 122:511, 1977.
8. Carlsson, E. Lipton MJ, Berninger WH, Doherty P, Redington RW: Selective left coronary myocardiography by computed tomography in living dogs. Invest Radiol 12:559, 1977.
9. Doherty PW, Lipton MJ, Berninger WH, Skioldebrand CG, Carlsson E, Redington RW: The detection and quantitation of myocardial infarction in vivo using transmission computed tomography. Circulation 63:597, 1981.
10. Gray H: The Heart. In Goss CM (ed): Anatomy of the Human Body, 28th ed. Philadelphia, Lea & Febiger, 1966, p 543.
11. Elliott LP, Schiebler GL: The X-ray Diagnosis of Congenital Heart Disease in Infants, Children, and Adults, 2nd ed. Springfield, Ill, Charles C Thomas, 1979, pp 28–34.
12. Silverman ME, Schlant RC: Anatomy of the heart and blood vessels. In Hurst JW, Logue RB, Schlant RC, Wenger NK (eds.): The Heart, 4th ed. New York, McGraw-Hill, 1978, p 19–32.
13. Walmsley R, Watson H: The outflow tract of the left ventricle. Br Heart J 28:435, 1966.
14. Berninger WH, Redington RW, Doherty P, Lipton MJ, Carlsson E: Gated cardiac scanning in normal and experimentally infarcted canines. J Comput Assist Tomogr 32:155, 1979.
15. Lipton MJ, Higgins CB: Evaluation of ischemic heart disease by computerized transmission tomography. Radiol Clin North Am 18:557, 1980.
16. Lackner K, Thurn P: Computed tomography of the heart: ECG-gated and continuous scans. Radiology 140:413, 1981.
17. Alfidi RJ, Haaga JR, MacIntyre WJ, Bacon KT, Ferrario CM: Gated computed tomography of the heart. Comput Tomogr 1:51, 1977.
18. Lipton MJ, Naple S, Brundage B, Tyberg J, Boyd D, Redington R: Electrocardiograph gated CT for regional myocardial motion analysis. Circulation 64:220, 1981.
19. Mattrey RF, Higgins CB: Detection of regional myocardial dysfunction during ischemia with computerized tomography. Invest Radiol 17:329, 1982.

20. Ringertz HG, Skioldebrand CT, Refsum H, Tyberg JV, Napel SA, Lipton MJ: A comparison between the information in gated and nongated cardiac CT images. J Comput Assist Tomogr 6:933, 1982.

21. Braunwald ED: Protection of the ischemic myocardium. Circulation (Suppl I) 53:1, 1976.

22. Herfkens RJ, Brundage BH, Kramer P, Goldstein J, Lipton MJ: Transmission computed tomography in acute myocardial infarction. In Proceedings of International Symposium: Advances in Noninvasive Cardiology. The Hague, Martinus Nijhoff Publishers (in press).

23. Sobel B, Shell W: Jeopardized, blighted and necrotic myocardium. Circulation 47: 215, 1973.

24. Gray W, Buja M, Hagler H, Parkey R, Willerson J: Computed tomography for localization and sizing of experimental acute myocardial infarcts. Circulation 58:497, 1978.

25. Abrams DL, Edelist A, Luria MH, Miller AJ: Ventricular aneurysm: A reappraisal based on a study of sixty-five consecutive autopsied cases. Circulation 27:164, 1963.

26. Schlicter J, Hellerstein HK, Katz LN: Aneurysm of the heart. Medicine 33:43, 1954.

27. Gay WA Jr, Ebert PA: Resection of postinfarction aneurysms of the left ventricle. In Coronary Artery Medicine and Surgery: Concepts and Controversies, Norman JC, Lawrence EP (eds.): New York, Appleton-Century-Crofts, 1975, pp 659–661.

28. Herfkens RJ, Goldstein J, Lipton MJ, Schiller NB, Ports TA, Brundage BH: Evaluation of left ventricular aneurysms with contrast enhanced computed tomography and two dimensional echocardiography, abstract. Invest Radiol 17:S10, 1982.

29. DeMaria AN, Bommer W, Neumann A, Grehl T, Weinart L, DeNardo S, Amsterdam EA, Mason DT: Left ventricular thrombi identified by cross-sectional echocardiography. Ann Intern Med 90:14, 1979.

30. Hurst JW, King SP: Coronary atherosclerotic heart disease. In Hurst JW, Logue RB, Schlant RC, Wenger NK (eds.): The Heart, 4th ed. New York, McGraw-Hill, 1978, pp 1129–1130.

31. Goldstein JA, Lipton MJ, Schiller NB, Ports TA, Brundage BH: Evaluation of intracardiac thrombi with contrast enhanced computed tomography and echocardiography. Am J Cardiol 49:972, 1982.

32. Godwin JD, Herfkens RJ, Skioldebrand CG, Brundage BH, Schiller NB, Lipton MJ: Detection of intraventricular thrombi by computed tomography. Radiology 138:717, 1981.

33. Tomoda H, Hoshiai M, Tagawa R, Koide S, Kawada S, Shotsu A, Matsuyama S: Evaluation of left atrial thrombus with computed tomography. Am Heart J 100:306, 1980.

34. Anderson RP: The prognosis of patients with coronary artery disease after coronary bypass operations. Time-related progress of 532 patients with disabling angina pectoris. Circulation 50:274, 1974.

35. Brundage BH, Lipton MJ, Herfkens RJ, Berninger WH, Redington RW, Chatterjee K, Carlsson E: Detection of patient coronary bypass grafts by computed tomography: A preliminary report. Circulation 61:826, 1980.

36. Moncada R, Salinas M, Churchill R, Love L, Reynes C, Demos T, Hale D, Schrieber R: Patency of saphenous aortocoronary bypass grafts demonstrated by computed tomography. N Engl J Med 303:503, 1980.

37. Guthaner DF, Brody WR, Ricci M, Oyer PE, Wesler L: The use of computed tomography in the diagnosis of coronary artery bypass graft patency. Cardiovasc Radiol 3:3, 1980.

38. Daniel WG, Dohring W, Lichtler PR, Stender HS: Noninvasive assessment of aortocoronary bypass graft patency by computed tomography. Lancet 1:1023, 1980.

39. Goldstein J, Brundage B, Herfkens RJ, Lipton MJ, McKay C: Evaluation of coronary bypass graft flow by contrast enhanced computed tomography. Circulation 64:182, 1981.

40. Axel L, Herfkens RJ, Lipton MJ, Berninger WH, Redington RW: Cardiac output determination by dynamic CT. Invest Radiol 14:389, 1979.

41. Thompson HH Jr, Starmer CF, Whalen RE, McIntosh HD: Indicator transit time considered as a gamma variate. Circ Res 14:502, 1964.

42. Goodwin JF: Clarification of the cardiomyopathies. Mod Concepts Cardiovasc Dis 41:41, 1972.

43. Abrams HL, Adams DF, Grant HA: The radiology of tumors of the heart. Radiol Clin North Am 9:299, 1971.

44. Meller J, Teichholz LE, Pichard AD, Matta R, Litwak R, Herman MV, Massie KF: Left ventricular myxoma: Echocardiographic diagnosis and review of the literature. Am J Med 63:816, 1977.

45. O'Neil M Jr, Grehl T, Hurley E: Cardial myxomas: A clinical diagnostic challenge. Am J Surg 138:68, 1979.

46. Prichard RW: Tumors of the heart: Review of the subject and report of one hundred and fifty cases. Arch Pathol 51:98, 1951.

47. Wenger NK: Cardiac tumors. In Hurst JW (ed): The Heart, Arteries, and Veins. New York, McGraw-Hill, 1978, pp 1668–1682.

48. Young JM, Goldman IR: Tumor metastasis to the heart. Circulation 9:220, 1954.

49. Hanfling SM: Metastatic cancer to the heart: Review of the literature and report of 127 cases. Circulation 24:474, 1960.

50. Herbut PA, Maisel AL: Secondary tumors of the heart. Arch Pathol 34:358, 1942.

51. Ports TA, Schiller NB, Strunk BL: Echocardiography of right ventricular tumors. Circulation 56:439, 1977.

52. Ports TA, Cogan J, Schiller NB, Rapaport E: Echocardiography of left ventricular masses. Circulation 58:528, 1978.

53. Huggins TJ, Huggins MJ, Schnapf DJ, Brott WH, Sinnott RC, Shawl FA: Left atrial myxoma: Computed tomography as a diagnostic modality. J Comput Assist Tomogr 4:253, 1980.

54. Norlindh T, Lilja B, Nyman U, Hellekant C: Left atrial myxoma demonstrated with CT. AJR 137:153, 1981.

55. Dunnick NR, Seibert K, Dramer HR Jr: Cardiac metastasis from osteosarcoma. J Comput Assist Tomogr 5:253, 1981.

56. Godwin JD, Axel L, Adams JR, Schiller NB, Simpson PC Jr, Gertz EW: Computed tomography: A new method for diagnosing tumor of the heart. Circulation 63:448, 1981.

57. Hidalgo H, Korobkin M, Sbreiman RS, Kisslo JR: CT of intracardiac tumor. AJR 137:608, 1981.

58. Spodick DH: Medical history of the pericardium. Am J Cardiol 26:447, 1970.

59. Holt JP: The normal pericardium. Am J Cardiol 26:455, 1970.

60. Bartle SH, Herman JH, Cavo JW, Moore RA, Costenbader JM: Effect of the pericardium or left ventricular

volume and function in acute hypervolemia. Cardiovasc Res 3:284, 1968.

61. Shabetai R, Mangiarde L, Bhargava V, Ross J Jr, Higgins CB: The pericardium and cardiac function. Prog Cardiovasc Dis 22:107, 1979.

62. Glantz SA, Misbach GA, Moores WY, Mathey DG, Lekven J, Stone DF, Pormley WN, Tyberg JV: The pericardium substantially affects the left ventricular diastolic pressure-volume relationship in the dog. Circ Res 42:433, 1978.

63. Refsum H, Junemann M, Lipton MJ, Skioldebrand CG, Carlsson E, Tyberg JV: Ventricular diastolic pressure-volume relations and the pericardium: Effects of changes in blood volume and pericardial effusion in dogs. Circulation 64:997, 1981.

64. Mursky, I, Ramkin JS: The effects of geometry, elasticity and external pressures on the diastolic pressure-volume and stiffness-stress relations: How important is the pericardium? Circ Res 44:601, 1979.

65. Shabetai R: The Pericardium. New York, Grune & Stratton, 1981, pp 1–3.

66. Moncada R, Baker M, Salinas M, Demos T, Churchill R, Love L, Reynes C, Hale D, Cardoso M, Pifame R, Gunnar RM: Diagnostic role of computed tomography in pericardial heart disease: Congenital defects, thickening, neoplasms and effusions. Am Heart J 103:263, 1982.

67. Houang MTW, Arozena X, Shaw SG: Demonstration of the pericardium and pericardial effusion by computed tomography. J Comput Assist Tomogr 3:601, 1979.

68. Doppman JL, Reinmuller R, Nissner J, Cyan J, Bolte HD, Stauer BE, Hellwig H: Computed tomography in constrictive pericarditis. J Comput Assist Tomogr 5:1, 1981.

69. Edwards JE: Congenital malformations of the heart and great vessels: F: Malformations of the pericardium. In Gould SE (ed): Pathology of the Heart and Blood Vessels, 3rd ed. Springfield, Ill, Charles C Thomas, 1968, pp 376–378.

70. Nassar WK: Congenital diseases of the pericardium. In Reddy PS, Leon DF, Shaver JA (eds): Pericardial Disease. New York, Raven Press, 1982, pp 93–111.

71. Tabakin BS, Hanson JS, Tampas JP, Caldwell EJ: Congenital absence of left pericardium. AJR 94:122, 1965.

72. Schuster B, Alejandrino S, Yavuz F, Imm CW: Congenital pericardial defect: Report of a patient with an associated patent ductus arteriosus. Am J Dis Child 110:199, 1965.

73. Mukerjee S: Congenital partial left pericardial defect with bronchogenic cyst. Thorax 19:176, 1964.

74. Nassar WK: Congenital absence of the left pericardium. Am J Cardiol 26:466, 1970.

75. Lajos TZ, Brunnell IL, Colkathis BP, Schmert G: Coronary artery insufficiency secondary to congenital pericardial defect. Chest 58:73, 1970.

76. Baum RS, MacDonald IL, Wise DJ, Lenkei SC: Computed tomography of absent left pericardium. Radiology 135:127, 1980.

77. Larrieu AJ, Wiener I, Alexander R, Wolma FJ: Pericardiodiaphragmatic hernia. Am J Surg 139:436, 1980.

78. Gomez MN, Hufnagel CA: Intrapericardial tracheal cysts. Am J Cardiol 36:817, 1975.

79. Pugatch RD, Braver JH, Robbins AH, Faling LJ: CT diagnosis of pericardial cysts. AJR 131:515, 1978.

80. Rogers CI, Seymour Q, Brock GJ: Atypical pericardial cyst location: The value of computed tomography. J Comput Assist Tomogr 4:683, 1980.

81. Miller AJ, Rick R, Johnson PJ: The production of acute pericardial effusion. Am J Cardiol 28:463, 1971.

82. Wong BYS, Kyo RL, McArthur R: Diagnosis of pericardial effusion by CT. Chest 81:177, 1982.

83. Tomoda H, Hoshiai M, Furuyu H, Oeda Y, Matsumoto S, Tamabe T, Tamachi H, Sasamoto H, Korde S, Kuribayashi S, Matsuyama S: Evaluation of pericardial effusion with computed tomography. Am Heart J 99:701, 1980.

84. Gibbons JE, Goldbloom RB, Dobill ARC: Rapidly developing pericardial constriction following nonspecific pericarditis. Am J Cardiol 15:863, 1965.

85. Wise DE, Contri RC: Constrictive pericarditis. Cardiovasc Clin 7:196, 1976.

86. Engle ME, Klein AA, Hepner S, Ehlers KH: The postpericardiotomy and other similar syndromes. Cardiovasc Clin 7:211, 1976.

87. Shapiro JH, Jacobson HG, Rubenstein BM, Poppel MH, Schwedel JB: Calcifications of the Heart. Springfield, Ill, Charles C Thomas, 1963, p 198.

88. Mathewson FAL: Calcification of the pericardium in apparently healthy people, electrocardiographic abnormalities found in tracings from apparently healthy persons with calcifications in the pericardium. Circulation 12:44, 1955.

89. Deloach JF, Haynes JW: Secondary tumors of the heart and pericardium: Review of the subject and report of 137 cases. Arch Intern Med 91:224, 1953.

90. Roberts WC, Glancy DL, DeVita VT: Heart in malignant lymphoma: A study of 196 autopsy cases. Am J Cardiol 22:85, 1968.

91. Posner MR, Cohen GI, Srarin AT: Pericardial disease in patients with cancer: The differentiation of malignant from idiopathic and radiation-induced pericarditis. Am J Med 71:407, 1981.

92. Society for Computed Body Tomography: New indications for computed body tomography. AJR 133:115, 1979.

93. Bove AA, Ziskin MC, Freeman E, Gimenez JL, Lynch PR: Selection of optimum cineradiographic frame rate: Relation to accuracy of cardiac measurements. Invest Radiol 5:329, 1970.

94. Higgins CB: Computed tomography of the heart. Radiology 140:525, 1981.

10 COMPUTED TOMOGRAPHY OF THE SPINE

Neil I. Chafetz

Harry K. Genant

John R. Mani

This chapter describes an approach to the planning, performance, and interpretation of spinal CT examinations using an advanced state-of-the-art scanner. Computed tomography of the lumbar spine has been particularly well received because it currently replaces, in most cases, an invasive procedure (myelography) with a noninvasive one. Consequently, special emphasis will be placed on this region and the technical considerations attendant to the planning of a lumbar CT scan. Technical factors and scanning options will be described in the context of the GE 8800 scanner, but these features can be readily extrapolated to other advanced high-resolution CT scanners.

Since most spinal CT exams are designed to assess the patient with a low back pain syndrome, interpretation of a lumbar scan for the patient suspected of having disc rupture, facet joint disease, or spinal stenosis will be addressed immediately following the discussion of the technical aspects of scanning. Special considerations for CT evaluation of cervical or thoracic disc disease will then be described. Additional suggestions for scanning the patient with tumor, infection, or trauma in the spine or the patient with sacroiliitis will follow.

TECHNICAL CONSIDERATIONS

The selection of technical factors and machine options available for CT scanning requires tradeoffs among image quality, patient dose,

The proliferation of high-resolution computed tomographic (CT) scanners in the world, having both a scout view and the capability of imaging the intervertebral discs, has focused attention on the use of this technique for evaluating the spine.

scanning time, and tube life.[1] Image quality can be evaluated by a quality assurance or resolving power phantom[2, 3] that contains graduated cylinders of high- and low-contrast material simulating bone and soft tissue, repectively. It has been shown that when statistical noise increases (decreasing photon flux), resolving power for low-contrast structures is more severely compromised than that for high-contrast structures.

The visibility of high-contrast objects is principally dependent upon spatial resolution, which in turn is a function of scanner geometry, collimator, detector and pixel size, and reconstruction algorithm.[4–6] The implication is that for scanning and detecting the soft-tissue contents of the spinal canal where density differences are small, the image must be optimized for low-contrast discrimination by using high milliamperage with resulting low noise.

In order to enhance spatial and density resolution and to reduce image artifacts, 9.6-second scans are obtained using the full 576 views.[7, 8] The standard 120 kVp is employed with relatively high milliamperage (300 to 400 mA) and 3-msec pulse width, which results in approximately 575 to 775 mA. When very thin sections (1.5 mm) are used, the maximum setting of 600 mA must be selected in order to partially offset the photon limitation (and quantum noise) that occurs with thin sections. To optimize image quality further, the pediatric calibration file with a 25-cm reconstruction circle may be used; it provides a pixel size of 0.8×0.8 mm rather than the medium body calibration file with a 35-cm reconstruction circle and a 1.1-mm pixel size.

The use of the small calibration file results in a slightly reduced radiation exposure of the patient (about 15 per cent reduction) because of the "bowtie filter," whereas the image quality is slightly improved. A significant shortcoming of this approach, however, is the potential for production of artifacts when soft tissues extend outside the reconstruction circle. The algorithm assumes that air is outside the reconstruction circle, and when significant amounts of soft tissue extend beyond the circle, particularly posteriorly in the region of the spine, streak artifacts and coarse granular noise combine to produce suboptimal images. Thus, when the small calibration file is used, centering becomes critical and the table must be elevated so that appreciable soft tissue does not lie outside the reconstruction circle in the posterior region. Such positioning is not always possible with large patients.

An alternative approach, and one that we recommend, is the application of reView or target imaging, replacing the standard display data image.[9] Rather than scanning with a 25-cm field of view, by using soft-tissue reView, the patient can be scanned with a 42-cm field of view that is prospectively reconstructed to a 20-cm field of view. The soft-tissue reView algorithm changes only the pixel size and results in a magnified image without the loss of resolution normally associated with pixel interpolation. The soft-tissue algorithm takes raw data from axial scans, recalculates each pixel, and produces a magnified image without the loss of resolution associated with magnification functions available at the display console. With a target factor of 2.1 used for the large calibration circle, the new pixel size becomes 0.64 mm with a 20-cm field of view. This new program permits uncompromised imaging of larger patients, yet maintains a normal reconstruction time of 35 to 40 seconds and an image quality comparable with or superior to that attainable with the small reconstruction circle and display data.

When osseous detail is of principal interest, however, a bone reView algorithm can be used in lieu of the soft-tissue reView program. This increases edge definition and improves spatial resolution, making the edges of hard bone stand out clearly against the increased noise of the high spatial resolution technique. With this program, the minimum magnification factor for maximum spatial resolution is 2.17 for the large body calibration, giving a pixel size of 0.6 mm and a field of 19.2 cm. The bone reView program combined with the newly available extended scale—permitting densities of $-1,000$ to $+3,000$ Hounsfield Units (H) to be displayed—results in optimal visualization of the osseous spinal canal. Either the soft-tissue or bone reView program can be performed prospectively or retrospectively, but the latter requires approximately 90 seconds for reconstruction, which may limit patient throughput if performed on-line. However, no additional time is required for the soft-tissue targeting program.

SCANNING OPTIONS

Any particular scanning regimen reflects a compromise weighted by the relative importance of the scanning parameters. In general terms, when other variables are held constant, the following principles hold true:

1. The smaller the slice thickness, the greater the milliamperage required for comparable image quality.

2. The higher the milliamperage, the fewer

slices that can be obtained before anode heat accumulation or "tube cooling" extends the interscan delay.

3. Reduction in milliamperage tends to be more detrimental to soft-tissue discrimination than to resolution of bony structures.

4. The higher the milliamperage, the greater the patient radiation exposure.

5. If reformations are to be obtained, continuous scans through a region with constant gantry angulation should be initially acquired (zero-degree angulation is optimal).

A discussion of our current approach follows. The reader should keep in mind that many similar protocols are currently and successfully in use. Furthermore, our own approach has evolved as our experience has widened. The protocol we use is designed to be adequate for CT diagnosis of soft tissue as well as bony abnormalities that cause low back pain syndromes. To help straighten the lumbar lordosis and reduce patient motion, we have found it helpful to support and immobilize the hips and knees in a flexed position using a special purpose foot board that is easily adapted to the scanning table (Fig. 10–1).

In all cases, an anteroposterior (Fig. 10–2) and lateral scout view (Fig. 10–3) should be obtained of the region of interest (ROI) before axial scanning. This technique provides precise anatomic localization for subsequent transverse scanning and, in addition, indicates the degree of angulation of the gantry necessary to maintain a transverse or nearly transverse orientation, particularly at the L5-S1 level. The anteroposterior view is useful for reviewing bony anatomy if plain films are not available; furthermore, if there is scoliosis or angulation, adjustments of the patient position on the table can be made before obtaining the lateral scout view. It is the latter technique, however, that is principally used for cursor localization in the scanning procedure.

From the lateral scout view, we initially obtain three 500-mA slices that are 5 mm thick at 4-mm intervals appropriately angled for the plane of the disc at the L5-S1 level (Fig. 10–3). The relatively high-milliamperage technique and overlapping scans are intended to compensate for the photon attenuation of the surrounding pelvis and the frequently narrowed disc space, respectively. Following these angled scans, we obtain scans that are 5 mm thick at 4-mm intervals from L3 to S1 with zero-degree angulation (Fig. 10–4). We are employing 320 mA for these scans as a compromise between the parameters of rapid exam time and adequate soft-tissue discrimination. The total scanning time is approximately 45 minutes.

CONTRAST ENHANCEMENT

Lumbar Spine

Intravenous or intrathecal contrast material is not routinely used for studies of the lumbar spine with advanced state-of-the-art scanners that have sufficient density resolution to differentiate the thecal sac from adjacent soft tissue structures, such as the intervertebral disc, ligamentum fla-

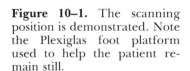

Figure 10–1. The scanning position is demonstrated. Note the Plexiglas foot platform used to help the patient remain still.

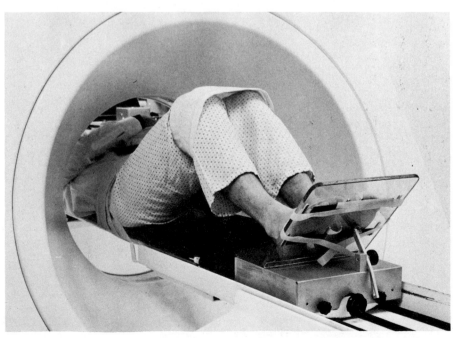

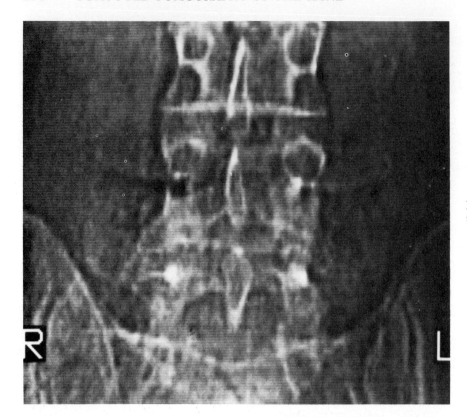

Figure 10–2. Digital anteroposterior scout image.

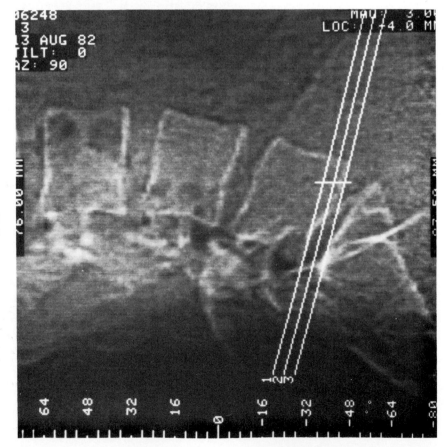

Figure 10–3. Digital lateral scout with cursor lines showing selection of angled scans at L5-S1.

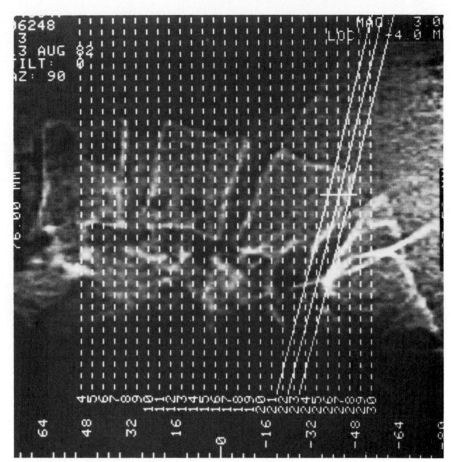

Figure 10–4. Digital lateral image demonstrates angled and unangled slices.

vum, and epidural fat.[10] In selected cases, however, intrathecal metrizamide combined with high-resolution CT scanning (reView or Target imaging) may provide additional helpful or essential information. This is particularly true in complicated postoperative cases in which extensive fibrosis obscures the normal soft-tissue planes.

It has been reported that postoperative fibrotic scar will enhance sufficiently to allow differentiation from a ruptured disc following intravenous administration.[11] However, a broader experience confirming this finding has not yet been obtained. Additionally, in the evaluation of intradural lesions, metrizamide-enhanced CT with high-resolution reView may be valuable. In this regard, the dense intrathecal contrast renders the thecal sac bonelike in x-ray attenuation; therefore, spatial resolution is more critical than density resolution, and the sharper, but noisier, image is optimal.

Cervical and Thoracic Regions

The abundance of epidural fat that provides soft-tissue contrast in the lumbar spine is generally absent in the cervical and thoracic regions. Nevertheless, CT without enhancement usually is

adequate for the diagnosis of metastases, fractures, infection, and dysplasia. However, metrizamide-assisted CT (CTMM) is suggested for assessment of disc disease of the cervical and thoracic spine. A complete water-soluble contrast myelogram may be performed prior to the CT scan or 3 to 5 ml of 170 mg/dl metrizamide may be injected specifically to assist CT interpretation.

When CT follows full-dose metrizamide myelography, the patient is left in an upright or semi-upright position for 4 to 6 hours between the two exams to reduce the incidence of adverse reactions. The partial resorption and dilution of the contrast medium that occur in this time interval leaves an intrathecal contrast concentration that is optimal for scanning. To avoid layering of contrast material, the patient should roll over several times just prior to the CT exam. Metrizamide will then outline the nerve roots and the normal oval contour of the spinal cord.

The spinal cord is located centrally in the cervical and lower thoracic regions but usually favors the anterior aspect of the spinal canal through the kyphotic midthorax. The ventral and dorsal nerve roots are usually visualized as focal defects

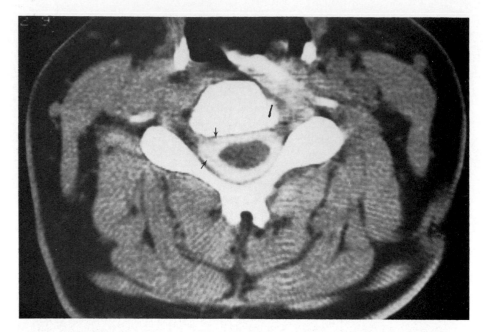

Figure 10–5. Normal metrizamide-assisted cervical CT demonstrating exiting nerve roots (arrows).

in the subarachnoid space (Fig. 10–5) before they leave the dura for the neural foramen where they join. As the spinal cord tapers in the lower thoracic or upper lumbar region, the nerve roots radiate around it (Fig. 10–6). Below the level of the cord individual nerve roots of the cauda equina lying in the dependent portion of the thecal sac can be visualized (Fig. 10–7). When CTMM is performed without myelography, 3 to 5 ml of 170 mg/dl of metrizamide is instilled by means of a lumbar route with a 22-gauge needle. A lateral C1-2 puncture may be employed in patients with severe spinal stenosis, paraspinal infection or any condition that precludes a lumbar puncture. The high-resolution bone reView reconstruction program with target imaging and extended scale generally proves optimal for CTMM. The cervical region is scanned with contiguous slices 1.5-mm or 5-mm thick overlapped at 2.5-mm intervals.

For the assessment of fractures of the cervical and thoracic spine, dynamic low-dose-scanning (100 mA at 3.3 msec) has the advantage of obviating the interscan delay, expediting the procedure, and reducing the absorbed radiation dose. With this scanning technique, projection data are generated during both clockwise and counterclockwise rotations with an interscan delay of approximately 1 second while the table is incremented.

DISPLAY AND PHOTOGRAPHIC OPTIONS

The factors to be considered in display and photographic options include anatomic sequence, optical magnification, window setting, reformations, and linear and area measurements.

In all cases, the anteroposterior and lateral scout views should be photographed in the magnification mode, i.e., approximately threefold, so that the cursor lines corresponding to the axial cuts obtained can be adequately displayed without obliterating the underlying anatomic landmarks. Additionally, the patient header file and scan parameters should be photographed so that the sequence, scanning procedures, and technical factors can be assessed while the case is being interpreted.

Generally, for photographing any scanning procedure, the window setting and the degree of magnification should be kept constant while the study is photographed in anatomic sequence from cephalad to caudad. This approach facilitates interpretations. For studies in which the osseous structures are of principal importance, i.e., spinal stenosis or postfusion cases, a window width of approximately 2000 H and a level of 200 to 300 H is selected. For studies in which the soft tissues, such as disc and thecal sac, are of principal interest, a window width of 500 H and a level of approximately 50 H are selected.

In practice, all scans can be photographed at both bone and soft-tissue windows. The use of narrow windows for this purpose, however, is advantageous only when the noise or statistical fluctuation is relatively low. For the relatively noisy, low-millamperage dynamic scan images, there is generally no advantage to using narrow windows, which merely enhance the perception of noise rather than increase contrast discrimination. In selected cases, identity or blink mode can be used to highlight density differences in relatively low-noise images. In these instances, the absence or extent of a disc rupture may be confirmed in an otherwise equivocal case.

When the newer soft-tissue reView program with a large body calibration file is being used, the disc and ligamentum flavum generally blink at one density (75 to 120 H), and the thecal sac and the nerve sheaths blink simultaneously at a lower density (0 to 50 H). When the subtle soft-tissue interfaces cannot be visualized because of very small density differences that are essentially "lost in the noise" of the image, the blink mode, unfortunately, will not enhance or uncover these subtle differences. Furthermore, by manipulating the

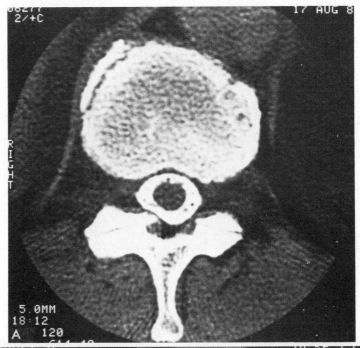

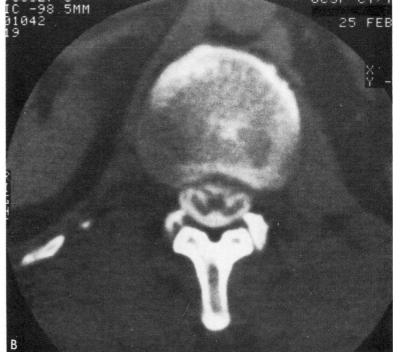

Figure 10–6. A Metrizamide-assisted CT (CTMM). The spinal cord surrounded by metrizamide in the subarachnoid space within which are numerous nerve roots seen as focal defects. Incidental note is made of the right superior articular facet impressing the right posterior aspect of the metrizamide column. **B** Normal CTMM of conus medullaris reveals "four-legged spider" configuration of the existing nerve roots.

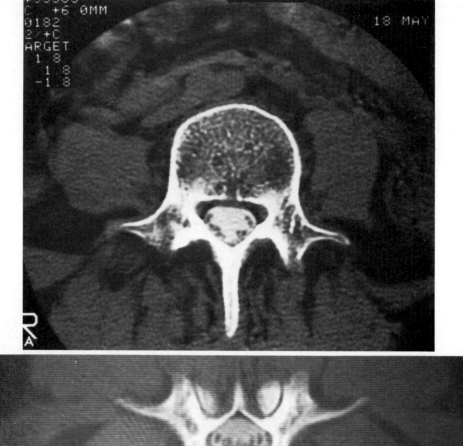

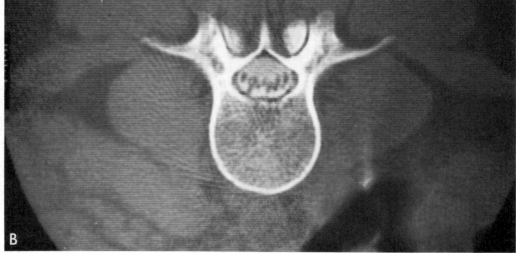

Figure 10–7. A Normal lumbar CTMM demonstrating normal array of cauda equina nerve roots. **B** Lumbar CTMM of patient in prone position demonstrating movement of cauda equina roots to dependent position.

blink mode levels, we can occasionally produce confusing information. Generally, for visual detection, the difference between the mean CT numbers of adjacent soft-tissue structures must be greater than the standard deviation of the means.[12]

For photographing hard copies with the multiformat camera, we have routinely used $1.8\times$ optical magnification on the video console for scans obtained with a 25-cm reconstruction circle. However, when the newer reView program with a large calibration circle and a target factor of 2.1 is being used, optical magnification of 1.3 to $1.4\times$ on the display console results in images of comparable size. With the standard photographic approach, a multiformat camera is used to obtain 12 images per 14×17-inch film.

It should be noted that in applying optical magnification at the display console, there is a delay of approximately 15 to 20 seconds to bring up each image, which results in an overall photographing time of 20 to 30 minutes. A recent adaptation permits faster photographing and requires fewer films. With this approach, the 12-on-1 format is used and four images are brought up, sequentially for each square, thus allowing a total of 48 images to be displayed on a single film. There is minimal delay for optical magnification since a smaller field is enlarged. Thus, a total of 48 images can be displayed and photographed in approximately one fourth of the time necessary for the standard approach and with the same resultant image size. Photographing the same four images at bone and soft-tissue windows above and below each other adds to convenience in diagnosis (Fig. 10–8).

Reformatted images may facilitate interpretation when applied to the assessment of complicated bone anatomy such as some cases of spinal fractures, spondylolytic defects, postfusion pseudarthrosis, and tumors. In this application, the

presentation of information in the sagittal, coronal, or oblique planes provides a new perspective but does not generate new pixel formation that is not present on the axial scans.

In general, however, reformations have relatively poor spatial resolution in the longitudinal or z-axis when derived from sections that are 5 mm thick and overlapped every 4 to 5 mm.[4] The spatial resolution in the longitudinal axis is greatly improved using 1.5-mm contiguous sections; however, such an approach is not feasible for studying large segments of the spine such as L3 to S1. In selected cases, when focal information concerning bony architecture is specifically sought, low-milliamperage dynamic scanning can be used with sections 1.5 mm thick. This results in relatively high spatial resolution images, including the longitudinal axis, although these im-

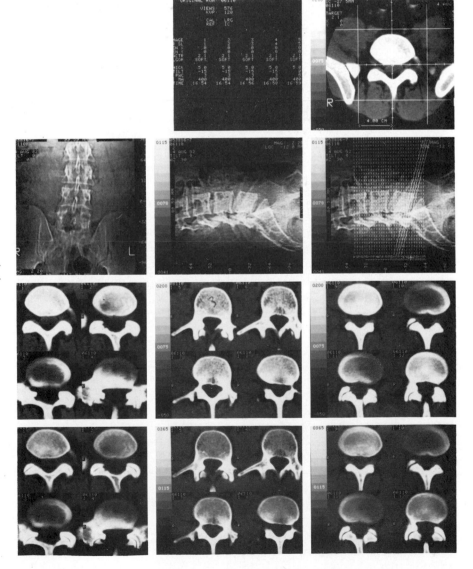

Figure 10–8. Radiograph demonstrating our current photographic format.

CT SCAN

Transverse images (___mm thick) from ___ to ___ at ___mm intervals; gantry angle_____
Transverse images (___mm thick) from ___ to ___ at ___mm intervals; gantry angle_____
Transverse images (___mm thick) from ___ to ___ at ___mm intervals; gantry angle_____
Sagittal images at _____
Coronal images at _____

Findings Graded on 0-3 Scale; 0 or blank=normal; 1=mild; 2=moderate; 3=severe

Levels scanned are bracketted

	Disc/Osteo-phyte bulge	Foramen stenosis	Central canal stenosis	Lat. recess stenosis	Artic. process Hypertrophy	Lamina or fusion mass hypertrophy
	Rt. Cen. Lt.	Rt. Lt.		Rt. Lt.	Rt. Lt.	Rt. Lt.
L1						
L1-2	__ __ __		___		___ ___	___ ___
L2						
L2-L3	__ __ __		___		___ ___	___ ___
L3						
L3-L4	__ __ __		___		___ ___	___ ___
L4						
L4-L5	__ __ __		___		___ ___	___ ___
L5						
L5-S1	__ __ __		___		___ ___	___ ___

Pantopaque or Metrizamide _____

Lam./Hemilam. _____

Fusion Levels: _____

Other: _____

_____

Summary: _____

_____

_____

_____

Interpretation by: _____

Figure 10–9. Reporting form used for systematic analysis and semiquantitative evaluation of lumbar CT findings. Form is modeled after one used by Glenn and associates (Spine 4:282, 1979).[13]

ages will be noisy and have poor density discrimination. As a general rule, however, in CT scanning for low back pain syndromes, the principal emphasis should be on obtaining the highest quality axial images and on diagnosis based upon the interpretation of axial images in which density discrimination is optimal.

SEMIQUANTITATIVE APPROACH

A systematic and semiquantitative method has been developed for interpretation of CT scans of the lumbar spine using a modification of a reporting form devised by Glenn.[13] The technical factors used for the examination, including scan thickness, angulation, and intervals, are recorded, and the findings are graded semiquantitatively on a scale of 0 for normal, 1 for mild, 2 for moderate, and 3 for severe. At each level the following findings are evaluated: disc bulge, central canal stenosis, foraminal stenosis, lateral recess stenosis, and ligamentum flavum hypertrophy. This reporting form permits a careful, thorough, and or-

ganized approach to the interpretation of lumbar CT scans and provides the clinician with a reproducible and readily understandable method of quantifying the severity of findings (Fig. 10–9). Such a form may be used in the process of interpreting the study or may be incorporated into a report form for the referring physician.

PATHOLOGY

FUNDAMENTALS OF INTERVERTEBRAL DISC DISEASE

Rupture of an intervertebral disc refers to a distortion in the normal anatomic configuration of the annulus. Two anatomic lesions comprise the category of disc rupture: disc protrusions and disc herniation.[14]

DISC PROTRUSION. Normally the annulus fibrosus forms a smooth continuous ring confining the nucleus pulposus. Occasionally a focal bulge develops after localized degenerative changes, although all of the annular fibers are still intact. With more generalized disc collapse, the annulus circumferentially protrudes beyond the peripheral rim of the vertebral bodies. Thus a disc protrusion may be a localized annular bulge or a diffuse annular bulge.

DISC HERNIATION. In contrast to protrusion, herniation refers to a disc in which some of the annular fibers are severed, allowing movement of at least some nucleus away from its normal central location. Three types of herniation can be recognized, depending on the extent of displacement of nuclear material: prolapsed, extruded, and sequestrated.

In the case of the prolapsed intervertebral disc, the displaced nuclear material is confined solely by the outermost fibers of the annulus. The extruded intervertebral disc is one in which the displaced nuclear material has burst through the posterior fibers of the annulus and lies under the posterior investing ligament. In the case of the sequestrated disc, nuclear material may be extruded through the posterior fibers of the annulus and through or around the posterior longitudinal ligament. The fragment lies free in the spinal canal. An extruded disc may therefore be associated with a sequestrated fragment that may remain trapped between nerve root and the disc or may migrate from the site of rupture. The sequestrated fragment may come to lie behind the vertebral body above or below the disc, in the axilla,

on the nerve root, in the intervertebral foramen, or in the midline anterior to the spinal cord or dural sac. On occasion, this unattached disc fragment may actually erode or burst through the dura.[14] The first seven of the cervical nerve roots exit above the associated vertebral body. The eighth cervical nerve exists below the C7 pedicle. Distal to the T1 vertebra the nerve roots exit just below the pedicle. In the region of the cauda equina, the nerve roots course obliquely over the intervertebral disc to emerge through the foramina of the vertebra below.

The L4 nerve root exits below the pedicle of L4 and usually escapes compression by the disc that lies between the L4 and L5 vertebrae. It is the L5 nerve root, however, that is most at risk from being compressed by the L4-5 disc.

Analogously, therefore, herniation of the L5-S1 disc will frequently compress the first sacral root. However, a lateral protrusion of the disc may distort the nerve exiting above the disc at the level of the foramen.

Compression of more than one nerve root may be seen when a large herniation compromises not only the nerve root crossing obliquely behind the disc, but also the nerve exiting through the foramen just cranial to it. Similarly, migration of a sequestrated fragment in either a cranial or caudal direction may involve more than one root. A massive central sequestration may involve several roots in the cauda equina with resulting bowel

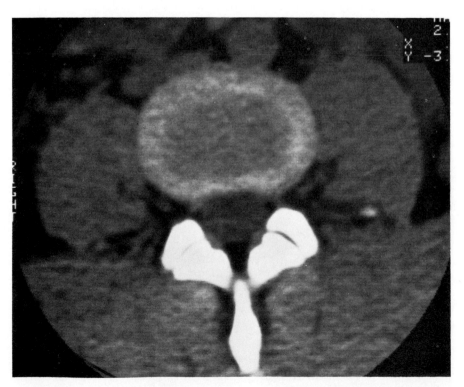

Figure 10–10. Normal L4-5 disc demonstrating posterior disc concavity.

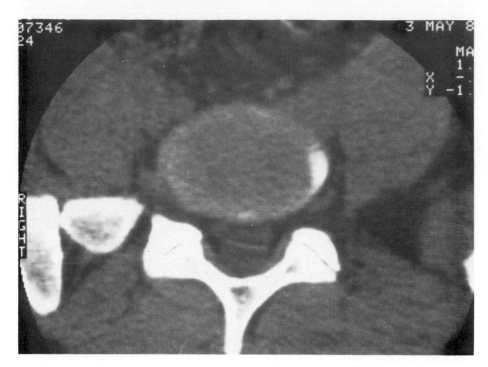

Figure 10–11. Normal L5-S1 disc demonstrates the greater amount of epidural fat seen at this level as well as visualization of the S1 roots adjacent to the thecal sac.

and bladder paralysis. This type of lesion is more commonly seen at the L4-5 level.[14]

ANATOMY OF THE LUMBAR DISC

The CT evaluation of the status of the lumbar disc and its relationship to the thecal sac and exiting nerve roots is made possible by the presence of the epidural fat in the spinal canal at the disc levels. The disc is of slightly higher CT density than the thecal sac, enabling the interface between the disc and the thecal sac to be distinguished on a CT scan in most cases. The normal configuration of the posterior aspect of the intervertebral disc at the L4-5 level is a slight concavity (Fig. 10–10), which becomes flattened with increasing age. In older patients, it is not uncom-

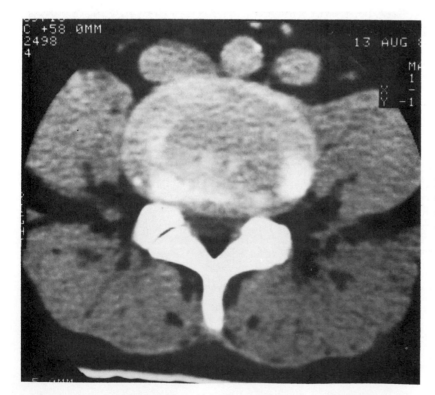

Figure 10–12. Diffuse annular bulge demonstrating mild flattening of the anterior aspect of the thecal sac at the L4-5 level.

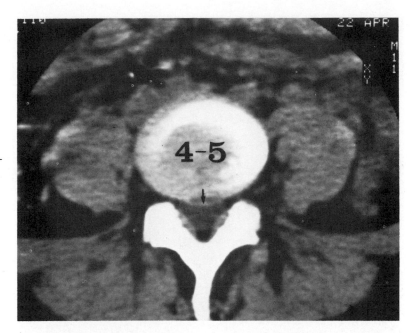

Figure 10–13. Mild, discrete central nodular disc bulge (arrow) at L4-5.

mon to see mild degrees of convexity representing a minor diffuse annular bulge that, if unassociated with obliteration of epidural fat, appears not to be of clinical significance. At the L5-S1 level, the posterior aspect of the normal intervertebral disc has a convex border (Fig. 10–11). However, abundant epidural fat frequently is present and the thecal sac and S1 roots, which generally are well demonstrated, are not normally impinged upon.[15]

DIAGNOSIS OF LUMBAR DISC DISEASE

Two patterns of discogenic impingement may be observed with CT. The first is a broad annular bulge presenting as a smooth curvilinear convexity impinging upon the thecal sac and obliterating epidural fat. This corresponds to a diffuse annular bulge type of disc protrusion (Fig. 10–12).

The second pattern is a discrete nodular or lumpy posterior bulge of the disc that when mild

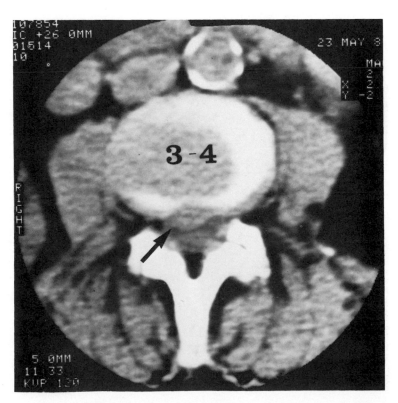

Figure 10–14. Extruded disc herniation at L3-4 (arrow).

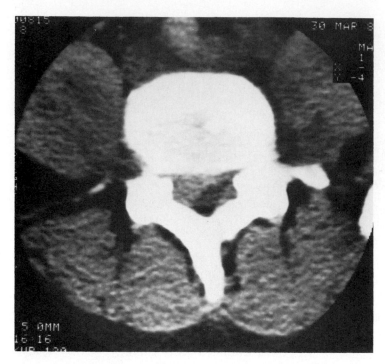

Figure 10–15. Large right-sided posterolateral extruded disc herniation.

in extent (Fig. 10–13) corresponds either to a localized annular bulge or to a prolapsed disc herniation. It is often not possible to distinguish between these two entities with CT.

When the posterior border of the disc has a focal lumpy or nodular bulge that is moderate or severe in posterior extent, an extruded disc herniation is diagnosed (Fig. 10–14). Such a disc her-

niation often impinges upon the thecal sac or nerve root with focal obliteration of the epidural fat. The fibers of the annulus are least abundant posteriorly, thereby predisposing toward a rupture in this direction. Because the posterior longitudinal ligament lends midline support to the posterior midline aspect of the annulus, rupture of the nucleus pulposus through a tear in the an-

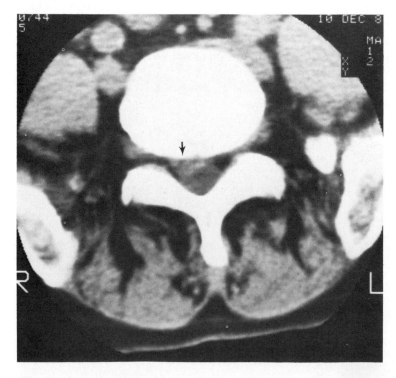

Figure 10–16. Right-sided, sequestrated disc herniation. The free fragment (arrow) is positioned superior to the disc space and distorts the right anterolateral aspect of the thecal sac.

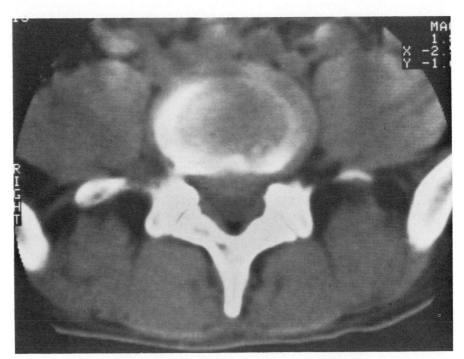

Figure 10–17. Flattening of the anterior aspect of the thecal sac by the ruptured disc.

nulus fibrosus generally occurs posterior and somewhat lateral of the midline (Fig. 10–15). When a nodular disc bulge is seen to extend above or below the level of the bulk of the disc or is noted to be separated, the CT diagnosis of sequestrated fragment is made (Fig. 10–16).

In the CT diagnosis of lumbar disc rupture, the obliteration of the anterolaterally located epidural fat is the most sensitive finding. The epidural fat that intervenes between the encroaching disc and either thecal sac or nerve root must first be sacrificed before contact between the disc and neural components can occur. The degree of distortion of the normal contour of the thecal sac (Fig. 10–17) by the disc or the degree of displacement of a nerve root by the disc (Fig. 10–18), or both, are

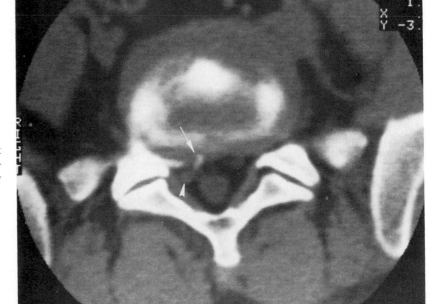

Figure 10–18. Posterior displacement of the swollen right S1 nerve root (arrowhead) by the right-sided partially calcified herniated disc (arrow).

of high diagnostic importance.[14] Obliteration of epidural fat in the absence of both of these signs is only a suspicious finding. When the epidural fat has been obliterated, an especially careful search for these additional findings should be made. Displacement of a nerve root is more commonly appreciated on a CT scan at L5-S1, where the S1 nerve root is normally easily distinguished from the thecal sac. The enlargement of the irritated nerve root may serve as a confirmatory finding.

The absolute size of the disc bulge itself has been found to be less meaningful.

It is important to trace the extent of an abnormal disc bulge both cephalad[16] (Fig. 10–19) and caudad to the disc level itself. Occasionally, a laterally bulging disc rupture encroaches upon the nerve root in the neural foramen just rostral to the disc space and will be detected in this manner (Fig. 10–20). Similarly, the caudal extent of a disc bulge or herniation may contribute to the com-

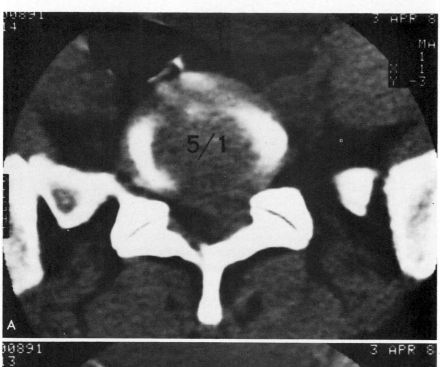

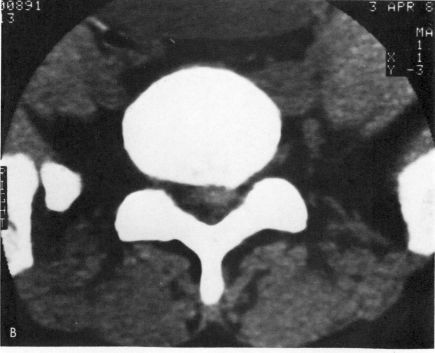

Figure 10–19. A Left-sided disc herniation at the L5-S1 level compressing the left S1 root and the left anterolateral aspect of the thecal sac. **B** Superior extent of the free fragment is shown by the higher-density disc anterior to and deforming the thecal sac.

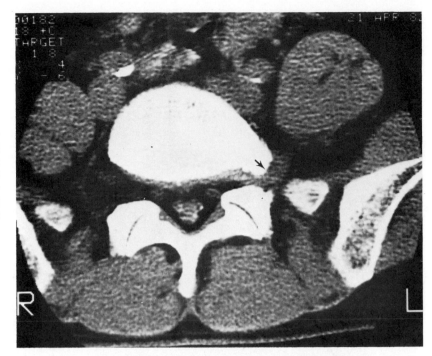

Figure 10–20. Far lateral, partially calcified disc rupture (arrow) is noted on the left. Although the thecal sac at this level and the S1 nerve roots within the central canal are unaffected by this disc herniation, the left L5 nerve root was impinged upon in the neural foramen.

promise of the central canal or lateral recess at the vertebral body level just distal to the disc space (Fig. 10–21).

Sometimes, calcification or ossification of the protruding broad-based annulus fibrosus is noted (Fig. 10–22). Less commonly, protrusion of a gas-containing disc into the central canal or neural foramen will be seen (Fig. 10–23). On the scout view or the conventional radiograph, such a disc may manifest a "vacuum" phenomenon.

The ROI may aid in the recognition of soft tissues within the spinal canal (Fig. 10–24). Similarly, this technique may be used to distinguish an anomalous neural element from a disc fragment. A conjoined nerve, for example, will have a CT number close to that of other nearby exiting

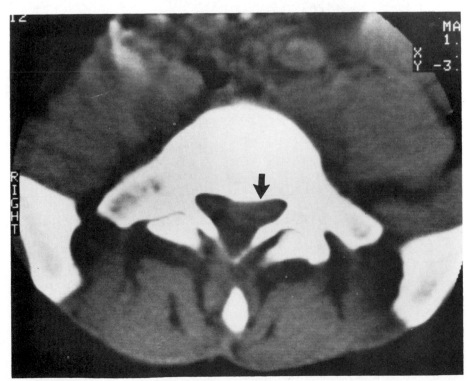

Figure 10–21. Caudal extent of a disc herniation (arrow) in the lateral recess.

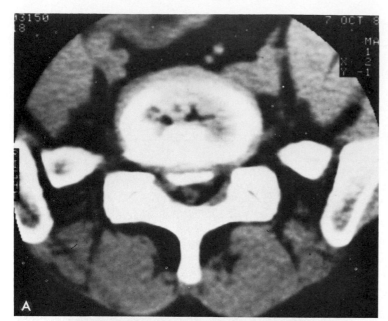

Figure 10–22. A Herniation of a calcified disc fragment into the central canal on the axial scan. **B** Sagittal reformation reveals the calcified disc (arrow) impinging upon the central canal at L5-S1.

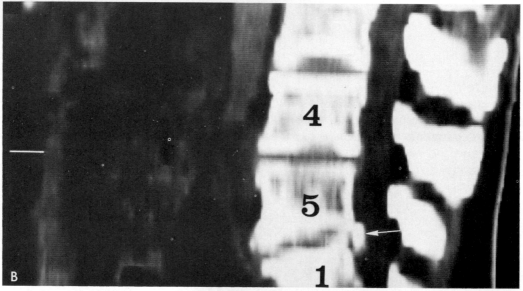

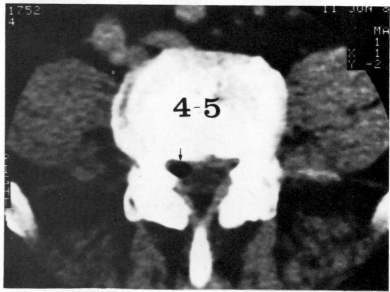

Figure 10–23. Protrusion of gas-containing disc (arrow) into the right L5 lateral recess.

nerves and different from that of a nearby disc (Fig. 10–25).[17]

A potential area of confusion is at L5-S1, where the prominent retrovertebral plexus should not be mistaken for a bulging disc. Close inspection, however, will reveal that this venous complex is composed of several small focal densities rather than only one mass (Fig. 10–26). It may be possible to show that the veins are different from a disc with the use of CT numbers and thereby to confirm the impression of epidural veins in a difficult case.

The postoperative patient whose epidural fat has been replaced by fibrosis can also be a diffi-

cult patient to evaluate (Fig. 10–27). Although in some cases no solution to this diagnostic dilemma may exist, it is important to recognize this potential problem and to indicate to the clinician that meaningful interpretation at this disc level is not possible. In some instances, the CT number may distinguish between scar, disc, and theca. In an individual patient, the disc has a higher CT number than that of scar tissue which in turn has a CT number greater than that of the thecal sac. We do not compare the CT numbers of a structure of unknown origin with average CT numbers of various tissues from a normal population. Instead, we use the same patient's CT numbers of the disc,

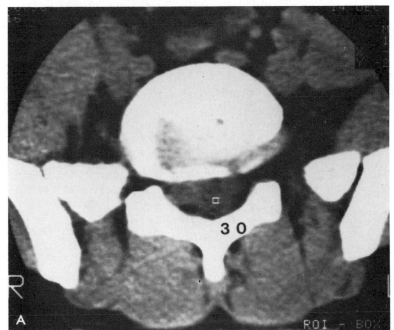

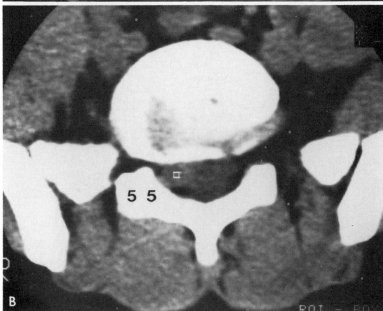

Figure 10–24. A Use of the region of interest (ROI) demonstrated the thecal sac to measure 30 H. **B** Right-sided herniated disc sequestration (free fragment) to measure 55 H—clearly different from the thecal sac and within the range of normal disc density.

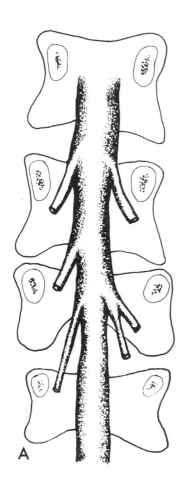

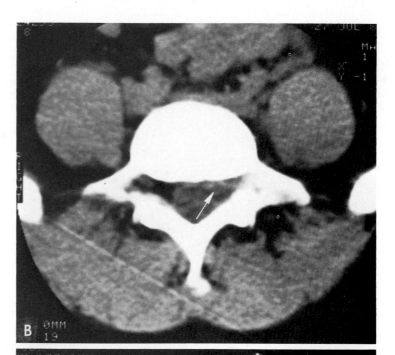

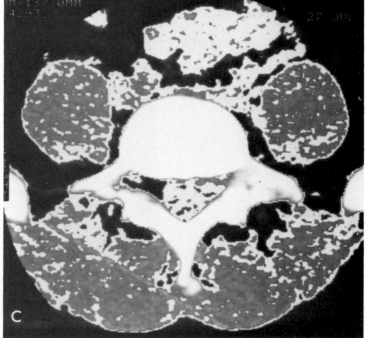

Figure 10–25. Conjoined nerve. **A** Schematically drawn. **B** Conjoined nerve shown on axial CT image (arrow). **C** Blink mode confirms that nerve has a CT density similar to that of the other nerve root and thecal sac.

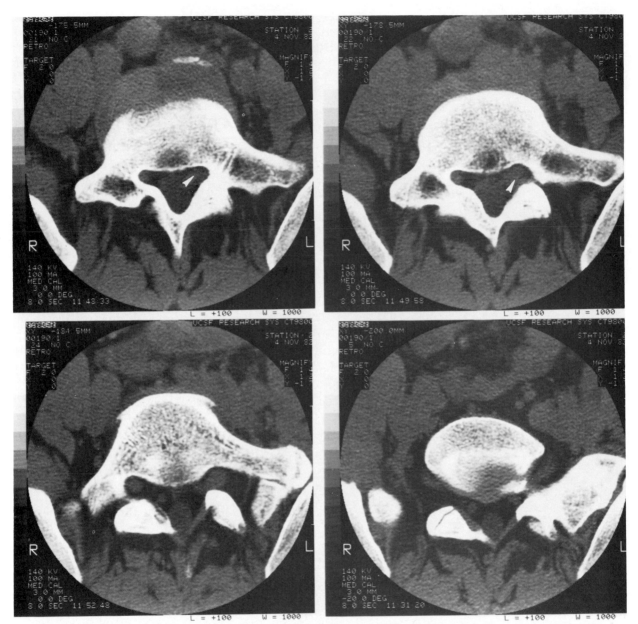

Figure 10–26. Conjoined nerves, craniocaudad sequence *(top left and right):* Soft-tissue density of conjoined nerves in the left L5 lateral recess (arrowheads) suggesting the presence of a "free disc fragment." *Bottom left and right:* The more caudad scans, however, reveal the separation of the conjoined nerves in the region of the left neural foramen.

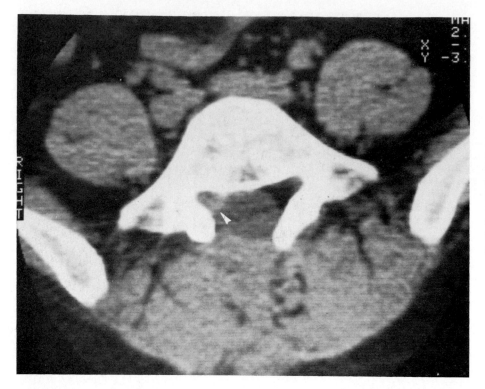

Figure 10–27. Postoperative fibrosis. Extensive posterior and right lateral recess fibrosis (arrowhead) obliterating the usual epidural fat. It would be difficult to exclude a free disc fragment in the right lateral recess under these circumstances.

nerve roots, and thecal sac as anatomically close as possible as a frame of reference. Metrizamide-assisted CT may also play a role in this setting.

The scan through the disc immediately caudal to a spondylolisthesis may show a factitious disc rupture. Generally, the body of the vertebra with bilateral defects in the pars interarticularis slips anteriorly. The adjacent distal intervertebral disc, however, usually retains its position relative to the vertebra below. The disc then lies posterior to the slipped vertebra above. Therefore, an axial scan through the vertebral body and the disc below

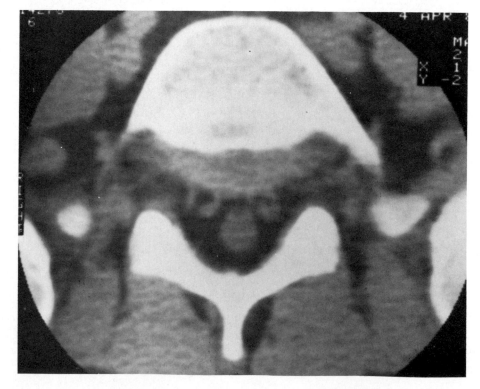

Figure 10–28. Axial scan through L5-S1 disc with L5 spondylolisthesis reveals large "pseudobulge" that is not affecting the thecal sac or S1 roots adversely.

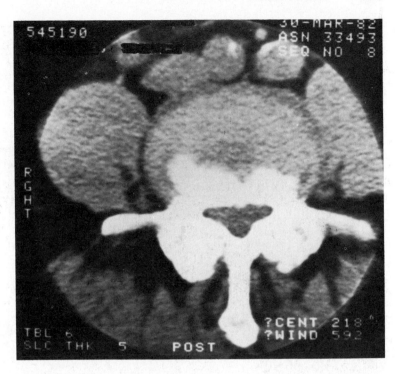

Figure 10–29. Axial CT scan of a patient with congenital spinal stenosis. Note the diminished anteroposterior dimension of the central spinal canal and the paucity of epidural fat.

will reveal an apparent posterior protrusion of the disc (Fig. 10–28). It is important to recognize that a large "pseudobulge" may be present under these circumstances. To determine the significance of a pseudobulge, close attention must be given to the overall contour of the disc and especially to its relationship to the nerve roots and thecal sac. The apparent size of the disc bulge should be disregarded. Reformations may assist in this assessment.

The sensitivity and specificity of CT diagnosis of the herniated nucleus pulposus are approximately 95 per cent, which is slightly superior to that of myelography.[18] It is increasingly apparent that CT is the first diagnostic radiologic procedure to follow conventional radiographs in evaluating the patient suspected of a ruptured lumbar disc.[19–21] It is a rapid, harmless, sensitive, and accurate method.[22] Myelography is reserved for patients whose clinical findings cannot be explained adequately by CT.[18]

SPINAL STENOSIS

Spinal stenosis may be defined as a condition involving any type of narrowing of the central spinal canal, lateral recesses or intervertebral foramen.

Central Canal Stenosis

Central spinal canal stenosis may be congenital (Figs. 10–29 and 10–30) or acquired (Fig. 10–31).

The congenital form may remain clinically quiescent until superimposed acquired stenosis renders the condition clinically symptomatic. The osteophytic changes of degenerative spondylosis, postoperative or post-traumatic bony overgrowth, and spondylolisthesis are the more common acquired causes.

The evaluation of spinal stenosis or congenital and acquired disorders compromising the spinal cord and nerve roots is an important application of computed tomography. In spinal stenosis, the cross-sectional display of CT permits precise definition of the critically important transverse configuration and size of the canal. Although CT measurements of the anteroposterior, transverse, and cross-sectional area of the lumbar spinal canal have been documented, the application and interpretation of such measurements can be difficult.[23, 24] There is wide biological variation in these measurements that makes discrimination between a given patient and a normal population difficult in many cases. In addition, as the window settings of a given scanner can affect the linear and area measurements, calibration of the scanner with a phantom of known dimension should be undertaken. In practice, one should not rely solely upon the measurement of the bony canal. A qualitative assessment based upon how tightly fitted the bony canal appears for the neural structures should determine the presence and severity of spinal stenosis. Ligamentum flavum hypertro-

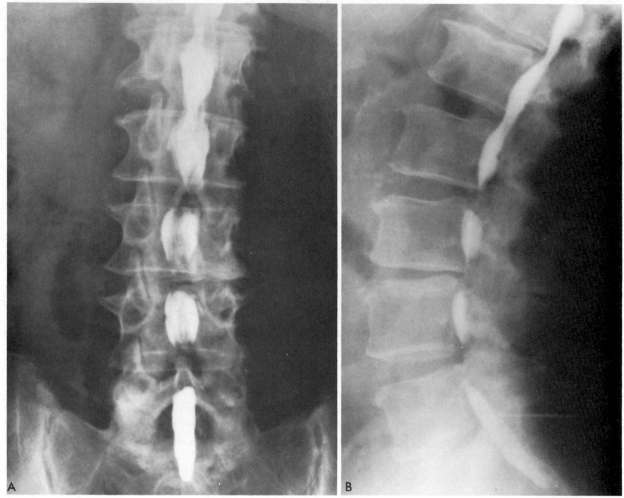

Figure 10–30. Congenital spinal stenosis. **A, B**   Anteroposterior and lateral views of the lumbar myelogram demonstrating multilevel congenital spinal stenosis, most marked at the intervertebral disc levels.

Illustration continued on opposite page

phy and consequent encroachment upon the dural sac may occur without osseous stenosis and is best evaluated with a soft-tissue CT window (Fig. 10–32). Similarly, a diffuse annular bulge with a broad-based posterior disc margin may result in central canal stenosis. In addition, when spinal stenosis is a result of hypertrophy of the superior articular facets, one may see a compressed or trefoil configuration of the spinal canal associated with encroachment of the lateral recesses and nerve root impingement.

Lateral Recess Stenosis

The lateral recess is an area bordered laterally by the pedicle, posteriorly by the superior articular facet, and anteriorly by the posterolateral surface of the vertebral body. The superior aspect of the pedicle marks the level where the lateral re-

cess is narrowest (Fig. 10–33). This is a consequence of the relatively anterior position of the horizontal portion of the superior articular facet at this point. Therefore it is at the more cephalad aspect of the superior articular facet that hypertrophy is likely to result in nerve root compression. It is here that the anteroposterior dimension of the lateral recess should be measured if measurements are being made.[24, 25]

Foraminal Stenosis

The evaluation of patency of the neural foramen requires a series of contiguous scans beginning at the level of the inferior surface of the pedicle and extending through the disc level. Generally, the nerve roots appear well outlined by epidural fat immediately adjacent to the inner aspect of the inferior pedicle in the region of the

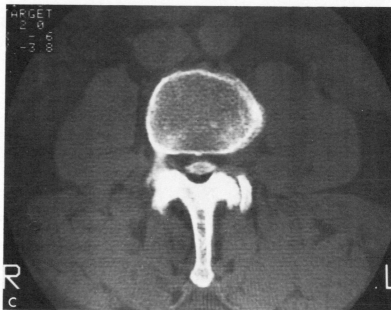

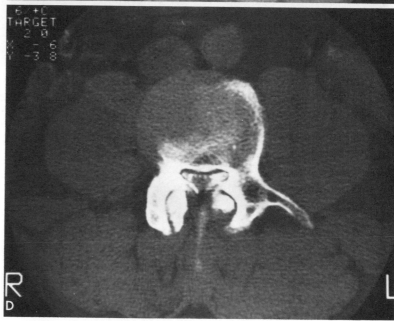

Figure 10–30. *Continued* **C, D** Metrizamide-assisted CT demonstrates diminutive size of thecal sac and central spinal canal.

lateral recess. In sections immediately caudad to the lower surface of the pedicle, one sees the neural foramen well and the nerve root surrounded by epidural fat. As one proceeds further caudad, the neural foramina generally become smaller and finally end at the level of the superior surface of the pedicle of the next adjacent vertebra. The finding of a narrow neural foramen at the level of the endplate and the disc does not by itself indicate significant neural foraminal encroachment with nerve root compression because the nerve has generally exited slightly superior to the level of the disc. The entire series of contig-

uous cuts needs to be evaluated in order to determine significant foraminal encroachment. Neurologically significant foraminal stenosis may be caused by any soft-tissue or bony space-occupying lesion that compresses the nerve root as it exits from the central canal. Bony encroachment may be caused by an osteophyte from the posteroinferior aspect of the vertebral body or the anterosuperior aspect of the superior articular facet (Figs. 10–34 and 10–35).

Occasionally, an important finding of lateral bulging or herniating disc encroaching upon the exiting nerve root laterally in the neural foramen

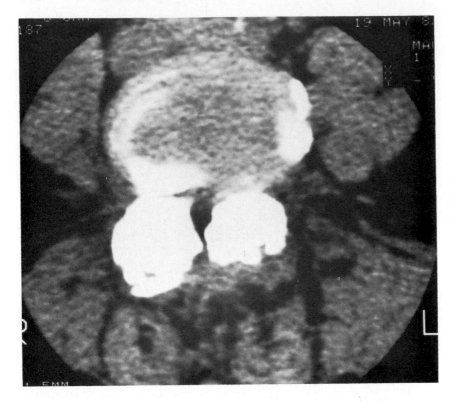

Figure 10–31. Marked postoperative facet hypertrophy, causing marked narrowing of the transverse dimension of the central canal.

may be encountered. The encroachment is often undetected by conventional myelography but is readily depicted by CT. In the evaluation of osseous neural foraminal encroachment, sagittal reformations occasionally provide additional useful information. Such reformations are of particular aid in assessing the presence of neural foraminal stenosis in the patient with spondylolisthesis.[26] The potential for entrapment of the exiting nerve by the articular pillar immediately superior to the pars defect is occasionally realized and most readily seen on sagittal reformations.

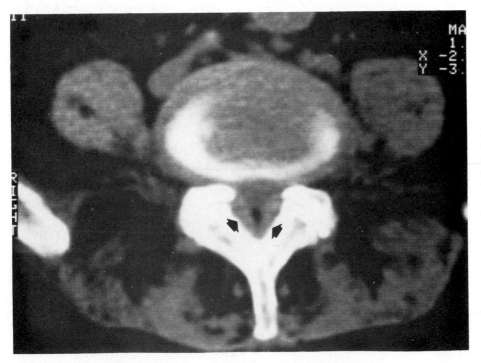

Figure 10–32. Ligamentum flavum hypertrophy (arrows) causing central spinal canal stenosis with narrowing of the transverse dimension of the central canal. A mild disc protrusion is incidentally noted.

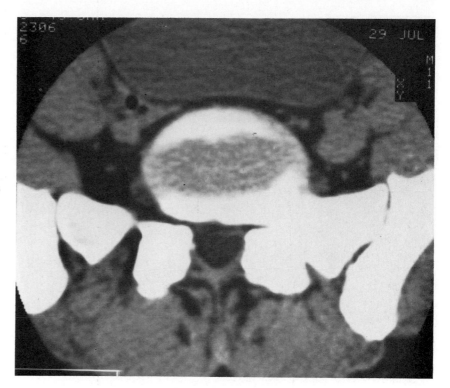

Figure 10–33. Left-sided recess stenosis is evident at the S1 level.

FACET JOINT DISEASE

Relatively recent radiologic[27, 28] and earlier orthopedic literature[29] has emphasized the role of the lumbar apophyseal joint in causing low back pain and sciatica that is clinically indistinguishable from that of a ruptured lumbar disc. The facets produce symptoms by impingement when hypertrophic bone or an osteophyte encroaches upon either a neural foramen or the central spinal canal, compromising either an exiting nerve root or the thecal sac, respectively (Fig. 10–36).

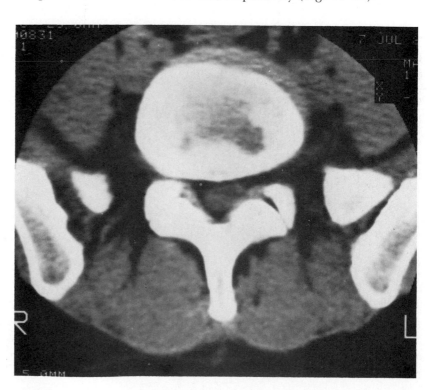

Figure 10–34. Severe right-sided neural foraminal stenosis.

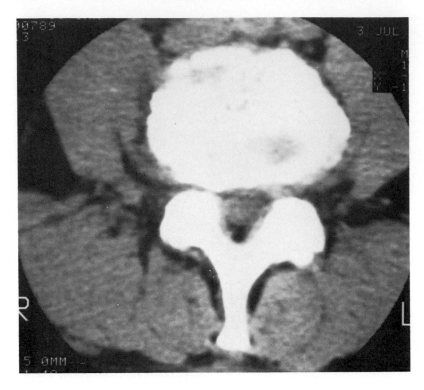

Figure 10–35. Foraminal stenosis and protruding disc. Severe right-sided neural foraminal stenosis is caused by osteophytic overgrowth; left-sided stenosis is caused by the soft-tissue density of the protruding disc.

The apophyseal joint is surrounded by a synovial capsule that is innervated by branches of the posterior primary ramus from the dorsal root ganglion with components from the level of the facet joint and the level immediately cranial to it. Inflammation and consequent destruction of the facet joint from osteoarthritis or another arthropathy have been shown to cause pain (Figs. 10–37 and 10–38). These synovial joints may fill with fluid and distend, leading to stimulation of the sensitive capsular nerve endings with subsequent pain. Additionally, enlargement of the medial

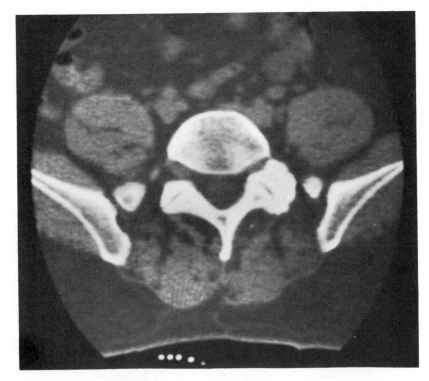

Figure 10–36. Hypertrophy of the left superior articular process of S1 is seen to cause severe left-sided neural foraminal encroachment.

tients may be studied by CT without the use of CTMM. A careful search for bony destruction and extradural soft-tissue densities should be made. For the majority of neoplasms that involve the spinal cord or are located in extradural sites and are associated with neurologic findings, CTMM is the modality of choice once the approximate level has been clinically determined. In those patients with neurologic findings whose level of in-volvement is in doubt, metrizamide myelography should precede CTMM. The upper and lower extent of the tumor may be seen by CTMM when an apparent block is seen at myelography.[30] The greater density resolution of CT allows visualization of tumor calcification and/or fat not otherwise seen (Figs. 10–45 through 10–47). The greatest role of CT, however, is defining the extradural or paraspinous extent of a tumor (Fig. 10–48).

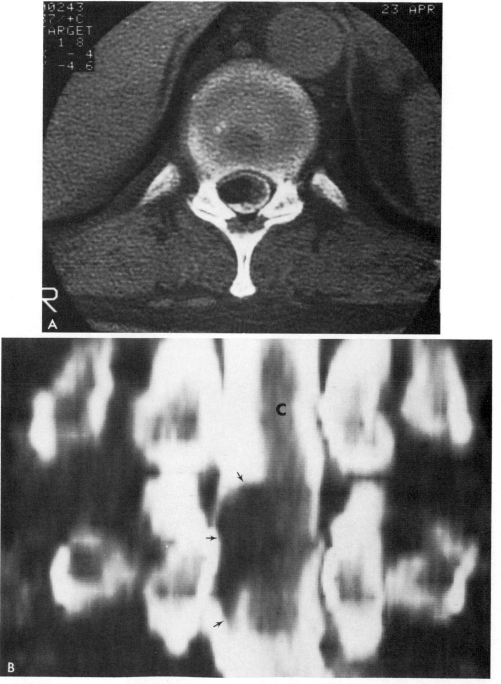

Figure 10–45. A Metrizamide-assisted CT (CTMM) at T12 level demonstrates intradural, extramedullary soft-tissue lesion typical of a lipoma. **B** Coronal CTMM at the T11-12 region delineates the relationship of the lipoma (arrows) to the spinal cord (C).

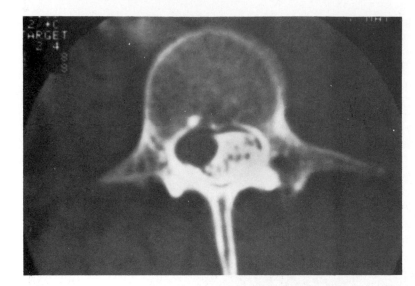

Figure 10–46. Intradural neurilemoma of the cauda equina.

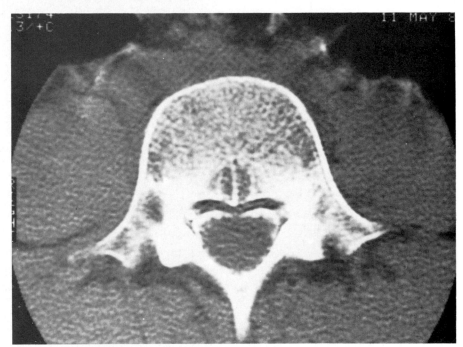

Figure 10–47. Metrizamide-assisted CT demonstrates intramedullary ependymoma with prominence of the epidural veins, which may indicate venous removal of metrizamide.

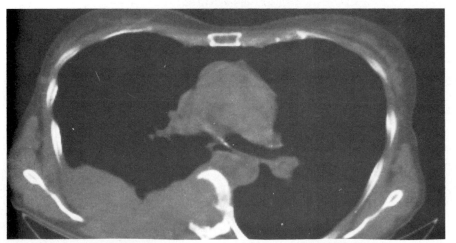

Figure 10–48. Solitary plasmacytoma with destruction of the soft-tissue, ribs, and T6 vertebral body.

INFLAMMATION

Arachnoiditis

Arachnoidal adhesions are a nonspecific inflammatory response to a variety of infectious or chemical irritants. Blood and iophendylate (Pantopaque) are the most common causes, and together they have a synergistic effect in producing adhesions.[30] Intrathecal metrizamide should be used to delineate the presence and degree of arachnoiditis.

Arachnoiditis is characterized by the deposition of immature collagen in the arachnoid and adjacent subarachnoid space.[31] The earliest findings are blunting of the axillary root sleeves seen at myelography. Slightly later nonfilling of the root sleeves can be discerned both at myelography and at CT. With progressively more severe adhesions, the roots begin to appear "clumped" and, in extreme cases, the coalescent roots resemble intradural and extradural masses (Fig. 10–49).

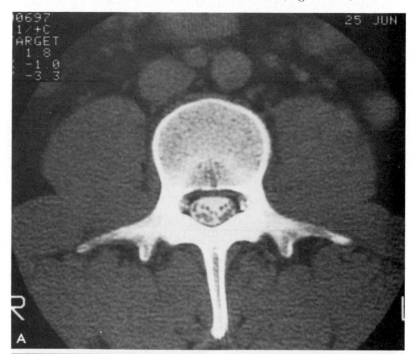

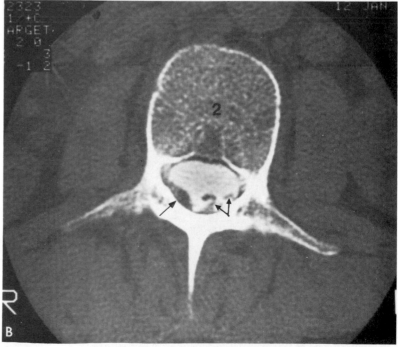

Figure 10–49. A Normal CTMM of L2 with metrizamide delineating the root sleeves in the lateral recesses. **B** Severe arachnoiditis with clumped nerve roots on the left (small branched arrows) and fixation of a portion of the cauda equina to the dura on the right (large arrows).

Infection

Computed tomography enables excellent study of involvement of the epidural and paraspinal regions as well as the vertebrae and discs by an infectious process (Fig. 10–50).[32] Only when edema and granulation tissue obscure the dural margins is intrathecal metrizamide suggested, and care must be exercised to perform the puncture at a site remote from the level of infection. The distortion of fascial planes that is apparent in the immediate postspinal operation patient renders CT scan interpretation difficult. Soft-tissue swelling often lasts 2 weeks. Postoperative infections generally become evident after this period. However, an increase in soft-tissue swelling beyond the first week may be regarded as suspicious of infection. Because both a resolving hematoma and an ab-

scess can appear as a paraspinal mass with a central lucency, needle aspiration may be required for definitive diagnosis (Figs. 10–51 through 10–53).[30]

SPINAL TRAUMA

Proper treatment of the patient with an acutely traumatized spine rests upon the rapid, accurate, and thorough assessment of the injury. The deployment of a high-resolution CT scanner for the evaluation of the patient with suspected spine injury will expedite the institution of appropriate therapy.

Conventional radiographs remain the primary mode of examinations following major spinal trauma. However, CT is the method of choice for

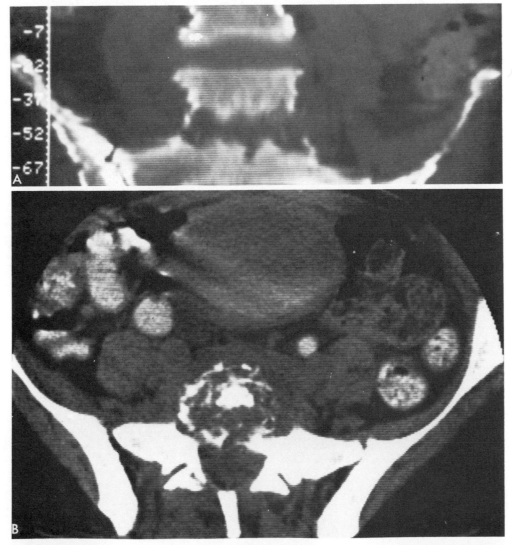

Figure 10–50. Disc space infection. **A** Coronal display of the lumbar spine demonstrates destruction of the adjacent L5 and S1 cortical endplates as well as an abnormal bilateral paraspinal soft-tissue mass. **B** Axial scan of superior aspect of the sacrum reveals bony destruction and a paravertebral soft-tissue mass. Note the replacement of the epidural fat on the left with the soft-tissue density.

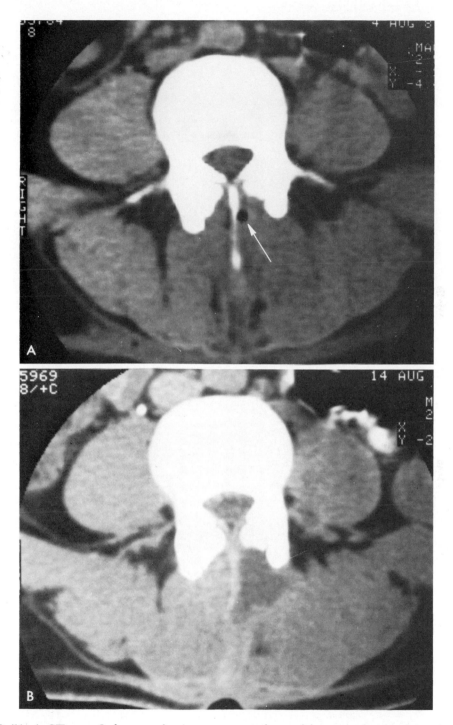

Figure 10–51. A CT scan 2 days postlaminectomy reveals suspicious gas density (arrow) on the left adjacent to the spinous process. **B** Repeat scan 10 days later reveals progression of paraspinal inflammatory process. Inflammation cleared with systemic antibiotic therapy.

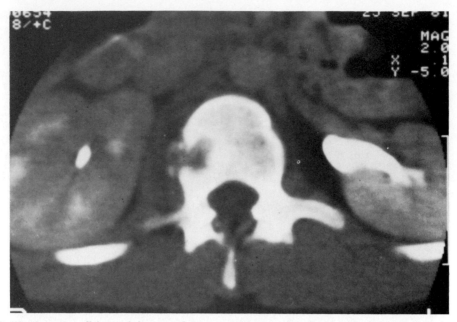

Figure 10–52. Osteomyelitis. Axial scan of 15-year-old boy with fever and right flank pain suspected of renal abscess. Right-sided L2 vertebral body destruction and adjacent paraspinous inflammatory mass are revealed by CT scan. Needle aspiration under CT guidance revealed salmonella osteomyelitis.

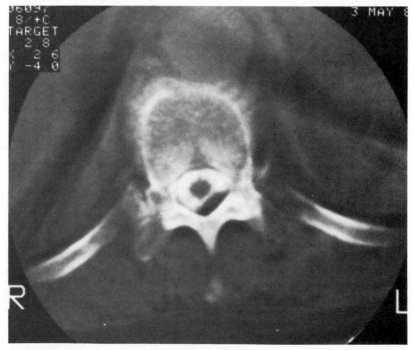

Figure 10–53. Epidural abscess. An 81-year-old man with fever and upper lumbar pain. Metrizamide-assisted CT at the T12 level reveals a typical epidural abscess with deformity of the metrizamide column.

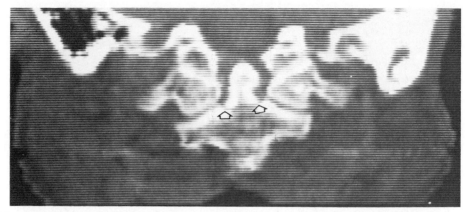

Figure 10–54. Fracture of dens. Coronal reformation from axial scans 1.5 mm thick displays the fracture (arrows) at the base of the dens to advantage.

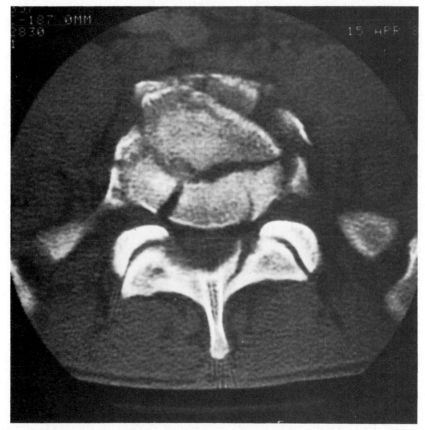

Figure 10–55. Unstable lumbar fracture with comminution of the vertebral body, central canal compromise, and laminar disruption.

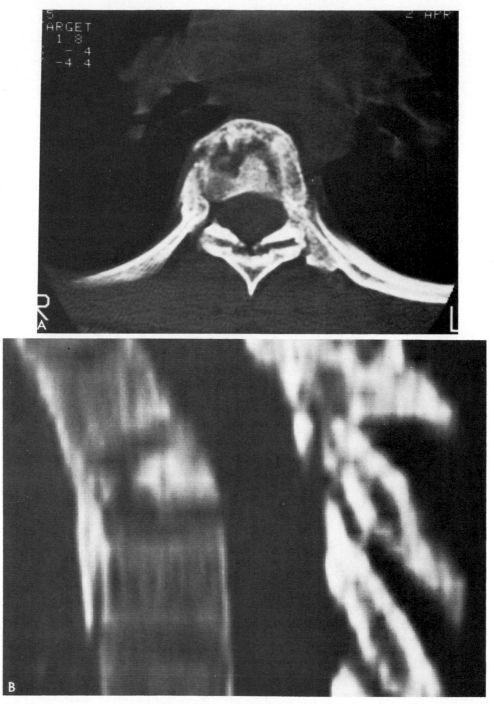

Figure 10–56. A, B Comminuted T7 fracture. Sagittal reformation shows no evidence of significant bony canal compromise.

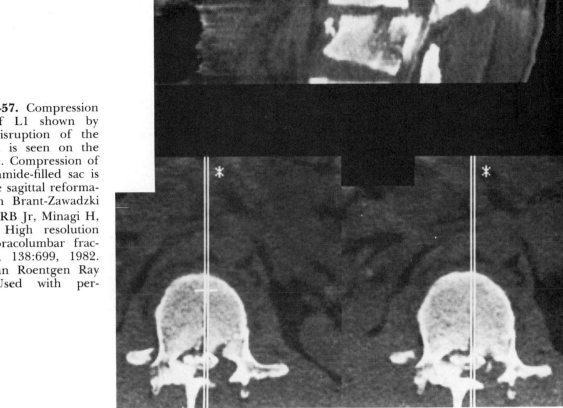

Figure 10–57. Compression fracture of L1 shown by CTMM. Disruption of the left lamina is seen on the axial image. Compression of the metrizamide-filled sac is seen on the sagittal reformation. (From Brant-Zawadzki M, Jeffrey RB Jr, Minagi H, Pitts LH: High resolution CT of thoracolumbar fractures. AJR 138:699, 1982. © American Roentgen Ray Society. Used with permission.)

studying integrity of the bony canal. Additionally, CT allows a patient to maintain one position (with or without traction) and to be quickly examined in multiple locations and planes. If neurologic signs are present, the subarachnoid instillation of 5 ml of 170 mg/dl of metrizamide is recommended.

In order to reformat the axial scans into high quality sagittal or coronal images, dynamic scanning with contiguous slices 1.5 mm thick may be used. At the anatomically complex C1-2 level, the thin contiguous 1.5-mm slices are especially helpful since correct diagnosis in this region often depends heavily on sagittal and coronal reformations. This is particularly true for the nondisplaced transverse fracture of the dens (Fig. 10–54).[33] Sagittal reformations are routine in the remainder of the spine.

Rapid-scanning software packages that allow for very small interscan delays require a low-milliamperage technique. High-contrast tissues such as bone or the metrizamide-containing subarachnoid space do not suffer significant spatial resolution degradation at lower milliamperage settings. Consequently, the dynamic scan mode with settings as low as 160 mA are generally used to expedite the scan.[34]

In this manner CT is an efficacious modality for the delineation of facet subluxation and fracture instability, the location of bony fragments within the spinal canal, and the existence of dural tears (Figs. 10–55 through 10–59).

SPINAL DYSRAPHISM

Myelography should, in most patients, follow conventional radiography in the assessment of a congenital spinal abnormality. After an overview has thereby been obtained, CTMM offers the opportunity to study a specific region more extensively. In particular, CTMM is well suited to the demonstration of the level and extent of the split spinal cord (Figs. 10–60 and 10–61) in diastematomyelia and the commonly associated fibrous or bony septum.[35] Meningocoeles (and syrinxes) (Fig. 10–62) are often best shown on a CTMM scan delayed to allow diffusion of metrizamide into the abnormal space. The lower concentration of contrast material not readily perceived at myelography may be easily detected by CT.

The size and position and point of attachment of a tethered spinal cord to the dura are also better shown by CTMM than metrizamide myelography.[36]

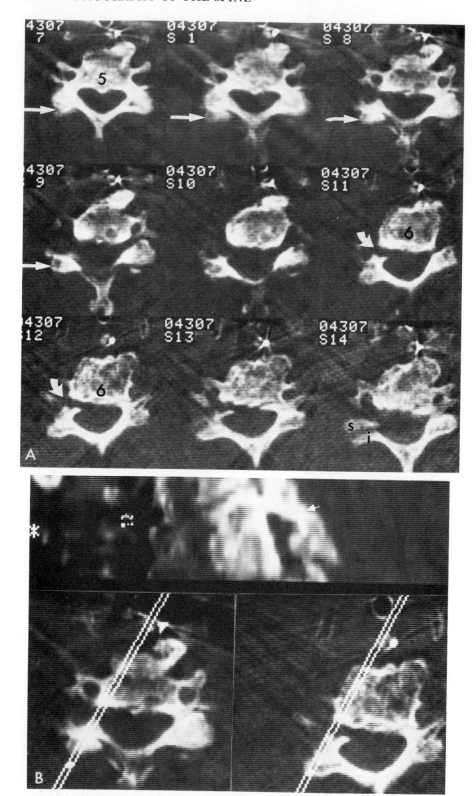

Figure 10–58. Subluxated cervical facet. **A**   Consecutive 1.5-mm axial sections starting at C5 and proceeding through C6 are shown. Note that a bony mass with a flat posterior surface progressively appears behind the inferior facet of C5 (arrows) and becomes contiguous with the posterior arch of C6. This is the posteriorly subluxed superior facet of C6. On the lower sections, a fracture through the right pedicle is shown (curved arrows), explaining the rotation of the C6 ring posteriorly on the right. Note the normal facet relationship shown in the lowest section, where the superior facet (S) of C7 articulates with the rotated inferior facet of C6 (i). **B**   Oblique reformation through the C5–6 facet (arrow). (Courtesy of Michael Brant-Zawadzki, M.D., University of California, San Francisco.)

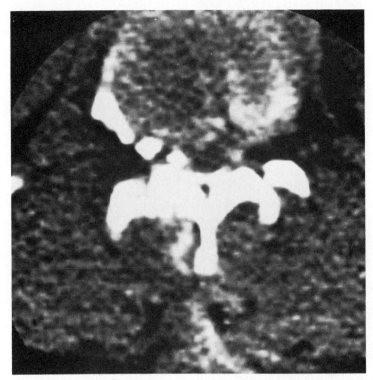

Figure 10–59. Dural tear demonstrated by the metrizamide in the posterior paraspinal musculature. Metrizamide was not injected at this site. (Courtesy of Michael Brant-Zawadzki, M.D., University of California, San Francisco.)

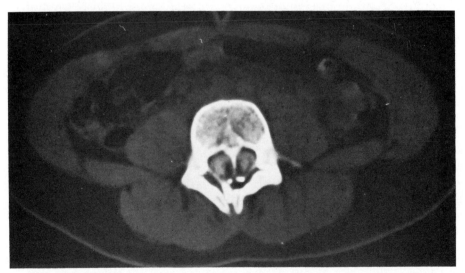

Figure 10–60. Axial scan of a patient with bony spur diastematomyelia.

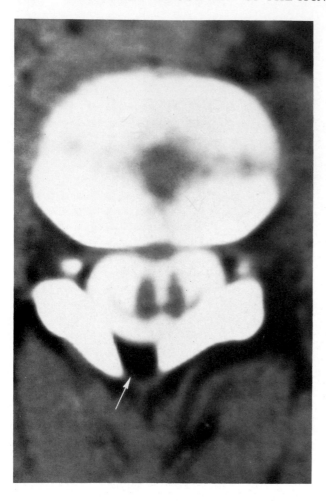

Figure 10–61. Spinal dysraphism demonstrating diplomyelia with a single dural sac, spina bifida, and a small posterior lipoma (arrow).

SACROILIITIS

Early diagnosis of the HLA-B27-associated spondyloarthropathies generally rests upon identification of bony changes at the sacroiliac joints. Both conventional radiographic and nuclear bone scanning techniques have shown disappointing sensitivity and specificity in this setting. Conventional tomographic assessment of sacroiliitis is associated with a radiation dosage that most regard as prohibitive. Additionally, the curved, oblique orientation of the sacroiliac joint and the overlying bony and soft-tissue structures render CT preferable for evaluation of these joints.[37–39]

The anatomy of this region is well displayed by CT images that are oriented either in the axial plane or through the long axis of the sacrum. Generally, 5-mm CT images obtained at 5-mm intervals suffice.

Computed tomography shows a normal synovial compartment that occupies the anterior half of the inferior two thirds of the sacroiliac joint to have symmetrical, parallel, and well-defined articular margins. In contrast, the ligamentous compartment occupying the dorsal half and all of the superior third of the sacroiliac joint is irregular and wider than the synovial compartment. A symmetrically escalloped contour of the articular surfaces marks the location of ligamentous attachments.

CT images are considered diagnostic for sacroiliitis when joint-space narrowing to less than 2 mm, sclerosis on both sides of the joint, erosions, or ankylosis are identified at the site of the synovial compartment (Fig. 10–63). When these criteria are observed, CT scanning has been shown to be more sensitive and equally specific in the diagnosis of sacroiliitis compared with conventional radiographs. As long as the relative monetary expense of CT remains high, CT for sacroiliitis is reserved only for those patients with normal or equivocal conventional radiographs and in whom spondyloarthropathy is highly suspect.

The identification of soft-tissue masses associated with sacroiliac osseous abnormalities often lead to definitive diagnosis (Fig. 10–64). Sacroiliac abnormalities seen on nuclear bone scans, when unexplained on conventional radiographs, are optimally assessed by CT (Fig. 10–65).

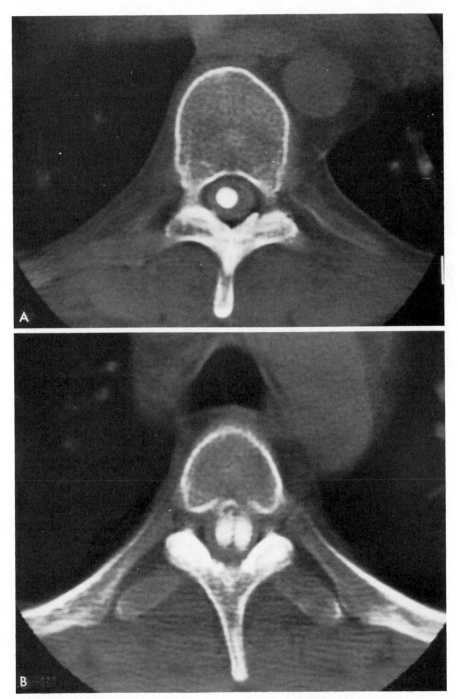

Figure 10–62. A Four hours after CTTM, dilated central canal, typical of a syrinx, is seen. **B** Two vertebral segments inferior to the one shown in Figure 10–63A reveals septated portion of the syrinx.

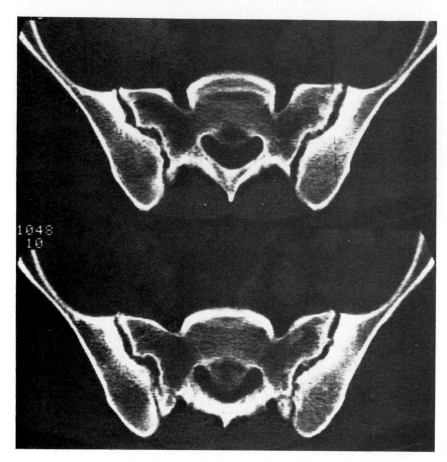

Figure 10–63. Bilateral subchondral iliac sclerosis and sacroiliac joint erosions are demonstrated on axial CT scans of a patient with early ankylosing spondylitis.

Figure 10–64. Tuberculous abscess. Marked destruction of the right sacroiliac joint was demonstrated on the conventional radiographs. The CT findings revealed an adjacent soft-tissue mass containing a central fluid density. This suggested infection as the etiology of the bony destruction. As a result of the CT findings, early drainage of the overlying tuberculous iliacus muscle abscess was made possible.

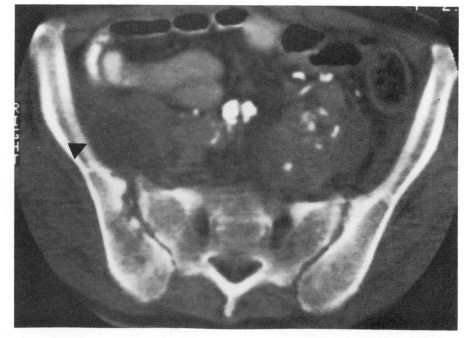

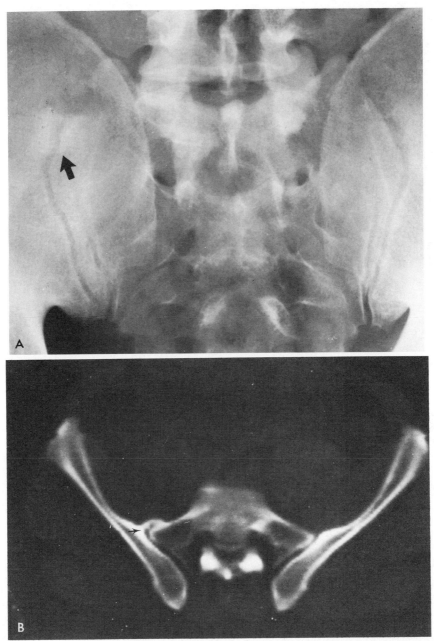

Figure 10–65. A This anteroposterior radiograph demonstrating sclerosis of the right sacroiliac joint in a patient with suspected metastatic disease was obtained to clarify a region of increased radionuclide activity on a bone scan. **B** The corresponding axial CT image demonstrates an osteophytic spur to correlate with the bone scan abnormality. No metastatic focus was demonstrated.

REFERENCES

1. Genant HK: Computed tomography of the lumbar spine: Technical considerations. In Genant HK, Chafetz N, Helms CA (eds): Computed Tomography of the Lumbar Spine. San Francisco, University of California, 1982, pp 23–52.
2. Hanson KM: Detectability in computed tomographic images. Med Phys 6:441, 1979.
3. Boyd DP, Margulis AR, Korobkin M: Comparison of translate-rotate and pure rotary computed tomography (CT) body scanners. SPIE. Optical Instrumentation in Medicine VI, 127:280, 1977.
4. Gould RG: Advanced CT instrumentation technology. In Genant HK, Chafetz N, Helms CA (eds): Computed Tomography of the Lumbar Spine. San Francisco, University of California, 1982, pp 15–22.
5. Hounsfield GN: Picture quality of computed tomography. AJR 127:3, 1976.
6. McCullough EC, Payne JT: Patient dosage in computed tomography. Radiology 129:457, 1978.
7. Axel L, Genant HK, Chafetz NI, Dorwart RH, Helms. CA, Cann CE, Moss AA: Analysis of imaging properties and scanning procedures for computed tomography of intervertebral discs (abstract). Radiological Society of North America, 66th Scientific Assembly. Dallas, Texas, Nov. 16–20, 1980.
8. General Electric Company: CT/T Continuum. Milwaukee General Electric Medical Systems Division, 1976.
9. General Electric Company: Application and Information Computed Tomography: Introduction to Review. Milwaukee, General Electric Medical Systems Division, 1981.
10. Naidich TP, King DG, Moran CJ, Sagel SS: Computed tomography of the lumbar thecal sac. J Comput Assist Tomogr 4:37, 1980.
11. Schubiger O, Valavanis A: CT differentiation between recurrent disc herniation and postoperative scar formation: The value of contrast enhancement. Neuroradiology 22:251, 1982.
12. Meaney TF, Raudkivi U, McIntyre WJ, Gallagher JH, Haaga JR, Havrilla TR, Reich NE: Detection of low contrast lesions in computed body tomography: An experimental study of simulated lesions. Radiology 134:149, 1980.
13. Glenn WV Jr, Rhodes ML, Altschuler EM, Wiltse LL, Lostanek C, Kuo YM: Multiplanar display computerized body tomography applications in the lumbar spine. Spine 4:282, 1979.
14. Macnab I: Backache. Baltimore: Williams & Wilkins, 1977.
15. Williams AL, Haughton VM, Daniels DL, Thornton RS: CT recognition of lateral lumbar disk herniation. AJR 139:345, 1982.
16. Chafetz N: Computed tomography of lumbar disk disease. In Genant HK, Chafetz N, Helms CA (eds): Computed Tomography of the Lumbar Spine. San Francisco, University of California, 1982, pp 125–138.
17. Helms CA, Dorwart RH, Gray M: The CT appearance of conjoined nerve roots and differentiation from a herniated nucleus pulposus. Radiology 144:803, 1982.
18. Fries JW, Abodeely DA, Vijungco JG, Yeager YL, Gaffey WR: Computed tomography of herniated and extruded nucleus pulposus. J Comput Assist Tomogr 6:874, 1982.
19. Haughton VM, Eldevik PO, Magnaes B, Amundsen P: A prospective comparison of computed tomography and myelography in the diagnosis of herniated lumbar disk. Radiology 142:103, 1982.
20. Williams AL, Haughton VM, Asbjorn S: Computed tomography in the diagnosis of herniated nucleus pulposus. Radiology 135:95, 1980.
21. Carrera GF, Williams AL, Haughton VM: Computed tomography in sciatica. Radiology 137:433, 1980.
22. Raskin SP, Keating JW: Recognition of lumbar disk disease: Comparison of myelography and computed tomography. AJR 139:349, 1982.
23. Ullrich CG, Binet EF, Sanecki MG, Kieffer SA: Quantitative assessment of the lumbar spinal canal by computed tomography. Radiology 134:137, 1980.
24. Mikhael MA, Ciric I, Tarkington JA, Vick NA: Neuroradiological evaluation of lateral recess syndrome. Radiology 140:97, 1981.
25. Ciric I, Mikhael MA, Tarkington JA, Vick NA: The lateral recess syndrome: A variant of spinal stenosis. J Neurosurg 53:433, 1980.
26. Helms CA, Vogler JB III: Computed tomography of spinal stenoses and arthroses. In Genant HK, Chafetz N, Helms CA (eds.): Computed Tomography of the Lumbar Spine. San Francisco, University of California, 1982, pp 187–200.
27. Carrera GF: Lumbar facet joint injection in low back pain and sciatica. Radiology 137:665, 1980.
28. Dory MA: Arthrography of the lumbar facet joints. Radiology 140:23, 1981.
29. Carrera GF, Haughton VM, Syvertsen A, Williams AL: Computed tomography of the lumbar facet joints. Radiology 134:145, 1980.
30. Goldthwait JE: The lumbosacral articulation: An explanation of many cases of "lumbago," "sciatica" and paraplegia. Boston Med Surg J 64:365, 1911.
31. Yeates AE, Newton TH: Applications of metrizamide in computed tomographic examination of the lumbar spine. In Genant HK, Chafetz N, Helms CA (eds): Computed Tomography of the Lumbar Spine. San Francisco, University of California, 1982, pp 67–86.
32. Haughton VM, Williams AL: Computed Tomography of the Spine. St. Louis: C.V. Mosby, 1982, pg 82.
33. Brant-Zawadzki M, Jeffrey RB Jr, Minagi H, Pitts LH: High resolution CT of thoracolumbar fractures. AJR 138:699, 1982.
34. Brant-Zawadzki M: Computed tomography in the evaluation of spinal trauma. In Genant HK, Chafetz N, Helms CA (eds.): Computed Tomography of the Lumbar Spine. San Francisco, University of California, 1982, pp 261–278.
35. Scotti G, Musgrave MA, Harwood Nash DC, Fitz CR, Chuang SH: Diastematomyelia in children: Metrizamide and CT metrizamide myelography. AJNR 1:403, 1980.
36. Kaplan JO, Quencer RM: The occult tethered conus syndrome in the adult. Radiology 137:387, 1980.
37. Kozin F, Carrera GF, Ryan LM, Foley D, Lawson T: Computed tomography in the diagnosis of sacroiliitis. Arthritis Rheum 24:1479, 1981.
38. Lawson TL, Foley WD, Carrera GF, Berland LL: The sacroiliac joints: Anatomic, plain roentgenographic, and computed tomographic analysis. Comput Assist Tomogr 6:307, 1982.
39. Carrera GF, Foley WD, Kozin F, Ryan L, Lawson TL: CT of sacroiliitis. AJR 136:41, 1981.

11 COMPUTED TOMOGRAPHY OF THE APPENDICULAR MUSCULOSKELETAL SYSTEM

Harry K. Genant
Clyde A. Helms

Computed tomography (CT) has a wide range of applications in the musculoskeletal system and is particularly effective in evaluating cases of trauma, soft-tissue and bony tumors, infection, low back pain syndromes, and metabolic bone dis-orders. For studying the soft tissues and areas of complex bony anatomy such as the spine, shoulder and hip joints, and the pelvis, CT may be superior to conventional radiographic techniques. It provides a cross-sectional view of the anatomy, has excellent density discrimination, and eliminates superimposed structures.

In an efficacy study at the Massachusetts General Hospital, Wittenberg and associates[1] showed that CT of the musculoskeletal system improved diagnostic understanding in 45 per cent of cases, increased precision of treatment in 52 per cent, and caused beneficial change in therapy in 5 per cent. As newer, more sophisticated applications are found, the percentage of patients in the latter category should increase. In a similar study at the University of California at San Francisco, Wilson and co-workers[2] showed that in 45 per cent of the patients CT added unique information establishing the correct diagnosis; in 78 per cent the location or extent of the lesion was better defined by CT than by the conventional imaging procedures; and also in 78 per cent, CT findings influenced treatment planning and therapeutic procedures.

In this chapter, we discuss the use of CT to assess the appendicular musculoskeletal system, including the technique of examination and specific applications to cases of trauma, neoplasm, and infection as well as miscellaneous applications.

TECHNICAL CONSIDERATIONS

With the continual upgrading of diagnostic computed tomographic procedures as new technical advances arise, CT is assuming a more important role in assessing musculoskeletal disorders, replacing many conventional techniques as well as invasive or time-consuming procedures. The advantages of this modality over conventional radiography are the capabilities for three-dimensional imaging, excellent contrast resolution, accurate measurement of tissue attenuation coefficient, noninvasive nature, and, in many instances, reduced radiation exposure to the patient.[3] All of these factors combine to make CT a powerful tool in the assessment of the musculoskeletal system.

Several scanners that are currently being marketed have the capability for submillimeter resolving power for high-contrast objects such as bone. This resolution, coupled with the use of thin sections (1 to 3 mm), means that high-quality images of fine bony structures can be readily obtained. The excellent contrast resolution of CT, always recognized as superior to that of conventional films, is approximately 0.3 per cent for most of the newer scanners. This image quality is obtained at a radiation dose of 1 to 3 rads, which is substantially lower than in older CT models.

The average scanning time for the newer systems is less than 5 seconds, eliminating most of the motion artifacts that were prevalent with the older machines. Rapid-sequence scanning in the dynamic mode greatly facilitates the performance of such studies, permitting 40 to 50 contiguous scans to be generated in 5 to 10 minutes. With dynamic scanning, back-to-back scans are obtained at relatively low millamperage with 1 to 2 seconds interscan delay for table incrementation.[4, 5] Thus, for high bone detail, contiguous stacked scans 1 to 3 mm thick provide not only excellent axial images but also the basis for high-quality sagittal, coronal, or multiplanar reformations,[6] supplanting conventional polytomography for delineating subtle structural changes in anatomically complex regions of the skeleton.

Variable reconstruction algorithms are now widely available that can be used to reconstruct original projection data to optimize high-contrast resolving power, low-contrast detectability, or other parameters. These options are especially useful for imaging bony structures.[3] The use of extended scales, −1000 to +3000 Hounsfield

Units (H), permits visualization of the entire range of densities in bone. Computed radiographic localization systems are also widely offered and greatly facilitate studies in musculoskeletal disease. The two-dimensional projection radiograph, indexed to the table location, can be used to specify precise scanning location and gantry angulation. The best external localization systems provide an accuracy of 0.5 to 1.0 mm in the table location, so that the limiting factor becomes patient motion between the time the computed radiograph is obtained and the time the axial scans are done.

Thus, the combination of projection computed radiography, high-resolution scanning, dynamic rapid-sequence scanning, thin-section capability, and multiplanar reformation has thus created an exciting array of possibilities for CT imaging of musculoskeletal system.

CT EVALUATION OF MUSCULOSKELETAL TRAUMA

Numerous publications[3, 4, 7–14] as well as general experience indicate an important role for computed tomography in evaluating fracture-disloca-

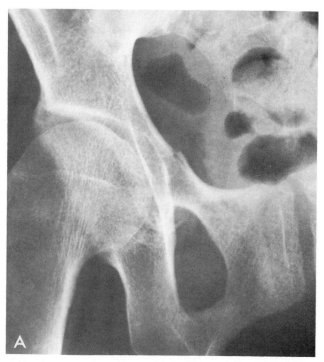

Figure 11–1. Determination of fracture extension. **A** Conventional radiograph demonstrates subtle pelvic fracture with questionable extension into acetabulum.

Illustration continued on opposite page

tions, particularly in anatomically complex regions such as the spine, sacrum, pelvis, and hip. Cross-sectional CT images optimally display the spatial relationships of fractures, the need for or adequacy of reduction, and the nature of associated articular and soft-tissue injuries.

PELVIC TRAUMA

Computed tomography is particularly useful in the evaluation of pelvic and hip trauma (Figs. 11–1 through 11–4). Surgical management of fracture-dislocations of the hip is based upon the stability of the joint-space, presence or absence of intra-articular fragments, congruity of fracture fragments, and the general condition of the patient.[13, 15, 16] In patients with hip trauma, the condition of the femoral head and acetabulum is frequently difficult to evaluate by means of conventional radiography or polytomography. Often, anteroposterior views are obtained using portable

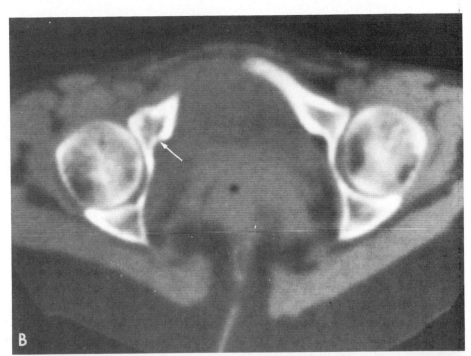

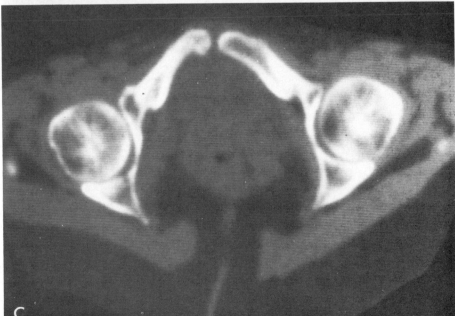

Figure 11–1. *Continued* **B, C** CT scans demonstrate anterior pubic fracture (arrow) but no involvement of the acetabulum.

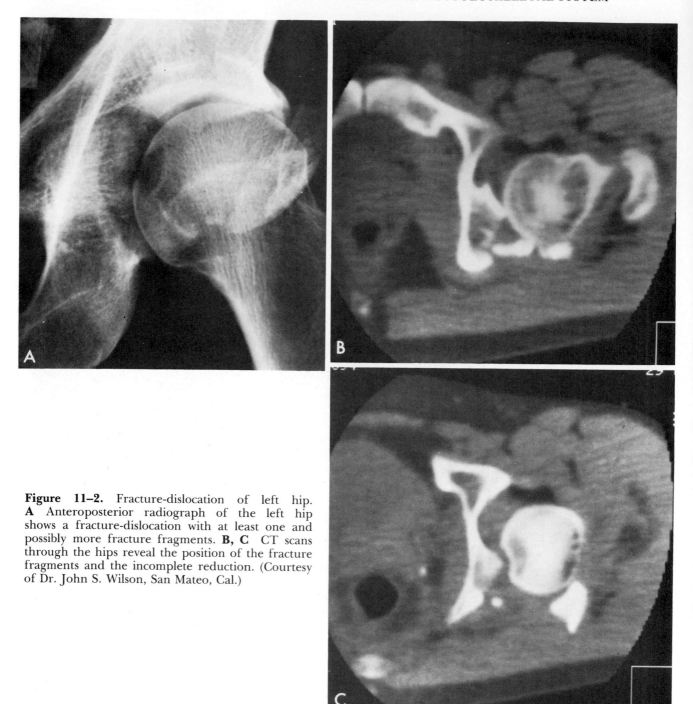

Figure 11–2. Fracture-dislocation of left hip. **A** Anteroposterior radiograph of the left hip shows a fracture-dislocation with at least one and possibly more fracture fragments. **B, C** CT scans through the hips reveal the position of the fracture fragments and the incomplete reduction. (Courtesy of Dr. John S. Wilson, San Mateo, Cal.)

apparatus, resulting in suboptimal image quality. Special views described by Judet,[17] including anterior and posterior oblique projections, provide additional important information but cannot always be obtained. Furthermore, they do not adequately define the joint-space or the integrity of the medial acetabulum.

Mack[12] analyzed the capability of CT for assessing acetabular fractures and showed that the tra-

ditional classification[18] of hip fractures into anterior column, posterior column, and complex two-column fractures was greatly facilitated by this modality. He indicated that the prognosis of acetabular fractures depends on the type of the fracture, the condition of the weight-bearing part of the joint, the persistence of displaced or intra-articular fragments, and additional fractures that further destabilize the pelvis. For each of these factors, CT provided essential and often unique information, so that appropriate surgical intervention could be undertaken and long-term prognosis could be improved. CT was particularly useful for evaluating two-column fractures providing information concerning the configuration of the fracture, integrity of acetabular dome and quadrilateral surface, and position of the stable fragment. Comparing conventional radiography with CT, Harley[11] found the two modalities comparable in the detection of fractures of the iliac wing, anterior pelvic column, posterior pelvic column, and the pubic rami, with high sensitivity and specificity for both examinations. CT, however, was more sensitive than plain radiography in detecting fractures involving the sacrum, quadrilateral surface of the acetabulum, the acetabular roof, and the posterior acetabular lip.

Finally, in the evaluation of complex pelvic fractures, the capability of CT to demonstrate, in cross-sectional array and with good contrast resolution, the surrounding muscle and soft-tissue

Figure 11–3. A Anteroposterior radiograph of the left hip shows a fracture-dislocation. **B** Following reduction, CT scan through the hip shows several fracture fragments, one of which is in the joint-space. (Courtesy of Dr. John S. Wilson, San Mateo, Cal.)

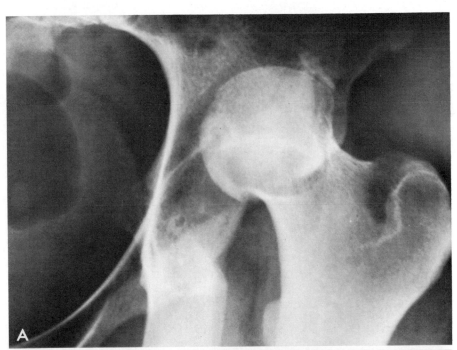

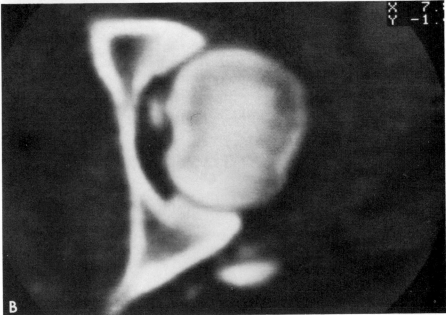

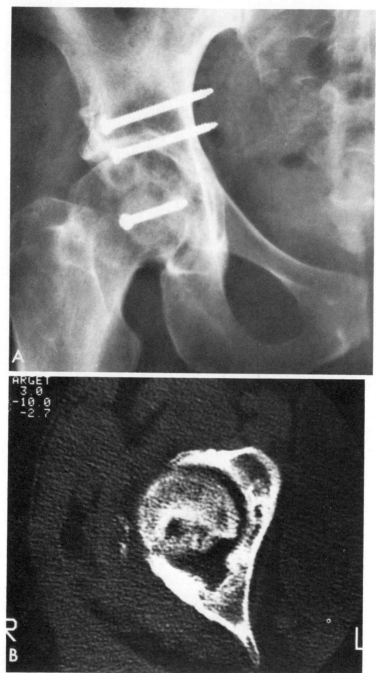

Figure 11–4. A   Conventional radiograph demonstrates abnormal right hip, 3 months following open reduction and internal fixation of an acetabular fracture. **B, C**   CT images demonstrate osseous and articular destruction, resulting from screw extending into hip joint. **D**   CT image using extended gray scale better displays the relationship of the screw to the hip joint.

Illustration continued on opposite page

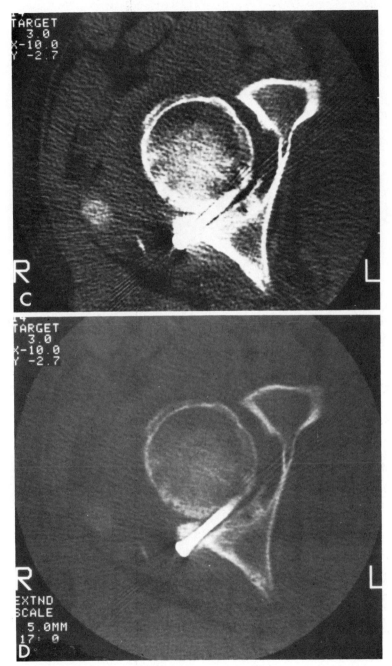

Figure 11–4. *Continued*

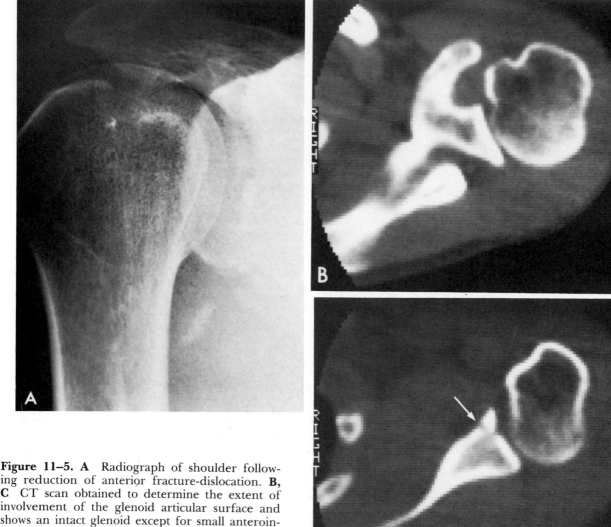

Figure 11–5. A Radiograph of shoulder following reduction of anterior fracture-dislocation. **B, C** CT scan obtained to determine the extent of involvement of the glenoid articular surface and shows an intact glenoid except for small anteroinferior fragment (arrow), obviating the need for exploration and open repair.

planes greatly facilitates the detection and evaluation of post-traumatic hematomas, which at times may be massive and life threatening.[3, 13, 17]

OTHER MUSCULOSKELETAL TRAUMA

Computed tomography may have importance in a wide spectrum of musculoskeletal trauma beyond pelvic and spinal fracture-dislocations. CT has been advocated for the evaluation of complex fracture-dislocations of the shoulder girdle including the glenohumeral (Figs. 11–5 and 11–6) and sternoclavicular articulations.[19, 20] CT may also be used to delineate subtle fracture planes extending into articular surfaces of the wrist, elbow, and ankle or to locate fragments associated with ballistic injuries (Fig. 11–7). Several studies[21, 22] have supported its use in the evaluation of stress fractures. Somer[21] reported that computed tomography was less sensitive than conventional radiographs in visualizing the cortical and periosteal changes; however, CT revealed endosteal callous formation of varying degrees even in cases with minor plain film findings. Two types of endosteal reaction were observed: a generalized endosteal thickening, and a slight local bridge-formed callous. The density of marrow cavity was generally increased, and soft-tissue edema around the lesion could also be observed.

SOFT-TISSUE STRUCTURES IN TRAUMA

The ability of CT to show subtle differences in tissue density generally allows one to distinguish among fat, muscle, blood (Fig. 11–8), serous and purulent fluids, and faint calcification not identifiable on plain radiographs (Fig. 11–9). Subtle circumferential ossification in the early stages of myositis ossificans can be diagnostic and therefore obviate additional workup. This ossification may or may not be visible on plain radiographs, and even if visualized, its circumferential nature can be difficult to ascertain (Fig. 11–10). Soft-tissue swelling that is due to a hematoma can occasionally be related to an adjacent vascular structure, which suggests it may be the source of the mass. Intravenous injection of contrast material enhances vascular areas and allows easy differentiation of some vascular masses, such as a pseudoaneurysm (Fig. 11–11). *Text continued on page 488*

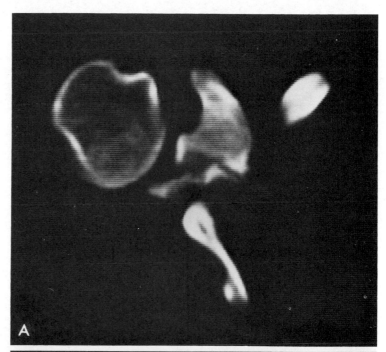

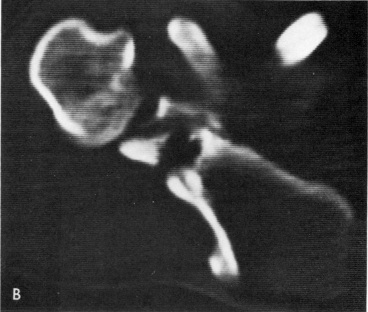

Figure 11–6. Fractured scapula. **A, B** CT scans demonstrate a complex comminuted fracture of the scapula with an intra-articular component.

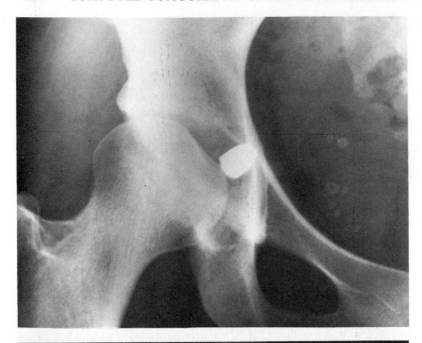

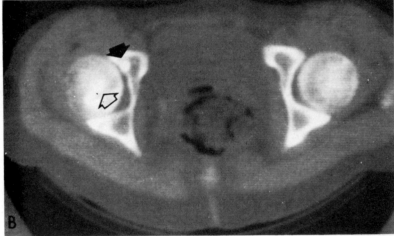

Figure 11–7. A Conventional radiograph demonstrates a bullet in the region of the right hip in a patient who sustained a gunshot wound to the right buttock several months earlier. The relationship of the bullet to the articular structures cannot readily be determined on conventional radiographs. **B** CT scan clearly defines the exact location of the bullet (solid arrow) in the subchondral bone of the acetabulum as well as the track where the bullet traversed the femoral head (open arrow).

Figure 11–8. Iliacus hematoma. CT scan of the pelvis in a patient taking sodium warfarin (Coumadin) who, following trauma developed femoral nerve palsy on the right side. The scan shows a soft-tissue mass (arrow) just anterior to the right ileum, which has a high CT density consistent with fresh hemorrhage into the iliacus muscle. The mass resolved with conservative treatment.

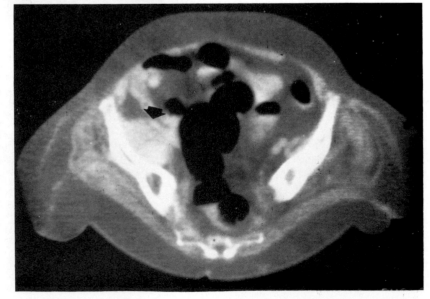

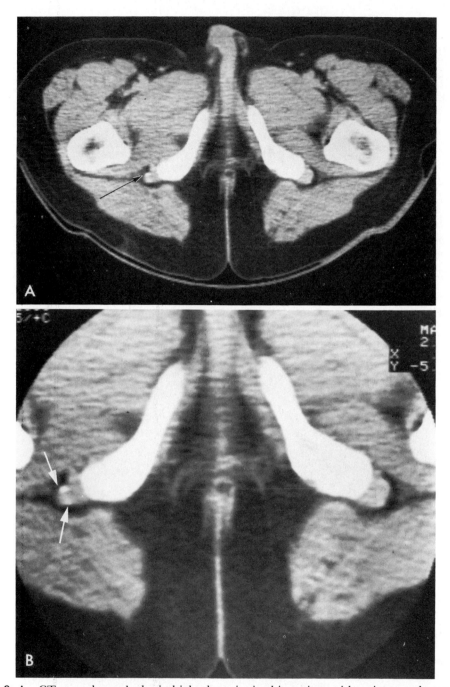

Figure 11–9. A   CT scan through the ischial tuberosity in this patient with pain, muscle atrophy, and reflex loss in the distribution of the right sciatic nerve. Scan shows faint calcifications (arrow) around the ischial tuberosity. **B**   Magnification shows better view of these calcifications (arrows). The sciatic nerve running adjacent to the ischial tuberosity on the right was found at surgery to be entrapped by a calcific inflammatory process of the ischial bursa caused by trauma from a paddle ball racquet.

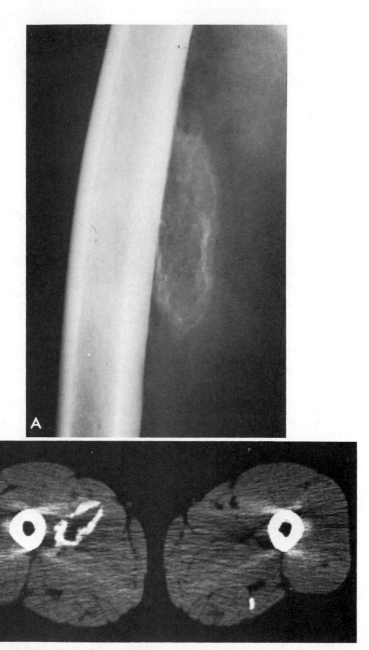

Figure 11–10. Myositis ossificans. **A** Radiograph of the femur in a patient with a slightly painful, enlarging mass in the thigh shows an ossified soft-tissue mass without definite bone destruction. A diagnosis of myositis ossificans was made, even though the history of trauma was equivocal. **B** CT scan through the mass shows peripheral ossification and an ill-defined centrum, the classic features of myositis ossificans. The CT findings made biopsy unnecessary.

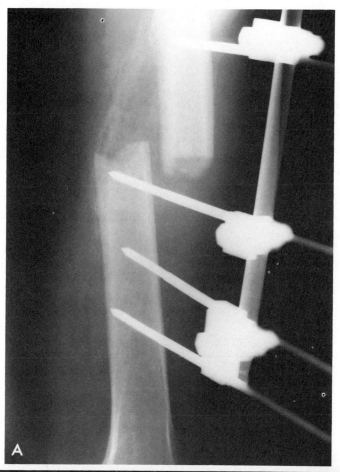

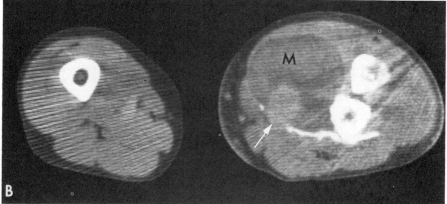

Figure 11–11. Post-traumatic pseudoaneurysm. **A** Radiograph of the femur taken 2 weeks after the fracture occurred shows internal traction pins and exuberant callous formation. This patient developed fever, pain, and swelling in his thigh over a 24-hour period and was considered to have an abscess. **B** Before the surgical drainage, a CT scan through the mass showed a large, low-density soft-tissue mass (M) surrounding a contrast-enhanced dilated artery (arrow). The diagnosis of pseudoaneurysm of the femoral artery with rupture, and bleeding in the soft-tissue was confirmed at surgery.

CT EVALUATION OF NEOPLASMS

A useful preoperative evaluation of musculoskeletal neoplasm should include elucidation of the following features: extent and depth of the process; involvement of vital adjacent structures; evidence of encapsulation or invasion; likelihood of aggressive or malignant nature; and finally, a meaningful differential diagnosis. Each parameter is of importance to the surgeon in planning the proper approach to the lesion. Many studies have shown that CT contributes valuable information concerning the nature, size, and extent of musculoskeletal tumors and that this information may influence patient management.

TYPES OF NEOPLASMS

Primary Bone Tumors

CT scanning of primary benign and malignant neoplasms of bone[2, 3, 23–32] is useful in localizing the lesion by cross-sectional display, determining the intramedullary and extraosseous extent, and defining the relationship between tumor and vital structures. Such assessment may have diagnostic or prognostic significance as, for example, in differentiating a solid from a cystic lesion, in demonstrating tumor invasion beyond the cortical confines, or in revealing a soft-tissue mass outside the ossified or calcified portions of a tumor, thereby suggesting malignancy.

Although the diagnosis of primary bone tumors is usually suggested by conventional radiography,

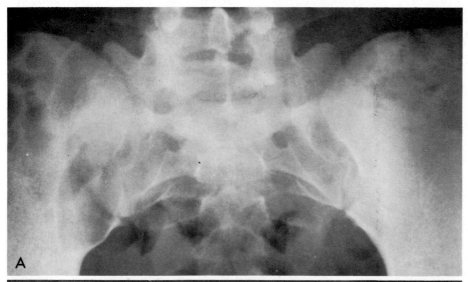

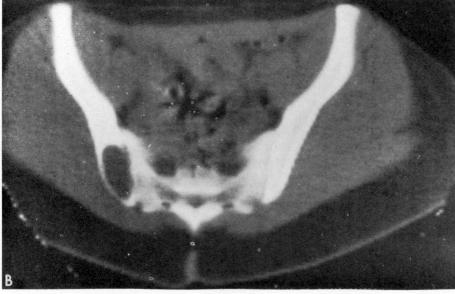

Figure 11–12. Unicameral bone cyst. **A** Conventional radiograph demonstrates a well-defined, lytic, expansile lesion in the right sacroiliac region. **B** CT scan with an early second-generation scanner demonstrates the precise posterior location and low-density fluid nature of the lesion.

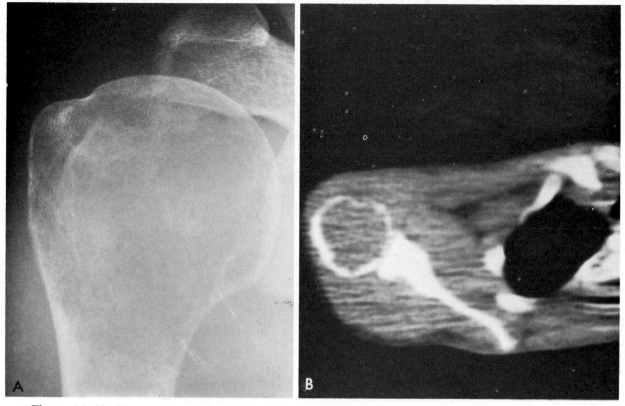

Figure 11–13. Giant cell tumor. **A** Conventional radiograph demonstrates a lytic, destructive lesion in the proximal humerus abutting the articular surface. **B** CT scan confirms the solid nature of this giant cell tumor, which is isodense with muscle. The integrity of the humeral cortex is also shown.

Figure 11–14. Fibro-osseous tumor of the mandible. CT scan shows an expansile lytic lesion of the mandible, which is isodense with muscle. Although there is focal cortical breakthrough, an appreciable extraosseous soft-tissue mass is not present in this benign fibro-osseous tumor. Such an accurate anatomic depiction of benign, but locally aggressive, bone tumors may alter the therapeutic approach from radical excision to simple curettage.

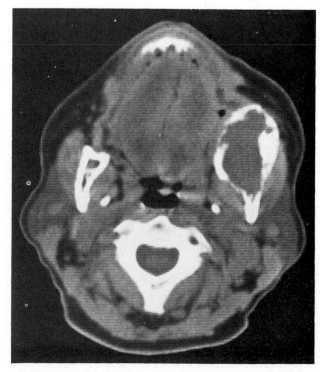

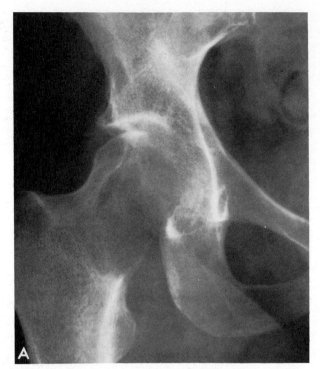

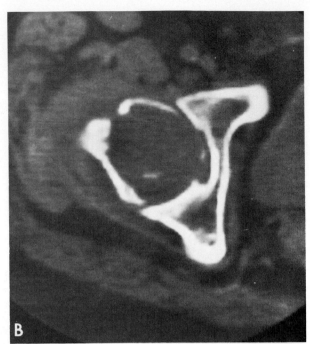

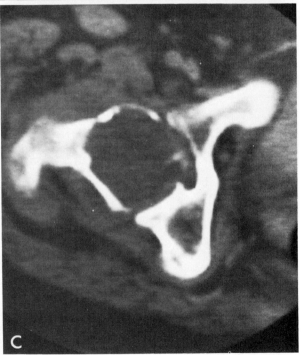

Figure 11–15. Fibrosarcoma. **A**   Conventional radiograph demonstrates a lytic destructive process involving the medial aspect of the femoral head and neck. **B, C**   CT scans demonstrate the intra-osseous rather than intra-articular nature of this process and shows several foci of dystrophic calcification and a mass lesion that is principally isodense with muscle. A fibrosarcoma was proven at biopsy.

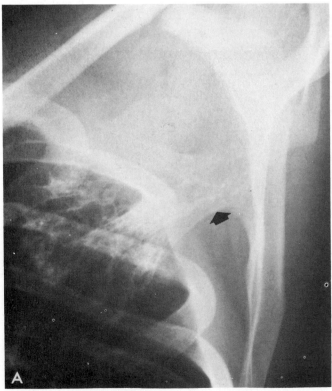

Figure 11–16. Osteochondroma. **A**   Trans-scapular view demonstrates an osteochondroma (arrow) projecting off the posterior surface of the scapula.

Illustration continued on opposite page

the CT differentiation of unicameral bone cyst[33] from similar-appearing processes is sometimes possible (Fig. 11–12). A unicameral bone cyst has a fluid-filled cavity, which has a density of about 20 H, whereas fibrous dysplasia, aneurysmal bone cysts, enchondromas and most malignant intraosseous neoplasms generally have higher CT numbers (Figs. 11–13 through 11–15).

CT also has been successfully used to differen-tiate osteochondromas from chondrosarcomas.[34, 35] In simple osteochondromas, CT scans readily show the attachment site of the tumor, even in complex joints where plain radiographs can be confusing. The absence of bone destruction and significant soft-tissue mass and the presence of well-circumscribed lobular surfaces are criteria for a benign osteochondroma (Figs. 11–16 through 11–18). Lesions with disorganized calcification,

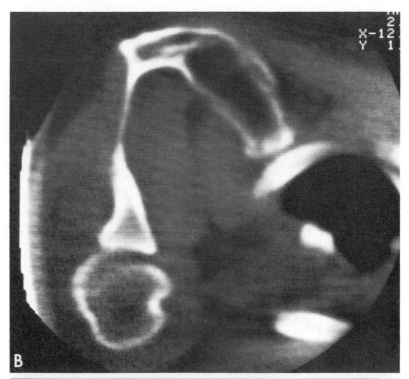

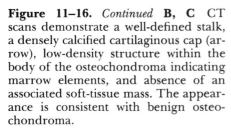

Figure 11–16. *Continued* **B, C** CT scans demonstrate a well-defined stalk, a densely calcified cartilaginous cap (arrow), low-density structure within the body of the osteochondroma indicating marrow elements, and absence of an associated soft-tissue mass. The appearance is consistent with benign osteochondroma.

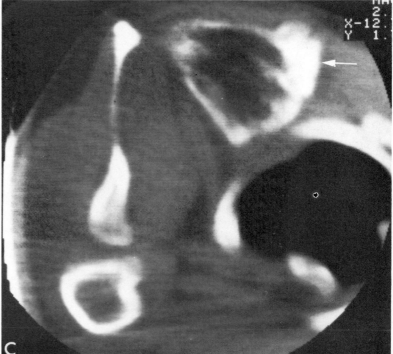

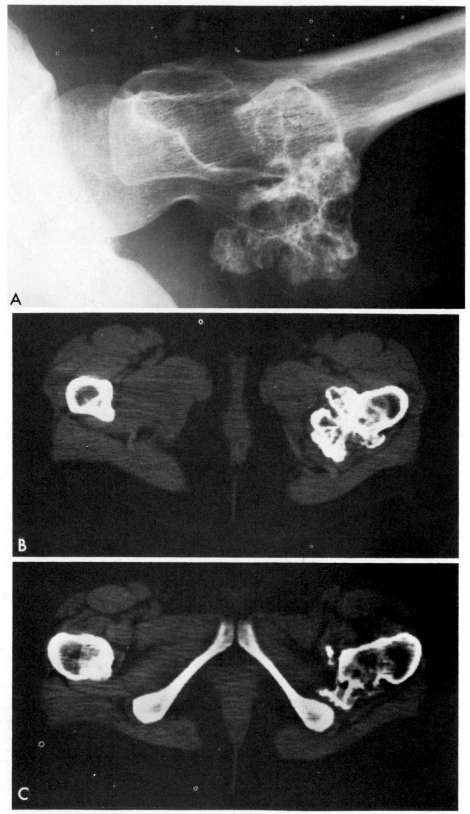

Figure 11–17. Osteochondroma. **A** Conventional radiograph demonstrates a deforming osteochondroma involving the proximal femur. **B, C** CT scans demonstrate the exact relationship of the stalk of the osteochondroma to the shaft of the femur, the proximity of the calcified cap to the ischium, and the absence of a significant soft-tissue mass, suggesting benignancy.

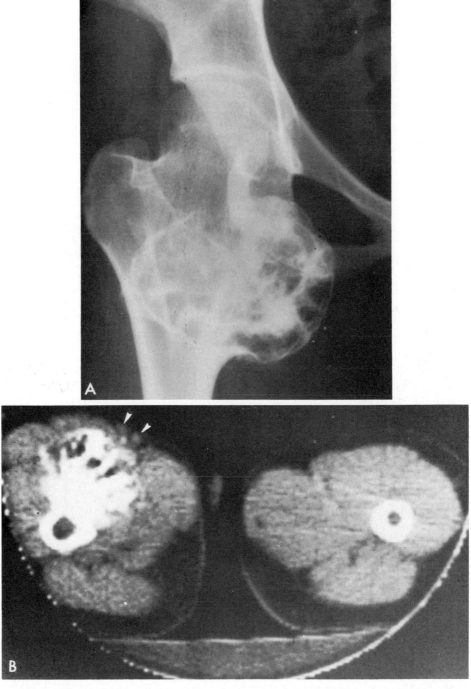

Figure 11–18. Osteochondroma. **A** Radiograph showing osteochondroma originating from the region of the lesser trochanter. **B** Computed tomography after intravenous injection of contrast medium shows the femoral artery and vein overlying the mass just beneath the skin (arrowheads) and the location of the base of the osteochondroma.

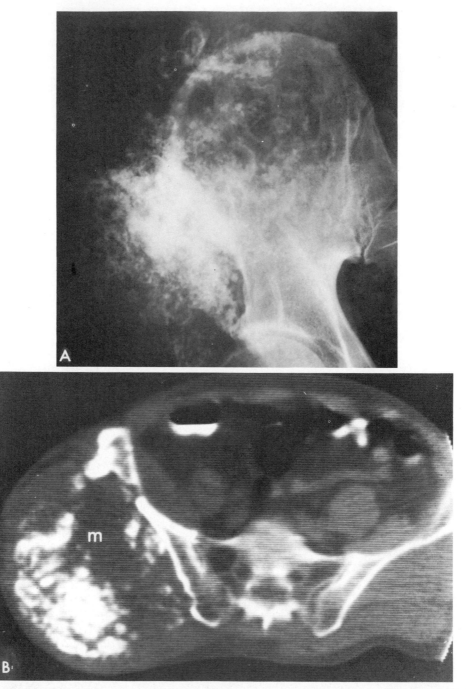

Figure 11–19. Chondrosarcoma. **A**   A plain radiograph of the pelvis shows a densely calcified cartilaginous mass in the region of the right buttock. **B**   CT scan of the pelvis accurately defines the extent
of the mass and reveals erosion of the ileum. A soft-tissue mass (m) located beyond the calcified portion of the mass has invaded the inner pelvic wall. These findings indicate malignancy and help to
determine an appropriate therapeutic approach. Chondrosarcoma was confirmed at surgery.

dense centers, and large soft-tissue masses are chondrosarcomas (Figs. 11–19 and 11–20). Kenney[34] found these criteria reliable in distinguishing six osteochondromas from six chondrosarcomas.

Although osteoid osteoma (Figs. 11–21 and 11–22) with its solid periosteal reaction and central lucent nidus is virtually diagnostic by CT, the appearance of osteoblastoma and osteosarcoma may be quite variable, depending upon the cellular nature and the degree of matrix ossification. Differentiation between osteosarcoma, periosteal sarcoma, and parosteal sarcoma (Figs. 11–23 through 11–26) may, in some cases, be facilitated by the axial orientation of CT and its elimination of superimposed structures.[3, 23, 25] Finally, tumor new-bone formation in the medullary space with osteosarcoma can be readily differentiated by CT (Fig. 11–27) as well as by conventional radiography, from the sclerotic intramedullary response to blastic metastases or Paget's disease (Fig. 11–28).

CT occasionally demonstrates tumor when the findings from radiographic techniques are minimal (Fig. 11–29) or normal.[3, 26, 27] This is especially true in round cell tumors, in which a large soft-tissue mass is often present and bone destruction minimal. These tumors are often radiosensitive, and CT, by defining tumor extent, is helpful in determining the size of the port used in therapy.

The therapeutic implications of computed tomography may be of greater importance than the diagnostic implications. For example, in the preoperative assessment of exophytic bone masses, CT may be helpful in defining the base of the lesion and its relationship to underlying bone; in indicating whether adequate bone will remain following resection to preserve structural integrity; and in identifying vascular structures, with the aid of intravenous contrast medium, to assess possible vessel entrapment within the tumor (Figs. 11–16 through 11–18). Finally, CT assessment may be important in evaluating benign but locally aggressive neoplasms in order to define tumor borders when the surgeon is considering an allograft or a custom prosthesis (Fig. 11–13).

Text continued on page 506

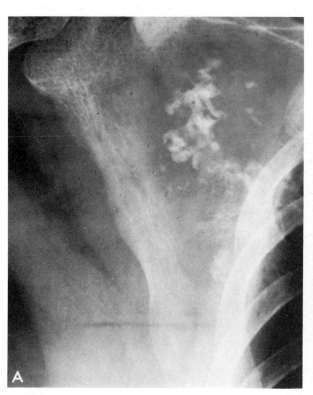
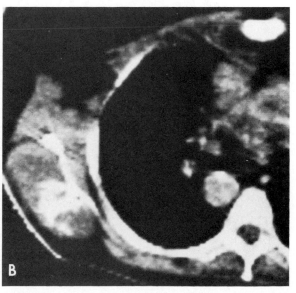

Figure 11–20. Chondrosarcoma of scapula. **A** Magnification radiograph of the shoulder demonstrates a calcified mass in the region of the scapula. **B** CT scan defines the precise posterior relationship of the stalk to the scapula and shows an extensive soft-tissue component beyond the calcified portion, suggesting a chondrosarcoma.

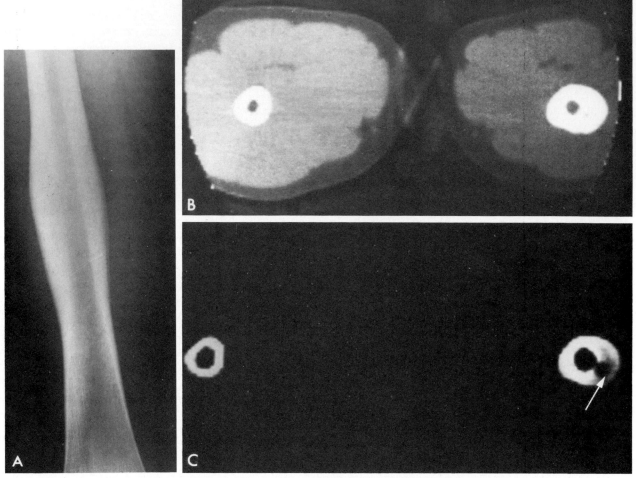

Figure 11–21. Osteoid osteoma. **A** Conventional radiograph of the femur demonstrates solid periosteal reaction circumscribing the femur. CT scans are shown at two different window settings, one optimal for soft-tissues **(B)** and one optimal for skeletal structures **(C)**. The lucent nidus (arrow), surrounded by dense bone on CT, is nearly diagnostic of an osteoid osteoma.

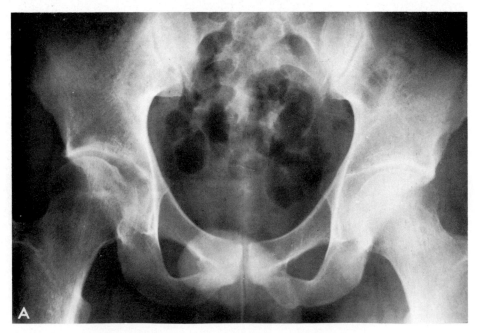

Figure 11–22. Osteoid osteoma of acetabulum. **A** Conventional radiograph of the pelvis of a young man with right hip pain reveals periarticular demineralization.

Illustration continued on opposite page

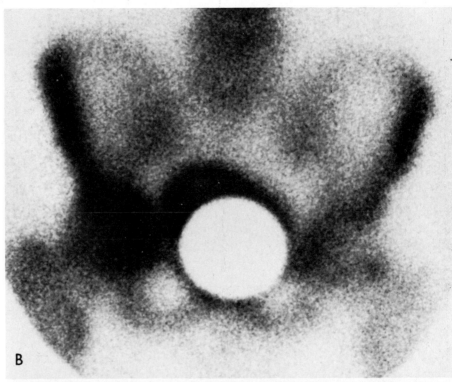

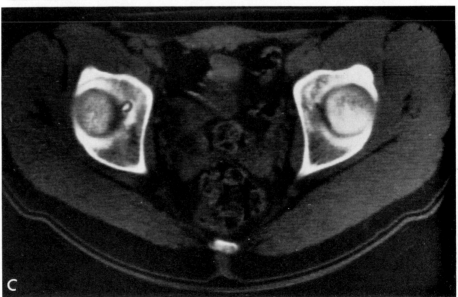

Figure 11–22. *Continued* **B** Bone scan shows increased radionuclide uptake in the acetabulum. **C** CT scan identified the nidus of an osteoid osteoma and defines its position in the acetabulum, facilitating surgical resection.

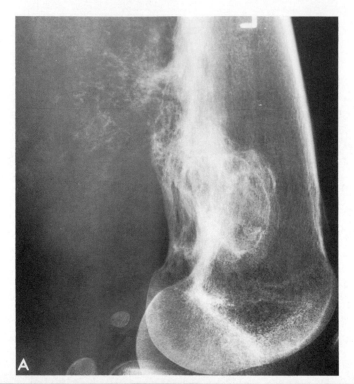

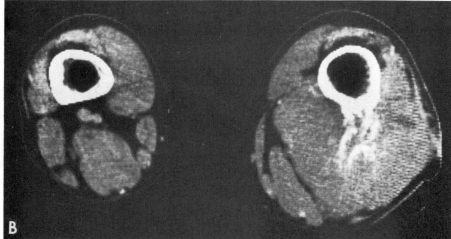

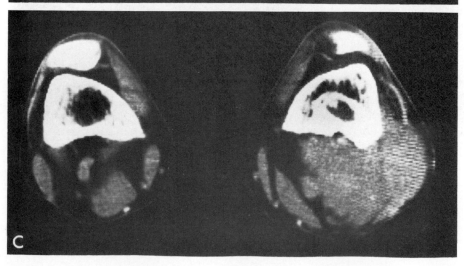

Figure 11–23. Osteosarcoma. **A** Lateral magnification radiograph of the left knee demonstrates a blastic sclerotic process involving the distal femoral metaphysis associated with aggressive periosteal reaction and a large soft-tissue mass. **B** CT scan defines the borders of the large soft-tissue component. **C** The CT scan was also useful in defining the intraosseous extent of the osteosarcoma.

Figure 11–24. Osteosarcoma. **A** In this adolescent with a painful right knee, minimal, patchy sclerosis is noted in the distal end of the femur and a subtle periosteal reaction is seen medially. **B** CT scan demonstrates osteosclerosis of the medullary space of the right knee, indicating a central osteosarcoma but showing no evidence of any extraosseous soft-tissue mass.

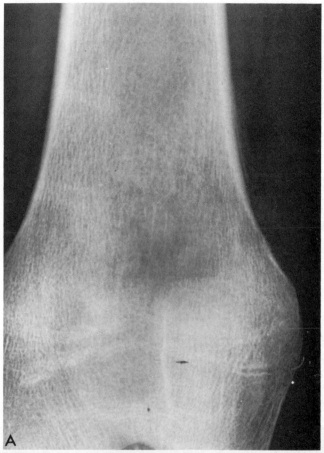

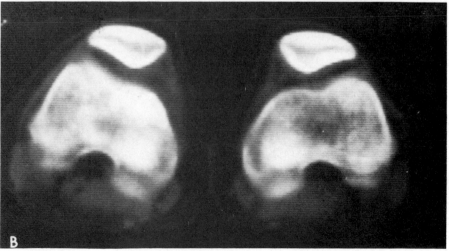

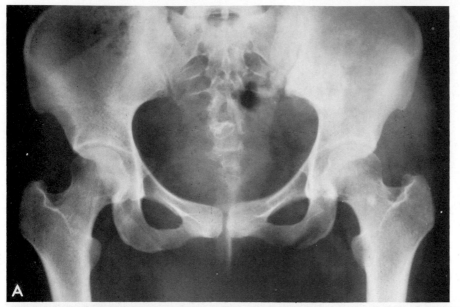

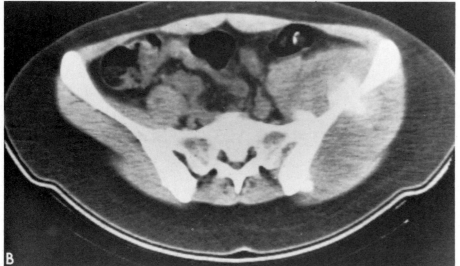

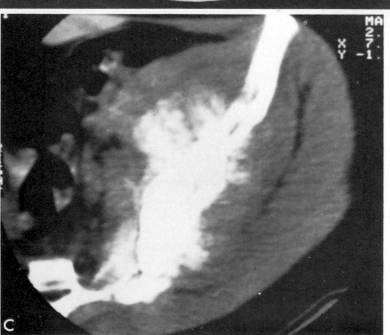

Figure 11–25. Osteosarcoma of ilium. **A** Conventional radiograph of the pelvis of a young adult reveals mixed sclerosis and destruction of the left ilium. **B, C** CT scans reveal osteoblastic activity with destruction of the ilium. This activity is accompanied by a large soft-tissue mass, suggesting osteosarcoma. In this case, the CT study yielded important diagnostic, prognostic, and therapeutic information.

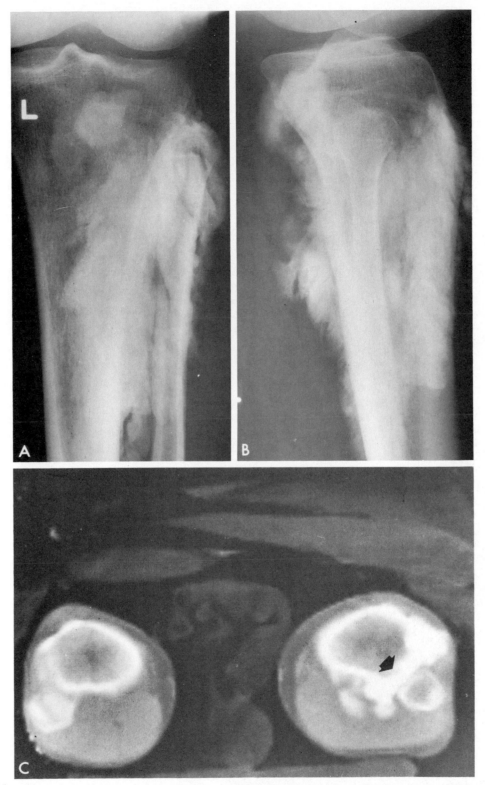

Figure 11–26. Parosteal osteosarcoma. **A, B** Anteroposterior and lateral radiograph of the proximal left tibia shows a typical parosteal osteosarcoma. **C** CT scan reveals intramedullary involvement (arrow) and also shows the exact location of the extraosseous component. The presence of intramedullary involvement with parosteal osteosarcoma carries prognostic and therapeutic importance.

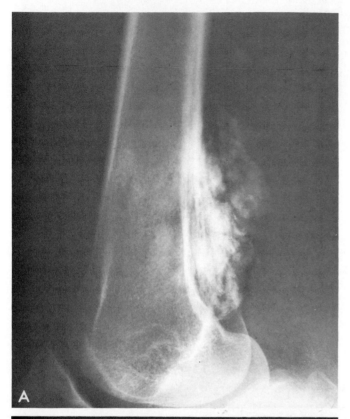

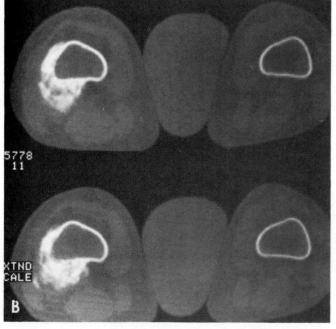

Figure 11–27. Parosteal osteosarcoma. **A** Lateral radiograph demonstrates a large ossifying mass encircling the posterior cortex of the distal femur. **B, C** CT scans demonstrate the intimate relationship of the ossifying mass to the underlying cortex and furthermore demonstrate sparing of the medullary space, supporting a diagnosis of parosteal sarcoma and bearing prognostic significance.

Illustration continued on opposite page

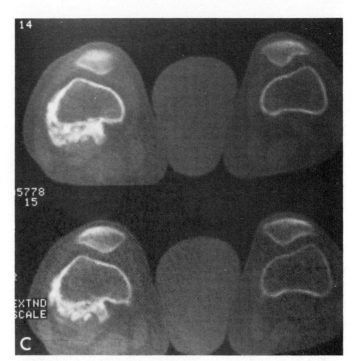

Figure 11–27. *Continued*

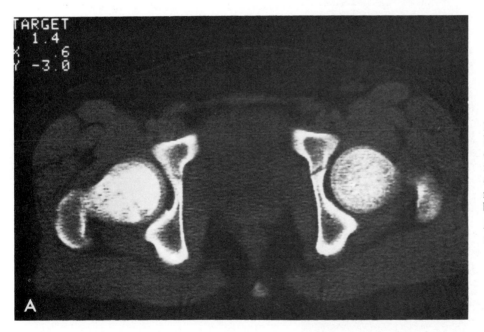

Figure 11–28. Patterns of blastic response. **A** CT scan demonstrates diffuse blastic intramedullary response to osteosarcoma of the proximal right femur. The trabeculae are not thickened.

Illustration continued on following page

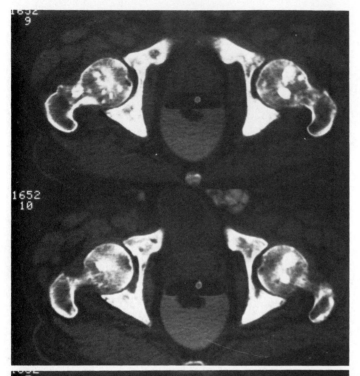

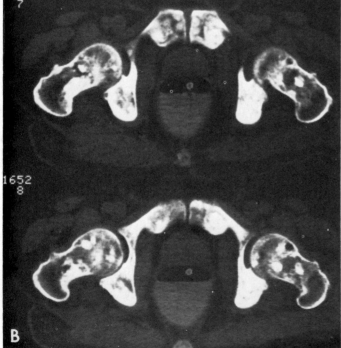

Figure 11–28. *Continued* **B** Discrete blastic foci characteristic of metastatic prostatic carcinoma are scattered throughout pelvis and hips.

Illustration continued on opposite page

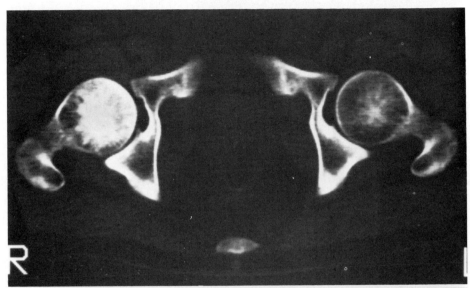

Figure 11–28. *Continued* **C**
Subtle blastic response to
early Paget's disease involving the right hip. The trabeculae are thickened. These
patterns of blastic response
are as readily distinguished
by CT as they generally are
by conventional radiography.

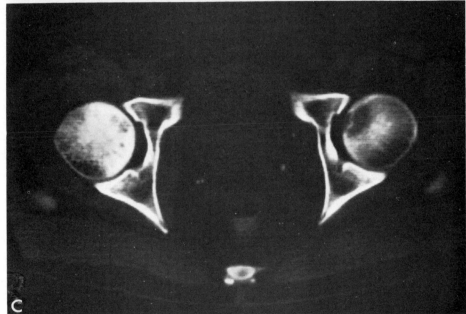

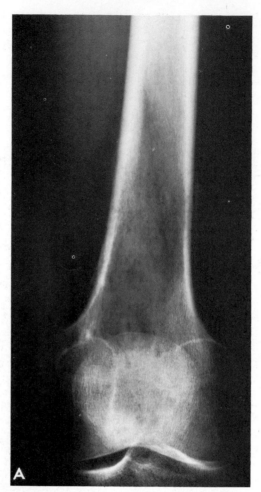

Figure 11–29. Intramedullary involvement by fibrous histiocytoma. **A** A plain radiograph of the left femur shows an ill-defined permeative lesion with minimal periostitis. This 35-year-old man had pain and a large soft-tissue mass in the left thigh.

Illustration continued on opposite page

Soft-Tissue Tumors

The role of CT as a primary imaging modality for assessing soft-tissue tumors is now well established.[2, 26, 31, 36–38] In such cases, CT not only determines the location and extent of the process, but also often provides a specific diagnosis. Routine radiography is confined to demonstrating the presence of a mass and gross changes such as osseous involvement and displacement of soft-tissue planes. Xeroradiography may provide additional information about the lesion because of its broad latitude and edge enhancement properties.[2] Any lucency or calcification detected may help to narrow the differential diagnosis. Angiography provides further information on extent of tumor by displacement of vessels and the presence of tumor vascularity; demonstration of vascular inva-

sion may give a clue to the neoplasm's biologic behavior. Assessment of malignancy is sometimes possible. However, angiography is nonspecific as far as diagnosis with the possible exception of lesions whose soft-tissue makeup (i.e., fat, calcium) is radiographically visible.[39–42]

The ability of CT to define anatomy in a cross-sectional scan is an obvious advantage in evaluating soft-tissue neoplasms. Furthermore, definition of tissue densities is a key feature of the method. Characteristic features of tissue density invisible on routine radiographs are readily detected by CT.[2, 31, 38, 43–46]

The lipoma presents as a well-defined lucent mass, avascular at angiography. CT (Fig. 11–30) demonstrates a homogeneous, sharply marginated low-density mass.[2, 31, 43, 44] Infiltrating lipoma is similar except for evidence of projections of fatty tissue into adjacent structures.[3] Both lipoma and normal subcutaneous fat demonstrate CT numbers in the − 100 H range, homogeneity and lack of significant contrast enhancement. These features correlate well with the known pathologic features.[37]

Liposarcoma (Fig. 11–31) presents as an ill-defined mass that is a heterogeneous mixture of fat and water density. The study by Kindblom and others[41] demonstrated a close radiologic-pathologic correlation between histologically demonstrable vascularity and gross and angiographic opacity. The denser lesions tend to occur in the more malignant types; less aggressive tumors have a higher fat content and a lower density. Of course, the cellular and myxoid elements in these types also contributes to their overall density. Such relative opacity is seen on CT as a heterogeneous mass of fat and water density; even if definite islands of fat are not demonstrated, the overall density of the lesion suggests the presence of fat. Contrast enhancement is generally found. Quantitative assessment of overall density and the degree of enhancement may prove useful in predicting the histologic category; such a relationship has been established angiographically in liposarcoma.[41] In addition to density, poor margination of the tumor and evidence of invasion further suggest malignancy. Angiolipoma (Fig. 11–32) may show features (heterogeneity, ill-defined margins, and contrast enhancement) quite similar to those of liposarcoma, yet is a benign lesion.[37]

Soft-tissue neoplasms other than fatty tumors may have densities less than surrounding muscle, which aids in their detection.[2, 26, 38] Neurogenic tumors such as neurofibroma (Fig. 11–33) and

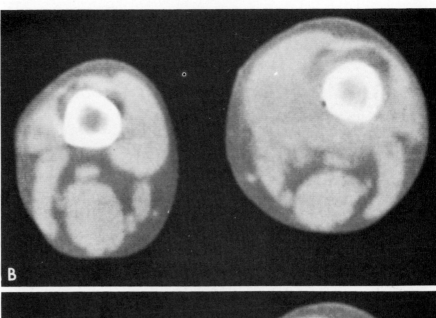

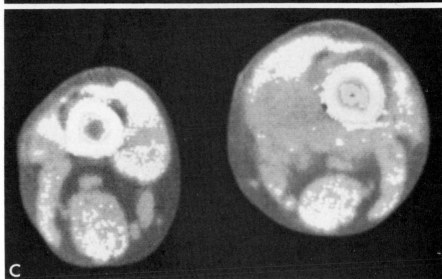

Figure 11–29. *Continued* **B** CT scan through this region shows a large soft-tissue mass with an increase in the intramedullary density on the left side. **C** The "blink mode" confirms the increased intramedullary density on the left side. A biopsy showed this mass to be a malignant fibrous histiocytoma. The CT scan showed the extent of the intramedullary involvement and influenced therapy.

schwannoma (Fig. 11–34) are often homogeneous, smoothly marginated cylindrical lesions having a density slightly lower than that of muscle. Their CT characteristics and location in the neurovascular bundle may strongly suggest a correct diagnosis.[3]

Soft-tissue neoplasms such as desmoid tumors (Fig. 11–35), fibrous histiocytoma (Figs. 11–36 and 11–37), rhabdomyosarcoma, and fibrosarcoma are of variable density, often isodense with muscle, but may have low-density areas related to tumor necrosis or high-density areas related to dystrophic calcification or ossification.[2, 26, 38] Even lesions that are isodense with muscle may be detected by CT if they are surrounded by fat, are superficial in location, or cause sufficient bulk anatomic displacement.

Other soft-tissue disorders of the appendicular musculoskeletal system that cause focal or generalized soft-tissue enlargement by CT, but are nonneoplastic in nature, include arteriovenous malformations (Fig. 11–38) and venous or lymphatic occlusive disease (Fig. 11–39).

Locally Recurrent Neoplasms

Locally recurrent neoplasms may best be evaluated by CT scanning.[3, 26] A baseline postoperative study may be performed when a tumor cannot be completely resected or when the aggressive nature of a tumor renders local recurrence a likely possibility. CT may be used in this setting to identify and to assess serially any recurrent disease (Fig. 11–40).

Text continued on page 521

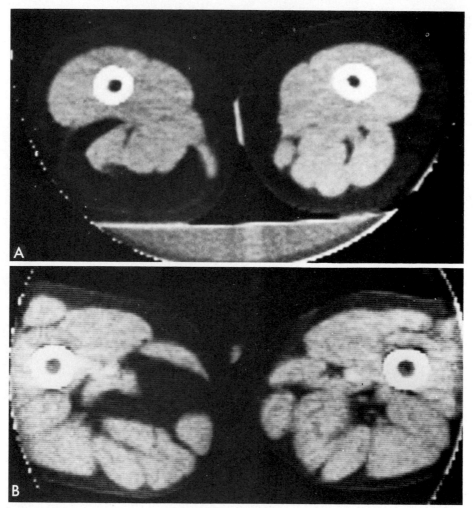

Figure 11–30. Lipoma. **A–D**   CT scans of four different cases reveal sharply marginated, homogeneous, low-density, soft-tissue masses diagnostic of lipomas.

Illustration continued on opposite page

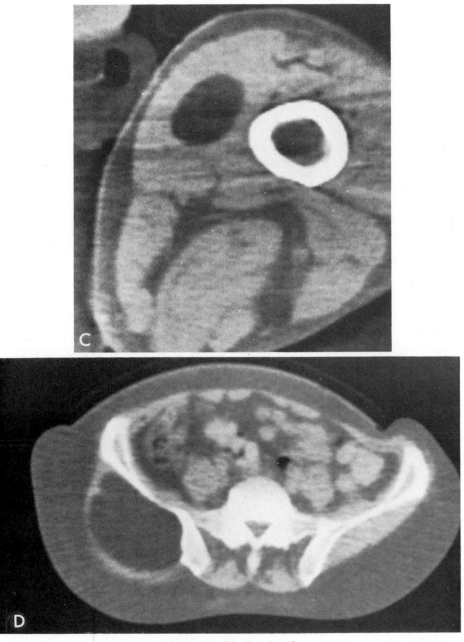

Figure 11–30. *Continued*

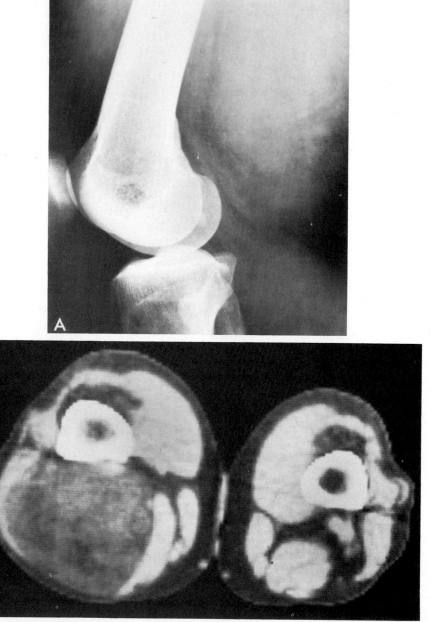

Figure 11–31. Liposarcoma. **A**   Radiograph demonstrates a bulky mass with areas of low-density in the right popliteal fossa. **B**   CT scan (without contrast) reveals a large, inhomogeneous mass of overall low-density located between the semimembranosus and semitendinosus muscles.

Illustration continued on opposite page

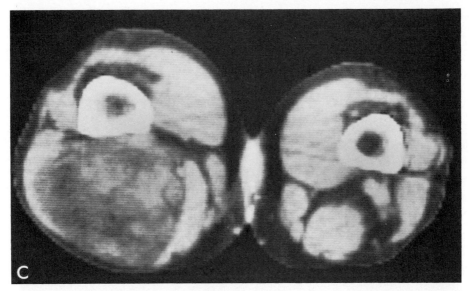

Figure 11–31. *Continued* **C**   Following intravenous contrast, areas of higher density are noted within the mass. These areas of enhancement correspond to vascular elements. Liposarcoma was found at surgery.

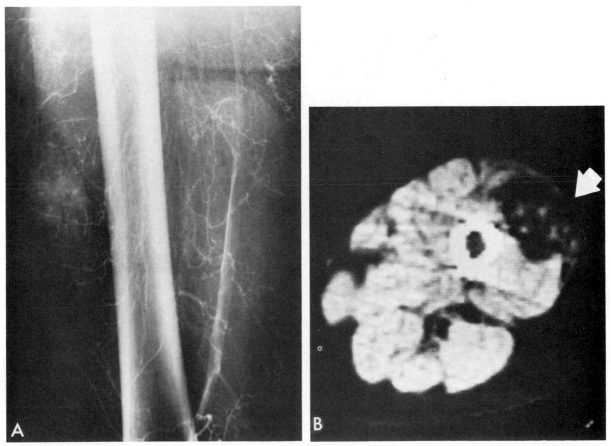

Figure 11–32. A   Angiolipoma, infiltrative, right thigh. A right femoral angiogram shows a tangle of irregular vessels and a tumor stain. **B**   CT scan (without contrast) demonstrates the mass (arrow) to have poorly defined margins and a heterogeneous mixture of fat and water and calcific density elements.

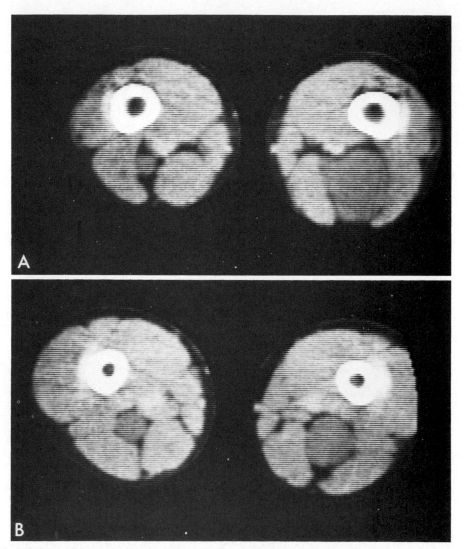

Figure 11–33. Neurofibroma. **A, B** CT scans in a patient with von Recklinghausen's disease and painful swelling of the left leg reveals a sharply marginated, low-density mass in the popliteal space. The mass extends, on contiguous sections, in a cylindrical fashion over many centimeters. Biopsy demonstrated the mass to be a neurofibroma. A second smaller neurofibroma was found incidentally in the right popliteal space.

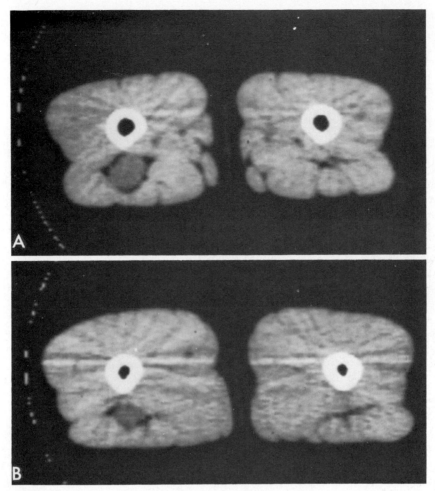

Figure 11–34. Schwannoma. **A, B** CT scans demonstrate a relatively low-density mass within the neurovascular bundle of the posterior thigh. This cylindric mass was shown by CT to extend over 15 cm, suggesting the correct diagnosis of schwannoma.

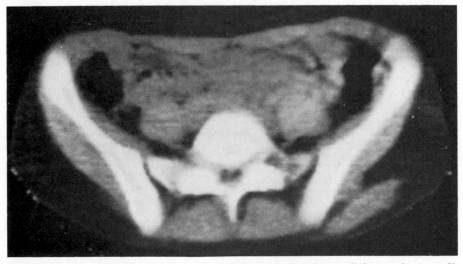

Figure 11–35. CT scan of desmoid tumor of buttock region showing pedicle attachment, dictating necessity of wide surgical resection of underlying gluteal muscle.

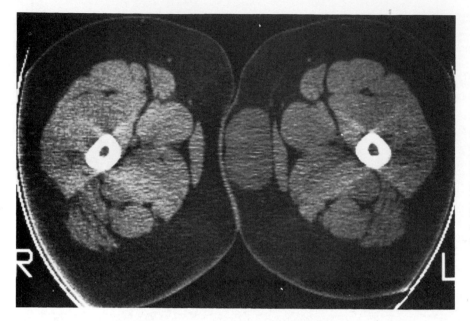

Figure 11–36. Fibrous histiocytoma. CT scan through the proximal thighs demonstrates a well-defined, smoothly marginated, homogeneous, soft-tissue mass of the left thigh. The mass has a density slightly lower than that of adjacent muscle, but well above that of subcutaneous fat. Precise localization by CT was helpful in planning surgical excision for this fibrous histiocytoma.

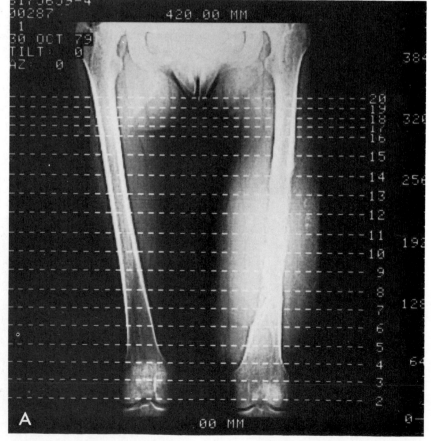

Figure 11–37. Malignant fibrous histiocytoma. **A** Scout view of the left thigh demonstrates the planes of sections obtained every 2 cm distally and through the main portion of the tumor and every 1 cm proximally to evaluate the extent of tumor.

Illustration continued on opposite page

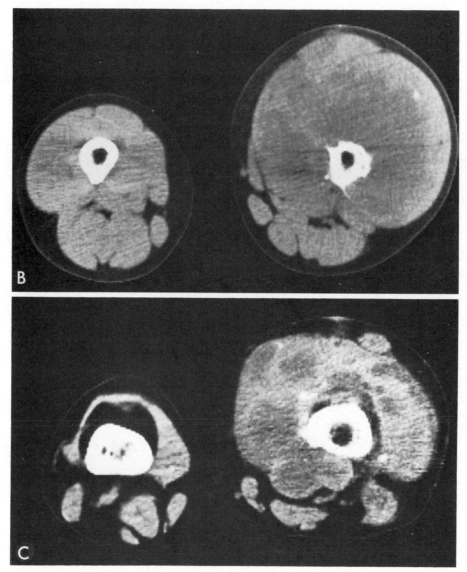

Figure 11–37. *Continued* **B, C**   CT scans with wide and narrow windows show a multilobulated, mixed-density soft-tissue mass with underlying bone involvement. The proximal borders of the tumor were identified in other planes, facilitating surgical planning.

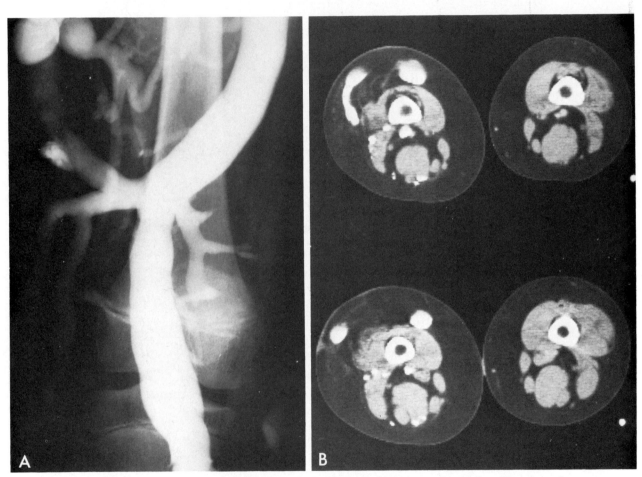

Figure 11–38. Arteriovenous malformation. **A** Angiogram demonstrates massive dilatation of venous channels in the left lower extremity due to extensive arteriovenous malformation. **B** CT scans delineate the spatial relationship of the enlarged vascular channels following intravenous contrast and fail to demonstrate a significant vascular neoplasm.

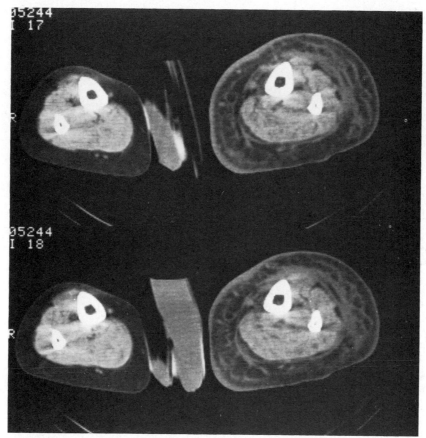

Figure 11–39. Filariasis. CT scans through the legs demonstrate massive enlargement of the left lower extremity due to involvement with filariasis. The CT study shows tremendous engorgement of lymphatic and venous channels with collections of fluid deep in the subcutaneous fat and marked thickening of the skin.

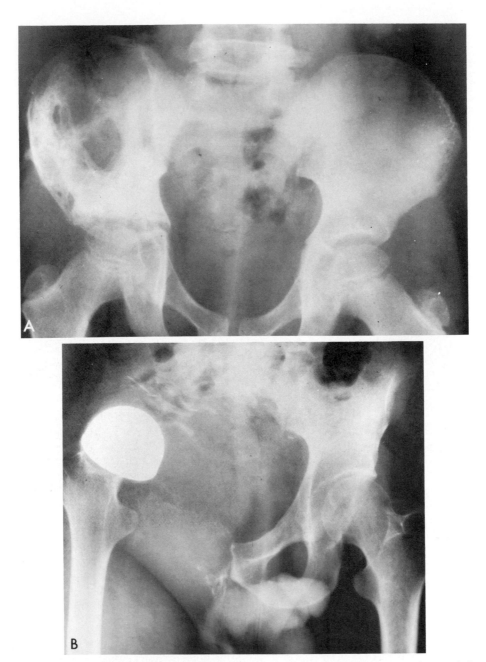

Figure 11–40. Desmoplastic fibroma. **A**   Conventional radiograph demonstrates advanced destruction of the right ilium due to desmoplastic fibroma. **B**   Ten years later, conventional radiograph shows only extensive postsurgical alterations.

Illustration continued on opposite page

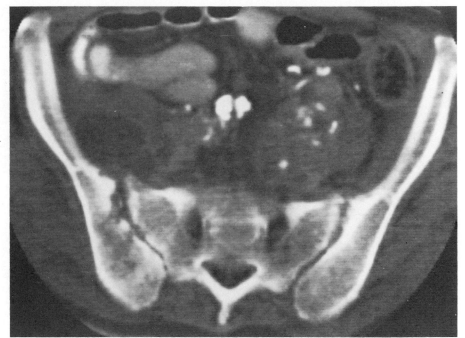

Figure 11–47. CT shows irregular destruction of the subchondral cortex of the right sacroiliac joint, focal lysis of the ilium, and a large presacral iliopsoas abscess.

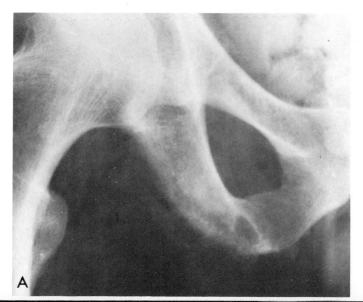

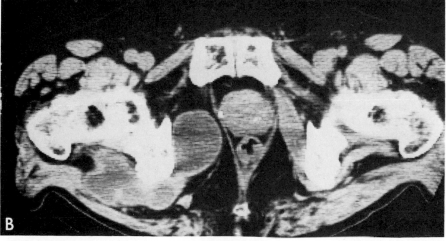

Figure 11–48. A Conventional radiograph demonstrates irregular destruction of the ischial tuberosity in a patient with chronic gluteal pain. **B** CT scan demonstrates massive enlargement of the ischial bursa owing to chronic indolent infection. CT-guided biopsy and aspiration were performed and tuberculous infection was found.

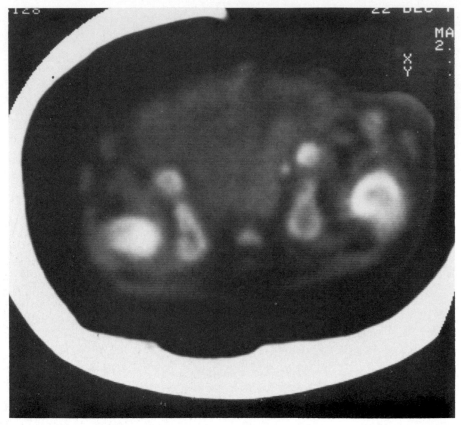

Figure 11–49. Computed tomography may be used to demonstrate the adequacy of reduction of congenital hip dislocations following placement in a spica cast. In this case, CT demonstrates lateral subluxation of the left proximal femur, indicating inadequate reduction.

observed in cases with capsular thickening, edema, and/or effusion.

Conventional tomography has traditionally been used to determine the position of the femoral head after placement of a child in an abduction cast for congenital dislocation of the hip. However, this technique involves considerable radiation to the gonads and often does not show whether the femoral head is covered by the acetabulum. Computed tomography[16, 55, 56] can locate the femoral head through the plaster cast occasionally, even if the femoral head has not completely ossified (Fig. 11–49).

The evaluation of complex patellofemoral compartment disorders by CT has been explored.[57–60] Chondromalacia patellae may be suggested by irregular imbibition of contrast material, roughening of cartilage surfaces, and generalized articular narrowing. Lateral subluxing and subtle tracking abnormalities may be evaluated by placing the knee in varying degrees of flexion-extension with and without quadriceps relaxation while axial images are taken through the midplane of the patella. Successful detection and classification of

plica syndromes also have been reported using axial CT images.[61]

Ligamentous injuries of the knees may be examined using CT. Direct off-axis scans or sagittally reformatted images derived from contiguous, axial CT scans can be used to evaluate the cruciate ligaments.[62, 63] Normal anterior and posterior cruciate ligaments should be visualized by reformatting several sagittal slices through the intercondylar notch.[64] A torn cruciate ligament is visible as either an interruption or an absence of the ligament (Fig. 11–50). CT has not proven useful in evaluation of the menisci with the current CT scanners.

The axial presentation provided by CT has made it a potentially valuable modality for assessing the complex articulations of the hindfoot (Fig. 11–51) and subtle tarsal coalitions, either fibrous or bony.[65] The anatomy of the hindfoot and the non-isoplanar orientation of its articulations provide a rationale for the use of CT with its capability for variable planar orientation. Similarly, the application of CT for assessing osseous and articular structures of the carpus has been explored.[66]

PROSTHESES

The evaluation of metallic prostheses by CT is significantly restricted by image artifacts that result from the presence of the x-ray opaque object in the field. Artifacts can be a deterrent, particularly for imaging structures in the immediate vicinity of the prosthesis. Nevertheless, advanced software methods for reducing scan artifacts in prosthetic hip (Fig. 11–52) and knee components have been explored.[67–69] The hope is that the axial representation of the cement-bone and cement-prosthesis interfaces may provide information of importance in biomechanical research, if not in the clinical practice of orthopedics.

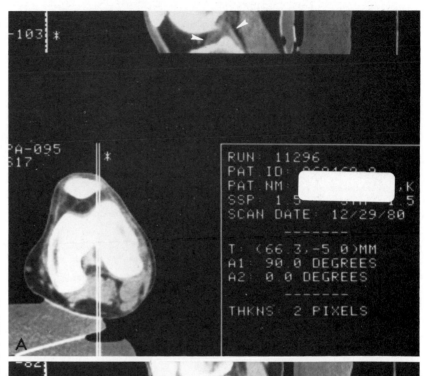

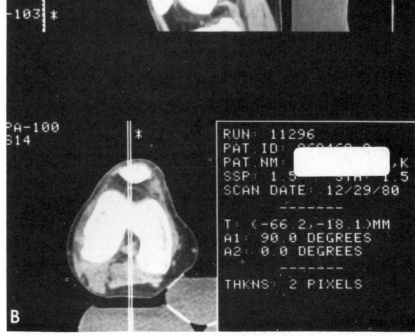

Figure 11–50. A CT scan through the left knee with sagittal reconstruction reveals a normal anterior and posterior cruciate ligament (arrowheads). **B** A similar scan through the right knee with sagittal reconstruction shows a normal posterior cruciate and an abnormal anterior cruciate ligament, later shown at surgery to be torn.

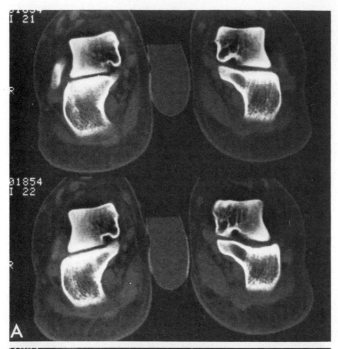

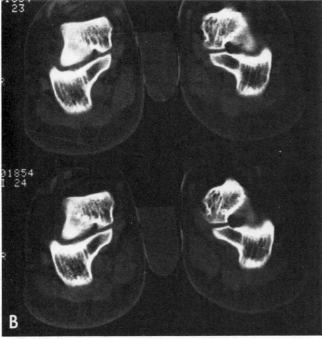

Figure 11–51. A, B CT scans through the hindfoot demonstrate to advantage the posterior and medial facets of the subtalar joint, without evidence of tarsal coalition.

MUSCLES

The normal and pathologic muscular system has been examined by Termote[70] using computed tomography. The normal size and density of muscle groups in the neck, shoulder, pelvis, thigh, and lower leg were determined and a series of patients with various neuromuscular diseases were evaluated. The study concluded that CT provided an important tool to study the nature of atrophy, hypertrophy, and other phenomena, such as pseudohypertrophy and denervation hypertrophy which previously had only been studied by biopsy or autopsy. Not only qualitative but also quantitative examination is possible, so that in addition to localization and evaluation of the extent of a lesion, the degree and progression can be measured. Other investigators[71, 72] have similarly found CT of value in studying the nature and extent of various muscular dystrophy syndromes. In general, these investigators have found that as muscle atrophies, it becomes smaller, infiltrated with fat and less dense. Consequently, in a given

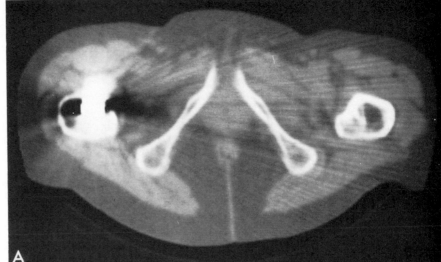

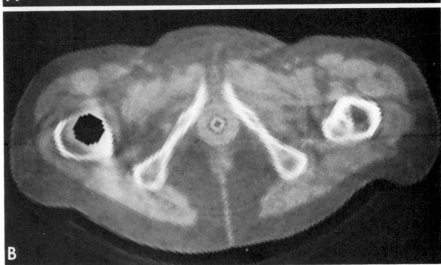

Figure 11–52. A CT slice through a metallic hip prosthesis reconstructed onto a 320 × 320 pixel matrix by the standard filtered back-projection software of a CT/T 7800 (General Electric) scanner has many streak artifacts. **B** Same CT slice, but projection data reconstructed onto a 160 × 160 pixel matrix by an algebraic reconstruction technique (ART) algorithm after just one 288 view iteration on the CDC 6400 computer eliminates the streak artifacts. The metallic prosthesis now appears black.

cross-sectional image, involvement of specific muscle groups and sparing of others can be readily determined.

REFERENCES

1. Wittenberg J, Fineberg HV, Ferucci JT Jr, Simeone JF, Mueller PR, Van Sonnenberg E, Kirkpatrick PH: Clinical efficacy of computed body tomography II. AJR 134:1111, 1980.
2. Wilson JS, Korobkin M, Genant HK, Bovil EG: CT of musculoskeletal disorders. AJR 131:55, 1978.
3. Genant HK, Cann CE, Chafetz NI, Helms CA: Advances in computed tomography of the musculoskeletal system. Radiol Clin North Am 19:645, 1981.
4. Brown BM, Brant-Zawadzki M, Cann CE: Dynamic CT scanning of spinal column trauma. AJNR 3:561, 1982.
5. Reese DF, McCullough EC, Balcer HL Jr: Dynamic sequential scanning with table incrementation. Radiology 140:719, 1981.
6. Glenn WV, Rhodes ML, Altschuler EM, Wiltse LL, Lostanek C, Kuo YM: Multiplanar display computerized body tomography applications in the lumbar spine. Spine 4:282, 1979.
7. Brant-Zawadzki M, Jeffrey RB, Jr, Minagi H, Pitts LH: High resolution CT of thoracolumbar fractures. AJNR 3:69, 1982.
8. Brant-Zawadzki M: Computed tomography in the evaluation of spinal trauma. In Genant HK, Chafetz NI, Helms CA (eds): Computed Tomography of the Lumbar Spine. San Francisco, University of California, Berkeley, Cal, 1982, pp 261–278.
9. Colley DO, Dunsler SB: Traumatic narrowing of the dorsolumbar spinal canal demonstrated by computed tomography. Radiology 129:95, 178.
10. Faerber E, Wolpert SM, Scott RM, Belkin SC, Carter LC: Computed tomography in spinal fractures. J Comput Assist Tomogr 5:657, 1979.
11. Harley JD, Mack LA, Winquist RA: CT of acetabular fractures: Comparison with conventional radiography. AJR 138:413, 1982.
12. Mack LA, Harley JD, Winquist RA: CT of acetabular fractures: Analysis of fracture patterns. AJR 138:407, 1982.
13. Shirkhoda A, Brashear HR, Staab EV: Computed tomography of acetabular fractures. Radiology 134:683, 1980.
14. Tadmor R, Davis KR, Roberson GH, New PRJ, Taveras

JM: Computed tomographic evaluation of traumatic spinal injuries. Radiology 127:827, 1978.

15. Lange TA, Alter AJ Jr.: Evaluation of complex acetabular fractures by CT. J Comput Assist Tomogr 4:849, 1980.

16. Lasda, NA, Levinsohn EM, Yuan HA, Bunnell WP: CT in disorders of the hip. J Bone Joint Surg 60A:1099, 1978.

17. Judet R, Judet J, Letournel E: Fractures of the acetabulum: Classification and surgical approaches for open reduction. J Bone Joint Surg. 46:1615, 1964.

18. Pennal GF, Davidson J, Garside H, Plewes J: Results of treatment of acetabular fractures. Clin Orthop 151:115, 1980.

19. Destout JM, Gilula LA, Murphy WA, Sagel SS: Computed tomography of the sternoclavicular joint and sternum. Radiology 138:123, 1981.

20. Levinsohn EM, Bunnell WP, Yuan HA: Computed tomography in the diagnosis of dislocation of the sternoclavicular joint. Clin Orthop 140:12, 1979.

21. Somer K, Meurman KOA: Computed tomography of stress fractures. J Comput Assist Tomogr 6:109, 1982.

22. Murcia M, Brennan RE, Edeiken J: Computed tomography of stress fracture. Skeletal Radiol 8:193, 1982.

23. De Santos LA, Bernardino ME, Murray JA: Computed tomography in the evaluation of osteosarcoma: Experience with 25 cases. AJR 132:535, 1979.

24. De Santos LA, Goldstein HM, Murray JA, Wallace S: Computed tomography in evaluation of musculoskeletal neoplasms. Radiology 128:89, 1978.

25. Destouet JM, Gilula LA, Murphy WA: Computed tomography of long bone osteosarcoma. Radiology 131:439, 1979.

26. Genant HK, Wilson, JS, Bovill EG, Brunelle FO, Murray WR, Rodrigo JJ: Computed tomography of the musculoskeletal system. J Bone Joint Surg 62A:1088, 1980.

27. Hardy DC, Murphy WA, Gilula LA: CT in planning percutaneous bone biopsy. Radiology 134:447, 1980.

28. Berger PE, Kuhn JP: Computed tomography of tumors of the musculoskeletal system in children: Clinical Applications. Radiology 127:171, 1978.

29. McLeod RA, Stephens DH, Beabout JW, Sheedy PF II, Hattery RR: Computed tomography of the skeletal system. Semin Roentgenol 13:235, 1978.

30. Levitt RG, Sagel SS, Stanley RJ, Evans RG: Computed tomography of the pelvis. Semin Roentgenol 13:193, 1978.

31. Schumacher TM, Genant HK, Korobkin MT, Bovill EG Jr: Computed tomography: Its use in space-occupying lesions of the musculoskeletal system. J Bone Joint Surg 60A:600, 1978.

32. Paul DF, Morrey BF, Helms CA: The role of computerized tomography in orthopaedic surgery. Clin Orthop 139:142, 1979.

33. Blumberg ML: CT of iliac unicameral bone cysts. AJR 136:1231, 1981.

34. Kenney PJ, Gilula LA, Murphy WA: The use of CT to distinguish osteochondroma and chondrosarcoma. Radiology 139:129, 1981.

35. Goldberg RR, Genant HK, Johnston WA: Case report: A case of differentiated chondrosarcoma of the scapula demonstrated on CT. Skeletal Radiol 3:179, 1978.

36. Genant HK: Advances in orthopedic diagnosis: The emergence of computed tomography. Presidents' Guest Lecture, presented at the Annual Assembly of the American Academy of Orthopedic Surgeons, San Francisco, February 24, 1979.

37. Hunter JC, Johnston WH, Genant HK: Computed tomography evaluation of fatty tumors of the somatic soft-tissues: Clinical utility and radiographic pathologic correlation. Skeletal Radiol 4:79, 1979.

38. Weinberger G, Levinsohn EM: Computed tomography in the evaluation of sarcomatous tumors of thigh. AJR 130:115, 1978.

39. Enzinger FM, Lattes R, Tarlone H: Histological typing of soft-tissue tumors. International classification of tumors, No. 3, Geneva, World Health Organization, 1969.

40. Hudson TM, Haas G, Enneking WF: Angiography in the management of musculoskeletal tumors. Surg Gynecol Obstet 141:11, 1975.

41. Kindblom L, Angervall L, Svendsen P: Liposarcoma: A clinicopathologic, radiographic and prognostic study, abstr. Acta Pathol Microbiol Scand Supplement No. 253, 1975.

42. Levin DC, Watson RC, Baltaxe HA: Arteriography in the diagnosis and management of acquired peripheral soft-tissue masses. Radiology 104:53, 1972.

43. Cohen WN, Seidelmann FE, Bryant JP: Computed tomography of localized adipose deposits presenting as tumor masses. AJR 128:1007, 1977.

44. Faer MJ, Burnam RE, Beck CL: Transmural thoracic lipoma: Demonstration by computed tomography. AJR 130:161, 1978.

45. Mategrano VC, Petasnick J, Clark J, Bin AC, Weinstein R: Attenuation values in computed tomography of the abdomen. Radiology 125:135, 1977.

46. Phelps ME, Hoffman EJ, Ter-Pogossian MM: Attenuation coefficients of various body tissues, fluids and lesions at photon energies of 18 to 136 keV. Radiology 117:573, 1975.

47. Helms CA, Cann CE, Brunelle FO, Gilula LA, Chafetz NI, Genant HK: Detection of bone-marrow metastases using quantitative CT. Radiology 140:745, 1981.

48. Orcutt J, Ragsdale BD, Curtis DJ, Levine MI: Misleading CT in parosteal osteosarcoma. AJR 136:1233, 1981.

49. Kuhn JP, Berger PE: Computed tomographic diagnosis of osteomyelitis. Radiology 130:503, 1979.

50. Azouz EM: Computed tomography in bone and joint infections. J de l'Assoc Canad des Radiol 32:102, 1981.

51. Bjersand AJ, Eastgate RJ: The accuracy of CT-determined femoral neck anteversion. Europ J Radiol 2:1, 1982.

52. Grote R, Elgeti H, Saure D: Bestimmung des Antertorsionswinkels am Femur mit der axialen Computertomographie. Roentgenblaetter 33:31, 1980.

53. Hernandez RJ, Tachdjian MO, Poznanski AK, Diaz LS: CT detection of femoral torsion. AJR 137:97, 1981.

54. Dihlmann W, Nebel G: CT for evaluation of the hip capsule. J Comput Assist Tomogr 7:278, 1983.

55. Padovani J, Faure, F, Devred P, Jacquemier M, Sarrat P: Use and advantages of tomodensitometry in testing congenital luxations of the hip. Ann Radiol 22:188, 1979.

56. Padovani FF, Devred MJ, Sarrat P: Intérêt et indications de la tomodensitométrie dans le bilan des luxations congénitales de la hanche. Ann Radiol 22:188, 1979.

57. Boven F, Bellemans MA, Geurts J, Potvliege R: A comparative study of the patellofemoral joint on axial roentgenogram, axial arthrogram, and computed to-

mography following arthrography. Skeletal Radiol 8:179, 1982.

58. Boven F, Bellemans MA, Geurts J, De Boeck H, Potvliege R: The value of computed tomography scanning in chondromalacia patellae. Skeletal Radiol 8:183, 1982.

59. Reiser M, Karpf P-M, Bernett P: Diagnosis of chondro-malacia patellae using CT arthrography. Europ J Radiol 2:181, 1982.

60. Delgado-Martins H: A study of the position of the patella using computerized tomography. J Bone Joint Surg 61B:443, 1979.

61. Boven F, De Boeck H, Potvlieg R: Synovial plicae of the knee on CT, abstr. Presented at the 68th Scientific Assembly and Annual Meeting of the Radiological Society of North America, Chicago, November 28–December 3, 1982.

62. Pavlov H, Hirschy JC, Torg JS: Computed tomography of the cruciate ligaments. Radiology 132:389, 1979.

63. Archer CR, Yeager V: Internal structures of the knee visualized by computed tomography. J Comput Assist Tomogr 2:181, 1978.

64. Chafetz NI, Marks AS, Helms CA, Glick J, Genant HK: CT of the menisci and cruciate ligaments, abstr. Invest Radiol 15:366, 1981.

65. Deutsch AL, Resnick D, Campbell G: Computed tomography and bone scintigraphy in the evaluation of tarsal coalition. Radiology 144:137, 1982.

66. Zucker-Pinchoff B, Hermann G, Srinivasan R: Computed tomography of the carpal tunnel: A radioanatomical study. J Comput Assist Tomogr 5:525, 1981.

67. Faul DD, Cough JL, Cann CE, Hoaglund FT, Genant HK: An ART approach to reconstructing CT slices through metallic prostheses. The Radiological Society of North America, 67th Annual Meeting, Chicago, Ill, November 15–19, 1981.

68. Hinderling TH, Ruegsegger P, Anliker M, Dietschi C: Computed tomography reconstruction from hollow projections: An application in vivo evaluation of artificial hip joints. J Comput Assist Tomogr 3:52, 1979.

69. Seitz P, Ruegsegger P: Bone densitometry in the vicinity of metallic implants, abstr. J Computed Assoc Tomogr 6:200, 1982.

70. Termote JL, Baert A, Crolla D, Palmers Y, Bulcke JA: Computed tomography of the normal and pathologic muscular system. Radiology 137:439, 1980.

71. Bulcke JA, Termote JL, Palmers Y, Crolla D: Computed tomography of the human skeletal muscular system. Neuroradiology 17:127, 1979.

72. O'Doherty DS, Schelling D, Raptopoulos V: Computed tomographic patterns of pseudohypertrophic muscular dystrophy: Preliminary results. J Comput Assist Tomogr 1:482, 1977.

12 COMPUTED TOMOGRAPHY OF THE GASTROINTESTINAL TRACT

Albert A. Moss
Ruedi F. Thoeni

Although barium radiography[1–3] and endoscopy[4] are safe and accurate initial diagnostic procedures for evaluating gastrointestinal abnormalities, neither assesses the extramucosal extent of disease. Angiography,[5] radionuclide scanning,[6] and ultrasonography[7, 8] have been employed as additional diagnostic and staging modalities, but because of the limitation of these techniques, surgical exploration has remained the only accepted method of assessing the true extent of disease accurately. Computed tomography displays the gastrointestinal tract in cross section and thus images both the inner and outer surfaces of the alimentary tube. In addition, by imaging both adjacent and distant organs, CT is capable of evaluating both local and distant spread of disease.[8–10] Thus, CT can provide the radiotherapist, surgeon, internist, and oncologist with a clearer understanding of the true extent of a gastrointestinal abnormality.

The Esophagus

ANATOMY

The esophagus connects the pharynx with the stomach and consists of extrathoracic, mediastinal, and abdominal segments. Throughout its length, the esophagus is intimately related to a variety of vital vascular, pulmonary, cardiac, lymphatic, and neural structures. The esophagus is surrounded throughout most of its length by periesophageal fat that permits ready differentiation of the esophagus from adjacent structures.

The thickness of the normal esophageal wall as measured by CT in a well-distended esophagus is usually less than 3 mm (Fig. 12–1)[11, 12] and any measurement above 5 mm should be considered abnormal.[11, 13] Air in the esophagus is present in 40 to 60 per cent of patients examined by CT[11, 14, 15] and should not be considered an abnormal finding. Air, when present in the normal esophagus, is centrally positioned, and an eccentric position of gas within the esophagus should raise the possibility of an esophageal abnormality.[11, 14]

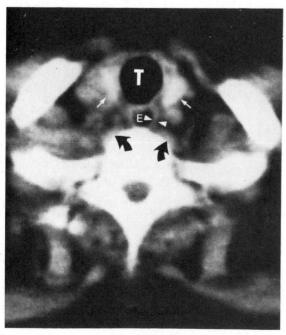

Figure 12–1. Normal esophagus—cervical region. Cervical esophagus (E) at level of thyroid gland (arrows) is positioned in the midline, just posterior to the trachea (T). The normal esophageal wall (arrowheads) is a thin, sharp structure outlined by air and mediastinal fat measuring less than 3 mm in diameter. Longus colli muscles are indicated by curved arrows.

UPPER ESOPHAGUS

The cervical esophagus is a midline structure, intimately related to the posterior tracheal wall (Fig. 12–1), which it indents in approximately 40 per cent of cases. A smooth, rounded esophageal impression on the trachea should not be interpreted as evidence of tracheal invasion by an esophageal mass. Lateral and dorsal to the esophagus on either side are the long muscles (longus colli) of the neck. The thyroid gland is seen as a high-density structure lying anterior and lateral to the trachea and esophagus. Air is present within the cervical esophagus more frequently than in any other part of the esophagus.

MIDDLE ESOPHAGUS

At the level just below the sternal notch, the trachea deviates slightly to the right of the esophagus with the esophagus remaining midline or shifting slightly to the left (Fig. 12–2).[11] The esophagus is closely applied to the thoracic spine, and no normal structure is found posterior to the esophagus at this level. A retrotracheal space of up to 4 mm can be present between the trachea and esophagus,[11] and a portion of lung can extend retrotracheally. The subclavian artery, common carotid artery, brachiocephalic artery, and brachiocephalic veins are also clearly identified at this level.

At the level of the aortic arch, the esophagus is closely related to the left posterolateral portion of the trachea (Fig. 12–3). The azygos vein is located to the right, posterior and lateral to the esophagus, and the arch of the azygos can be identified at this level (Fig. 12–3). The lung is in direct contact with the right side of the esophagus, forming the azygoesophageal recess, which is identified on 77 per cent of mediastinal CT scans.[14] Just below the carina, the esophagus is closely related to the left mainstem bronchus, separated only by a small amount of mediastinal fat (Fig. 12–4).[11, 14] At this level, a lung recess is present in 10 to 20 per cent between the esophagus and the left pulmonary artery.[14]

LOWER ESOPHAGUS

Below the left mainstem bronchus, the esophagus comes in contact with the pericardium surrounding the posterior wall of the left atrium. The esophagus is positioned near the left pulmonary vein as it enters into the left atrium, and the azygos vein is visible as a midline structure (Fig.

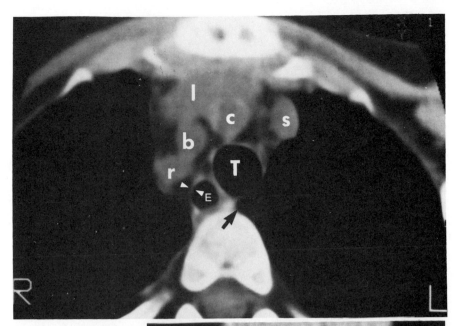

Figure 12–2. Normal esophagus—level of sternal notch. In this patient the trachea (T) is slightly to the left of the esophagus (E). The retrotracheal extension of lung (arrow) is a normal finding. The left subclavian artery (s), common carotid artery (c), brachiocephalic artery (b), right (r) and left (l) bracheocephalic veins and thin wall (arrowheads) of the normal esophagus are clearly identified.

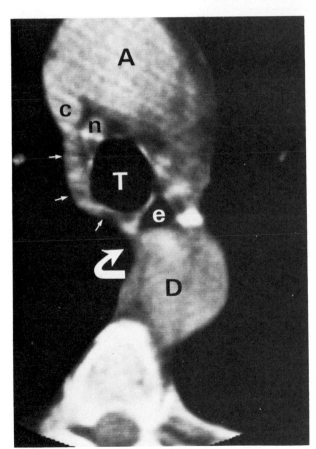

Figure 12–3. Normal esophagus—level of aortic arch. The esophagus (e) is slightly to the right of the trachea (T) and the ascending (A) and descending (D) aorta, arch of the azygos vein (arrows) entering the superior vena cava (c) and azygoesophageal recess (curved arrow) are identified at this level. n = Normal sized pretracheal lymph node.

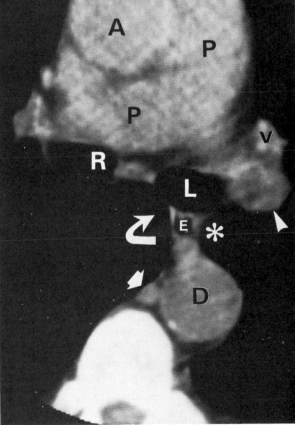

Figure 12–4. Normal esophagus—level just below carina. A scan at this level demonstrates the relationships of the right (R) and left (L) main stem bronchi, esophagus (E), descending aorta (D), azygos vein (arrow), pulmonary artery (P), ascending aorta (A), and azygoesophageal recess (curved arrow). The left lung recess (asterisk) is shown abutting on the left main stem bronchus, esophagus and left pulmonary artery (arrowhead). V = Left pulmonary vein.

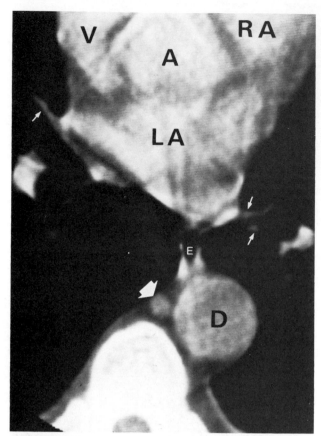

Figure 12–5. Normal esophagus—level of left atrium. The esophagus (E) is in contact with pericardium surrounding the left atrium (LA). Pulmonary veins (small arrows), right ventricle (V), right atrium (RA), ascending aorta (A), descending aorta (D), and azygos vein (large arrow) are also seen. At this level the esophagus is separated from lung by only the thickness of the esophageal wall and pleura.

12–5). Below the level of the left atrium, the esophagus moves slightly to the left of midline just anterior to the descending aorta (Fig. 12–6) with only mediastinal fat separating the esophagus from the pericardium.

Just after the esophagus passes through the diaphragm, it turns left and courses in a horizontal plane to enter the gastric fundus (Fig. 12–7). On CT scans, the region of the gastroesophageal junction appears as a thickening or mass along the medial cephalic aspect of the stomach in approximately one third of patients.[11, 16, 17] The apparent mass is produced as a result of the transverse plane of axial CT sections passing through the horizontally directed normal esophagogastric junction (Fig. 12–7).

Knowledge of the anatomy of this region usu-

ally permits a distinction of a true mass from a normal gastroesophageal junction. The gastrohepatic ligament courses between the lesser curvature of the stomach and liver, and the distal esophagus is enveloped by the cranialmost aspect of the ligament (Fig. 12–8).[16] The gastrohepatic ligament fuses with the fissure of the ligamentum venosum to pass anterior to the caudate lobe. Thus the cleft seen on transverse CT images separating the caudate lobe from the lateral segment of the left lobe points directly to the region of the esophagogastric junction (Fig. 12–7).[16]

When a soft-tissue mass is noted high along the lesser curvature of the stomach, its relation to the fissure plane anterior to the caudate lobe should be studied. If the mass and fissure plane are present on the same or adjoining sections, a pseudotumor should be suspected.

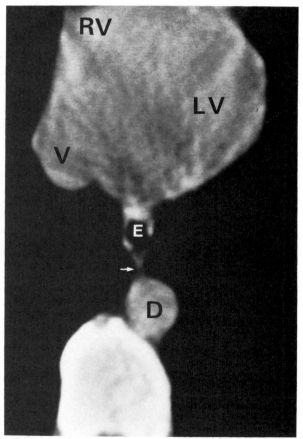

Figure 12–6. Normal esophagus—level of left ventricle. The esophagus (E) is just to the left of midline, closely related to the left ventricle (LV) and separated from the descending aorta (D) by the posterior junction line (arrow). V = Inferior vena cava; RV = right ventricle.

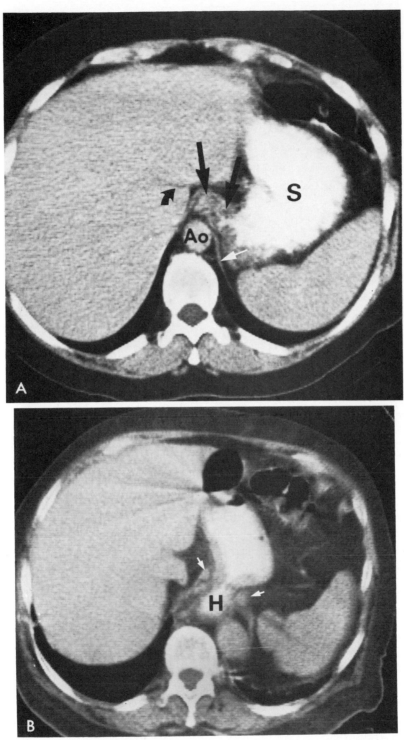

Figure 12–7. Normal esophagus—level of gastroesophageal junction. **A** The normal esophagus (large arrows) courses in a horizontal plane to enter the fundus of the stomach (S). The cleft above the caudate lobe (curved arrow) points to gastroesophageal junction. Left diaphragmatic crus (small arrow) is closely applied to the abdominal aorta (AO). (From Marks WM, Callen PW, Moss AA: Gastroesophageal region: Source of confusion on CT. AJR 136:359, 1981. © 1981, American Roentgen Ray Society. Reprinted by permission.) **B** Hiatus hernia (H) producing a mass in region of gastroesophageal junction. Note that the crura of the diaphram (arrows) at the level of the esophageal hiatus are widely separated instead of tightly surrounding the descending aorta and esophagus.

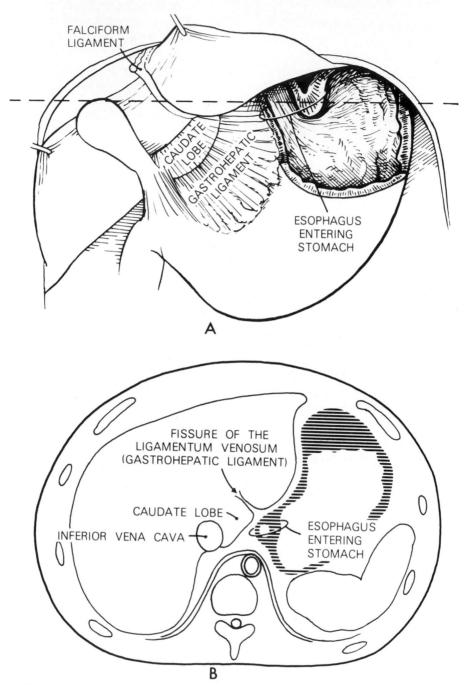

Figure 12–8. Diagram of anatomic relationships at the gastroesophageal junction. **A** Relation of esophageal entrance into stomach and gastrohepatic ligament (lesser omentum). **B** Illustration of CT scan at level of esophageal entrance into stomach (dashed line in **A**) demonstrating the location of the gastroesophageal junction to be opposite the fissure of ligamentum venosum (gastrohepatic ligament). (From Marks WM, Callen PW, Moss AA: Gastroesophageal region: Source of confusion on CT. AJR 136:359, 1981. © 1981, American Roentgen Ray Society. Reprinted by permission.)

TECHNIQUES OF EXAMINATION

Patients are routinely fasted, except for water by mouth, from midnight until the CT examination in the morning. CT scans 1 cm in thickness are taken contiguously at 1-cm intervals from the sternal notch to the umbilicus with the patient in the supine position. The examination is extended to the umbilicus to detect abdominal lymphadenopathy commonly found in esophageal carcinoma. CT scans of the neck are obtained if barium esophagography or endoscopy suggests a cervical esophageal lesion. Scans are obtained using the shortest scan time available with the scanner gantry at 0° angulation. CT sections thinner than 1 cm are routinely employed through areas of esophageal abnormality to better define the relationship of the esophagus to adjacent structures. In certain instances, placement of a nasogastric tube or decubitus positioning is employed to evaluate the esophagogastric junction more accurately.

An intravenous infusion of 150 ml of 60 per cent methylglucamine diatrizoate is administered during the scanning procedure to define the mediastinal vascular structures. When additional opacification of mediastinal vascular structures is needed, a 50- to 80-ml intravenous bolus of 60 per cent methylglucamine diatrizoate is administered. Patients are not routinely given oral contrast media to drink, but in some patients additional CT scans are obtained during or immediately following a swallow of a 1 to 2 per cent solution of Gastrografin or barium sulfate in order to identify the esophageal lumen or distend the esophagus.

CT scans of the cervical esophagus are reconstructed using the infant or cranial reconstruction file, and the rest of the esophagus is displayed on the appropriate adult whole body reconstruction file. The CT images of the esophagus and adjacent mediastinal structures are magnified 1.5 to 2.5 times prior to filming to ensure optimal display of the esophagus and paraesophageal tissues.

PATHOLOGY

MALIGNANT ESOPHAGEAL TUMORS

Malignant esophageal tumors outnumber benign tumors more than 4 to 1.[18] The majority of malignant esophageal tumors are squamous cell carcinomas, although there are scattered examples of primary esophageal adenocarcinoma, carcinosarcoma, lymphoma, sarcoma, and mela-

noma.[19-21] Carcinoma of the esophagus is rarely diagnosed prior to extraesophageal spread to the mediastinum, abdomen, or liver,[19-22] and as a result of the usually advanced state of the disease at the time of diagnosis, the overall 5-year survival rate is less than 10 per cent. Moreover, the survival rate has remained essentially unchanged over the past two decades despite more aggressive surgical and radiation therapy regimens.[19, 21, 23-27] With the esophagus lacking a serosa, esophageal carcinoma can spread rapidly by way of lymphatic channels to regional lymph nodes and directly to contiguous structures such as the trachea, bronchi, and pericardium.[19, 20, 25, 26, 28]

DIAGNOSIS. An accurate diagnosis of esophageal carcinoma is made in over 90 per cent of patients by esophagography and/or endoscopy. Chest radiography, mediastinal tomography, azygous venography, mediastinoscopy, and bronchoscopy have been used to assess the extent of disease,[28-34] although they have not proved accurate in staging carcinoma of the esophagus.[19, 20, 28, 34] As computed tomography accurately displays the anatomy and relationships between the esophagus and mediastinal structures,[11-15, 35-37] CT is the imaging procedure of choice to stage and assess the degree of the spread of carcinoma into extraesophageal tissues and to determine the effect of therapy.[12, 13, 35]

CT STAGING. Based upon the CT findings, esophageal carcinoma can be classified into one of four stages (Table 12–1):

1. Esophageal carcinoma producing an intraluminal mass without esophageal wall thickening, mediastinal extension, or distant metastasis is classified as Stage I.

2. Stage II esophageal malignancy thickens the esophageal wall to greater than 5 mm, but there is no evidence of metastatic disease or mediastinal tumor extension (Fig. 12–9).

3. Stage III carcinomas thicken the esophageal

Table 12–1.   CT STAGING OF ESOPHAGEAL CARCINOMA

Stage I	Intraluminal polypoid mass without thickening of esophageal wall, no mediastinal extension or metastasis
Stage II	Thickened esophageal wall (greater than 5 mm) without invasion of adjacent organs or distant metastasis
Stage III	Thickened esophageal wall with direct extension into surrounding tissue; local or regional mediastinal adenopathy may or may not be present; no distant metastasis
Stage IV	Any tumor stage with distant metastatic disease

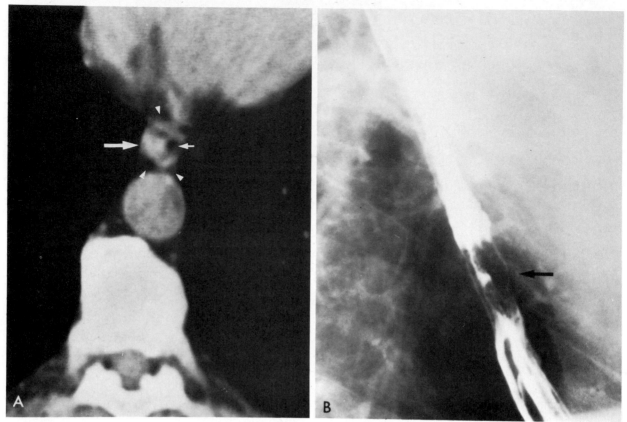

Figure 12–9. Stage II esophageal carcinoma. **A** CT scan showing focal thickening of the right lateral esophageal wall (large arrow), which causes the esophageal lumen (small arrow) to have an eccentric position. Fat planes (arrowheads) surrounding the esophagus are preserved. **B** Esophagogram of focal nonobstructing mass (arrow) in distal third of esophagus. (From Moss AA, Schnyder P, Thoeni RF, Margulis AR: Esophageal carcinoma: Pre-therapy staging by computed tomography. AJR 136:1051, 1981. © 1981, American Roentgen Ray Society. Reprinted by permission.)

wall to more than 5 mm and have extended directly into the surrounding tissue (Fig. 12–10). Local or regional mediastinal lymphadenopathy may be present, but distant metastasis has not occurred.

4. Evidence of distant metastatic spread classifies an esophageal carcinoma as Stage IV (Fig. 12–11).

CT FINDINGS. Accurate determination of extraesophageal tumor extension can be difficult and demands excellent technique and careful evaluation of the periesophageal tissues. One of the most useful CT findings in determining extraesophageal spread of esophageal carcinoma is the loss of tissue fat planes between an esophageal

mass and contiguous mediastinal structures (Fig. 12–10). When direct extension of esophageal carcinoma has occurred, normal fat planes are invariably lost; however, in patients with sparse mediastinal fat, it can be difficult to determine if esophageal carcinoma has invaded or is just contiguous with an adjacent mediastinal structure. Administration of intravenous contrast material is often helpful in determining whether actual obliteration of the periesophageal fat plane has occurred (Fig. 12–12).

Interpretation that direct tumor extension has occurred requires CT to reveal loss of the periesophageal fat and a definite mass extending into an adjacent structure. Identification of a polypoid

Fig. 12–11. Stage IV esophageal carcinoma. **A** CT scan at level of tumor (t) demonstrates circumferential thickening of the esophagus and narrowing of the esophageal lumen (arrow). **B** Scan through upper abdomen. Spread of esophageal cancer to the celiac lymph nodes (arrow). (From Moss AA, Schnyder P, Thoeni RF, Margulis AR: Esophageal carcinoma: Pre-therapy staging by computed tomography. AJR 136:1051, 1981. © 1981, American Roentgen Ray Society. Reprinted by permission.)

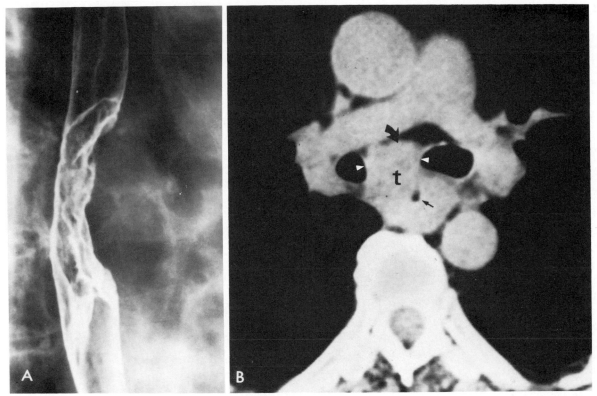

Figure 12–10. Stage III esophageal carcinoma. **A** Esophagogram of large infiltrating carcinoma of the midesophagus. **B** CT scan of a tumor mass (t) causing thickening of the esophageal wall and narrowing of the esophageal lumen (arrow) and invading the subcarinal space (curved arrow). Tumor obliterates the fat plane (arrowheads) between the esophagus and bronchial wall of the right and left main stem bronchi. (From Moss AA, Schnyder P, Thoeni RF, Margulis AR: Esophageal carcinoma: Pre-therapy staging by computed tomography. AJR 136:1051, 1981. © 1981, American Roentgen Ray Society. Reprinted by permission.)

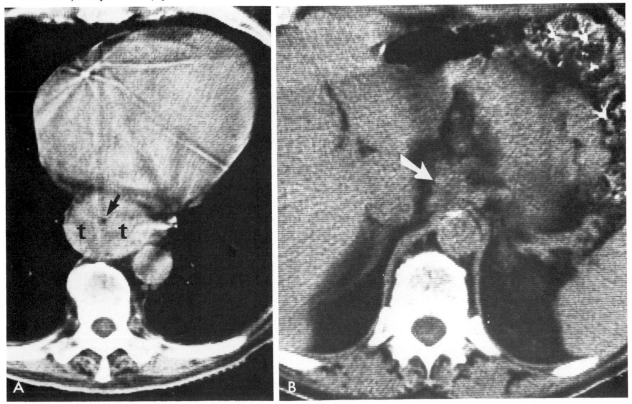

Figure 12–11. *See legend on opposite page*

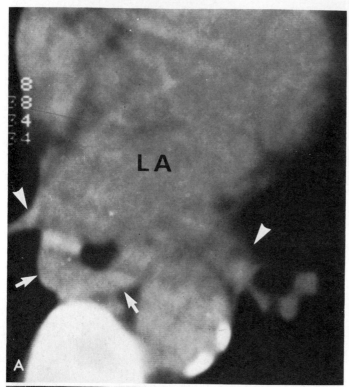

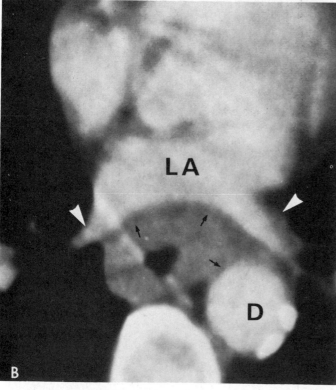

Figure 12–12. Value of intravenous contrast medium administration. **A** Scan performed prior to rapid infusion of contrast material. There is circumferential thickening of the esophageal wall (arrows) and apparent obliteration of the fat plane between the tumor and the left atrium. Pulmonary veins are indicated by arrowheads. **B** Scan during rapid contrast infusion. A normal fat plane (arrows) is now apparent between the thickened esophageal wall, the left atrium (LA), and the descending aorta (D). Pulmonary veins are indicated by arrowheads.

mass extending from the esophagus into the trachea or bronchi (Fig. 12–13) or demonstration of an esophagobronchial fistula (Fig. 12–14) prior to therapy has proved to be an accurate indicator of extraesophageal tumor spread.[12, 35] CT identification of hepatic, pulmonary, abdominal lymphatic

(Fig. 12–11), or bony metastasis is also evidence of extraesophageal disease.

In staging esophageal carcinoma, care must be taken in evaluating mediastinal adenopathy. Mediastinal lymphadenopathy (nodes larger than 1.5 cm in diameter), especially in nodal groups close

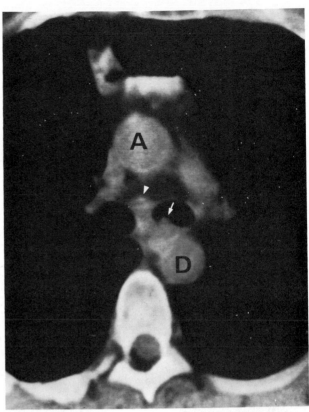

Figure 12–13. Extraesophageal spread of esophageal carcinoma. CT scan at level of tracheal bifurcation demonstrates a polypoid mass (arrow) extending into the left main stem bronchus. Tumor also involves the subcarinal space (arrowhead) and has obliterated the fat plane surrounding the descending aorta (D). A = Ascending aorta. (From Moss AA, Schnyder P, Thoeni RF, Margulis AR: Esophageal carcimona: Pre-therapy staging by computed tomography. AJR 136;1051, 1981. © 1981, American Roentgen Ray Society. Reprinted by permission.)

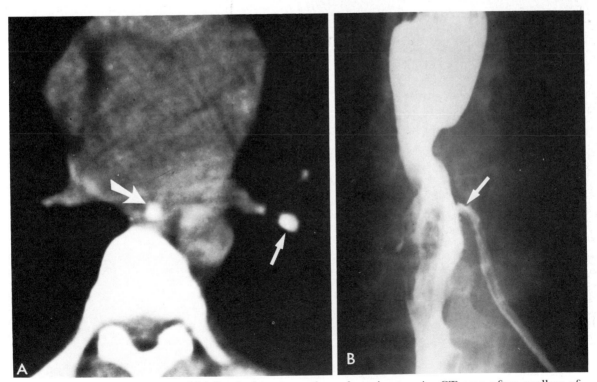

Figure 12–14. Esophagobronchial fistula due to esophageal carcinoma. **A**   CT scan after swallow of 2 per cent barium sulfate. Esophageal lumen (large arrow) and left bronchial tree (small arrow) are opacified by barium. **B**   Esophagogram of esophagobronchial fistula (arrow). (From Moss AA, Schnyder P, Thoeni RF, Margulis AR: Esophageal carcinoma: Pre-therapy staging by computed tomography. AJR 136:1051, 1981. © 1981, American Roentgen Ray Society. Reprinted by permission.)

to an esophageal carcinoma, usually is secondary to metastatic spread of esophageal carcinoma. However, reactive hyperplasia or lymphadenopathy resulting from prior inflammatory disease can produce CT findings that cannot be distinguished from metastatic disease. If clinically indicated, histologic sampling by means of mediastinoscopy or CT-directed biopsy can be performed to determine whether the enlarged lymph nodes are due to benign or malignant disease.

A variety of CT findings are encountered in patients with esophageal carcinoma. Most commonly found are focal esophageal wall thickening, which produces an eccentrically positioned esophageal lumen (Fig. 12–9) and large esophageal masses that obliterate the esophageal lumen (Fig. 12–15). Subtle eccentricities of the esophageal lumen may be indicators of early esophageal carcinomas (Fig. 12–9), although detection may be impossible with-

out a prior endoscopic or radiologic examination. A dilated esophagus above an obstructing carcinoma is evidence that an advanced malignancy is present (Fig. 12–15). The length of esophageal carcinoma as judged by CT closely correlates with tumor lengths measured by esophagography,[12] and CT measurement of tumor thickness permits accurate esophageal tumor volumes to be calculated.

Computed tomography detects direct extension of esophageal carcinoma into a variety of mediastinal structures and identifies metastatic disease to the liver, adrenal gland, lung, and cervical, retrocrural, celiac, retroperitoneal, and mediastinal lymph nodes (Table 12–2).[12] Extraesophageal spread of carcinoma was found in 87 per cent of patients studied by Moss and co-workers.[12] Most frequently involved by direct extension were the trachea, bronchi, and aorta, whereas spread to ab-

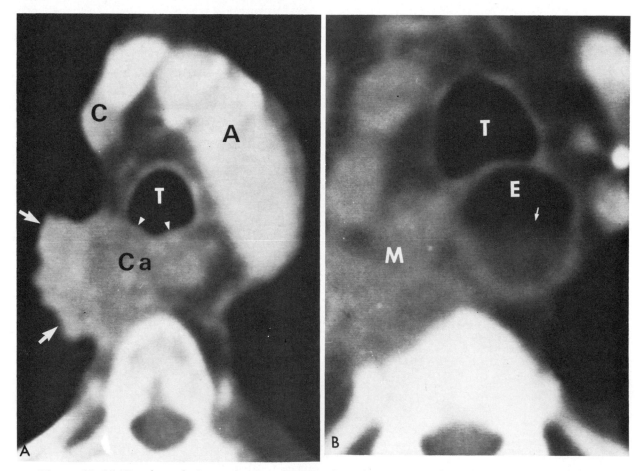

Figure 12–15. Esophageal obstruction by esophageal carcinoma. **A** A large esophageal cancer (Ca) obliterates the esophageal lumen and extends into the right paraesophageal soft tissues (arrows). The tumor invades the trachea (T), causing the posterior wall to have an irregular appearance (arrowheads). A = Aortic arch; C = superior vena cava. **B** Scan 2 cm cephalad from **A** demonstrates a dilated esophagus (E) with an air-fluid-food level (arrow). The spread of esophageal cancer has produced a mass (M) in the right paraesophageal soft tissues. T = Trachea.

Table 12–2. EXTRAESOPHAGEAL EXTENT OF ESOPHAGEAL CARCINOMA IN 52 PATIENTS*

Direct Invasion		Metastatic Disease	
Trachea	24	Liver	3
Carina	12	Adrenals	1
Bronchi		Lung	1
Right main	6	Pleura	2
Left main	14	Lymph nodes	
Fistula	2	Right paratracheal	5
Left atrium	8	Left paratracheal	3
Aorta	17	Pulmonary aortic window	4
Pulmonary vessels		Pretracheal space	3
Artery	3	Cervical	1
Veins	2	Retrocrural	1
Azygos vein	3	Celiac	7
Vertebra	1	Para-aortic, paracaval	3
		Jugular	2
		Superior mediastinum	1

*Adapted from Moss AA, Schnyder P, Thoeni RF, Margulis AR: Esophageal carcinoma: Pre-therapy staging by computed tomography. AJR: 136:1051, 1981. ©1981, American Roentgen Ray Society. Used with permission.

dominal lymph nodes was the most frequent site of distant metastasis.

Based on results to date, several investigators advocate that CT be routinely employed prior to surgery or radiation therapy in patients with esophageal carcinoma.[12, 34] Moss and colleagues[12] found a 100 per cent correlation between CT and surgery; Daffner and associates[35] reported a CT accuracy of more than 96 per cent in detecting extraesophageal spread of esophageal carcinoma. The high accuracy rate of CT in detecting and defining extraesophageal extension of esophageal carcinoma permits a more accurate preoperative determination of resectability; the assessment of location, extent and volume of tumor to be treated permits for the planning of an optimal regimen of radiation therapy. Following therapy, CT can be used to evaluate the effectiveness of the radiation therapy on the primary tumor and involved adjacent structures or detect recurrent esophageal carcinoma following esophageal-enteric anastomosis (Fig. 12–16).

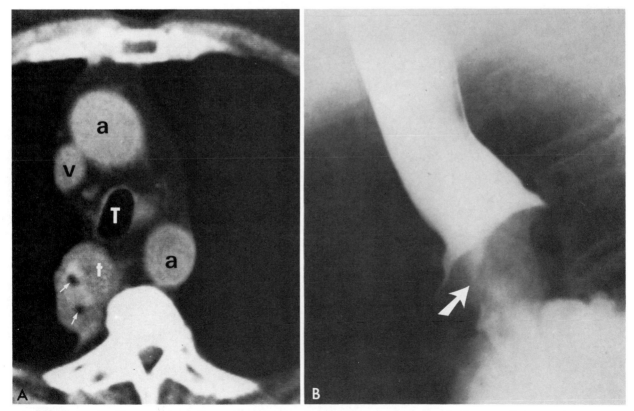

Figure 12–16. Recurrent esophageal carcinoma. **A** CT scan showing that the lumen of the esophagus (arrows) is narrowed and there is a solid tumor mass (t) that does not fill with contrast material. v = Superior vena cava; a = aorta; T = trachea. **B** Esophagogram. A tumor mass (arrow) is present at the esophageal-enteric anastomosis.

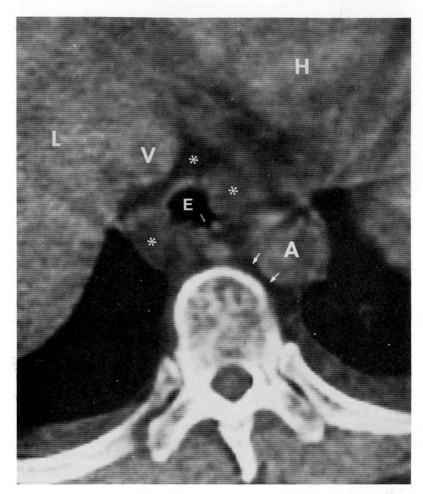

Figure 12–17. Liposarcoma of the esophagus. Air is seen in the esophageal lumen (E), surrounded by a mass lesion (asterisks) that has a density only slightly greater than periaortic fat (arrows). L = Liver; V = inferior vena cava; H = heart; A = aorta.

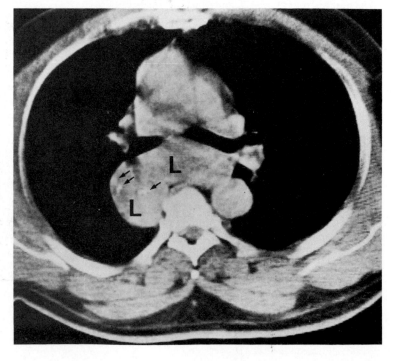

Figure 12–18. Leiomyoma of the esophagus. A large esophageal leiomyoma (L) extending primarily to the right has a sharp, rounded, well-defined outer margin and multiple foci of calcification (arrows).

Differentiating between an esophageal squamous cell carcinoma and less frequent adenocarcinomas, melanomas, or sarcomas on the basis of CT findings alone is usually not possible. Squamous cell carcinoma and esophageal adenocarcinoma are solid lesions without calcification that have a CT number close to or identical with adjacent soft tissues. All other esophageal malignancies except liposarcomas (Fig. 12–17), which can have a CT attenuation value close to periesophageal fat, also appear similar to squamous cell carcinoma of the esophagus. The administration of intravenous contrast material has not aided in differentiating between various forms of primary esophageal malignancy.

BENIGN ESOPHAGEAL TUMORS

Benign esophageal tumors are relatively rare lesions found in less than 1 per cent of autopsies performed at the Mayo Clinic.[38] The esophageal leiomyoma accounts for 45 to 73 per cent of all benign esophageal tumors.[38, 39] Most frequently, esophageal leiomyomas occur in the lower third of the esophagus (60 per cent) and are detected in early or middle adult life.[39] Most leiomyomas are solitary tumors, but occasionally multiple tumors are present.[39] Leiomyomas usually present no symptoms, but when lesions become large, they can produce dysphagia.

Diagnosis by esophagography is usually straightforward; an intramural lesion producing a smooth crescent-shaped defect in the barium column is found. CT typically reveals an esophageal mass, which may contain calcium (Fig. 12–18). Preservation of adjacent fat planes and calcification distinguish a benign leiomyoma from a malignant carcinoma.

The Stomach

ANATOMY

The stomach joins the esophagus to the duodenum and is usually divided into fundal, body, and antral segments. The normal gastric wall as measured by CT in a well-distended stomach usually ranges from 2 to 5 mm thick, and any measurement above 1 cm is considered abnormal.[40–42] Rugal thickness varies greatly, but the normal gastric wall when measured at the depth of a rugal fold is usually less than 1 cm thick.

GASTRIC FUNDUS

As the esophagus becomes an intra-abdominal organ and joins the stomach, it may produce either a focal thickening involving the cranial aspect of the medial gastric wall or an apparent mass projecting into the gastric lumen (Figs. 12–6, 12–7, 12–19).[16, 17] Marks and colleagues[16] found either of these features in 38 per cent of patients retrospectively reviewed and in 33 per cent of those studied in a prospective manner. The configuration seen on CT relates to the transverse

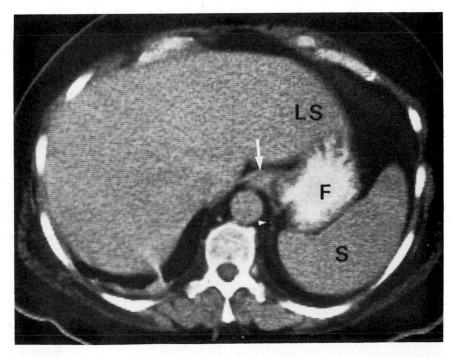

Figure 12–19. Normal stomach—level of fundus. The normal gastric fundus (F) is related to the spleen (S), lateral segment of the left lobe of the liver (LS), and left diaphragmatic crus (arrowhead). The intra-abdominal portion of the esophagus (arrow) can simulate a mass lesion at the gastroesophageal junction.

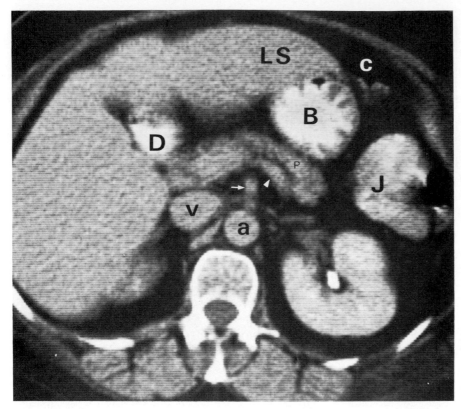

Figure 12–20. Normal stomach—level of body. CT scan is through body of the stomach (B) at a level just below the spleen. The lateral segment of the left lobe of the liver (LS), tail of the pancreas (P), splenic flexure of the colon (C), and proximal jejunum (J) are adjacent structures. D = Duodenum; v = inferior vena cava; a = aorta; arrow = superior mesenteric artery; arrowhead = splenic vein.

anatomic plane section through the normal esophagogastric junction and cardia and should not be interpreted as a mass lesion. Variations in anatomic configuration and gastric distention most likely are responsible for the different CT profiles of this anatomic region.

The stomach at the level of the gastroesophageal junction is also related intimately to the spleen, the lateral segment of the left lobe of the liver, and the diaphragmatic crus (Fig. 12–19). Frequently, an air fluid level is present in the fundus, which can produce streak artifacts making

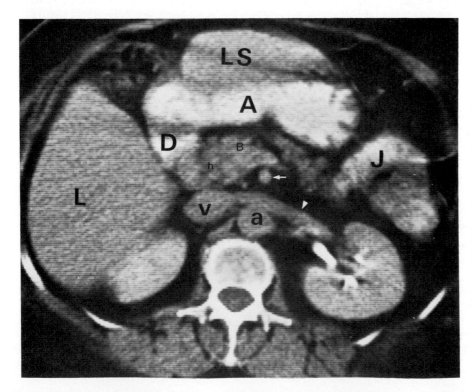

Figure 12–21. Normal stomach (level of antrum) and proximal duodenum. The gastric antrum (A) crosses the midline of the body and appears contiguous with the proximal duodenum (D). Important adjacent or nearby organs are the lateral segment of left hepatic lobe (LS), body of pancreas (B), superior mesenteric artery (arrow), head of the pancreas (h), inferior vena cava (V), aorta (a), left renal vein (arrowhead), right lobe of liver (L), and jejunum (J).

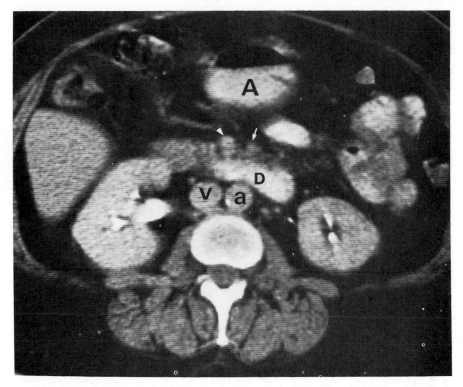

Figure 12–22. Normal stomach (level of antrum) and third portion of duodenum. In this patient the gastric antrum (A) is present at the same level as the third portion of the duodenum (D) which is shown crossing the midline of the body anterior to the aorta (a) and inferior vena cava (V) and posterior to the superior mesenteric artery (arrow) and vein (arrowhead).

evaluation of the lateral segment of the left hepatic lobe difficult. When this occurs, scanning in the lateral decubitus position helps to eliminate the problem.

BODY OF THE STOMACH

The body of the stomach is related to the spleen, lateral segment of the left hepatic lobe, jejunum, tail of the pancreas, and in some patients to the splenic flexure of the colon (Fig. 12–20). The lesser and greater curvatures of the stomach are depicted in cross section, and frequently either the celiac or superior mesenteric artery can be identified.

ANTRUM

The gastric antrum is an anteriorly positioned horizontal structure crossing the midline of the body. It is contiguous with the first portion of the duodenum and frequently receives an impression from the left lobe of the liver and/or gallbladder (Fig. 12–21). The body of the pancreas lies immediately dorsal to the antrum and the head of the pancreas just medial to the duodenum. The superior mesenteric artery is seen in cross section as it arises from the aorta, and the splenic vein is identified dorsal to the pancreas. The antrum and duodenal sweep surround the head of the pancreas, and in some patients the antrum often can still be identified at the level where the third portion of the duodenum crosses the spine dorsal to

the superior mesenteric artery and vein (Fig. 12–22).

TECHNIQUES OF EXAMINATION

In order to ensure that the stomach is empty of solid food prior to the CT examination, patients are allowed water but no food from midnight until the CT scan in the morning. Thirty minutes before the CT examination, 480 to 500 ml of a 0.5 to 1 per cent solution of Gastrografin is given orally. This contrast material rapidly passes into the proximal small bowel; thus 200 to 300 ml of a 1 per cent barium sulfate mixture is administered just prior to the patient's being placed on the CT scan table. The barium sulfate mixture coats the stomach and duodenum better than Gastrografin and tends to move more slowly out of the stomach. The use of large volumes of dilute contrast media ensures the stomach will be fully distended during the CT scan. Foaming agents and hypotonic agents are not routinely administered, but are employed in instances of rapid gastric emptying.

The scanner gantry is positioned at 0° and a CT scan 1 cm thick is taken at 1-cm intervals from the xyphoid to the umbilicus with the patient supine. Prone and/or lateral decubitus scans are performed if better delineation and distention of

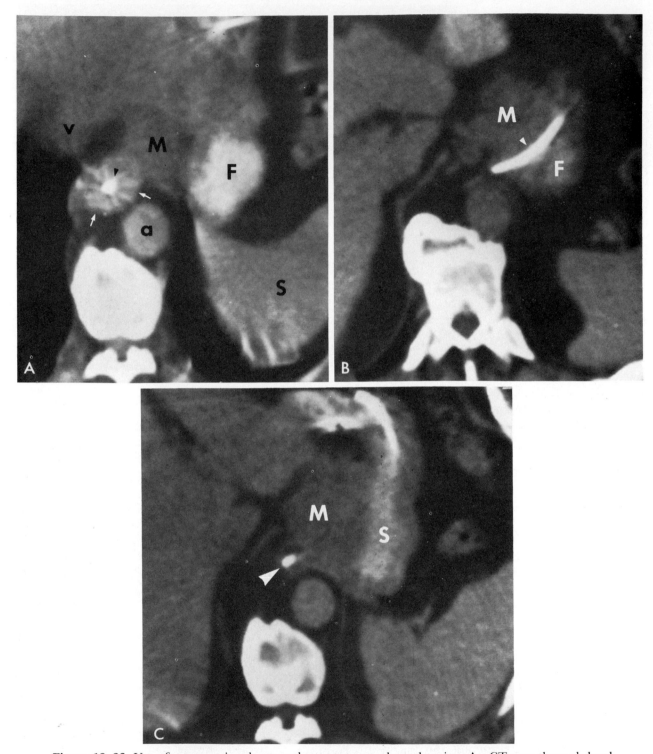

Figure 12–23. Use of nasogastric tube to evaluate gastroesophageal region. **A**   CT scan through level of distal esophagus: A nasogastric tube (arrowhead) passes through the esophagus, which has a thickened wall (arrows). A questionable mass (M) is present between the esophagus and gastric fundus (F). S = Spleen; a = aorta; v = inferior vena cava. **B**   CT scan 1 cm lower than in **A** shows nasogastric tube (arrowhead) passing into gastric fundus (F). The nodular mass (M) is displacing the nasogastric tube and therefore cannot represent a pseudotumor. **C**   CT scan 1 cm lower than in **B**. A large tumor mass (M) is present along the lesser curvature of the stomach (S), separate from the nasogastric tube (arrowhead) in the distal esophagus. Diagnosis: gastric adenocarcinoma spreading up the esophagus.

the antrum and duodenal sweep are required. Intravenous contrast material is not routinely administered, but a rapid intravenous bolus of 70 to 80 ml of Hypaque 60 followed by a dynamic scan sequence has been of value in determining vascularity of mass lesions and in demonstrating associated lower esophageal and upper abdominal varices.

Whenever a mass lesion is demonstrated, it is useful to confirm that the mass is not a pseudotumor by giving additional contrast material and rescanning the patient in the decubitus or left posterior oblique position. These maneuvers will help distinguish true masses from pseudotumors because the additional contrast and change in position combine to distend the stomach, particularly in the antral and gastroesophageal regions. Pseudotumors, but not true pathologic lesions, are usually obliterated by such positional changes. Passage of a nasogastric tube also can be of help in evaluating the gastroesophageal junction (Fig. 12–23).

All CT scans are analyzed for gastric wall thickness, contour of the inner and outer gastric margins, ulcerations, extension of a mass into adjacent organs, and distant metastasis. Vascular anatomy and change in the CT density of a mass are best evaluated after intravenous contrast administration.

The criteria employed to determine direct tu-

Table 12–3.   CT STAGING OF GASTRIC ADENOCARCINOMA

Stage I	Intraluminal gastric mass without gastric wall thickening, no evidence of local or distant spread of disease
Stage II	Thickened gastric wall (greater than 1 cm) without invasion of adjacent organs or distant metastasis
Stage III	Thickened gastric wall with direct extension into adjacent organs; no distant metastasis
Stage IV	Any tumor stage with distant metastatic disease

mor extension include loss of the fat plane between a gastric mass and the pancreas, liver, spleen, mesocolon or duodenum; a mass extending anterior and posterior to the pancreas; thickening of the esophageal wall; and obliteration of the periportal fat in the liver hilum. Ascites and metastasis to the liver, adrenal glands, mesentery, lymph nodes, kidney, or peritoneal cavity are shown by computed tomography as features of extensive spread of gastric tumors.

PATHOLOGY

MALIGNANT GASTRIC TUMORS

Adenocarcinoma

Gastric adenocarcinoma is the most common form of primary gastric malignancy, with more than 23,000 new cases encountered yearly in the

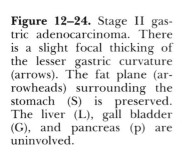

Figure 12–24. Stage II gastric adenocarcinoma. There is a slight focal thicking of the lesser gastric curvature (arrows). The fat plane (arrowheads) surrounding the stomach (S) is preserved. The liver (L), gall bladder (G), and pancreas (p) are uninvolved.

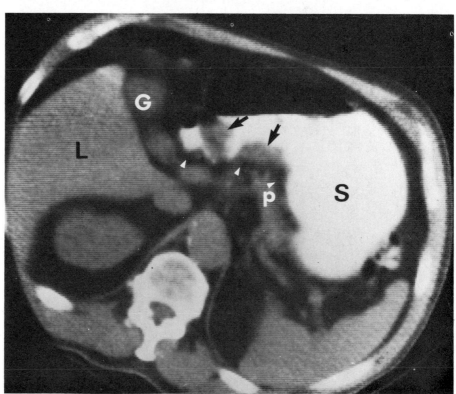

United States.[43] Preoperative evaluation of gastric adenocarcinoma has been largely dependent upon radiography and endoscopy of the upper gastrointestinal tract despite the limitations of these techniques in detecting local, regional, or distant spread.[44, 45] Arteriography,[5] radionuclide imaging,[6] and ultrasonography[8] have been used to detect tumor spread, but each has serious limitations as a staging technique. In contrast, CT has been shown capable of accurately detecting and staging gastric adenocarcinoma.[8, 40–42, 46–49]

Based upon the CT findings, gastric adenocar-cinoma can be classified into one of four stages (Table 12–3):

1. A Stage I gastric adenocarcinoma produces an intraluminal mass without gastric wall thickening or evidence of spread to distant or adjacent organs. Stage I adenocarcinomas are rare, and we have not encountered one case in more than 50 cases of gastric adenocarcinoma.

2. Stage II gastric cancers show gastric wall thickening to greater than 1 cm but have not spread beyond the stomach (Fig. 12–24).

3. Thickening of the gastric wall with direct ex-

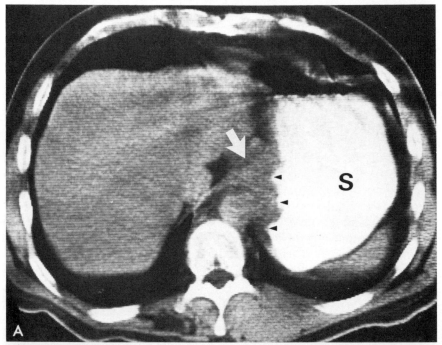

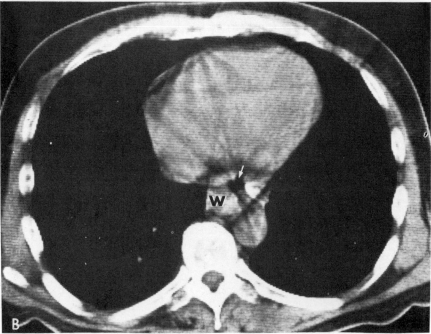

Figure 12–25. Stage III gastric adenocarcinoma. **A** Scan reveals a mass (arrow) along the lesser curvature of the stomach; The stomach (S) has an irregular inner margin due to multiple ulcerations (arrowheads). **B** Scan through lower esophagus demonstrates a thickened esophageal wall (W) due to gastric tumor extension which is causing the lumen (arrow) of the esophagus to be eccentrically positioned.

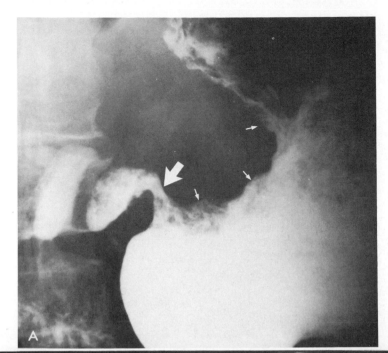

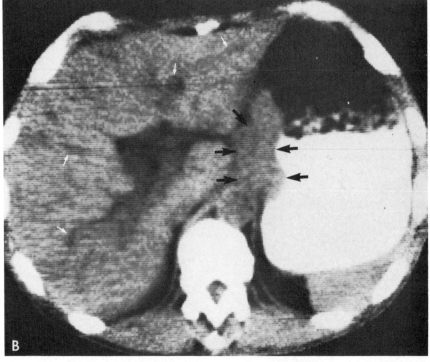

Figure 12–26. Stage IV gastric adenocarcinoma. **A** Upper gastrointestinal examination: A tumor (large arrow) narrows the gastric antrum and infiltrates the lesser curvature of the stomach (small arrows). **B** CT scan of a lesser curve gastric mass (large arrows) causing focal thickening of the wall of the stomach. The tumor has metastasized to the porta hepatis, producing obstructive jaundice and dilated bile ducts (small arrows).

tension of tumor into adjacent organs but without evidence of distant metastatic disease is classified as Stage III (Fig. 12–25).

4. Distant spread of tumor is evident in Stage IV disease (Fig. 12–26).

The most frequently demonstrated CT abnormality is focal gastric wall thickening (Figs. 12–24 through 12–27), but diffuse gastric wall thickening can also be encountered. Other abnormalities frequently demonstrated by CT are: an irregular outer and inner gastric margin (Fig. 12–27), ulcerated masses (Fig. 12–27), and gastric outlet obstruction. Direct invasion of gastric adenocarcinoma into the pancreas, esophagus (Fig. 12–25), spleen, liver, and transverse mesocolon and metastatic involvement of the liver, adrenal glands, lymph nodes, kidneys, ovaries, and peritoneal cavity are also frequently demonstrated by CT (Table 12–4). Correlation of CT staging with surgical, laparoscopic, or autopsy findings has sub-

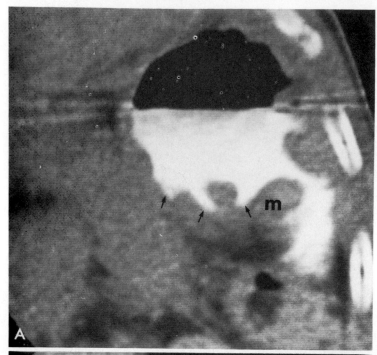

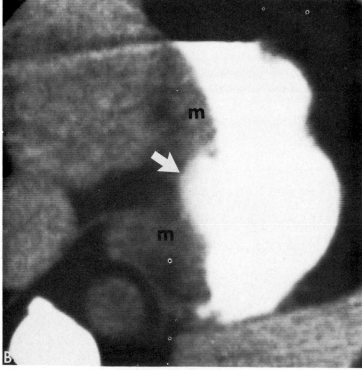

Figure 12–27. Ulcerating gastric adenocarcinoma. **A** Gastric adenocarcinoma producing marked irregularity of the inner gastric margin due to multiple ulcerations (arrows) penetrating into the gastric mass (m). **B** Gastric mass (m) along lesser curvature with large single gastric ulcer (arrow).

stantiated the accuracy of CT staging of gastric adenocarcinoma.[40] Preoperative CT studies have correctly predicted patients who had locally confined gastric adenocarcinoma and those whose gastric adenocarcinoma had spread to adjacent or distant structures. In addition to preoperatively staging gastric adenocarcinoma, CT has also been shown to be valuable in planning radiation fields, assessing tumor response to therapy and in detecting tumor recurrence.

Lymphoma

Gastric lymphomas represent 1 to 5 per cent of the malignant tumors of the stomach. They occur either as part of a generalized lymphomatous process, or in 10 per cent of instances arise as an

Table 12–4. EXTRAGASTRIC EXTENT OF GASTRIC ADENOCARCINOMA IN 22 PATIENTS*

Direct Invasion		Metastatic Disease	
Spleen	2	Peritoneum	2
Pancreas	6	Liver	9
Transverse mesocolon	2	Paraaortic nodes	4
Esophagus	3	Adrenal	1
Duodenum	2	Kidney	1
Gastrohepatic ligament	1	Ovary	1

*From Moss AA, Schnyder P, Marks W, Margulis AR: Gastric adenocarcinoma: A comparison of the accuracy and economics of staging by computed tomography and surgery. Gastroenterology 80:45, 1981.

isolated primary gastric malignancy.[50–51] The lymphomatous process usually extends submucosally, producing thickening of the gastric wall and rugal folds without mucosal abnormalities until ulceration occurs. As a result of the submucosal pattern of spread, barium sulfate studies of the upper gastrointestinal tract often reveal only thickened gastric folds; endoscopy and mucosal biopsy are frequently nondiagnostic and even if positive are unable to determine the extent of spread.[52–54] By directly imaging the entire gastric wall and adjacent structures, CT has proved capable of diagnosing and determining the extent of spread of gastric lymphoma with a high degree of accuracy.[55–56]

In our experience, gastric wall thickening greater than 1 cm has been seen in all patients with gastric lymphoma[41, 46, 47, 55] (mean gastric wall thickness 4 cm, range 1.1 to 7.7 cm) (Fig. 12–28). Most commonly, gastric lymphoma results in thickening of the wall of the entire stomach (50 per cent of cases) or thickening of the antrum and body or fundus and body of the stomach. The abnormally thickened portion of the gastric wall typically involves greater than half the circumference of the stomach (Fig. 12–29).

The CT attenuation value of the gastric wall measured at the site of maximum width of the lymphoma varies from patient to patient within a range of 34 to 74 Hounsfield Units (H). However, there are areas within lymphomatous tissue that have lower CT attenuation values than the major portion of the gastric mass. Most commonly, these hypodense regions are located just below the inner surface of the lymphoma and give the tumor an inhomogeneous appearance (Fig. 12–30). Whether these areas of low attenuation represent true tissue inhomogeneity of the lymphomatous tissue versus necrosis hemorrhage, submucosal edema, or artifact has not been proven. However, pathologic studies commonly reveal areas of necrosis and hemorrhage within gastric lymphoma with a distribution similar to the hypodense lesions detected by CT.[57, 58]

The outer gastric margin is smooth or lobulated in approximately two thirds of patients with gastric lymphoma, and the fat plane between the outer wall of the stomach and adjacent abdominal organs is preserved in a similar percentage of patients (Figs. 12–28, 12–29, and 12–31). The inner gastric wall is frequently irregular (Fig. 12–29). In

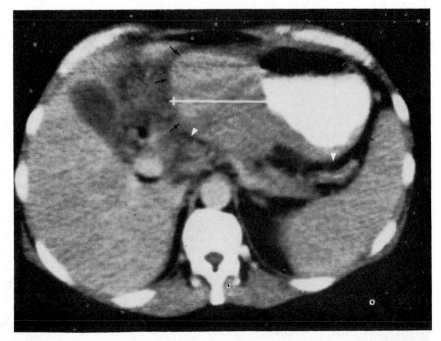

Figure 12–28. Gastric lymphoma producing thickening of the gastric wall (measured distance 7.7 cm). The outer margin of the thickened gastric wall (arrows) is smooth and the perigastric fat plane (arrowheads) is preserved. (From Buy J-N, Moss AA: Computed tomography of gastric lymphoma. AJR 138:859, 1982. © 1982, American Roentgen Ray Society. Reprinted by permission.)

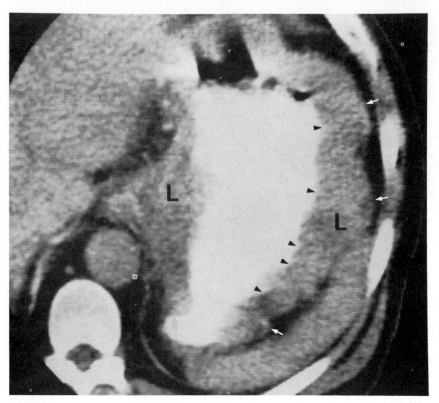

Figure 12–29. Gastric lymphoma: There is diffuse thickening of entire gastric wall by gastric lymphoma (L). The outer margin of the gastric wall is smoothly lobulated (arrows); the inner contour is diffusely irregular (arrowheads). (From Buy J-N, Moss, AA: Computed tomography of gastric lymphoma. AJR 138:859, 1982. © 1982, American Roentgen Ray Society. Reprinted by permission.)

one third of patients, at least a portion of the outer gastric margin is ill defined and the perigastric fat plane is lost. Although preservation of the perigastric fat plane is strong evidence for lack of extension of lymphoma into adjacent organs, obliteration of the fat plane is found to be secondary to direct invasion in only 70 to 75 per cent of instances.[53] Most frequently, gastric lymphoma invades the pancreas, but extension to the spleen (Fig. 12–32), transverse mesocolon, and pleura is also found.

Perigastric lymphadenopathy is most frequent,

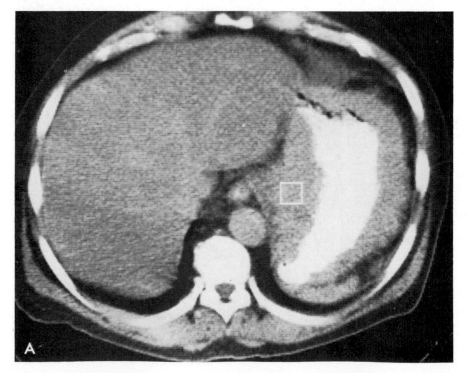

Figure 12–30. Diffuse gastric lymphoma with inhomogeneity of tumor: **A** Region-of-interest square in major part of gastric wall measured 62 H.

Illustration continued on opposite page

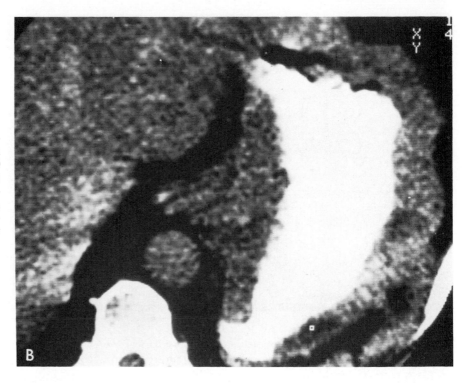

Figure 12–30. *Continued* **B**   Region-of-interest square in area of low attenuation measured 10 H. (From Buy J-N, Moss AA; Computed tomography of gastric lymphoma. AJR 138:859, 1982. © 1982, American Roentgen Ray Society. Reprinted by permission.)

but lymph node enlargement both above and below the renal hilum is also common. Lymphadenopathy in patients with gastric lymphoma usually indicates disseminated disease, but lymphadenopathy can be secondary to reactive hyperplasia; thus care must be exercised in equating lymph node enlargement with lymphomatous involvement, even in patients with proven gastric lymphoma.

As in gastric adenocarcinoma, CT scanning is useful in following the effects of radiation and/or chemotherapy on gastric lymphomas. In success-

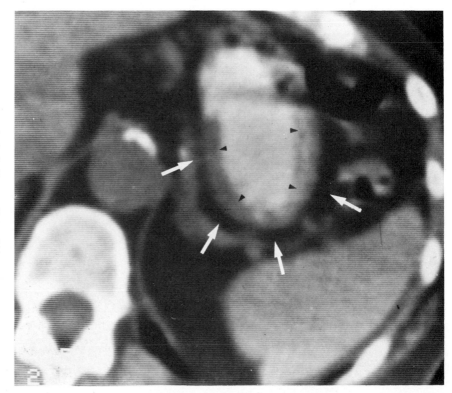

Figure 12–31. Gastric lymphoma. There is thickening of the body of the stomach (arrowheads) with preservation of the perigastric fat plane (arrows). (From Buy J-N, Moss AA: Computed tomography of gastric lymphoma. AJR 138:859, 1982. © 1982, American Roentgen Ray Society. Reprinted by permission.)

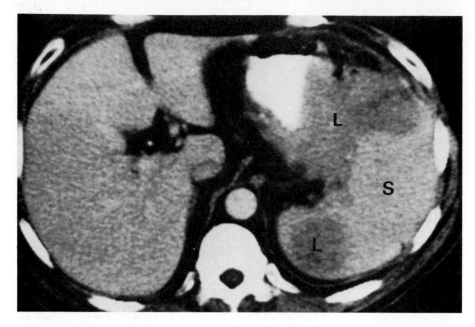

Figure 12–32. Primary gastric lymphoma. The lymphoma (L) is extending to obliterate the fat plane between the stomach and spleen (S). Surgery confirmed direct lymphomatous extension into spleen. (From Buy J-N, Moss AA: Computed tomography of gastric lymphoma. AJR 138:859, 1982. © 1982, American Roentgen Ray Society. Reprinted by permission.)

ful treatment, disappearance of the gastric mass is documented; recurrent disease may be detected by CT prior to recurrence of symptoms (Fig. 12–33).

The individual CT features of gastric carcinoma and gastric lymphoma overlap, but the pattern of gastric involvement, incidence of particular CT findings, and location of extragastric metastasis vary enough to permit a differentiation to be made in some patients (Table 12–5). CT features highly suggestive of a diagnosis of gastric lymphoma include the following:

1. Gastric wall thickening, which diffusely involves the entire circumference of the gastric lumen or encompasses an entire region of the stomach (such as the antrum or body) and the outer contour of the gastric wall, which is smooth or slightly lobulated.

2. Preservation of the fat plane between the stomach and adjacent organs.

3. Lymphadenopathy above and below the renal pedicle and/or massive periaortic lymph node enlargement.

4. Gastric wall thickening greater than 3 cm.

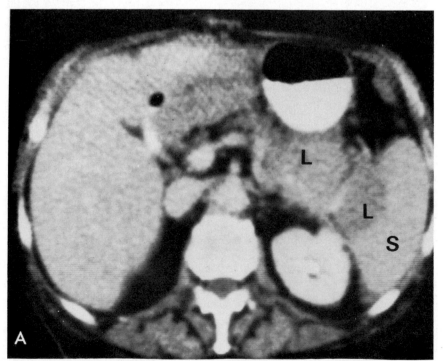

Figure 12–33. Histiocytic lymphoma. **A** Before treatment. There is marked thickening of the gastric wall by lymphoma (L), which has invaded the spleen (S) and pancreas.

Illustration continued on opposite page

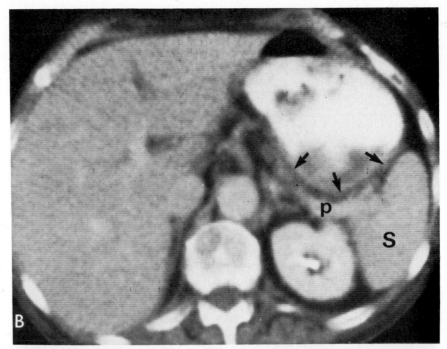

Figure 12–33. *Continued* **B** Two months after chemotherapy. Gastric wall now is of normal thickness; restoration of fat planes (arrows) between stomach and spleen (S) and stomach and pancreatic vein (p) can be seen. **C** CT scan one year after chemotherapy, while patient was asymptomatic. Note thickening of the gastric fundus (small arrows) and evidence of an extragastric mass (large arrow). After another course of therapy, the mass and gastric thickening again resolved. (Case courtesy of Dr. J. Kaiser.) (From Buy J-N, Moss AA: Computed tomography of gastric lymphoma. AJR 138:859, 1982. © 1982, American Roentgen Ray Society. Reprinted by permission.)

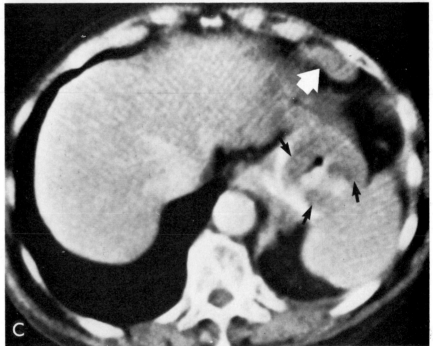

Table 12–5. FEATURES OF GASTRIC LYMPHOMA AND ADENOCARCINOMA AS SHOWN BY COMPUTED TOMOGRAPHY

CT Findings	Lymphoma	Carcinoma
Wall thickness		
Mean	4.0 cm	1.8 cm
Range	1.1–7.7 cm	1.1–3.2 cm
Contour	Regular—42%	Regular—27%
	Irregular—58%	Irregular—73%
Extent	Diffuse—83%	Focal—91%
Direct spread to adjacent organs	42%	73%
Lymphadenopathy above, below renal hilum	42%	0%

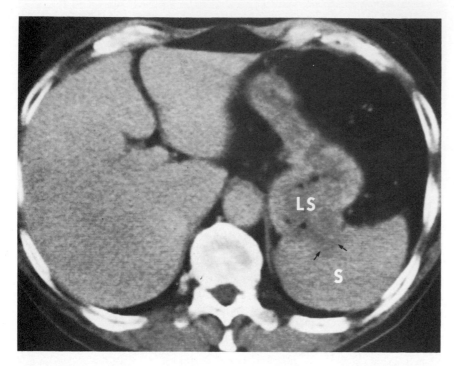

Figure 12–34. Leiomyosarcoma of the stomach. Leiomyoma of the stomach (LS) appears as a large, pedunculated, extraluminal tumor, which has obliterated the perigastric fat plane (arrows) and invaded the spleen (S).

Leiomyosarcoma

Leiomyosarcomas are malignant tumors arising from smooth muscle of the gastrointestinal tract. Of these, 60 per cent arise in the stomach, but gastric leiomyosarcomas make up only 0.5 per cent of gastric neoplasms.[59] Leiomyosarcomas are often large (50 per cent are greater than 10 cm), and growth tends to be extraluminal with often only a small mural or luminal component (Fig. 12–34).[59] Central tumor necrosis is common, and calcification does occur. Metastasis to the liver is common and, when present, typically shows areas of necrosis within the metastatic deposits.

BENIGN GASTRIC TUMORS

Benign gastric tumors are usually asymptomatic but occasionally cause obstruction, bleeding, and epigastric pain.

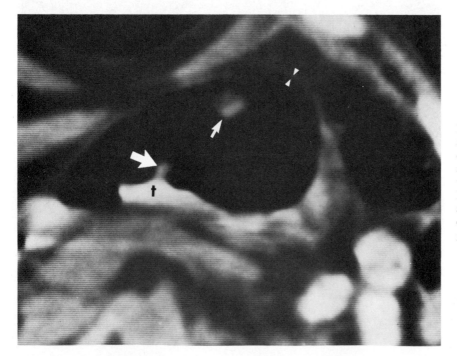

Figure 12–35. Adenomatous polyp and polypoid carcinoma. A pedunculated adenomatous polyp (small arrow) produces no thickening of the adjacent gastric wall (arrowheads). The polypoid mass (large arrow) with adjacent thickening (t) of the gastric wall proved to be gastric adenocarcinoma.

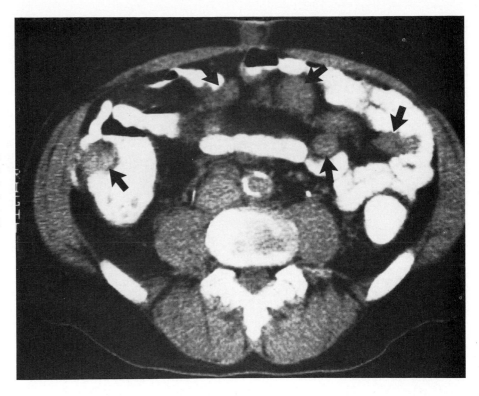

Figure 12–52. Metastatic melanoma to the small bowel. The tumor (arrows) forms soft-tissue masses located in the mesentery adjacent to the wall of the small intestine.

DIVERTICULA

When duodenal or small bowel diverticula fill with air or contrast material, the CT diagnosis is apparent. However, diverticula may not fill when the patient is supine, and unfilled diverticula may simulate neoplastic or inflammatory masses.[84, 88] In these cases, additional scans with the patient in the decubitus or prone position usually will opacify the diverticulum adequately.

OBSTRUCTION

Small bowel obstruction produces dilated loops of small intestine which have thin walls (Fig. 12–

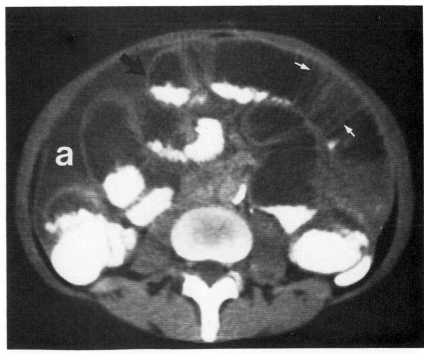

Figure 12–53. Small bowel obstruction. There is a dilated, fluid-filled small bowel with oral contrast medium in the dependent portion of the bowel. The bowel wall (large arrow) and valvulae conniventes (small arrows) are of normal thickness. a = Ascites. Diagnosis: Metastatic gastric carcinoma.

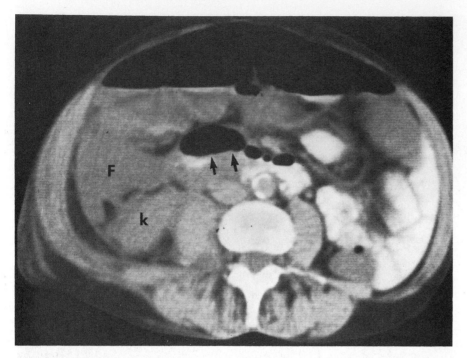

Figure 12–54. Duodenal perforation secondary to endoscopic sphincterotomy. CT scan is through lower pole of right kidney (k). Fluid (F) and gas (arrows) are present in anterior perirenal space. Note the dilated transverse colon with long air-fluid level in the anterior abdomen. At surgery 800 ml of fluid was drained.

53). The obstructed small bowel maybe fluid-filled or contain air-fluid levels. Orally administered contrast medium often layers in the most dependent portions of the dilated small intestine (Fig. 12–53). An obstructed afferent loop can be demonstrated as a U-shaped cystic mass located caudal to the superior mesenteric artery and in direct contiguity with the biliary system.[89, 90] CT cholangiography permits differentiation from a pancreatic pseudocyst by proving contiguity of the afferent loop with the biliary system.

Intussusception of a bypassed jejunoileal segment occurs in 4 per cent of patients following jejunoileal bypass for morbid obesity.[91] As conventional radiographic studies do not visualize the bypassed segment of small bowel, the diagnosis is often missed. CT can identify the intussuscepted bypassed segment of small bowel as a rounded, oval abdominal mass with a "targetlike" appearance.[91, 92] The mass has a well-defined enhancing rim and a low-density center,[91, 92] which does not fill with oral contrast.

The mechanism and CT appearance of intussusception has been described.[80] Three concentric circles are formed as the small bowel invaginates. The central portion is the entering layer of the intussusceptum. Just peripheral to this is the entrapped mesentery. Beyond the mesentery is the intussusceptum and intussuscipiens. Features demonstrated by CT include a soft-tissue mass containing an eccentric crescent of mesenteric fat, contrast material peripheral to the intussuscep-

tum, and evidence of a leading lesion that is responsible for the intussusceptum.[80]

TRAUMA

Blunt abdominal trauma can injure the small bowel, resulting in bleeding which produces a mass that has intraluminal, intramural and/or mesenteric components.[93] The duodenum is the most frequently injured segment of small bowel, with obstruction secondary to a duodenal hematoma being the most common sequela. More severe injury can result in the duodenum's rupturing into either the peritoneal cavity or retroperitoneal space.[94]

The duodenal bulb and small segment of duodenum near the ligament of Treitz lie intraperitoneally, and perforation of these portions of the duodenum usually produces a pneumoperitoneum detectable by conventional radiologic studies. Retroperitoneal rupture of the duodenum is often not apparent on abdominal radiographs,[95, 96] but is on computed tomographic studies.[94, 97]

Gas and fluid liberated from retroperitoneal duodenal rupture are most frequently confined to the right anterior pararenal space (Fig. 12–54). Trauma can result in rupture of the fascial planes and permits gas to be found either intraperitoneally or in other retroperitoneal spaces. Right perirenal gas usually occurs from a rent in the anterior renal fascia that allows gas to escape from the anterior pararenal space into the perirenal space. The anterior and posterior pararenal spaces join below the apex of the cone of renal fascia at about the level of the iliac crest; below the apex, gas can escape the anterior pararenal space and proceed up to the flank into the properitoneal fat. Because of its greater contrast resolution and tomographic nature, CT can detect small amounts of retroperitoneal gas that are not seen on plain film examinations.

CT is recommended in patients with blunt abdominal trauma who do not require immediate surgery and in patients with suspected iatrogenic trauma resulting from endoscopic duodenal biopsy or sphincterotomy. In this subset of patients, the increased sensitivity of CT to retroperitoneal abnormalities permits the most accurate nonsurgical assessment of the duodenum and surrounding organs.

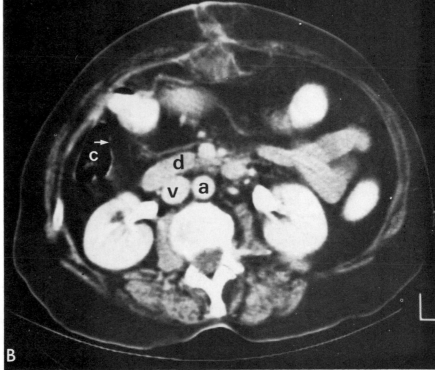

Figure 12–55. Normal colon. **A** Rectosigmoid colon: The wall of the colon (white arrows) is less than 1 cm thick. The outer colonic margin is surrounded by pericolonic fat (f), and a clear tissue plane is seen between the colon and seminal vesicles (black arrows). **B** The ascending colon (c) has a thin wall (arrow) and is filled with air. A bolus injection of contrast material demonstrates the normal anatomy of inferior vena cava (v) and aorta (a). d = Duodenum.

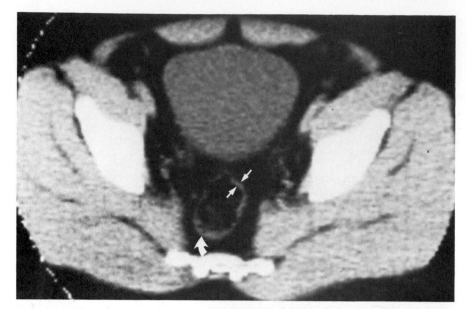

Figure 12–56. A normal recto-sigmoid anastomosis 14 months following resection of carcinoma. The colonic wall is thin (arrows), with only a slight posterior irregularity (curved arrow) owing to a plication defect at the surgical anastomosis. (From Moss AA, Thoeni RF, Schnyder P, Margulis AR: The value of computed tomography in detecting recurrent rectal carcinomas. J Comput Assist Tomogr 5:870, 1981. Reprinted by permission.)

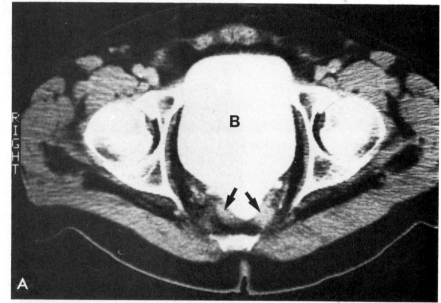

Figure 12–57. A Male pelvis following abdominal-perineal resection. The bladder (B) extends posteriorly and the seminal vesicles (arrows) are displaced dorsally. No scar tissue is present. **B** Symmetric streaky linear densities (arrows) are seen in the presacral space in a patient following an abdominal-perineal resection. No recurrent tumor was found on subsequent studies.

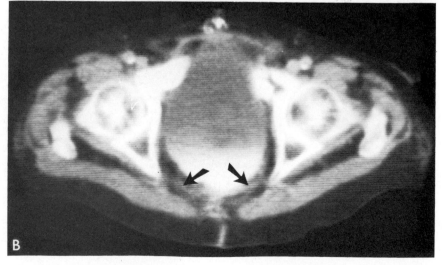

The Colon

ANATOMY

The thickness of the wall of the normal colon (Fig. 12–55) ranges from 0.3 to 0.5 cm in diameter.[98, 99] Walls thicker than 0.5 cm in diameter are considered suspicious; if they are 1 cm or thicker in diameter, they are definitely considered abnormal unless it can be determined that the colonic wall was scanned obliquely or that the colon was partially collapsed. The luminal margin is usually smooth, being well outlined on the mucosal side by contrast or air. The outer colonic margin is sharply outlined by surrounding pericolonic fat (see Fig. 12–55). Inflammation adjacent to the colonic wall obliterates the sharpness of the outer colonic margin by increasing the density of the pericolonic fat.

CT scans after resection of a rectal or rectosigmoid tumor and reanastomosis demonstrate a shorter rectosigmoid area and can reveal a slight thickening or irregularity at the anastomotic site (Fig. 12–56). It therefore is important to obtain a baseline CT scan following surgery to avoid interpreting slight anastomotic irregularity as evidence of recurrence of tumor on later examinations. We

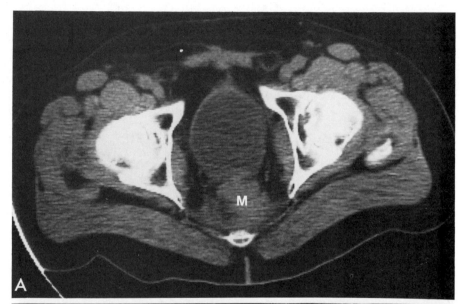

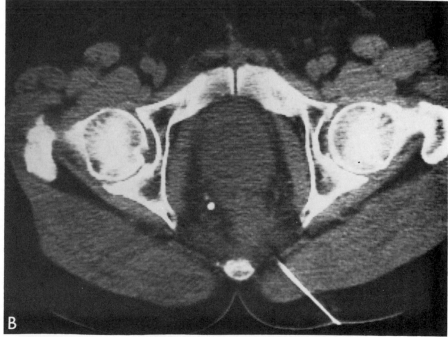

Figure 12–58. Scar tissue simulating recurrent tumor: **A** A globular soft-tissue mass (M) is present in the presacral space of a patient 9 months following total abdominal-perineal resection of a primary rectosigmoid carcinoma. **B** A CT-guided biopsy of the mass revealed extensive scar tissue but no evidence of recurrent tumor. Biopsy findings were confirmed at surgery.

delay baseline CT studies for 6 to 8 weeks after surgery to permit obliteration of fascial tissue planes related to edema, radiation change, and hemorrhage to resolve. In patients having total abdominal perineal resections, the bladder extends far posteriorly (see Fig. 12–57) and the pelvic fat may be normal or contain linear, streaky densities representing scar tissue (Fig. 12–57B). The linear nature of scar tissue usually permits scar tissue to be distinguished from tumor recurrence, which generally appears as a globular soft-tissue mass.[100, 101] However, scar tissue can be asymmetric, have a rounded shape, and simulate a tumor mass (Fig. 12–58).

TECHNIQUES OF EXAMINATION

CT scans of patients with suspected colonic tumors are obtained from the dome of the liver to the anal verge. The entire abdomen is scanned because even though most patients will have colonic adenocarcinoma limited to only one area of the colon, a significant number (25 per cent) will prove to have disease elsewhere in the abdomen.[98, 102] The entire abdomen and pelvis are also examined after surgery because liver and lymph node metastases can be detected while the site of the primary tumor remains normal.[103] In patients with suspected inflammatory disease, the area of concern and immediate surrounding region are scanned, but the rest of the abdomen and pelvis is not usually examined.

CT sections are taken from the dome of the liver through the liver at 1.0-cm intervals, from the lower liver margin to the aortic bifurcation at 2-cm intervals, and at 1-cm intervals from the aortic bifurcation to the anal verge. Routine scanning is done with the patient supine, but decubitus or prone scans are occasionally performed. Approximately 30 to 45 minutes prior to the examination patients drink 400 to 600 ml of a 1 per cent solution of Gastrografin. Immediately prior to CT study, another 200 to 500 ml of a 1 per cent Hypaque solution is given as an enema in order to distend the colon and avoid interpreting a normal but collapsed colon as being thickened by tumor or inflammation. In some patients, 400 to 600 ml of a 10 per cent solution of Gastrografin is given the evening before the CT study to ensure good filling of the distal small and proximal large bowel (Fig. 12–59). Intravenous contrast material is not routinely given, but fluids (at least 400 to 600 ml 1 hour before the examination) are forced to ensure that the bladder is adequately distended. The bladder is distended with unopacified urine rather than with intravenous contrast material because the density of contrast material can obscure slight thickening of the wall of the bladder. A vaginal tampon is inserted to better identify the vagina and cervix in female patients.

An injection of 1 mg of glucagon permits maximum distention of the rectum and rectosigmoid colon, ensuring accurate delineation, measurement, and staging of small tumors prior to endocavitary radiation.[104] In these patients, a rapid

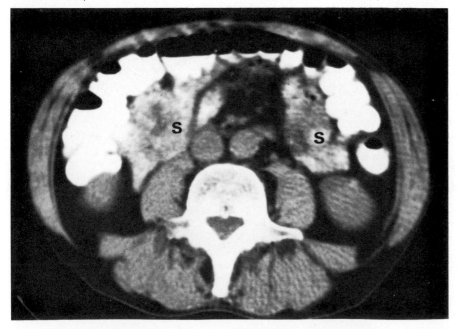

Figure 12–59. Oral contrast material given the night before the examination ensures good filling of proximal and transverse colon. Small bowel contrast (S) is still present.

drip infusion of iodinated contrast material permits better delineation of tumor and bowel wall thickening. Tumors of the transverse colon, colonic flexures, and incompletely distended areas of the large bowel are also better examined following an intravenous injection of glucagon.

PATHOLOGY

CARCINOMA OF THE COLON

Over 100,000 new cases of carcinoma of the colon are identified each year in the United States.[105] Endoscopic and double-contrast radiographic examinations are the primary modalities used to evaluate patients who are suspected of having colonic tumors. Although both of these techniques afford high accuracy, neither permits an assessment of the depths of tumor infiltration or detection of the spread of tumor to distant sites. CT cross sections of the abdomen and pelvis permit precise measurements of the thickness of the colonic wall, determination of the relationship of abdominal and pelvic organs, and detection of the presence or absence of metastases to lymph nodes, adrenal glands, liver, bony structures, or adjacent musculature. The rectum and rectosigmoid are easily evaluated by CT because of the fixed position of these organs in the pelvis; the ascending and descending colon also can be readily assessed because of their fixed retroperitoneal positions. Tumors in the flexures and transverse colon are less readily examined by CT because colonic peristalsis and diaphragmatic excursion make these parts of the colon more difficult to evaluate.

Although CT offers many advantages for obtaining information about the extent of tumor in and beyond the colonic wall,[106] CT is not the primary modality for evaluating patients with suspected tumors of the colon. Early and subtle changes of the mucosal surface and lesions less than 1 cm in diameter are usually not detected by CT because of retained fecal material and incomplete distention of parts of the large bowel. However, an aggressive diagnostic approach that includes pretherapy staging of colonic malignancies can enable the most appropriate treatment regimen to be planned. Pretherapy staging is particularly useful in patients in whom resection of the tumor is not immediately feasible but may become possible after irradiation and also in patients who may benefit from local endocavitary irradiation.[98, 104]

Following surgery, evaluation of the surgical site is important as local recurrence of colonic carcinoma after surgery is not uncommon.[107] In a study of 280 patients with complete resection of primary adenocarcinoma of the colon, Cass and associates[108] showed that 105 patients (37 per cent) had recurrence of the tumor within the first 2 years after surgery. Among these 105 patients, 60 per cent had local recurrence alone, 14 per cent had concomitant local recurrence and distant metastases, and 26 per cent had isolated distant metastases. In 92 per cent of the patients with local recurrences, the recurrent tumor was contiguous to the operative area of incision. In postsurgical patients CT has proved to be most valuable in assessing the success of therapy, in determining the presence or absence of recurrence, and in designing radiation ports for patients having recurrent tumors that are unresectable.[99, 100, 103, 106, 107]

Owing to the high frequency of tumor recurrence in the first 24 months after surgery, a series of follow-up CT examinations is obtained to detect early tumor recurrence. We currently recommend a baseline CT scan 6 to 8 weeks after surgery and then every 6 to 8 months for 2 to 3 years. In addition, a CT scan is obtained whenever a patient is found to have a rising carcinoembryonic antigen (CEA) titer.

The staging of colonic tumors has been most frequently based on Dukes' classification[109] or a modification thereof.[110] However, as CT is unable to determine whether a tumor is localized to the mucosa or extends to the muscularis, CT staging is based on an analysis of thickness of the colon wall and the presence or absence of tumor spread to adjacent and distant organs.[111] The size of a recurrent or primary colon tumor can be measured, and the tumor placed into one of four stages depending upon the CT findings[111] (Table 12–6):

1. An intramural mass without thickening of the wall of the colon is classified as a Stage I tumor (Fig. 12–60).

Table 12–6. CT STAGING OF PRIMARY AND RECURRENT COLONIC TUMORS

Stage I	Intraluminal polypoid mass without thickening of colonic wall
Stage II	Thickened colonic wall (>1.0 cm) or pelvic mass without invasion of adjacent organs or extension to pelvic sidewalls
Stage IIIA	Thickened colonic wall or pelvic mass with invasion of adjacent muscles and/or organs
Stage IIIB	Thickened colonic wall or pelvic mass extending to pelvic sidewalls and/or abdominal wall
Stage IV	Metastatic disease with or without local abnormality

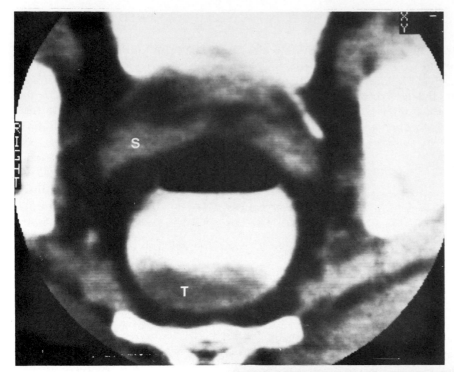

Figure 12–60. Stage I rectal carcinoma. An intraluminal tumor mass (T) without thickening of the bowel wall is present in a patient with a primary adenocarcinoma of the rectum. S = Seminal vesicles.

Figure 12–61. Stage II rectal carcinoma. **A** Thickening of the posterolateral rectal wall (arrows) and an intraluminal mass (M) is present in a patient with primary adenocarcinoma of the rectum. The perirectal fat planes are preserved. The levator muscle (arrowheads) is not invaded. The prostate (P) is slightly enlarged. b = Bladder; O = internal obturator muscle. **B** Recurrent rectal carcinoma detected three months post resection. A polypoid mass 2 × 2 cm in dimensions (arrow) is demonstrated along the right posterolateral wall of the rectum. The thickness of the uninvolved rectal wall is normal. There is no invasion of adjacent organs or pelvic sidewalls.

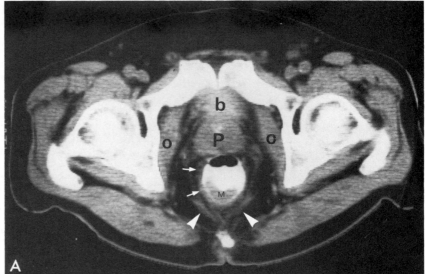

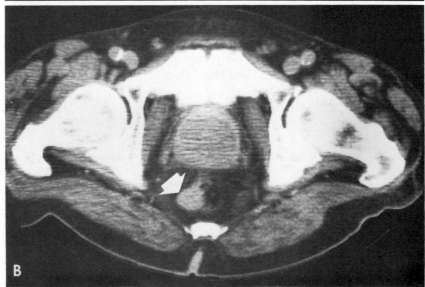

2. A Stage II carcinoma produces thickening of the colonic wall to greater than 1 cm without invasion of adjacent organs (Fig. 12–61).

3. Tumors invading adjacent pelvic muscles or organs but not extending to the pelvic sidewalls are staged as IIIA (Fig. 12–62). If a rectal or sigmoid carcinoma reaches the pelvic sidewalls, it is staged as IIIB (Fig. 12–63).

4. Stage IV colonic carcinoma has spread to distant sites within the body (Fig. 12–64).

Extracolonic tumor spread is suggested by loss of tissue fat planes between the large bowel and

surrounding muscles (levator ani, obturator internus, piriform, coccygeal, and gluteus maximus). However, invasion is definite only when a tumor mass extends directly into an adjacent muscle, obliterating the fat plane and enlarging the individual muscle (Figs. 12–62A, 12–63, and 12–65). Spread to contiguous organs in the pelvis can be simulated by the absence of tissue planes between the viscera and the tumor mass without actual invasion. Therefore, invasion should be cautiously diagnosed and considered definite only if a major portion of the viscera is enveloped or if an ob-

Figure 12–62. Stage IIIA colonic carcinoma. **A** A circumferential mass (M) invading and thickening the levator ani muscle (arrows). The mass has not yet extended to the sacrum. (From Thoeni RF, Moss AA, Schnyder P, Margulis AR: Staging of primary rectal and rectosigmoid tumors by computed tomography. Radiology 141:135, 1981. Reprinted by permission.) **B** Recurrent sigmoid carcinoma producing a mass (M) that extends beyond the bowel wall to invade the mesentery (arrows).

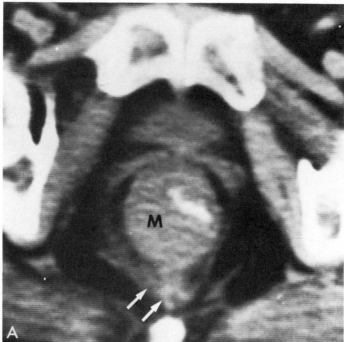

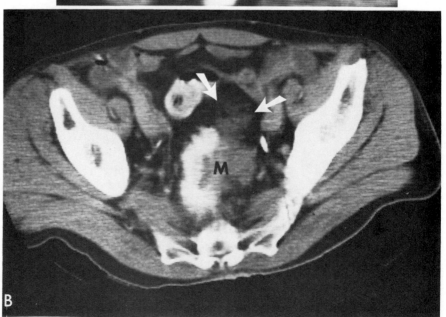

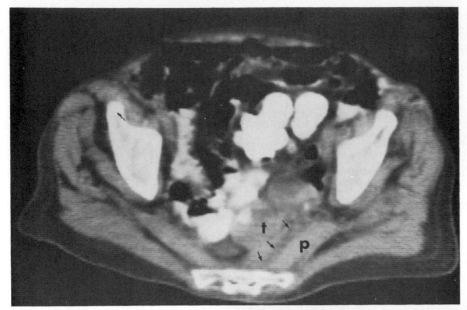

Figure 12–63. Stage IIIB colonic carcinoma. There is extension of a primary colonic tumor (t) to the pelvic sidewalls with obliteration of fat planes (arrows) and invasion of the left piriformis muscle (p). (From Thoeni RF, Moss AA, Schnyder P, Margulis AR: Staging of primary rectal and rectosigmoid tumors by computed tomography. Radiology 141:135, 1981. Reprinted by permission.)

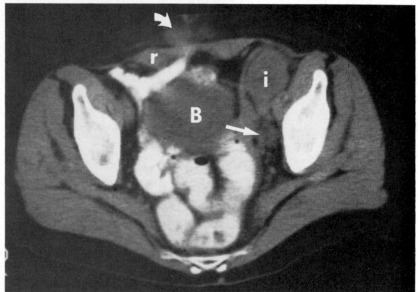

Figure 12–64. Stage IV colonic carcinoma. Metastatic spread of recurrent rectal carcinoma (curved arrow) has occurred to the subcutaneous tissue, abdominal rectus muscle (r), obturator (arrow), and external iliac lymph nodes (i). B = Bladder. Liver metastasis was seen on scans at a more cephalad level.

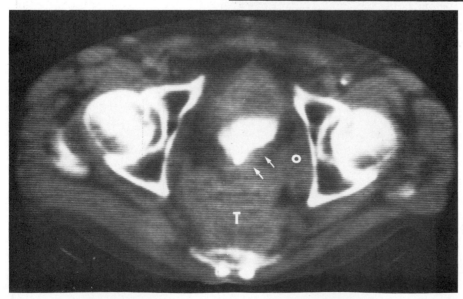

Figure 12–65. Recurrent rectal carcinoma (T) is present in the presacral space and extends into the left obturator internus muscle (o) and base of the bladder (arrows).

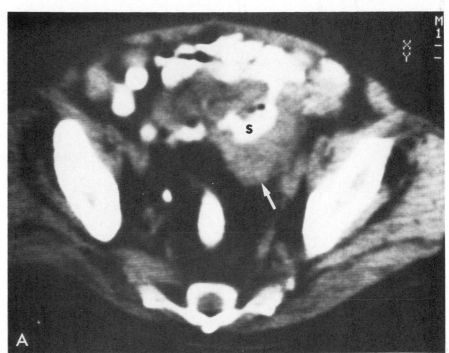

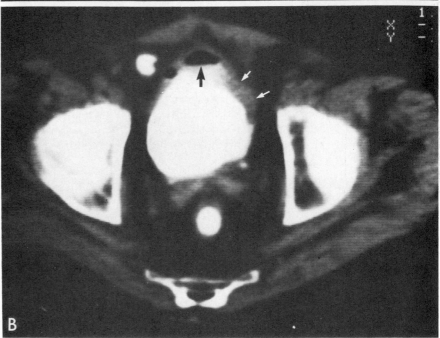

Figure 12–66. Sigmoid carcinoma producing colovesical fistula. **A** A large carcinoma (arrow) of the sigmoid colon (s) extends beyond the bowel wall. **B** The bladder wall is thickened (small arrows) by tumor, and an air-fluid level is present (large arrow) in the bladder. Surgery confirmed a colovesical fistula.

vious mass involves an adjacent organ (Figs. 12–65 and 12–66).

Primary and recurrent colonic cancer can invade the seminal vesicles, sciatic nerves, prostate, bladder, uterus, and ovaries and can produce hydronephrosis by obstructing the ureters. Occasionally, tumors of the prostate, uterus, or ovaries that invade or are contiguous with the rectum or sigmoid colon can be indistinguishable from an invasive colonic neoplasm. Tumor necrosis is suggested by areas of low attenuation within the

mass, and tumor calcifications indicate a mucinous adenocarcinoma.

Colonic tumors can destroy adjacent bone. Destruction most frequently involves the sacrum and coccyx, but large tumors can involve the ilium (Fig. 12–67). When advanced, invasion of bone is easily diagnosed by identifying destruction of bone and evidence of a soft-tissue mass adjacent to and within bone. However, minor invasion of bone can be diagnosed only if cortical destruction is seen.

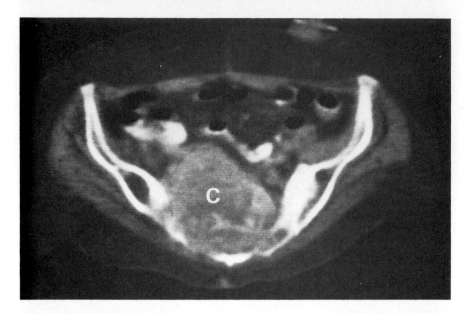

Figure 12–67. Recurrent rectal carcinoma (C) destroying the sacrum and a portion of the right ilium.

Liver metastases are usually recognized as areas of low attenuation before contrast enhancement, although foci of calcification can be seen within metastatic mucinous adenocarcinomas (Fig. 12–68). Following a bolus injection of contrast material, the CT density of hepatic colonic metastasis can change rapidly. The metastatic deposits often show early rim enhancement or become uniformly hyperdense, go through an isodense phase and finally again become low-density lesions. If only a solitary hepatic metastasis is detected, an aggressive approach appears warranted because an improved 5-year survival rate has been demonstrated after removal of isolated hepatic metastatic foci.[112] Adrenal metastasis occurs in up to 14 per cent of patients with colon carcinoma, producing enlarged, often inhomogeneous adrenal glands (Fig. 12–68).

Generally, rectal or rectosigmoid carcinoma metastasizes to lymph nodes along the external iliac arteries and to the inguinal and para-aortic chains (Fig. 12–64). Occasionally, metastasis to portal hepatic nodes occurs.

Lymph nodes measuring larger than 1.5 cm in

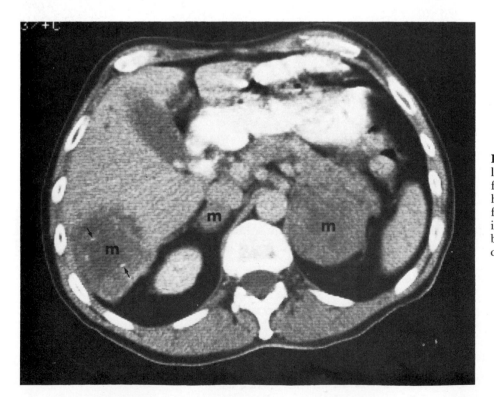

Figure 12–68. Liver and bilateral adrenal metastasis (m) from colonic carcinoma. The hepatic metastasis has a few foci of calcification (arrows), indicating the metastasis to be from a mucinous adenocarcinoma.

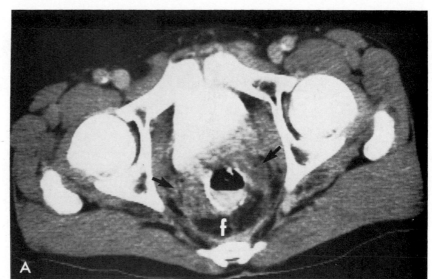

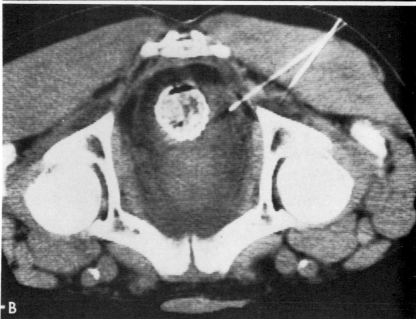

Figure 12–69. Radiation change simulating recurrent tumor. **A** There is an increased density in the anterior perirectal soft tissue (arrows), which cannot be distinguished from recurrent tumor. f = Posterior perirectal fat. **B** CT-guided biopsy of perirectal tissues. Final diagnosis: Fibrofatty proliferation due to radiation damage.

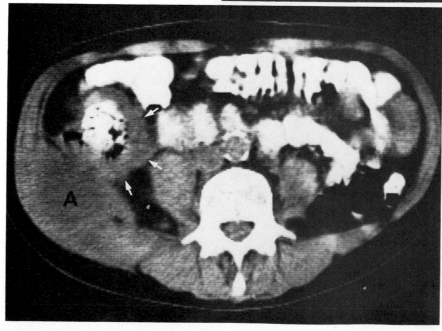

Figure 12–70. Perforation of colonic carcinoma. Right flank abscess (A) secondary to perforated carcinoma of the ascending colon. The diagnosis of colonic carcinoma is suggested by the presence of a markedly thickened colonic wall (arrows).

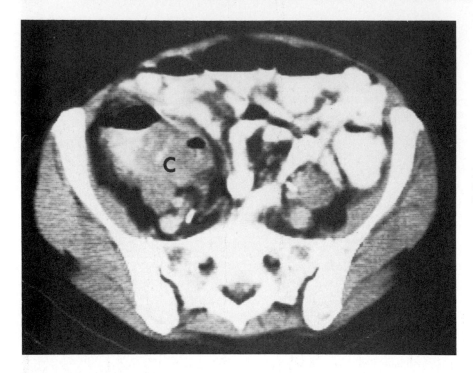

Figure 12–71. Carcinoma of the cecum (C) producing a large soft-tissue mass.

diameter are considered abnormal, but although asymmetry and size can be used to determine lymph node abnormality, the pathologic nature of the enlargement cannot be absolutely determined by computed tomography.[113] Benign as well as malignant disease can produce lymphadenopathy, and only lymphangiography or guided biopsy can give a definitive diagnosis.

Although interpretation of CT scans in patients with colonic tumors is usually not difficult, there are potential pitfalls to accurate interpretation.[114] CT scans obtained during or soon after surgery or irradiation can demonstrate edema of the pelvic structures that simulates recurrent neoplasm. Chronic radiation changes in the pelvis[100, 101, 114] may be difficult or impossible to distinguish from colonic tumors without CT-guided biopsies (Fig. 12–69). Benign bony defects can simulate meta-

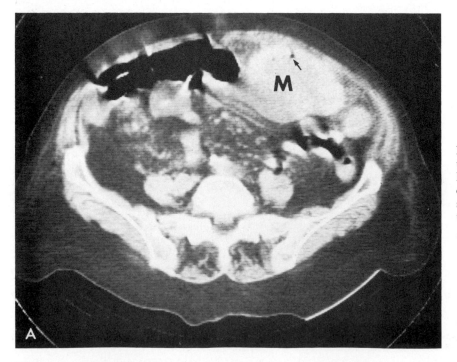

Figure 12–72. Carcinoma of the transverse colon. **A** CT reveals large soft-tissue mass (M), which contains a focus of gas (arrow). At surgery a perforated carcinoma of the transverse colon was found.

Illustration continued on opposite page

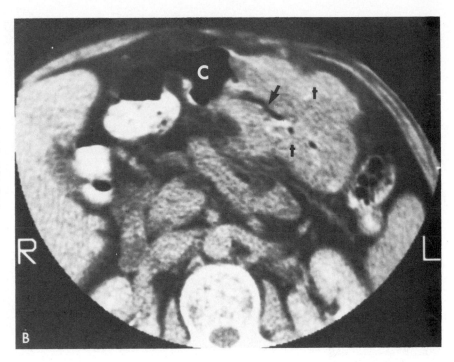

Figure 12–72. *Continued* **B**   A large tumor mass (t) thickens the wall and narrows the lumen (arrow) of the distal portion of the transverse colon. The wall of the proximal transverse colon (C) is normal.

static foci and nonopacified bowel loops can be mistaken for a tumor mass. Perforation of a colonic cancer can result in an inflammatory mass or abscess, which makes diagnosis of the underlying cancer difficult (Fig. 12–70).[115]

Little information is available about the detection and staging of tumors in the cecum and ascending, transverse, and descending colon.[102, 103] Most tumors in these areas are easily demonstrated (Figs. 12–71 and 12–72), but no investigation has analyzed these lesions in detail.

CT Accuracy

Computed tomography has shown a high degree of accuracy in detecting and staging primary and recurrent rectal and rectosigmoid tumors.[98, 99, 103, 106, 107, 116, 117] At the University of California in San Francisco, 40 patients with primary tumors (24 rectal, 16 rectosigmoid) had abnormal CT scans (sensitivity, 100 per cent), but three examinations were misinterpreted (accuracy, 93 per cent).[98, 99, 117] In one patient, a benign enlarged

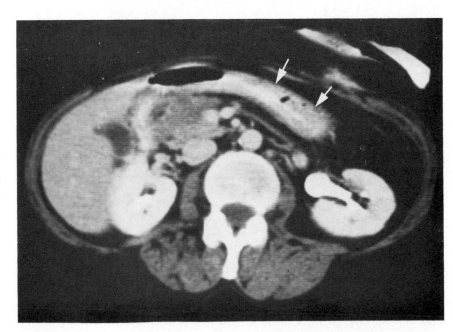

Figure 12–73. Granulomatous colitis: Thickening of the wall of the transverse colon (arrows) in a patient with long-standing Crohn's disease and an ileotransverse colonic anastomosis.

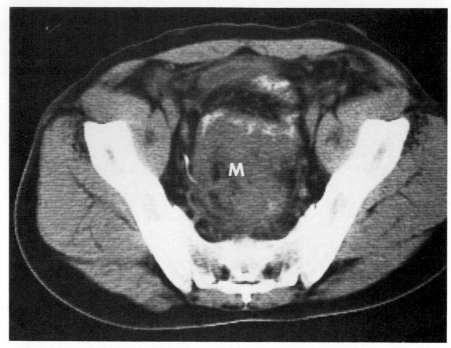

Figure 12–74. Amebiasis producing a large soft-tissue mass (M) in the presacral space. The wall of the colon appears irregular and cannot be separated from the mass. Differentiation from a primary adenocarcinoma or a paracolic abscess due to diverticulitis is not possible. Final diagnosis: Paracolonic abscess due to amebiasis.

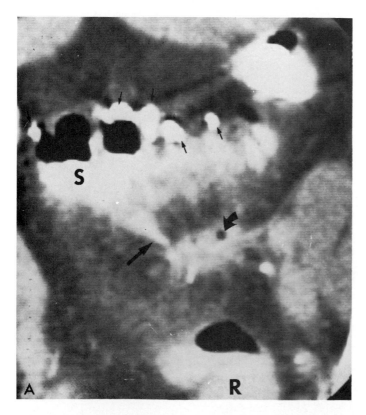

Figure 12–75. Diverticulitis with sigmoid-vesicle fistula. **A** CT scan demonstrates multiple diverticula (small arrows) in the sigmoid colon and a fistula tract (large arrow) leading to a small mass containing a focus of gas (curved arrow). R = Rectum; S = sigmoid colon.

Illustration continued on opposite page

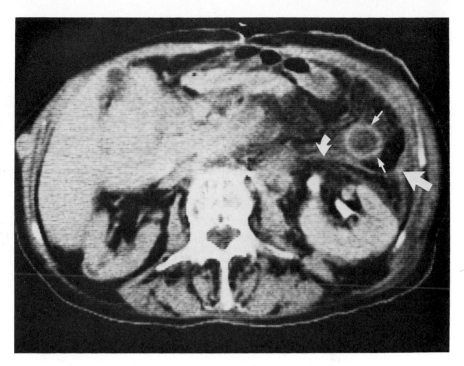

Figure 12–79. Pancreatitis spreading into the anterior pararenal space, thickening Gerota's fascia (curved arrow), the lateral conal fascia (large arrow), and the wall of the colon (small arrows).

REFERENCES

1. Laufer I, Mullens JE, Hamilton J: The diagnostic accuracy of barium studies of the stomach and duodenum: Correlation with endoscopy. Radiology 115:569, 1975.

2. Herlinger H, Glanville JN, Kreel L: An evaluation of the double contrast barium meal (DCBM) against endoscopy. Clin Radiol 28:307, 1977.

3. Moss AA, Beneventano TC, Gohel V, Laufer I, Margulis AR: The current status of upper gastrointestinal radiography. Invest Radiology 15:92, 1980.

4. Moule EB, Cochrane KM, Sokhi GS: A comparative study of the diagnostic value of upper gastrointestinal endoscopy and radiography. Gut 16:411, 1975.

5. Efsen F, Fisherman K: Angiography in gastric tumors. Acta Radiol (Diagn) 15:193, 1974.

6. Marsden DS, Alexander CH, Yeung PK: The use of ⁹⁹ᵐTc to detect gastric malignancy. Am J Gastroenterol 59:410, 1973.

7. Walls WJ: The evaluation of malignant gastric neoplasms by ultrasound B scanning. Radiology 118:159, 1976.

8. Komaiko MS: Gastric neoplasm: Ultrasound and CT evaluation. Gastrointest Radiol 4:131, 1979.

9. Kressel HY, Callen PW, Montagne JP, Korobkin M, Goldberg HI, Moss AA, Arger PH, Margulis, AR: Computed tomographic evaluation of disorders affecting the alimentary tract. Radiology 129:451, 1978.

10. Parienty RA, Smolarski N, Pradel J, Ducellier R, Lubrano JM: Computed tomography of the gastrointestinal tract: Lesion recognition and pitfalls. J Comput Assist Tomogr 3:615, 1979.

11. Halber MD, Daffner RH, Thompson WM: CT of the esophagus: 1. Normal appearance. AJR 133:1047, 1979.

12. Moss AA, Schnyder P, Thoeni RF, Margulis AR: Esophageal carcinoma: Pre-therapy staging by computed tomography. AJR 136:1051, 1981.

13. Moss AA, Schnyder P, Margulis AR: Computed tomographic evaluation of esophageal and gastric tumors. In Goldberg HI (ed): Interventional Radiology and Diagnostic Imaging Modalities. San Francisco, University of California Press, 1982, pp 215–225.

14. Goldwin RL, Heitzman ER, Proto AV: Computed tomography of the mediastinum: Normal anatomy and indications for the use of CT. Radiology 124:235, 1977.

15. Jost RG, Sagel SS, Stanley RJ, Levitt RG: Computed tomography of the thorax. Radiology 126:125, 1978.

16. Marks WM, Callen PW, Moss AA: Gastroesophageal region: Source of confusion on CT. AJR 136:359, 1981.

17. Kaye MD, Young SW, Hayward R, Castellino RA: Gastric pseudotumor on CT scanning. AJR 135:1980.

18. Plachta A: Benign tumors of the esophagus: Review of literature and report of 99 cases. Am J Gastroenterol 38:639, 1962.

19. Drucker, MH, Mansour KA, Hatcher CR Jr, Symbas PN: Esophageal carcinoma: An aggressive approach. Ann Thorac Surg 28:133, 1979.

20. Guerney JM, Knudsen DF: Abdominal exploration in evaluation of patients with carcinoma of the thoracic esophagus. J Thorac Cardiovasc Surg 59:62, 1970.

21. Beatty JD, DeBoer G, Rider ND: Carcinoma of the esophagus: Pretreatment assessment, correlation of radiation treatment parameters with survival, and identification and management of radiation treatment failure. Cancer 43:2254, 1979.

22. Cukingnan RA, Casey JS: Carcinoma of the esophagus. Ann Thorac Surg 26:274, 1978.

23. Van Andel JG, Dees J, Dijkhuis CM: Carcinoma of the esophagus: Results of treatment. Ann Surg 190:684, 1979.

24. Nakayama K, Hirota K: Experience of about 3000 cases with cancer of the esophagus and the cardia. Aust NZ J Surg 31:222, 1962.

25. Cederquist C, Nielsen J, Berthelsen A, Hansen HS:

Cancer of the esophagus: I: 1002 cases survey and survival. Acta Chir Scand 144:227, 1978.

26. Cederquist C, Nielsen J, Berthelsen B, Hansen HS: Cancer of the esophagus: II: Therapy and outcome. Acta Chir Scand 144:233, 1978.

27. Schuchmann GF, Heydorn WH, Hall RV: Treatment of esophageal carcinoma: A retrospective review. J Thorac Cardiovasc Surg 79:67, 1980.

28. Mori S, Kasai M, Watanabe T, Shibuya I: Preoperative assessment of resectability for carcinoma of the thoracic esophagus. Ann Surg 190:100, 1979.

29. Daffner RH, Postlethwait RW, Putman CE: Retrotracheal abnormalities in esophageal carcinoma. Prognostic implications. AJR 130:719, 1978.

30. Akiyama H, Kogure T, Itai Y: The esophageal axis and its relationship to resectability of carcinoma of the esophagus. Ann Surg 176:30, 1972.

31. Segarra MS, Cardus JC: The value of azygography in carcinoma of the esophagus. Surg Gynecol Obstet 141:248, 1973.

32. Saito J: Submucosal esophagography: A new method for demonstrating the depth of invasion of, esophageal cancer. Jpn J Surg 9:37, 1979.

33. Yamada A: Radiologic assessment of resectability and prognosis in esophageal carcinoma. Gastrointest Radiol 4:213, 1979.

34. Murray GF, Wilcox BR, Stareck PJK: The assessment of operability of esophageal carcinoma. Ann Thorac Surg 23:393, 1977.

35. Daffner RH, Halber MD, Postlethwait RW, Korobkin M, Thompson WM: CT of the esophagus: II. Carcinoma. AJR 133:1051, 1979.

36. Heitzman ER, Goldwin RL, Proto AV: Radiologic analyis of the mediastinum utilizing computed tomography. Radiol Clin North Am 15:309, 1977.

37. Crowe JK, Brown LR, Muhm JR: Computed tomography of the mediastinum. Radiology 128:75, 1978.

38. Moersch HJ, Harrington SW: Benign tumors of the esophagus. Ann Otol 53:800, 1944.

39. Godard JE, McCranie D: Multiple leiomyomas of the esophagus. AJR 117:259, 1973.

40. Moss AA, Schnyder P, Marks W, Margulis AR: Gastric adenocarcinoma: A comparison of the accuracy and economics of staging by computed tomography and surgery. Gastroenterology 80:45, 1981.

41. Balfe DM, Koehler RE, Karstaedt MB, Stanley RJ, Sagel SS: Computed tomography of gastric neoplasms. Radiology 140:431, 1981.

42. Moss AA, Schnyder P, Candardjis G, Margulis AR: Computed tomography of benign and malignant gastric abnormalities. J Clin Gastroenterol 2:401, 1980.

43. Silverberg E: Cancer Statistics 1980. CA—A Cancer Journal for Clinicians 30:23, 1980.

44. Friedland GW: Stomach. In Steckel RJ, Kugan AR (eds): Diagnosis and Staging of Cancer: A Radiologic Approach. Philadelphia, WB Saunders Company, 1976, pp 129–155.

45. Frik W: Neoplastic diseases of the stomach. In Margulis AR, Burhenne HJ (eds): Alimentary Tract, Vol. I, 2nd ed. St. Louis, CV Mosby, 1973, pp 662–709.

46. Lee KR, Levine E, Moffat RE, Bigongiari LR, Hermreck AS: Computed tomographic staging of malignant gastric neoplasms. Radiology 133:151, 1979.

47. Yeh H-C, Rabinowitz JG: Ultrasonography and computed tomography of gastric wall lesions. Radiology 141:147, 1981.

48. Phatak MG, Dobben GD, Asselmeir GH: CT demonstration of scirrhous carcinoma of stomach: A case report. Comput Radiol 6:31, 1982.

49. Freeny PC and Marks WM: Adenocarcinoma of the gastroesophageal junction. Barium and CT examination. AJR 138:1077, 1982.

50. Rosenberg SA, Diamond HD, Jaslowitz B, Craver LF: Lymphosarcoma: A review of 1296 cases. Medicine 40:31, 1961.

51. Brady LW, Asbell O: Malignant lymphoma of the gastrointestinal tract. Radiology 137:291, 1980.

52. Sherrick DW, Hudson JR, Dockerty MB: The roentgenologic diagnosis of primary gastric lymphoma. Radiology 86:925, 1965.

53. Nelson RS, Lanza FL: The endoscopic diagnosis of gastric lymphoma: Gross characteristics and histology. Gastrointest Endos 21:66, 1976.

54. Katz S, Klein MS, Winawer SJ, Sherlock P: Disseminated lymphoma involving the stomach: Correlation of endoscopy with directed cytology and biopsy. Am J Dig Dis 18:370, 1973.

55. Buy J-N, Moss AA: Computed tomography of gastric lymphoma. AJR 138:859, 1982.

56. Krudy AG, Dunnick NR, Magrath IT, Shawker TH, Doppman JL, Spiegel R: CT of American Burkitt lymphoma. AJR 136:747, 1981.

57. Hertzer NR, Hoerr SO: An interpretive review of lymphoma of the stomach. Surg Gynecol Obstet 143:113, 1976.

58. Ellis HA, Lannigan R: Primary lymphoid neoplasms of the stomach. Gut 4:145, 1963.

59. Clark RA, Alexander ES: Computed tomography of gastrointestinal leiomyosarcoma. Gastrointest Radiol 7:127, 1982.

60. Kriss N: Some unusual features of gastric adenomas. Am J Dig Dis 15:103, 1970.

61. Palmer ED: Benign intramural tumors of the stomach: A review with special reference to gross pathology. Medicine 30:81, 1951.

62. Kleyn KA, Mandell GH, Sakawa S, Kobernick SD: Glomus tumor of the stomach. Arch Surg 97:111, 1968.

63. Keshishian JM, Alford TC: Granular cell myoblastoma of the esophagus: Report of a case. Am Surg 30:263, 1964.

64. Stout AP: Tumors of the stomach. Washington, DC, Armed Forces Institute of Pathology, 1953.

65. Heiken JP, Forde KA, Gold RP: Computed tomography as a definitive method for diagnosing gastrointestinal lipomas. Radiology 142:409, 1982.

66. Coin CG, Coin JT, Howiler WE, Phillips CA, Tart JA: Computed tomography in peptic ulcer: A preliminary report. Comput Tomogr 5:225, 1981.

67. Omojola MF, Hood IC, Stevenson GW: Calcified gastric duplication. Gastrointest Radiol 5:235, 1980.

68. Goldberg HI: Computed tomographic evaluation of the gastrointestinal tract in diseases other than primary adenocarcinoma. In Goldberg HI (ed): Interventional Radiology and Diagnostic Imaging Modality. San Francisco, University of California Press, 1982, pp 236–250.

69. Megibow AJ, Bosniak MA: Dilute barium as a contrast agent for abdominal CT. AJR 134:1273, 1980.

70. Kreel L: Computerized tomography using the EMI general purpose scanner. Br J Radiol 50:2, 1977.

71. Ruijs SHJ: A simple procedure for patient preparation in abdominal CT. AJR 133:551, 1979.

72. Marks WM, Goldberg HI, Moss AA, Koehler FR, Federle MP: Intestinal pseudotumors: A problem in abdominal computed tomography solved by direct techniques. Gastrointest Radiol 5:155, 1980.

73. Goldberg HI, Gore RM, Margulis AR, Moss AA, Baker EL: Computed tomography in the evaluation of Crohn disease. AJR 140:277, 1983.

74. Schnor MJ, Winer SN: The "String Sign" in computerized tomography. Gastrointest Radiol 7:43, 1982.

75. Megibow AJ, Bosniak MA, Ambos MA, Redmond PE: Crohn's disease causing hydronephrosis. J Comput Assist Tomogr 5:909, 1981.

76. Seigel RS, Kuhns LR, Borlaza GS: Computed tomography and angiography in ileal carcinoid tumor and retractile mesenteritis. Radiology 134:437, 1980.

77. Pagani JJ, Bernardino ME: CT-radiographic correlation of ulcerating small bowel lymphomas. AJR 136:998, 1981.

78. Schaefer PS, Friedman AC: Nodular lymphoid hyperplasia of the small intestine with Burkitt's lymphoma and dysgammaglobulinemia. Gastrointest Radiol 6:325, 1981.

79. Parienty RA, Lepreux Jf, Gruson B: Sonographic and CT features of ileocolic intussusception. AJR 136:608, 1981.

80. Donovan AT, Goldman SM: Computed tomography of ileocecal intussusception. Mechanism and appearance. J Comput Assist Tomogr 6:603, 1982.

81. Megibow AJ, Redmond PE, Bosniak MA, Horowitz L: Diagnosis of gastrointestinal lipomas by CT. AJR 133:743, 1979.

82. Cohen WN, Seidelmann FE, Bryan PJ: Computed tomography of localized adipose deposits presenting as tumor masses. AJR 128:1007, 1977.

83. Diamond RT, Greenberg HM, Boult IF: Direct metastatic spread of right colon adenocarcinoma to duodenum—barium and computed tomographic findings. Gastrointest Radiol 6:339, 1981.

84. Ginaldi S, Zornosa J: Large duodenal diverticulum simulating a pancreatic mass by computed tomography. Comput Tomogr 4:169, 1980.

85. Fisher JF: Computed tomographic diagnosis of volvulus in intestinal malrotation. Radiology 140:145, 1981.

86. Hoyt TS: Malrotation of small bowel simulating a neoplastic mass in the right upper quadrant. Computerized Radiol 6:27, 1982.

87. Li DKB, Rennie CS: Abdominal computed tomography in Whipple's disease. J Comput Assist Tomogr 5:249, 1981.

88. Downey EF Jr, Pyatt RS Jr, Vincent M, Evans DR, Daye S: Upper gastrointestinal diverticula. J Comput Assist Tomogr 6:193, 1982.

89. Kuwabara Y, Nishitani H, Numaguchi Y, Kamoi I, Matsuura K, Saito S: Afferent loop syndrome. J Comput Assist Tomogr 4:687, 1980.

90. Robbins AH: CT appearance of afferent loop obstruction. AJR 138:1085, 1982.

91. Billimoria PE, Fabian TM, Schulz EE: Computed tomography of intussusception in the bypassed jejuno-ileal segment. J Comput Assist Tomogr 6:86, 1982.

92. Lo G, Fisch AE, Brodey PA: CT of the intussuscepted excluded loop after intestinal bypass. AJR 137:157, 1981.

93. Federle MP, Goldberg HI, Kaiser JA, Moss AA, Jeffrey RB, Mall JC: Evaluation of abdominal trauma by computed tomography. Radiology 138:637, 1981.

94. Glazer GM, Buy J-N, Moss AA, Goldberg HI, Federle MP: CT detection of duodenal perforation. AJR 137:333, 1981.

95. Toxopeus MD, Lucas CE, Krabbenhoft KL: Roentgenographic diagnosis in blunt retroperitoneal duodenal rupture. Radiology 115:281, 1972.

96. Kelly G, Norton L, Moore G, Eiseman B: The continuing challenge of duodenal injuries. J Trauma 18:160, 1978.

97. Karnaze GC, Sheedy PF II, Stephens DH, McLeod RA: Computed tomography in duodenal rupture due to blunt abdominal trauma. J Comput Assist Tomogr 5:267, 1981.

98. Thoeni RF, Moss AA, Schnyder P, Margulis AR: Staging of primary rectal and rectosigmoid tumors by computed tomography. Radiology 141:135, 1981.

99. Moss AA, Thoeni RF, Schnyder P, Margulis AR: The value of computed tomography in detecting recurrent rectal carcinomas. J. Comput Assist Tomogr 5:870, 1981.

100. Lee JKT, Stanley RJ, Sagel SS, Levit RG, McClennan BL: CT appearance of the pelvis after abdomino-perineal resection for rectal carcinoma. Radiology 14:737, 1981.

101. Doubleday LC, Bernardino ME: CT findings in the perirectal area following radiation therapy. J Comput Assist Tomogr 4:634, 1980.

102. Mayers GB, Zornoza J: Computed tomography of colon carcinoma. AJR 135:43, 1980.

103. Ellert J, Kreel L: The value of CT in malignant colonic tumors. CT 4:225, 1980.

104. Hamlin DJ, Burgener FA, Sischy B: New techniques to stage early rectal carcinoma by computed tomography. Radiology 141:539, 1981.

105. Silverberg E: Cancer statistics 1977. CA—A Cancer Journal for Clinicians 27:26, 1977.

106. Husband JE, Hodson NJ, Parsons CA: The use of computed tomography in recurrent rectal tumors. Radiology 134:677, 1980.

107. Grabbe E, Winkler R: Radiologische Diagnostik nach abdomino-perinealer Rektumamputation. ROEFO 131:127, 1979.

108. Cass AW, Million RR, Pfaff WW: Patterns of recurrence following surgery alone for adenocarcinoma of the colon and rectum. Cancer 37:2861, 1976.

109. Dukes CE: The classification of cancer of the rectum. J Pathol and Bacteriol 35:232, 1932.

110. Astler VB, Coller FA: The prognostic significance of direct extension of carcinoma of the colon and rectum. Am Surg 139:846, 1954.

111. Moss AA, Margulis AR, Schnyder P, Thoeni RF: A uniform, CT-based staging system for malignant neoplasms of the alimentary tube, editorial. AJR 136:1251, 1981.

112. Wilson SM, Adson MA: The surgical treatment of hepatic metastases from colorectal cancers. Arch Surg 111:330, 1976.

113. Lee KT, Stanley RJ, Sagel SS, McClennan BL: Accuracy of CT in detecting intra-abdominal and pelvic lymph node metastases from pelvic cancers. AJR 131:675, 1978.

114. Zaunbauer W, Haertel M, Fuchs WA: Computed tomography in carcinoma of the rectum. Gastrointest Radiol 6:79, 1981.

115. Colley DP, Farrell JA, Clark RA: Perforated colon carcinoma presenting as a suprarenal mass. Comput Tomogr 5:55, 1981.

116. Grabbe E, Buurman R, Winkler R, Buechler E, Shreiber HW: Computer-tomographische Befunde nach Rektumamputation. ROEFO 131:135, 1979.

117. Thoeni RF: Computed tomography of rectosigmoid tumors. In Goldberg HI (ed): Interventional Radiology and Diagnostic Imaging Modalities. San Francisco, University of California Press, 1982, pp 227–236.

118. Walsh JW, Amendola MA, Hall D, Tisnado J, Goplerud DR: Recurrent carcinoma of the cervix: CT diagnosis. AJR 136:117, 1981.

119. Goodman PC, Federle MP: Pseudomembranous colitis. J Comput Assist Tomogr 4:403, 1980.

120. Hoddick W, Jeffrey RB, Federle MP: CT differentiation of portal venous air from biliary air. J Comput Assist Tomogr 6:633, 1982.

121. Frick MP, Feinberg SB, Stenlund RR, Gedgaudas E: Evaluation of abdominal fistulas with computed body tomography (CT). Comput Radiol 6:17, 1982.

122. Alexander ES, Weinberg S, Clark RA, Belkin RD: Fistulas and sinus tracts radiologic evaluation, management and outcome. Gastrointest Radiol 7:135, 1982.

13 COMPUTED TOMOGRAPHY OF THE HEPATOBILIARY SYSTEM

Albert A. Moss

Computed tomography (CT) has been utilized to detect hepatic abnormalities since its introduction in 1974.[1-3] Initial reports demonstrated that a variety of diseases affecting the hepatobiliary system produced sufficient alteration in hepatic morphology or attenuation value to permit accurate localization and precise diagnosis.[1-11] Advances in CT technology have permitted high-resolution, motionless images of the liver to be routinely obtained, permitting more exact display of normal and abnormal hepatic anatomy. As in other areas of the body, accurate interpretation of hepatobiliary CT scans depends on a thorough knowledge of normal anatomy.

ANATOMY

GROSS MORPHOLOGY

Cross-sectional computed tomographic images readily display most border-forming perihepatic structures, including the anterior abdominal wall, posterior diaphragm, right kidney, stomach, in-

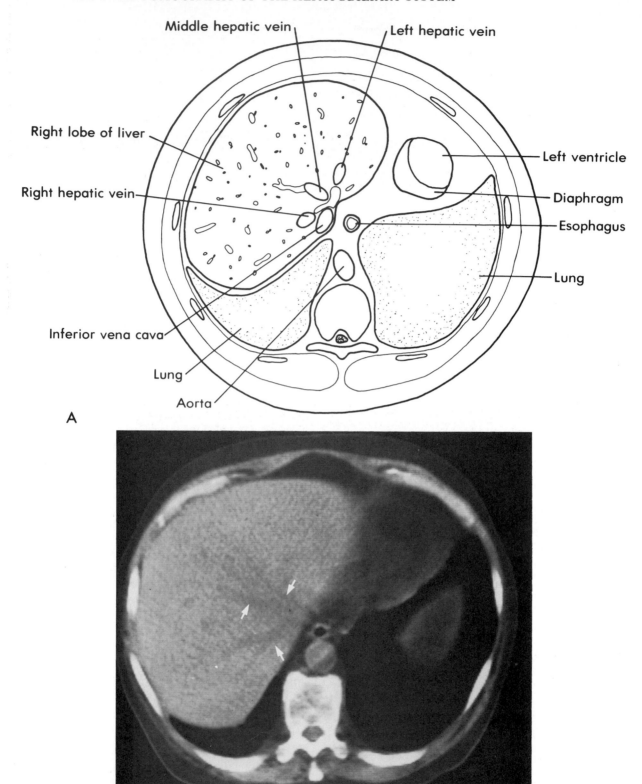

Figure 13–1. Normal liver anatomy. **A**   Diagram of cross section of liver near dome of diaphragm. **B**   CT scan taken at approximately the same level, demonstrating the right, middle, and left hepatic veins (arrows).

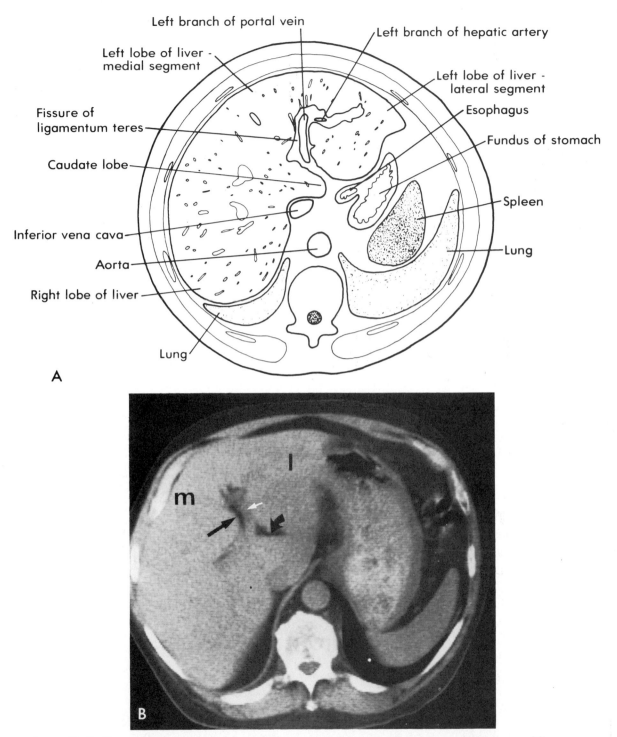

Figure 13–2. Normal liver anatomy. **A** Diagram of cross section of liver through fissure of ligamentum teres and branch of left portal vein. **B** CT scan taken at approximately the same level. Fissure of ligamentum teres (black arrow), branch of left portal vein (white arrow), fissure of ligamentatum venosum (curved arrow), and medial (m) and lateral (l) segments of left lobe of liver are shown.

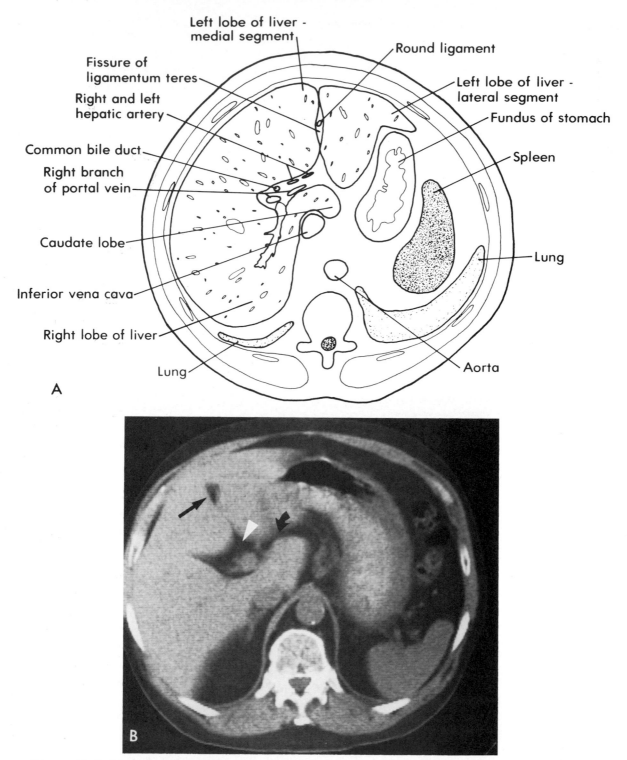

Figure 13–3. Normal liver anatomy. **A** Diagram of cross section of liver through porta hepatis. **B** CT scan taken at approximately the same level. The juncture (arrowhead) of the fissures of the ligamentum teres (arrow) and ligamentum venosum (curved arrow) is shown.

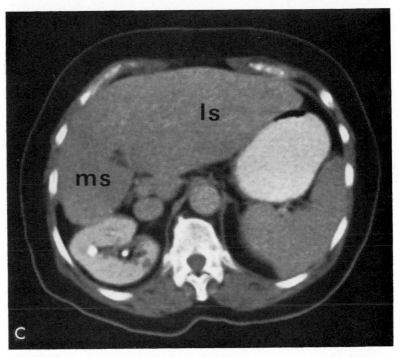

Figure 13–5. *Continued* **C** Total right hepatectomy. The lateral segment of the left lobe of the liver (ls) has enlarged to occupy the entire midabdomen. ms = Medial segment of left hepatic lobe.

tions. An approximation of its location may be made by drawing a line that bisects the liver parenchyma between the anterior and posterior branches of the right portal vein (Fig. 13–7).[14]

HEPATIC VASCULATURE

Consistent identification of intrahepatic vascular structures on CT images generally requires administration of iodinated contrast material either as a rapid intravenous infusion or as an intravenous bolus. However, intrahepatic vessels in patients with fatty infiltration of the liver are displayed as high-density structures surrounded by low-density hepatic parenchyma on CT scans without or following slow intravenous infusion of contrast material (Fig. 13–8). Noncontrast scans in normal patients may occasionally demonstrate

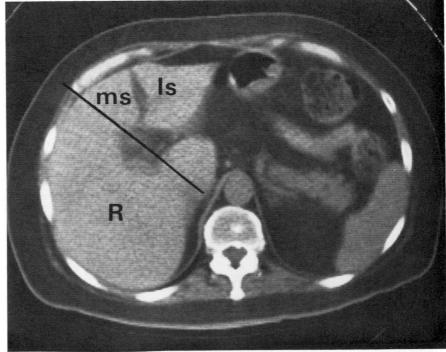

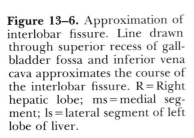

Figure 13–6. Approximation of interlobar fissure. Line drawn through superior recess of gallbladder fossa and inferior vena cava approximates the course of the interlobar fissure. R = Right hepatic lobe; ms = medial segment; ls = lateral segment of left lobe of liver.

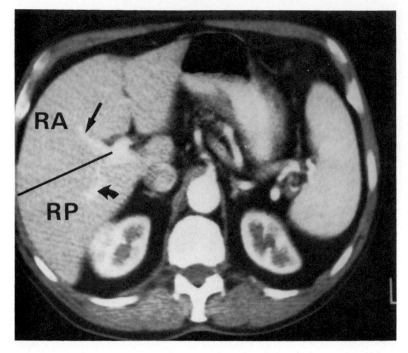

Figure 13–7. Approximation of right intersegmental fissure. Line bisecting anterior (arrow) and posterior (curved arrow) branches of right portal vein approximates course of right intersegmental hepatic fissure. RA = Anterior right segment; RP = posterior right segment of right lobe of liver.

poorly defined, low-density portal venous structures surrounded by higher attenuation liver parenchyma.[19]

The hepatic veins comprise the efferent vascular system of the liver. Three major hepatic vein trunks—the right, middle, and left—drain into the inferior vena cava at the posterior superior margin of the liver (Figs. 13–1 and 13–9). The hepatic veins are all intersegmental or interlobar in position. The right hepatic vein runs in a coronal plane at the superior aspect of the right intersegmental fissure and enters the right lateral margin of the inferior vena cava. The middle hepatic vein is located at the top of the interlobar fissure between the right and left hepatic lobes and enters the left anterior aspect of the inferior

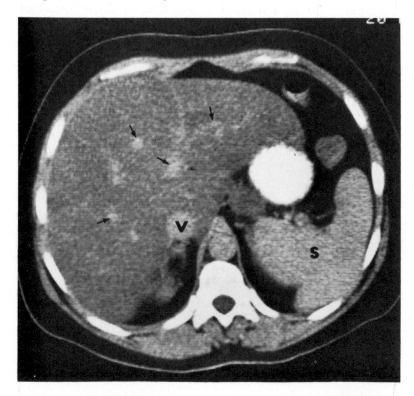

Figure 13–8. Hepatic vasculature. Fatty liver due to hypertriglyceridemia. Noncontrast–enhanced CT scan demonstrates liver to have a lower density than the spleen (s). The intrahepatic segment of the inferior vena cava (v) and portal vein branches (arrows) appear as high-density structures against the background of the fatty liver. The hepatic vessels have the same CT density as the aorta. The prominent splenic foot is a normal variant.

vena cava. The left hepatic vein courses in the left intersegmental fissure and enters the anterior left portion of the inferior vena cava alone or after being joined by the middle hepatic vein. Multiple short hepatic veins drain the caudate lobe directly into the inferior vena cava from the posterior margin of the caudate lobe.[12–16]

The right, middle, and left hepatic veins are routinely displayed as they drain into the inferior vena cava at the superior aspect of the liver (Figs. 13–1 and 13–9). Axial images show a somewhat variable angulation of each hepatic vein at its juncture with the inferior vena cava. Caudate lobe veins are not seen on CT scans. The positions of the right, middle, and left hepatic veins on axial CT images provide landmarks for distinguishing the anterior and posterior segments of the right hepatic lobe, the right and left hepatic lobes, and the medial and lateral segments of the left hepatic lobe. Axial CT scans obtained more caudally may demonstrate the right hepatic vein ascending within the right intersegmental fissure between the anterior and posterior right portal vein limbs and the middle hepatic vein in the interlobar fissure (Fig. 13–9B,C). The course of the longitudinal right hepatic vein may be identified in profile on reformatted images in order to define the inferior extension of the right intersegmental fissure (Fig. 13–9D). Reformatted images through the smaller middle and left hepatic veins are generally not helpful because of limitations of spatial resolution. Thus the margins of the four major hepatic segments usually can be delineated on axial CT images by using the landmarks provided by the hepatic fissures and principal hepatic venous trunks (Figs. 13–9 and 13–10).

The main portal vein extends in a relatively straight course from its retropancreatic origin at the confluence of the superior mesenteric vein and splenic vein, through the gastrohepatic ligament at the anterior margin of the inferior vena cava into the porta hepatis, where it bifurcates into the right and left portal vein (Figs. 13–10 and 13–11). The main portal vein always lies posterior to the main hepatic artery and common bile duct.

At its origin the initial portion of the left portal vein, or pars transversa, extends anteriorly, leftward and cranial over the anterior surface of the caudate lobe giving off small caudal lobe branches. At the left intersegmental fissure, the left portal vein turns sharply craniad and ascends as the second portion, or umbilical segment (Fig. 13–12) of the left portal vein within the left intersegmental fissure. The umbilical segment gives horizontal branches to the medial and lateral segments of the left hepatic lobe (Fig. 13–11). The undivided right portal vein courses rightward and craniad, giving several small caudal lobe branches. Within the substance of the right hepatic lobe, the right portal vein divides into anterior and posterior branches, which supply the corresponding segments of the right hepatic lobe (Figs. 13–9C and 13–10). Unlike the hepatic venous trunks that run in fissures between major hepatic segments, portal veins run within the parenchyma of major hepatic segments.[12–16] The angulation of the venous branches relative to the axial plane appears to determine the likelihood of visualization of these vessels on transverse CT scans. Horizontally oriented vessels (right portal vein) and vertically oriented vessels (right hepatic vein, inferior vena cava, and the umbilical segment of the left portal vein) are more readily identified on axial CT sections than obliquely directed vessels (middle hepatic vein and pars transversa of the left portal vein).

The proper hepatic artery usually arises from the celiac axis, continues as the common hepatic artery after giving off the gastroduodenal artery, and branches into the right and left arteries in the porta hepatis. The common and proper hepatic arterial trunks are readily identified after an intravenous bolus of contrast medium (Fig. 13–13A).[20] Unlike the proximal portal veins, the initial hepatic arterial trunks display considerable variability in their origins and proximal course. In up to 45 per cent of cases, anomalous origins of the common, left, and other hepatic arteries are present with replacement either to the superior mesenteric or left gastric arteries (Fig. 13–13B).[13] Smaller intrahepatic arteries are identified only infrequently unless a hepatic arterial bolus of contrast is administered. As with the portal venous system, every distal hepatic artery supplies a definite hepatic segment.

BILIARY SYSTEM

Two main bile ducts (right and left hepatic) exit from the liver and join in the right side of the porta hepatis to form the common hepatic duct.

The common hepatic duct is a thin-walled structure 3 to 5 mm in size located anterolateral to the portal vein in the porta hepatis, better appreciated after intravenous contrast administration and detectable in about 22 per cent of normal patients (Fig. 13–13B).[18, 21]

The common bile duct is approximately 3

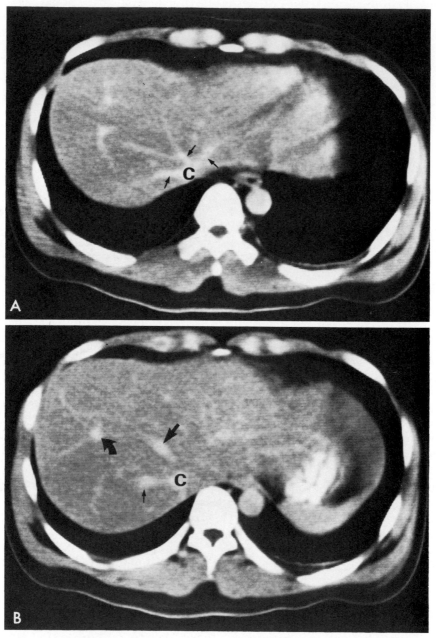

Figure 13–9. Hepatic venous anatomy. **A** The right, middle, and left hepatic veins (arrows) drain into the inferior vena cava (C) at the posterior superior margin of the liver. In this patient the middle hepatic vein has two major branches. **B** Scan at a more caudal level. The right (small arrow) and middle hepatic veins (large arrow) are clearly shown. Portal vein (curved arrow) is imaged in cross section. C = Inferior vena cava.

Illustration continued on opposite page

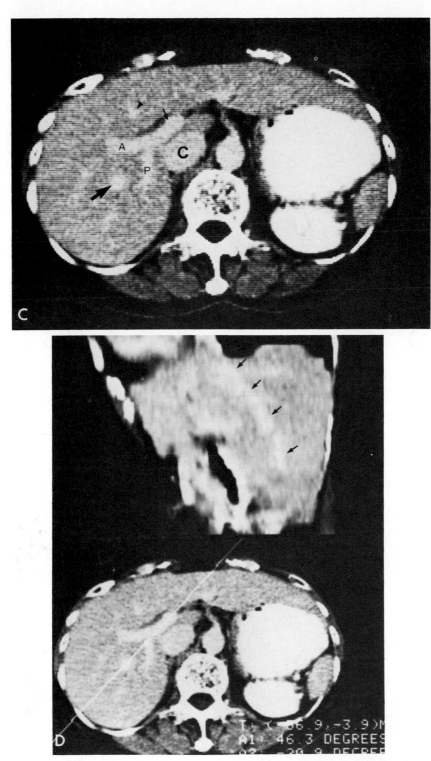

Figure 13–9. *Continued* **C** CT scan demonstrating anterior (A) and posterior (P) branches of right portal vein (small arrow). The right hepatic vein (large arrow) ascends in the right intersegmental fissure between the two branches of the right portal vein. The middle hepatic vein (arrowhead) is also identified and marks the interlobar fissure. **D** Oblique CT reformation through right hepatic vein demonstrates the course of the right hepatic vein (arrows) from its inferior extent until it joins the inferior vena cava near the diaphragm.

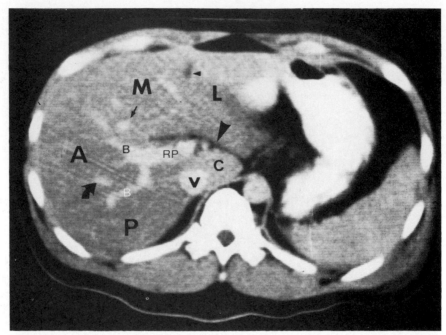

Figure 13–10. Hepatic segmental anatomy. The lateral segment (L) and medial segment (M) of the left hepatic lobe are separated by the left intersegmental fissure (small arrowhead). The middle hepatic vein (small arrow), coursing in the interlobar fissure, divides the left and right hepatic lobes, and the right hepatic vein (curved arrow) separates the anterior (A) and posterior (P) right hepatic segments. C = Caudate lobe; large arrowhead = fissure for ligament venosum; V = inferior vena cava; RP = right portal vein; black B = anterior branch, white B = posterior branch, of right portal vein.

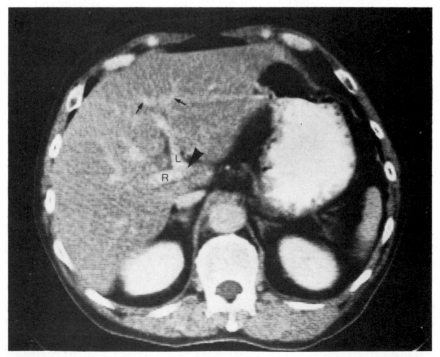

Figure 13–11. Portal vein anatomy. CT scan demonstrates main portal vein (arrowhead) branching into right (R) and left (L) portal veins in the porta hepatis. The ascending portion of the left hepatic vein is called the umbilical segment and gives branches to the medial and lateral segments of the left hepatic lobe (arrows).

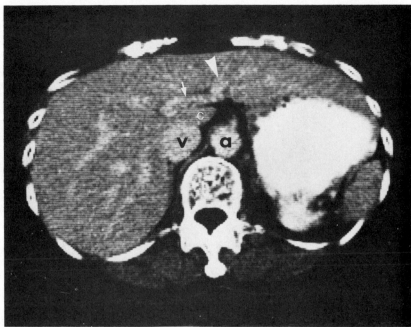

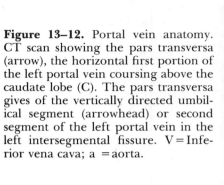

Figure 13–12. Portal vein anatomy. CT scan showing the pars transversa (arrow), the horizontal first portion of the left portal vein coursing above the caudate lobe (C). The pars transversa gives of the vertically directed umbilical segment (arrowhead) or second segment of the left portal vein in the left intersegmental fissure. V = Inferior vena cava; a = aorta.

inches long and has a slightly larger diameter. The initial third courses in the free edge of the lesser omentum, the second lies behind the first duodenum, sloping away from the portal vein, and the third lies in a deep groove on the posterior surface of the pancreas, where it joins the main pancreatic duct in the ampulla of Vater.[12] The common bile duct is detectable in 30 per cent of normal patients.[21]

Intrahepatic bile ducts are not seen on CT scans unless there is biliary obstruction, a biliary enteric anastomosis, or biliary contrast administration.[22] This is due to the small size of the intrahepatic ducts and the oblique direction of the ducts relative to the axial CT scan, which results in partial volume averaging with adjacent hepatic parenchyma.

The gallbladder is well seen when distended as an oval sac of water density lying in a fossa on the inferior hepatic surface. The wall of the gallbladder is thin (1 to 2 mm) when seen in profile and may enhance after intravenous contrast administration. The relationship of the gallbladder to the liver, anterior abdominal wall, duodenum, colon, right kidney, and stomach are readily displayed by axial CT images (Fig. 13–4D–F).

HEPATIC PARENCHYMA

The mean CT density of normal adult liver is reported to vary between 54 and 68 H[23–26] with normal liver CT attenuation values ranging from 38 to 76,[24] 38 to 80,[25] 33 to 74,[26] 50 to 70,[18] and 40 to 80[6] H. However, the range in the individual patient is much narrower, causing the normal liver to appear relatively homogeneous. The broad range of reported hepatic CT numbers is largely due to attenuation values being obtained on different CT scanners, using different scanning energies, and methods of calibration. In addition, varying amounts of liver glycogen in fasting and recently fed patients may affect hepatic CT attenuation values[27] and CT numbers may vary with patient size: obese patients will have lower CT numbers because of the greater amount of fat in the liver.[27, 28]

Although a wide range of hepatic attenuation values is found, the normal liver has a higher density than that of the pancreas and kidneys and always has as great or greater density than the spleen.[26] The average liver-spleen difference is 7 to 8 H, with high normal hepatic CT numbers always associated with high normal splenic attenuation values; the converse is also true (Fig. 13–14).[26]

When the hepatic parenchyma has a greater attenuation than that of blood, the portal and hepatic venous systems are seen as low-density branching structures within the liver on non-contrast–enhanced CT scans. Distinction can usually be made between dilated bile ducts and normal vascular structures by anatomic position and CT density. However, differentiation of venous structures from dilated bile ducts is best accomplished by intravenous administration of contrast media; this increases the density of the hepatic venous structures above the hepatic parenchyma but has no effect on a dilated biliary system.

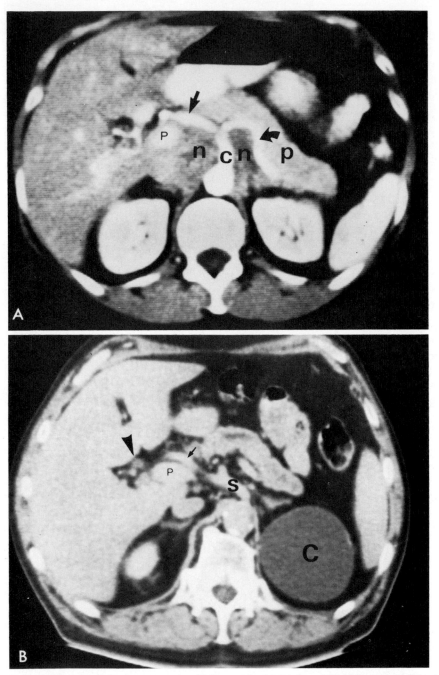

Figure 13–13. Hepatic arterial anatomy. **A**   Celiac axis (c) giving off proper hepatic (arrow) and splenic artery (curved arrow). The hepatic artery lies ventral to the portal vein (P). n = Enlarged celiac nodes due to lymphoma; p = pancreas. **B**   Replaced right hepatic artery (arrow) arising from superior mesenteric artery (S). P = Portal vein; c = renal cyst; arrowhead = common hepatic duct. A dilated pancreatic duct is present.

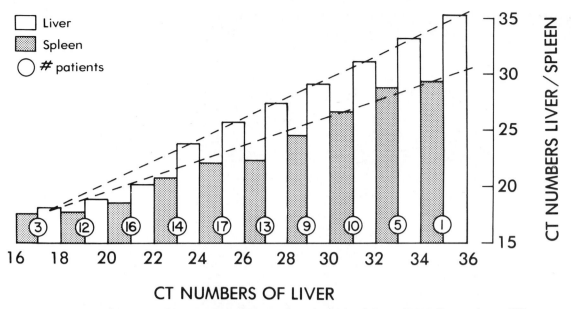

Figure 13–14. Relationship of liver-spleen CT numbers in 100 adults, relating liver-spleen difference at specific hepatic CT number. CT number scale ranges from +500 to −500. (From Piekarski J, Goldberg HI, Royal RA, Axel L, Moss AA: Difference between liver and spleen CT numbers in the normal adult: Usefulness in predicting the presence of diffuse liver disease. Radiology 137:727, 1980. Reprinted by permission.)

TECHNIQUES OF EXAMINATION

The majority of patients are scanned in the supine position without angulation of the scanner gantry. The right lateral decubitus position is useful when streak artifacts from the gastric air-fluid level project across the liver (Fig. 13–15). With the patient in the decubitus position, streak artifacts are not as likely to degrade the hepatic CT image because they are projected away from the hepatic parenchyma.

If the liver is the primary organ of interest, the entire liver is scanned using transverse images 1 cm thick at 1-cm intervals. A 2-cm interval is employed if the liver is being examined only as a part of a more generalized whole body survey. Contiguous thin section scans (5 mm or less) are utilized only when additional resolution is required to characterize a particular abnormality (i.e., common bile duct calculi).

Our routine procedure is to scan the liver initially without intravenous contrast media. The scans are evaluated, and it is determined whether the examination is adequate or administration of contrast material, change in patient position, or more finely collimated scans are needed to establish the diagnosis. In making this determination, the images must be viewed at varying window width and height levels to optimize focal differences in CT density. If contrast material is to be administered, the type, volume, rate, method of delivery, and most appropriate CT scan protocol is selected. The choice is dependent upon the particular clinical question to be answered and also on the restraints of equipment specifications, time, radiation dose, and technical support.

CONTRAST ENHANCEMENT

Detection of hepatic abnormalities by computed tomography is dependent upon differentiating between normal and pathologically altered hepatic tissue. Abnormalities in hepatic contour may permit detection of hepatic disease, but most abnormalities are identified by CT on noncontrast scans as regions of altered hepatic density. Attempts to increase the difference in CT density between normal liver and hepatic abnormalities have focused on the administration of various intravenous contrast media,[29–43] upon timing of contrast administration, and performance of the CT scan.[29, 44–58] Obtaining maximum contrast enhancement of the liver involves:

1. Selection of the most effective contrast media.

2. Administration of the media in the most efficacious manner.

3. Performing the scan in a manner ensuring that maximum hepatic contrast enhancement is realized on the CT images.

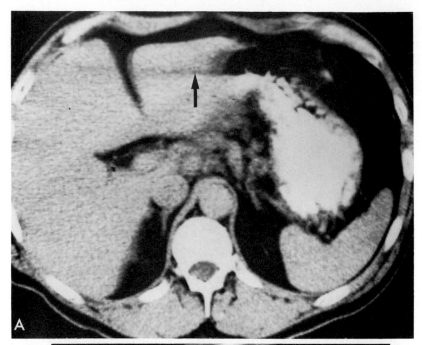

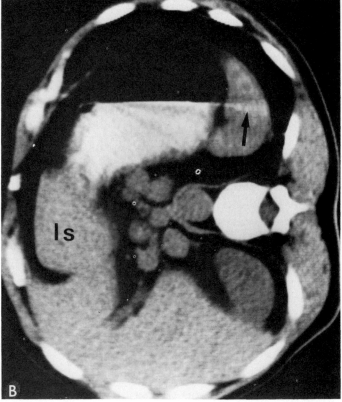

Figure 13–15. A CT scan done in supine position demonstrates a streak artifact (arrow) originating from the air-fluid level in the stomach. The streak artifact makes evaluation of the lateral segment of the left lobe of the liver difficult. **B** CT scan done in right lateral decubitus position projects the streak (arrow) off the lateral segment (ls) of the left lobe of the liver and clearly demonstrates the liver to be normal.

Urographic Contrast

Hepatic contrast enhancement is most frequently accomplished by the administration of water-soluble urographic contrast material. Urographic contrast agents enhance the hepatic vascular compartment and rapidly diffuse into the extravascular space.[29, 50, 53, 55, 59] Although injection of urographic contrast material increases the den-sity of the liver, the degree of increase in attenuation value is related in part to hepatic blood flow, tumor vascularity, volume of distribution, and interstitial space variations. Contrast dose, rapidity of injection, and timing of the CT scan following contrast administration all have an important effect on the degree of hepatic contrast enhancement obtained following intravenous administration of urographic contrast media.[29, 50, 53, 55, 59] The ability to enhance the vascular compartment of the liver, low toxicity, ready availability, and lack of dependence on hepatic function are advantages of urographic contrast material for contrast enhancement in hepatic CT scanning.

Iodolipids

Iodolipids are iodinated, emulsified fat globules which are being investigated as hepatosplenic CT contrast agents.[32–37, 60] Injection of iodolipids, 1 to

7 μ in diameter, produces a selective, homogeneous increase in the density of the hepatic and splenic parenchyma (Fig. 13–16). Iodolipids opacify the hepatic reticuloendothelial space, and following an intravenous injection of 0.2 to 0.3 ml/kg (40 to 60 mgI/kg) produce an increase in hepatic density averaging about 20 H with a range of 8 to 48 H.[33, 35]

Two advantages of iodolipids as hepatic CT contrast agents are *selectivity* (only functioning hepatic tissue enhances) and *persistence* (contrast enhancement remains for several hours). Persist-

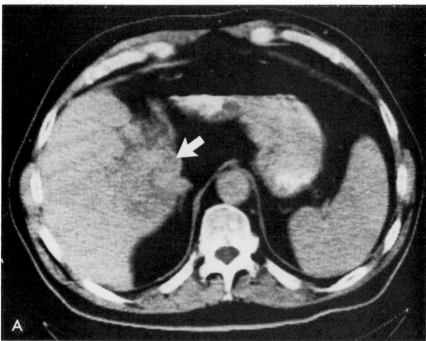

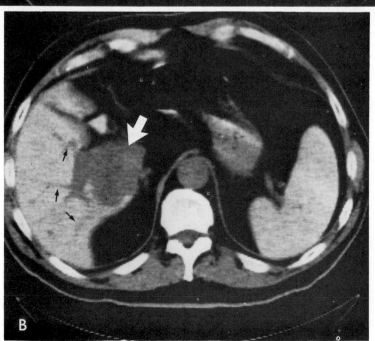

Figure 13–16. Iodolipid hepatic contrast material. **A** CT scan prior to administration of contrast material demonstrates an ill-defined solid mass (arrow) in the caudate lobe. **B** After administration of the iodolipid EOE-13 in a dose of 0.2 ml/kg the density of the normal liver and spleen has increased by 20 to 30 H. The metastatic carcinoma (arrow) in the caudate lobe is sharply delineated from the normal liver. The portal venous branches stand out as low-density, branching structures (small arrows) in the hepatic parenchyma. (Case courtesy of M. Bernardino, M.D.)

ence of contrast enhancement makes timing of the CT scan less critical than following administration of urographic contrast agents.

Although iodolipids possess many desirable features, they require a 20- to 60-minute period of infusion to administer, are more toxic than urographic agents, provide no information about hepatic and tumor vascularity, are as nonspecific as radionuclide particulate scanning agents, and are difficult to manufacture.[32–37, 60]

Biliary Contrast Media

Intravenous biliary contrast media rarely are employed as contrast agents for CT scanning.[2, 22]

Such materials are rapidly cleared from the blood and hepatic parenchyma into the biliary tree and have not proven superior to urographic contrast agents in providing differential enhancement of normal liver from lesions of the liver parenchyma.[2] The higher toxicity of intravenous biliary contrast media also limits widespread use. When employed, the rate of contrast administration must be slower and the total dose lower, thereby ensuring that biliary contrast agents will not be capable of providing information about the vascularity of hepatic lesions.

Recently, Koehler and associates[30] and Moss and Brito[31] demonstrated potential usefulness of

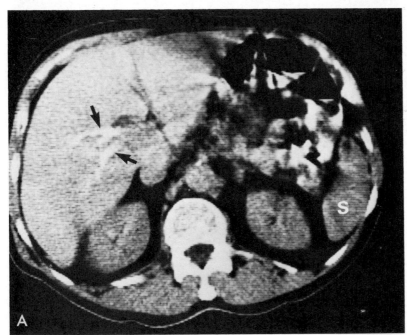

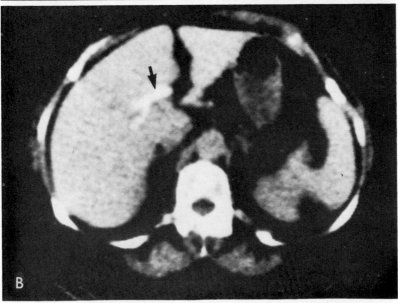

Figure 13–17. Biliary contrast. **A** Iosefamate meglumine. CT scan 45 minutes after injection of 150 mg I/kg demonstrates a 30 H increase in hepatic attenuation value. The spleen (S), lacking functioning hepatocytes, does not enhance. Normal-sized biliary radicles (arrows) are clearly shown. **B** Iodipamide meglumine. Slightly dilated right biliary tree (arrow) is well opacified by iodipamide meglumine (Cholografin).

Illustration continued on opposite page

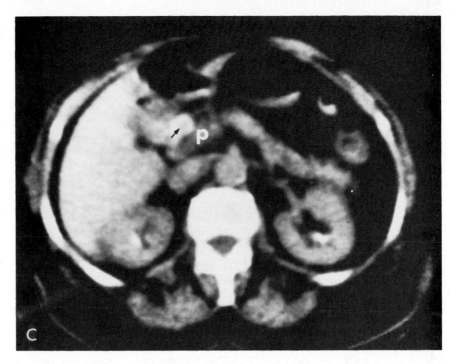

Figure 13–17. *Continued* **C** Scan at more caudal level demonstrates a dilated common bile duct containing a low-density calculus (arrow). The relationship of the common bile duct to the head of the pancreas (p) is shown.

a new cholecystocholangiographic agent, iosefamate meglumine, as a hepatic CT contrast medium. The biliary system was readily opacified and a 30 to 42 H increase in the CT density of the liver was noted which persisted for over 2 hours (Fig. 13–17A).[30, 31] However, isosefamate is more toxic than urographic agents and contrast enhancement proved to be highly dependent upon hepatic function.

Although biliary contrast agents are limited in their usefulness, they are capable of opacifying the normal biliary tree and defining the relationships of the common bile duct to the pancreatic head (Fig. 13–17).[22] Excretion of biliary contrast opacifies the duodenum, permitting separation of the duodenum from the head of the pancreas in patients whose duodenum does not fill after oral contrast administration. Administration of biliary contrast agents has proven useful to define the anatomy of some patients who have had a Billroth II or Roux-en-Y gastroenterostomy.

Methods of Contrast Medium Administration

Contrast enhancement of the liver is to a great extent dependent upon the method of contrast administration. Contrast medium can be given as a slow or rapid infusion, an intravenous or arterial bolus, or a combination of infusion and bolus techniques.[1–3, 6–9, 19, 29, 44–46, 48–54, 56–59, 61–70] Each method of contrast administration results in a different peak and duration of effective contrast enhance-

ment and requires selecting the CT scan protocol that optimizes hepatic contrast enhancement. Complicating the selection is the fact that different hepatic abnormalities show peak enhancement at different times following contrast administration.

INTRAVENOUS INFUSION. The effect of contrast infusion upon normal and abnormal hepatic tissue is variable. Some investigators believe contrast medium infusion is almost always helpful and perform hepatic CT scans only after intravenous contrast infusion[69]; others have found that a small percentage of hepatic abnormalities become less detectable following contrast infusion and recommend that hepatic CT scans be performed initially without contrast administration.[2, 51, 61, 67, 71] Itai and co-workers[61] found an overlap between the CT density of normal liver, metastatic, and primary hepatic abnormalities on precontrast CT scans and noted that the overlap remained after contrast infusion of urographic contrast. Moss and colleagues[67] found that the majority of focal hepatic lesions were equally well detected on precontrast contrast CT scans and 13 per cent of lesions were much less well delineated following intravenous infusion of contrast media.

An infusion of 300 ml of 30 per cent contrast material increases the average difference in attenuation value between normal liver and malignant tissue by only 5 H (Table 13–1).[72] The large range of attenuation value change after contrast media infusion makes it impossible to predict the effect of contrast infusion in any one patient. However,

Table 13–1. CT VALUES OF MALIGNANT HEPATIC TISSUE: 61 CASES

	Mean	Range	Average Difference (Normal–Malignant Hepatic Tissue)
Precontrast infusion	27.2 H	0–60 H	18.4 H
Postcontrast infusion	36.0 H	0–84 H	23.4 H

it is becoming clear that performing hepatic CT scanning only after infusion of contrast material will result in some hepatic lesions becoming isodense or less detectable when compared with that of normal liver.[51, 67]

When an infusion technique is employed for hepatic CT scanning, the contrast medium should be infused as rapidly as possible; CT scanning is initiated shortly after the start of the infusion and scanning completed just before the infusion finishes. It is important to ensure that CT scans are obtained prior to contrast material becoming equilibrated between normal liver and hepatic lesions as hepatic CT scans performed during the nonequilibrium phase of contrast enhancement are least likely to obscure a hepatic lesion.[51] In order to reach satisfactory blood contrast levels at the start of the CT study, a 50 ml bolus of 60 per cent contrast material is given immediately before the start of the contrast infusion. Either 300 ml of 30 per cent or 150 ml of 60 per cent urographic contrast material is employed for the intravenous infusion.

INTRAVENOUS BOLUS. Administration of contrast material as a bolus injection produces a very rapid rise of blood iodine level, followed by a rapid diffusion of contrast material from the intravascular to the extravascular compartment.[46, 49, 51, 55, 59] CT scanners with scan times longer than 5 seconds cannot adequately capture the rapid change in the degree of vascular and parenchymal contrast enhancement that occurs following a bolus injection of contrast material. The development of dynamic CT scanning techniques has enabled CT density changes to be followed sequentially. Both experimental and clinical studies have shown that a bolus injection of contrast media coupled with dynamic CT scanning is the method of choice for evaluating the rapid density changes that can occur in hepatic abnormalities.[29, 56, 57]

Our current hepatic CT technique is to initially scan the liver without contrast administration. An appropriate level is selected from the noncontrast scan and a 80- to 100-ml bolus of 60 per cent urographic contrast material is rapidly injected by way of an antecubital vein with an 18-gauge needle; following this, 150 ml of 60 per cent urographic contrast is rapidly infused. A series of 6 to 12 CT scans is taken within 1 minute following the bolus injection at the preselected level. The rapid sequence of the CT scans allows density changes to be closely related to time and results in better delineation of tumor vascularity and vascular supply of hepatic abnormalities (Fig. 13–18). Following the dynamic sequence of CT scans, the entire liver can be rescanned if necessary while contrast is being rapidly infused. The combination of bolus and rapid infusion permits the examination to be completed while there is a high level of blood and tissue iodine.

INTRA-ARTERIAL BOLUS. CT scanning following intrahepatic arterial injection of contrast material (computed tomographic angiography) detects smaller lesions and better demonstrates the vascularity of the normal and abnormal liver.[44, 56, 73] Prando and associates[44] injected 300 ml of 30 per cent methylglucamine diatrizoate at a rate of 3 to 5 ml/sec, whereas we perform a dynamic scan sequence after rapid intrahepatic arterial injection of 12 to 20 ml of contrast material containing 400 mgI/ml.[56] After an intrahepatic arterial contrast injection, some lesions demonstrate rim enhancement, others become uniformly hyperdense, and occasional lesions show no evidence of contrast enhancement (Fig. 13–19).[56] Changes in CT density from hypodense to hyperdense to isodense and back to hypodense can occur rapidly, and a variety of patterns of contrast enhancement can be seen in a liver containing multiple lesions of the same histologic type (Fig. 13–19). CT following intrahepatic arterial contrast injection is not a routine procedure; however, should an intrahepatic arterial catheter be in place for therapeutic purposes, a CT scan after an intrahepatic arterial injection of contrast provides optimum information concerning size, number, location, and vascularity of hepatic abnormalities.

HEPATIC VOLUME

CT can measure hepatic volume (Fig. 13–20) to within 5 per cent accuracy.[74, 75] The technique requires no special equipment other than a method

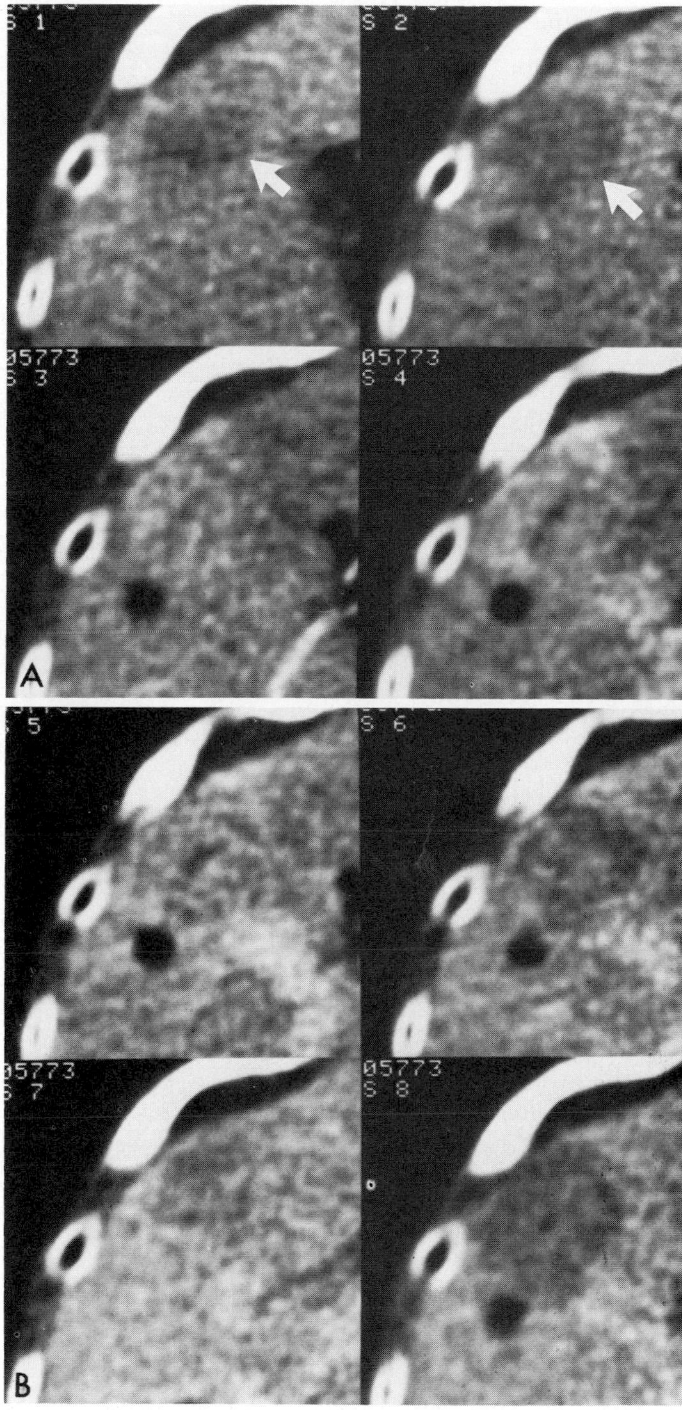

Figure 13–18. Pattern of rapid density change following intravenous bolus injection. **A, B** A series of eight CT scans taken after rapid intravenous bolus of 70 ml of 60 per cent contrast medium. Total elapsed time, scan 1 to scan 8, is 28.4 seconds. A hypodense metastasis (arrow) is demonstrated on scan 1, which becomes hyperdense (scans 3, 4), almost isodense (scan 5), and finally again hypodense (scan 8) with regard to the surrounding normal liver. (From Moss AA, Dean PB, Axel L, Goldberg HI, Glazer GM, Friedman MA: Dynamic CT of hepatic masses with intravenous and intraarterial contrast material. AJR 138:847, 1982. © 1982, American Roentgen Ray Society. Reprinted by permission.)

of tracing an area of interest within a particular CT slice. Contiguous axial CT scans are obtained through the entire liver. The liver margin is traced on all scans and the volumes within the traced areas summated. It is important that patients be instructed to respire at the same level throughout the examination, and whenever possible, dynamic CT scanning techniques with table incrementation are employed. Determination of the volume of the liver is important in planning radiation therapy, quantitating the effect of therapy, and providing a more accurate measurement of liver size than "eyeballing" or simply measuring hepatic length and width.

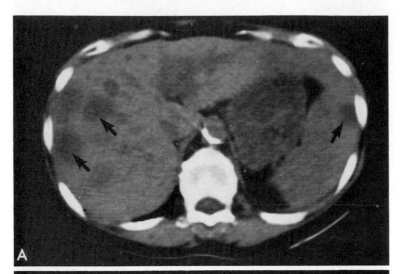

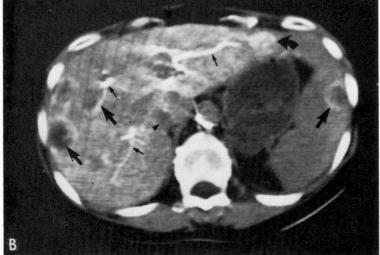

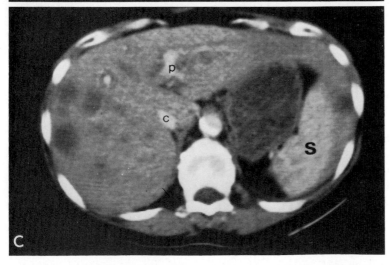

Figure 13–19. Patterns of density change following intrahepatic arterial bolus injection of 15 ml of contrast material. **A** Precontrast CT scan demonstrates multiple hypodense hepatic metastasis (arrows). **B** Scan immediately after injection reveals hepatic arterial branches to all hepatic lobes (small arrows). Some metastatic lesions exhibit a pattern of rim enhancement (large arrows), while a lesion in the left lobe (curved arrow) is uniformly hyperdense. The inferior vena cava (arrowhead) is not opacified at this time. **C** Scan 30 seconds later shows the inferior vena cava (c) and portal vein (P) to be opacified. The rim enhancement has almost disappeared, and the uniformly hyperdense lesion is now isodense with normal liver. S = Spleen. (From Moss AA, Dean PB, Axel L, Goldberg HI, Glazer GM, Friedman MA: Dynamic CT of hepatic masses with intravenous and intraarterial contrast material. AJR 138:847, 1982. © 1982, American Roentgen Ray Society. Reprinted by permission.)

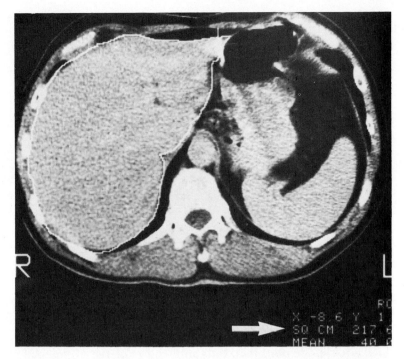

Figure 13–20. CT measurement of hepatic volume. The outline of the liver has been traced with a cursor. The area within the tracing measures 217.6 cm² (arrow). As the scan section is 1 cm thick, a volume of 217.6 cu cm is represented. Summation of liver volumes on sequential continuous scans gives an accurate measure of total liver volume.

HEPATIC PATHOLOGY

The appearance of hepatic CT scans in patients with diffuse hepatocellular disorders ranges from normal to grossly abnormal with readily apparent alterations in hepatic size, shape, or density. Normal CT scans are usually found in patients with amyloidosis, sarcoidosis, hepatitis, Hodgkin's disease, and early cirrhosis.[6, 9, 19, 27, 69, 76] These limitations have relegated CT to a secondary role as compared with ultrasound and radionuclide scanning in the detection and evaluation of diffuse hepatocellular disorders. Despite the limitations of CT in patients with hepatocellular diseases, a variety of specific CT patterns has been found in such processes as fatty infiltration, cirrhosis, and hemochromatosis, which permit identification and in some instances quantitation of the extent of the disease process.

FATTY INFILTRATION OF THE LIVER

Fatty infiltration of the liver is the result of excessive deposition of triglycerides, which occurs in a variety of hepatic disorders (Table 13–2).[27, 69, 77–80] Fatty infiltration appears to be a nonspecific response of the liver cells to certain metabolic insults,[81] and although indicative of significant hepatic abnormality, is reversible.[66]

The degree of fat normally found in the liver appears to be directly related to body weight. In morbid obesity, the liver fat content rises with weight gain and decreases with weight loss.[82] The normal triglyceride level ranges from 1 to 5 mg/gm of wet weight liver, whereas obese patients may have more than 100 mg/gm.[27] Increase in hepatic fat content is manifested by a decrease in mean hepatic CT attenuation value (Fig. 13–21).

Experimental work in rabbits[77] and dogs[83] has shown that for each milligram of triglyceride deposited in a gram of liver, there is a decrease in hepatic attenuation of 1.6 H. Knowledge of the relationship between triglyceride deposition and change in CT density permits estimation of the amount of fat within the liver.[27]

The method for estimating hepatic fat is based upon the known relationship between hepatic and splenic CT density and the fact that the spleen

Table 13–2. DISEASES CAUSING FATTY INFILTRATION OF THE LIVER

Alcoholic cirrhosis
Cushing's disease
Diabetes mellitus
Intravenous hyperalimentation
Iatrogenic corticosteroidism
Reyes syndrome
Kwashiorkor
A-beta-lipoproteinemia
Morbid obesity
Jejunoileal bypass surgery
Radiation hepatitis
Carbon tetrachloride ingestion
Congenital hypertriglyceridemia
Glycogen storage disease

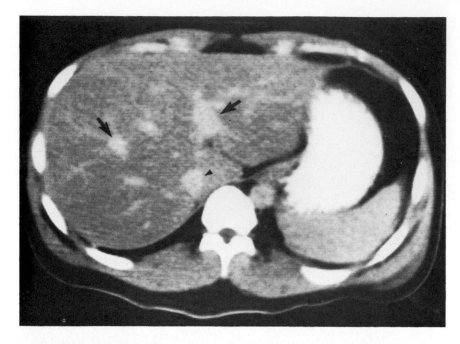

Figure 13–21. Diffuse fatty infiltration of the liver resulting from congenital hypertriglyceridemia. Precontrast CT scan demonstrates the liver to have a lower attenuation value than the spleen. The inferior vena cava (arrowhead) and portal veins (arrows) stand out as high-density structures.

does not change density in fatty infiltration of the liver. Piekarski and co-workers[26] demonstrated that the mean normal liver CT number was 7 to 8 H greater than the spleen, was never lower and that high normal CT values were always associated with high normal spleen CT numbers. This relationship is useful for estimating whether a liver having a CT density of 20 H is normal or contains a large or small amount of intrahepatic fat. For example, if the CT number of the spleen is 50 H, the liver should be at least 50 H and probably nearer 57 to 58 H. Assuming the base-line CT number of the liver was 58 H and it now measures 20 H, a fatty liver is present, containing as much as 23.75 mg of fat per gram of liver [58 − 20 = 38 H: 1.6 H/mg fat = 23.75 mg/gm]. An estimation of the amount of hepatic fat can indicate the severity of the underlying disease process and afford a way of monitoring the effect of therapy without resorting to hepatic biopsy.

In many patients, deposition of fat in the liver is uniform and diffuse. The portal veins in a diffusely fatty liver appear as high-density structures surrounded by the background of low density

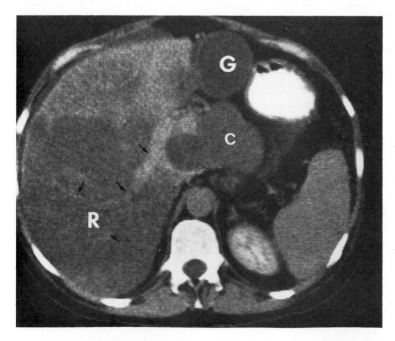

Figure 13–22. Patchy fatty infiltration of the liver resulting from cirrhosis. The right (R) and caudate (c) lobes of the liver are replaced by fat to a degree that makes their density almost equal to that of the gallbladder (G). The medial segment of the left hepatic lobe has a higher CT density but contains foci of low attenuation. The spleen is large, and the caudate lobe is prominent. The portal vein (arrows) courses normally through the center of the right hepatic lobe, distinguishing fatty infiltration from a low-density tumor.

caused by hepatic fat (Fig. 13–21).[6, 18, 27, 69, 84, 85] Diffuse fatty infiltration most frequently occurs in patients who are obese, are on corticosteroid therapy, have Cushing's disease, or have diabetes mellitus.[27]

In some patients, fatty infiltration of the liver occurs in a focal or nonuniform manner (Fig. 13–22).[78, 80] Nonuniform fatty infiltration occurs commonly in alcoholism and cirrhosis[78, 80] but also in patients on intravenous hyperalimentation. Diabetes, starvation, and exogenous steroids also have been reported to cause focal hepatic fatty infiltration.[27, 80]

Occasionally, localized collections of hepatic fat can produce a CT appearance that resembles either a primary tumor or metastases. The observation that normal portal vessels traverse the areas of fatty infiltration usually permits distinction of fatty infiltration from tumorous masses (Fig. 13–22). Radionuclide uptake is often normal in areas of fatty infiltration,[78] and a fine-needle aspiration biopsy will provide definitive proof of focal fatty infiltration.

CIRRHOSIS

Cirrhosis resulting from a variety of etiologies can produce changes in the liver that are detectable by CT scanning. However, the basic pathologic process characterizing cirrhosis, that of extensive collagen deposition with replacement of hepatocytes and distortion of the normal hepatic lobular architecture, does not increase the mean CT number above normal.[24] Therefore, measurement of CT density is of little value in identifying the presence of cirrhosis.

Although there may be no hepatic CT abnormalities detectable in patients with proven cirrhosis,[18, 27, 86] frequently there are changes either in liver contour, size, or homogeneity of CT number.[87] A small liver with a nodular contour resulting from focal atrophy, fibrosis and/or regenerating nodules (Fig. 13–23) is seen in advanced cirrhosis.[18, 27, 87] A prominence of the caudate lobe associated with shrinkage of the right lobe (Figs. 13–22 and 13–23) has been noted.[87] The ratio of the transverse caudate lobe width to the transverse right hepatic lobe width, increased from a mean of 0.37 in a normal population to 0.83 in patients with cirrhosis.[87] No normal liver had a value above 0.55, and only one cirrhotic liver had a ratio less than 0.6.[87] The increase in caudate lobe/right lobe ratio in cirrhotic livers results both from actual caudate lobe enlargement and greater fibrotic scarring and shrinkage of the right he-

patic lobe. One possible explanation for caudate lobe hypertrophy is that the caudate lobe receives blood from both the right and left portal veins and hepatic arteries and thus its blood supply is relatively spared until late in cirrhosis. A similar caudate lobe prominence is found with the Budd-Chiari syndrome, in which the caudate lobe draining veins are spared from the thrombosis that affects the right, middle, and left hepatic veins.[87, 88]

Fatty infiltration is most commonly identified as a mixture of low-density areas irregularly interspersed with areas of fibrosis and nodular regeneration[69, 71] (Figs. 13–22 and 13–23B). Occasionally, a diffusely enlarged liver with a homogeneous low-density background may be seen.

Other CT findings in cirrhosis are ascites (Figs. 13–23A and 13–24), liver masses representing regenerating nodules or hepatomas, and portal hypertension manifested by enlarged collateral vessels (Figs. 13–23 and 13–24). Collateral vessels produce numerous round, serpiginous soft-tissue densities in the porta hepatis, perigastric, umbilical, and splenic regions that increase in CT number after an intravenous bolus or rapid infusion of contrast material (Figs. 13–23B and 13–24). Regenerating nodules are usually of normal CT density (Fig. 13–23A), whereas hepatomas have a spectrum of densities. Hepatomas are particularly likely to occur in patients with hepatitis B surface antigen-positive cirrhosis.[89]

Although radionuclide scans can detect abnormalities resulting from cirrhosis prior to computed tomography,[2, 6, 86] radionuclide abnormalities are not specific for cirrhosis. CT scans are often helpful to differentiate between regenerating nodules, focal fatty infiltration, and focal hepatic masses (hepatoma, abscess, or metastasis).

HEMOCHROMATOSIS

Excessive total body iron stores can result from either a primary process (idiopathic hemochromatosis) or develop as a secondary disorder in patients with congenital or acquired anemia who receive repeated blood transfusions. Patients with idiopathic hemochromatosis have increased iron absorption due to a defect in intestinal mucosal cells and usually present with cirrhosis, diabetes mellitus, and hyperpigmentation.[90] Secondary hemochromatosis is most frequently seen in patients having thalassemia, sickle cell anemia, and sideroblastic anemia.[90–93]

The diagnosis of primary or secondary hemochromatosis is readily made by CT when scans re-

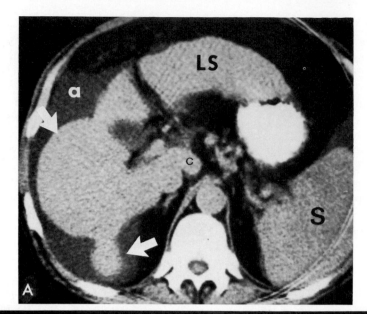

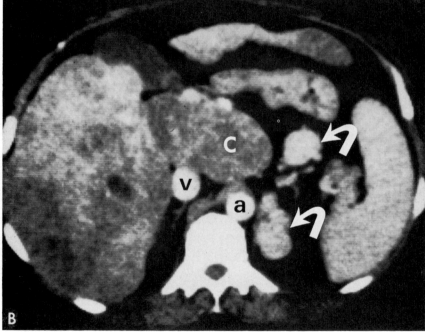

Figure 13–23. Advanced cirrhosis. **A** The overall liver size is small, but there is prominence of the lateral segment (LS) of the left hepatic lobe and caudate lobe (c). Regenerating nodules (arrows) give the liver an irregular contour. Splenomegaly (S) and ascites (a) are present. **B** There is patchy fatty infiltration of the liver and a markedly enlarged caudate lobe (c). Vascular masses (curved arrows) represent collateral vessels from a spontaneous splenorenal shunt. a = Aorta; v = inferior vena cava.

veal an overall increase in density of the hepatic parenchyma. At scanning energies of 120 kVp, the average CT density of the liver in patients with either primary or secondary hemochromatosis ranges between 75 and 132 H.[27, 84, 90, 92–95] As a result of the diffuse increase in hepatic CT density, the portal venous structures appear as low-density tubular branching structures against the background of the hyperdense liver (Figs. 13–25 and 13–26). Patients with increased hepatic iron also have increased iron deposited in the spleen, pancreas, lymph nodes, pituitary, heart, adrenals, bowel wall, parathyroid, and thyroid glands (Fig. 13–26).[90–92] The lymph nodes accumulate great

amounts of iron in secondary hemochromatosis, some having attenuation values greater than 200 H.[92] Endocrine dysfunction and cardiac abnormalities are frequently encountered in hemochromatotic patients.[90–92] The differential diagnosis of hemochromatosis is limited but includes patients receiving thorium oxide (Thorotrast) (Fig. 13–27).

By using dual-energy scanning techniques (Fig. 13–28), computed tomography is capable of quantitating the amount of iron present within the liver.[27, 94, 96] The use of dual-energy scanning is based on the fact that iron produces its increase in density by virtue of its high atomic number. In the range of energies used in clinical CT scan-

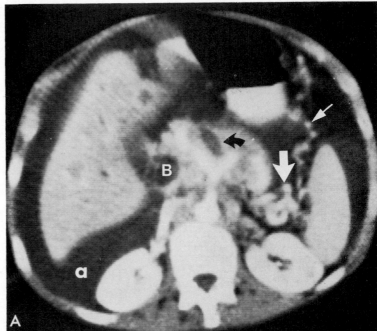

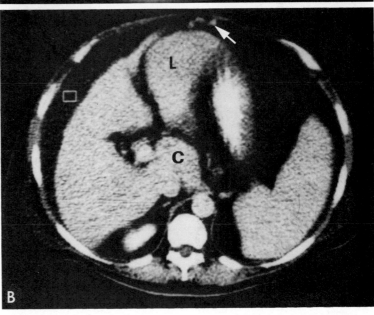

Figure 13–24. Two patients with advanced cirrhosis and portal hypertension. **A** There is ascites (a) and marked enlargement of collateral vessels in the hilum of the spleen (large arrow), which also ascend along the greater curvature of the stomach (small arrow). An enlarged distal common bile duct (B) and pancreatic duct (curved arrow) are present. Scans at a lower level revealed pancreatitis with a pseudocyst obstructing the common bile duct. **B** Ascites (box), slight prominence of the caudate lobe (c) and lateral segment of the left lobe of the liver (L), and a patent enlarged umbilical vein (arrow) are present. Patient has Cruveilhier-Baumgarten syndrome.

ning, the CT density is related to the third power of the atomic number (Z^3) but only to the single power of physical density (gm/ml). Thus, changing the CT scanning energy from 120 kVp to 80 kVp will result in a large change in the CT number of the liver if an excessive amount of a high atomic number element such as iron is present (Fig. 13–26). Experimental work has shown there to be a constant change in CT attenuation value for each gram of iron present within the liver[27, 94, 96] (see chapter 23). Dual-energy scanning for liver densitometry is applicable not only in detecting hemochromatosis but also in following the prog-

ress of therapy of the disease without the need to perform liver biopsies to obtain tissue for iron measurement.

GLYCOGEN STORAGE DISEASE

Glycogen storage diseases are autosomal genetic disorders of carbohydrate metabolism categorized into six groups on the basis of the specific enzyme defect.[97] Various enzymatic defects in all forms of glycogen storage disease result in faulty glycogenolysis and excessive storage of glycogen. The liver is a site of excessive glycogen storage in

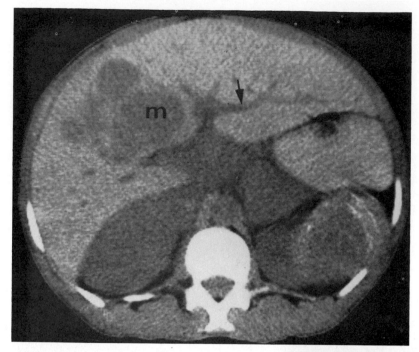

Figure 13–25. Secondary hemochromatosis in a patient with sickle cell disease. The liver is diffusely hyperdense, measuring 78H. Hepatic vessels (arrow) are seen as low-density, branching structures. The spleen is partially calcified. The large low-density mass (m) in the liver was biopsied and represented old hemorrhage.

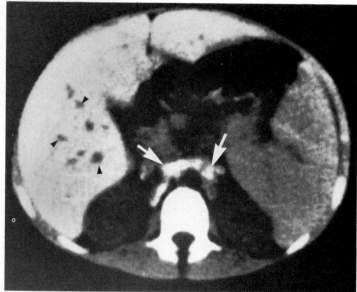

Figure 13–26. Primary hemochromatosis. The liver is hyperdense, with portal vessels appearing as low-density structures (arrowheads). There is accumulation of iron in para-aortic lymph nodes (arrows). CT number in cursor square = 124 H.

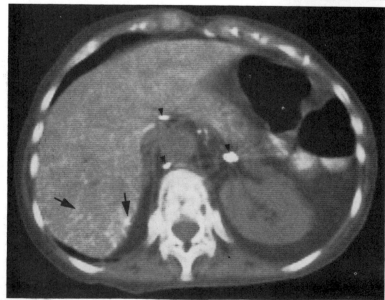

Figure 13–27. Hyperdense liver (arrows) resulting from thorium oxide (Thorotrast) administration. The distribution is patchy and the overall density of the liver is less than with hemochromatosis. Lymph nodes also have an increased density (arrowheads).

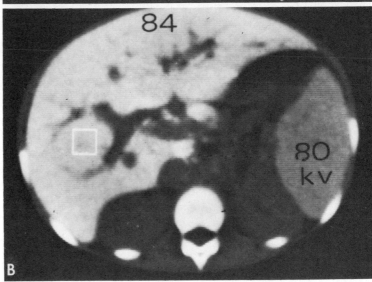

Figure 13–28. Dual-energy CT scan in patient with hemochromatosis. **A** Scan at 120 kVp reveals density of the liver in the cursor box to be 50 (scale +500 to −500). **B** Scan at 80 kVp demonstrates the measured liver density to have increased to 84 (scale +500 to −500). The increase in measured liver density at 80 kVp is due to excessive iron deposition in the liver. A linear relationship between CT number change and iron content permits quantitation of hepatic iron.

Types I, II, III, IV, and VI glycogen storage diseases.[97] Although the diseases are present at birth, except for Type IV, they may not be detected until late childhood when hepatomegaly is discovered. CT scans in patients with glycogen storage disease have revealed both an increased hepatic density (Figs. 13–29 and 13–30),[94, 98] and a low-density liver.[85, 98] Livers having CT attenuation values greater than normal are more common. The excessive amount of glycogen packed into the liver produces an increased hepatic attenuation value, which is related to the single power of the physical density of the glycogen. CT densities of 55 to 90 H are seen on conventional hepatic CT scans, and these values overlap with those seen in hemochromatosis. Separation of the two entities is usually not difficult clinically, but when there is debate, dual-energy CT scanning can be employed to determine whether the high hepatic

CT density is due to iron or glycogen.[94] As opposed to the great increase in hepatic CT number observed in hemochromatosis when the liver is scanned at 80 kVp compared with 120 kVp, the glycogen-laden liver has a much smaller attenuation value change. Dual-energy CT scanning can be employed to quantitate the amount of glycogen present in the liver without biopsy (see chapter 23).

Glycogen storage disease may produce a liver having a low attenuation value as a result of the fatty infiltration that occurs in long-standing glycogen storage disease.[85, 98] The areas of fatty infiltration can be nonhomogeneous with foci of normal hepatic density scattered throughout the liver. These areas of normal density may be difficult to distinguish from foci of tumor or hyperplasia. Additional abnormalities that may be identified by CT in glycogen storage disease are

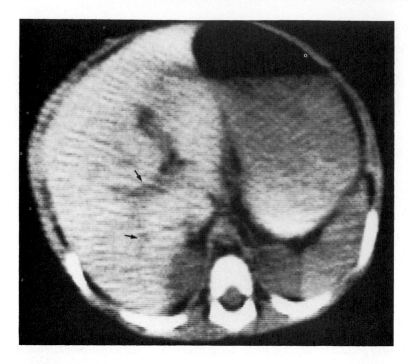

Figure 13–29. Glycogen storage disease Type II. A diffuse increased hepatic density, CT number = 66 H, in a child with glycogen storage disease producing hepatomegaly. Portal vessels (arrows) appear as low-density structures within the high-density liver. The kidneys and spleen are normal.

renomegaly with increased cortical density (Type I), splenomegaly (Types I, III and VI), renal calculi (Type I) and adenoma or hepatoma (Type I) (Fig. 13–30).[85]

RADIATION INJURY

Hepatocellular damage induced by radiation therapy can result in a focal hypodense area of the liver having attenuation values similiar to those found in focal fatty infiltration of the liver.[99, 100] Typically, the low-density region has a sharp, straight border corresponding to the radiation port (Fig. 13–31).[99, 100] Clinically, the acute form of radiation damage has its onset 2 to 6 weeks after therapy and is generally not seen in patients receiving less than 3500 rad (35 Gy) to the liver.[101] Histologically, acute hepatic injury is characterized by panlobular congestion, hemorrhagic foci, decreased numbers of hepatocytes, variable amounts of fatty change, lipofuscin-laden

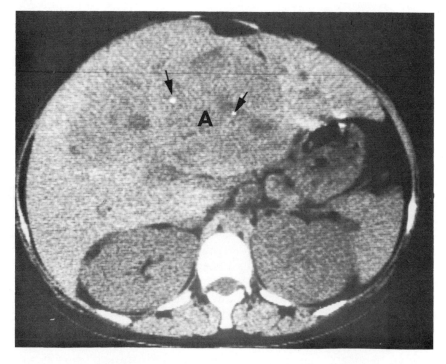

Figure 13–30. Glycogen storage disease Type I. The liver has an increased density and there is a large low-density mass containing foci of calcification (arrows), which proved to be a hepatic adenoma (A). The kidneys are enlarged and have a density slightly higher than normal.

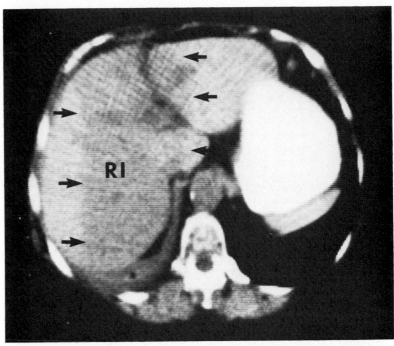

Figure 13–31. Radiation injury (RI) producing a zone of low attenuation within the liver, having straight margins (arrows) which correspond to the radiation port. Radiation had been given for carcinoma of the gallbladder. A small right pleural effusion is present. (From Jeffrey RB Jr, Moss AA, Quivey JM, Federle MP, Wara WM: CT of radiation-induced hepatic injury. AJR 135:495, 1980. © American Roentgen Ray Society. Used with permission.)

macrophages, and marked venous occlusion.[100] The changes resolve by 3 to 5 months and follow-up scans are usually normal.

FOCAL HEPATIC MASSES

Focal hepatic masses can be classified into one of several categories (Table 13–3). Space-occupying hepatic lesions are detectable by computed tomography when the density of the mass differs

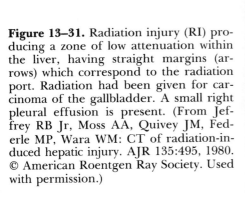

Table 13–3. FOCAL HEPATIC MASSES

Congenital
  Unifocal cyst
  Polycystic liver disease
Neoplastic
  Primary benign
    Hemangioma
    Adenoma
    Focal nodular hyperplasia
    Mesodermal tumors
  Primary malignant
    Hepatocellular carcinoma
    Cholangiocarcinoma
    Lymphoma
    Mesodermal tumors
  Metastatic disease
Inflammatory
  Pyogenic abscess
  Parasitic infection
  Fungal abscess
Traumatic
  Hematoma
  Biloma
  Arterial-venous fistula
  Pseudoaneurysm

significantly from normal liver tissue either prior to or following contrast medium administration.[2, 6, 18, 65, 69, 72] Rarely will an isodense hepatic mass be detected solely by an alteration in hepatic contour. Masses containing calcium or fresh hemorrhage can appear as high-density lesions, but the vast majority of intrahepatic masses of any etiology have attenuation values less than normal hepatic parenchyma.[6, 18, 72] The vast majority of lesions 1 cm or greater in size will be diagnosed by CT.[6, 18]

The CT attenuation value of non-gas–containing hepatic masses varies from that of water (OH) to bone (200+ H). Although the CT density of a hepatic mass usually permits distinction between neoplasm, abscess, and cyst,[2, 3, 6, 18, 65, 76] there is an overlap of CT densities between various hepatic masses of differing etiologies.[6, 18, 76] In smaller lesions the overlap is principally due to the partial volume effect of overlying tissue in the Z axis (Fig. 13–32). However, solid tumors can undergo necrosis and appear cystlike[6, 102–104] and cysts may have high CT numbers as a result of hemorrhage, high protein content, or debris.[104]

Thus, correct differentiation of hepatic masses does not rely primarily on measurement of the CT density of the lesion but more on the clinical data and response to contrast media. Even after contrast administration, overlap between cysts, tumors and infections may exist, requiring additional diagnostic imaging procedures or needle biopsy to make a definitive diagnosis.[6, 102–104]

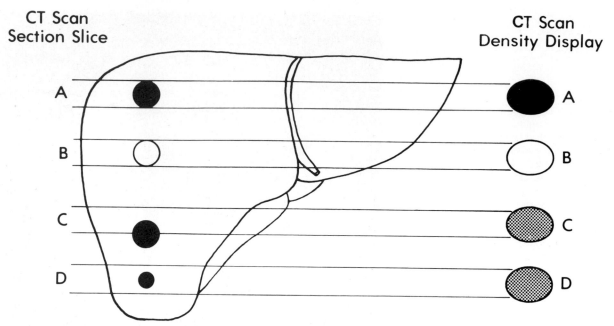

Figure 13–32. Diagram illustrating partial volume effect. **A** Hepatic cyst completely in the scan section has low CT density. **B** Hepatic solid mass completely in the scan section has high CT density. **C** Large hepatic cyst only partially within the CT section has intermediate CT density. **D** Hepatic cyst smaller than the CT slice thickness also has intermediate CT density.

CYSTS

Hepatic cysts vary in size from a few millimeters to several centimeters in diameter and appear as sharply delineated, round, or oval low-density lesions. The CT density of cysts ranges from 0 to 15 H,[69] with smaller cysts measuring higher be-cause of partial volume averaging with adjacent parenchyma (Fig. 13–32). There are no internal septations, and the cyst wall is very thin. Administration of intravenous contrast material enhances the normal liver but does not change the CT attenuation value of hepatic cysts.[18, 69] Hepatic

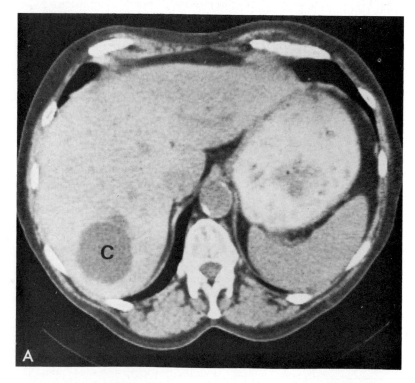

Figure 13–33. Hepatic cystic disease. **A** Single hepatic cyst (c) in right hepatic lobe has sharp margins and a low attenuation value.

Illustration continued on opposite page

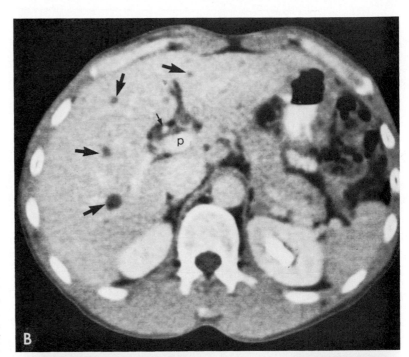

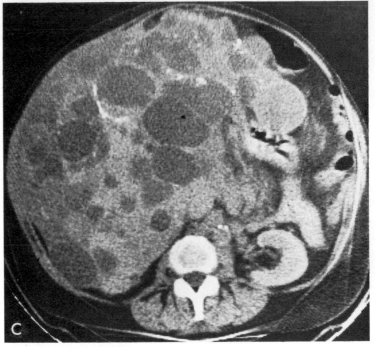

Figure 13–33. *Continued* **B** Several small, round, simple hepatic cysts of water density (large arrows) found incidentally. No renal or pancreatic cysts were present, and there was no family history of polycystic liver disease. The relationship of the portal vein (p) to the hepatic artery (small arrow) is clearly shown. Density of cysts varies because of partial volume effect. **C** Polycystic liver disease producing multiple rounded, sharply margin-ated hepatic cysts. Some cysts have partially calcified walls. No renal or pancreatic cysts were present.

cysts can occur singly, in small numbers, or as innumerable multifocal cysts in polycystic liver disease (Fig. 13–33).

Differentiation of hepatic cysts from other hepatic mass lesions is usually straightforward because of the characteristic appearance, density, and response to contrast administration (Fig. 13–33). However, cystic neoplasms (Fig. 13–34)[102–105] and old hematomas (Fig. 13–35) may have atten-uation values identical to simple hepatic cysts. In these cases, ultrasonography may permit differentiation by demonstrating internal septations and irregularities of the inner margin of the wall of cystic tumors, characteristics not seen in non-neoplastic hepatic cysts.[102] In rare instances, a percutaneous fine-needle biopsy may be needed to differentiate a simple cyst from a necrotic, cystic metastasis.[103]

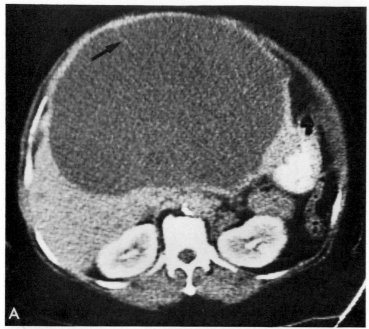

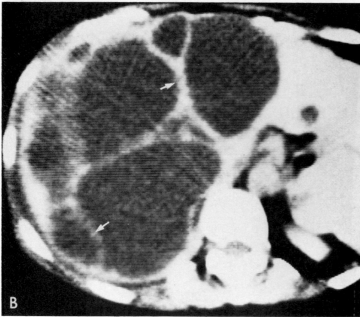

Figure 13–34. Neoplasms simulating hepatic cysts. **A** Large single hepatic metastasis from an ovarian carcinoma having a CT density of 6 H. The rim around the lesion is slightly thick, and there is a single internal septum (arrow). **B** Lung carcinoma producing multiple large metastatic lesions, having a CT density of 4 H. The walls of the lesions (arrows) are thick, and the inner content of the metastasis is slightly inhomogeneous. (From Federle MP, Filly RA, Moss AA: Cystic hepatic neoplasms: Complementary role of CT and sonography. AJR 136:345, 1981. © 1981, American Roentgen Ray Society. Reprinted by permission.)

NEOPLASMS

Primary Benign Tumors

CAVERNOUS HEMANGIOMA. This is the most common benign tumor of the liver, occurring in 0.4 to 7.3 per cent of patients in autopsy examinations.[107–111] Greater than 70 per cent of cavernous hemangiomas occur in women,[111, 112] and although all ages are affected, it is rarely diagnosed before adulthood.[111, 113] Histologically, cavernous hemangiomas are composed of multiple, endothelium-lined cystic blood-filled spaces that are separated by fibrous septa of variable thickness.[108, 110] Calcifications occur but phleboliths are rare.[108, 109] The majority of hemangiomas are single lesions less than 5 cm in diameter, but multiple hemangiomas and larger lesions are not uncommon.[107–110]

Most cavernous hemangiomas are asymptomatic and are found incidentally at surgery, autopsy, or angiography. Symptomatic cavernous hemangiomas are usually found to be "giant hemangiomas"[107, 114, 115] presenting with symptoms of an abdominal mass due to hepatomegaly and/or

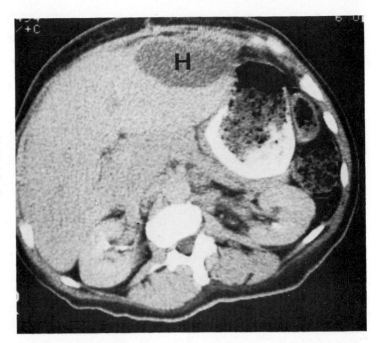

Figure 13–35. Hematoma simulating hepatic cyst. An isolated low-density mass (5H) in the lateral segment of the left hepatic lobe proved to be an intrahepatic hematoma (H) secondary to a liver biopsy performed 5 weeks prior to the CT scan.

abdominal discomfort related to pressure on adjacent organs.[114, 115] Cavernous hemangiomas may enlarge during pregnancy and rarely spontaneous rupture with massive hemorrhage and death occurs.[111, 116, 117] Percutaneous biopsy of a cavernous hemangioma with any size needle is extremely dangerous, with serious hemorrhage and deaths being reported.[114, 118–120]

Ultrasonography[107, 121–123] and scintigraphy[86, 120–126] can detect most hemangiomas larger than 2 cm in diameter. However, the echographic features of cavernous hemangiomas are variable, ranging from hypoechoic to hyperechoic lesions with discrete to irregular margins.[107, 123] Radionuclide scintigraphy also suffers from a lack of specificity. On ^{99m}Tc sulfur colloid scans, hemangiomas produce cold areas that cannot be differentiated from other hepatic mass lesions.[108, 120] Dynamic radionuclide scintigrams using blood pool imaging agents may reveal the increased vascularity of a hemangioma,[108, 109, 120, 121] but hemangiomas have varying degrees of hypervascularity and both false-positive and false-negative results have been reported.[120] [67]Gallium citrate accumulates in pyogenic abscesses and some metastatic lesions but not in cavernous hemangiomas.[108, 109, 120, 121]

Prior to computed tomography, hepatic angiography was the only diagnostic imaging procedure that could successfully differentiate cavernous hemangiomas from other hepatic mass lesions. The angiographic features of hepatic hemangiomas—prominent lakes of contrast persisting well into the venous phase, absence of arteriovenous shunting, a normal portal vein, a normal-sized hepatic artery, and feeding vessels that are stretched around the lesion—permit differentiation of benign hemangiomas from malignant hepatic lesions in virtually every instance.[112, 127–131] Angiography can detect lesions as small as 0.5 cm and still is regarded as the most sensitive, specific, and accurate imaging procedure of heptic hemangioma.[109, 129]

Detection and differentiation of cavernous hemangiomas from other solid hepatic lesions using computed tomography are possible in greater than 90 per cent of instances.[6, 47, 64, 72, 86, 105, 107–110, 123, 124, 132] Prior to the injection of contrast material, cavernous hemangiomas are usually identified as hypodense, well-circumscribed, homogeneous lesions (Figs. 13–36A and 13–37A). Central low-density foci are not uncommon (Fig. 13–36A)[109, 110] but calcification is rare.[109] Occasionally, a hemangioma will appear isodense with normal liver on precontrast scans.[86, 110]

After intravenous contrast administration, hemangiomas show an increase in CT density of all or part of the rim of the lesion that exceeds the enhancement of the normal liver (Fig. 13–36B and 13–37B). CT numbers can exceed 140 H in the rim of the hemangioma within the first minute after a rapid intravenous bolus of contrast material (Figs. 13–36C and 13–37C).[108] Delayed CT scans reveal progressive contrast enhancement of the more central parts of the hemangioma (Fig. 13–37D) owing to gradual accumulation and slow washout of contrast material.

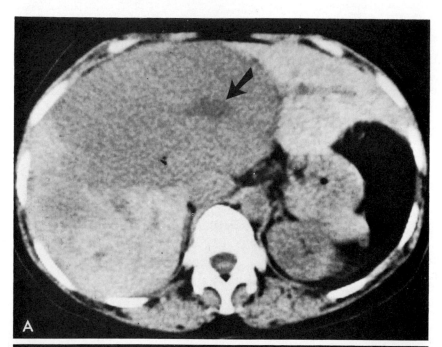

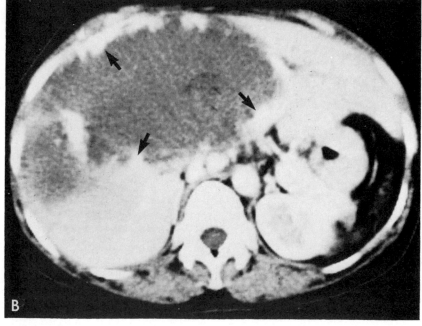

Figure 13–36. Cavenous hemangioma. **A** Precontrast CT scan demonstrates a large, hypodense, well-circumscribed lesion in the liver, which contains a central focus of decreased density (arrow). **B** Scan performed after bolus injection of contrast material reveals the periphery of the lesion to enhance dramatically (arrows) and become hyperdense with respect to normal liver.

Illustration continued on opposite page

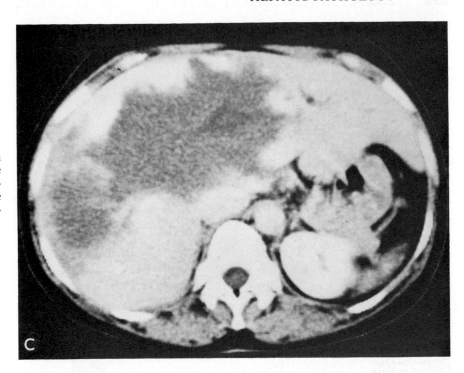

Figure 13–36. *Continued* **C** Scan 1 minute later. The hyperdense rim persists but has spread toward the central portion of the hemangioma. The central low-density cleft remains unchanged.

Although the edge of the hemangioma typically has its peak contrast enhancement within the first minute, contrast transit time through the lesion is slow and the center of the hemangioma can continue to increase in CT density for 15 minutes or more.[108] In many hemangiomas larger than 3 cm, central clefts that do not enhance are seen on delayed CT scans (Fig. 13–36C). As the periphery of a hemangioma becomes isodense, the hemangioma appears smaller (Fig. 13–37D) and it is only after the contrast is washed out that it assumes its original size.[109] Smaller hemangiomas can rapidly become totally hyperdense and may not show peripheral enhancement (Figs. 13–38 and 13–39). The persistence of contrast indicating slow transit of contrast usually permits distinction of a small hemangioma from a hypervascular metastasis, which typically has a rapid change in CT density following contrast administration.

Hepatic hemangiomas are best distinguished from other solid hepatic masses by administering contrast material as a 60- to 100-ml bolus and performing a dynamic CT sequence with delayed scans at 1 to 4 minutes. Although the CT appearance of hemangiomas is somewhat variable, in the vast majority of instances the CT features are sufficiently unique to permit a diagnosis of a hepatic hemangioma to be made without angiographic confirmation. Hepatic angiography need be performed only when the CT findings are indeterminate or when surgery or biopsy is planned.

HEPATIC ADENOMA. Liver cell adenomas are benign, well-encapsulated, true hepatic neoplasms composed entirely of hepatocytes.[105, 133–136] The hepatocytes and capsule may be vacuolated by fat globules,[134] but fibrous septations, bile ducts and Kupffer cells are not found. Liver cell adenomas are usually solitary tumors that arise in women taking oral contraceptives but also arise in men on hormonal therapy.[105, 134–138] Clinically, liver cell adenomas are usually asymptomatic until growth of the tumor produces an abdominal mass or tumoral hemorrhage results in abdominal pain; if the hemorrhage is massive, shock and even death may result.[105, 135, 136] Liver cell adenomas can regress or completely disappear following withdrawal of oral contraceptives or hormonal therapy.[137, 139, 140] However, hemorrhage and growth of liver cell adenomas may occur despite stoppage of oral contraceptives[136] and therefore surgical resection remains the therapy of choice for symptomatic liver cell adenomas.

The angiographic and radionuclide features of liver cell adenomas permit a diagnosis to be made in the majority of patients. Radionuclide colloid hepatic scans always demonstrate a cold, space-occupying lesion. Angiography reveals either a hypovascular mass in 50 per cent of cases with displacement and draping of hepatic arteries around the tumor or a hypervascular tumor mass with tortuous vessels coursing through the lesion.[105, 136] A dense capillary blush is usually not

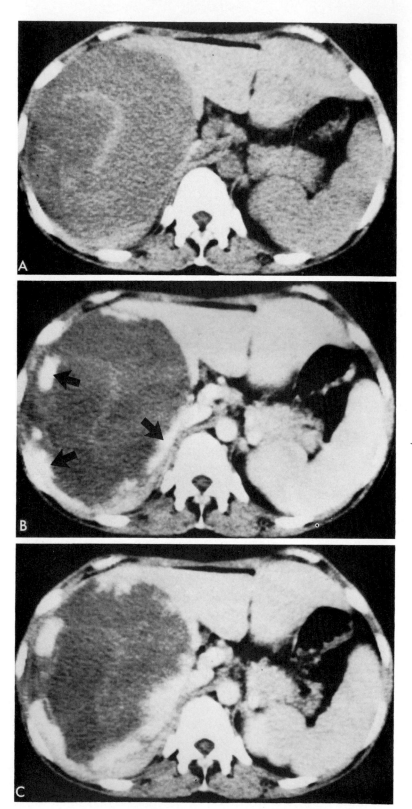

Figure 13–37. Cavernous hemangioma. **A** Large low-density hemangioma of the right lobe of the liver. **B** Scan 30 seconds after a bolus injection demonstrates typical intense peripheral enhancement (arrows). **C** Scan 1 minute after contrast injection shows gradual spread of contrast material toward the center of the hemangioma.

Illustration continued on opposite page

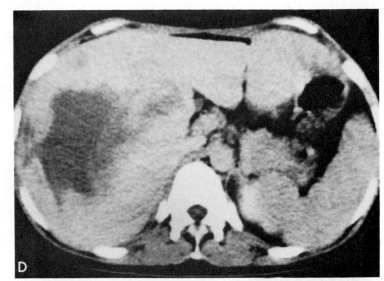

Figure 13–37. *Continued* **D** Scan 4 minutes later reveals continued progressive contrast enhancement of the center of the hemangioma. The peripheral part of the hemangioma is almost isodense, with the normal liver making the hemangioma appear smaller than on the initial scan. **E** Arterial phase of hepatic arteriogram, demonstrating typical features of a large cavernous hemangioma.

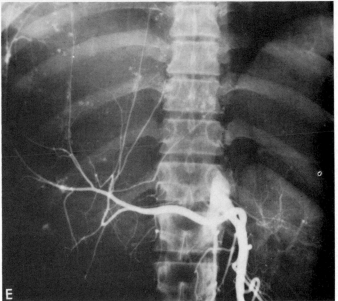

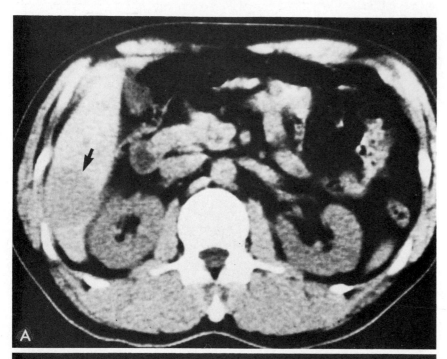

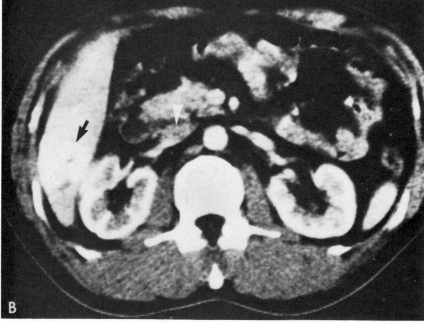

Figure 13–38. Cavernous hemangioma. **A** Precontrast CT scan demonstrates a 4-cm hemangioma (arrow) in the right lobe of the liver. **B** The hemangioma (arrow) becomes uniformly hyperdense during peak hepatic arterial inflow. At this time, there is sharp cortical-medullary differentiation and opacification of the renal arteries, but no filling of the inferior vena cava (arrowhead) has occurred.

Illustration continued on opposite page

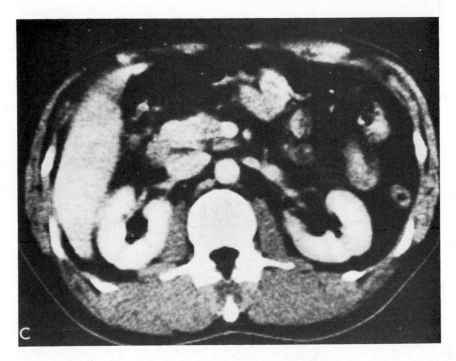

Figure 13–38. *Continued* **C** The hemangioma is almost isodense with the liver by the time the inferior vena cava is well opacified.

seen and septations are not identified.[105] Feeding vessels may enter from the periphery or center of the tumor.

Ultrasonography has demonstrated liver cell adenomas to be sonodense,[134, 136, 141] but the findings are nonspecific as similar sonographic features have been found in a variety of malignant and benign hepatic lesions.

Computed tomography can detect liver cell adenomas.[6, 7, 69, 134, 136, 137, 142] Most frequently, a solid mass of low attenuation is identified on scans performed without intravenous contrast material (Figs. 13–30 and 13–40),[134, 136, 137] but isodense liver cell adenomas, detectable only by contour abnormalities, have been described.[66, 142] While the CT density of liver cell adenomas does not permit differentiation from other solid hepatic masses,[66, 134] the capsule may contain an excess of lipid-laden hepatocytes, permitting a low-density peripheral ring to be identified around the adenoma.[134] Following drip infusion or bolus injection of contrast material, liver cell adenomas have not shown marked contrast enhancement. When hepatic adenomas are treated with hepatic arterial ligation CT may demonstrate gas within the infarcted liver cell adenoma (Fig. 13–41), which should not be mistaken for an hepatic abscess.

FOCAL NODULAR HYPERPLASIA.   This is a rare, benign liver lesion composed of Kupffer cells, hepatocytes, and bile ducts.[105, 143–145] It is usually well circumscribed but not encapsulated[105] and is subdivided into nodules by a central fibrous core and radiating septa containing arterial and venous channels, and proliferating bile ducts.[105, 143]

Focal nodular hyperplasia occurs in all age groups and in both sexes and is associated with oral contraceptives in only 11 per cent of the cases reported in females.[143] The lesion arises in an otherwise normal liver, is most frequently subcapsular rather than pedunculated, is multiple in 20 per cent of cases, and typically is 4 to 7 cm in diameter. Hemorrhage, necrosis, or malignant degeneration is very rare and the vast majority of patients remain entirely asymptomatic. As a result of the benign nature of focal nodular hyperplasia, no therapy is recommended unless tortion, infarction, or lesion size forces surgical resection.

Diagnosis is usually possible by correlating the findings of the radionuclide colloid scintigram and hepatic angiography (Fig. 13–42A,B). Radionuclide colloid scintigrams most frequently are normal as the Kupffer cells in the area of focal nodular hyperplasia concentrate colloid normally.[143] Rarely there is hyperconcentration of colloid and in 35 per cent of patients the region of focal nodular hyperplasia is photopenic.[105, 143] Angiographically, the lesions are hypervascular with fine radiating septations identifiable in the parenchymal stain (Fig. 13–42C).[143–145] As in liver cell adenomas, the vascular supply may appear to arise centrally and radiate in a spoke-wheel fashion or enter from the periphery of the mass.[143] The combination of a normal radionuclide scan and a hypervascular mass or masses usually allows

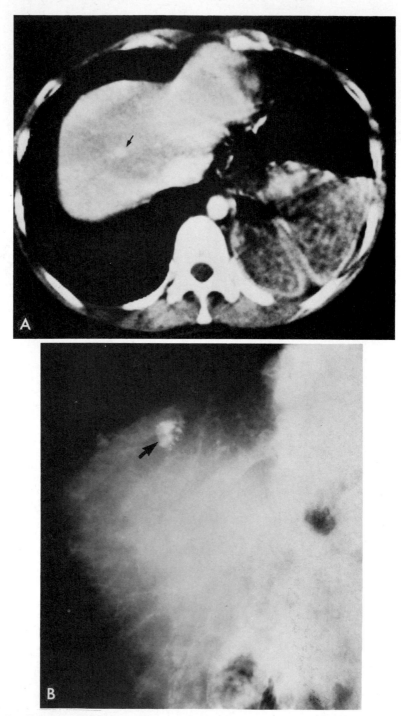

Figure 13–39. Small hepatic hemangioma. **A** A small, totally hyperdense lesion (arrow) seen in the dome of the liver following a bolus injection of contrast material. **B** Delayed film from hepatic angiogram confirms the presence of a small hepatic hemangioma (arrow).

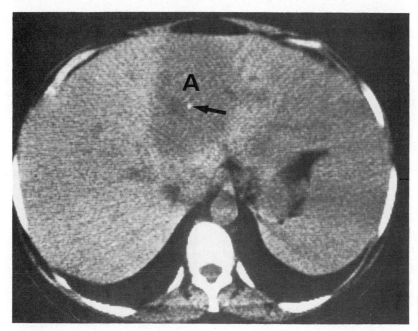

Figure 13–40. Hepatic adenoma (A) containing a focus of calcification (arrow) produces a large, low-density mass in a liver, which is hyperdense owing to glycogen storage disease.

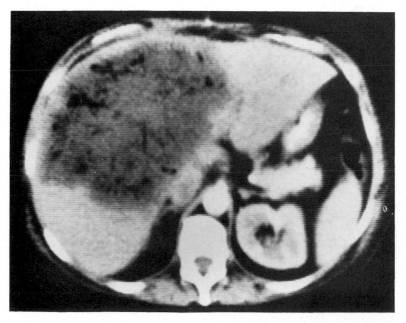

Figure 13–41. Hepatic adenoma. CT scan after treatment of hepatic adenoma by hepatic artery ligation demonstrates gas within tubular structures, thought to be vessels within the adenoma. Patient was asymptomatic.

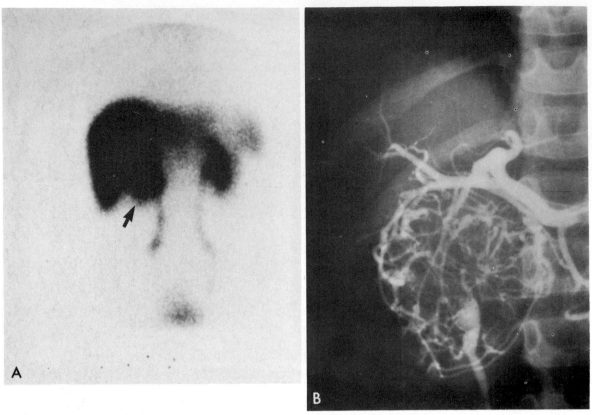

Figure 13–42. Focal nodular hyperplasia. **A**   Radionuclide colloid scintigram demonstrates a mass lesion arising in the right lobe of the liver, which concentrates colloid normally. **B**   A hypervascular mass with vessels entering from the periphery is present on angiography.

Illustration continued on opposite page

focal nodular hyperplasia to be distinguished from liver cell adenoma. A biopsy may have to be performed when the radionuclide scan is photopenic or the angiographic features are not typical.

Sonography and computed tomography can detect focal nodular hyperplasia, but the findings are nonspecific. Hypoechoic, hyperechoic, and a mixed echo pattern have been reported in proven cases.[143] Computed tomography has demonstrated the lesion to be hypodense or isodense on nonenhanced scans (Fig. 13–42D); after infusion of intravenous contrast material, hypodense lesions have become hyperdense or isodense or have exhibited no change in attenuation value.[6, 86, 143] Isodense lesions have not become visible after intravenous infusion, but the density change after intravenous bolus injection has not been reported.[143] The CT features of focal nodular hyperplasia are similar to those seen in many solid hepatic mass lesions; therefore it appears it will be difficult for CT to differentiate focal nodular hyperplasia from other hepatic masses without a biopsy.[124, 143]

MISCELLANEOUS BENIGN TUMORS. Rare pri-

mary benign hepatic tumors may arise from mesodermal derivatives or lymphangiomatous elements.[104] The CT appearance of unusual hepatic tumors such as lipomas, fibromas, lymphangiomas, or leiomyomas has only rarely been described (Fig. 13–43).[104] Single cases of a cystic hamartoma and a lymphangioma both resembled multiloculated hepatic cysts (Fig. 13–44).[6, 104] It is likely that the CT appearance of benign mesodermal tumors will be nonspecific and not permit differentiation from other benign and malignant solid hepatic masses.

Primary Malignant Tumors

HEPATOCELLULAR CARCINOMA (HEPATOMA). This is the most common primary malignant tumor of the liver, representing over 80 per cent of all primary hepatic malignancies.[69] Hepatomas can occur as solitary tumors (50 per cent of the time), multinodular tumors (16 to 20 per cent of the time) or diffuse lesions (30 to 35 per cent of the time).[71, 146] Hepatocellular carcinoma is more prevalent in patients with pre-existing liver dis-

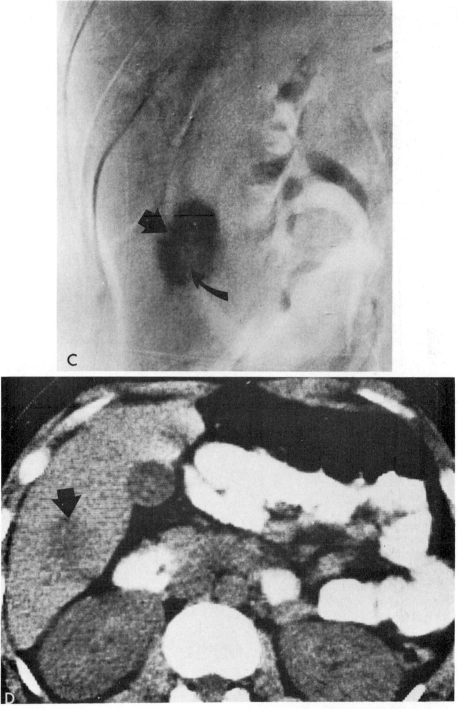

Figure 13–42. *Continued* **C**   Hepatic angiogram demonstrating typical hypervascular lesion (arrow). A septum (curved arrow) is present in the center of the lesion, which was confirmed pathologically. **D**   A CT scan performed without contrast reveals the zone of focal nodular hyperplasia as an area of low attenuation (arrow), which is indistinguishable from a primary or secondary hepatic neoplasm. The lesion became isodense following contrast administration.

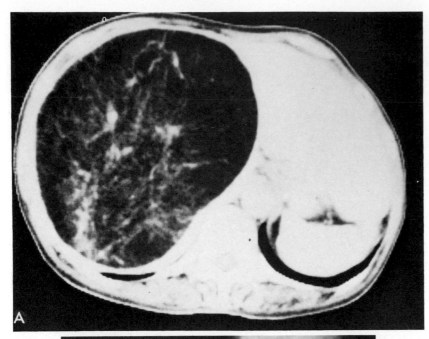

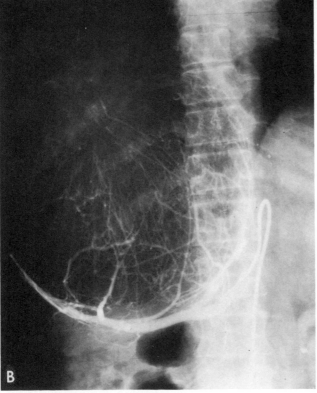

Figure 13–43. Benign hepatic tumor composed almost entirely of fat. It is sharply marginated from the normal liver and contains multiple linear densities, which enhanced after contrast administration. **B** Hepatic angiogram showing displacement of the hepatic artery and a number of small, thin vessels entering the center of the tumor from the periphery.

ease such as cirrhosis or hemochromatosis (Fig. 13–45), in patients with positive hepatitis B surface antigen levels, and in the oriental population.

Pathologically, hepatomas are characterized by a tendency toward intravascular growth into the hepatic veins and portal system.[147] The usual angiographic appearance of a hepatocellular carcinoma is that of a hypervascular mass being supplied by an enlarged hepatic artery, having prominent tumor neovascularization, arteriovenous shunting, capillary staining, arterial encasement, and portal vein occlusion.[146, 148–151] Although hypervascularity is the most frequent finding, hypovascular hepatomas and hepatomas having a mixed hypovascular-hypervascular pattern occur.[146, 148] Avascular areas result from vas-

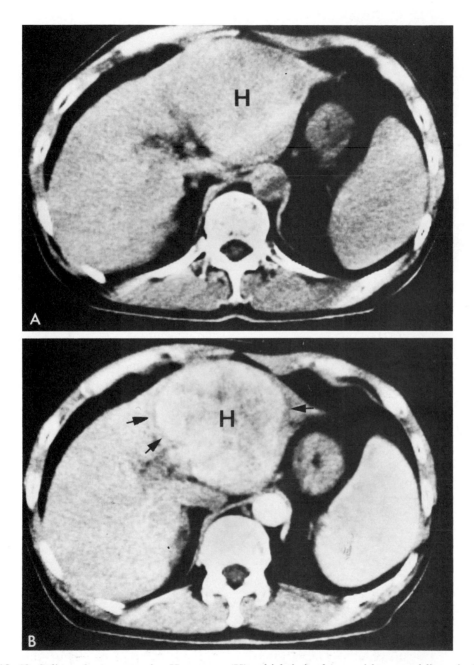

Figure 13–49. Solitary hepatoma. **A**   Hepatoma (H), which is isodense with normal liver, is detected by CT owing to alteration in the normal contour of the lateral segment of the left lobe of the liver. **B**   The hepatoma (H) becomes hyperdense 30 seconds after an intravenous bolus injection of contrast media. A low-density pseudocapsule (arrows) surrounds the hepatoma.

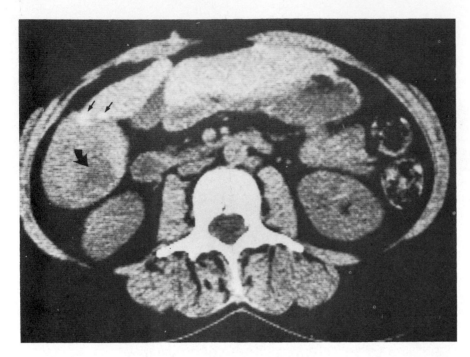

Figure 13–50. Pedunculated hepatoma containing foci of calcification (arrows) and necrosis (curved arrow).

for hepatomas have varied from 79 per cent[55] to 94 per cent[64] with an overall detection rate of 89 per cent for 155 reported hepatomas.[1, 18, 44, 46, 61, 65, 67, 69, 70, 71, 105, 124, 148–153]

The effect of intravenous contrast media on the CT appearance of hepatocellular carcinoma is variable.[56, 61, 70, 71, 146, 152] Following an intravenous infusion of contrast material, hepatomas may become better visualized (Fig. 13–46), less well visualized, or exhibit no change in detectability. Although the average difference in density between hepatocellular carinoma and normal liver is marginally improved by intravenous contrast infusion, in certain instances hepatomas become isodense with surrounding hepatic parenchyma and thus are undetectable after contrast administration.[61, 72] For this reason, precontrast as well as postcontrast CT scans should be performed when searching for a hepatocellular carcinoma (Fig. 13–51).

Administration of contrast material as a bolus injection of 80 to 150 ml of 60 per cent diatrizoate or iothalamate followed by dynamic CT scanning results in improved delineation of tumor vascularity (Figs. 13–47, 13–49, and 13–52), venous shunting (Fig. 13–53), venous occlusion (Fig. 13–54) and hepatic lobar or segmental flow abnormalities (Figs. 13–53 and 13–55).[46, 71, 148, 151, 153, 154] Hepatomas, being supplied by hepatic arterial branches, become maximally hyperdense during the arterial phase of a dynamic scan sequence and then rapidly become less dense as portal inflow to the liver becomes dominant (Fig. 13–52).

Arteriovenous shunting is common in hepatomas but rare in other types of primary and metastatic tumors. The best demonstration of arteriovenous shunting is after a bolus injection of contrast medium and a dynamic scan sequence (Fig. 13–53). Portal vein or inferior vena cava thrombosis is usually detected as a filling defect in the portal vein or inferior vena cava (Figs. 13–53 and 13–54); in some instances the thrombosis is surrounded by a thin hyperdense ring of contrast material after a bolus injection (Fig. 13–54B). In some patients, a segmental attenuation difference can be identified on dynamic CT scans obtained after a bolus injection of contrast material (Figs. 13–53 and 13–55).[153, 154]

Intrahepatic arterial injection of contrast in a 10- to 15-ml bolus or a 300-ml rapid infusion[41] produces greater contrast enhancement[154] and detects more lesions than intravenous contrast infusion or bolus injection (Fig. 13–56).[44, 56] Changes in CT density occur very rapidly, lesions changing from hypodense to hyperdense to isodense to hypodense within 60 seconds. As with intravenous bolus injections, some hepatomas show no contrast enhancement and others only a slight increase in density after intrahepatic arterial contrast injection (Fig. 13–56). Intrahepatic arterial contrast administration is not recommended as a routine technique but can be employed if an hepatic arterial line is in place for chemotherapy or if arteriography fails to delineate completely the location and number of tumors prior to surgery.

CT is useful for following the effects of radia-

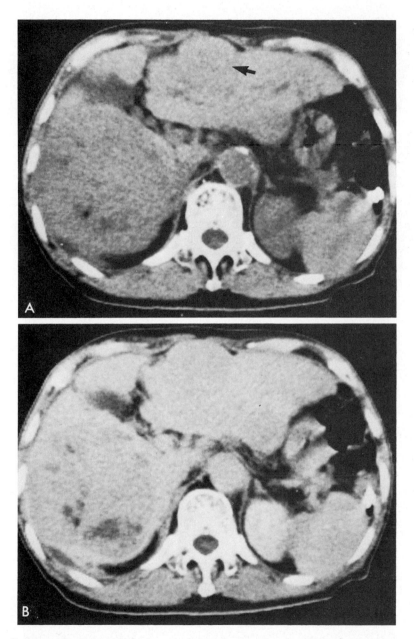

Figure 13–51. Failure of contrast infusion to detect hepatoma. **A** Precontrast scan reveals a small, slightly hypodense mass in lateral segment of the left hepatic lobe (arrow) and a larger tumor in the right lobe of the liver. **B** Following contrast infusion, the hepatomas and normal liver enhance to a similar degree: The differential between the margin of the tumor in the lateral segment of the left lobe of the liver and normal liver has not been increased, and the lesion is now less well demonstrated.

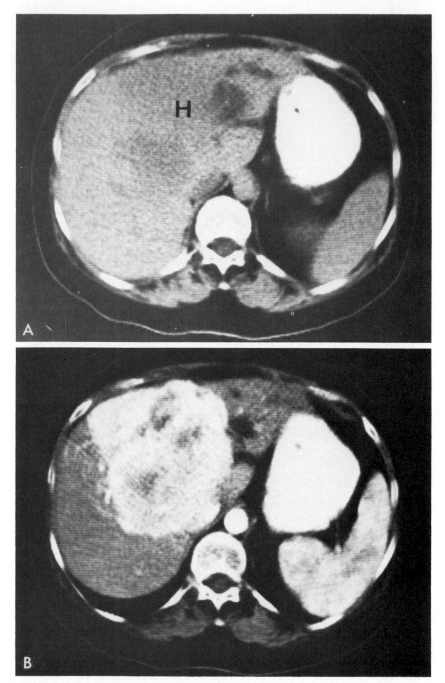

Figure 13–52. Hepatoma—dynamic CT scan technique. **A**   Precontrast scan. The hepatoma (H) appears as an ill-defined, low-density mass. **B**   CT scan during peak arterial contrast. The hepatoma dramatically enhances to become a well-circumscribed, hyperdense mass.

Illustration continued on opposite page

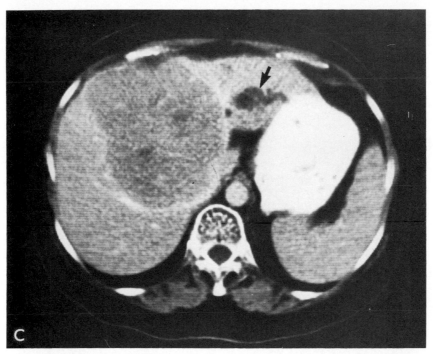

Figure 13–52. *Continued* **C**   CT scan 30 seconds later reveals the hepatoma to have a hyperdense rim, but the tumor itself is now hypodense with respect to normal liver. The left biliary system (arrow) is dilated.

tion therapy, chemotherapy, or embolic therapy on hepatocellular carcinoma.[71, 155, 156] Following embolization, air can be identified[155] in an infarcted but not infected tumor (Fig. 13–57). Bubbles of gas more typical of an abscess are seen if a tumor treated with chemotherapy becomes infected.[71] Most frequently, CT is utilized to demonstrate whether tumor size and volume have changed.[156]

CHOLANGIOCARCINOMA.   This slow-growing tumor is most frequently located in the common bile duct between the cystic duct and ampulla of Vater but may involve the porta hepatis, common hepatic duct and intrahepatic ducts.[105, 157, 158] Jaundice, usually painless, is the most common presenting symptom. The tumors are frequently small when discovered, since the bile duct lumen permits little narrowing before it becomes obstructed. Although cholangiocarcinomas may be small when first detected, invasion into adjacent vessels or viscera usually is present at the time of diagnosis. Thus although complete surgical removal is only rarely possible, prolonged survival can be expected if adequate biliary drainage is provided by surgical or percutaneous methods.[158]

The CT findings in cholangiocarcinoma are nonspecific, with similar findings being produced by a variety of neoplastic and benign diseases.

The most common CT finding in primary carcinoma of the biliary ductal system is either focal or generalized biliary obstruction (Fig. 13–58).[157-163] The level of the obstruction can be determined by noting the point at which the dilated biliary system becomes obliterated.[164] The CT density of a cholangiocarcinoma may not differ greatly from normal surrounding hepatic parenchyma on precontrast CT scans.[158, 159] Cholangiocarcinomas also can appear as solid, hypodense lesions in the periphery of the liver (Fig. 13–59) or infiltrating centrally located tumors which enhance following contrast administration (Fig. 13–60).[159]

LYMPHOMA.   This tumor only rarely arises in the liver as a primary malignancy[165] but is found as a secondary site of involvement in 60 per cent of patients with Hodgkin's disease and in 50 per cent of those with non-Hodgkin's lymphoma. Diffuse infiltration is more frequent in Hodgkin's disease, whereas diffuse and nodular hepatic involvement are equally frequent in non-Hodgkin's lymphoma.

CT is able to detect hepatic involvement in only 4 per cent of patients with lymphoma,[165] and thus currently CT is an insensitive method of screening for hepatic involvement in lymphoma. The low rate of detection is due to the fact that foci of lymphomatous infiltration are commonly less than

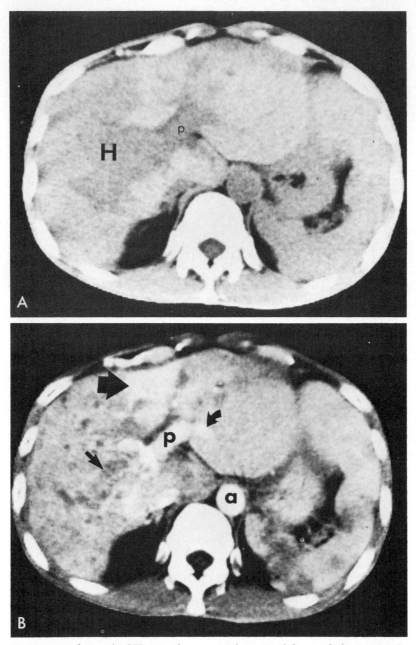

Figure 13–53. Hepatoma: dynamic CT scan demonstrating arterial-portal shunt. **A** Precontrast scan. A large hepatoma (H) appears as an ill-defined, low-density mass contiguous with the portal vein (p). **B** CT scan during peak arterial contrast. There is simultaneous filling of the main portal vein (p) and left portal vein branch (curved arrow) while the aorta (a) is maximally enhanced, indicating an arterial-portal vein shunt. The thrombosed right portal vein is seen as a low-density structure (small arrow). A portion of the left lobe of the liver is normally enhanced (large arrow), indicating a segmental flow abnormality.

Illustration continued on opposite page

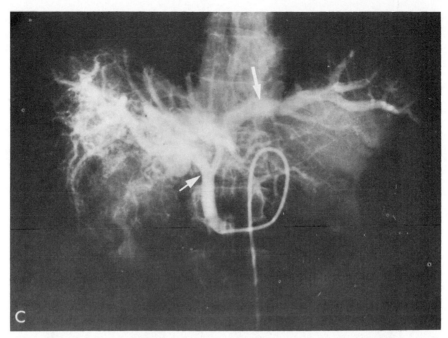

Figure 13–53. *Continued* **C**   Hepatic angiogram confirming presence of hepatic artery (small arrow) to portal vein (large arrow) shunt. The thrombosed right portal vein branch does not opacify.

0.5 cm in diameter.[152] When positive, CT usually demonstrates solid, hepatic masses having a lower density than surrounding hepatic parenchyma (Fig. 13–61). Diffuse hepatic involvement is more difficult to detect because the density differential between normal and abnormal tissue on precontrast and postcontrast studies is small. The use of intravenous liposoluble contrast better demonstrates hepatic involvement with lymphoma[35] and raises hope that the diagnosis of hepatic lymphoma can be significantly improved.

CT demonstration of hepatomegaly alone should not be interpreted as evidence of lymphomatous involvement of the liver, as lymphoma is histologically absent in 43 per cent of patients with non-Hodgkin's lymphoma and hepatomegaly.[166] Although the CT detection rate is low, the liver should be included in every abdominal CT study of a patient with known or suspected lymphoma as an additional aid in staging the lymphoma. The demonstration of spread of lymphoma to the liver indicates advanced disease (Stage III or IV) and has important implications in therapy planning.

MISCELLANEOUS PRIMARY TUMORS. A variety of rare primary hepatic tumors can be detected by computed tomography. The tumors are detected as low-density, solid, circumscribed mass lesions usually indistinguishable from other primary or metastatic tumors.

Neurosecretory tumors arising from the amine precursor uptake and decarboxylation (APUD) cells within the liver resemble carcinoid tumors, but the patients do not have the carcinoid syndrome.[105] Angiosarcoma can arise in the liver and present with solitary or multiple hepatic low-density mass lesions that dramatically enhance after a contrast bolus injection (Fig. 13–62).[167] Malignancies derived from mesodermal tissues (such as fibrosarcoma and liposarcoma) are extremely rare primary hepatic malignancies.

Secondary Malignant Tumors (Metastases)

Taken as a group, metastases are the most common malignant tumors of the liver. The accuracy of computed tomography in detecting focal or multifocal metastatic lesions has ranged from 77 to 96 per cent. The accuracy of CT is comparable with that achieved using ultrasonography[86, 124, 133] and radionuclide scintigraphy[124, 168–170] despite the fact that most comparison studies employed CT scanners with scan times longer than 18 seconds.[2, 86, 124, 142, 168] Comparison studies utilizing finely collinated, high-resolution CT scanners capable of dynamic CT imaging are not yet available but should improve sensitivity to above 90 per cent. False-negative CT studies range from 2 to 12 per cent primarily because of streak artifacts, partial volume averaging of small masses

Text continued on page 665

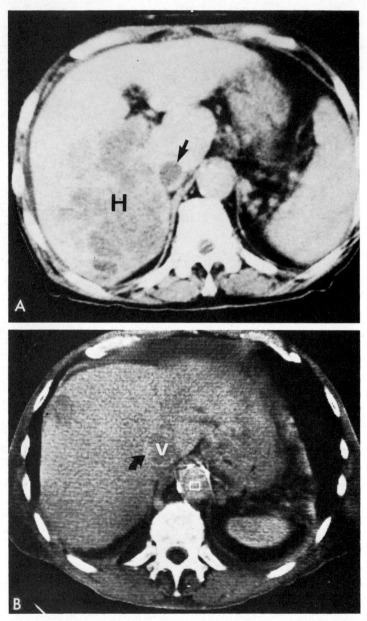

Figure 13–54. Venous occlusion produced by hepatoma. **A** Large right hepatic lobe hepatoma (H) invading and occluding the inferior vena cava (arrow). The inferior vena cava contains tumor thrombi and does not enhance after contrast administration. **B** Hepatoma producing inferior vena cava obstruction, shown as an enlarged vena cava (v) containing a tumor thrombus surrounded by a rim of contrast material (arrow).

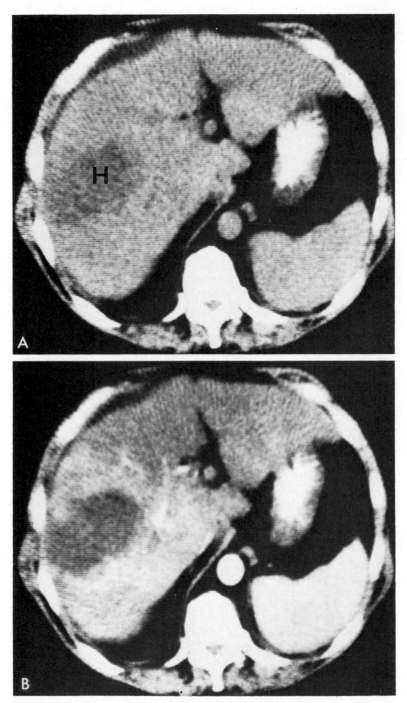

Figure 13–55. Segmental hepatic flow abnormality produced by hepatoma. **A**   Precontrast scan shows a solitary hepatoma (H) surrounded by a normal-appearing liver. **B**   At time of maximum aortic opacification, the right lobe of the liver has dramatically enhanced, while the hepatoma and left lobe of the liver have barely increased in density. A possible explanation is that the hepatoma "steals" blood, resulting in more arterial inflow to the hepatic lobe containing the tumor. The density of the lobes equalizes as portal inflow arrives.

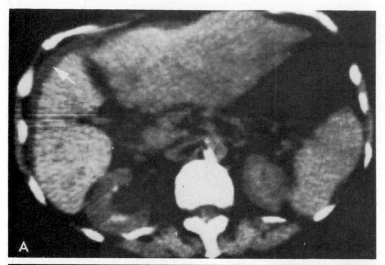

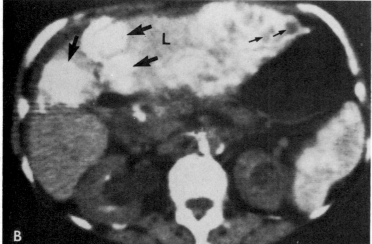

Figure 13–56. Multifocal hepatoma: intrahepatic arterial versus intravenous injection of contrast material. **A** Precontrast scan demonstrates ascites (arrow) and an enlarged left lateral segment without focal defects. **B** CT scan at peak hepatic arterial contrast. There are multiple focal hepatomas, which are dramatically enhanced (large arrows), whereas other lesions (small arrows) appear as hypodense lesions. The uninvolved liver (L) enhances normally. **C** CT scan 30 seconds after **B**. The hyperdense hepatomas (large arrows) have become hypodense with respect to the normal liver, which now has a greater attenuation value than the tumors. The low-density hepatomas (small arrows) have not changed during the scan sequence.

Illustration continued on opposite page

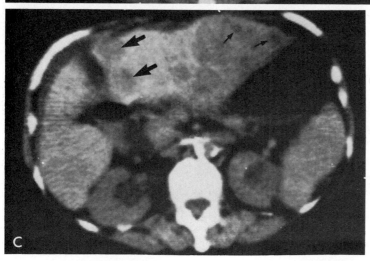

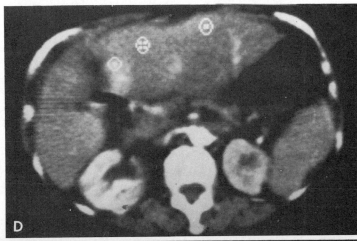

Figure 13–56. *Continued* **D** CT scan performed during peak enhancement of hepatoma after intravenous bolus injection of contrast material demonstrates that contrast enhancement is less and fewer lesions are seen. The small hypodense tumors demonstrated in **B** and **C** are not visible. **E** Time-density curve of three areas indicated in **D**. The maximum hepatoma density was 72 whereas the density of liver increased slowly, as did other foci of hepatoma. Time-density curve was plotted on a scale of +500 to −500. **F** Time-density curve of same areas after intrahepatic arterial injection. Hepatomas reach greater density: 116 and 96. The liver increases more rapidly and exceeds the hepatoma density 24 seconds after the injection. Time density curve plotted on a scale of +500 to −500. (From Moss AA, Dean PB, Axel L, Goldberg HI, Glazer GM, Friedman MA: Dynamic CT of hepatic masses with intravenous and intraarterial contrast material. AJR 138:847, 1982. © 1982, American Roentgen Ray Society. Reprinted by permission.)

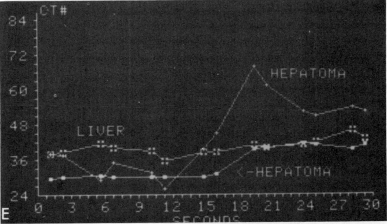

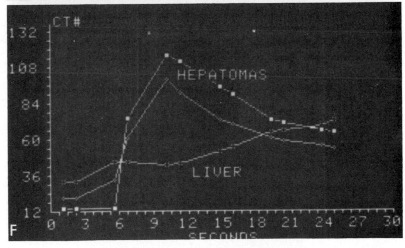

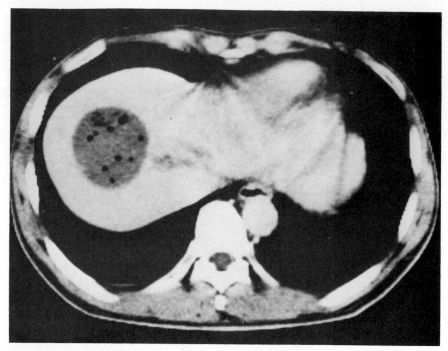

Figure 13–57. Infarcted hepatoma. Gas bubbles are present in a solitary hepatoma treated four weeks previously by hepatic artery ligation. Patient had no signs of sepsis.

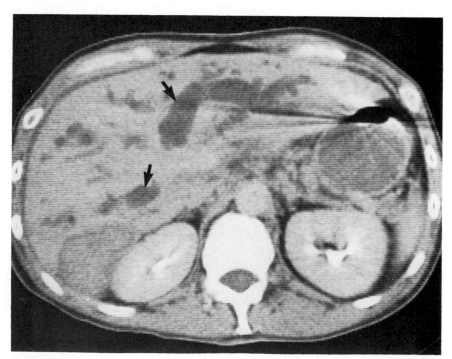

Figure 13–58. Cholangiocarcinoma producing obstructive jaundice. There is marked dilatation of the left and right intrahepatic ducts (arrows) due to a small intraductal cholangiocarcinoma.

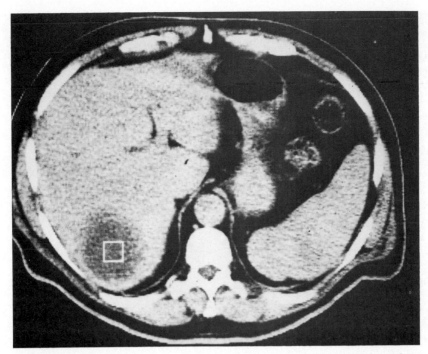

Figure 13–59. Peripheral cholangiocarcinoma (box) appearing as solid hypodense mass.

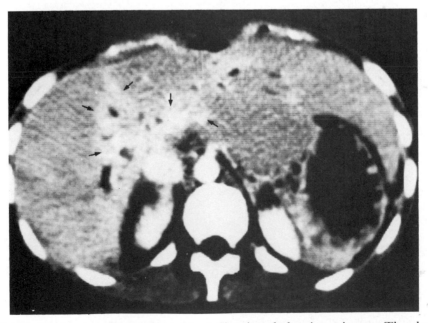

Figure 13–60. Obstructive jaundice produced by infiltrating cholangiocarcinoma. The cholangiocarcinoma (arrows) becomes hyperdense after bolus injection of contrast medium. The cholangiocarcinoma surrounds the bile ducts and extends directly into adjacent liver parenchyma.

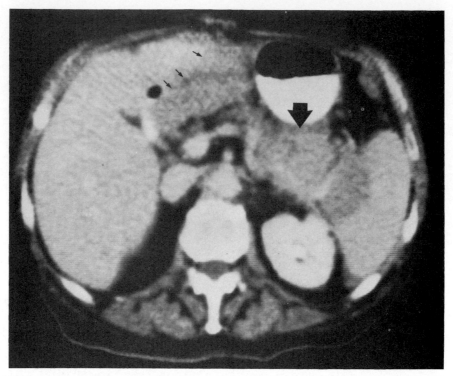

Figure 13–61. Gastric lymphoma (large arrow) invading the pancreas, spleen, and liver (small arrows). The lymphoma has a lower CT density than the surrounding liver parenchyma. (From Buy J-N, Moss AA: Computed tomography of gastric lymphoma. AJR 138:859, 1982. © 1982, American Roentgen Ray Society. Reprinted by permission.)

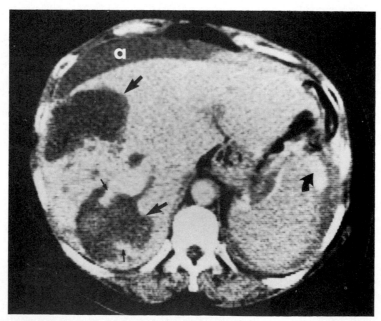

Figure 13–62. Hepatic angiosarcoma. Two foci of angiosarcoma (large arrows) are present in the right hepatic lobe. The periphery of the lesions (small arrows) enhances after contrast administration in a similar pattern to that found in hepatic hemangiomas. Bloody ascites (a) due to rupture of tumor is present. Angiosarcoma of spleen (curved arrow) is also present. (From Mahony B, Jeffrey RB, Federle MP: Spontaneous rupture of hepatic and splenic angiosarcoma demonstrated by CT. AJR 138:965, 1982. © 1982, American Roentgen Ray Society. Reprinted by permission.)

and lesions becoming isodense after contrast infusion.[124, 142, 168] The 4 to 12 per cent false-positive rate has been due to the inability of CT to distinguish inflammatory, regenerative, or fatty infiltrative lesions from metastatic deposits.[86, 124, 142, 168]

Noncontrast CT scans usually demonstrate metastases as single or multiple mass lesions having a CT density lower than surrounding normal hepatic parenchyma (Fig. 13–63A). Occasionally, metastatic disease will have a higher density than that of the surrounding liver (Fig. 13–63B). Most metastatic lesions appear as well-circumscribed, solid masses having attenuation numbers in the range of 15 to 45 H units; however, metastatic tumors can appear cystlike, have thin walls and a CT density close to zero (Fig. 13–34).[69, 102–104] Metastatic mucinous ovarian or colonic carcinoma, melanoma, leiomyosarcoma, lung, and carcinoid tumors are responsible for most cystic or necrotic hepatic metastasis (Figs. 13–34, 13–63A and 13–64).[69, 102–104, 171] Rarely, fluid-fluid levels can be identified in necrotic hepatic metastasis (Fig. 13–65)[171] and some metastatic lesions contain foci of calcification (Fig. 13–66).[69, 172, 173] Most frequently,

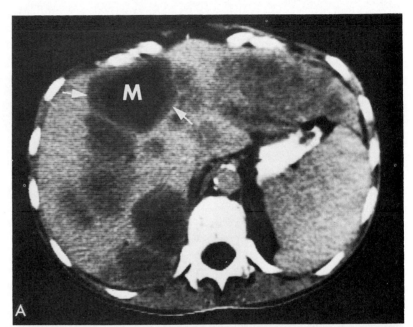

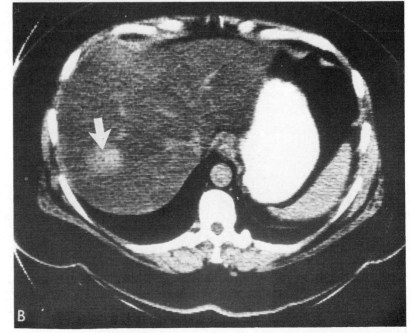

Figure 13–63. A Hepatic metastasis from leiomyosarcoma. There are multiple low-density hepatic masses, which appear well circumscribed. One metastasis (M) has a thick, irregular rim (arrows) and a very low density center due to tumor necrosis. **B** Metastatic carcinoid. The carcinoid metastasis (arrow) has a higher density than the surrounding liver, which is diffusely infiltrated by fat and has a CT density of 1 H.

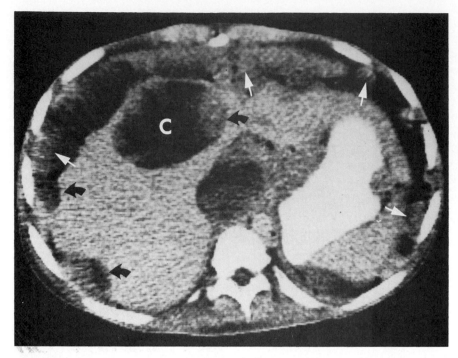

Figure 13–64. Ovarian carcinoma producing cystic (C) appearing hepatic metastasis. Typical of ovarian carcinoma is the subcapsular location (curved arrows) of the liver metastasis and the presence of peritoneal metastasis (arrows).

the foci of calcification are surrounded by a larger noncalcified zone of tumor, which permits distinction from benign calcified masses such as calcified granulomas.

The most commonly encountered metastatic tumor to the liver containing calcific deposits is mucinous colonic carcinoma. However, metastatic deposits from ovarian, breast, renal, pancreatic islet cell, neuroblastoma, leiomyosarcoma and melanoma may also be partially calcified.[69, 172, 173] As any tumor that undergoes necrosis may calcify, it is anticipated that additional calcified metastasis will be detected.

In screening for hepatic metastases, the CT examination should be initially performed without contrast administration, since a small percentage of metastatic lesions will be masked by the use of intravenous contrast.[67, 69] Intravenous infusion of

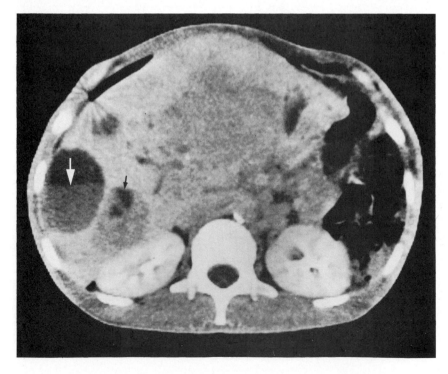

Figure 13–65. Hepatic metastasis with fluid-fluid level. A fluid-fluid level (large arrow) is present in a hepatic metastasis that has undergone necrosis. Other hepatic lesions have various densities from solid to partially cystic (small arrow). Primary tumor was adenocarcinoma of the colon.

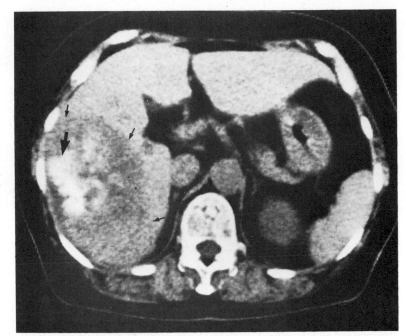

Figure 13–66. Mucinous colonic carcinoma metastatic to the liver. The calcified portion of the metastasis (large arrow) is surrounded by a larger, noncalcified zone of tumor (small arrows).

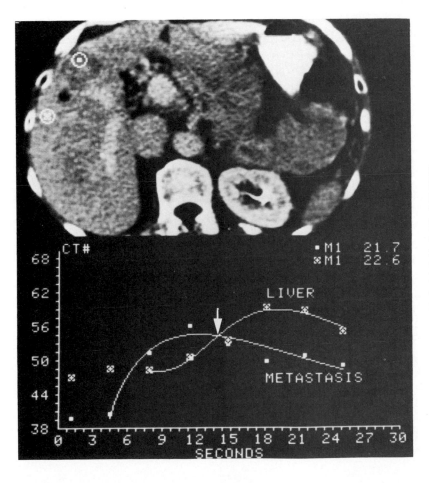

Figure 13–67. Time-density curve of hepatic metastasis and normal liver following an intravenous bolus injection. The colonic metastasis initially has a lower CT number than the liver. Its density increases rapidly to exceed normal liver 9 to 15 seconds after injection, becomes isodense (arrow) with liver, and then decreases in CT density as the attenuation of liver continues to increase.

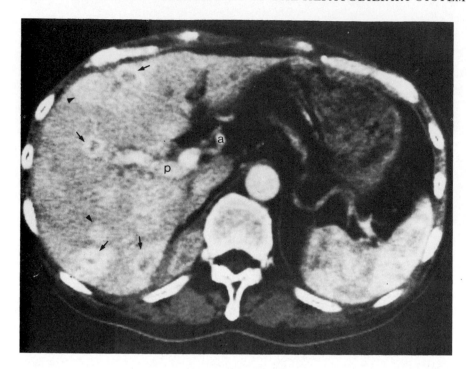

Figure 13–68. Renal cell carcinoma metastatic to liver. Dynamic CT scan demonstrates multiple metastatic foci (arrows), which have a rim of contrast enhancement. Other lesions are uniformly hyperdense (arrowheads). The inhomogeneity of the spleen is normal. p = Portal vein; a = hepatic artery.

contrast material will make some lesions more detectable (26 per cent), but in the majority (58 per cent), the lesions will be equally well demonstrated before and after the contrast infusion.[67] In fewer than 5 per cent of metastatic tumors, the lesion will be detected only following contrast infusion.[45, 67]

The value of dynamic CT scanning in detecting hepatic metastasis has not been determined. In a report by Marchal and associates, 44 of 46 lesions could be seen on precontrast CT scans, and in only two patients was contrast enhancement by bolus technique necessary to identify lesions.[62] The same authors reported minimal contrast enhancement in 68 per cent of patients, positive contrast enhancement in 9 per cent, and a mixed pattern in 23 per cent of 68 noncystic hepatic lesions.[45] In both reports, lesions were also noted to become isodense following bolus injections. A bolus of contrast material will have a varied effect on the detectability of liver metastasis,[45, 47, 48] depending on tumor cell type, vascularity, presence of necrosis, the ratio of tumor intracellular and extracellular compartments, and intravascular and interstitial fluid volumes.

A major limitation of current CT scanners is the restriction of being able to scan only a single level at one time. Thus, in order to survey the entire liver, a series of sequential dynamic scans at different levels must be performed. Because this is impractical, initial scans are performed without contrast medium, an appropriate level is selected and an 80- to 150-ml contrast bolus is injected, followed by a dynamic scan series at the preselected level. This is followed by a rapid infusion of contrast, and the entire liver is rapidly scanned before contrast equilibrium has been reached.

Despite the limitations of dynamic scan techniques for detection of metastatic lesions, rapid scanning procedures have provided better characterization of the patterns of time-density change of liver metastases (Figs. 13–18 and 13–67). The most common pattern identified by CT following a bolus injection of contrast material is a rim of contrast enhancement around a less dense central zone (Fig. 13–68). The rim of increased density may exist for only several seconds or persist for 30 seconds or longer. Other lesions become uniformly hyperdense (Figs. 13–18 and 13–67), and some metastatic foci exhibit no contrast enhancement (Fig. 13–34). The initial density of the lesion, cell type, and size are not consistently related to the degree or nature of the pattern of contrast enhancement.

Intra-arterial contrast injection produces an intensified pattern of contrast enhancement and may show metastatic deposits to be hyperdense when CT studies after intravenous bolus or infusion of contrast material demonstrate the metastasis to show little if any contrast enhancement (Fig. 13–69).[56, 72] The detection of hepatic metastatic disease is greatest following the administra-

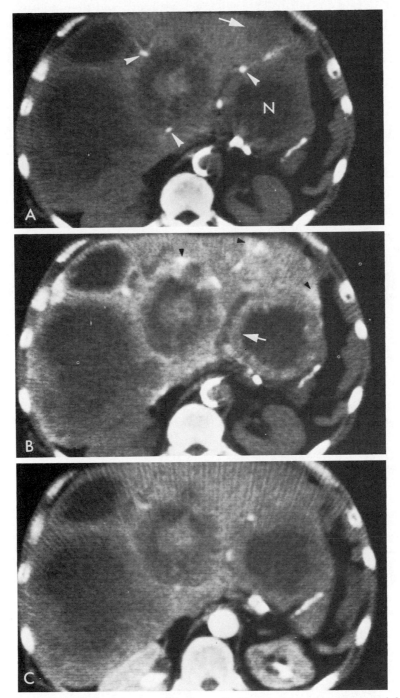

Figure 13–69. Metastatic leiomyosarcoma. **A**   Immediately after intrahepatic arterial injection, arterial vessels (arrowheads) are opacified. Hypodense metastatic lesions are identified, of which some appear necrotic (N) and some solid (arrow). **B**   Scan during peak arterial contrast demonstrates the rim of the necrotic metastasis (arrow) to have become isodense with normal liver while other foci of metastatic disease are intensely hyperdense (arrowheads). **C**   CT scan at peak arterial enhancement after intravenous bolus injection demonstrates hepatic arterial vessels but little evidence of marked contrast enhancement of the tumor.

tion of liposoluble contrast material (Fig. 13–16). Smaller lesions are detected with greater certainty, and the long period liposoluble material remains in the liver permits the entire liver to be thoroughly evaluated during peak contrast enhancement.

INFLAMMATORY MASSES

Pyogenic Abscess

Patients having a pyogenic liver abscess usually present with fever and abdominal pain, occasionally hepatomegaly, and rarely jaundice. Hepatic abscesses are readily detected as low-density masses with attenuation values typically between those of hepatic cysts and solid tumors (Fig. 13–70A).[18, 69]

This distinction between abscesses and cysts is not absolute as there is overlap between low-density neoplasms and high-density cysts. Approximately 20 to 30 per cent of pyogenic abscesses contain gas (Fig. 13–70B),[159] whereas amebic abscesses (Fig. 13–71) do not contain gas unless they have become secondarily infected.[174] Hepatic abscesses frequently have a well-defined outer margin, may have a thick capsule or irregular inner margins, and are most frequently located in the posterior aspect of the right hepatic lobe. Abscesses located in the subphrenic and subhepatic spaces or falciform ligament are also readily demonstrated by CT.[175, 176]

The wall of an hepatic abscess may enhance following intravenous contrast, but the central por-

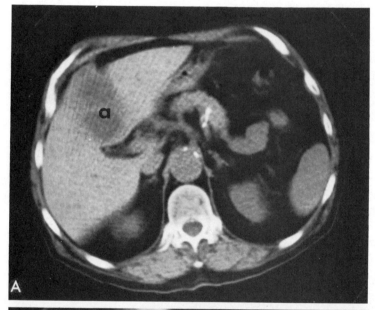

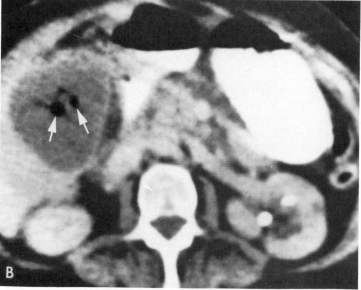

Figure 13–70. Hepatic abscess—pyogenic. **A** Typical hepatic abscess (a) appearing as low-density mass having an attenuation value of 20 H. **B** Hepatic abscess containing gas (arrows) following gallbladder surgery.

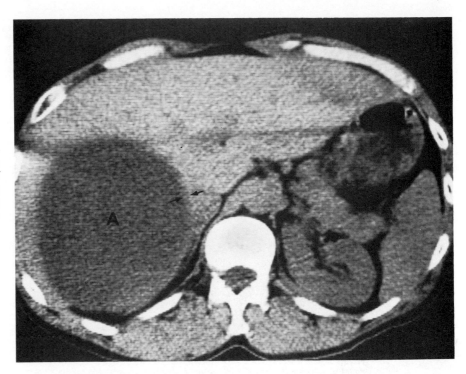

Figure 13–71. Hepatic abscess—amebic. A large amebic abscess (A) in the posterior aspect of the right hepatic lobe has a smooth outer margin, does not contain gas, and has a measurable capsule (arrows).

tion of a liquid abscess does not increase in density. When a low-density hepatic mass lesion enhances uniformly, it usually proves to be a focal area of inflammation[18] or a neoplasm and not a hepatic abscess. Re-formation of axial images into coronal or sagittal planes aides in distinguishing subphrenic and subhepatic abscesses from intrahepatic lesions.

CT has become the imaging procedure of choice for directing percutaneous drainage of hepatic abscesses (Fig. 13–72), obtaining material for culture, and determining the number and exact location of abscesses and degree of resolution of a medically treated abscess.

Hydatid Disease

Hydatid disease is caused by the larval stage of either *Echinococcus granulosus* or *Echinococcus alveolaris*.[177–180] Infection by *E. granulosus* is prevalent in Australia, New Zealand, southern Europe, North Africa, South America, and the Near and Middle East. *E. alveolaris* infection is found in central Europe, Russia, Alaska, Japan, and the United States. In both forms, the liver is the most frequently involved organ.[179]

Echinococcus involvement of the liver produces a variety of clinical symptoms including epigastric and right upper abdominal pain, hepatomegaly, fever, and fixed or intermittent jaundice. Usually, the general condition of patients is good, and the

diagnosis in nonendemic areas is suspected only when plain abdominal radiographs reveal a calcified cyst.

E. granulosus produces lesions that tend to form well-delineated cysts that grow by gradual expansion. On CT scans, *E. granulosus* lesions appear as sharply marginated single or multiple cystic masses having a CT density varying between 3 and 30 H (Fig. 13–73).[177–180] The surrounding wall of the cyst frequently is partially or entirely calcified (Fig. 13–73); when not calcified, it is identified as a rim of higher density. Daughter cysts can be seen within the interior of the larger cysts as miniature cysts, each surrounded by its own cyst wall. Although the identification of daughter cysts is virtually pathognomonic for *E. granulosus* infestation, other multiloculated cystic masses may simulate hepatic echinococcosis.[181] Air fluid levels may be found in echinococcal cysts that have become secondarily infected or have ruptured into the gastrointestinal tract.[179, 180]

The CT appearance of hydatid disease due to *E. alveolaris* is different from that caused by *E. granulosus*. *E. alveolaris* produces geographic, infiltrating lesions without sharp margins or dense rims.[179] The lesions have the appearance and attenuation values (14 to 38 H) of low-density, solid mass lesions rather than cysts. True cystic structures are rare. Calcification is amorphous or nodular, never ringlike, and the infection frequently extends by direct extension to the abdominal wall,

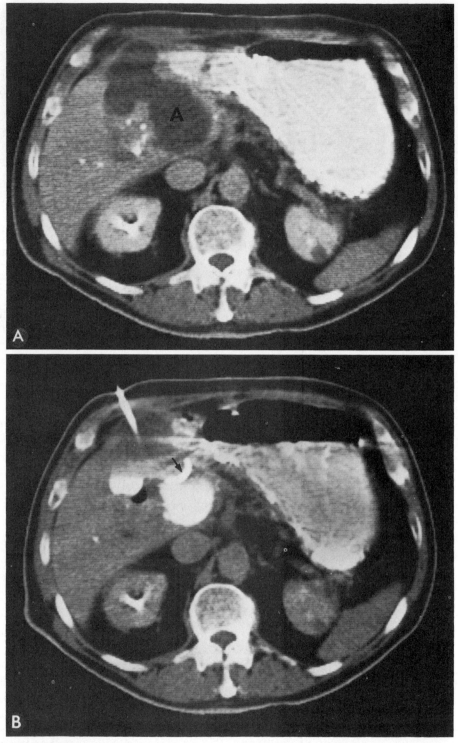

Figure 13–72. Drainage of intrahepatic abscess. **A** CT scan demonstrating an irregularly shaped hepatic abscess (A). **B** Pigtail catheter (arrow) was placed under CT guidance into the abscess for therapeutic drainage. Contrast material injected into the abscess fills the entire abscess cavity, excluding loculations of pus that do not communicate with the main abscess cavity.

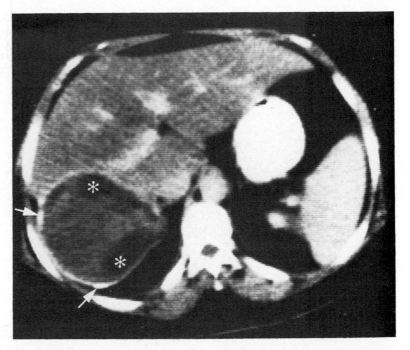

Figure 13–73. Echinococcal disease of the liver. A well-marginated, single cystic lesion with a partially calcified cyst wall (arrows) due to *Echinococcus granulosus* is present in the right hepatic lobe. The noncalcified portion of rim enhances after contrast administration. Daughter cysts (asterisk) are present along the inner margin of the echinococcal abscess.

diaphragm, or porta hepatis. The CT appearance of hepatic *E. alveolaris* infection is not pathognomonic, since it closely resembles an infiltrating hepatic malignancy.

Schistosomiasis japonica

Infestation with *Schistosoma japonicum* results from ova penetrating and obstructing the portal vein branches. The ova are deposited in the larger radicals and produce a fine or coarse hepatic fibrosis in the smaller portal tracts.[182] Marked fibrosis can result in a geographic pattern of calcification. The linear bandlike calcifications are more prevalent in the other third of the liver and are not usually seen on conventional radiographs.

Fungal Abscesses

Hepatic abscesses resulting from fungal infections are uncommon and usually occur in patients who have compromised immunologic systems. Although large single or multiple hepatic abscesses due to fungal infections occur, a pattern of multiple microabscesses has been more frequently observed in patients with acute myelogenous and lymphocytic leukemia.[183]

CT scans demonstrate multiple small, rounded, low-density lesions, some of which have a central higher density foci, thus giving the abscess a target appearance (Fig. 13–74A). The abscesses are scattered rather uniformly throughout the liver, spleen, and in some cases the kidneys. Blood cultures are usually negative, but smears of CT guided aspirates will demonstrate hyphae typical of the fungus *Candida albicans*. CT scans after therapy have demonstrated resolution of the abscesses in some patients (Fig. 13–74B) and progression in others. Although pyogenic hepatic abscesses in immunosuppressed patients are not rare, when multiple microabscesses are found scattered throughout the entire liver, infection with *Candida albicans* should be strongly considered as the etiologic agent.

TRAUMA

Traumatic injuries to the liver can occur as the result of blunt or penetrating abdominal trauma and as complications of surgery, percutaneous cholangiography, biopsy, portography, or biliary drainage procedures.[69, 184–192] Injuries include intrahepatic and subcapsular hematoma, laceration, frank hepatic fracture, hepatic necrosis, bile pseudocyst, pseudoaneurysm, arteriovenous and arterioportal fistula, and intraperitoneal hemorrhage.

The most common hepatic injuries are lacerations and subcapsular and intrahepatic hematomas resulting from blunt abdominal trauma, percutaneous transhepatic cholangiography, or liver biopsy (Figs. 13–35 and 13–75).[184, 186, 189–192] Subcapsular hematomas usually appear as crescentic- or lenticular-shaped, well-marginated, low-density fluid collections, located just beneath the hepatic capsule (Fig. 13–75A). Intrahepatic hematomas produce round-to-oval collections within the he-

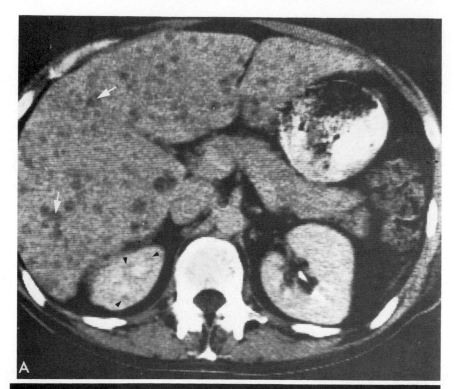

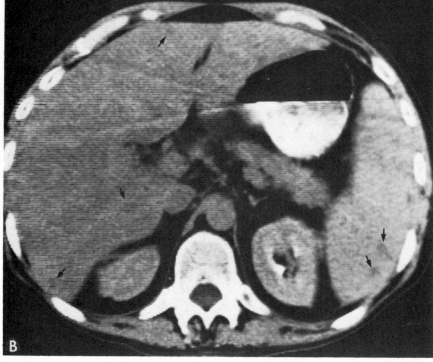

Figure 13–74. Fungal abscesses in immunosuppressed patient with leukemia. **A** Multiple small, rounded abscesses are present throughout the liver (arrows) and kidneys (arrowheads) and, at a higher level, the spleen. Some abscesses have a central focus of higher density (arrows), giving the abscess a target or bull's-eye appearance. **B** CT scan following treatment demonstrates resolution of most of the abscesses. Several small abscesses are still present in the spleen and liver (arrows).

patic parenchyma (Fig. 13–35).[184, 186, 190] Hepatic lacerations appear as irregular-shaped clefts or masses with the liver parenchyma, which often extend to the periphery of the liver (Fig. 13–75B). As elsewhere in the body, recent hemorrhage and clot have a higher density than older hematomas that have matured.

Diffuse hepatic necrosis produces an irregular mottled, parenchymal defect that enhances slightly after intravenous contrast.[184] Bile pseudocysts result from biliary duct disruption and resemble extrapancreatic pseudocysts (Fig. 13–76).

Hepatic artery pseudoaneurysm[185] and arteriovenous[187] or arterioportal[188] fistulae are all potential sequelae of hepatic vascular injury. The CT diagnosis of a traumatic pseudoaneurysm may be suggested by identifying a mass which markedly enhances after a bolus injection of contrast mateial.[185] However, the diagnosis should be confirmed by a hepatic arteriogram.

Identification of arteriovenous and arterioportal fistulae is usually not possible on unenhanced CT scans.[187, 188] A dynamic scan sequence following a bolus injection of contrast material will best demonstrate the arterial communication with the hepatic venous or portal system (Fig. 13–77).

Traumatic hepatic injuries are less frequent than those of the kidney or spleen, but they have a higher mortality. If a patient's condition does not demand immediate surgery, CT should be performed to accurately define the nature and extent of the hepatic injury. Certain types of limited hepatic injuries such as small subcapsular hematomas can be managed conservatively, whereas most lacerations, pseudoaneurysms, large fistulae, and intrahepatic hematomas are best treated surgically.

BILIARY TRACT ABNORMALITIES

Jaundice is a common clinical problem with a variety of etiologies. Most frequently, jaundice is due to hepatocellular disease (medical—nonob-

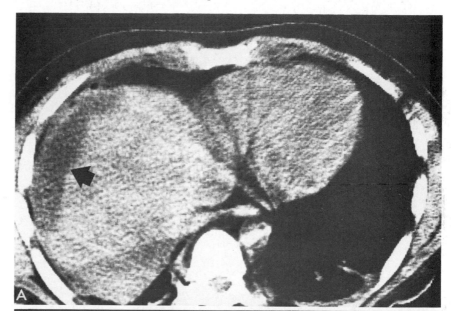

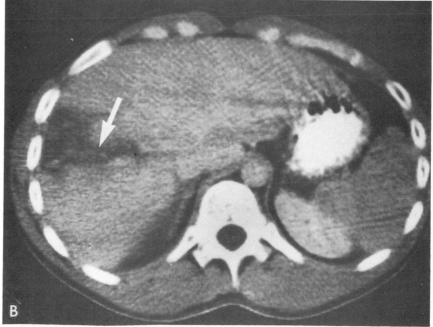

Figure 13–75. A Hepatic subcapsular hematoma producing a crescent-shaped, low-density mass (arrow) conforming to lateral margin of liver. **B** Hepatic laceration and intrahepatic hematoma demonstrated as a horizontal, irregularly shaped, low-density lesion (arrow).

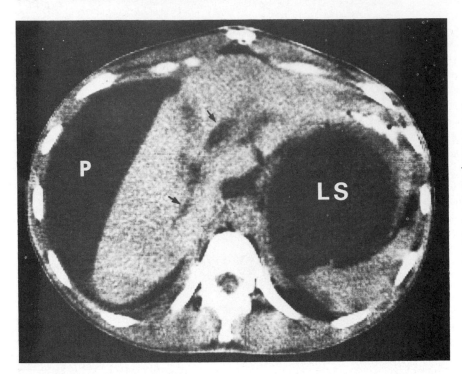

Figure 13–76. Blunt abdominal trauma. There is bile in the lesser sac (LS) and peritoneal cavity (P) resulting from bile duct injury. Dilated bile ducts (arrows) are due to clot obstructing the distal common bile duct. (From Federle MP, Goldberg HI, Kaiser JA, Moss AA, Jeffrey RB, Mall JC: Evaluation of abdominal trauma by computed tomography. Radiology 138:637, 1981. Used with permission.)

structive jaundice), but biliary tract obstruction (surgical—obstructive jaundice) secondary to neoplasm, calculi, trauma, or inflammation is also common. Distinction between obstructive and nonobstructive causes of jaundice can usually be made on the basis of history, physical examination and laboratory studies. However, there remains a group of patients in whom the differentiation is difficult and requires an additional diagnostic procedure for definitive diagnosis.

Both ultrasonography and computed tomography have been advocated as the initial procedure for evaluating the icteric patient.[18, 164, 193, 194] Because both modalities have proved to be equally accurate in separating obstructive from nonobstructive jaundice,[164, 193] the choice of which to employ is best made on the basis of availability and accessibility of equipment and upon the skill and experience of the radiologist. When both ultrasound and computed tomography are available, ultrasound is preferred as the initial screening procedure because of its low cost, lack of ionizing radiation, and high accuracy in detecting gallstones. CT is employed whenever the ultrasonographic findings are in question, when a mass lesion is suspected, when the distal common duct is not clearly shown, when a segmental obstruction is suspected, or when a hepatic parenchymal abnormality is identified.

The reported accuracy of computed tomography in differentiating obstructive from nonobstructive jaundice has ranged from 87 to more

than 98 per cent.[18, 65, 163, 193] False-negative CT studies occur in patients with normal-sized intrahepatic ducts and only minimal dilatation of the common bile duct.[162, 193] Typically, this occurs in patients with cirrhosis or sclerosing cholangitis, when periductal fibrosis restricts the ease with which intrahepatic bile ducts can dilate.

Normal portal venous structures can simulate dilated bile ducts.[19] Distinction of portal venous structures from dilated biliary radicles can usually be made by observing the density of the branching structures and comparing it with those of the aorta and inferior vena cava. The attenuation value of a dilated biliary system will be lower than the aorta and vena cava, whereas the portal vein will have a CT density virtually identical with the great vessels. In difficult cases, injection of contrast material produces pronounced enhancement of the intrahepatic vascular system, thus permitting easy differentiation between vascular structures and dilated bile ducts.

The biliary tract dilates to the point of obstruction; thus intrahepatic biliary radicles, the common hepatic duct, common bile duct and gallbladder may be enlarged, depending upon the location and severity of obstruction. Dilated intrahepatic biliary radicles appear as multiple, branching, low-density structures within the liver (Fig. 13–78A). The dilated left biliary system is often horizontal and linear in configuration, whereas the right biliary radicles, seen more in cross section, appear round or oval in

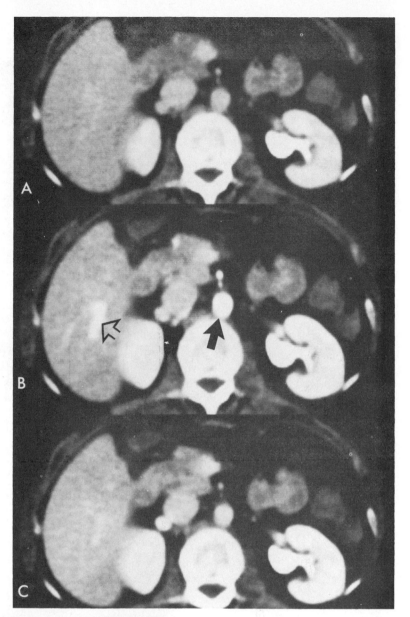

Figure 13–77. Hepatic artery–portal vein fistula secondary to liver biopsy. Composite of selected images from dynamic CT scan sequence through right lobe of liver at level of hepatic arterio-portal vein fistula. **A** Baseline scan just prior to injection reveals normal liver. **B** Scan during peak aortic enhancement (solid arrow) reveals right portal vein (open arrow) to be opacified at the same moment. **C** Twenty-four seconds after the bolus is administered the liver again appears normal (From Axel L, Moss AA, Berninger W: Dynamic computed tomography demonstration of hepatic arteriovenous fistula. J Comput Assist Tomogr 5:95, 1981. Reprinted by permission.)

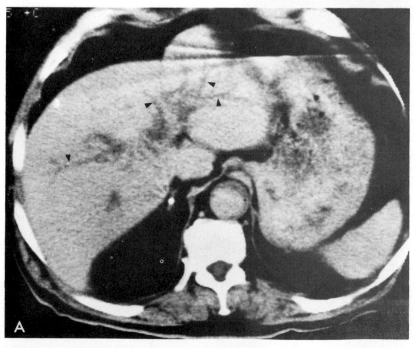

Figure 13–78. Obstructive jaundice CT scans at various levels. **A** Intrahepatic level: Dilated intrahepatic ducts (arrowheads) are demonstrated as multiple, branching, low-density tubular structures.

Illustration continued on following page

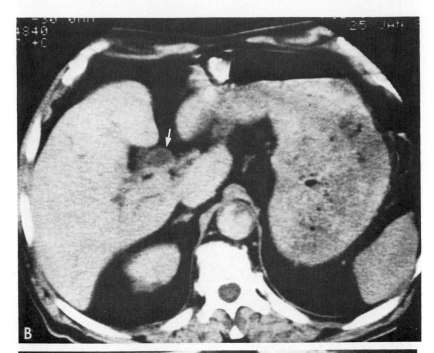

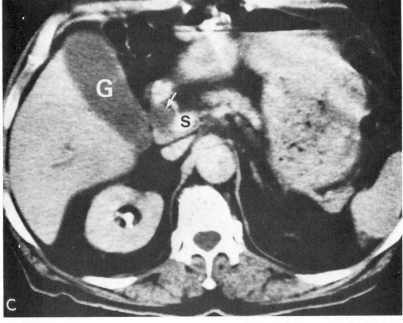

Figure 13–78. *Continued* **B** CT scan above the level of the gallbladder. A dilated common hepatic duct (arrow) is seen in the porta hepatis. **C** Scan at the level of the gallbladder (G) demonstrates a dilated common bile duct (arrow) just lateral to the superior mesenteric vein (S) in the head of the pancreas.

Illustration continued on opposite page

shape.[18, 162, 164, 195] The dilated common hepatic and common bile duct are identified as round or oval low-density structures in the region of the porta hepatis or head of the pancreas (Fig. 78*B*–*E*).[164] Although absolute measurements are often meaningless, an extrahepatic bile duct larger than 1 cm should be considered to be dilated[162, 195] and a duct less than 6 mm to be normal.[21, 162] A CT measurement of 10 mm has been shown to be equal to a direct cholangiographic measurement of 12 mm.[162] A definitive diagnosis of extrahepatic biliary obstruction is usually not possible in patients having an extrahepatic bile duct measurement of between 6 mm to 10 mm unless the intrahepatic bile ducts are dilated.

CT has an accuracy of 80 to 97 per cent in determining the level of obstruction in patients with obstructive jaundice.[161, 162, 164, 193, 195–198] Pedrosa and colleagues,[164] using contiguous sections 1 cm thick, divided the dilated biliary system into four anatomic segments: hepatic, suprapancreatic, pancreatic, and ampullary. The level of obstruction could be accurately determined in 97 per cent of cases by counting the number of contig-

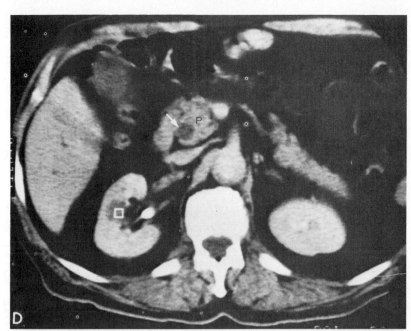

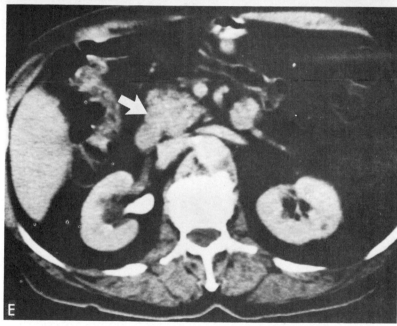

Figure 13–78. *Continued* **D** Scan 2 cm distal to **C**. The dilated common bile duct (arrow) is still seen in the head of the pancreas (P). **E** Scan 1 cm distal to **D** reveals a solid mass (arrow) in the head of the pancreas producing an abrupt obstruction of the dilated common bile duct. Diagnosis: Pancreatic carcinoma.

uous CT sections in which a dilated common hepatic and common bile duct could be identified. Obstruction in the porta hepatis just distal to the junction of the right and left hepatic ducts produces localized dilation of the intrahepatic ducts[161, 164] and proximal common hepatic duct (Fig. 13–79). Suprapancreatic obstruction results in one or two scans showing a dilated common hepatic duct or common bile duct. Biliary obstruction present on three to six sections indicates obstruction at the level of the distal common bile duct (Fig. 13–78) and if detected on seven or

eight sections, the obstruction is at the ampullary level.[164]

In daily practice, continuity between the common bile duct, common hepatic duct and intrahepatic radicles can usually be demonstrated on serial CT scans in cases of distal common bile duct obstruction (Fig. 13–78) and only rarely will an obstruction of the common bile duct be present without intrahepatic ductal dilatation.[18, 198, 164, 196] Demonstration of an enlarged gallbladder (greater than 5 cm in diameter) usually indicates obstruction distal to the cystic duct,

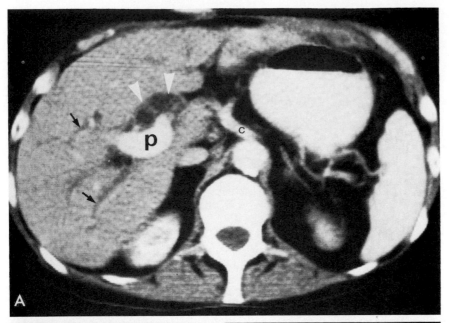

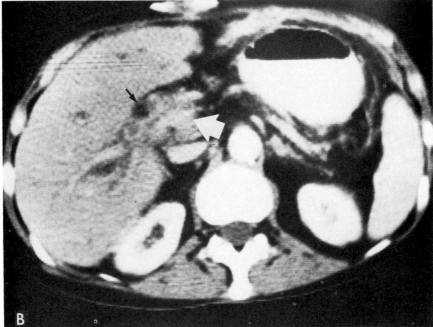

Figure 13–79. Obstructive jaundice secondary to obstruction in porta hepatis. **A** Dilated intrahepatic (arrows) and common hepatic duct (arrowheads). The common hepatic duct appears as a tubular horizontal structure because it is sectioned along its longitudinal axis. P = portal vein; c = celiac axis. **B** Scan at slightly more caudal level demonstrates the top of the mass in the porta hepatis (large arrow) and the dilated common hepatic duct (small arrow). **C** Transhepatic cholangiogram confirms biliary obstruction at level of common hepatic duct. Diagnosis: Pancreatic carcinoma spreading to hilus of the liver.

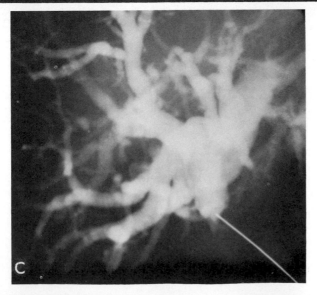

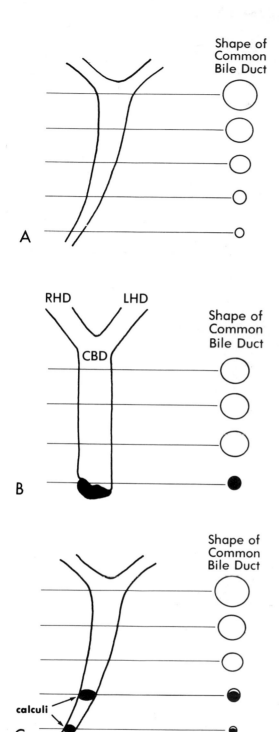

and lack of gallbladder enlargement in patients with intrahepatic ductal dilatation points to a level of obstruction above the cystic duct (Fig. 13–79).

In addition to demonstrating bile duct obstruction and determining the level of obstruction, CT can determine the cause of obstructive jaundice in 75 to 94 per cent of cases.[163, 164, 199] The detection of bile duct calculi, the size of the dilated bile duct, the shape of the distal end of the obstructed duct, and the level of obstruction aid in determining the cause of obstructive jaundice. Multiplanar

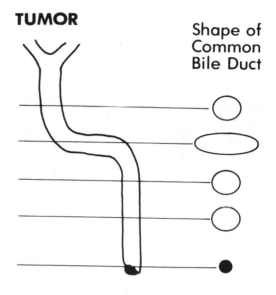

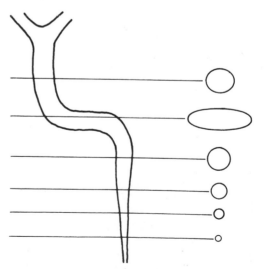

Figure 13–80. Diagrams of CT findings in obstructive jaundice due to different etiologic factors. **A** Pancreatitis produces a moderately dilated biliary system and a common bile duct which tapers gradually. **B** Tumor causes marked biliary dilatation and a common bile duct which does not taper but abruptly changes caliber. The distal margin of the common bile duct is often irregular. **C** A bile duct calculus usually results only in mild biliary dilatation and a common bile duct that tapers gradually until the level of the calculus. The calculus is seen as a high-density, rounded mass giving a crescent-shaped appearance to the distal bile duct.

Figure 13–81. Diagram of the course of the extrahepatic biliary system when markedly dilated due to tumor or pancreatitis. The common hepatic or common bile duct can assume a horizontal course, which causes the duct to have an oval or elliptical shape on axial CT scans.

reconstruction adds information concerning the cause of obstruction in 27 per cent of cases.[200] The most frequent lesions producing obstructive jaundice are biliary duct calculi, chronic pancreatitis, and either pancreatic or biliary ductal carcinoma. Each produces a typical appearance of the extrahepatic bile duct (Fig. 13–80).

Pancreatitis typically produces a minimally to moderately dilated common bile duct that smoothly tapers to a fusiform distal duct (Fig. 13–80A). Associated findings are evidence of calcific pancreatitis (50 per cent) and a normal-size gallbladder (71 per cent).[160]

An abrupt change in caliber of a markedly dilated bile duct to one that is undetectable is most often due to a malignant lesion (Figs. 13–78 and 13–80B). The terminal bile duct may be rounded, irregular, or nipple-shaped. Associated CT features of malignant lesions are porta hepatis (Fig. 13–79) or pancreatic masses (Fig. 13–78), gallbladder dilatation, dilatation of the common hepatic or common bile duct which is so marked that it courses in a horizontal plane for part of its length (Figs. 13–79 and 13–81), and invasion of vessels and retroperitoneal structures.[160]

An impacted common bile duct calculus also results in an abrupt occlusion of the common bile duct. However, the dilatation is usually only mild to moderate, with the duct tapering slightly, and in 82 to 90 per cent of cases, the calculi are visible (Figs. 13–80C and 13–82).[160, 200a, 201] Common duct calculi can be densely calcified or can have a den-

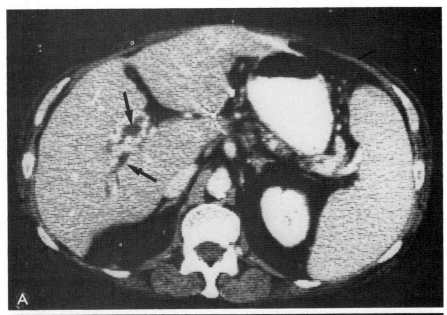

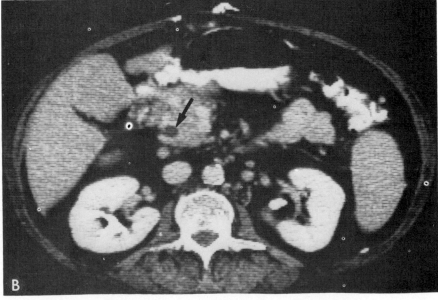

Figure 13–82. Obstructive jaundice resulting from common bile duct calculi. **A** Scan through the porta hepatis demonstrates dilated intrahepatic bile ducts (arrows). **B** A dilated distal common bile duct (arrow) is identified in the head of the pancreas.

Illustration continued on opposite page

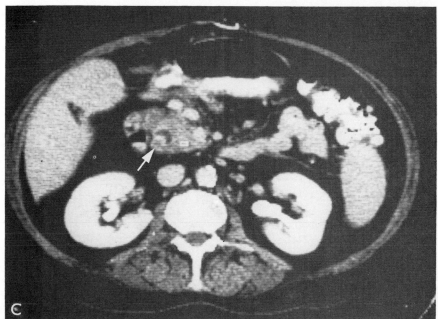

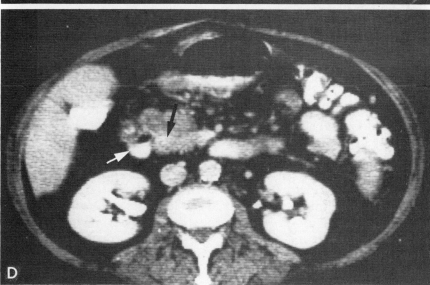

Figure 13–82. *Continued* **C** Scan just distal to **B** demonstrates crescent sign produced by common bile duct calculi (arrow) partially blocking the common bile duct. Cursor box=head of pancreas. **D** Scan 1 cm below **C**. The calculus (black arrow) is seen as a high-density structure impacted and totally occluding the distal common bile duct. The relationship of the distal calculi to the duodenum (white arrow) is also shown.

sity just barely above the adjacent structures.[160, 200a] A pure cholesterol calculi produces an obstruction having a lower attenuation value than that of bile.

Segmental biliary obstruction is most frequently caused by calculi, primary hepatic and biliary tumors, metastatic disease, gallbladder carcinoma, surgical mistakes, chronic or recurrent pyogenic cholangitis, abscesses and traumatic injury.[193, 197, 201, 202, 202a] Intrahepatic calculi are rare in the United States but common in Japan and China.[201, 202a] Intrahepatic calculi appear as high-density, rounded lesions in dilated intrahepatic ducts (Fig. 13–83).

Primary hepatic (Fig. 13–52)[193] and metastatic tumors[197] can produce dilated biliary radicles pe-

ripheral to the area of neoplastic involvement. The remaining liver and common bile duct are normal and these patients may or may not be jaundiced. In long-standing segmental biliary obstruction, atrophy of the obstructed part of the liver and hypertrophy of the normal liver can occur.[202] Crowding together of dilated bile ducts is a clue that atrophy of the obstructed segment of liver has occurred.[202]

CONGENITAL ABNORMALITIES
Choledochal Cyst

Choledochal cyst is a congenital dilatation of the common bile duct and is most frequently seen in females of oriental races.[159] It predisposes to cholangitis, biliary calculi, and cholangiocarci-

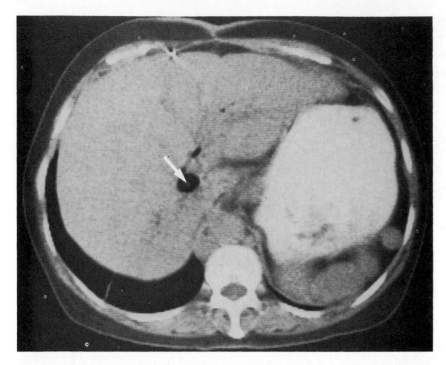

Figure 13–83. Retained intrahepatic biliary calculi shown as a high-density structure (arrow) within air-filled dilated biliary radicle following surgery.

noma and classically presents with jaundice, pain, and a palpable abdominal mass.[159, 203] However, because few patients present with the complete triad, a choledochal cyst should be considered in all patients having right upper-quadrant pain or a mass with or without jaundice.

In patients with a choledochal cyst, CT can demonstrate the nature of the cyst and display the size and extent of the abnormality. The extrahepatic biliary ducts are always dilated,[159, 203] and cystic dilatation of the central part of the left and right main hepatic ducts is also common. Intrahepatic duct dilatation is present in 60 per cent of patients with choledochal cysts. In contrast to acquired dilatation, there is absence of peripheral duct dilatation, gradual tapering toward the hepatic periphery, and abrupt changes in duct caliber at the junction with normal ducts. As cholangiocarcinoma develops in 4 to 7 per cent of patients with a choledochal cyst, a careful search for a solid mass lesion should be performed in all patients and, in particular, in those having evidence of intrahepatic duct obstruction.[159]

Communicating Cavernous Ectasia (Caroli's Disease)

Caroli's disease is a rare congenital abnormality of the biliary tract. It is characterized by either sacular dilatation of the intrahepatic bile ducts, cholangitis, and calculi formation, with absence of cirrhosis and portal hypertension or proliferation of small intrahepatic canaliculi, fibrosis, cirrhosis, portal hypertension, and absence of cholangitis, stone formation and ductal dilation.[204]

Renal tubular abnormalities are almost invariably present, ranging from benign tubular ectasia to severe ectasia resulting in medullary sponge kidney. Cysts of varying sizes can be present in the medulla, cortex, and corticomedullary region. The abnormality is inherited as an autosomal recessive trait in contrast to polycystic liver and renal disease, which is transmitted as an autosomal dominant. The clinical manifestations of Caroli's disease depend on whether the predominant lesion is fibrosis or bile duct dilatation. Portal hypertension, cirrhosis, and variceal bleeding occur when hepatic fibrosis is predominant, and fever, pain and jaundice occur when intrahepatic biliary dilatation, bile stasis, and cholangitis predominate.[204]

In patients with the dilated ductal form of Caroli's disease, CT can make the diagnosis in virtually every case. CT demonstrates multiple-branching, low-density, tubular structures that extend to the periphery of the liver and communicate with localized, ectatic cystic areas (Fig. 13–84).[204] Distinction from polycystic liver disease is possible when the cystic lesions can be shown to directly communicate with the biliary system. In polycystic liver disease, the cysts deform but do not communicate with the bile ducts. Differentiation from biliary obstruction is usually possible because biliary obstruction results in dilatation of the bile ducts, which is more pronounced centrally and does not produce areas of biliary ectasia.

When hepatic fibrosis predominates, the CT findings are those of cirrhosis. Depending on the severity of the disease, the liver may be small, normal or enlarged. Splenomegaly, ascites, and dilated portal and splenic veins may be present. The diagnosis of Caroli's disease should be suggested when cirrhosis in association with renal cystic disease occurs in a young patient who is not an alcoholic.[204]

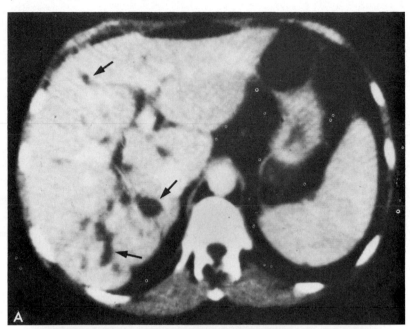

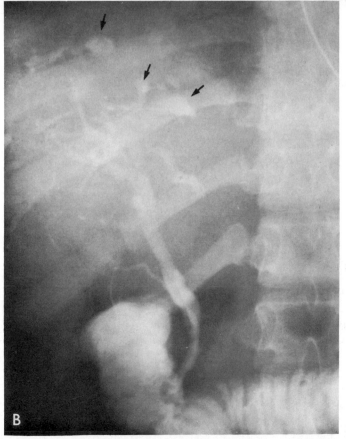

Figure 13–84. Caroli's disease. **A** CT scan demonstrating multiple branching, low-density tubular structures that extend to the periphery of the liver and communicate with localized, ectatic cystic areas (arrows). **B** Percutaneous transhepatic cholangiogram confirms presence of dilated communicating saccular intrahepatic bile ducts (arrows) typical of Caroli's disease. The extrahepatic biliary tract is normal. (Case courtesy of J. Kaiser, M.D.) (From Kaiser JA, Mall JC, Salmen BJ, Parker JJ: Diagnosis of Caroli disease by computed tomography: Report of two cases. Radiology 132:661, 1979. Reprinted by permission.)

MISCELLANEOUS ABNORMALITIES

Portal Vein Thrombosis

Thrombosis of the portal vein may be secondary to neoplasm (Figs. 13–53 and 13–85), infection, cirrhosis, or trauma. Chronic portal vein thrombosis often produces perihepatic portal hypertension and results in splenomegaly, enlarged collateral venous channels and gastroesophageal varices.[205] CT demonstrates portal vein thrombosis as a rounded filling defect within the portal vein that does not enhance after administration of contrast media.[205, 206] The thrombus is frequently surrounded by a peripheral ring of enhancement following contrast administration (Fig. 13–85), and enlarged collateral venous channels and varices are often demonstrated. CT may also reveal extension of the thrombus back into the splenic and superior mesenteric veins. In incomplete or branch occlusion of the portal vein, following a bolus injection of contrast material, there may be a transient segmental decrease in hepatic enhancement to the segment or segments of liver that are supplied by the occluded portal vein branches.

Cruveilhier-Baumgarten Syndrome

The Cruveilhier-Baumgarten syndrome is characterized by an enlarged spleen, distended paraumbilical veins, and esophageal varices.[207] The syndrome is a reflection of portal hypertension secondary to many etiologies, the most common being cirrhosis. There is recanalization of the umbilical vein, and blood is shunted from the portal system to superficial epigastric veins in the abdominal wall leading to formation of a caput medusa.[207] CT clearly demonstrates the enlarged patent umbilical vein and caput medusa following intravenous contrast injection (Fig. 13–24).[207]

ARTERIOVENOUS SHUNTS

Either hepatic artery–hepatic vein or hepatic artery–portal vein shunts occur in disorders such as hepatomas (Fig. 13–53), hemangiosarcomas, vascular metastasis, angiodysplastic malformations,[208] and as sequelae of percutaneous transhepatic procedures, needle biopsy and blunt abdominal trauma. In patients with hereditary hemorrhagic telangiectasia, CT demonstrates enlarged hepatic arteries and filling of the hepatic veins prior to portal filling without evidence of an hepatic tumor.[208] Most other causes result in hepatic masses (hepatoma, metastases, sarcomas, lacerations) that are detected in addition to the rapid arteriovenous shunting of contrast material. Dynamic CT scan techniques best display the rapid shunting of blood, and dynamic flow curve analysis is useful for displaying the rapid chain of events.[187]

Hepatic Arterial Occlusion

Usually, hepatic arterial occlusion is idiopathic, but it has been associated with surgery, trauma, embolization, generalized occlusive vascular disease, mycotic aneurysms, periarteritis nodosa, and metastatic carcinoma.[209] Rarely, hepatic arterial thrombosis occurs following pregnancy.

Abrupt central hepatic arterial occlusion can result in massive hepatic infarction, which CT demonstrates as hepatomegaly with numerous, sharply

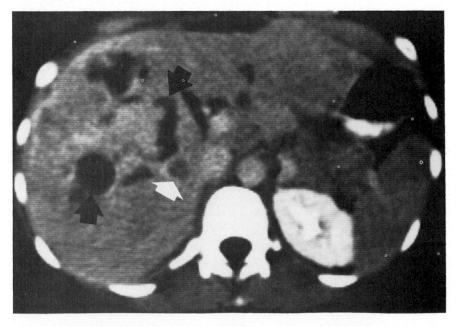

Figure 13–85. Portal vein thrombosis. Hepatoma producing bile duct obstruction (black arrows) and thrombosis of the posterior branch of the right portal vein (white arrow). Note the ring of contrast enhancement surrounding the thrombosed portal vein.

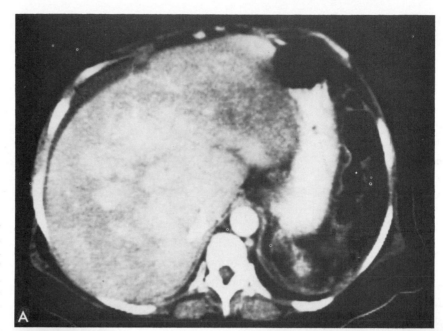

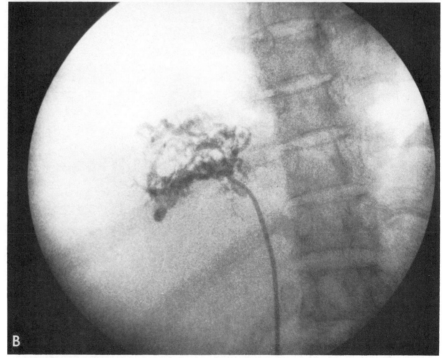

Figure 13–86. Budd-Chiari syndrome: hepatic vein obstruction secondary to polycythemia rubra vera. **A** CT scan following 60 ml bolus of contrast material demonstrates a patchy, fan-shaped, enhancing pattern typical of hepatic vein obstruction. Flow through the liver is slow and consistent with venous outflow obstruction. **B** Hepatic venogram demonstrating hepatic venous occlusion and pattern of collateral veins. (From Harter LP, Gross B, St Hilaire J, Filly RA, Goldberg HI: Computed tomographic and ultrasonic appearance of hepatic vein obstruction. AJR 139:176, 1982. © 1982, American Roentgen Ray Society. Reprinted by permission.)

demarcated areas of reduced density that do not enhance after contrast injection.[209] If the patient survives, the hepatic artery usually recanalizes and the liver returns to normal. Doppman and co-workers[210] reported bile cysts in a patient with periarteritis nodosa and multiple occlusions of peripheral hepatic arteries. A causative relationship was postulated and substantiated when experimental occlusion of peripheral hepatic arterial branches in rhesus monkeys led to focal hepatic infarction and subsequent bile cyst formation. The cysts communicated with the biliary tree and closely resembled the bile cysts seen in Caroli's disease.

Hepatic Venous Occlusion (Budd-Chiari Syndrome)

Budd-Chiari syndrome is a rare clinical entity associated with hypercoagulopathy states, oral contraceptives, leukemia, invading tumors, and congenital hepatic webs.[211] Clinically, patients are frequently asymptomatic presenting only with hepatosplenomegaly. CT reveals a patchy area of increased attenuation radiating from the retrohepatic portion of the inferior vena cava in a fanlike distribution (Fig. 13–86). The early scans in a dynamic CT scan sequence demonstrate poor contrast enhancement in the central portion of the liver. Later scans reveal increased attenuation in unobstructed collateral veins, which persist as high-density structures (Fig. 13–86). The enhancement pattern in the central portion of the liver has the same time-course as seen in hepatic hemangiomas. The caudate lobe that drains directly into the inferior vena cava is usually not involved in the Budd-Chiari syndrome and has a normal pattern of contrast enhancement.

GALLBLADDER DISEASE

GALLBLADDER CARCINOMA

Carcinoma of the gallbladder ranks fifth in incidence among malignant tumors of the accessory digestive organs.[212, 213] It occurs primarily in the sixth and seventh decades of life and is fourfold more common in women. Gallstones and chronic cholecystitis are found in 65 to 95 per cent of patients with carcinoma of the gallbladder. Oral cholecystography will demonstrate nonopacification of the gallbladder but cannot make a definite

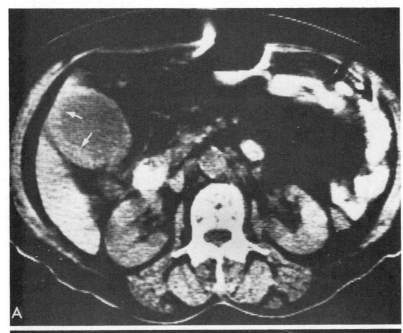

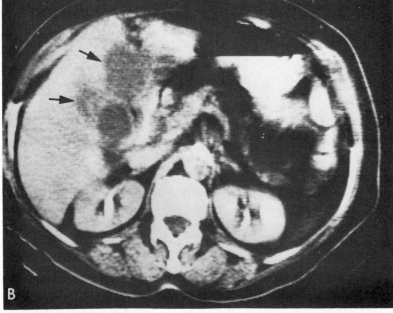

Figure 13–87. Carcinoma of the gallbladder. **A** The wall of the gallbladder is asymmetrically thickened (arrows). **B** Postcontrast CT scan at more cephalic level demonstrates an irregular mass (arrows) that extends into the liver.

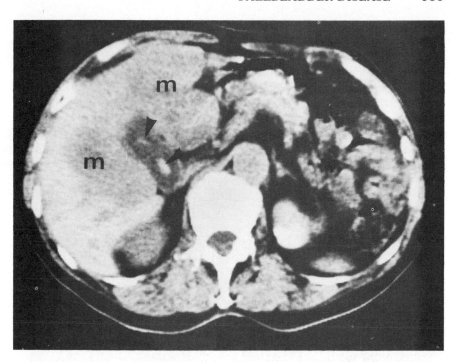

Figure 13–88. Carcinoma of the gallbladder. Gallbladder containing calculi (arrowheads) is surrounded by a large intrahepatic mass (m) representing extension of carcinoma into the liver. The wall of the gallbladder is thickened.

diagnosis of carcinoma of the gallbladder. Angiography and ultrasonography are more accurate in making a diagnosis,[212, 213] but angiography is an invasive procedure and ultrasonographic distinction of carcinoma from chronic cholecystitis is frequently difficult.

CT appears to be highly accurate in diagnosing gallbladder carcinoma and in determining the extent of intrahepatic and extrahepatic spread. Itai and colleagues correctly diagnosed 89 per cent of gallbladder carcinomas and found hepatobiliary

abnormalities suggesting a gallbladder lesion in every case.[213] Carcinoma of the gallbladder most frequently produces thickening of the gallbladder wall and a mass in the gallbladder fossa, which has irregular ill-defined margins (Fig. 13–87) that enhance after intravenous contrast administration.[213] Invasion into the liver is found in over 75 per cent of cases and produces an area of low density within the liver immediately adjacent to the tumor (Figs. 13–87B and 13–88). Less common findings are an irregular or smooth thicken-

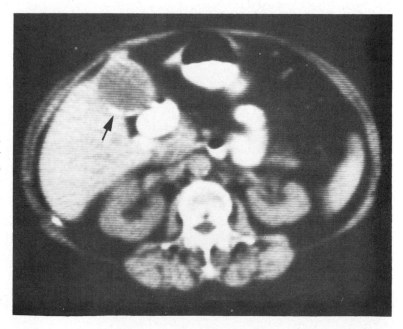

Figure 13–89. Carcinoma of the gallbladder. The wall of the gallbladder is partially calcified (arrow) but no intrahepatic mass is present. Carcinoma confined to the gallbladder was found at surgery.

ing of the gallbladder wall (22 per cent), calcification of the gallbladder wall (Fig. 13–89), and an intraluminal mass (15 per cent).[213] Commonly associated findings are gallstones, biliary tract obstruction, and hepatic metastasis.

Differentiation of gallbladder carcinoma, which produces only a thickened wall, from cholecystitis is not possible in every instance. Thickening of the gallbladder wall to greater than 1 cm and dis-

continuous or focal thickening of the wall of the gallbladder strongly favor carcinoma (Fig. 13–87A), but less advanced carcinoma can appear similar to cholecystitis. Contrast enhancement is of little help as the wall of the gallbladder markedly enhances after contrast injection in both carcinoma and cholecystitis.[212–215]

At times, a solitary hepatic tumor arising adjacent to the gallbladder can mimic a gallbladder

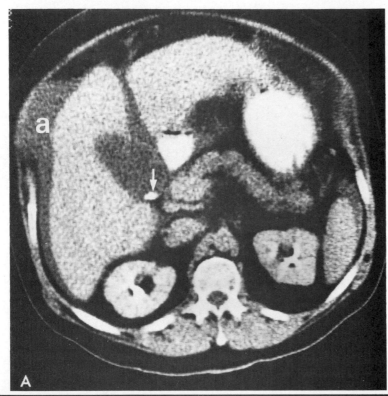

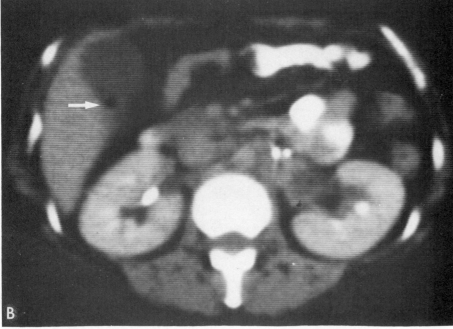

Figure 13–90. The varied CT appearance of gallstones **A** Cirrhosis, ascites (a), and a high-density gallstone (arrow) are seen. **B** Cholesterol gallstone is demonstrated as a low-density filling defect (arrow) in the bile-filled gallbladder. (From Moss AA, Filly RA, Way LW: In vitro investigation of gallstones with computed tomography. J Comput Assist Tomogr 4:827, 1980. Reprinted by permission.)

carcinoma that has spread into the liver. However, primary and metastatic hepatic tumors usually do not produce biliary obstruction or cause focal thickening of the gallbladder wall. As gallbladder cancer spreads into the liver, the wall of the gallbladder often becomes necrotic and perforates, producing an abscess in the liver or gallbladder bed. Identification of gallstones located within an area of abscess fluid should suggest the diagnosis of gallbladder carcinoma.

CHOLELITHIASIS AND CHOLECYSTITIS

Although CT has not been widely used for evaluating patients with suspected gallbladder dis-

ease, the gallbladder is routinely displayed on abdominal CT scans and gallstones are frequently identified. Gallstones are usually seen as high-density filling defects within the gallbladder (Fig. 13–90A),[214–219] but gallstones having attenuation values less than that of surrounding bile can also be detected (Fig. 13–90B).[216, 219–221] Pure cholesterol gallstones have a CT density approximating that of fat,[219] whereas gas-containing gallstones have attenuation values close to that of air.[220]

The accuracy of CT in detecting gallstones is not known with certainty. Havrilla and co-workers[216] detected 78 per cent of gallstones prospectively and 94 per cent retrospectively; Toombs[217] detected 87 per cent of calculi proven by surgery

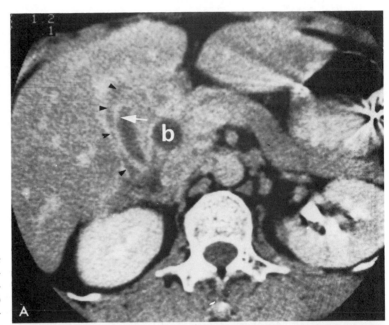

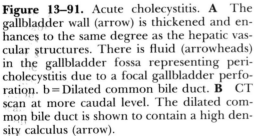

Figure 13–91. Acute cholecystitis. **A** The gallbladder wall (arrow) is thickened and enhances to the same degree as the hepatic vascular structures. There is fluid (arrowheads) in the gallbladder fossa representing pericholecystitis due to a focal gallbladder perforation. b = Dilated common bile duct. **B** CT scan at more caudal level. The dilated common bile duct is shown to contain a high density calculus (arrow).

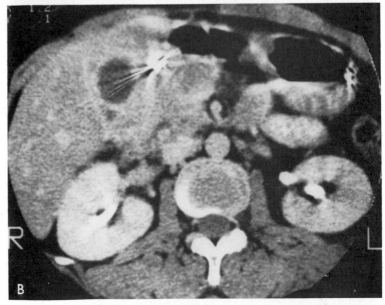

or ultrasound. When positive CT is virtually 100 per cent accurate, however, lack of demonstration of a gallstone by CT does not mean a calculi does not exist, as small noncalcified calculi may be missed.[218]

Acute and chronic cholecystitis (Fig. 13–91) can be detected by CT.[215] Acute cholecystitis produces a thickened gallbladder wall (greater than 3 mm) which enhances after intravenous contrast (Fig. 13–91). An important associated CT finding is the presence of fluid in the gallbladder bed (Fig. 13–91).[214] CT can diagnose emphysematous cholecystitis by demonstrating gas in the wall of the gallbladder[222] and a porcelain gallbladder by showing the gallbladder wall to be calcified (Fig. 13–89). Chronic cholecystitis can produce a thickened gallbladder wall[216] but most frequently gallstones are the only abnormality demonstrated by CT.

The density of normal bile ranges from 0 to 20 H.[214, 216] An increase in the density of bile can be due to hemorrhage,[223] pus,[214] milk of calcium, or a sludge-filled hydropic gallbladder.[224] Abnormally dense bile is strong evidence of gallbladder pathology and warrants further investigation.

REFERENCES

1. Alfidi RJ, Haaga J, Meaney TF, MacIntyre WJ, Gonzalez L, Tarar R, Zelch MG, Boller M, Cook SA, Kelden G: Computed tomography of the thorax and abdomen: A preliminary report. Radiology 117:257, 1975.
2. Alfidi RJ, Haaga JR, Havrilla TR, Pepe RG, Cook SA: Computed tomography of the liver. AJR 127:69, 1976.
3. Stephens DH, Hattery RR, Sheedy PF II: Computed tomography of the abdomen. Radiology 119:331, 1976.
4. Twigg HL, Axelbaum SP, Schellinger D: Computerized body tomography with the ACTA scanner. JAMA 234:314, 1975.
5. Schellinger D, DiChiro G, Axelbaum SP, Twigg HL, Ledley RS: Early clinical experience with the ACTA scanner. Radiology 114:257, 1975.
6. Stephens DH, Sheedy PF II, Hattery RR, MacCarty RL: Computed tomography of liver. AJR 128:579, 1977.
7. Sagel SS, Stanley RJ, Evens RG: Early clinical experience with motionless whole-body computed tomography. Radiology 119:321, 1976.
8. Sheedy PF II, Stephens DH, Hattery RR, Muhm JR, Hartman GW: Computed tomography of the body: Initial clinical trial with the EMI prototype. AJR 127:23, 1976.
9. Stanley RJ, Sagel SS, Levitt RG: Computed tomography of the body: Early trends in application and accuracy of the method. AJR 127:53, 1976.
10. Harell GS, Marshall WH Jr, Breiman RS, Seppi EJ: Early experience with the Varian six second body scanner in the diagnosis of hepatobiliary tract disease. Radiology 123:355, 1977.
11. Philips RL, Stephens DH: Computed tomography of liver specimens. Radiology 115:43, 1975.
12. Healey JE Jr, Schroy PC: Anatomy of the biliary ducts within the human liver. Arch Surg 66:599, 1953.
13. Michels NA: Normal anatomy of the liver and its variant blood supply and collateral circulation. Am J Surg 112:337, 1966.
14. Marks WM, Filly RA, Callen PW: Ultrasonic anatomy of the liver: A review with new applications. J Clin Ultrasound 7:137, 1979.
15. Starzal TE, Bell RH, Beart RW, Putman CW: Hepatic trisegmentectomy and other liver resections. Surg Gynecol Obstet 141:429, 1975.
16. Covinaud C, Le Foie: Etudes Anatomiques et Chirurgicales. Paris: Masson, 1957.
17. Halber MD, Daffner RH: Fat in the intrahepatic fissure. AJR 132:842, 1979.
18. Sagel SS, Stanley RJ: Computed tomography. In Margulis AR, Burhenne HJ (eds): Alimentary Tract Radiology, Vol. 3: Abdominal Imaging, St. Louis, CV Mosby Company, 1979, pp 163–182.
19. Kressel HY, Korobkin M, Goldberg HI, Moss AA: The portal venous tree simulating dilated biliary ducts on computed tomography of the liver. J Comput Assist Tomogr 1:169, 1977.
20. Moncada R, Reynes C, Churchill R, Love L: Normal vascular anatomy of the abdomen on computed tomography. Radiol Clin North Am 17:25, 1979.
21. Foley WD, Wilson CR, Quiroz FA, Lawson TL: Demonstration of the normal extrahepatic biliary tract with computed tomography. J Comput Assist Tomogr 4:48, 1980.
22. Arndt RD, Joyce PW, Gray RK, Haveson SB, Bos CJ: Iodipamide-enhanced computed tomography of the pancreas. Radiology 139:491, 1981.
23. Schmitt WG, Hübener KH: Attenuation values of normal and pathological liver tissues as a basis for computed tomographic densitometry of fatty livers. ROEFO 129:555, 1978.
24. Ritchings RT, Pullman BR, Lucas SB, Fawcitt RA, Best JJK, Isherwood I, Morris AI: An analysis of the spatial distribution of attenuation values in computed tomographic scans of liver and spleen. J Comput Assist Tomogr 3:36, 1979.
25. Mategrano VC, Petasnick J, Clark J, Bin AC, Weinstein R: Attenuation values in computed tomography of the abdomen. Radiology 125:135, 1977.
26. Piekarski J, Goldberg HI, Royal SA, Axel L, Moss AA: Difference between liver and spleen CT numbers in the normal adult: Usefulness in predicting the presence of diffuse liver disease. Radiology 137:727, 1980.
27. Goldberg HI: Recognition of hepatocellular disorders by computed tomography. In Moss AA, Goldberg HI, Norman D (eds): Interventional Radiologic Techniques: Computed Tomography and Ultrasonography. New York, Academic Press, 1981, pp 265–274.
28. Holzbach RT, Weiland RG, Lieber CS, DeCarli LM, Koepke KR, Green SG: Hepatic lipid in morbid obesity assessment at and subsequent to jejunoileal bypass. N Engl J. Med 290:296, 1974.

29. Dean PB, Violante MR, Mahoney JA: Hepatic CT contrast enhancement: Effect of dose, duration of infusion, and time elapsed following infusion. Invest Radiol 15:158, 1980.

30. Koehler RE, Stanley RJ, Evens RG: Iosefamate Meglumine: An iodinated contrast agent for hepatic computed tomography scanning. Radiology 132:115, 1979.

31. Moss AA, Brito AC: Computed tomography of the liver in rhesus monkeys following iosefamate meglumine administration. Radiology 141:123, 1981.

32. Lamarque JL, Bruel JM, Dondelinger R, Vendrell B, Pelissier O, Rovanet JP, Michel JL, Boulet P: The use of iodolipids in hepatosplenic computed tomography. J Comput Assist Tomogr 3:21, 1979.

33. Vermess M, Doppman JL, Sugarbaker P, Fisher FI, Chatterji DC, Luetzeler J, Grimes G, Girton M, Adamson RH: Clinical trials with a new intravenous liposoluble contrast material for computed tomography of the liver and spleen. Radiology 137:217, 1980.

34. Vermess M, Adamson RH, Doppman JL, Girton M: Computed tomographic demonstration of hepatic tumor with the aid of intravenous iodinated fat emulsion: An experimental study. Radiology 125:711, 1977.

35. Vermess M, Bernardino ME, Doppman JL, Fisher RI, Thomas JL, Velasquez WS, Fuller LM, Russo A: Use of intravenous liposoluble contrast material for the examination of the liver and spleen in lymphoma. J Comput Assist Tomogr 5:709, 1981.

36. Alfidi R, Laval-Jeantet M: AG 60.99: A promising contrast agent for computed tomography of the liver and spleen. Radiology 121:491, 1976.

37. Vermess M, Chatterji DC, Doppman JL, Grimes G, Adamson RH: Development and experimental evaluation of a contrast medium for computed tomographic examination of the liver and spleen. J Comput Assist Tomogr 3:25, 1979.

38. Havron A, Seltzer SE, Davis MA, Shulkin P: Radiopaque liposomes: A promising new contrast material for computed tomography of the spleen. Radiology 140:507, 1981.

39. Havron A, Davis MA, Seltzer SE, Paskins-Hurlburt AJ, Hessel SJ: Heavy metal particulate contrast materials for computed tomography of the liver. J Comput Assist Tomogr 4:642, 1980.

40. Seltzer SE, Adams DF, Davis MA, Hessel SJ, Havron A, Judy PF, Paskins-Hurlburt AJ, Hollenberg NK: Hepatic contrast agents for computed tomography: High atomic number particulate material. J Comput Assist Tomogr 5:370, 1981.

41. Cohen A, Seltzer SE, Davis MA, Hanson RN: Iodinated starch particles: new contrast material for computed tomography of the liver. J Comput Assist Tomogr 5:843, 1981.

42. Cassel DM, Young SW, Brody WR, Muller HH, Hall AL: Radiographic blood pool contrast agents for vascular and tumor imaging with projection radiography and computed tomography. J Comput Assist Tomogr 6:141, 1982.

43. Young SW, Enzmann DR, Long DM, Muller HH: Perfluoroctylbromide contrast enhancement of malignant neoplasms: Preliminary observations. AJR 137:141, 1981.

44. Prando A, Wallace S, Bernardino ME, Lindell MM Jr: Computed tomographic arteriography of the liver. Radiology 130:697, 1979.

45. Marchal GJ, Baert AL, Wilms GE: CT of noncystic liver lesions: Bolus enhancement. AJR 135:57, 1980.

46. Tada S, Fukuda K, Aoyagi Y, Harada J: CT of abdominal malignancies: Dynamic approach. AJR 135:455, 1980.

47. Araki T, Itai Y, Furui S, Tasaka A: Dynamic CT densitometry of hepatic tumors. AJR 135:1037, 1980.

48. Koehler PR, Anderson RE: Computed angiotomography. Radiology 137:843, 1980.

49. Young SW, Noon MA, Nassi M, Castellino RA: Dynamic computed tomography body scanning. J Comput Assist Tomogr 4:168, 1980.

50. Young SW, Turner RJ, Castellino RA: A strategy for the contrast enhancement of malignant tumors using dynamic computed tomgraphy and intravascular pharmacokinetics. Radiology 137:137, 1980.

51. Burgener FA, Hamlin DJ: Contrast enhancement in abdominal CT: Bolus vs. infusion. AJR 137:351, 1981.

52. Young SW, Enzmann D, Marglin SI: Computed tomography of rabbit V2 carcinoma after intraarterial contrast enhancement. J Comput Assist Tomogr 3:185, 1979.

53. Dean PB, Kivisaari L, Kormano M: The diagnostic potential of contrast enhancement pharmacokinetics. Invest Radiol 13:533, 1978.

54. Young SW, Noon MA, Marincek B: Dynamic computed tomography time-density study of normal human tissue after intravenous contrast administration. Invest Radiol 16:36, 1981.

55. Newhouse JH, Murphy RX Jr: Tissue distribution of soluble contrast: Effect of dose variation and changes with time. AJR 136:463, 1981.

56. Moss AA, Dean PB, Axel L, Goldberg HI, Glazer GM, Friedman MA: Dynamic CT of hepatic masses with intravenous and intraarterial contrast material. AJR 138:847, 1982.

57. Rossi P, Rivighi L, Tipaldi L, Bompiani C, Simonetti G: High contrast enhancement of the liver in CT by repeated doses of contrast medium. Europ J Radiol 1:126, 1981.

58. Berland LL, Lawson TL, Foley WD, Melrose BL, Chintapalli KN, Taylor AJ: Comparison of pre- and postcontrast CT in hepatic masses. AJR 138:853, 1982.

59. Kormano M, Dean PB: Extravascular contrast material: The major component of contrast enhancement. Radiology 126:807, 1978.

60. Vermess M, Doppman JL, Sugarbaker PH, Fisher RI, O'Leary TJ, Chatterji DC, Grimes G, Adamson RH, Willis M, Edwards BK: Computed tomography of the liver and spleen with intravenous lipoid contrast material: Review of 60 examinations. AJR 138:1063, 1982.

61. Itai Y, Nishikawa J, Tasaka A: Computed tomography in the evaluation of hepatocellular carcinoma. Radiology 131:165, 1979.

62. Marchal G, Wilms G, Baert AL: Evaluation of contrast enhancement by bolus technique in the study of liver metastasis (abstract). Symposium on the diagnosis of liver metastasis. AJR 133:976, 1979.

63. Korobkin M, Kressel HY, Moss AA, Koehler RE: Computed tomographic angiography of the body. Radiology 126:807, 1978.

64. Parienty R: Computed tomography in the diagnostic approach to cavernous hemangioma of the liver. Radiology 134:553, 1980.

65. Stanley RJ, Sagel SS, Levitt RG: Computed body tomography of the liver. Radiol Clin of North Am 15:331, 1977.

66. Kreel L: Computerized tomography and the liver. Clinical Radiol 28:571, 1977.

67. Moss AA, Schrumpf J, Schnyder P, Korobkin M, Shimshak RR: Computed tomography of focal hepatic lesions: A blind clinical evaluation of the effect of contrast enhancement. Radiology 131:427, 1979.

68. Kirkpatrick RH, Wittengerg J, Schaffer DL, Black EB, Hall DA, Braitman BS, Ferrucci JT Jr: Scanning techniques in computed body tomography. AJR 130:1069, 1978.

69. Liver and hepatobiliary system. In Haaga J, Reich NE (eds): Computed Tomography of Abdominal Abnormalities. St Louis, CV Mosby, 1978, pp 39–85.

70. Itai Y, Araki T, Furui S, Tasaka A: Differential diagnosis of hepatic masses on computed tomography, with particular reference to hepatocellular carcinoma. J Comput Assist Tomogr 5:834, 1981.

71. Kunstlinger F, Federle MP, Moss AA, Marks W: Computed tomography of hepatocellular carcinoma. AJR 134:431, 1980.

72. Moss AA: CT contrast enhancement of the liver. In Fuchs WA (ed): Contrast Enhancement in Body Computerized Tomography. Stuttgart, Verlag, 1981, pp 95–110.

73. Young SW, Enzmann D, Marglin SI: Computed tomography of rabbit V2 carcinoma after intraarterial contrast enhancement. J Comput Assist Tomogr 3:185, 1979.

74. Moss AA, Friedman MA, Brito AC: Determination of liver, kidney, and spleen volumes by computed tomography: An experimental study in dogs. J Comput Assist Tomogr 5:12, 1981.

75. Heymsfield SB, Fulenwiler T, Nordling B: Accuracy of measurements of liver, kidney and splenic volumes and masses by computed axial tomography. Ann Intern Med 90:185, 1979.

76. Stanley RJ, Sagel SS: Computed tomography of the liver and biliary tract. In Berk RN, Clemett AR (eds): Radiology of the Gallbladder and Bile Ducts. Philadelphia, WB Saunders Company, 1977, p 352.

77. Ducommun JC, Goldberg HI, Korobkin M, Moss AA, Kressel HY: The relation of liver fat to computed tomography numbers: A preliminary experimental study in rabbits. Radiology 130:511, 1979.

78. Scott WW Jr, Sanders RC, Siegelman SS: Irregular fatty infiltration of the liver: Diagnostic dilemmas. AJR 135:67, 1980.

79. Cunningham DG, Churchill RJ, Reynes CJ: Computed tomography in the evaluation of liver disease in cystic fibrosis patients. J Comput Assist Tomogr 4:151, 1980.

80. Mulhern CB Jr, Arger PH, Coleman BG, Stein GN: Nonuniform attenuation in computed tomography study of the cirrhotic liver. Radiology 132:399, 1979.

81. Leevy CM: Fatty liver: A study of 270 patients with biopsy proven fatty liver and a review of the literature. Medicine 41:249, 1962.

82. Westwater JO, Fainer D: Liver impairment in the obese. Gastroenterology 34:686, 1958.

83. Goldberg HI, Cann C, Moss AA: Unpublished data.

84. Scherer U, Santos M, Lissner J: CT studies of the liver in vitro: A report on 82 cases with pathological correlation. J Comput Assist Tomogr 3:589, 1979.

85. Biondetti PR, Fiore D, Muzzio PC: Computed tomography of the liver in Von Gierke's disease. J Comput Assist Tomogr 4:685, 1980.

86. MacCarty RL, Wahner HW, Stephens DH, Sheedy PF, Hattery RR: Retrospective comparison of radionuclide scans and computed tomography of the liver and pancreas. AJR 129:23, 1977.

87. Harbin WP, Robert NJ, Ferrucci JT Jr: Diagnosis of cirrhosis based on regional changes in hepatic morphology: A radiological and pathological analysis. Radiology 135:273, 1980.

88. Tavill AS, Wood EJ, Kreel L, Jones EA, Gregory M, Sherlock S: The Budd-Chiari syndrome: Correlation between hepatic scintigraphy and the clinical, radiological, and pathological findings in nineteen cases of hepatic venous outflow obstruction. Gastroenterology 68:509, 1975.

89. Omata M, Ashcovai M, Liew C-T, Peters RL: Hepatocellular carcinoma in the USA: Etiological considerations. Gastroenterology 76:279, 1979.

90. Mills SR, Doppman JL, Nienhuis AW: Computed tomography in the diagnosis of disorders of excessive iron storage of the liver. J Comput Assist Tomogr 1:101–104, 1977.

91. Long JA Jr, Doppman JL, Nienhuis AW, Mills SR: Computed tomographic analysis of beta-thalassemic syndromes with hemochromatosis: Pathologic findings with clinical and laboratory correlations. J Comput Assist Tomogr 4:159, 1980.

92. Mitnick JS, Bosniak MA, Megibow AJ, Karpatkin M, Feiner HD, Kutin N, Van Natta F, Piomelli S: CT in B-thalassemia: Iron deposition in the liver, spleen and lymph nodes. AJR 136:1191, 1981.

93. Jovana MTW, Arozena X, Skalicka A, Huehns ER, Shaw DG: Correlation between computed tomographic values and liver iron content in thalassemia major with iron overload. Lancet 1:1322, 1979.

94. Royal SA, Beiderman BA, Goldberg HI, Koerper MM, Thaler MM: Detection and estimation of iron, glycogen and fat in liver of children with hepatomegaly using computed tomography (CT). Pediatr Res 13:408, 1979.

95. Chapman RWG, Williams G, Bydder G: Computed tomography for determining liver iron content in primary hemochromatosis. Br Med J 280:4, 1980.

96. Goldberg HI, Cann CE, Moss AA, Ohto M, Brito A, Federle M: Noninvasive quantitation of liver iron in dogs with hemochromatosis using dual energy CT scanning. Invest Radiol 17:375, 1982.

97. Miller JH, Stanley P, Gates GF: Radiography of glycogen storage diseases. AJR 132:379, 1979.

98. Doppman JL, Cornblath M, Dwyer AJ, Adams AJ, Girton ME, Sidbury J: Computed tomography of the liver and kidneys in glycogen storage disease. J Comput Assist Tomogr 6:67, 1982.

99. Kolbenstvedt A, Kjolseth I, Klepp O, Kolmannskog F: Postirradiation changes of the liver demonstrated by computed tomography. Radiology 135:391, 1980.

100. Jeffrey RB Jr, Moss AA, Quivey JM, Federle MP, Wara WM: CT of radiation-induced hepatic injury. AJR 135:445, 1980.

101. Ingold J, Reed GB, Kaplan HS, Bagshaw MA: Radiation hepatitis. AJR 93:200, 1965.

102. Federle MP, Filly RA, Moss AA: Cystic hepatic neoplasms: Complementary roles of CT and sonography. AJR 136:345, 1981.

103. Wooten WB, Bernardino ME, Goldstein HM: Computed tomography of necrotic hepatic metastases. AJR 131:839, 1978.

104. Barnes PA, Thomas JL, Bernardino ME: Pitfalls in the diagnosis of hepatic cysts by computed tomography. Radiology 141:129, 1981.

105. Freeny PC: Radiologic diagnosis of focal hepatic masses: An integrated approach. In Moss AA, Goldberg HI, Norman D (eds): Interventional Radiologic Techniques: Computed Tomography and Ultrasonography. New York, Academic Press, 1981, pp 253–264.

106. Gesundheit N, Kent DL, Fawcett HD, Effron MK, Maffly RH: Infected liver cyst in a patient with polycystic kidney disease. West J Med 136:246, 1982.

107. Freeny PC, Vimont TR, Barnett DC: Cavernous hemangioma of the liver: Ultrasonography, arteriography and computed tomography. Radiology 132:143, 1979.

108. Barnett PH, Zerhouni EA, White RI Jr, Siegelman SS: Computed tomography in the diagnosis of cavernous hemangioma of the liver. AJR 134:439, 1980.

109. Itai Y, Furui S, Araki T, Yashiro N, Tasaka A: Computed tomography of cavernous hemangioma of the liver. Radiology 137:149, 1980.

110. Johnson CM, Sheedy PF II, Stanson AW, Stephens DH, Hattery RR, Adson MA: Computed tomography and angiography of cavernous hemangiomas of the liver. Radiology 138:115, 1981.

111. Ishak KG, Rabin L: Benign tumors of the liver. Med Clin North Am 59:995, 1975.

112. Abrams RM, Berhbaum ER, Santos JS, Lipson J: Angiographic features of cavernous hemangioma of the liver. Radiology 92:308, 1969.

113. Moss AA, Clark RE, Palubinskas AJ, DeLorimer AA: Angiographic appearance of benign and malignant hepatic tumors in infants and children. AJR 113:61, 1971.

114. Adam YG, Huvos AG, Fortner JG: Giant hemangiomas of the liver. Ann Surg 172:239, 1970.

115. Wilson H, Tyson WT: Massive hemangioma of the liver. Ann Surg 135:765, 1952.

116. Sewell JH, Weiss K: Spontaneous rupture of hemangioma of the liver. Arch Surg 83:729, 1961.

117. Stayman JW, Polsky HS, Blamm L: Ruptured cavernous hemangioma of the liver. Pa Med 79:62, 1976.

118. Kato M, Sugawara I, Okada A, Kuwata K, Satani M, Okamoto E, Manabe H: Hemangioma of the liver: Diagnosis with combined use of laparoscopy and hepatic arteriography. Am J Surg 129:698, 1975.

119. Muehlbauer MA, Farber JG: Hemangioma of the liver—Some interesting clinical and radiological observations. Am J Gastroenterol 45:355, 1966.

120. Good LI, Alavi A, Trotman BW, Oleuga JA, Eymontt MJ: Hepatic hemangiomas: Pitfalls in scintigraphic detection. Gastroenterology 74:952, 1978.

121. Taylor RD, Anderson PM, Winston MA, Blahd SW: Diagnosis of hepatic hemangioma using multiple-radionuclide and ultrasound techniques. J Nucl Med 17:362, 1976.

122. McArdle CR: Ultrasonic appearances of a hepatic hemangioma. J Clin Ultrasound 6:124, 1978.

123. Wiener SN, Parulekar SG: Scintigraphy and ultrasonography of hepatic hemangioma. Radiology 132:149, 1979.

124. Snow JH Jr, Goldstein HM, Wallace S: Comparison of scintigraphy sonography and computed tomography in the evaluation of hepatic neoplasms. AJR 132:915, 1979.

125. Front D, Hardoff R, Israel O, Schneck SO: Perfusion vascularity mismatch in liver hemangiomas. Clin Nucl Med 3:212, 1978.

126. Freeman LM, Bernstein RG, Hoyt DB: Diagnosis of hepatic hemangioma with combined scanning technique. Radiology 95:127, 1970.

127. Pantoja E: Angiography in liver hemangioma. AJR 104:874, 1968.

128. Pollard JJ, Fleishli DJ, Nebesar RA: Angiography of hepatic neoplasms. Radiol Clin North Am 8:31, 1970.

129. McLoughlin MJ: Angiography in cavernous hemangioma of the liver. AJR 113:50, 1971.

130. Olmsted WW, Stocker JT: Cavernous hemangioma of the liver. Ann Surg 172:239, 1970.

131. Pollard JJ, Nebesar RA, Mattoso: Angiographic diagnosis of benign disease of the liver. Radiology 86:276, 1966.

132. Newmark H III, Horn NL, Silberman EL: Postradiation-treated hemangioma of the liver seen on a computed tomogram scan. Comput Tomogr 5:65, 1981.

133. Casarella WJ, Knowles DM, Wolff M, Johnson PM: Focal nodular hyperplasia and liver cell adenoma: Radiologic and pathologic differentiation. AJR 131:393, 1978.

134. Angres G, Carter JB, Velasco JM: Unusual ring in liver cell adenoma. AJR 135:172, 1980.

135. Benedict KT Jr, Chen PS, Janower ML, Farmelant MH, Howard JT, McDermott W: Contraceptive-associated hepatic tumor. AJR 132:452, 1979.

136. Mariani AF, Livingstone AS, Pereiras RV Jr, VanZuiden PE, Schiff ER: Progressive enlargement of an hepatic adenoma. Gastroenterology 77:1319, 1979.

137. Penkava RR, Rothenberg J: Spontaneous resolution of oral contraceptive-associated liver tumor. J Comput Assist Tomogr 5:102, 1981.

138. Brum JK, Bookstein JJ, Holtz F, Klein EW: Possible association between benign hepatomas and oral contraceptives. Lancet 2:926, 1973.

139. Andersen PH, Packer JT: Hepatic adenoma: Observations after estrogen withdrawal. Arch Surg 111:898, 1976.

140. Edmondson HA, Reynolds TB, Henderson B, Benton B: Regression of liver cell adenomas associated with oral contraceptives. Ann Intern Med 86:180, 1977.

141. Sandler MA, Petrocelli RD, Marks DS, Lopez R: Ultrasonic features and radionuclide correlation in liver cell adenoma and focal nodular hyperplasia. Radiology 135:393, 1980.

142. Scherer U, Rothe R, Eisenburg J, Schildberg F-W, Meister P, Lissner J: Diagnostic accuracy of CT in circumscript liver disease. AJR 130:711, 1978.

143. Rodgers JV, Mack LA, Freeny PC, Johnson ML, Sones PJ: Hepatic focal nodular hyperplasia: Angiography, CT, sonography, and scintigraphy. AJR 137:198, 1981.

144. McLoughlin MJ, Colapinto RF, Filday DL, Hobbs BB, Korobkin MT, McDonald P, Phillips MJ: Focal nodular hyperplasia of the liver angiography and radioisotope scanning. Radiology 170:257, 1973.

145. McMullen CT, Montgomery JL: Arteriographic findings of focal nodular hyperplasia of the liver and review of the literature. AJR 117:380, 1973.

146. Inamoto K, Sugiki K, Yamasaki H, Nakao N, Miura T: Computed tomography and angiography of hepatocellular carcinoma. J Comput Assist Tomogr 4:832, 1980.

147. Vigo M, DeFaveri D, Biandetti PR Jr, Benedetti L: CT demonstration of portal and superior mesenteric vein thrombosis in hepatocellular carcinoma. J Comput Assist Tomogr 4:627, 1980.

148. Inamoto K, Sugiki K, Yamasaki H, Miura T: CT of hepatoma: Effects of portal vein obstruction. AJR 136:349, 1981.

149. Freeny PC: Portal vein tumor thrombus: Demonstration by computed tomographic arteriography. J Comput Assist Tomogr 4:263, 1980.

150. Zerhouni EA, Barth KH, Siegelman SS: Computed tomographic demonstration of inferior vena cava invasion in a case of hepatocellular carcinoma. J Comput Assist Tomogr 2:363, 1978.

151. Pauls CH: Ultrasound and computed tomographic demonstration of portal vein thrombosis in hepatocellular carcinoma. Gastrointest Radiol 6:281, 1981.

152. Dunnick NR, Ihde DC, Doppman JL, Bates HR: Computed tomography in primary hepatocellular carcinoma. J Comput Assist Tomogr 4:59, 1980.

153. Nishikawa J, Itai Y, Tasaka A: Lobar attenuation difference of the liver on computed tomography. Radiology 141:725, 1981.

154. Itai Y, Moss AA, Goldberg HI: Transient hepatic attenuation difference of lobar or segmental distribution detected by dynamic computed tomography. Radiology 144:835, 1982.

155. Bernardino ME, Chuang VP, Wallace S, Thomas JL, Soo C-S: Therapeutically infarcted tumors: CT findings. AJR 136:527, 1981.

156. Moss AA, Cann CE, Friedman MA, Marcus FS, Resser KJ, Berninger W: Volumetric CT analysis of hepatic tumors. J Comput Assist Tomogr 5:714, 1981.

157. Levine E, Maklad NF, Wright CH, Lee KR: Computed tomographic and ultrasonic appearances of primary carcinoma of the common bile duct. Gastrointest Radiol 4:147, 1979.

158. Oleaga JA, Ring EJ, Freiman DB, McLean GK, Rosen RJ: Extension of neoplasm along the tract of a transhepatic tube. AJR 135:841, 1980.

159. Araki T, Itai Y, Tasaka A: CT of choledochal cyst. AJR 135:729, 1980.

160. Pedrosa CS, Casanova R, Lezana AH, Fernandez MC: Computed tomography in obstructive jaundice: Part II: The cause of obstruction. Radiology 139:635, 1981.

161. Araki T, Itai Y, Tasaka A: Computed tomography of localized dilatation of the intrahepatic bile ducts. Radiology 141:733, 1981.

162. Shimizu H, Ida M, Takayama S, Seki T, Yoneda M, Nakaya S, Yanagi T, Bando B, Sato H, Uchiyama M, Okumura T, Miura S, Fujisawa M: The diagnostic accuracy of computed tomography in obstructive biliary disease: A comparative evaluation with direct cholangiography. Radiology 138:411, 1981.

163. Havrilla TR, Haaga JR, Alfidi RJ, Reich NE: Computed tomography and obstructive biliary disease. AJR 128:765, 1977.

164. Pedrosa CS, Casanova R, Rodriguez R: Computed tomography in obstructive jaundice: Part I: The level of obstruction. Radiology 139:627, 1981.

165. Zornoza J, Ginaldi S: Computed tomography in hepatic lymphoma. Radiology 138:405, 1981.

166. Rosenberg SA, Diamond HD, Jaslowitz B, Craver LF: Lymphosarcoma: A review of 1269 cases. Medicine (Baltimore) 40:31, 1961.

167. Mahony B, Jeffrey RB, Federle MP: Spontaneous rupture of hepatic and splenic angiosarcoma demonstrated by CT. AJR 138:965, 1982.

168. Biello DR, Levitt RG, Siegel BA, Sagel SS, Stanley RJ: Computed tomography and radionuclide imaging of the liver: A comparison evaluation. Radiology 127:159, 1978.

169. Sullivan DC, Taylor KJW, Gottschalk A: The use of ultrasound to enhance the diagnostic utility of the equivocal liver scintigraph. Radiology 128:727, 1978.

170. Bryan PJ, Dinn WM, Grossman ZD, Wistow BW, McAfee JG, Kieffer SA: Correlation of computed tomography, gray scale ultrasonography, and radionuclide imaging of the liver in detecting space-occupying processes. Radiology 124:387, 1977.

171. Noon MA, Young SW, Castellino RA: Leiomyosarcoma metastatic to the liver: CT appearance. J Comput Assist Tomogr 4:527, 1980.

172. Bernardino ME: Computed tomography of calcified liver metastases. J Comput Assist Tomogr 3:32, 1979.

173. Federle MP, Jeffrey RB Jr, Minagi H: Calcified liver metastasis from renal cell carcinoma. J Comput Assist Tomogr 5:771, 1981.

174. Hoffman E, McCort JJ: Pyogenic liver abscess with walled off intraperitoneal perforation. CT/T Clinical Symposium Volume 2, Number 8, 1979.

175. Sones PJ Jr, Thomas BM, Masand PP: Falciform ligament abscess: Appearance on computed tomography and sonography. AJR 137:161, 1981.

176. Harbin WP, Wittenberg J, Ferrucci JT Jr, Mueller PR, Ottinger LW: Fallibility of exploratory laparotomy in detection of hepatic and retroperitoneal masses. AJR 135:115, 1980.

177. Kirschner LP, Ferris RA, Mero JA, Moss ML: Hydatid disease of the liver evaluated by computed tomography. J Comput Assist Tomogr 2:229, 1978.

178. Newmark H III, Smith JJ, Burrows R, Silberman EL: Echinococcal cyst of the liver seen on computed tomography. J Comput Assist Tomogr 2:231, 1978.

179. Scherer U, Weinzierl M, Sturm R, Schildberg F-W, Zrenner M, Lissner J: Computed tomography in hydatid disease of the liver: A report of 13 cases. J Comput Assist Tomogr 2:612, 1978.

180. Gonzalez LR, Marcos J, Illanas M, Hernandez-Mora M, Picouto JP, Cienfuegos JA, Alvarez JLR: Radiologic aspects of echinococcosis. Radiology 130:21, 1979.

181. Schnyder PA, Candardjis G: Extreme hydronephrosis versus echinococcal cyst of the liver: Computed tomography evaluation. J Comput Assist Tomogr 3:126, 1979.

182. Hamada M, Ohta M, Yasuda Y, Fukae S, Fukishima M, Nakayama S, Akagawa H, Ohtake H: Hepatic calcification in schistosomiasis japonica. J Comput Assist Tomogr 6:76, 1982.

183. Callen PW, Filly RA, Marcus FS: Ultrasonography and computed tomography in the evaluation of hepatic

microabscesses in the immunosuppressed patient. Radiology 136:433, 1980.

184. Federle MP, Goldberg HI, Kaiser JA, Moss AA, Jeffrey RB, Mall JC: Evaluation of abdominal trauma by computed tomography. Radiology 138:637, 1981.

185. Foley WD, Berland LL, Lawson TL, Maddison FE: Computed tomography in the demonstration of hepatic pseudoaneurysm with hemobilia. J Comput Assist Tomogr 4:863, 1980.

186. Tylen U, Hoevels J, Nilsson U: Computed tomography of iatrogenic hepatic lesions following percutaneous transhepatic cholangiography and portography. J Comput Assist Tomogr 5:15, 1981.

187. Axel L, Moss AA, Berninger W: Dynamic computed tomography demonstration of hepatic arteriovenous fistula. J Comput Assist Tomogr 5:95, 1981.

188. Hoiem L, Kvam G: Arterio-portal fistula diagnosed by computerized tomography (CT). Europ J Radiol 1:57, 1981.

189. Moss AA: Abdominal trauma: Computed tomography. In Moss AA, Goldberg HI (eds): Computed Tomography, Ultrasound and X-ray: An Integrated Approach. San Francisco, University of California Press, 1979, pp 271–282.

190. Federle M: Evaluation of abdominal trauma by CT. In Moss AA, Goldberg HI, Norman D (eds): Interventional Radiologic Techniques: Computed Tomography and Ultrasonography. New York, Academic Press, 1981, pp 299–311.

191. Toombs BD, Sandler CM, Rauschkolb EN, Strax R, Harle TS: Assessment of hepatic injuries with computed tomography. J Comput Assist Tomogr 6:72, 1982.

192. Federle MP: Abdominal trauma: the role and impact of computed tomography. Invest Radiology 16:260, 1981.

193. Goldberg HI, Filly RA, Korobkin M, Moss AA, Kressel HY, Callen PW: Capability of CT body scanning and ultrasonography to demonstrate the status of the biliary ductal system in patients with jaundice. Radiology 129:731, 1978.

194. Taylor KJU, Rosenfield AT, Spiro AM: Diagnostic accuracy of gray scale ultrasonography for the jaundiced patient. Arch Intern Med 139:60, 1979.

195. Levitt RG, Sagel SS, Stanley RJ, Jost RG: Accuracy of computed tomography of the liver and biliary tract. Radiology 124:123, 1977.

196. Shanser JD, Korobkin M, Goldberg HI, Rohlfing BM: Computed tomographic diagnosis of obstructive jaundice in the absence of intrahepatic ductal obstruction. AJR 131:389, 1978.

197. Thomas JL, Bernardino ME: Segmental biliary obstruction: Its detection and significance. J Comput Assist Tomogr 4:155, 1980.

198. Zeman RK, Dorfman GS, Burrell MI, Stein S, Berg GR, Gold JA: Disparate dilatation of the intrahepatic and extrahepatic bile ducts in surgical jaundice. Radiology 138:129, 1981.

199. Fawcitt RA, Forbes WSC, Isherwood I, Morris AI, March MN, Turnberg LA: Computed tomographic scanning in liver disease. Clin Radiol 29:251, 1978.

200. Pedrosa CS, Casanova R, Rodriguez R: CT cholangiography: Multiplanar reconstruction in obstructive jaundice. J Comput Assist Tomogr 5:503, 1981.

200a. Jeffrey RB, Federle MP, Laing FC, Wall SD, Rego J,

Moss AA: CT of choledocholithiasis (in press).

201. Itai Y, Araki T, Furui S, Tasaka A, Atomi Y, Kuroda A: Computed tomography and ultrasound in the diagnosis of intrahepatic calculi. Radiology 136:399, 1980.

202. Myracle MR, Stadalnik RC, Blaisdell FW, Farkas JP, Martin P: Segmental biliary obstruction: Diagnostic significance of bile duct crowding. AJR 137:169, 1981.

202a. Federle MP, Cello HP, Laing FC, Jeffrey RB: Recurrent pyogenic cholangitis in Asian immigrants. Radiology 143:151, 1982.

203. Jakata H, Nobe T, Takahashi M, Maeda T, Koga M: Choledochal cyst. J Comput Assist Tomogr 5:99, 1981.

204. Kaiser JA, Mall JC, Salmen BJ, Parker JJ: Diagnosis of Caroli disease by computed tomography: Report of two cases. Radiology 132:661, 1979.

205. Vujic I, Rogers CI, LeVeen HH: Computed tomographic detection of portal vein thrombosis. Radiology 135:697, 1980.

206. Parienty R: Computed tomography in venocclusive liver disorders. AJR 136:842, 1981.

207. Park SC, Glanz S, Gordon DH, Johnson M: Computed tomography and angiography in the Cruveilhier-Baumgarten syndrome. J Comput Assist Tomogr 5:19, 1981.

208. Henderson JM, Liechty EJ, Jahnke RW: Liver involvement in hereditary hemorrhagic telangiectasia. J Comput Assist Tomogr 5:773, 1981.

209. Dammann HG, Hagemann J, Runge M, Klöppel G: In vivo diagnosis of massive hepatic infarction by computed tomography. Dig Dis Sci 27:73, 1982.

210. Doppman JL, Dunnick NR, Girton M, Fauci AS, Popovsky MA: Bile ducts cysts secondary to liver infarcts: Report of a case and experimental production by small vessel hepatic artery occlusion. Radiology 130:1, 1979.

211. Harter LP, Gross B, St Hilaire J, Filly RA, Goldberg HI: Computed tomographic and ultrasonic appearance of hepatic vein obstruction. AJR 139:176, 1982.

212. Yeh HC: Ultrasonography and computed tomography of carcinoma of the gall bladder. Radiology 133:167, 1979.

213. Itai Y, Araki T, Yoshikawa K, Furui S, Yashiro N, Tasaka A: Computed tomography of gallbladder carcinoma. Radiology 137:713, 1980.

214. Solomon A, Kreel L, Pinto D: Contrast computed tomography in the diagnosis of acute cholecystitis. J Comput Assist Tomogr 3:585, 1979.

215. Pedrosa CS, Casanova R, Rodriguez R: CT findings in subacute perforation of the gallbladder: Report of 5 cases. Europ J Radiol 1:137, 1981.

216. Havrilla TR, Reich N, Haaga JR, Seidelmann FE, Cooperman AM, Alfidi RJ: Computed tomography of the gallbladder. AJR 130:1059, 1978.

217. Toombs BD, Sandler CM, Conoley PM: Computed tomography of the nonvisualizing gallbladder. J Comput Assist Tomogr 5:164, 1981.

218. Sarva RP, Farivar S, Fromm H, Foller W: Study of the sensitivity and specificity of computerized tomography in the detection of calcified gallstones which appear radiolucent by conventional roentgenography. Gastrointest Radiol 6:165, 1981.

219. Moss AA, Filly RA, Way LW: In vitro investigation of gallstones with computed tomography. J Comput Assist Tomogr 4:827, 1980.

220. Dunne MG, Johnson ML: Gas within gallstones on CT. AJR 134:1065, 1980.
221. Suzuki M, Takashima T, Funaki H, Kanno S, Ushitani K, Tabuchi M: Low-density stone of the gallbladder on computed tomography. Gastrointest Radiol 7:65, 1982.
222. Poleynard GD, Harris RD: Diagnosis of emphysematous cholecystitis by computed tomography. Gastrointest Radiol 4:153, 1979.
223. Berland LL, Doust BD, Foley WD: Acute hemorrhage into the gallbladder diagnosed by computed tomography and ultrasonography. J Comput Assist Tomogr 4:260, 1980.
224. Ferris RA, Kirschner LP, Mero JH, Chung DH: Increased attenuation value in hydropic gallbladder. J Comput Assist Tomogr 3:545, 1979.

14 COMPUTED TOMOGRAPHY OF THE PANCREAS

Michael P. Federle

Henry I. Goldberg

ANATOMY

The pancreas is located in the most ventral of the three retroperitoneal compartments, the anterior pararenal space. The space is defined ventrally by the posterior parietal peritoneum and dorsally by the anterior renal (Gerota's) fascia. Laterally, the anterior pararenal space is separated from the posterior pararenal space by the lateral conal fascia (Fig. 14–1).[1] In all but the thinnest or most emaciated patients, the pancreas is surrounded by fat that clearly defines its margins. In asthenic individuals and young children, peripancreatic fat is often minimal, making the margins difficult to discern, especially along the anterior margin of the pancreas.

The pancreas is commonly divided descriptively into head, neck, body, and tail segments. The *head* is the broad right end of the gland lying within the curve of the duodenum (Figs. 14–2 and 14–3). The uncinate process is the prolongation of the left and the caudal border of the head and extends to the superior mesenteric vessels. The *neck* is the constricted portion to the left of the head, lying ventral to the superior mesenteric vessels. The *pancreatic body* lies behind the lesser sac (omental bursa) and stomach, and its dorsal surface is indented by the splenic vein, the course of which generally parallels that of the pancreatic body and tail. The pancreatic tail is usually at the same level or cephalad to the body of the pancreas and follows the splenic vessels into the splenic hilum. The most distal part of the gland lies within the splenorenal ligament, where it becomes an intraperitoneal structure.[1]

The position and configuration of the pancreas are quite variable and these variations may simulate disease states.[2] For example, the pancreatic head has no fixed anatomic relationships, being limited only by the confines of the anterior pararenal space. Although the splenic vein usually marks the dorsal margin of the body and tail, the tip of the gland may rarely curve dorsal to the splenic vein to simulate adrenal pathology.[1, 3] Occasionally, even in normal persons, the pancreatic tail may be anteromedial to the kidney, where it may appear as a pseudomass on excretory urography. Congenital or surgical absence of the left kidney alters the retroperitoneal compartments and the pancreatic tail may be displaced into the empty renal fossa, simulating recurrent tumor or a primary retroperitoneal lesion.[2]

Several attempts have been made to determine normal limits of pancreatic size on axial CT sections in the expectation that this would permit more accurate determination of pathologic states

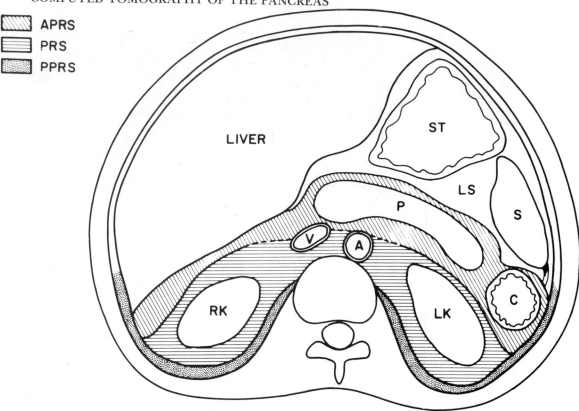

Figure 14–1. Retroperitoneal compartments. Pancreas (P) lies in anterior pararenal space (APRS), the borders of which are the posterior parietal peritoneum ventrally, the anterior renal (Gerota's) fascia dorsally, and lateral conal fascia laterally. Other important structures in the APRS are the duodenal loop (not shown) and the ascending and descending colon (C). ST=Stomach; LS=lesser sac; S= spleen; RK and LK=right and left kidney; V=vena cava; A=aorta.

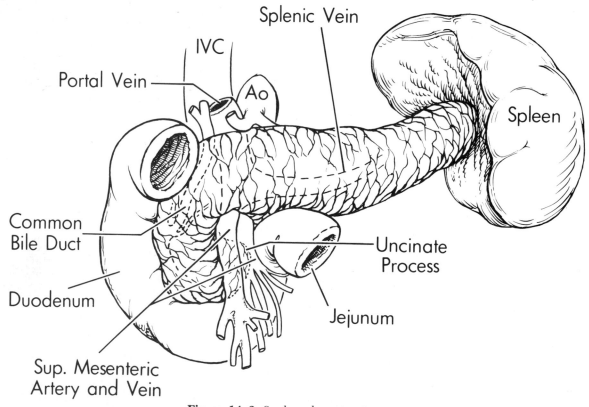

Figure 14–2. *See legend on opposite page*

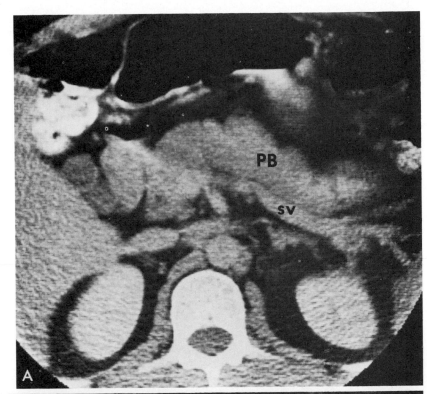

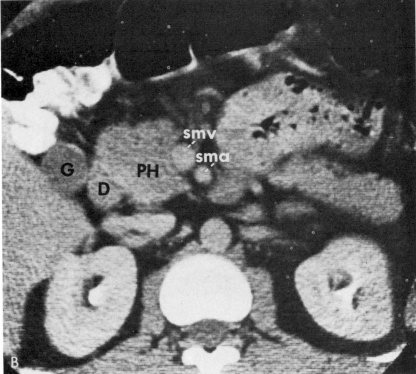

Figure 14–3. Normal pancreas. Patient is a 30-year-old man. **A** The pancreatic body (PB) lies just ventral to the splenic vein (sv). **B** CT scan 2 cm caudal to **A**. Pancreatic head (PH) lies between the superior mesenteric vessels and second portion of duodenum. The uncinate process lies behind superior mesenteric vein and has a beaklike medial margin. G = Gallbladder;   D = duodenum; smv = superior mesenteric vein; sma = superior mesenteric artery.

Figure 14–2. Pancreatic anatomy. The pancreatic head lies between the superior mesenteric vessels and second portions of the duodenum. The uncinate process lies behind the mesenteric vessels, while the neck lies ventral to them. The body lies ventral to the splenic vein. The tail constitutes the last few centimeters of the gland, lies intraperitoneally, and inserts into the splenic hilum within the leaves of the splenorenal ligament.

such as pancreatitis, tumor, or atrophy. Using different 20-second scanners, Haaga[4] and Stanley[5] published somewhat different criteria, though each group related the anteroposterior diameter of the pancreas to the transverse diameter of the adjacent vertebral body. In general, the pancreatic head dimension does not exceed the width of the vertebral body, averaging about 0.7 when expressed as a ratio. The pancreatic body-tail/vertebral ratio is usually about 0.33. However, these authors[4,5] noted a broad overlap between the upper and lower limits of normal and the abnormal

gland. Kreel and colleagues[6] published a set of in vivo and in vitro measurements of pancreatic dimensions and concluded that the "normal" diameter of the head was up to 3 cm, neck and body up to 2.5 cm, and tail up to 2 cm. In assessing these values, the authors noted the importance of assuring that adjacent structures—such as the portal and splenic veins, superior mesenteric vein, and duodenum—are not included in the measurements.

All experienced CT observers have noted that the size, shape, and position of the normal pan-

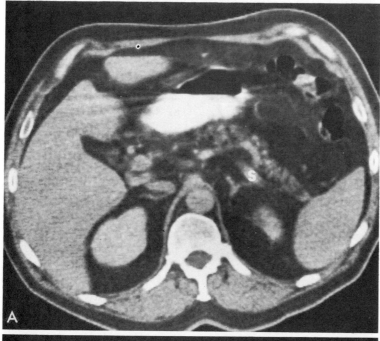

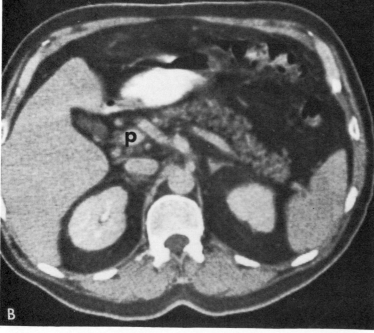

Figure 14–4. Normal pancreas. Patient is a obese 65-year-old-woman. **A–C** Pancreatic width is reduced and the gland is lobulated. These findings are common and normal, particularly with advanced age and obesity.

Illustration continued on opposite page

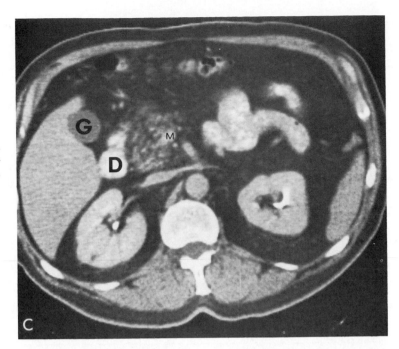

Figure 14–4. *Continued* The pancreas retains its relationship to important vascular landmarks.   G = Gallbladder;   D = duodenum;   s = splenic vein;   p = portal vein,   M = superior mesenteric vein.

creas are highly variable. Rigid adherence to any ratio or absolute measurements, without consideration of other factors, will lead to interpretive error. In general, there is a gradual tapering from the head to the tail without abrupt alterations in size or contour. There is also a gradual diminution in pancreatic size with advancing age, sometimes becoming quite marked beyond the seventh decade. The contour of the pancreas is smooth (Fig. 14–3) in about 80 per cent of cases and lobulated in 20 per cent.[6] Fatty lobulations are more commonly observed in obese and elderly subjects (Fig. 14–4). Such lobulations are not indicative of disease; to the contrary, the observation of evenly distributed lobulations may help exclude underlying inflammation or tumor.

TECHNIQUES OF EXAMINATION

Because the pancreas has essentially the same attenuation coefficient as unopacified bowel and blood vessels, techniques of examination are mainly directed toward identifying all adjacent structures by use of oral and intravenous contrast media.

Oral contrast medium administration is almost always indicated because the stomach, duodenum, and proximal small bowel must be distinguished from the pancreas and because these structures are commonly involved by pancreatic lesions. The two oral contrast agents in common use are dilute

(1 to 3 per cent) meglumine and sodium diatrizoate (Gastrografin and Gastroview) and barium (E-Z CAT). Preliminary attempts[7] to introduce a "negative" oral contrast medium, polyunsaturated oil, met with little enthusiasm because of poor patient acceptance and medical contraindications in pancreatitis, cholecystitis, and other conditions.

When the stomach is collapsed, jejunal segments are commonly interposed between the pancreas and stomach[8] and may simulate a tumor or lesser sac abnormality or result in a distorted impression of pancreatic size.[5] The fundus of the collapsed stomach may itself give rise to a pseudotumor in the pancreatic tail.[6, 9] Full distention of the stomach with dilute oral contrast medium effectively eliminates both these potential pitfalls by outlining the gastric lumen and displacing small bowel loops away from the ventral surface of the pancreatic body and tail.[10] Gastric distention serves the additional purpose of orienting the pancreas more transversely as a result of caudal displacement of the spleen, allowing complete visualization on several contiguous sections.

Intravenous contrast administration is frequently useful to distinguish pancreatic parenchyma from adjacent blood vessels and to better delineate normal structures (e.g., pancreatic and common bile ducts) and abnormal conditions (pseudocysts, peripancreatic edema). An intense pancreatogram can be obtained by rapid bolus infusion of 60 to 100 ml of 60 per cent contrast medium followed by rapid consecutive CT sections ("dynamic CT," "CT angiography"). Following a

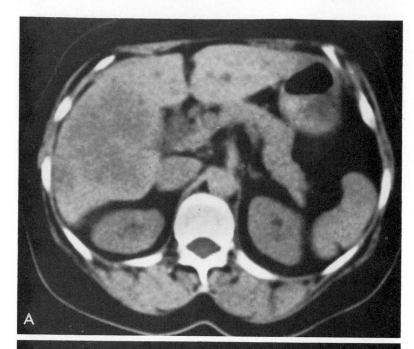

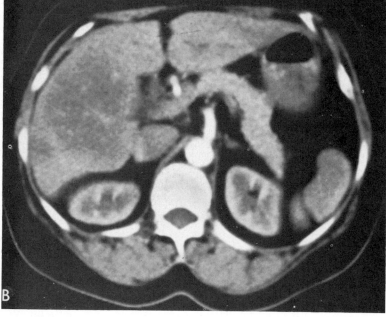

Figure 14–5. Normal pancreas—dynamic CT scans. **A** Before intravenous injection of a bolus of 60 ml of iodinated contrast material. The CT scan shows a normal pancreas which had a CT density of 44 H. A large metastasis is present in the liver. **B** CT scan during maximum aortic enhancement. The pancreas has increased in CT density to 66 H. The aorta and celiac artery are enhanced, as are the hepatic artery and renal cortex.

Illustration continued on opposite page

bolus injection of contrast medium, the normal pancreas enhances uniformly (Fig. 14–5); during the brief pancreatogram phase (lasting less than 2 minutes), the distinction between normal pancreatic parenchyma and intrinsic or extrinsic lesions is more evident than with the drip infusion method of contrast administration.[11] In theory, such specific pathologic entities as splenic vein occlusion, pseudoaneurysms, and vascular tumors should be more easily detected, though clinical experience is limited to date.

Variation from the usual supine positioning may be useful in selected cases. Right decubitus positioning helps to distend the duodenum with oral contrast medium and, indirectly, to better define the pancreatic head. Prone positioning is useful when food and secretions in the dependent position of the stomach blur the distinction between gastric and pancreatic borders. However, this problem is better avoided by withholding solid food for several hours prior to the CT study.

The collimation and spacing of CT sections vary somewhat, depending on the indication for the study and the findings on preliminary sections. For most purposes, 8 to 10 mm collimation

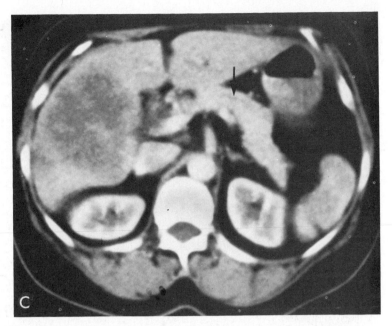

Figure 14–5. *Continued* **C** CT scan 10 seconds later: the pancreas has reached a CT density of 84 H. The faint outlines of a normal pancreatic duct (arrow) are evident; it is detected as the result of enhancement of surrounding pancreatic parenchyma.

(section thickness) is adequate, although 3 to 5-mm collimation through the pancreatic parenchyma is extremely useful in detecting small masses and abnormalities of the pancreatic or distal common bile ducts.[12] Spatial resolution is also improved if scanning time is increased in conjunction with collimation (Fig. 14–6). Contiguous sections are usually obtained, although spacing may be increased to 1.5 or even to 2.0 cm through the peripancreatic area in most cases of widespread inflammation or tumor.

PATHOLOGY

ACUTE PANCREATITIS

Acute pancreatitis may result from numerous etiologies including alcohol, trauma and surgery, cholelithiasis, penetrating peptic ulcer, hyperlipoproteinemia, hypercalcemia, and infection. Regardless of the etiology, the pathologic and radiographic findings are similar and represent a spectrum of changes. It has not been established that acute and chronic pancreatitis are different stages of the same disease. The international symposium held at Marseilles in 1963 defined acute pancreatitis as inflammation with the potential for complete healing, whereas chronic pancreatitis is associated with residual permanent damage. Either form may be marked by relapses of acute inflammation. Duration of the disease is not considered in this classification.[13]

Acute pancreatitis can be subdivided into somewhat overlapping clinical categories reflecting the underlying process of interstitial (edematous)

pancreatitis or hemorrhagic (necrotizing) pancreatitis. In some cases, however, it may be difficult to differentiate these two types of pancreatitis except by their clinical course, with a more prolonged complicated course felt to be indicative of hemorrhagic pancreatitis.[14, 15] Interstitial pancreatitis accounts for 75 to 95 per cent of cases, with most patients showing clinical improvement within 48 to 72 hours on supportive management. The incidence of hemorrhagic pancreatitis varies with the criteria for diagnosis, ranging from 5 to 25 per cent, but results in a disproportionate amount of morbidity and mortality.[14–16]

Indications for CT Scanning

In many cases of acute pancreatitis, diagnosis and management are reasonably straightforward and simple. If a young patient with a recent history of heavy alcoholic intake presents with stabbing upper abdominal pain radiating to the back and with hyperamylasemia, acute pancreatitis is the probable diagnosis and neither CT nor any other imaging modality is necessary at this point. The acute process usually resolves with conservative management within a few days without complication or further diagnostic evaluation. However, computed tomography, in addition to selected complementary imaging tests, is very helpful in at least three clinical settings:

1. Uncertainty about the diagnosis of acute pancreatitis in an acutely ill patient.

2. Suspicion of complications, such as abscess or hemorrhage, in patients believed clinically to have acute pancreatitis.

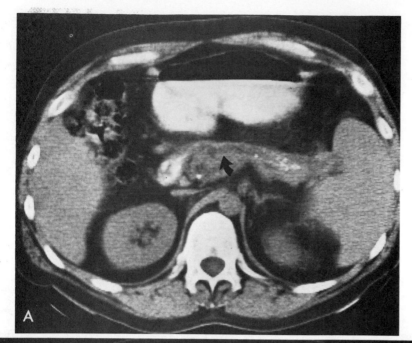

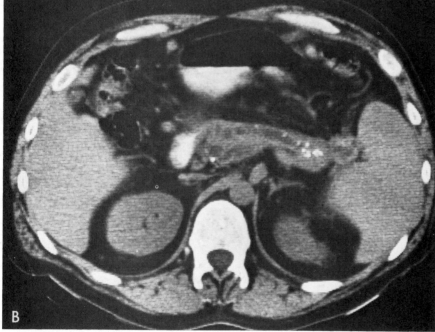

Figure 14–6. Effect of narrowing collimation and increasing scanning times on resolution of pancreatic anatomy. **A** CT scan through the body and tail of the pancreas in a patient with chronic pancreatitis, using 10-mm collimation and a scan time of 4.8 seconds. Dilatation of the pancreatic duct (arrow) and calcifications in the duct are seen. **B** Using 5-mm collimated section and scan time of 9.6 seconds, the ductal structures are more clearly seen.

Illustration continued on opposite page

3. Clinical deterioration or failure to respond to supportive therapy.[17]

Although acute pancreatitis is generally a clinical diagnosis made on the basis of patient history and physical examination, it has a wide range of manifestations and the diagnosis may not be considered. Peterson and Brooks[18] noted that in 40 patients dying of severe pancreatitis, a premortem diagnosis was not made in 43 per cent. Other diseases may exactly simulate the clinical, laboratory, and radiographic manifestations of acute pancreatitis, including acute cholecystitis, peptic ulcer disease, and bowel infarction. Patients may be subjected to a nontherapeutic laparotomy because of misdiagnosis; laparotomy is generally contraindicated in acute interstitial pancreatitis. Even more serious is delaying surgical intervention in cases of bowel infarction misdiagnosed as acute pancreatitis.

Prior to CT, no imaging test had been sufficiently sensitive or specific to have a substantial effect in resolving difficult diagnostic dilemmas. In a prospective study of all patients with a clinical diagnosis of acute pancreatitis, Silverstein and co-workers[19] found that 98 per cent of cases had diagnostic CT studies. Only 62 per cent had di-

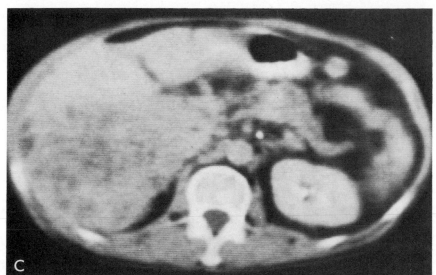

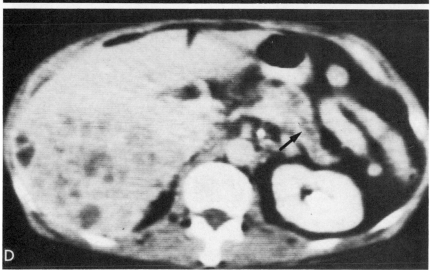

Figure 14–6. *Continued* **C**   Patient with carcinoma of the body of the pancreas, dilated pancreatic duct, and liver metastasis. A 1-cm thick section was obtained after contrast material was given by drip infusion. **D**   A scan through the same region as in **C,** obtained with a 5-mm collimated slice and following an intravenous bolus of contrast material, more clearly demonstrates the tumor, a dilated pancreatic duct (arrow), and metastasis.

agnostic ultrasonographic studies, and of these only 20 per cent were judged to be of good quality. Even in these cases, portions of the pancreas and retroperitoneum were not clearly seen. In many cases, pathology was demonstrated in these areas on CT. In 27 per cent of patients with acute pancreatitis, the CT examination results were normal.[19] It is clear that CT scans should not be performed on every patient with acute pancreatitis, but should be generally obtained in patients who are severely ill and/or who are not responding to supportive therapy. In such a setting, CT will detect abnormalities in virtually every instance.[17, 20]

CT Findings

The manifestations of acute pancreatitis on CT are varied, and there is not a close correlation between the extent of disease as shown by CT and the clinical severity of the attack. The most common finding in acute interstitial pancreatitis is swelling of the gland, though this finding must be interpreted with caution in light of the normal variability of pancreatic size. The swelling is diffuse in the majority of cases, though focal swelling of the head and tail is seen in approximately 48 per cent of cases.[19] The pancreas does not have a firm capsule, and pancreatic secretions commonly break through the thin layer of connective tissue that surrounds the gland (Fig. 14–7). When pancreatic or peripancreatic fluid collections become loculated and fixed by a dense fibrous capsule, they are called *pseudocysts.*

Siegelman and associates[20] chose to designate as "fluid collections" all manifestations of extrapancreatic spread of inflammation. Most investigators prefer the term *phlegmon* to indicate an inflammatory mass arising from the pancreas or diffuse spreading inflammation which goes on to suppu-

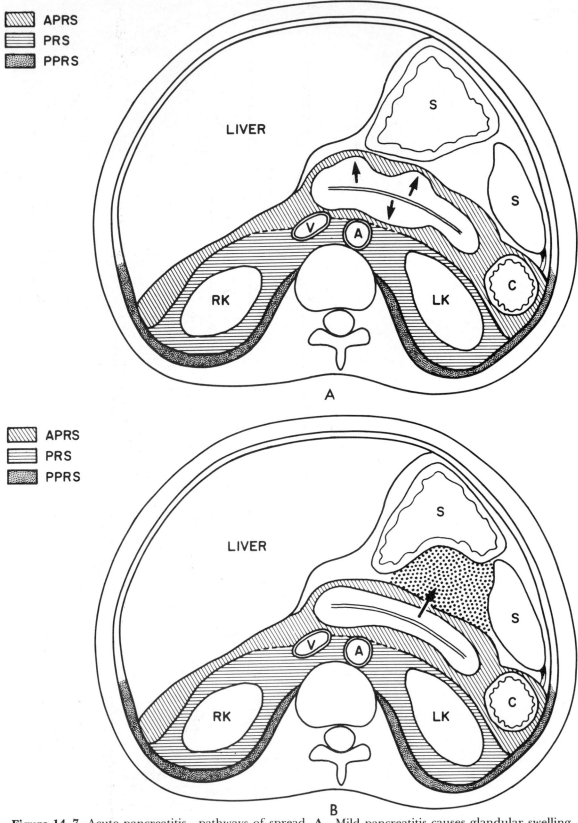

Figure 14–7. Acute pancreatitis—pathways of spread. **A** Mild pancreatitis causes glandular swelling limited by the thin capsule (**B–D**). More extensive inflammation commonly breaks through the capsule to spread within the lesser sac (**B**), anterior pararenal space (**C**), or both (**D**).

Illustration continued on opposite page

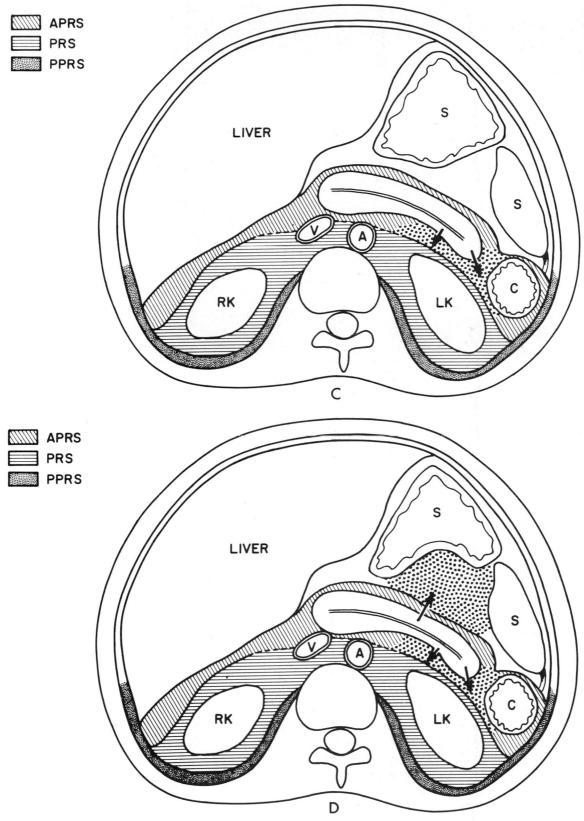

Figure 14–7. *Continued* Spread into the transverse mesocolon and small bowel mesentery is also common.

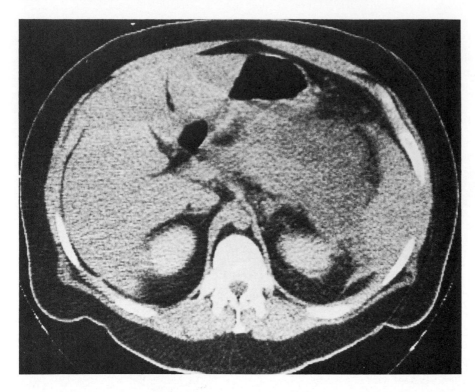

Figure 14–8. Acute pancreatitis. The pancreas is diffusely enlarged, and the margins are obscured by extensive infiltration of peripancreatic fat.

rate or resolve spontaneously.[19, 21] Proof that pancreatic phlegmons are not fluid collections is obtained by sonography and the results of attempted needle aspiration. Although the attenuation value of a pancreatic phlegmon may be near 0 Hounsfield Units (H), pathologically, phlegmons are boggy, edematous soft-tissue masses composed of an admixture of inflammation, exudate, and retroperitoneal fat.

Phlegmonous extension is demonstrable in 18 per cent of unselected cases of pancreatitis[19] and well over 50 per cent of patients with more severe disease.[17, 20] The most common sites of involvement are the lesser sac and left anterior pararenal space; less frequently involved are the transverse mesocolon and small bowel mesentery.

Commonly encountered CT signs of pancreatitis are diffuse pancreatic enlargement, blurring of the pancreatic margins, and thickening of the renal (Gerota's) fascia (Figs. 14–8 through 14–11). Thickening of the renal fascia is a strong indicator of local inflammation and is not seen in normal individuals or those with focal intrapancreatic neoplasms (Figs. 14–9 through 14–11).[22, 23] Infiltration of the pararenal spaces with sparing of the perirenal space can result in the "renal halo sign" on either plain radiographs or CT (Fig. 14–9).[24] Focal thickening of the gastric wall (Fig. 14–9) is seen in 70 per cent of cases of acute pancreatitis in which accurate measurements are possible,[25] and although focal thickening has been described

as a sign of gastric carcinoma or lymphoma,[26, 27] pancreatitis is a more common etiology in some patient populations.

Complications

The morbidity and mortality associated with acute pancreatitis can be attributed largely to the development of hemorrhage, pseudocyst, or abscess.

HEMORRHAGIC PANCREATITIS. The diagnosis of "hemorrhagic pancreatitis" is based on clinical criteria such as a falling hematocrit, hypocalcemia, and failure to respond quickly to resuscitative measures. Significant hemorrhage occurs in 2 to 5 per cent of patients with acute pancreatitis.[15, 16, 28] The mortality in cases of acute hemorrhagic pancreatitis varies from 33 to 100 per cent, depending on the criteria for diagnosis.[16, 29] Prompt surgical intervention has been advocated in patients with hemorrhagic pancreatitis.[16, 29, 30]

The accuracy of CT in detecting hemorrhagic pancreatitis is not known, but pancreatic hemorrhage is identified in about 5 per cent of cases of acute pancreatitis[31] as a collection of high attenuation (greater than 60 H) in the pancreatic area (Fig. 14–12). However, the CT diagnosis of hemorrhagic pancreatitis is not simple because it is difficult to differentiate diffuse peripancreatic hemorrhage from hemorrhage into a pre-existing pseudocyst; moreover, there is no correlation of CT evidence of hemorrhage with the clinical diagnosis of hemorrhagic pancreatitis.[31] Since CT reveals hemorrhage in some patients with a benign clinical course, surgical management is not generally indicated unless clinical factors dictate otherwise.

PSEUDOCYSTS.   Data on the true incidence and natural history of pancreatic pseudocysts are dif-

ficult to compare because of varying criteria and modalities employed for diagnosis. We use the term "pseudocyst" to indicate a collection of necrotic tissue, old blood, and secretions that have escaped from the pancreas damaged by pancreatitis.[32] These secretions, rich in proteolytic enzymes, may become loculated in the lesser sac or they may extend along retroperitoneal tissue

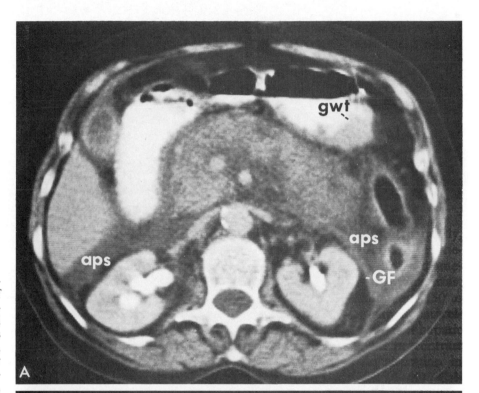

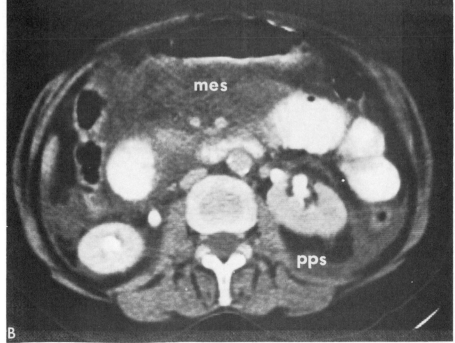

Figure 14–9. Acute pancreatitis. **A,B** Typical pathways of spread of pancreatic inflammation include the left and right anterior pararenal spaces (aps), transverse mesocolon, and small bowel mesentery (mes). Note also focal thickening of the gastric wall (gwt), thickening of Gerota's (anterior renal) fascia (GF), and involvement of the posterior pararenal space (pps) on the left, with sparing of the perirenal space. This is the origin of the "renal halo" sign.

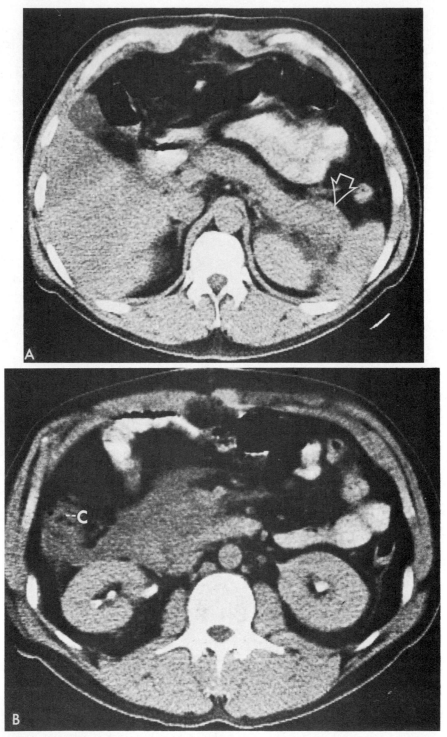

Figure 14–10. Acute pancreatitis simulating appendicitis. Patient is a young man studied by CT after laparotomy for presumed appendicitis. **A**   Pancreatic body is normal in size, but inflammation (open arrow) surrounds the pancreatic tail. **B**   Pancreatic head is swollen and surrounded by inflammation, which spreads within the right anterior pararenal space to involve the ascending colon (C). Symptoms of appendicitis produced by pericolonic inflammation.

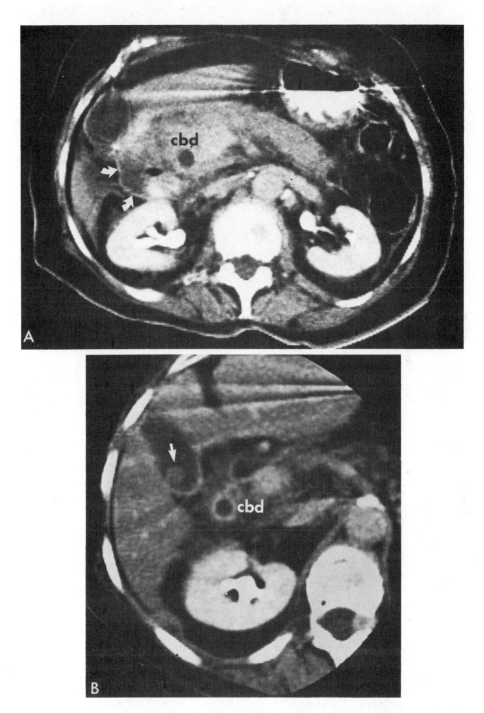

Figure 14–11. Acute pancreatitis. Elderly female clinically suspected of having bowel infarction of cholecystitis. **A**   CT scan reveals the pancreatic head and body to be mildly enlarged. Head of pancreas and duodenum are surrounded by inflammation (curved arrows). Common bile duct (cbd) is enlarged within the pancreatic head. **B**   Gallstone (straight arrow) within gallbladder. The periampullary common bile duct (cbd) is dilated.

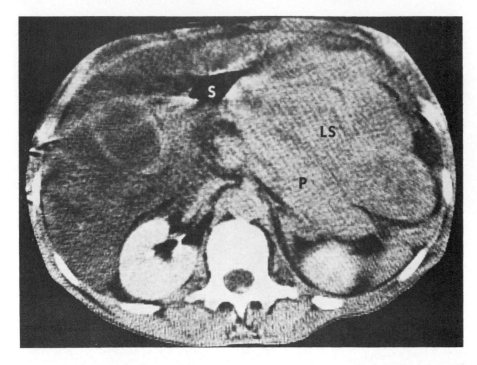

Figure 14–12. Hemorrhagic pancreatitis. Pancreas (P) is enlarged. The stomach (S) is displaced medially by a large mass in the lesser sac (LS) having an attenuation coefficient of 60 H. At surgery 2 liters of blood and necrotic tissue were drained from the lesser sac.

planes in any direction. Pseudocysts may remain within the pancreatic capsule (Fig. 14–13), but more commonly they are found in an extrapancreatic location. They may dissect up into the mediastinum[33] as far as the neck or retroperitoneally until they reach the groin. Pseudocysts may burrow into the wall of the duodenum and simulate intramural or obstructing masses (Fig. 14–14)[34] or may dissect into the liver or spleen. Pseudocysts

extending into the liver along portal tracts may simulate dilated bile ducts (Fig. 14–15).[35]

The wall of the pseudocyst is initially formed by whatever tissue structures first limit its spread. Gradually, the evoked inflammatory reaction encapsulates the contents of the pseudocyst with granulation tissue and then with a fibrous wall; when this has occurred, the pseudocyst is called mature.[32, 36]

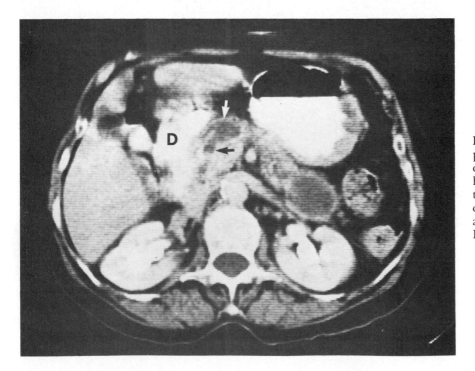

Figure 14–13. Intrapancreatic pseudocysts. Two intrapancreatic pseudocysts, one in the head (white arrow) and one in the tail. Note the slightly dilated common bile duct (black arrow) adjacent to pseudocyst. D = Duodenum.

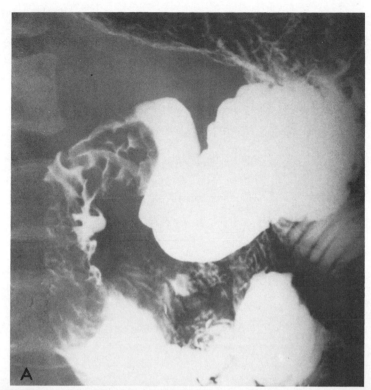

Figure 14–14. Intramural pseudocyst of the duodenum. **A** Upper gastrointestinal series shows intramural mass in the duodenum producing thickening of the mucosal folds, and a partial gastric outlet obstruction. **B** A CT scan demonstrates that the duodenum (D) is compressed medially by a pseudocyst (PC). The pancreatic head is enlarged, and peripancreatic inflammatory infiltrate is present (arrow).

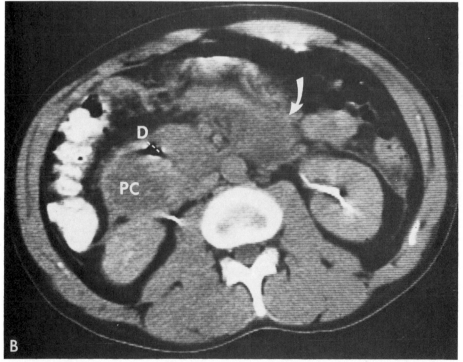

The incidence of pseudocyst following acute pancreatitis in the pre-ultrasound and CT era was estimated as only 2 to 3 per cent.[37, 38] Using CT, Bradley[39] found "fluid collections" in 56 per cent of patients with moderately severe pancreatitis, and Siegelman[20] found "fluid collections" complicating pancreatitis in 54 per cent of patients.

However, both these studies are somewhat misleading, since they grouped all peripancreatic exudates, whether phlegmonous or truly cystic, under the same designation and excluded patients with mild pancreatitis. In a prospective CT study of consecutive patients with pancreatitis, pseudocysts were detected in 10 per cent and extrapan-

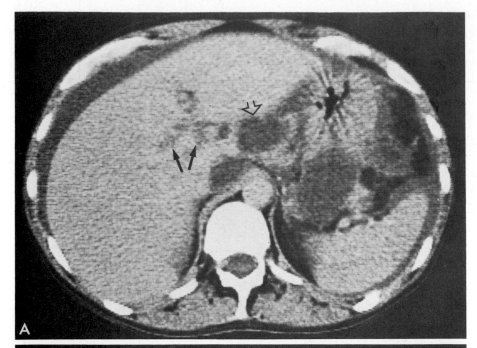

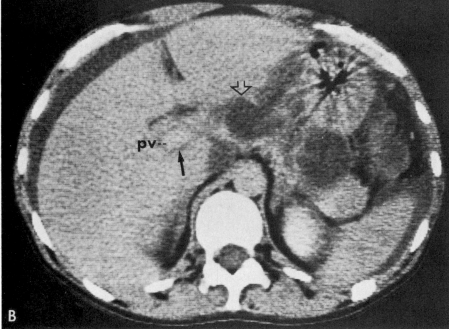

Figure 14–15. Intrahepatic extension of pseudocyst. **A,B** Multiple intra- and peripancreatic pseudocysts, including one in porta hepatis (open arrow). Portal vein (pv) and its branches are surrounded by a region of low density (closed arrows) simulating dilated bile ducts. Ascites surrounds the liver. Ultrasonography demonstrated fluid around the portal venous branches but normal bile ducts.

creatic phlegmons in 18 per cent,[16] figures that are comparable with others using sonography for diagnosis.

It is important to understand the clinical implications of pancreatic inflammation despite the differences in semantics used to describe pancreatic inflammatory lesions. A phlegmon is a pancreatic inflammatory mass or a spreading diffuse inflammation that may resolve completely or may go on to liquify or suppurate.[21, 32] The inflammatory mass may be indistinguishable from neoplasm by CT,[40] but a presumptive diagnosis is usually possible when clinical and biochemical findings are considered. CT scans and sonography can demonstrate evolution of a phlegmon into a pseudocyst by showing progressive liquefaction of the contents and development of a well-defined fibrous capsule (Fig. 14–16). A pseudocyst may simulate a solid mass early in its formation as blood and proteinaceous necrotic debris elevate the attenuation value (Fig. 14–17). Ultrasonography is useful in confirming the fluid nature of the contents of the developing cyst.[41]

Both CT and ultrasonography are useful in following the course of phlegmons and pseudocysts. Twenty to 44 per cent of pseudocysts resolve spontaneously within 6 weeks,[39, 40] but beyond 6 weeks further resolution is rare as a firm fibrous capsule has usually formed.[42] Although CT can be used to follow the maturation of a pseudocyst, sonography is preferred because of its low cost and lack of ionizing radiation. However, prior to surgery, a CT scan should be performed, since CT reveals the number, size, and location of cysts relative to pertinent gastrointestinal structures to better advantage than sonography.[17, 19]

Percutaneous drainage of pseudocysts is becoming a feasible alternative to surgery. However, care must be taken because a variety of pancreatic cystic tumors including cystadenocarcinoma and necrotic carcinoma may mimic the CT appearance of a pseudocyst.[41, 43] Hancke and Pederson[44] reported 14 cases of single percutaneous pseudocyst aspirations using an 18-gauge needle, and had initial success in all 14. Although half of these patients had recurrent pseudocysts within a year, Anderson[45] reported no recurrences in eight patients following single-needle aspirations. Percutaneous placement of multi-holed catheters offers more complete drainage of cysts and thus is becoming preferred over single-needle aspiration.[46–48] Whether catheter drainage will be as effective as internal drainage (cystgastrostomy or jejunostomy) is unknown at present, but it is evident that percutaneous drainage of pancreatic pseudocysts is a safe alternative for surgery in certain patients.

ABSCESSES. Pancreatic abscesses are collections of pus and necrotic tissue within the pancreatic parenchyma that may extend into the lesser sac and retroperitoneum. They are usually the result of secondary infection of devitalized pancreatic and retroperitoneal tissue following necrotizing pancreatitis. Some pseudocysts become infected and are converted into abscesses. Abscesses develop in 4 per cent of all patients with pancreatitis, but the incidence increases with the severity of the attack; abscesses are found in 50 to 70 per cent of fatal cases of necrotizing pancreatitis.[49–52] Survival without surgical drainage is very rare but increases to 66 per cent following surgical drainage.[50–52]

There are a variety of CT findings in pancreatic abscesses[53–55], although the CT findings may not permit a specified diagnosis to be made in all cases. The most diagnostic CT finding is the demonstration of pancreatic or peripancreatic gas, which is usually produced by gas-forming coliform bacteria (Figs. 14–18 and 14–19). However, gas is found in only 30 to 50 per cent of proven abscesses,[55, 56] and caution must be exercised to exclude extraneous sources of gas such as cutaneous or enteric fistulae, ruptured duodenum, or prior surgical intervention. If doubt exists, water-soluble contrast studies of the upper and lower gastrointestinal tract should be obtained, particularly in stable patients, to detect fistulous communications and to avoid unnecessary surgery.[57] Spontaneous rupture of a pseudocyst into stomach or duodenum may be associated with clinical improvement (Fig. 14–20), but spontaneous communication with the distal small bowel or colon usually results in bacterial contamination and necessitates surgery. Half of pseudocysts that rupture spontaneously do so into the peritoneal cavity; these patients have a mortality rate of 70 per cent.[58]

If gas is not present, abscesses are indistinguishable from noninfected phlegmons or pseudocysts (Fig. 14–21).[55, 59] When persistent fever and leukocytosis are present in combination with the CT findings of an inflammatory mass or fluid collection, a percutaneous thin-needle aspiration of the fluid for bacteriologic studies is strongly recommended. CT or sonography is helpful in planning an approach that avoids needle puncture of bowel, thus minimizing the danger of contaminating a sterile collection.

Even when surgery is planned on the basis of a strong clinical suspicion of abscess, CT is valuable in demonstrating the full extent of spread.[55, 60] Multiple abscesses occur in about a third of patients and often are far removed from the pancreatic bed.[51, 60] The preoperative information provided by CT can optimize surgical drainage.

CT scans of patients who have had previous surgical drainage for necrotizing pancreatitis or abscess are also useful. One third of patients require repeated operations for drainage of pancreatic abscesses, and recurrent infection is particularly difficult to diagnose in the postoperative patient.[49, 51] In our experience,[55] CT has been 100 per cent accurate in postoperative patients in con-

Text continued on page 722

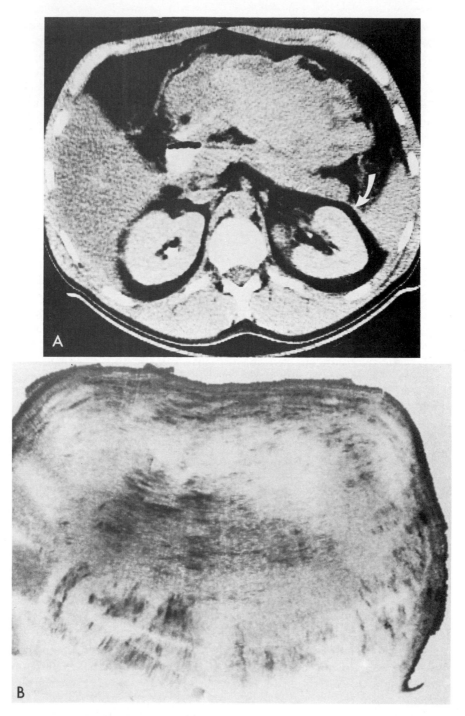

Figure 14–16. Evolution of pancreatic phlegmon into a pseudocyst. **A** CT scan initially shows a peripancreatic mass with irregular borders and nonhomogeneous density (mean, 40 H). Note slight thickening of renal fascia (arrow), a clue to the origin of the mass. **B** Ultrasonogram on same day as initial CT. A poorly defined mass is present which has many internal echoes and limited through-transmission.

Illustration continued on opposite page

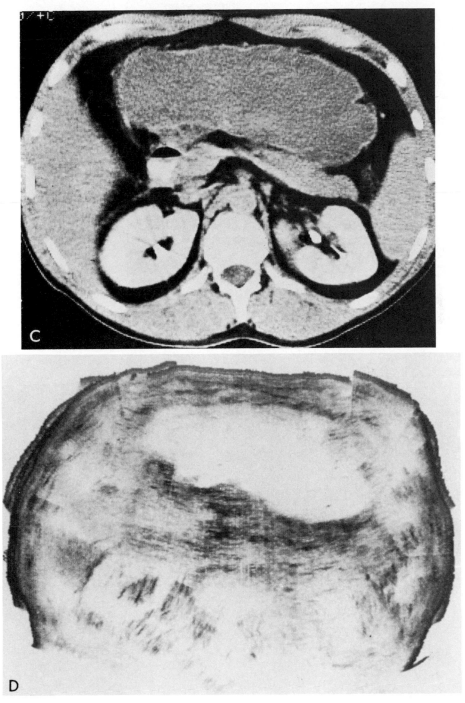

Figure 14–16. *Continued* **C,D**   Repeat CT and sonogram 10 days later. The mass now has an attenuation coefficient of 10 H and has the typical appearance of a pseudocyst with well-defined margins. The ultrasonogram reveals the pseudocyst to have only a few internal echoes and demonstrates enhanced through-transmission.

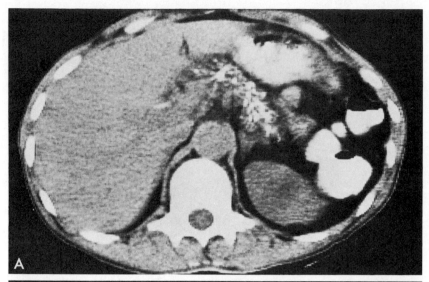

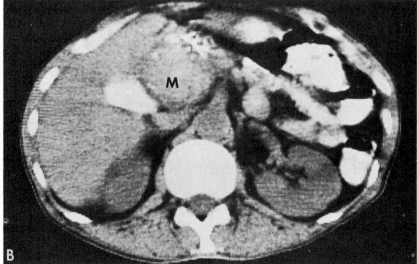

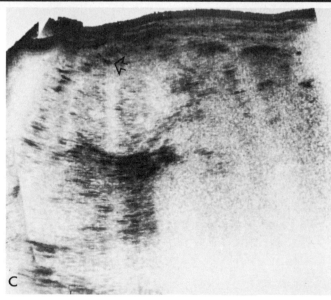

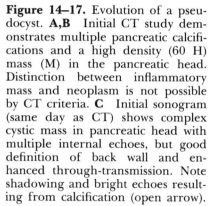

Figure 14–17. Evolution of a pseudocyst. **A,B** Initial CT study demonstrates multiple pancreatic calcifications and a high density (60 H) mass (M) in the pancreatic head. Distinction between inflammatory mass and neoplasm is not possible by CT criteria. **C** Initial sonogram (same day as CT) shows complex cystic mass in pancreatic head with multiple internal echoes, but good definition of back wall and enhanced through-transmission. Note shadowing and bright echoes resulting from calcification (open arrow).

Illustration continued on opposite page

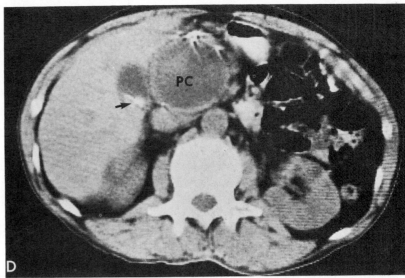

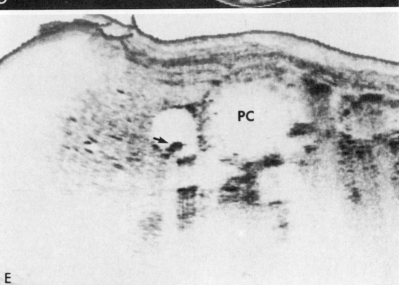

Figure 14–17. *Continued* **D,E** Repeat CT scan and sonogram 10 days later show typical pseudocyst (PC) with well-defined wall, low-density contents (12 H), and few internal echoes. Gallstones are noted incidentally (closed arrow). Complex, high-density characteristics of earlier pseudocyst (**B** and **C**) are due to blood and necrotic debris.

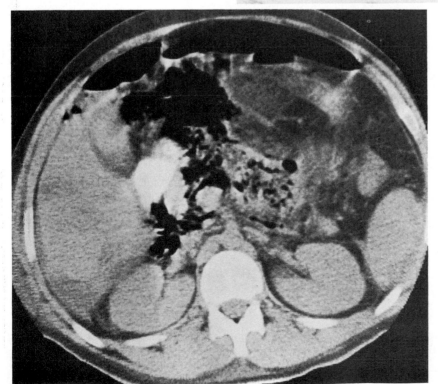

Figure 14–18. Gas-forming pancreatic abscess. The pancreatic parenchyma contains a large amount of gas. There is also gas in the mesentery, retroperitoneum, and peritoneal cavity.

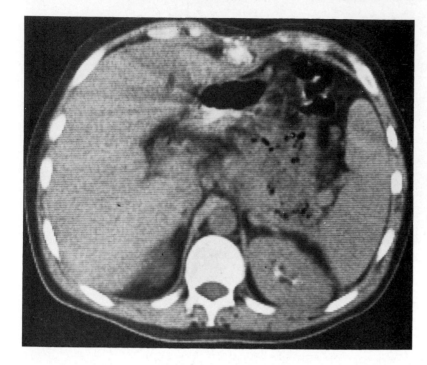

Figure 14–19. Pancreatic abscess. There is extensive gas in pancreatic and peripancreatic region produced by coliform bacteria. The abscess has extended into the anterior pararenal space and lesser sac.

firming the presence or absence of a pancreatic abscess.

CHRONIC PANCREATITIS

Chronic pancreatitis is an irreversible inflammatory disease of the pancreas associated with a number of predisposing factors. Although patients frequently give a history of multiple prior attacks of acute pancreatitis, some patients present with the metabolic, radiographic, and pathologic changes associated with "chronic pancreatitis" during their first acute attack or even without any episodes of pain.[61] Chronic pancreatitis may be clinically manifested as chronic abdominal pain, weight loss, steatorrhea and diabetes. These clinical features and various laboratory determinations are nonspecific, and concern about possible pancreatic carcinoma or other pathology often ultimately requires extensive, expensive, and invasive investigation.

CT Findings

Standard radiographic modalities including plain abdominal radiographs and barium studies may reveal pancreatic calcifications and/or evidence of a mass. Calcifications strongly suggest a diagnosis of chronic alcohol-related pancreatitis, although other etiologies have been rarely implicated.[62] CT can detect calcifications not evident on plain radiographs (Fig. 14–22), dilatation of the pancreatic and common bile duct, and atrophy of the gland and can better delineate and characterize

pancreatic mass lesions (Figs. 14–6 and 14–22 through 14–24).[63]

The diameter of the main pancreatic duct is usually maximum in the head of the pancreas, ranging from 2.0 to 6.5 mm (average 3.9 mm), and gradually decreases in caliber toward the tail.[64] With the use of thin-section (5-mm) collimation and bolus contrast injection with rapid-sequence scanning, normal-sized pancreatic ducts can be identified by CT in 70 per cent of pancreatic studies.[65] (Fig. 14–5). Using optimal CT technique, dilated pancreatic ducts are detectable in all instances.

Neither the diameter nor the degree of irregularity of the lumen of the pancreatic duct is a reliable distinguishing feature between benign and malignant causes of duct obstruction.[12, 65–68] However, in our series of 73 cancers and 46 cases of chronic pancreatitis, the degree of dilatation was less with pancreatitis than with cancer, and the contour was more irregular. Similarly, dilatation of both the pancreatic and common bile ducts (double-duct sign) is found in both chronic pancreatitis and carcinoma (Fig. 14–24).[69] CT can display the anatomy of the pancreatic duct when it is obstructed to retrograde contrast injection and can disclose the underlying cause of ductal obstruction. When endoscopic retrograde cholangiopancreatography (ERCP) fails, CT is useful for determining whether the failure is technical or whether it resulted from a distal duct obstruction.[65]

Several technical and anatomic points must be considered in interpretation of pancreatic duct

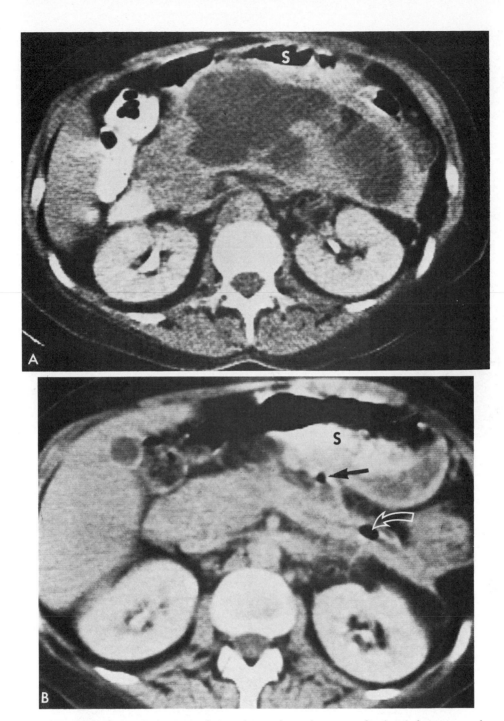

Figure 14–20. Spontaneous rupture of pseudocyst into the stomach. **A** A large pseudocyst in the lesser sac is displacing the stomach (S) forward. **B** One day after a sonogram documented the existence of the large pseudocyst, the patient reported voluminous vomiting and diarrhea. The CT scan demonstrates decompression of the pseudocyst into the stomach. Gas bubbles are noted within a dilated pancreatic duct (open arrow) and within a fistula (closed arrow) between the pancreas and stomach. Patient had an uneventful recovery without surgery.

pathology. CT is technically capable of detecting normal ducts, but streak artifacts may obscure a normal-sized duct. A low-attenuation linear structure mimicking a pancreatic duct may be produced by the margins between the pancreas and splenic vessels (Fig. 14–24),[68, 70] or by alignment of fatty septa within the gland.[65]

Atrophy of the pancreas is a common consequence of chronic inflammation of the pancreas. The CT diagnosis is somewhat subjective but can be suggested when the pancreas is small, the parenchyma is thin, and there are signs of chronic pancreatitis (Figs. 14–22 through 14–25).

Text continued on page 728

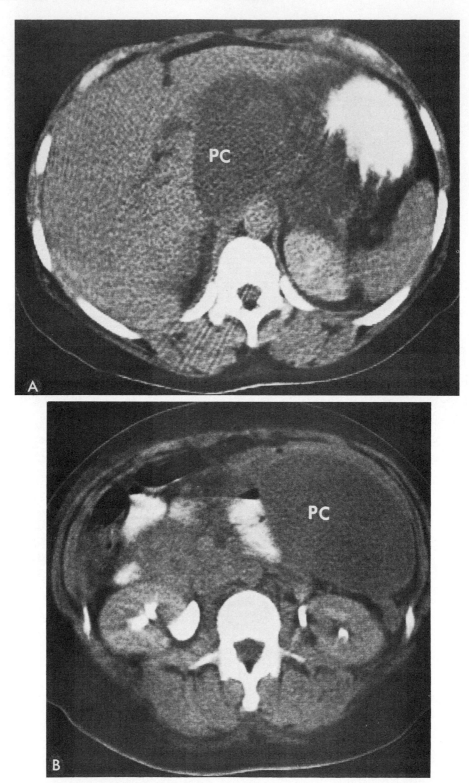

Figure 14–21. Infected pseudocysts. Two large infected pseudocysts (PC) in the upper **(A)** and lower **(B)** recesses of the lesser sac which cannot be distinguished from noninfected pseudocysts. Percutaneous thin-needle aspiration of fluid revealed turbid fluid, which was Gram-stain and culture positive for coliform bacteria. The infected pseudocysts were drained at surgery.

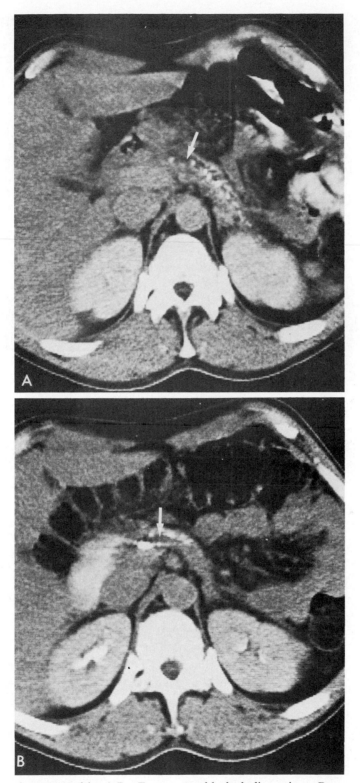

Figure 14–22. Chronic pancreatitis. **A,B**   Forty-year-old alcoholic patient. Pancreatic atrophy is evident along with multiple intraductal calculi and dilatation of the pancreatic duct (arrow). Calcifications are not seen on plain radiograph.

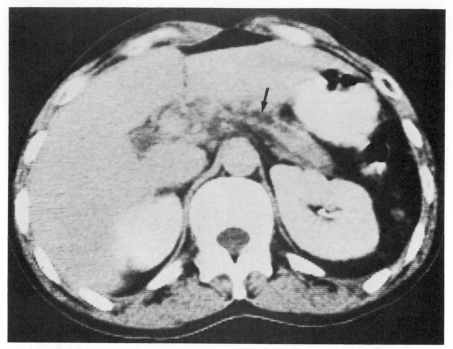

Figure 14–23. Chronic pancreatitis. There is pancreatic atrophy and a dilated pancreatic duct (arrow) but no evidence of pancreatic calcification.

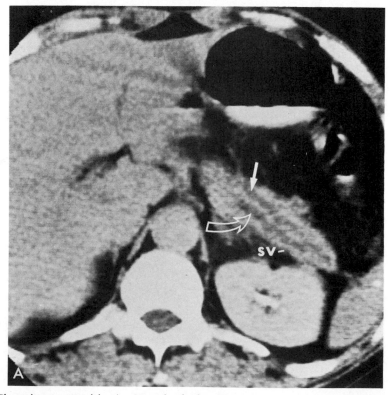

Figure 14–24. Chronic pancreatitis. **A** Note both the dilated slightly irregular pancreatic duct (closed arrow) and the "pseudoduct" (open arrow) owing to the blurred margin between the pancreas and the splenic vessels (sv).

Illustration continued on opposite page

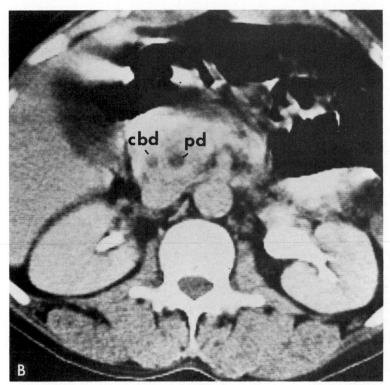

Figure 14–24. *Continued* **B** CT section through the pancreatic head demonstrating the double duct sign. The pancreatic duct (pd) and common bile duct (cbd) are dilated as a result of chronic pancreatitis.

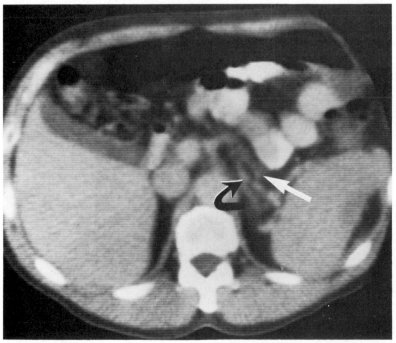

Figure 14–25. Pancreatic atrophy. This patient with chronic pancreatitis has a shrunken pancreas (straight arrow), which is about the same size as the splenic vein (curved arrow).

Pancreatic size and shape vary considerably between normal individuals, and there is a decrease in size with advancing age, sometimes becoming quite marked beyond the sixth decade.[71] Parenchymal atrophy is often accompanied by mild dilatation of the pancreatic duct. However, there is little correlation between the CT appearance of "senile atrophy" and clinical evidence of pancreatic insufficiency.

During an acute exacerbation of chronic pancreatitis, the gland may appear small, normal, or enlarged.[63, 72] Focal enlargements of the gland, accompanied by signs of duct dilatation, may closely mimic pancreatic carcinoma (Fig. 14–26). Chronic

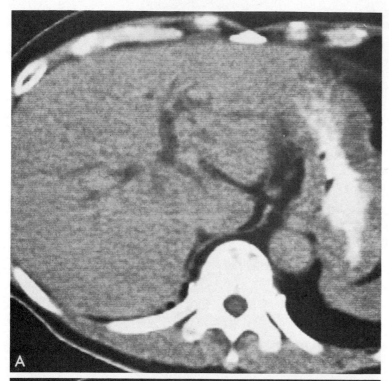

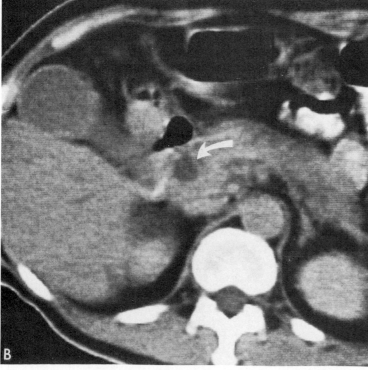

Figure 14–26. Chronic pancreatitis simulating carcinoma. Patient is a 57-year-old man with painless jaundice and no history of alcohol abuse. **A** CT scan demonstrating dilated intrahepatic ducts, **B** CT scan at level on pancreatic head reveals the common bile duct (arrow) to be dilated as it enters the pancreas. The pancreatic body and tail appear normal.

Illustration continued on opposite page

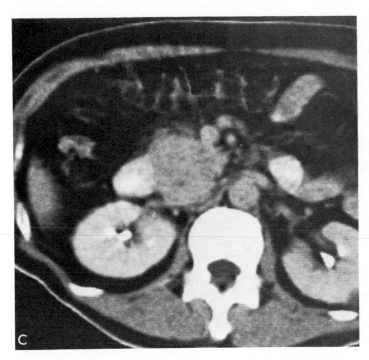

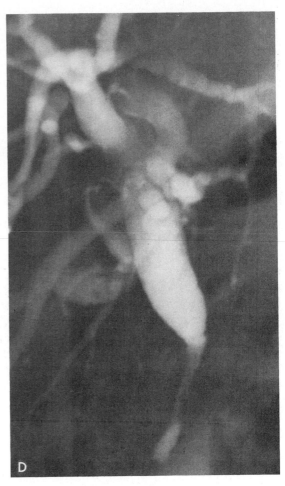

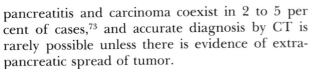

Figure 14–26. *Continued* **C**   Focal enlargement of head and uncinate process of pancreas with obliteration of common bile duct. **D**   A transhepatic cholangiogram demonstrating a focal stricture and angulation of common bile duct within the pancreatic head, with proximal dilatation of the intrahepatic ducts. At surgery, a focal hard mass was found in the pancreatic head and a total pancreatectomy was performed. Multiple pathologic sections revealed only chronic inflammatory changes.

pancreatitis and carcinoma coexist in 2 to 5 per cent of cases,[73] and accurate diagnosis by CT is rarely possible unless there is evidence of extrapancreatic spread of tumor.

At this time, the ability of real-time ultrasonography to detect normal or enlarged pancreatic ducts exceeds that of CT in most cases. However, CT appears to detect other morphologic features such as duct calculi, parenchymal atrophy, and associated inflammatory or neoplastic masses to better advantage than sonography.[61, 74] False-positive and false-negative studies for chronic pancreatitis occur with CT, ultrasonography, and ERCP. Currently, patients suspected of having chronic pancreatitis or pancreatic carcinoma are initially examined with CT. Further investigation by ERCP is indicated if CT is negative but a high clinical index of suspicion remains, or if CT reveals changes of chronic pancreatitis and surgical therapy is being considered.[75]

NEOPLASMS

Initial interest in the capabilities of CT scanning for the detection of pancreatic cancer was based on the results of CT scanning using slower scanners (18 seconds and longer).[4, 5, 76, 77] During the past few years, the availability of fast, high-resolution CT scanners has permitted the demonstration of finer details of the pancreas and surrounding tissues. The application of CT scanning and ultrasound to guidance of transabdominal needles for obtaining histologic and cytologic samples has provided new dimensions to the detection of pancreatic cancer. The development of rapid-sequence, contrast-enhanced scanning techniques has permitted evaluation of vasculature surrounding and supplying the pancreas as well as vascularity of pancreatic tumors. Thus, technologic advances have resulted in greater potential for the detection of pancreatic tumors and have decreased false-negative determinations.[78]

Indications for CT Scanning

Symptoms or signs suggestive of cancer of the pancreas often reflect the location of the tumor. In cancer of the head of the pancreas, the most common features are jaundice and weight loss. If the tumor is confined to the tail or body, frequently no symptoms are present until the lesion is very large, at which time weight loss, back pain, and occasionally a palpable mass may be present. Peripheral thrombophlebitis may indicate an underlying carcinoma. In these clinical situations, CT scanning of the pancreas is indicated. Pancreatic CT scans are also indicated in the presence of a metastatic lesion detected in the lungs or liver, in the absence of a known primary site, and in patients with biochemical evidence of a functioning islet cell tumor.

Primary Pancreatic Tumors

PANCREATIC ADENOCARCINOMA. Change in the size and shape of the pancreas, along with abnormalities in CT attenuation values, obliteration of peripancreatic fat and loss of boundaries with surrounding structures, involvement of vessels and regional lymph nodes, pancreatic ductal dilatation, pancreatic cysts, and obstruction of the common bile duct are all features that indicate possible presence of a pancreatic malignancy.

Change in the Size of the Pancreas. Pancreatic cancer may produce either focal or diffuse pancreatic enlargement. Focal enlargement is most common and is usually confined to specific anatomic areas such as the tail, body, head, or uncinate process or at the interface between these boundaries. Diffuse enlargement of the pancreas resulting from an underlying cancer is uncommon and most often the result of an associated pancreatitis rather than diffuse neoplastic infiltration. However, with cystic neoplasms of the pancreas, the majority of the pancreas may be diffusely involved.

Pancreatic enlargement is common in pancreatic carcinoma, but enlargement is a nonspecific finding and cannot be used as the sole criterion to diagnose carcinoma because an enlarged pancreas can be due to an anatomic variation, inflammation, or benign disease. On the other hand, aging and chronic pancreatitis can result in an atrophic pancreas that may also harbor a small cancer. Measurements have not aided in the detection of small pancreatic masses because of the wide variation in size of the normal pancreas. Usually by the time the pancreatic width is abnormal, an advanced neoplasm is present and other features of malignancy are evident (Fig. 14–27).

Change in Shape and Contour of the Pancreas. This feature is frequently more important than the actual size of the suspected mass. Pancreatic cancer may produce a focal, eccentric mass involving only one surface of the gland, focal rounding of the posterior and anterior surfaces, smooth or lobulated enlargement of the uncinate process, or diffuse enlargement of the head of the pancreas. Even in the absence of absolute enlargement of the head of the pancreas, a focal bulge on one surface may indicate an underlying tumor (Fig. 14–28).[78]

The most difficult area for detecting focal pancreatic enlargement is in the head of the pancreas, whereas such changes in shape and contour are most readily detected in the tail or anterior surface of the pancreatic body. Focal alterations in shape and contour are frequently encountered in the patient with pancreatic carcinoma, but occasionally focal lobulations prove to be normal anatomic variations. With high-resolution CT scan-

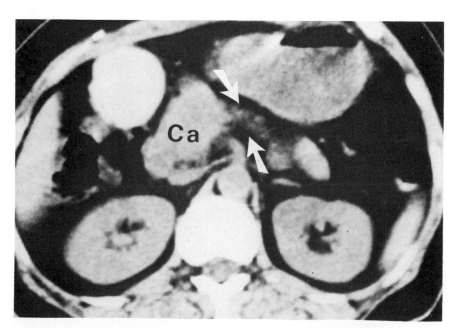

Figure 14–27. Carcinoma of the head of the pancreas. A CT scan demonstrating focal enlargement of the head of the pancreas due to pancreatic carcinoma (Ca). The carcinoma produces an abrupt change in shape from the body of the pancreas (arrows).

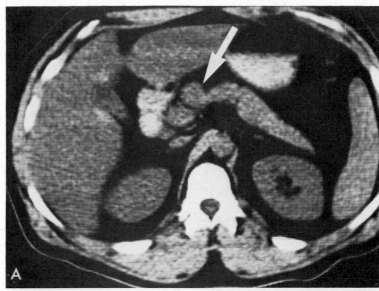

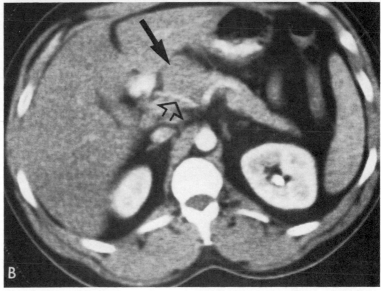

Figure 14–28. Rapid growth of small pancreatic carcinoma. **A** CT scan demonstrating a focal change in shape of the ventral contour of the pancreas at the junction of the body and head (arrow). No enlargement of pancreatic tissue is present. This was initially interpreted as representing an anatomic variation. **B** Three months later, a repeat CT scan shows a focal tumor mass (closed arrow) in the location of the focal contour abnormality seen in **A**. A dynamic CT scan after intravenous bolus injection demonstrates splenic and hepatic arteries at the base of the tumor. The hepatic artery (open arrow) has an irregular contour. Arteriography showed encasement by tumor.

ners, it is possible to detect the fatty interstices frequently seen in the normal pancreas (Fig. 14–4). If fatty interstices enter an area of focal enlargement, then the underlying tissue is more likely to be normal, whereas if the focal enlargement is solid without fatty lobulations, it is most likely to be abnormal and should be the subject of a CT-guided needle biopsy (Fig. 14–29). Diffuse enlargement of the head of the pancreas may result in either a smooth or lobulated contour. When the uncinate process is involved, the sharp, tongue-like contour of the process is lost, replaced by a blunted enlargement projecting between the superior mesenteric vein and the renal vein or duodenum (Fig. 14–30). Change in the size and change in the shape or contour together are the most frequent features of pancreatic cancer, occurring in 95 per cent of patients.[79]

Abnormalities in CT Attenuation Values. The normal mean CT attenuation value of the pancreas ranges from 30 to 50 H,[6] and most pancreatic tumors do not have CT numbers significantly different from those of the surrounding pancreatic parenchyma (Fig. 14–28).[5, 9, 79] Pancreatic tumors undergoing necrosis have lower CT numbers, but usually the decrease in CT attenuation has an irregular distribution without sharply defined margins. However, in some cases a necrotic tumor simulates a pseudocyst by having well-defined borders and a uniform low density (Fig. 14–31). The term "pseudo-pseudocyst" has been used to describe these necrotic, cystic pancreatic carcinomas.[43] Necrotic pancreatic carcinomas must be differentiated from true pseudocysts secondary to pancreatitis and from massively dilated pancreatic ducts containing mucin. Gener-

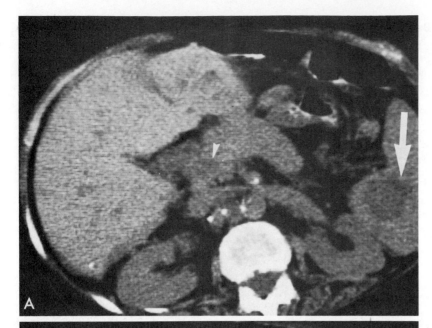

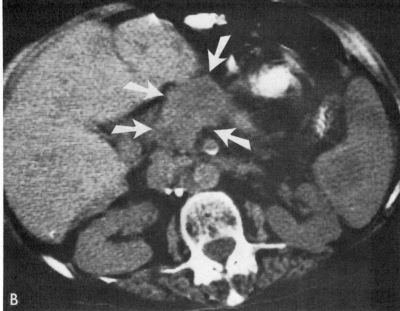

Figure 14–29. Carcinoma of pancreatic head with CT guided percutaneous needle biopsy. **A** CT scan of the pancreas in a 38-year-old patient with weight loss and mild jaundice shows a normal body, with an ill-defined, low-density mass in the pancreatic head (arrowhead). A metastatic lesion is also present in the spleen (arrow). **B** CT scan 2 cm caudal to **A**. Focal enlargement of the pancreatic head is seen (arrows).

Illustration continued on opposite page

ally, necrotic pancreatic neoplasms have thicker walls and central attenuation values greater than seen in inflammatory pseudocysts. However, a CT-guided biopsy may be needed to confirm or exclude the diagnosis of a necrotic pancreatic tumor.

The usefulness of intravenous contrast medium administration to detect pancreatic carcinoma is still being clarified. In one series of tumors studied before and after intravenous infusion of contrast material, the tumors were noted to enhance to the same degree as the normal pancreas.[80] However, by giving an intravenous bolus of 70 to 80 ml of contrast material and performing rapid-sequence scanning, some solid pancreatic tumors do not increase or increase less in density than the surrounding normal pancreatic parenchyma, and thereby appear as relatively low-density lesions (Figs. 14–32 and 14–33). The difference in CT attenuation value of pancreatic tumor and normal pancreatic tissue can be very transient, being undetectable minutes after contrast agent injection (Fig. 14–34). Not all pancreatic neoplasms are demonstrated as hypodense areas after a contrast bolus, but fewer are identified after a slow infusion of contrast material. Therefore, our proce-

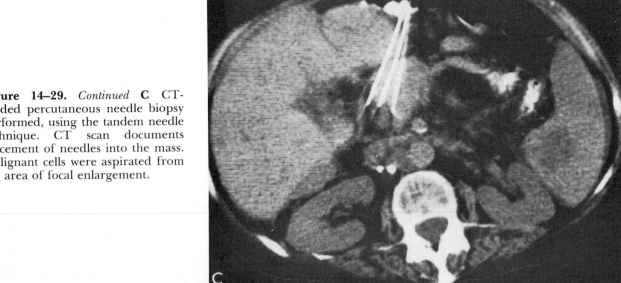

Figure 14–29. *Continued* **C** CT-guided percutaneous needle biopsy performed, using the tandem needle technique. CT scan documents placement of needles into the mass. Malignant cells were aspirated from the area of focal enlargement.

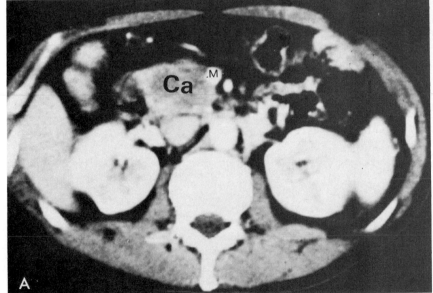

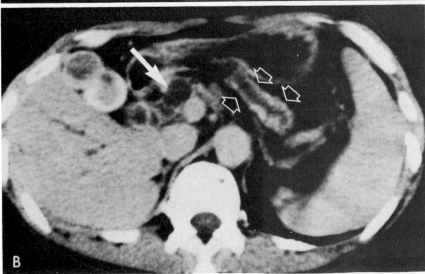

Figure 14–30. Cystadenocarcinoma of the uncinate process. **A** CT scan demonstrates a nonenhancing tumor (Ca) of the uncinate process. There is enlargement and rounding of the uncinate process. The tumor has a round shape as it extends beneath the inferomedial border of the superior mesenteric vein (M). The normal uncinate process tapers as it passes beneath the superior mesenteric vein (see Figs. 14–3*B* and 14–4*B*). **B** The pancreatic duct distal to the cystadenocarcinoma is dilated (open arrows), appears slightly tortuous and has a generally smooth contour. A dilated common bile duct (solid arrow) is present adjacent to the portal vein–superior mesenteric vein confluence.

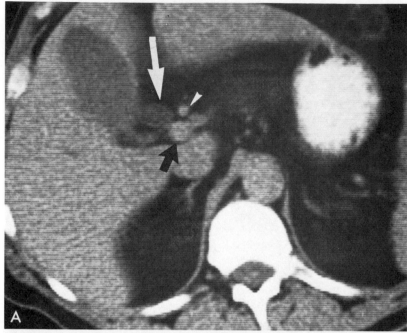

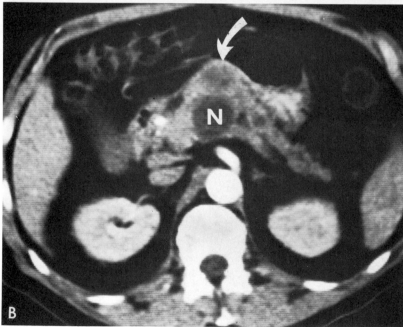

Figure 14–31. Necrotic pancreatic carcinoma associated with cystic dilatation of the obstructed pancreatic duct. **A** CT scan through the porta hepatis of a cirrhotic patient with jaundice and weight loss demonstrates a mildly dilated common hepatic duct (white arrow) with the portal vein (black arrow), and hepatic artery (arrowhead) just ventral to it. **B** CT section through the body of the pancreas demonstrates a necrotic lesion (N) with a low-density area which simulates a pseudocyst. Ventral to the mass is the dilated pancreatic duct (arrow) which has a rounded appearance. The dilated duct in the tail of the pancreas is somewhat beaded in appearance. (From Itai Y, Moss AA, Goldberg HI: Pancreatic cysts caused by carcinoma of the pancreas: A pitfall in the diagnosis of pancreatic carcinoma. J Comput Assist Tomogr 6:772, 1982. Used with permission.

Illustration continued on opposite page

dure is to give a bolus injection of contrast media and perform a dynamic CT scan sequence through any area of suspected pancreatic abnormality.

Obliteration of Peripancreatic Fat. As pancreatic carcinoma extends from the substance of the gland, peripancreatic fat is invaded resulting in an increase in CT number and obliteration of the normally detected fat. Peripancreatic spread of carcinoma may take the form of subtle irregularity in the pancreatic margin, or it may be seen as a diffuse change in part or all of the peripan-

creatic fat. Obliteration of some portion of the fat is one of the most common findings in pancreatic cancer,[9, 79, 81] occurring in 84 per cent of one series.[79] Changes in the CT appearance of the fat are almost always the result of tumor invasion.[5, 9] However, pancreatitis associated with cancer may contribute to the change in fat density.

Pancreatic carcinoma can extend to obliterate the fat planes between the pancreas and the spleen, splenic flexure of the colon, posterior gastric wall, gastric antrum, duodenum, transverse

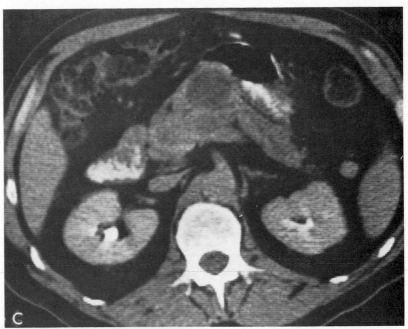

Figure 14–31. *Continued* **C** The tumor has spread into the head of the gland. The obstructed pancreatic duct now also simulates a pancreatic pseudocyst.

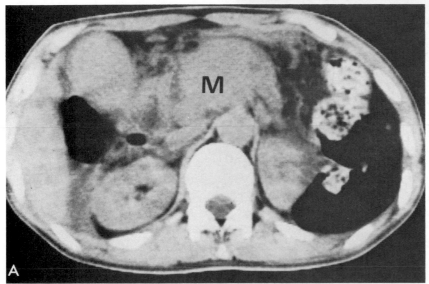

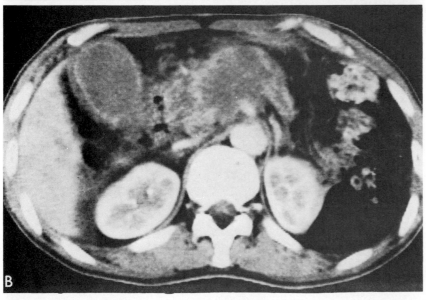

Figure 14–32. Intravenous bolus injection of contrast material and dynamic scan technique for outlining pancreatic carcinoma. **A** CT scan prior to intravenous contrast material administration demonstrates a homogeneous mass (M) in the body of the pancreas. **B** CT scan after an intravenous bolus of contrast material. Sequential scans were obtained every 5 seconds for 1 minute. Scan at time of maximum aortic contrast reveals the surrounding vascular structures and normal pancreatic parenchyma to enhance while the pancreatic carcinoma remains unchanged and thereby appears as a low-density mass.

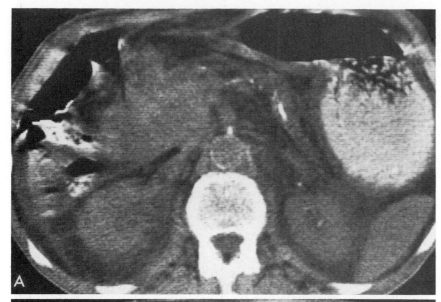

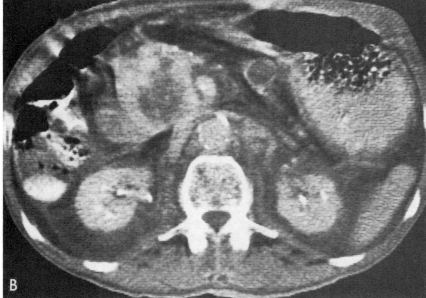

Figure 14–33. Pancreatic cancer after bolus injection of contrast material. **A** A large mass in the head of the pancreas appears isodense with kidney and spleen prior to administration of intravenous contrast material. **B** After a bolus intravenous injection, the center of the tumor remains unenhanced, while the periphery and surrounding pancreatic parenchyma increase in CT density.

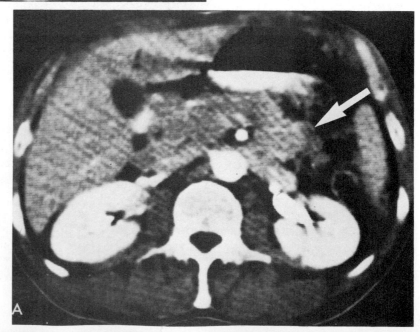

Figure 14–34. Transient enhancement of a functional islet cell carcinoma after intravenous bolus injection of contrast material. **A** After a 50-ml intravenous bolus of contrast material, a CT scan shows a focal hyperdense bulge in the tail of the pancreas (arrow).

Illustration continued on opposite page

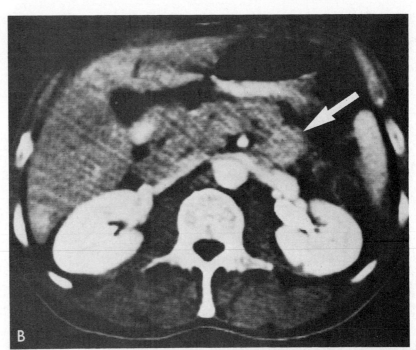

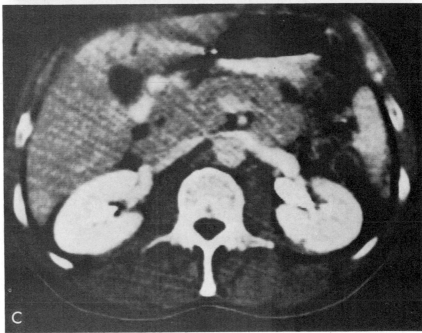

Figure 14–34. *Continued* **B**   A CT scan obtained 6 seconds after **A** demonstrates greater enhancement of the tumor (arrow). **C**   A CT scan obtained 6 seconds after **B** shows the tumor has become isodense with normal pancreatic parenchyma.

mesocolon, and porta hepatis (Figs. 14–35 through 14–39).[4, 5, 9, 76, 78, 81] Although a mass in the porta hepatis is readily detected on CT scans, extension of tumor along the gastrohepatic ligament may be difficult to detect.

When no fat plane is seen separating a pancreatic mass from an adjacent organ or structure, usually it is assumed that pancreatic tumor has invaded the adjacent organ by direct extension. However, obliteration of the peripancreatic fat plane indicates that the pancreatic mass is touching a surrounding organ but is not proof that the pancreatic mass has actually extended into the adjacent structures. Caution must therefore be exercised in reporting direct pancreatic invasion into adjacent structures unless the peripancreatic fat plane is obliterated and the pancreatic tumor is seen to directly replace or invade the parenchyma of nearby organs. Caution must also be exercised in interpreting preservation of the peripancreatic fat planes as absolute proof that no direct extension has occurred as microscopic invasion may occur without obliteration of peripancreatic fat.

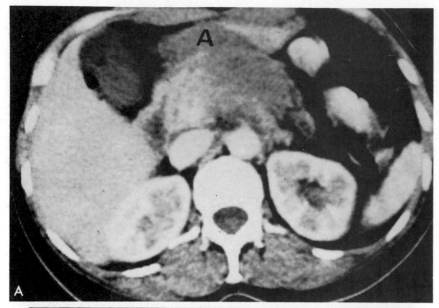

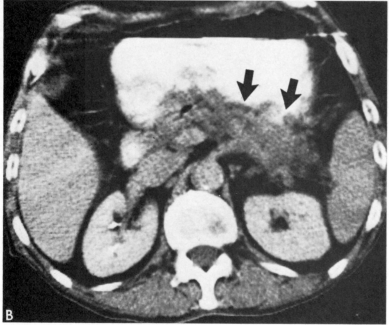

Figure 14–35. Pancreatic carcinoma invading the stomach. **A** There is invasion of the antrum of the stomach (A) by an adjacent pancreatic cancer, causing thickening of the antral wall and obliteration of fat between the antrum and pancreas. **B** Direct invasion of the greater curvature of the stomach by pancreatic cancer originating in the body and tail (arrows). (From Itai Y, Moss AA, Golberg HI: Pancreatic cysts caused by carcinoma of the pancreas: A pitfall in the diagnosis of pancreatic carcinoma. J Comput Assist Tomogr 6:772, 1982. Used with permission.)

When a very thin fat plane exists between the mass and the organ, it is also possible that small fingerlike extensions of tumor may be present and not detected by CT scanning. Despite these limitations, evidence from studies on extension of rectal, gastric and esophageal carcinoma to adjacent structures indicate that when tumor obliterates adjacent fat planes and appears on CT scans to extend into adjacent organs, tumor extension is confirmed by surgical examination.[26, 82]

When adjacent organs are directly invaded by pancreatic tumor, the CT number of the tumor may be the same as that of the involved organ, thereby rendering the actual amount of the tumor indistinguishable from the invaded tissue. In other instances, the tumor has a lower CT number than that of the involved organ and can readily be identified and distinguished from normal tissue. Intravenous contrast injections help to accentuate the difference between pancreatic tumor and surrounding normal tissue.

Involvement of Vessels and Regional Lymph Nodes. Pancreatic malignancies frequently extend to involve adjacent vascular structures. Angiographic techniques reveal that the splenic and portal vein, as well as the celiac, superior mesenteric, splenic, and hepatic arteries can be narrowed, displaced, or occluded by pancreatic tumors (Figs. 14–28, 14–38, 14–40, and 14–41). Computed tomography using bolus injection techniques can also

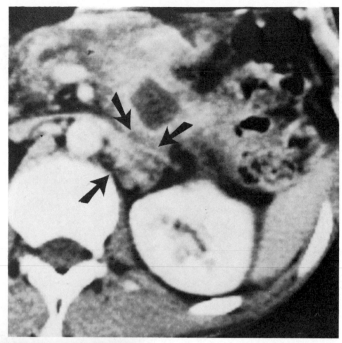

Figure 14–36. Pancreatic carcinoma involving the renal vasculature. A CT scan demonstrating direct extension of carcinoma from the tail of the pancreas to the left renal vein and artery (arrows). The fat ordinarily separating these structures has been obliterated.

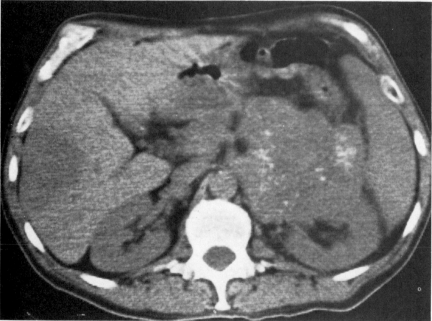

Figure 14–37. Renal invasion by a pancreatic malignancy. There is invasion of the left kidney by a large functioning islet call carcinoma (gastrinoma) of the tail of the pancreas. Foci of calcium are present within the tumor.

Figure 14–38. Pancreatic carcinoma invading the porta hepatis. A CT scan demonstrates a direct extension of carcinoma of the head of the pancreas into the porta hepatis (small arrows), encasing the hepatic arteries and common bile duct (large arrow). (Case courtesy of General Electric Medical Systems Division, Milwaukee, Wis.)

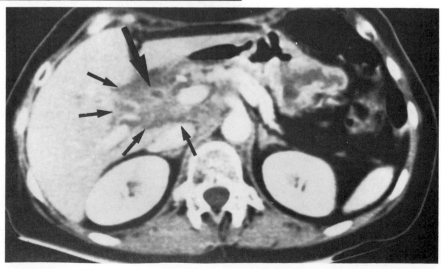

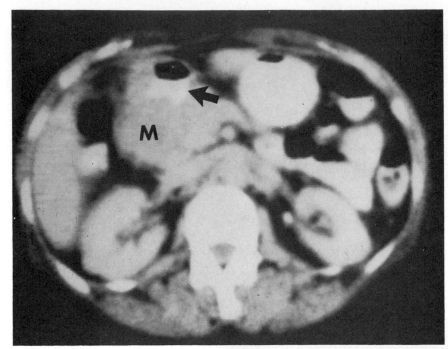

Figure 14–39. A large carcinoma of the head of the pancreas (M) invading and encasing the duodenum (arrow).

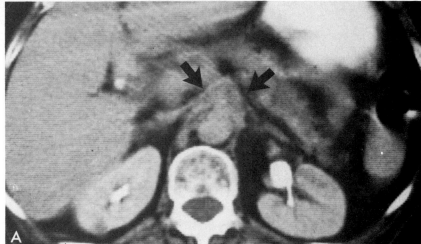

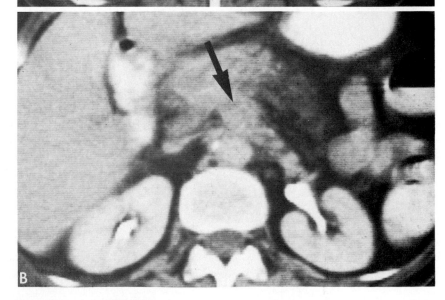

Figure 14–40. Extension of pancreatic tumor to involve the origin of the celiac and superior mesenteric arteries. **A** Obliteration of the fat ordinarily surrounding the celiac artery, with replacement by tumor tissue resulting in a triangle of density (arrows). No pancreatic tumor is seen in this section. Tumor in lymph nodes surrounding the artery was confirmed in specimens obtained by a CT-guided fine-needle aspiration biopsy and at surgery. **B** CT scan at level of origin of superior mesenteric artery. The pancreatic tumor at the junction of the body and head is extending directly to the root of the superior mesenteric artery (arrow).

Illustration continued on opposite page

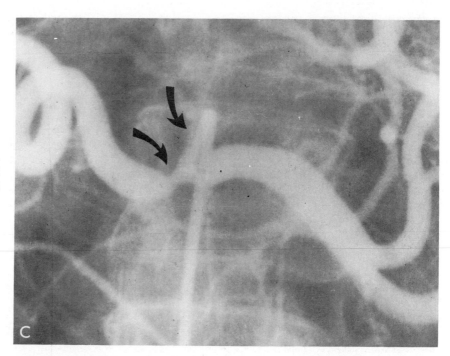

Figure 14–40. *Continued* **C** Encasement of the celiac artery and origin of hepatic artery (arrows) confirmed by angiography.

demonstrate abrupt obstruction, narrowing, or displacement of peripancreatic vessels (Figs. 14–28 and 14–42). Venous occlusion is often accompanied by collateral venous circulation which is manifest on contrast-enhanced CT scans as a plethora of vessels located in and around the gastric wall and splenic hilum (Fig. 14–43). Loss of the perivascular fat plane around the celiac or superior mesenteric artery is evidence that a pancreatic tumor is probably unresectable.

Tumor spread to regional lymph nodes is frequently detected by CT scans. In a series of 73 cases reviewed at the University of California, San Francisco, 23 (32 per cent) had evidence of regional lymph node involvement, and in another series, 65 per cent of patients had similar spread.[79]

Tumor commonly metastasizes to the group of lymph nodes around the celiac and superior mesenteric artery. Ordinarily, lymph nodes occurring in this area are too small to produce significant soft-tissue densities in the background of perivascular fat. However, when tumor is present, the fat surrounding the celiac or superior mesenteric artery becomes the same density as the unenhanced artery, producing a triangle of soft-tissue density (Fig. 14–40). The increased density may be caused by enlargement of regional lymph nodes, or by direct extension of tumor into the fat ordinarily surrounding these vessels. Angiography may demonstrate encasement of the involved artery when this finding is present on CT scans (Fig. 14–40). Occasionally, the appearance of a soft-tissue

Figure 14–41. Flattening of superior mesenteric vein (arrows) by a small pancreatic tumor.

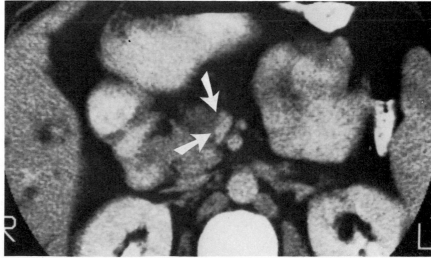

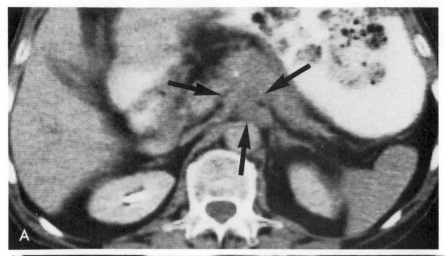

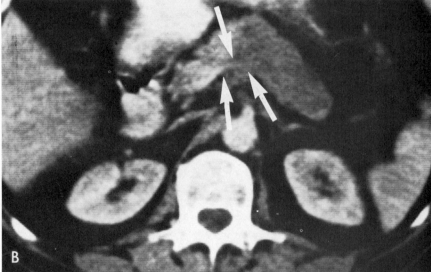

Figure 14–42. Involvement of vessels by pancreatic cancer. **A** A tumor in the body of the pancreas has extended dorsally to encase the celiac artery (arrows). **B** A bolus injection obtained on a section 1 cm lower than in **A** shows the tumor narrowing the splenic vein (arrows).

Figure 14–43. Compression of splenic vein by tumor. **A** A carcinoma of the head of the pancreas (Ca) producing ostructive jaundice.

Illustration continued on opposite page

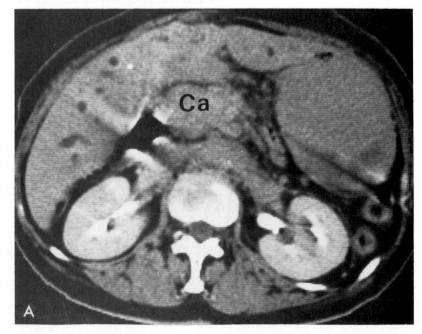

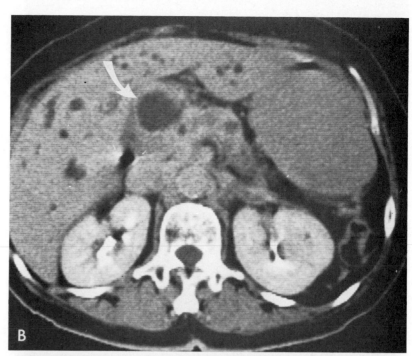

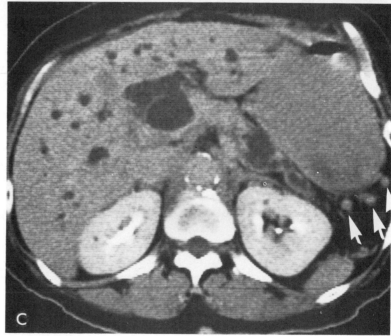

Figure 14–43. *Continued* **B** CT scan at higher level demonstrates pancreatic ductal dilatation and dilatation of the common bile duct (arrow). **C** CT scan 2 cm cephalad to the one in **B** reveals dilated gastric venous collaterals (arrows) resulting from splenic vein compression.

Illustration continued on following page

density around the celiac and superior mesenteric arteries occurs in the absence of a definable pancreatic mass. In one study, obliteration of perivascular fat around these arteries was present in one third of patients with pancreatic cancer studied by CT scanning,[83] and in our series of 73 pancreatic cancers, 34 per cent had this finding. Enlargement of lymph nodes in the para-aortic, pericaval, retrocrural, and porta hepatis regions owing to metastasis can also be detected on CT scans

The overall occurrence of regional lymph node spread has been reported to vary between 38 and 65 per cent.[79, 83]

Metastases to the liver are common in pancreatic cancer, occurring in 17 to 55 per cent of patients.[79, 80] Hepatic metastases from pancreatic adenocarcinoma usually appear as low-density lesions in the unenhanced liver and only rarely dramatically enhance after administration of the intravenous contrast material. They may be isolated,

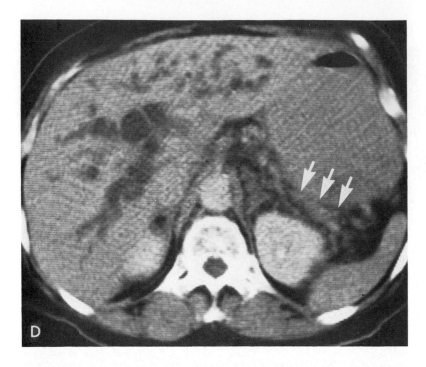

Figure 14–43. *Continued* **D** CT scan 1 cm cephalad to the one in **C** confirms patency of the splenic vein (arrows).

single or multiple metastases and can occur in all lobes of the liver. Splenic metastases are rare (Fig. 14–29).

Association of Pancreatic Cancer with Pseudocysts, Pancreatic and Biliary Ductal Dilatation, and Chronic Pancreatitis. Pancreatic cancer, which invariably originates from ductal epithelium, often results in obstruction of the pancreatic duct with resultant dilatation.[12, 67, 84–87] With the utilization of high-resolution, rapid-sequence CT scanning, dilated and even normal pancreatic ducts can be readily detected. (Figs. 14–5 and 14–6).[12, 65, 88] A massively enlarged pancreatic duct can easily be detected with the older-generation scanners having slow scan speeds, but detection of slight to moderate enlargement is dependent upon adequate technique and newer scanners. Sagittal and coronal reconstructed images can also aid in the evaluation of the pancreatic duct.[88] Using appropriate techniques, linear low-density structures of 3 mm are clearly seen in phantoms of the pancreas,[65] and short segments of normal pancreatic ducts can be identified in vivo (Fig. 14–5).

The incidence of pancreatic ductal dilatation in the presence of pancreatic cancer is difficult to ascertain. In a study of 500 CT scans of the pancreas,[67] a dilated duct was found in ten patients (2 per cent) and in half of these associated pancreatic cancer was present. In our series of 73 pancreatic cancers, the pancreatic duct was detected in 72 per cent of patients, and was dilated in 66 per cent. In another series[81] of 15 cases of cancer of the pancreatic head, the duct was dilated in 11 patients (73 per cent). The size of the

dilated duct resulting from pancreatic carcinoma ranged from 5 to 10 mm and was either smooth or beaded (Figs. 14–30, 14–31, and 14–44 through 14–46). The contour of the dilated duct in pancreatic cancer is more often smooth or beaded, whereas in chronic pancreatitis it is more often irregular. However, there is an overlap in these features. It is important to detect ductal dilatation because it may represent the major pancreatic abnormality in pancreatic cancer in which the tumor is too small to be identified by CT scanning (Fig. 14–46). In our series, five of ten pancreatic carcinomas without a demonstrable mass had a dilated pancreatic duct.

Pancreatic Cysts. Cystic lesions in the body and tail of the pancreas are occasionally found in association with carcinoma of the head of the pancreas. Although these cystic lesions may be pseudocysts associated with chronic pancreatitis, they can also represent cysts secondary to pancreatic cancer. These secondary cysts are relatively uncommon, occurring in one series in 8 per cent of 73 documented pancreatic cancers.[89] The cysts, which on CT scans may be indistinguishable from pseudocysts associated with pancreatitis, are always located distal to the tumor (Figs. 14–31, 14–47, and 14–48). Differentiation of a secondary cyst from a true pseudocyst or a congenital cyst occurring as part of polycystic renal-liver disease or von Hippel-Lindau disease may depend on analysis of the fluid content after CT-guided needle aspiration. Even examination of pathologic specimens may not permit differentiation between true pseudocysts and retention cysts sec-

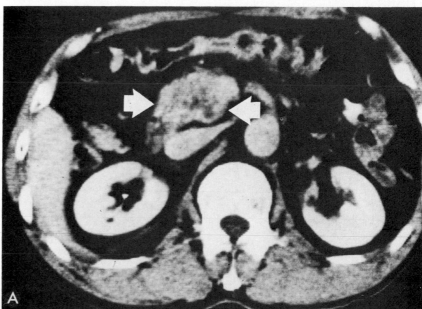

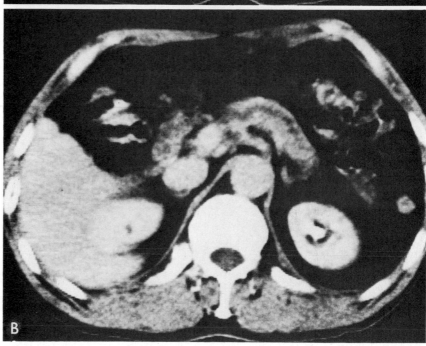

Figure 14–44. Pancreatic duct dilatation produced by carcinoma in the head of the gland. **A** Low-density focal carcinoma in the head of the pancreas (arrows). **B** The main pancreatic duct is dilated. The duct has a smooth contour in the body and a slightly irregular contour in the tail.

ondary to cancer. When a pseudocyst is encountered in a patient without a history of predisposing factors for pancreatitis, further investigation is necessary to determine whether an underlying tumor is present.

Association with Chronic Pancreatitis. An increased incidence of carcinoma of the pancreas has been noted in chronic calcific pancreatitis.[73, 90] However, the CT detection of carcinoma in a gland which has undergone the changes of chronic inflammation depends on whether the tumor is hypodense, is larger than the rest of the pancreas,

has spread to adjacent lymph nodes and organs, or metastasized to the liver. In the absence of these findings, the detection of a carcinoma is often not possible in the chronically inflamed, enlarged, inhomogeneous pancreas containing a dilated duct and calcification. Except for rare malignant islet cell tumors (Fig. 14–37),[91] most pancreatic cancers do not contain calcification. In pancreatitis with pancreatic atrophy, the presence of a tumor may be suggested by detection of a focal mass associated with pancreatic ductal dilatation (Fig. 14–44). In some patients with pancreatitis

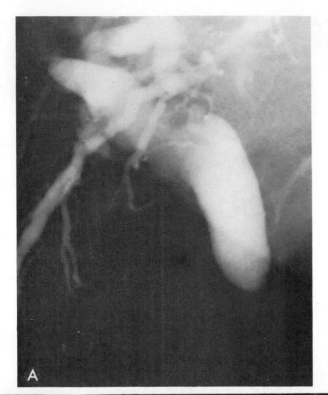

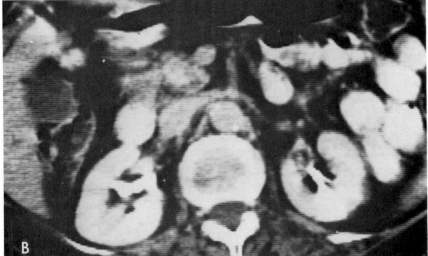

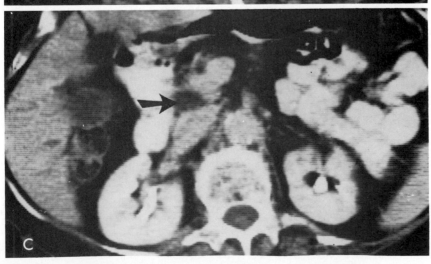

Figure 14–45. Carcinoma of the papilla of Vater causing biliary and pancreatic duct dilatation. **A** Percutaneous transhepatic cholangiogram demonstrates dilatation of the common bile duct with obstruction in the distal, intrapancreatic portion. **B** CT scan through the head of the pancreas and uncinate process shows no tumor mass and no common bile duct dilatation. **C** CT scan 1 cm cephalad to **B** shows the dilated distal common bile duct (arrow) and defines the point of obstruction in the head of the pancreas. No tumor mass is demonstrated.

Illustration continued on opposite page

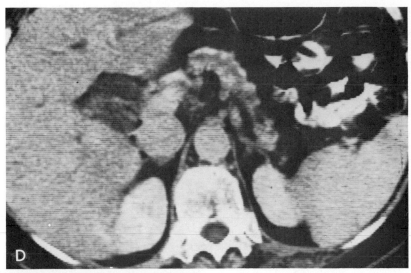

Figure 14–45. *Continued* **D**   The main pancreatic duct is dilated proximal to the papillary tumor. Although the contour is undulating, it does not have the beaded appearance typical of chronic pancreatitis.

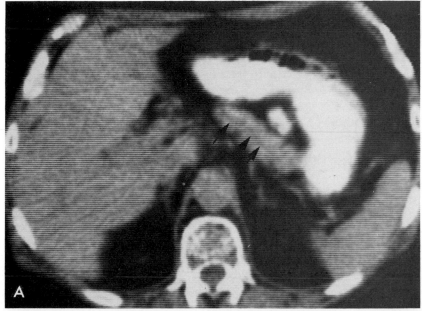

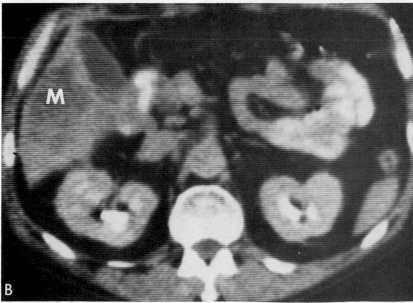

Figure 14–46. Pancreatic ductal dilatation in the absence of a definable pancreatic cancer. **A** Mild pancreatic ductal dilatation is present in the tail and body (arrows). No pancreatic mass or density abnormality is noted. **B** CT scan of head and uncinate process fails to demonstrate the 2-cm carcinoma that was found at surgery. Even though the tumor was small, extensive liver metastasis were already present (M).

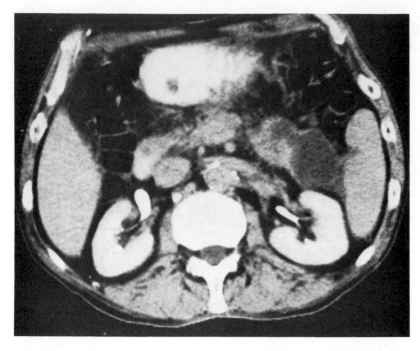

Figure 14–47. Cystic changes in the tail of the pancreas occurring distal to the carcinoma of the body of the pancreas shown in Figure 14–35*B*. (From Itai Y, Moss AA, Goldberg HI: Pancreatic cysts caused by carcinoma of the pancreas: A pitfall in the diagnosis of pancreatic carcinoma. J Comput Assist Tomogr 6:772, 1982. Used with permission.)

and pancreatic carcinoma, CT-guided percutaneous needle aspiration biopsy of the pancreas has documented a pancreatic tumor. However, experience in detecting pancreatic cancer in the presence of chronic pancreatitis has not been encouraging unless signs of advanced malignancy are present.

Association with Dilatation of the Biliary Tract. Cancer of the head of the pancreas is frequently associated with obstructive jaundice. Biliary ductal

dilatation was detected in 43 of 47 (91 per cent),[79] 8 of 17 (47 per cent),[80] and 16 of 36 (44 per cent) cases.[92] The dilated gallbladder, common bile duct, common hepatic duct, and intrahepatic ducts caused by cancer of the pancreas can be demonstrated (Figs. 14–31, 14–43, and 14–45). When a large pancreatic mass causes the obstruction, it will often displace the common bile duct anteriorly and medially. When the tumor is small and located near the papilla of Vater, the dilated

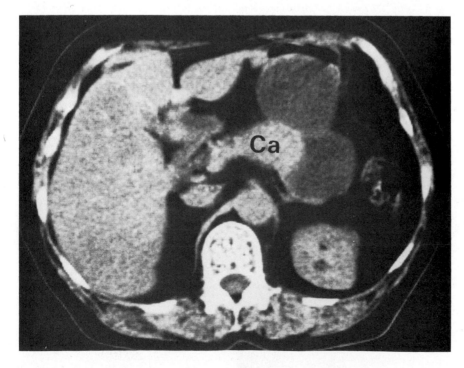

Figure 14–48. Carcinoma of the body of the pancreas (Ca) with two large cysts distal to the tumor. (From Itai Y, Moss AA, Goldberg HI: Pancreatic cysts caused by carcinoma of the pancreas: A pitfall in the diagnosis of pancreatic carcinoma. J Comput Assist Tomogr 6:772, 1982. Used with permission.)

duct appears as a low-density, round structure medial to the duodenum in the region of the head of the pancreas (Fig. 14–45). Accuracy in detecting a malignant obstruction of the biliary tract by CT scanning ranges from 90 to 95 per cent.[93]

Ascites. Although malignant ascites occurs in some patients with pancreatic cancer, it is not a common feature. Ascites can be the result of spread of pancreatic cancer throughout the lesser sac with the induction of fluid or distant spread to the greater peritoneal cavity. In one series[79] ascites was found in 13 per cent of patients with pancreatic cancer, most frequently in patients with far advanced disease.

Detection of the Pancreatic Tumor 3 cm in Size or Less. By the time most pancreatic cancers are clinically suspected, the carcinoma is greater than 3 cm in size. An early report[77] found that only a third of the pancreatic tumors detected by CT were less than 10 cm. Subsequent studies found only 3 of 24 (12.5 per cent),[80] 3 of 18 (16.66 per cent)[78] and 4 of 50 (8 per cent)[5] of pancreatic cancers were 3 cm or less in size. Functioning islet cell tumors of the pancreas are an exception to this rule because many of these are smaller than 3 cm in size.[94–96] In most instances, large tumors are inoperable.[94]

Rarely is a tumor less than 3 cm in diameter detected on the basis of an abnormality in size or shape of the pancreas.[97, 98] In Sanger's series[94] only 50 per cent of small, operable tumors were detected by CT scans. More likely, a small lesion will be suspected because of secondary signs, such as metastasis to regional lymph nodes or liver, obliteration of a portion of the peripancreatic fat plane, dilation of pancreatic duct, or obstructive jaundice.

In Ariyama's series,[99] 14 of 62 patients (22 per cent) with resectable pancreatic cancer had tumors 3 cm in size or less. Survival was prolonged in this group, compared with a group of patients who had resection of tumor larger than 3 cm, indicating that it is worthwhile to attempt to detect pancreatic tumors when they are small. However, the detection of a small lesion, even one in which no mass is seen and only secondary findings of ductal dilatation are present, does not assure prolongation of life as a result of resection. Even though the tumor may be resectable, local spread to organs or metastasis to regional lymph nodes and the liver may already have occurred (Fig. 14–46). In ten pancreatic cancers less than 3 cm in size diagnosed at the University of California,

San Francisco, four already had evidence of metastasis. Nonetheless, a CT scan of the pancreas showing a dilated pancreatic or bile duct should stimulate the further evaluation by ERCP and possibly angiography to detect small pancreatic tumors. Ariyama's experience indicates that when some small pancreatic tumors are resected, there is prolonged survival as compared with patients with large pancreatic tumors.[99]

Islet Cell Tumors of the Pancreas. Pancreatic islet cell tumors are either secretory or nonfunctioning. The tumors that actively secrete one or more hormones produce clinical and biochemical abnormalities that signal their underlying presence. The insulin-secreting tumors are the most common islet cell tumors and account for 60 to 75 per cent of all islet cell neoplasms.[100] Next in frequency (20 per cent) are the gastrin-secreting alpha-1 islet cell tumors that cause the Zollinger-Ellison syndrome. Rarer islet cell tumors are those producing glucagon (alpha-2 cell), vasoactive intestinal peptide (VIP) (non-beta cell), and somatostatin (d-cell).[101] In addition, APUDomas* of the pancreas are occasionally encountered, particularly in association with other endocrine-secreting tumors such as pituitary adenomas, pheochromocytomas, medullary carcinoma of the thyroid, and bronchial and intestinal carcinoids. APUDomas produce endocrine peptides of various types and are thought to originate from neural crest derivatives. These tumors in the pancreas produce adrenocorticotropic hormone (ACTH), antidiuretic hormone (ADH), and VIP.[101] As all secretory pancreatic islet cell tumors produce clinically apparent abnormalities due to excessive hormone secretion, they are often detected at a smaller size than nonfunctioning islet cell lesions or pancreatic adenocarcinomas. Because functioning islet cell tumors tend to be referred for diagnosis while tumors are small, CT demonstration of islet cell tumors is often difficult.[75, 96]

No specific CT features separate the islet cell tumors from solid adenocarcinomas. The smaller islet cell lesions are usually isodense with the uninvolved pancreas (Fig. 14–34 and 14–49), although larger tumors can have low-density areas due to foci of tumor necrosis (Fig. 14–50). The location of the tumor determines whether the common bile duct or pancreatic ducts are obstructed and which adjacent organ is likely to be involved.

---

*Tumors composed of *a*mine *p*recursor *u*ptake and *d*ecarboxylation cells.

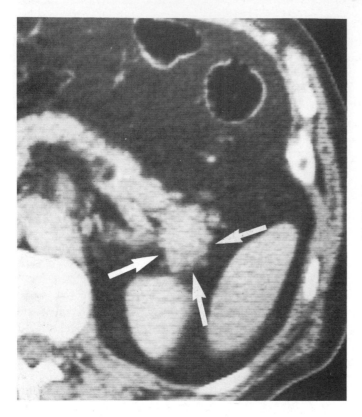

Figure 14–49. Focal enlargement of the tail of the pancreas (arrows) is due to the presence of an insulinoma. The lesion is isodense with the adjacent pancreatic tissue.

Calcification has been noted in malignant islet cell tumors (Figs. 14–37 and 14–51),[91] a finding almost never seen in adenocarcinomas.

As a result of the small size of some primary tumors, it is frequently easier to detect evidence of metastatic disease than to locate the primary neoplasm. In one series of 25 patients, hepatic metastases were detected in 40 per cent, whereas the primary lesion was detected by CT in only 33 per cent.[96] Moreover, the tumors detected by CT scanning were large, ranging from 4 to 10 cm in diameter. In another series of insulinomas studied by CT scanning,[95] only 6 of 14 tumors (43 per cent) were detected. However, both of these studies were carried out using second-generation 18-second CT scanners. Studies at the University of California, San Francisco, using high-resolution, fast scanners demonstrated that 70 per cent of 20 patients with functioning islet cell tumors had tumors demonstrated by CT scans.

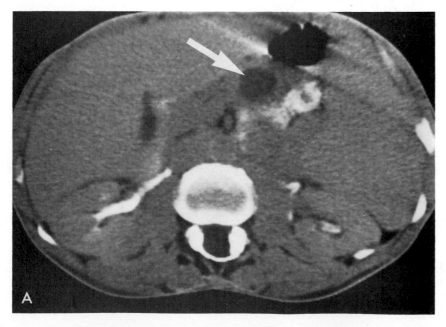

Figure 14–50. Large gastrin-secreting islet cell tumor of the pancreas. **A** The tumor occupies the entire body and tail of the pancreas and encases a segment of contrast-filled jejunum. An area of low density (arrow) is present in the tumor, as a result of tumor necrosis.

Illustration continued on opposite page

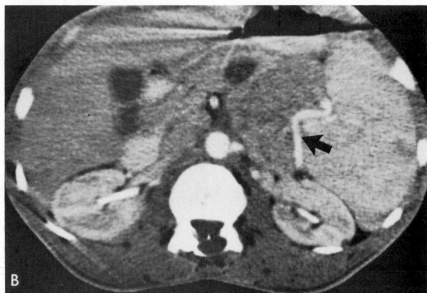

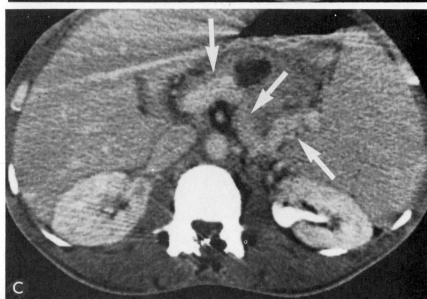

Figure 14–50. *Continued* **B** A CT scan from a dynamic scan sequence clearly shows the splenic artery (arrow) displaced by the tumor. **C** A CT obtained later in the dynamic scan sequence. Although the spleen is enlarged and the tumor is in a location to obstruct the splenic vein, the dynamic CT scan shows a large, patent splenic vein (arrows) surrounded by tumor.

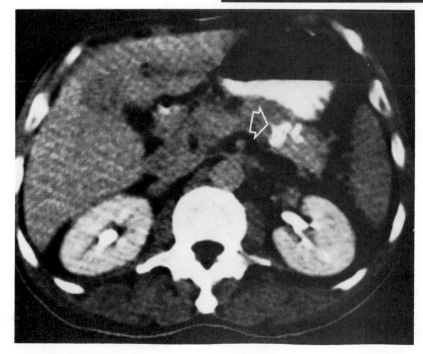

Figure 14–51. Pancreatic APUDoma. Coarse calcifications (arrow) are demonstrated in tail of the pancreas.

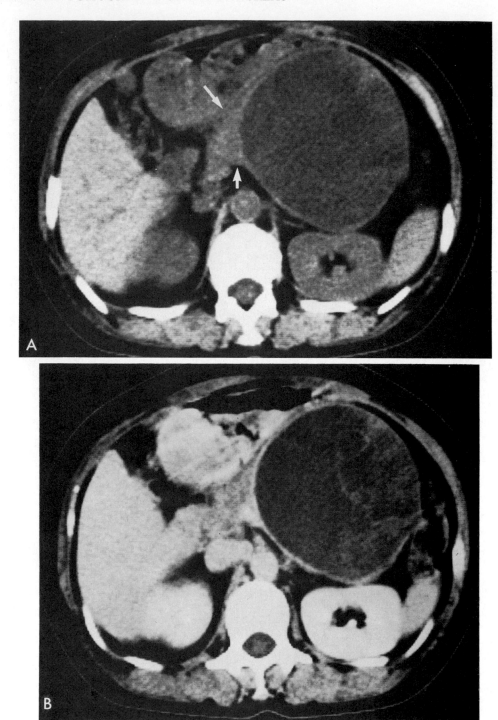

Figure 14–52. Mucinous cystadenoma of the pancreas. **A** A precontrast scan reveals a large, low-density, well-circumscribed mass in the left abdomen. Its pancreatic origin is shown by the extension of pancreatic tissue (arrows) over the medial border of the mass. **B** After administration of intravenous contrast material, the capsule and the internal septa are shown more clearly. (From Itai Y, Moss AA, Ohtomo K: Computed tomography of cystdenoma and cystadenocarcinoma of the pancreas. Radiology 145:419, 1982. Used with permission.)

CYSTIC PANCREATIC NEOPLASMS. Primary cystic neoplasms of the pancreas are categorized as nonmucinous, glycogen-rich microcystic or serous adenomas, and mucinous cystadenomas and cystadenocarcinomas. These two types of cystic neoplasms make up only about 10 to 15 per cent of all cystic pancreatic lesions[102–104] and account for only a few per cent of all pancreatic tumors.[102, 103]

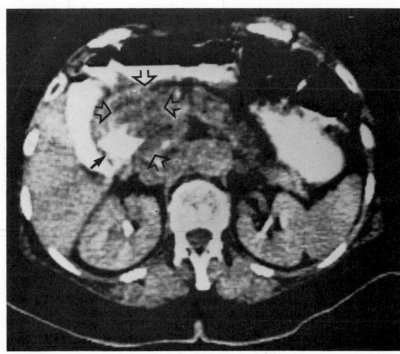

Figure 14–53. Cystadenocarcinoma. A postcontrast scan reveals a large, lobulated mass in the head of the pancreas (open arrows), which has multiple irregular cystic portions. The dense area (solid arrow) is contrast material in a a duodenal diverticulum. (From Itai Y, Moss AA, Ohtomo K: Computed tomography of cystadenoma and cystadenocarcinoma of the pancreas. Radiology 145:419, 1982. Used with permission.)

Mucinous lesions arise from ductal epithelium and are either obviously malignant or in the case of cystadenomas considered to be premalignant.[102, 104] On the other hand, nonmucinous microcystic adenomas have no malignant potential.[102–104] Complete surgical resection is recommended for patients with any mucinous cystic pancreatic tumor, whereas microcystic adenomas may be safely followed or have local surgical resection.

Mucinous Cystic Tumors. The vast majority of these neoplasms occur in the body and tail of the pancreas,[102] whereas solid adenocarcinomas occur more frequently in the head of the pancreas. Mucinous neoplasms are almost always greater than 2 cm in size, usually exhibiting areas of low CT density and appearing as fluid-filled cysts. As a result of their large size and low CT density, almost all cystic pancreatic neoplasms are readily detected by CT. Many tumors are multiloculated but usually contain less than ten cystic components (Fig. 14–52). Well-defined margins are usually present but in some, multiple, irregular cystic masses are surrounded by normal pancreatic tis-

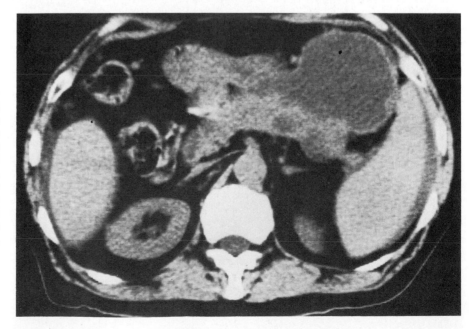

Figure 14–54. Cystadenocarcinoma. A large cystic mass protrudes from the tail of the pancreas. The thick wall is thickened and smaller cysts are present in the enlarged body and tail of the pancreas. (From Itai Y, Moss AA, Ohtomo K: Computed tomography of cystadenoma and cystadenocarcinoma of the pancreas. Radiology 145:419, 1982. Used with permission.)

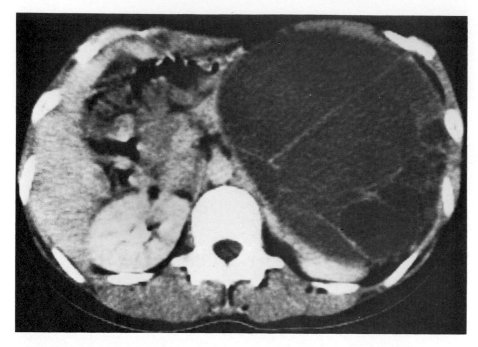

Figure 14–55. Mucinous cystadenoma. Postcontrast scan demonstrates a large, rounded mass with thin straight and curvilinear septa. (From Itai Y, Moss AA, Ohtomo K: Computed tomography of cystadenoma and cystadenocarcinoma of the pancreas. Radiology 145:419, 1982. Used with permission.)

sue (Fig. 14–53). In others, only a portion of the tumor is connected to the pancreas (Figs. 14–52 and 14–54). Cyst walls are often thin but may be thickened locally. The degree of thickening does not correlate with the presence of malignancy.[104] Septa and local projections into the cyst are frequently seen, and these undergo CT enhancement after delivery of contrast material (Figs. 14–52 and 14–55). Occasionally, the septa contain small collections of calcification. In cystadenocarcinomas, typically there is a large solid component to the tumor, along with small daughter cysts immediately adjacent to one of the large cystic masses (Figs. 14–53 and 14–54). Although stomach, spleen, colon, and small bowel may be displaced by these large tumors, adjacent organs are not usually invaded.

Serous Cystic Tumors. Serous or microcystic adenomas occur in all areas of the pancreas and are usually made up of multiple small cysts, less than 2 cm in size (Fig. 14–56).[103, 104] Often a mass that appears to be made up of many small cysts inter-

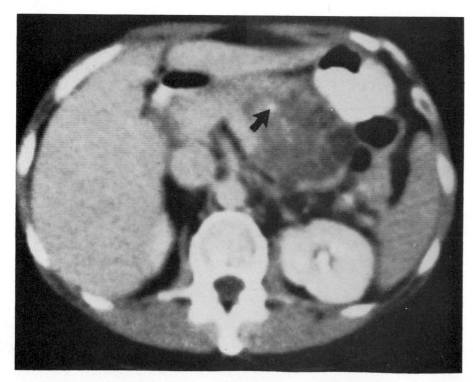

Figure 14–56. Serous cystadenoma. Postcontrast CT scan demonstrates an oval mass in the tail of the pancreas, which has multiple central septa, giving the mass a honeycomb appearance. A small focus of calcification (arrow) is seen. (From Itai Y, Moss AA, Ohtomo K: Computed tomography of cystadenoma and cystadenocarcinoma of the pancreas. Radiology 145:419, 1982. Used with permission.)

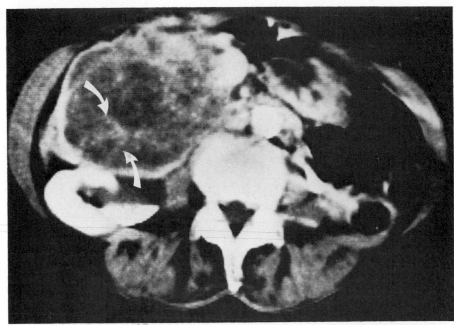

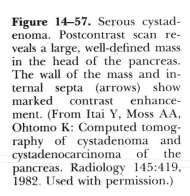

Figure 14–57. Serous cystadenoma. Postcontrast scan reveals a large, well-defined mass in the head of the pancreas. The wall of the mass and internal septa (arrows) show marked contrast enhancement. (From Itai Y, Moss AA, Ohtomo K: Computed tomography of cystadenoma and cystadenocarcinoma of the pancreas. Radiology 145:419, 1982. Used with permission.)

mixed with solid portions is identified. These cysts may contain central connective tissue with radiating strands, giving a stellate or honeycomb appearance (Figs. 14–56 and 14–57),[103, 104] and foci of calcification may be seen in the center of the cyst. In some cases, the CT features of microcystic or serous adenomas appear to be sufficiently different from the mucinous cystadenoma-carcinoma to permit differentiation on the basis of CT scans alone. However, the premalignant cystadenoma cannot be distinguished from the frankly malignant cystadenocarcinoma by CT unless there is evidence of local invasion or metastatic lesions.

Metastatic Tumors

As a result of its strategic location in the abdomen, the pancreas is susceptible to invasion or displacement by neoplasms from adjacent organs and lymph nodes. Carcinoma of the stomach, gallbladder, and hepatomas may invade pan-

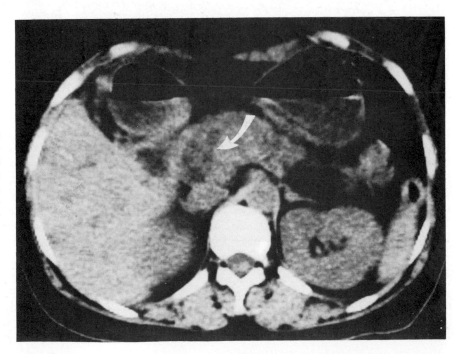

Figure 14–58. Carcinoma of the gallbladder invading the pancreas. Scan demonstrating a mass in the head of the pancreas proven to be the result of spread from carcinoma of the gallbladder. The mass has caused pancreatic duct dilatation (arrow).

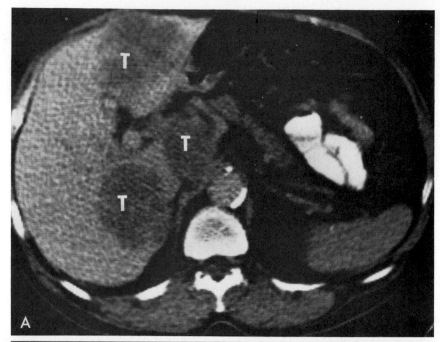

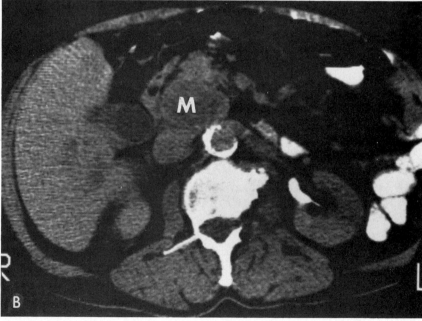

Figure 14–59. Hepatoma invading the pancreas. **A** Three foci of tumor (T) are present in the liver. **B** The caudate lobe mass extends into the pancreas, causing the pancreatic head (M) to be enlarged.

creatic tissue (Figs. 14–58 and 14–59). In these patients, CT scans demonstrate that the fat normally separating the pancreas from the stomach or the liver is obliterated and tumor extends directly into the pancreatic substance, producing indistinct margins between pancreas and adjacent organs. In addition, lesions of the left adrenal and kidney may displace the tail of the pancreas, destroy surrounding fat, and occlude the splenic vein (Fig. 14–60).

Involvement of peripancreatic lymph nodes, particularly those in and around the celiac and mesenteric arteries, may simulate pancreatic tu-

mors (Fig. 14–61). Enlargement of peripancreatic lymph nodes resulting from metastatic tumor, infection, or lymphoma can result in lobulated masses that impinge on the pancreas. However, the boundary of fat between the pancreas and the nodal mass is often preserved. Differentiating a primary pancreatic tumor from peripancreatic lymphadenopathy may not be possible if the fat planes are totally obliterated. However, if the fat planes are intact, a diagnosis of peripancreatic lymph node enlargement can be suggested on CT. Occasionally, the differentiation between a lymph node mass simulating a lesion in the head and/or body of the pancreas and a true pancreatic mass is possible by enhancement of the pancreatic parenchyma as a result of an intravenous bolus of contrast material. A lymph node mass that does not enhance can be more clearly seen and the actual boundary between the lymph node mass and the pancreas more readily discerned.

Accuracy of CT in Detection of Pancreatic Carcinoma

The accuracy of computed tomography in detecting pancreatic cancer has been determined in several studies using various scanners and techniques (Table 14–1). In some studies, false-negative and false-positive results have been also reported, providing a measure of sensitivity and specificity. In a total of 537 cases of pancreatic tumor reported in Table 14–1, the overall CT accuracy ranged from 71 to 91 per cent with a sensitivity of 71 to 95 per cent and specificity, when reported, of 83 to 90 per cent. It is obvious that the type of scanning equipment, technique, use of contrast material, amount of natural peripancreatic fat, and density of the pancreatic lesion all affect detection by CT techniques. To date, the few false-positive CT studies that have been reported were mostly due to pancreatic lobulations, pancreatic cysts, chronic pancreatitis, or peripancreatic lymphoma.

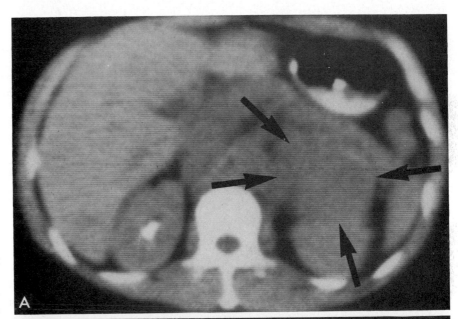

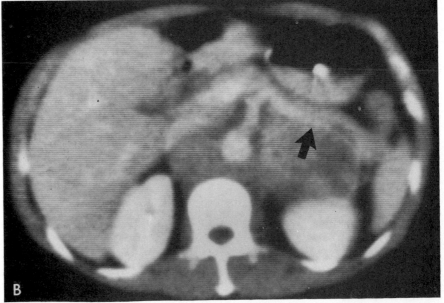

Figure 14–60. Large left adrenal tumor simulating a carcinoma of the tail of the pancreas. **A** A large mass (arrows) occupies the region between pancreas and left kidney. **B** After an intravenous bolus injection, the mass is seen to displace the splenic vein (arrow) and tail of pancreas. The splenic vein is narrowed and was invaded by the adrenal tumor.

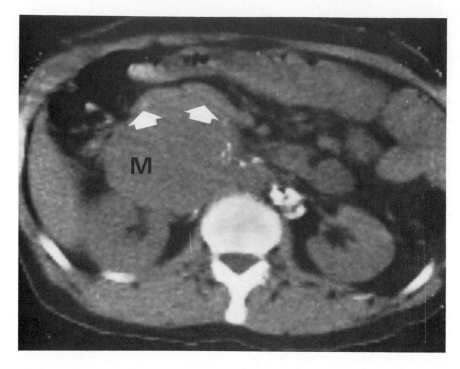

Figure 14–61. Enlarged pericaval lymph nodes due to lymphoma simulating the CT appearance of a mass (M) in the head of the pancreas. Several contrast-enhanced lymph nodes are present as a result of a prior lymphangiogram. The pancreas is displaced and stretched over the top of the mass (arrows).

The use of fine-needle percutaneous CT-guided biopsy has greatly increased the overall accuracy of computed tomography in diagnosing pancreatic disease. This technique, discussed in Chapter 22, has been applied effectively in establishing the presence of pancreatic cancer. In Mitty's series,[105] fine-needle aspiration of 43 patients with clinically diagnosed pancreatic carcinoma revealed cancer in 37, with six false-negatives, for an accuracy of 88.7 per cent. We achieved a 95 per cent accuracy in patients with pancreatic tumor biopsied by fine needle aspiration technique. In our series of 32 needle biopsies performed because of the presence of either a pancreatic mass or peripancreatic lymph nodes, 21 gave true-positive and 28 gave true-negative results, with only one false-negative and one inadequate sample.

RELATIONSHIP OF CT TO OTHER IMAGING MODALITIES

In a hospital or clinical radiology department setting having modern radiographic, CT, and ultrasound equipment, several imaging techniques are available for evaluating pancreatic cancer. We first utilize a noninvasive technique and depend

Table 14–1.   ACCURACY OF CT IN DETECTION OF PANCREATIC CANCER

Author	No. Cases Tumor/Normal	TP	TN	FP	FN	Sensitivity	Specificity	Accuracy (%)
Foley[74]	7/13	5	—	—	2	—	0.71	71
Freeny[110]	77/146	62	135	17	15	0.82	0.88	88
Gmelin[111]	10	6	—	0	2	0.75	—	80
Haaga[4]	32/12	28	11	0	4	0.87	1.00	88
Haertel[79]	75	71	—		4	0.95	—	—
Hessel[114]	52	—	—	—	—	0.84	—	—
Inamoto[81]	43/235	37	195	40	6	0.86	0.83	83
Itai[84]	62	54	—	—	8	0.87	—	—
Lackner[107]	41	—	—	—	—	0.93	—	—
Levitt[78]	18/150	15	147	0	1	0.93	1.00	88
Moss[112]	8/32	6	27	1	1	0.85	0.90	84
Pistolesi[92]	36/39	33	—	—	3	0.84	—	—
Stanley[5]	52	36	—	4	12	0.75	—	—

upon invasive techniques such as ERCP, PTC, and angiography only when CT scanning or ultrasound fails to provide adequate diagnostic information.

Currently CT is considered the imaging procedure of choice for evaluating the pancreas for suspected pancreatic cancer. Pancreatic CT scanning is recommended in all patients with suspected pancreatic cancer on the basis of back and/or epigastric pain and weight loss. CT is ideally suited for patients with sufficient retroperitoneal fat because of its ability to outline abnormalities in the pancreas and other structures within the retroperitoneal fat. Emaciated patients, on the other hand, are studied best with ultrasound. Current-generation CT scanners are almost always capable of imaging the entire pancreas and providing important information concerning peripancreatic spread and distant metastatic disease.

If a patient presents with jaundice and it is suspected that a pancreatic mass in the head or uncinate process is the cause, ultrasound is usually performed as the initial imaging procedure. Ultrasonography and CT have identical rates of detection of dilated bile ducts and in detecting lesions in the head of the pancreas.[75, 106] Ultrasonography is also the imaging procedure of choice in emaciated jaundiced patients. Overall, ultrasound detection rates for pancreatic carcinoma have been reported to be similar to those of CT scanning (85 to 94 per cent).[107–109] However, although overall detection rates for pancreatic cancer may be similar, CT better demonstrates peripancreatic tumor spread and more completely images the tail of the pancreas.

If a mass or definite contour abnormality is detected in the pancreas, fine-needle aspiration biopsy should be performed by using either CT or ultrasound guidance at the time of initial detection. This additional technique greatly enhances the usefulness of CT or ultrasound because direct cytologic or histologic confirmation may be obtained without resorting to further diagnostic imaging tests or exploratory laparotomy. If the mass detected proves to be adenocarcinoma, CT is used to stage the pancreatic carcinoma. If any question remains about the extent of the tumor or if the tumor appears on the basis of CT scanning to be possibly resectable, selected pancreatic angiography is performed to provide information about encasement of adjacent vascular structures.[75, 110] If CT or ultrasonograms of the pancreas appear normal but a strong clinical suspicion of pancreatic disease remains, endoscopic

retrograde pancreatography (ERP) should be performed. When the pancreatic duct is successfully cannulated, and most studies show ERP to be more accurate than CT in detecting pancreatic cancer.[74, 111–113] However, because of cannulation failures, overall accuracy rates for ERP are lower than with CT or ultrasound.[112]

The overall impact of CT scanning of the pancreas for suspected pancreatic disease was studied by Freeny and colleagues.[110] The study showed that when CT scanning was used in the evaluation of pancreatic disease, additional examinations such as ERP and angiography were not necessary in 74 per cent of cases. Using CT as the initial screening process, ERP utilization decreased 68 per cent and angiography 54 per cent. This indicates that ERP and angiography have important but secondary roles in the overall evaluation of suspected pancreatic cancer and should act as complementary studies to computed tomography whenever the CT findings are nonspecific or equivocal.

REFERENCES

1. Meyers MA: Dynamic radiology of the abdomen: Normal and pathologic anatomy. New York, Springer, 1976.
2. Neumann CH, Hessel SJ: CT of the pancreatic tail. AJR 135:741, 1980.
3. Callen PW, Breiman RS, Korobkin M, DeMartini WJ, Mani JR: Carcinoma of the tail of the pancreas: An unusual CT appearance. AJR 133:135, 1979.
4. Haaga JR, Alfidi RJ, Havrilla TR, Tubbs R, Gonzales L, Meaney TF, Corsi MA: Definitive role of CT scanning of the pancreas: The second year's experience. Radiology 124:723, 1977.
5. Stanley RJ, Sagel SS, Levitt RG: Computed tomographic evaluation of the pancreas. Radiology 124:715, 1977.
6. Kreel L, Haertel M, Katy D: Computed tomography of the normal pancreas. J Comput Assist Tomogr 1:290, 1977.
7. Baldwin CN: Computed tomography of the pancreas: Negative contrast medium. Radiology 128:827, 1978.
8. Jeffrey RB, Federle MP, Goodman PC: Computed tomography of the lesser peritoneal sac. Radiology 141:117, 1981.
9. Sheedy PF, Stephens DH, Hattery RR, MacCarty RL, Williamson B Jr: Computed tomography of the pancreas. Radiol Clin North Am 15:349, 1977.
10. Stuck KJ, Kuhns LR: Improved visualization of the pancreatic tail after maximum distention of the stomach. J Comput Assist Tomogr 5:509, 1981.
11. Marchal G, Baert AL, Wilms G: Intravenous pancreatography in computed tomography. J Comput Assist Tomogr 3:727, 1979.
12. Callen PW, London SS, Moss AA: Computed tomographic evaluation of the dilated pancreatic duct: The value of thin-section collimation. Radiology 134:253, 1980.
13. Etiology and pathological anatomy of chronic pancrea-

titis. Symposium of Marseilles, April 1963. Bibl Gastroenterol, 1965.

14. Spiro HM: Pancreatic disorders. In Clinical Gastroenterology, 1st ed. London, McMillan, 1970, pp 813–823.

15. Jordan GL, Spjut HJ: Hemorrhagic pancreatitis. Arch Surg 104:489, 1972.

16. Lawson DW, Daggett WM, Civetta JM, Corry RJ, Bartlett MK: Surgical treatment of acute necrotizing pancreatitis. Ann Surg 172:605, 1970.

17. Jeffrey RB, Federle MP, Cello JP, Crass RA: Early computed tomographic scanning in acute severe pancreatitis. Surg Gynecol Obstet 154:170, 1982.

18. Peterson LM, Brooks JR: Lethal pancreatitis, a diagnostic dilemma. Am J Surg 137:491, 1979.

19. Silverstein W, Isikoff MB, Hill MC, Barkin J: Diagnostic imaging of acute pancreatitis: Prospective study using CT and sonography. AJR 137:497, 1981.

20. Siegelman SS, Copeland BE, Saba GP, Cameron JL, Sanders RC, Zerhouni EA: CT of fluid collections associated with pancreatitis. AJR 134:1121, 1980.

21. Robbins SL: Inflammation and repair. In Pathology. Philadelphia, WB Saunders Company, 1967, p 58.

22. Dembner AG, Jaffe CC, Simeone J, Walsh J: A new computed tomographic sign of pancreatitis. AJR 133:477, 1979.

23. Nicholson RL: Abnormalities of the perinephric fascia and fat in pancreatitis. Radiology 139:125, 1981.

24. Susman N, Hammerman AM, Cohen E: The renal halo sign in pancreatitis. Radiology 142:323, 1982.

25. Brown BM, Federle MP, Jeffrey RB: Gastric wall thickening and extragastric inflammatory processes. J Comput Assist Tomogr 6:762, 1982.

26. Moss AA, Schnyder P, Marks W, Margulis AR: Gastric adenocarcinoma: A comparison of the accuracy and economics of staging by computed tomography and surgery. Gastroenterology 80:45, 1981.

27. Balfe DM, Koehler RE, Karstaedt MB, Stanley RJ, Sagel SS: Computed tomography of gastric neoplasms. Radiology 140:431, 1981.

28. Yeh H-C, Rabinowitz JG: Ultrasonography and computed tomography of gastric wall lesions. Radiology 141:147, 1981.

29. Waterman NC, Walsky BA, Kasdan ML, Abrams BL: The treatment of acute hemorrhagic pancreatitis by sump drainage. Surg Gynecol Obstet 126:963, 1968.

30. Norton L, Eiserman B: Near total pancreatectomy for hemorrhagic pancreatitis. Am J Surg 127:191, 1974.

31. Isikoff MB, Hill MC, Silverstein W, Barkin J: The clinical significance of acute pancreatic hemorrhage. AJR 136:679, 1981.

32. Warshaw AL: Inflammatory masses following acute pancreatitis. Surg Clin North Am 54:621, 1979.

33. Owens GR, Arger PH, Mulhern CB, Coleman BG, Gohel V: CT evaluation of mediastinal pseudocyst. J Comput Assist Tomogr 4:256, 1980.

34. Bellon EM, George CR, Schreiber H, Marshall JB: Pancreatic pseudocysts of the duodenum. AJR 133:827, 1979.

35. Nacianceno SE, Gross SC, Rajn JS, Song SH, Joseph RR: Pancreatic pseudocyst simulating dilated biliary duct system in computed tomography. Radiology 134:165, 1980.

36. Trapnel J: The natural history and management of acute pancreatitis. Clin Gastroenterol 1:147, 1972.

37. Rosenberg IK, Kahn JA, Walt JA: Surgical experience with pancreatic pseudocysts. Am J Surg 117:11, 1969.

38. Trapnel J: Management of the complications of acute pancreatitis. Ann R Coll Surg Engl 49:361, 1971.

39. Bradley EL III, Clements JL Jr, Gonzalez AC: The natural history of pancreatic pseudocysts: A unified concept of management. Am J Surg 137:135, 1979.

40. Sarti DA: Rapid development and spontaneous regression of pancreatic pseudocysts documented by ultrasound. Radiology 125:789, 1977.

41. Kolmannskog F, Kolbenstvedt A, Aakhus T: Computed tomography in inflammatory mass lesions following acute pancreatitis. J Comput Assist Tomogr 5:169, 1981.

42. Federle MP: Pancreatitis and its complication: The role of computed tomography and ultrasound. In Margulis AR, Gooding CA (eds): Diagnostic Radiology 1982. San Francisco, University of California Press, 1982.

43. Kaplan JO, Isikoff MB, Barkin J, Livingstone AS: Necrotic carcinoma of the pancreas: "The pseudo-pseudocyst." J Comput Assist Tomogr 4:166, 1980.

44. Hancke S, Pedersen JF: Percutaneous puncture of pancreatic cysts guided by ultrasound. Surg Gynecol Obstet 142:551, 1976.

45. Andersen BN, Hancke S, Neilsen SA, Schmidt A: The diagnosis of pancreatic cyst by endoscopic retrograde pancreatography and ultrasonic scanning. Ann Surg 185:286, 1977.

46. Gerzof SG, Robbins AH, Birkett DH, Johnson WC, Pugatch RD, Vincent ME: Percutaneous catheter drainage of abdominal abscesses guided by ultrasound and computed tomography. AJR 133:1, 1979.

47. Gronvall J, Gronvall S, Hegedvs V: Ultrasound-guided drainage fluid-containing masses using angiographic catheterization techniques. AJR 129:997, 1977.

48. Karlson KB, Martin EC, Fankuchen EI, MaHern RF, Schultz RW, Casarella WJ: Percutaneous drainage of pancreatic pseudocysts and abscesses. Radiology 142:619, 1982.

49. Attemeier WA, Alexander JW: Pancreatic abscess: A study of 32 cases. Arch Surg 87:80, 1963.

50. Bolooki H, Jaffe B, Gleidiman ML: Pancreatic abscesses and lesser omental sac collections. Surg Gynecol Obstet 126:1301, 1968.

51. Warshaw AL: Pancreatic abscess. N Engl J Med 287:1234, 1972.

52. Miller TA: Pancreatic abscess. Arch Surg 108:545, 1974.

53. Pistolesi GF, Marzoli GP, Quarta Colosso P, Pederzoli P, Procacci C: Computed tomography in surgical pancreatic emergencies. J Comput Assist Tomogr 2:165, 1978.

54. Mendez G, Isikoff MB: Significance of intrapancreatic gas demonstrated by CT: A review of nine cases. AJR 132:59, 1979.

55. Federle MP, Jeffrey RB, Crass RA, Van Dalsem V: Computed tomography of pancreatic abscesses. AJR 136:879, 1981.

56. Woodard S, Kelvin FM, Rice RP, Thompson WM: Pancreatic abscess: Importance of conventional radiology. AJR 136:871, 1981.

57. Torres WE, Clements JL Jr, Sones PJ, Knopf DR: Gas in the pancreatic bed without abscess. AJR 137:1131, 1981.

58. Clements JL, Bradley EL, Eaton SB: Spontaneous internal drainage of pancreatic pseudocysts. AJR 126:985, 1976.

59. Mendez G Jr, Isikoff MB, Hill MC: CT of acute pancreatitis: Interim assessment. AJR 135:463, 1980.

60. Hubbard TB Jr, Eilber FR, Okdroyd H: The retroperitoneal extension of necrotizing pancreatitis. Surg Gynecol Obstet 134:927, 1972.

61. Benson JA Jr: Chronic pancreatitis. In Sleisenger MH, Fordtran JS (eds): Gastrointestinal Disease. Philadelphia, WB Saunders Company, 1973 pp 1185–1197.

62. Ring EJ, Eaton SB, Ferrucci JT Jr, Short WF: Differential diagnosis of pancreatic calcification. AJR 117:446, 1973.

63. Ferrucci JT Jr, Wittenberg J, Black EB, Kirkpatrick RH, Hall DA: Computed body tomography in chronic pancreatitis. Radiology 130:175, 1979.

64. Ohto M, Ono T, Tsuchiya Y, Saisho H: Cholangiography and Pancreatography. Tokyo, Igaku-Shoin, 1978, p 82.

65. Berland LL, Lawson TL, Foley D, Greenan JE, Stewart ET: Computed tomography of the normal and abnormal pancreatic duct: Correlation with pancreatic ductography. Radiology 141:715, 1981.

66. Gold RP, Seaman WB: Computed tomography and the dilated pancreatic duct: An ominous sign. Gastrointest Radiol 6:35, 1981.

67. Fishman A, Isikoff MB, Barkin J, Friedland JT: Significance of a dilated pancreatic duct on CT examination. AJR 133:225, 1979.

68. Hauser H, Bettikha JG, Wettstein P: Computed tomography of the dilated pancreatic duct. J Comput Assist Tomogr 4:53, 1980.

69. Freeny PC, Bilbao MK, Katon RM: "Blind" evaluation of endoscopic retrograde cholangiopancreatography (ERCP) in the evaluation of pancreatic carcinoma: The "double duct" and other signs. Radiology 119:271, 1976.

70. Seidelmann FE, Cohen WN, Bryan PJ, Brown J: CT demonstration of the splenic vein-pancreatic relationship: The pseudodilated pancreatic duct. AJR 129:17, 1977.

71. Kreel L, Sadin B: Changes in pancreatic morphology associated with aging. Gut 14:962, 1973.

72. Ponetti E, Pringot J, Baert AL: Computerized tomography and ultrasonography in pancreatitis. Acta Gastroenterol Belg 39:402, 1976.

73. Johnson JR, Zintel HA: Pancreatic calcification and cancer of the pancreas. Surg Gynecol Obstet 117:585, 1963.

74. Foley WD, Stewart ET, Lawson TL, Geenan J, Longuidice J, Maker L, Unger G: Computed tomography, ultrasonography, and endoscopic retrograde cholangiopancreatography in the diagnosis of pancreatic disease: A comparative study. Gastrointest Radiol 5:29, 1980.

75. Simeone JF, Wittenberg J, Ferrucci JT Jr: Modern concepts of imaging of the pancreas. Invest Radiol 15:6, 1980.

76. Haaga JR, Alfidi RJ, Qeich MA, Meaney TF, Baller M, Gonzalez L, Jelden GL. Computed tomography of the pancreas. Radiology 120:589, 1976.

77. Wiggans G, Schein PS, MacDonald JS: Computerized axial tomography for diagnosis of pancreatic cancer. Lancet 2:233, 1976.

78. Levitt RG, Stanley RJ, Sagel SS, Lee JKT, Weyman PJ: Computed tomography of the pancreas: 3 second scanning vs 18 second scanning. J Comput Assist Tomogr 6:259, 1982.

79. Haertel M, Zaunbauer W, Fuchs WA: Die computertomographische morphologische Morphologie des Pankreaskarzinoms. ROEFO 133:1, 1980.

80. Takekawa S: Comparison study in the diagnosis of pancreatic carcinoma by CT and angiography. Presented at 40th annual meeting of the Japanese Society of Radiology, Tokyo, 1981.

81. Inamoto K, Yamazaki H, Kuwata K, Okamoti E, Kotoura Y, Ishikawa Y: Computed tomography of carcinoma in the pancreatic head. Gastrointest Radiol 6:343, 1981.

82. Thoeni RF, Moss AA, Schnyder P, Margulis AR: Detection and staging of primary rectal and rectosigmoid cancer by computed tomography. Radiology 141:135, 1981.

83. Meyerbow AJ, Roxniak MA, Ambios MA, Berenbaum ER: Thickening of the celiac axis and/or superior mesenteric artery: A sign of pancreatic carcinoma on computed tomography. Radiology 141:449, 1981.

84. Itai Y: Progress of imaging diagnosis for cancer: Computed tomography of abdominal malignancy. Jpn J Cancer Clin 26:1029, 1980.

85. Gosink BB, Leopold GR: The dilated pancreatic duct: Ultrasonic evaluation. Radiology 126:475, 1978.

86. Weinstein DP, Weinstein BJ: Ultrasonic demonstration of the pancreatic duct: An analysis of 41 cases. Radiology 130:729, 1979.

87. Ohto M, Saoteme S, Saisho H, Tsuchiya Y, Ono T, Okuda K, Karasawa E: Real-time sonography of the pancreatic duct: Application to percutaneous pancreatic ductography. AJR 134:647, 1980.

88. Foley DW, Lawson TL, Quiroz F. Sagittal and coronal image reconstruction: Application in pancreatic computed tomography. J Comput Assist Tomogr 3:717, 1979.

89. Itai Y, Moss AA, Goldberg HI. Pancreatic cysts caused by carcinoma of the pancreas: A pitfall in the diagnosis of pancreatic carcinoma. J Comput Assist Tomogr 6:772, 1982.

90. Paulino-Netto A, Dreiling DA, Baronofsky ID: The relationship between pancreatic calcification and cancer of the pancrcas. Ann Surg 151:530, 1960.

91. Imhof H, Frank P: Pancreatic calcifications in malignant islet cell tumors. Radiology 122:333, 1977.

92. Pistolesi GF, Procacci C, Fugazzola C, Marzoli GP, Pederzoli P, Quarta Colosso P: Place of computed tomography in pancreatic disease: comparison with other radiological methods. Comput Tomogr 5:115, 1981.

93. Goldberg HI, Filly RA, Korobkin M, Moss AA, Kressel HY, Callen PW: Capability of CT body scanning and ultrasonography to demonstrate the status of the biliary ductal system in patients with jaundice. Radiology 129:731, 1978.

94. Sager, WD, zur Nedden D, Lepuschütz H, Zalaudek G, Bodner E, Fotter R, Lammer J: Computertomographische Diagnostik der Pankreatitis und des Pankreaskarzinoms. Computertomographie 1:52, 1981.

95. Dunnick NR, Long JA, Kridy A, Shawker TH, Doppman JL: Localizing insulinomas with combined radiographic methods. AJR 135:747, 1980.

96. Dunnick NR, Doppman JL, Mills SR, McCarthy DM: Computed tomographic detection of nonbeta pancreatic islet cell tumors. Radiology 135:117, 1980.

97. Stanley RJ, Sagel SS, Evens RG: The impact of new im-

aging methods on pancreatic arteriography. Radiology 136:251, 1980.

98. Levin DG, Wilson R, Abrams HL: The changing role of pancreatic arteriography in the era of computed tomography. Radiology 136:245, 1980.

99. Ariyama J: Radiology in Disorders of the Liver, Biliary Tract, and Pancreas. Tokyo, Igaku-Shoin, 1981, pp 147–149.

100. Arky RA, Knopf RH: Evaluation of islet-cell function in men. N Engl J Med 285:1130, 1971.

101. Tischler AS, Dichter MA, Bilaes B, Greene LA: Neuroendocrine neoplasms and their cells of origin. N Engl J Med 296:919, 1977.

102. Logan SE, Boet RL, Tompkins RK: The malignant potential of mucinous cysts of the pancreas. West J Med 136:157, 1982.

103. Wolfman NT, Ramquest NA, Karstaedt N, Hopkins MB: Cystic neoplasms of the pancreas: CT and sonography. AJR 138:37, 1982.

104. Itai Y, Moss AA, Ohtomo K: Computed tomography of cystadenoma and cystadenocarcinoma of the pancreas. Radiology 145:419, 1982.

105. Mitty HA, Efrimidis SC, Heh H-C: Impact of fine-needle biopsy on management of patients with carcinoma of the pancreas. AJR 137:1119, 1981.

106. Taylor KJW, Rosenfeld AT: Grey scale ultrasonography in the differential diagnosis of jaundice. Arch Surg 112:820, 1970.

107. Lackner K, Frommhold H, Grauthoff H, Modder I, Heuser L, Braun G, Burman R, Scherer K: Wertigkeit der Computertomographie und der Sonographie in-

nerhalb der Pankreasdiagnostik. ROEFO 132:509, 1980.

108. Taylor KJW, Buchin PJ, Biscomi GN, Rosenfeld AT: Ultrasonographic scanning of the pancreas. Radiology 138:211, 1981.

109. Freeny PC, Ball TJ: Rapid diagnosis of pancreatic carcinoma. Radiology 127:627, 1978.

110. Freeny PC, Marks WM, Ball TJ: Impact of high-resolution computed tomography of the pancreas on utilization of endoscopic retrograde cholangiopancreatography and angiography. Radiology 142:35, 1982.

111. Gmelin Von E, Weiss HD, Fuchs HD, Reiser M: Vergleich der diagnostischen Treffsicherheit von Ultraschall, Computertomographie und ERPC bei der chronischen Pankreatitis und beim Pankreaskarzinom. ROEFO 134:136, 1981.

112. Moss AA, Federle M, Shapiro H, Ohto M, Goldberg H, Korobkin M, Clemett A: The combined use of computed tomography and endoscopic retrograde cholangiopancreatography in the assessment of suspected pancreatic neoplasm: A blind clinical evaluation. Radiology 134:159, 1980.

113. Cotton PB, Denyer ME, Kreel L, Husband J, Meire HB, Lees W: Comparative clinical impact of endoscopic pancreatography, grey-scale ultrasonography and computed tomography (EMI scanning) in pancreatic diseases: Preliminary report. Gut 19:679, 1978.

114. Hessel SJ, Siegelman SS, McNeil BJ, Sanders R, Adams DF, Alderson PO, Finberg HJ, Abrams HL: A prospective evaluation of computed tomography and ultrasound of the pancreas. Radiology 143:129, 1982.

15 COMPUTED TOMOGRAPHY OF THE KIDNEYS

Albert A. Moss

Computed tomography (CT) provides valuable diagnostic information in various renal and ureteral lesions.[1–13] Although excretory urography is still the principal uroradiologic imaging procedure, CT has enlarged the capacity to image the genitourinary tract noninvasively. CT is a rapid, easily performed, safe diagnostic imaging procedure that is independent of renal function, provides unique cross-sectional anatomic information, and is unsurpassed in evaluating lesions containing fat or calcium. The only complications are reactions to contrast media; however, a satisfactory examination can usually be obtained without intravenous administration of contrast material. The combination of unique information, safety, and high diagnostic yield make CT a vital component of uroradiologic diagnosis.

ANATOMY

Basic to an understanding of the anatomy of the kidney and ureters is a detailed knowledge of the extraperitoneal fascial planes, which divide the extraperitoneal region into three compartments, and the relationships among the renal fascia, the extraperitoneal compartments, and the organs within the extraperitoneal region. By its ability to differentiate between fat and fascial tissue, CT demonstrates the three extraperitoneal compartments in all but the most emaciated patients.[2, 3, 14–17]

The extraperitoneal region is divided into the anterior pararenal, the perirenal, and the posterior pararenal compartments by the anterior and posterior layers of renal fascia (Fig. 15–1).[14–17] The kidney and its blood vessels are surrounded by a mass of fatty tissue, or perirenal fat, which is enveloped by the dense, collagenous renal fascia. The renal fascia is connected to the kidney by numerous trabeculae that cross the fatty tissue. The anterior and posterior layers of the renal fascia fuse behind the descending colon into the single lateroconal fascia which continues around the flank to blend with the posterior peritoneal reflection.[14, 15, 18, 19]

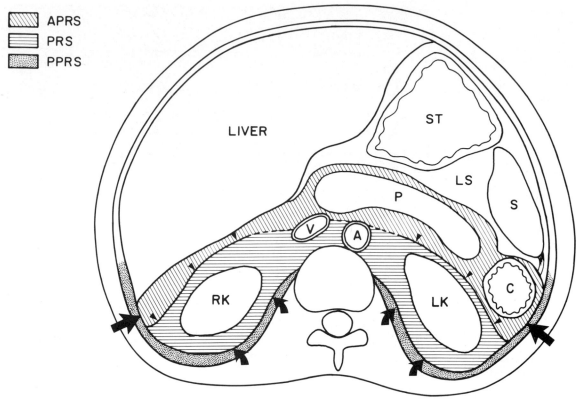

Figure 15–1. Diagram of extraperitoneal compartments. The relationships of the anterior (arrow-heads) and posterior (curved arrows) renal fascia to the anterior (APRS), perirenal (PRS) and posterior pararenal (PPRS) compartments are shown. Arrows = Lateroconal fascia; dashed lines = anterior renal fascia where debate exists over degree of fusion to great vessels; P = pancreas; ST = stomach; LS = lesser sac; S = spleen; C = splenic flexure of colon; V = inferior vena cava; A = aorta.

ANTERIOR PARARENAL COMPARTMENT

The anterior pararenal compartment lies between the anterior renal fascia and posterior parietal peritoneum (Figs. 15–1 and 15–2). The lateral border is defined by the lateroconal fascia, and the compartment is potentially contiguous across the midline.[14, 15, 19]

The anterior pararenal compartment contains the pancreas; the descending, horizontal, and terminal portions of the duodenum; the ascending and descending colon; and the splenic, hepatic, pancreatic, and duodenal vascular supply. Medially the second portion of the duodenum descends immediately in front of the right kidney, and inferiorly the extraperitoneal colon courses obliquely over the lower pole of the right kidney. The extraperitoneal left colon is adjacent to the anterior surface of the left renal fascia and to the lateroconal fascia formed by the fusion of the two layers of the renal fascia.

Abnormalities of any structures within the anterior pararenal compartment can produce thick-ening of the anterior renal and lateroconal fascia (Fig. 15–3).[14–17, 19–20] The most common sources of abnormalities in the anterior pararenal space are lesions arising in the colon, pancreas, or appendix. Renal abnormalities only rarely are the cause of anterior pararenal space lesions.

PERIRENAL COMPARTMENT

The perirenal compartment is limited by the cone of renal fascia formed by the fusion of the anterior renal fascia (Zuckerkandl's fascia) and the posterior renal fascia (Gerota's fascia) (Figs. 15–1, 15–3, 15–4). The renal fascia fuses superiorly with the diaphragmatic fascia and laterally with the lateral conal fascia; inferiorly the layers of renal fascia fuse weakly with the iliac fascia and blend loosely with the periureteric connective tissue.[14–16] The inferior apex of the compartment remains open toward the iliac fossa,[14, 15, 21] and the weakest point of the perirenal compartment through which perirenal effusions escape most easily is at the inferomedial angle adjacent to the ureter.[14, 22, 23] The posterior renal fascia fuses me-

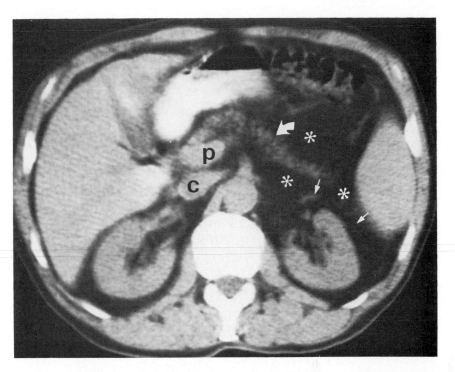

Figure 15–2. CT scan through normal kidneys demonstrating that the pancreas (curved arrow) lies in the anterior pararenal compartment (asterisk). The posterior parietal peritoneum is not visible, but portions of the anterior renal fascia (arrows) are demonstrated. c = Inferior vena cava; p = portal vein.

dially with the psoas and quadratus lumborum fascia.[4, 14]

There is disagreement concerning the continuity of the perirenal space anteriorly. Meyers[14] claimed that the anterior renal fascia fused with the connective tissue around the great vessels in the root of the mesentery, prohibiting any "actual or potential direct communication" between the right and left perirenal compartments. However, Gerota[23] reported that the anterior layer of the renal fascia continued across the midline to fuse with the fascia on the opposite side. Using CT, Somogyi and colleagues demonstrated a communication between the right and left perirenal compartments in a patient after blunt abdominal trauma.[21]

The perirenal compartment contains the adrenal gland, the kidney, the renal vasculature, peri-

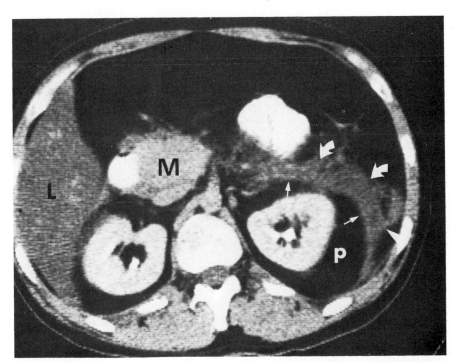

Figure 15–3. Pancreatitis producing a mass (M) that simulates a pancreatic carcinoma. Pancreatitis also has caused a diffuse increase in density of fat in the anterior pararenal space (curved arrows). The anterior renal fascia (arrows) and lateroconal fascia (arrowhead) are also thickened. The perirenal space (p) is normal. The liver (L) contains excessive fat.

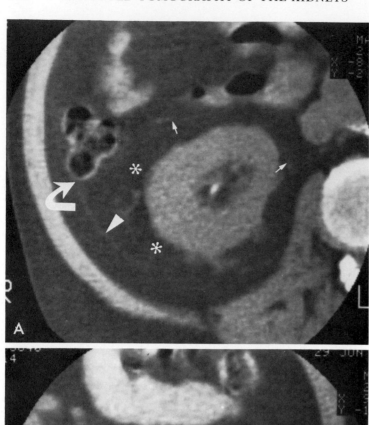

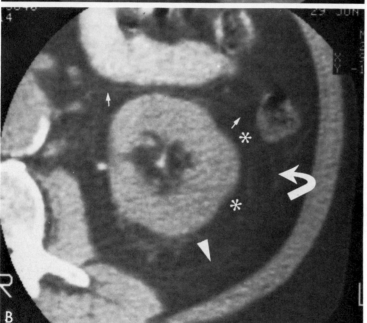

Figure 15–4. Normal CT anatomy of renal fascia and perirenal space. **A,B** Scans through right **(A)** and left **(B)** kidney demonstrate the anterior (arrows) and posterior (arrowheads) pararenal fasciae, which join to form the lateroconal fascia (curved arrows). The perirenal space (asterisk) contains fat and is limited by the renal fascia.

renal fat, and the proximal part of the renal collecting system. Abnormalities of these organs can extend into the perirenal compartment, thicken the renal fascia, and obliterate the perirenal fat (Fig. 15–5).[14]

POSTERIOR PARARENAL COMPARTMENT

The posterior pararenal compartment lies between the posterior renal fascia and the transversalis fascia (Figs. 15–1 and 15–4). It contains no organs other than fatty tissue and continues lat-

erally as the properitoneal fat stripe. The space is open inferiorly at the iliac crest, but medially the transversalis fascia fuses with the psoas fascia and prevents communication between the right and left posterior pararenal compartments.

The posterior pararenal compartment contains no major organs; therefore, diseases rarely arise and are only infrequently confined solely within this compartment. Abnormalites of the posterior pararenal compartment are associated with diseases involving other extraperitoneal compartments or contiguous structures.[14] Traumatic or spontaneous retroperitoneal hemorrhage, retroperitoneal lymphatic extravasation, posterior spread of pancreatitis, infection as a complication of rib or spinal osteomyelitis, or, rarely, a neoplasm can selectively involve the posterior pararenal compartment.[14] Also, pelvic lesions can spread upward to involve the posterior pararenal space because it is open inferiorly.[14]

INTERCOMPARTMENTAL COMMUNICATION

Although the three extraperitoneal compartments are anatomically well defined, there are pathways by which a process involving one space can spread to the others. Commonly, a process originating caudally in the anterior pararenal space spreads around the inferior border of the cone of renal fascia and extends cephalad into the posterior pararenal compartment.[15] Pelvic disease can spread cephalad directly into the three extraperitoneal compartments. Rectal and sigmoid diseases are particularly likely to spread into the extraperitoneal spaces. Abnormalities arising in any of the extraperitoneal compartments can spread directly through the lateroconal fascia or Gerota's fascia into the other extraperitoneal compartments, usually after pus, pancreatic enzymes, or tumors have eroded and destroyed the limiting fascial planes.[15]

KIDNEYS

CT directly displays axial cross-sectional renal anatomy and permits reconstruction of renal anatomy into coronal, sagittal, and oblique planes (Fig. 15–6). The kidneys are surrounded by abundant perirenal fat which permits sharp delineation of the renal margins in almost every patient. The transverse contour of the kidneys is smooth, except where the vascular pedicle points anteromedially toward the aorta and the inferior vena cava.[1] The renal parenchyma in a given patient has a relatively uniform density of 30 to 50 Hounsfield Units (H). The cortex and medial portions of the kidney cannot be distinguished by density differences on precontrast CT scans.[1] Segments of the urine-filled calices have a CT attenuation value of water; fat in the perirenal space and renal hilum has a CT density less than that of water and can therefore be identified by density differences. The size and volume of the kidneys can be measured by CT (Fig. 15–7). These measurements correlate closely with direct measurements of resected specimens.[24]

In most patients, the renal arteries and veins are demonstrated as linear structures joining the aorta or inferior vena cava (Fig. 15–8). The renal arteries arise posterior (dorsal) to the renal veins and CT scans frequently demonstrate accessory renal arteries. The renal veins are usually larger

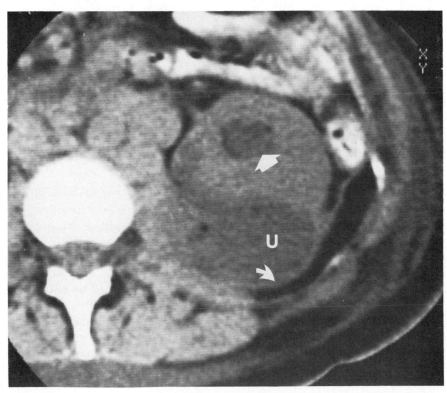

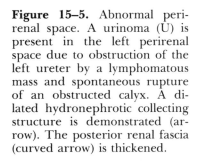

Figure 15–5. Abnormal perirenal space. A urinoma (U) is present in the left perirenal space due to obstruction of the left ureter by a lymphomatous mass and spontaneous rupture of an obstructed calyx. A dilated hydronephrotic collecting structure is demonstrated (arrow). The posterior renal fascia (curved arrow) is thickened.

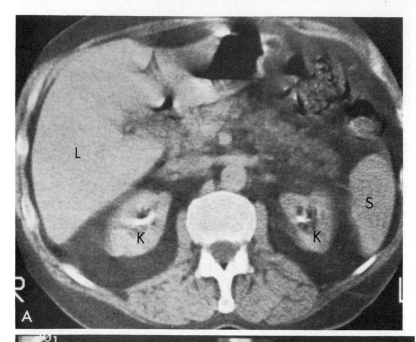

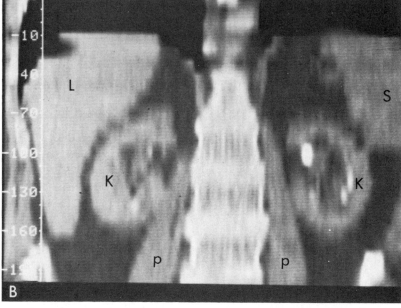

Figure 15–6. Normal kidneys. **A–D** Axial **(A)**, coronal **(B)**, right sagittal **(C)**, and left sagittal **(D)** CT scans demonstrating the relationships of the kidneys to adjacent organs. K = Kidney; L = liver; S = spleen; p = psoas muscle.

Illustration continued on opposite page

than the corresponding artery, and the longer left renal vein crosses ventral to the aorta and enters the inferior vena cava at the level of the uncinate process of the pancreas. The aorta and superior mesenteric artery pinch the left renal vein, which causes the left renal vein to appear larger than the right.[25]

The CT appearance of the renal parenchyma after the administration of contrast medium depends on the amount and concentration injected, the rapidity of injection, and the timing of the scan. If a dynamic scan series of six to 12 CT scans is obtained after a bolus injection of contrast medium, the first CT images usually demonstrate the renal arteries or renal veins (Fig. 15–9). The contrast effect in the renal cortex increases rapidly and reaches a peak of 55 to 120 H at 30 to 50 seconds,[26, 27] permitting a clear differentiation of the renal cortex from the renal medulla (Fig. 15–9). The thickness of the renal cortex measured by CT is 0.48 ± 0.02 cm and decreases with age.[26]

Dynamic CT is useful for displaying the change in attenuation value versus time (time-density curves) in various portions of the kidney (Figs. 15–9 and 15–10).[26, 27] The attenuation value of the renal medulla increases more slowly but ultimately rises to a higher level than that of the

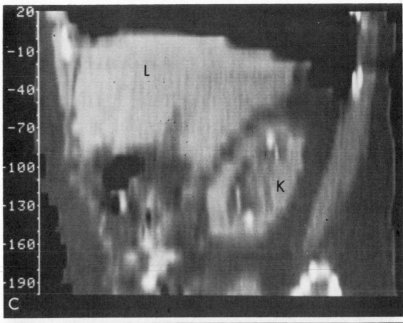

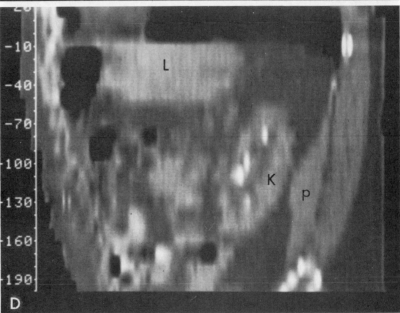

Figure 15–6. *Continued*

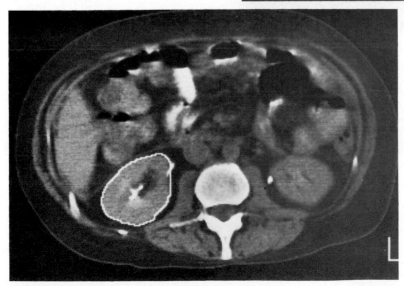

Figure 15–7. Renal size and volume determination. The kidney margin has been traced, and the calculated area within the trace is 23.3 cm². As the slice thickness is 1 cm, a volume of 23.3 cm³ is contained within the outline of the kidney. Summation of individual slice volumes provides a measure of total renal volume.

769

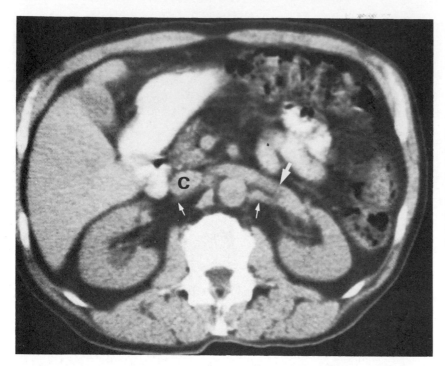

Figure 15–8. Normal renal arterial and venous anatomy. The renal arteries (small arrows) arise from the aorta dorsal to the renal veins. In this patient the left renal vein (large arrow) is seen crossing over the aorta to join the inferior vena cava (C). On CT the renal veins usually appear larger than the renal arteries.

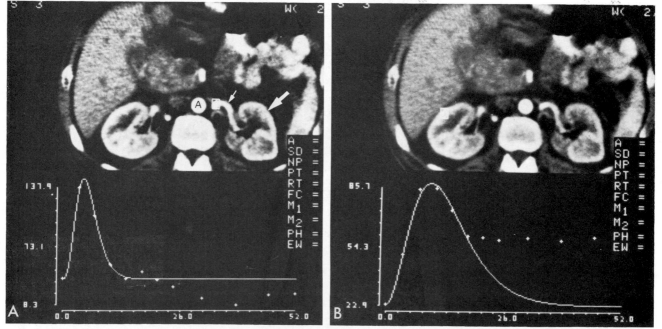

Figure 15–9. Dynamic CT scan following bolus injection of contrast material. **A**   The left renal artery (small arrow) is maximally opacified during peak aortic (A) contrast enhancement. The renal cortex (large arrow) is shown as a densely opacified peripheral zone. The time-density curve plots the increase in CT density with time and shows a rapid rise and fall in CT density of the left renal artery. **B**   Time-density plot of right renal cortex (box). Curve demonstrates a rapid increase in the CT density of the renal cortex of 85.7 H and then a gradual decline. The rise in attenuation value of the cortex parallels that of the renal artery, but there is a slower rise to a lower peak and then a more gradual decline in CT density. The curve is not corrected for recirculation.

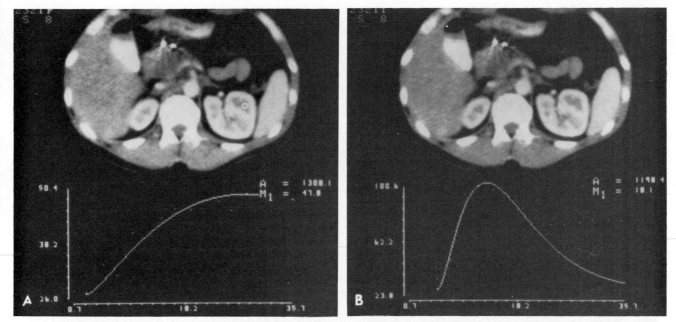

Figure 15–10. Time-density curve of the renal cortex and medulla following a bolus injection of contrast material. **A**   The cursor box ⊙ is in the renal medulla. There is a gradual increase in the CT density of the renal medulla to 50 H by 25 to 30 seconds and no evidence of a decline in attenuation value. **B**   Plot of renal cortex reveals a rapid increase to 100 H by 15 seconds, followed by a decline. The curve is not corrected for recirculation.

renal cortex (Fig. 15–10). The crossover of medullary and cortical values typically occurs about 65 seconds after a bolus injection of contrast medium. This component of the time-density curve, the corticomedullary junction, may reflect renal glomerular function.[26]

Following a bolus injection, prominent columns of Bertin are shown as structures having a density equal to that of the surrounding cortex (Fig. 15–11). The attenuation value of the medulla increases for 1 to 5 minutes; then the density of the renal parenchyma becomes uniform and the cal-

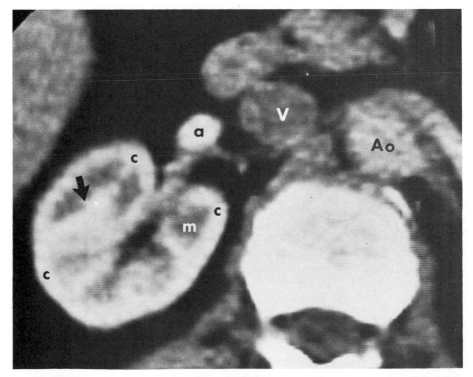

Figure 15–11. Column of Bertin. Dynamic CT scan through the right kidney was obtained after a bolus injection of contrast material. There is sharp demarcation between the renal cortex (c) and renal medulla (m). The column of Bertin (arrow) has a density equal to that of the renal cortex and extends into the renal medulla. a = Renal artery; V = vena cava; Ao = aorta.

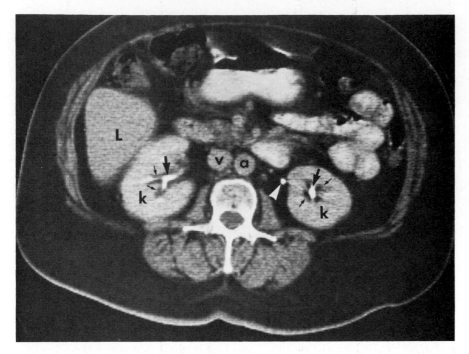

Figure 15–12. Normal kidneys (k) following a drip infusion of contrast material. The renal parenchyma is homogeneous without distinction of the renal cortex and medulla. The attenuation value of the kidneys is greater than that of the liver (L), aorta (a), or inferior vena cava (v). The renal pelvic collecting structures (large arrows) are surrounded by fat (small arrows). The left ureter (arrowhead) is shown as a dot of high density.

ices and renal pelvis are sharply delineated. On delayed CT scans, fetal lobulations are shown to have the same attenuation value as the rest of the functioning renal parenchyma.[1] After an intravenous infusion of contrast medium, renal parenchymal density increases uniformly and the sharp delineation of the corticomedullary junction seen after a bolus injection is absent (Fig. 15–12).

TECHNIQUES OF EXAMINATION

Ideally, every CT study should be monitored by a radiologist and modified to meet the clinical problem being addressed. Renal or ureteral CT is usually performed to clarify a suspected abnormality detected on an excretory urogram or an ultrasonogram. Localization of the CT scan has been guided by a preliminary plain abdominal radiograph, a radiograph with a lead grid[1] or a catheter-marking device taped on the abdomen.[28] Intravenous pyelograms and computerized radiographs obtained by CT scanner have also been used to localize the kidneys before the CT examination[3] although in most patients, a preliminary abdominal or computerized radiograph is not necessary. The usual anatomic location of the kidneys is from T12 to L3, or roughly from the xiphoid to the umbilicus.[2]

We perform an initial CT scan at the level of the xiphoid process, and the technician adjusts the scan level according to the location of the kidneys on the scan. A trained and experienced technician can precisely position the patient for a renal CT scan by viewing the initial baseline CT scan obtained from external anatomic landmarks.

The entire kidney is routinely scanned using contiguous CT sections 1 cm thick during suspended respiration with the patient supine. Scans are continued down through the pelvis if a distal ureteral abnormality is suspected. Technical factors should be appropriate to the patient's size. Scan times are selected to ensure that high-resolution CT images are obtained, permitting the maximal amount of information to be extracted from the CT study. Oral contrast medium—480 ml of 1 per cent meglumine diatrizoate (Gastrografin) or barium sulfate 30 minutes before the CT scan and another 240 ml 5 minutes before the examination—is administered to ensure that the gastrointestinal tract is adequately opacified. Adequate opacification is particularly important when the ureter is examined for expected abnormality, as unopacified bowel may simulate a solid periureteral mass lesion. Occasionally, prone or decubitus positioning is useful in evaluating juxtarenal pathology[3] or obstructive uropathy[4]; CT scans less than 1.0 cm thick or overlapping scans can be used to better delineate small abnormalities. Reformatting axial CT images into coronal, sagittal, or various oblique planes provides additional information for evaluating the extent of renal abnormalities and aids in determining the organ from which a right upper abdominal mass lesion originates.

Scanning the kidneys before and after administration of intravenous contrast medium[1-4] ensures the greatest diagnostic yield, but the patient receives twice the radiation exposure, the examination is longer, and frequently the precontrast scans provide no unique information.

Engelstad and co-workers[5] studied 176 patients to determine the role of precontrast CT scans of the kidney. All 152 mass lesions were detected, accurately classified as a simple cyst or a solid renal mass, and characterized as to size and extent from the contrast-enhanced CT scans alone. In no patient with a renal mass lesion, hydronephrosis, or polycystic disease was the diagnosis hindered by administration of contrast medium. Precontrast CT images added diagnostic information in only 9 per cent of 176 patients; i.e., when contrast medium obscured calcification in the renal parenchyma or collecting system, or in cases of renal or perirenal hemorrhage.

Unless CT is performed to detect renal calcification, extravasation of contrast medium or perirenal hemorrhage, we obtain contrast-enhanced CT scans of the kidneys as the initial scan procedure. However, faster CT scanners with low exposure rates allow both enhanced and nonenhanced scans to be obtained with little additional time, expense, or radiation exposure.

Intravenous contrast medium may be given as a drip infusion or as a bolus injection, or the two methods can also be used in combination.[1-5] Most commonly, either a 50- to 100-ml bolus of standard diatrizoic acid salts (Renografin 60 or Conray 400) or a 300-ml infusion of 30 per cent contrast medium is administered over 10 to 15 minutes.[1-5] We administer 150 ml of 60 per cent contrast medium, which enables the contrast to be infused more quickly and provides greater enhancement of major vessels during the infusion. Contrast is usually administered through an antecubital vein and CT scanning is begun when two thirds of the contrast medium has been administered. An additional 25- to 40-ml bolus injection can be combined with a rapid sequence of CT scans at the level of the renal pedicle to better define renal vasculature.[29]

Dynamic CT scanning permits sequential CT images of the kidneys and renal vasculature to be obtained rapidly.[11, 26, 27, 30] After intravenous bolus injection of 40 to 60 ml of contrast medium, a series of dynamic CT scans can differentiate the renal cortex from the renal medulla (Fig. 15–9).[2, 26, 27, 31–33] Dynamic renal CT can demonstrate renal vascular anatomy, the vascularity of mass lesions, renovascular hypertension, the relationship of the great vessels to the ureters, and time-density curves of the renal cortex and medulla (Fig. 15–10).[2, 26, 27, 30, 31, 32, 33]

The best dynamic CT images are obtained when a bolus of contrast is given after a nonenhanced baseline CT study. If contrast medium has been administered, satisfactory results can be obtained by waiting 10 to 15 minutes and then injecting the contrast bolus. Repeated 40- to 50-ml bolus injections can be given to evaluate different anatomic regions of the kidney if enough time is allowed for the contrast medium to be excreted. Dynamic CT scanning to detect renal hypoperfusion in patients with renal vascular hypertension has not been adequately studied, but it may be a useful screening modality when technical advancements permit the entire kidney to be imaged simultaneously after a bolus injection.[34]

PATHOLOGY

RENAL MASSES

CT has proved valuable for detecting, localizing, and characterizing renal mass lesions. CT has been used to determine the extent and stage of a renal tumor, to plan and evaluate the response to therapy, and to detect tumor recurrence after therapy.

Renal masses are detected by CT because:

1. They have an attenuation value different from that of normal renal parenchyma.

2. They alter the normal contour of the kidney.

3. They are enhanced to a different degree after intravenous contrast administration.

4. They distort the renal collecting structures.

5. They cause hydronephrosis.

6. They produce filling defects in the renal pelvis or caliceal system.

Cystic Renal Masses

BENIGN RENAL CYSTS. Simple cysts are extremely common lesions of the kidney. They are present in more than 50 per cent of patients over the age of 50 years[2, 35, 36] and vary greatly in number, size, and location. The cause of renal cysts is unknown, although tubular obstruction or vascular compromise has been suggested.[7, 37]

The simple renal cyst originates in the renal parenchyma and usually produces an abnormal renal outline that is readily detected by CT. A typical benign renal cyst has the following characteristics:

1. It is round or slightly oval mass with a smooth outer margin.

2. The cyst wall has no measurable thickness.

Table 15–1.   CT DIFFERENTIATION OF RENAL MASSES

CT Feature	Cyst	Neoplasm
Shape	Round, slightly oval	Irregular, lobulated
Margin	Smooth	Lobulated
Wall	Thin, no measurable thickness	Thick, can measure thickness
Interface with parenchyma	Sharp, distinct	Indistinct, irregular
Density	Homogeneous	Inhomogeneous
	Close to water (0–15 H)	Close to renal parenchyma (30 + H)
Contrast enhancement	No	Yes
Vascular invasion	No	Yes

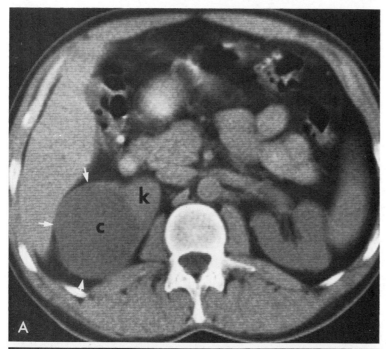

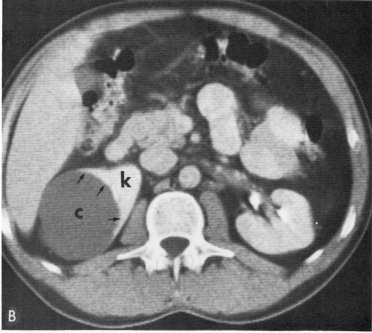

Figure 15–13. Benign renal cyst. **A** Pre-contrast CT scan demonstrates the cyst (c) to be round and to have a smooth outer margin (arrows). The density of the cyst is uniform and measures 2 H. k = Normal kidney. **B** Scan after contrast injection reveals the cyst (c) to have a sharp interface (arrows) with normal renal parenchyma, no increase in attenuation value, and a cyst wall that has no measurable thickness.

3. The attenuation value is uniform and close to that of water and does not increase after intravenous contrast administration.

4. The interface with normal renal parenchyma is distinct and sharp.

5. It may abut but does not obliterate renal sinus fat.

6. It is confined wholly within the renal fascia and does not invade renal veins (Table 15–1 and Figs. 15–13 and 15–14).

When a renal mass meets all the criteria of a renal cyst, the accuracy of the CT diagnosis approaches 100 per cent.[1, 4, 38] Applying strict criteria, McClennan and associates[32] found no erroneous CT interpretations in 56 proved benign renal cysts; Sagel and associates[1] found none in

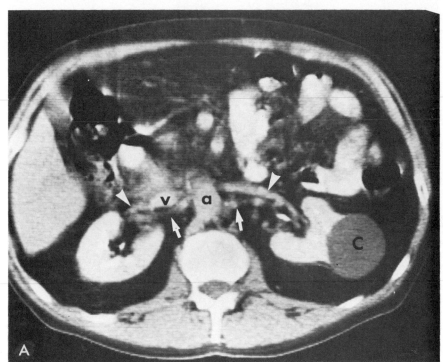

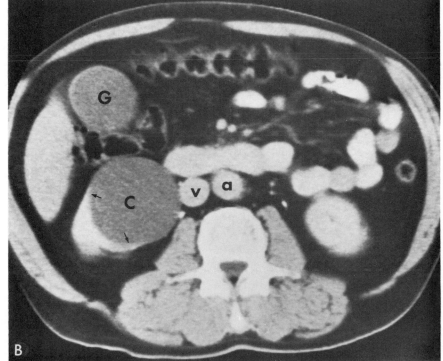

Figure 15–14. Typical renal cysts following contrast infusion. **A** Peripheral cyst (C) of water density in left kidney with a sharp cyst-parenchymal junction. **B** Large right renal cyst (C) has the same CT density as the gallbladder (G). Junction with renal parenchyma is sharp and tapers into a beaklike configuration (arrows). a = Aorta; v = vena cava; arrows = renal artery; arrowheads = renal veins.

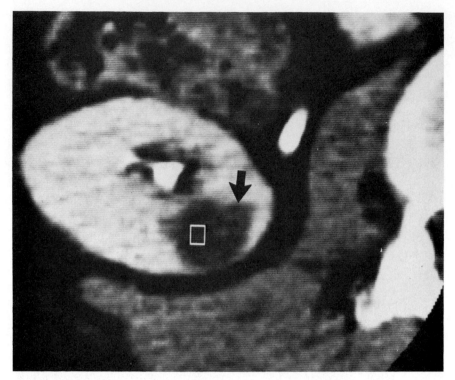

Figure 15–15. Intrarenal cyst (box) which has slightly irregular margins (arrow) and a measured density of 24 H. Aspiration proved the lesion to be a simple cyst. Partial volume averaging was responsible for the spuriously high attenuation value.

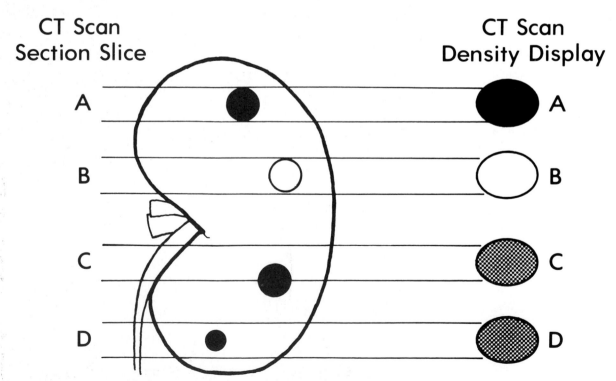

Figure 15–16. Diagram of partial volume averaging effect on measured density of renal masses. **A** Renal cyst entirely in CT section appears as low-density lesion. **B** Solid renal mass entirely in the section of the scan appears as a mass of soft-tissue density. **C,D** Large renal cyst partially in the scan section and a renal cyst smaller than the slice thickness both have intermediate CT densities.

104 cysts (22 proved), and Hattery's group[4] found none in 60 cysts in 20 patients. There is no evidence that a renal lesion meeting all the CT criteria of a renal cyst has ever developed into a solid renal mass.[2] Thus, a renal cyst puncture is not necessary to exclude malignancy when strict CT criteria for a benign renal cyst have been met.[38] Because renal cysts are so common and the CT diagnosis so secure, we no longer advocate

further examination or follow-up to confirm the CT diagnosis of a simple renal cyst.

Although CT can accurately detect and characterize a renal mass as a benign cyst, there are potential pitfalls to avoid. Depending upon the size and location of a renal cyst, its measured attenuation value may be greater than that of water (Fig. 15–15). Unless a cyst occupies the entire thickness of the CT slice, partial volume averag-

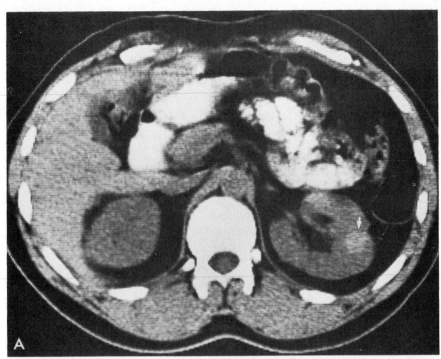

Figure 15–17. Patient with von Hippel–Lindau disease and multiple renal cysts. **A** Precontrast CT scan. A high-density, round mass (arrow) is present in the left kidney. CT number = 32 H. **B** Postcontrast CT scan. The renal parenchyma has increased in density so that the mass (arrow) now appears as a low-density lesion that has same characteristics as that of a renal cyst. At surgery, fresh hemorrhage into a simple renal cyst was found. The top of a right parapelvic cyst (c) is also identified.

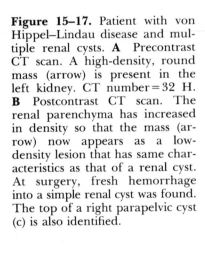

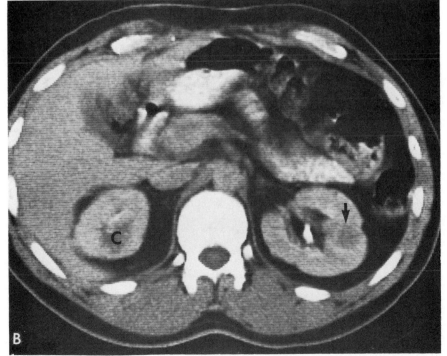

ing with the normal adjacent renal parenchyma may spuriously raise the displayed attenuation value of the renal cyst (Fig. 15–16). Cysts smaller in diameter than the CT slice thickness always undergo partial volume averaging, and multiloculated and parapelvic cysts may have erroneously elevated attenuation values resulting from adjacent cysts, septa, or hilar structures.[1, 2, 11] The magnitude of partial volume averaging can be reduced by using thinner CT scan sections; how-

ever, this requires more CT sections to image the entire kidney and should be used only when renal mass lesions are small or indeterminate.

High attenuation values of renal cysts may also be produced by these conditions:

1. Hemorrhage into the cyst (Fig. 15–17).

2. Contrast medium leaking into the cyst by a communication with the collecting system[23] or by diffusion.[39]

3. Calcification of the cyst wall (Fig. 15–18).

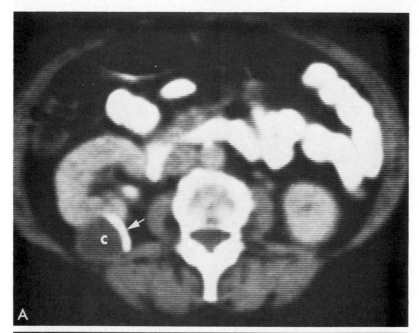

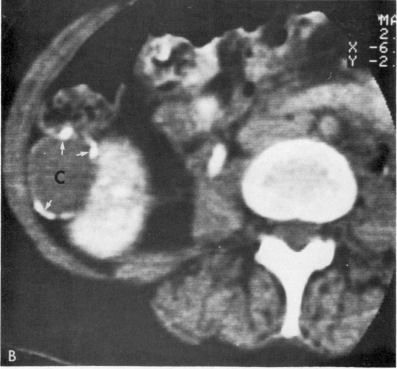

Figure 15–18. Renal cysts with peripheral calcification and hemorrhage. **A** Posteriorly directed right renal cyst (c), which has a density of 20 H and a cyst wall that is partially calcified (arrow). Surgery revealed a cyst containing old hemorrhage. **B** Laterally positioned right renal cyst (c) with partial cyst wall calcification (arrows) and a CT density of 34 H. Diagnosis: simple cyst with recent hemorrhage. Rim calcification is more common in cysts than in carcinoma, but it occurs in both. Evidence for benign cyst is the lack of any associated soft-tissue mass.

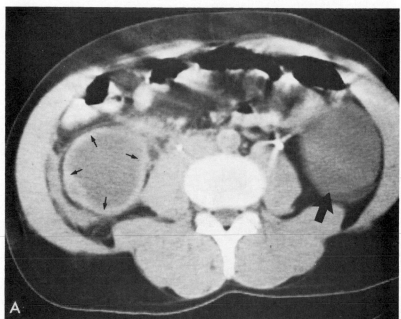

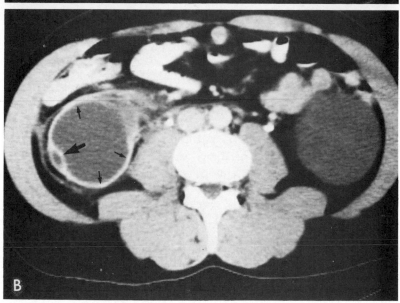

Figure 15–19. Infected right renal cyst. **A** CT scan: After contrast infusion, a large left renal cyst (large arrow) is seen without a measurable cyst wall. A thick cyst wall (small arrows) is noted around a right renal cyst. The density of the right cyst is slightly higher than that of the left renal cyst. **B** Dynamic CT study after bolus injection of contrast material demonstrates marked contrast enhancement of the wall (small arrows) of right renal cyst. The cyst also contains a septation (large arrow). The wall of the left renal cyst does not enhance.

4. Infection (Fig. 15–19).

5. Image degradation by high-density streak artifacts.

Infection can also produce thickening of the rim of a cyst and can cause the rim to dramatically enhance after contrast administration (Fig. 15–19).

A CT diagnosis of a benign renal cyst should never be based solely on the attenuation value of the renal mass but only after all of the CT characteristics of the lesion have been appraised. If the attenuation value of a renal mass exceeds 15 Hounsfield Units (H) or if the mass has other atypical features, we consider the mass to be in-

determinate (Fig. 15–20) and recommend additional studies to determine its true nature.

PARAPELVIC CYSTS. These masses have all the features of simple benign renal parenchymal cysts but are located adjacent to the renal sinus. Parapelvic cysts have an attenuation value close to that of water but are difficult to distinguish from a dilated or an extrarenal pelvis on nonenhanced CT scans. After contrast medium is administered, the unenhanced parapelvic cyst is readily detected adjacent to the contrast-filled hilar collecting structures. (Fig. 15–21A). CT can easily distinguish between a parapelvic cyst and pelvic fibrolipomatosis (Figs. 15–21B, C).[40] The attenuation value of fi-

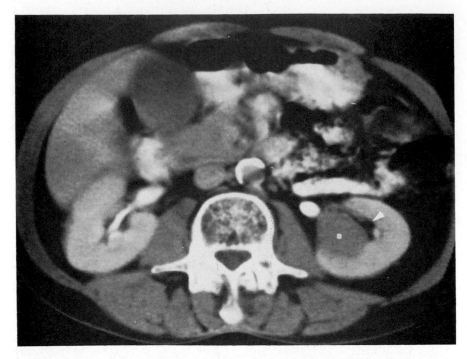

Figure 15–20. CT scan of indeterminate renal mass. A parapelvic mass (box), present in the left kidney, has a CT density of 74 H. There is no evidence of obstruction, and the hilar fat (arrowhead) is well preserved. The interface between mass and renal parenchyma is slightly blurred. Surgical findings: Benign parapelvic cyst containing hemorrhage, mucinous material, and debris.

brolipomatous tissue ranges from −5 to −100 H and is always less than that of a parapelvic cyst.

POLYCYSTIC DISEASE.   Polycystic disease is commonly classified into infantile and adult types. In the infantile form, the kidneys are bilaterally large but retain a reniform shape. Cystic lesions in the liver, spleen, and pancreas are common. The kidneys are riddled with small cysts (a few millimeters in size), which usually do not produce caliceal or pelvic distortion.[37] Renal function is poor and most infants die shortly after birth. Other children survive into young adult life with signs of renal insufficiency, chronic pyelonephritis, portal hypertension, progressive portal fibrosis, and gastroesophageal varices.

Adult polycystic kidney disease is characterized by multiple cysts of varying sizes in both the cortex and medulla. Both kidneys are involved but

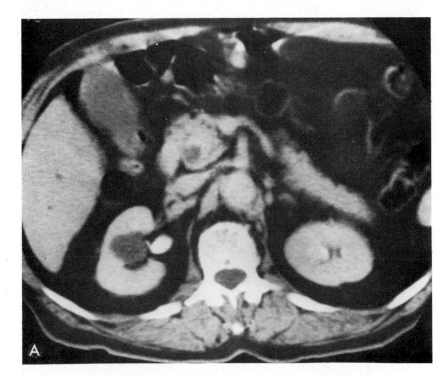

Figure 15–21. Parapelvic cysts. **A** A single cystic structure of water density adjacent to the renal sinus is seen.

Illustration continued on opposite page

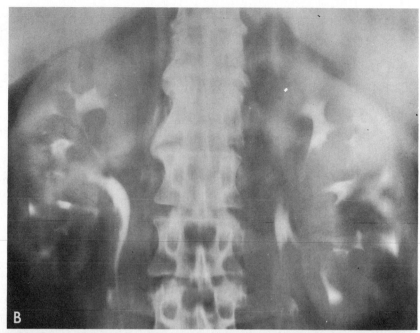

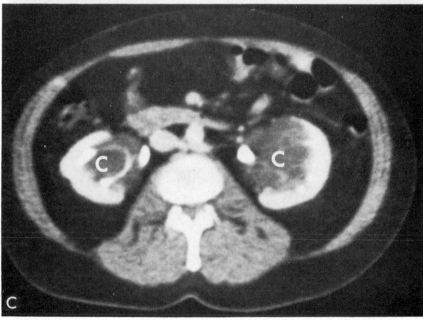

Figure 15–21. *Continued* **B** Excretory urogram demonstrating splaying of the renal collecting structures by low-density masses, which suggests polycystic renal disease or renal fibrolipomatosis. **C** CT scan reveals bilateral parapelvic cysts (c) without evidence of polycystic disease or renal pelvic fibrolipomatosis.

usually not symmetrically. The intervening renal tissue appears grossly normal but contains numerous very small renal cysts. Cysts are often present in the liver and occur less frequently in the spleen, lung, and pancreas.[37] Progressive renal failure and hypertension usually become evident in the fourth decade, but the adult form of polycystic renal disease may be seen in children and young adults.[37]

The CT appearance of adult polycystic disease consists of bilateral renal enlargement, splaying and distortion of the collecting system, and multiple renal cysts (Fig. 15–22).[1–4, 41] The renal contour is lobulated and a multitude of small and large cysts that appear benign give the kidneys a honeycomb or "Swiss cheese" appearance. In one third of patients, CT also demonstrates hepatic or pancreatic cystic disease (Figs. 15–22 and 15–23).[37] The CT diagnosis of polycystic kidney is usually straightforward; confusion occurs only in distinguishing patients with multiple simple cysts (Figs. 15–24 and 15–25) from those with polycystic disease. Patients with multiple simple renal cysts have many fewer renal cysts, show no family history of polycystic renal or liver disease, and are not predisposed to hypertension and renal failure.

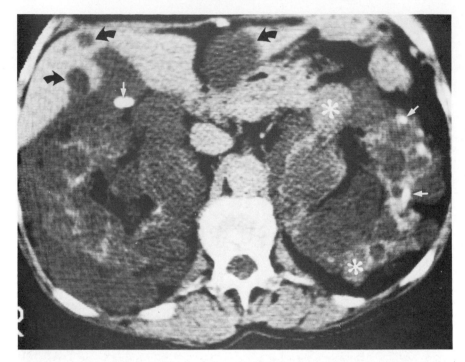

Figure 15–22. Polycystic kidney disease with hemorrhage. A CT scan demonstrates bilateral renal enlargement with multiple renal cysts. There are foci of calcification (arrows) in both kidneys and marked distortion of the renal contour. Several cysts (asterisk) have a higher CT density, which proved to be the result of hemorrhage into the cyst. Multiple hepatic cysts (curved arrows) are also present.

CT is particularly valuable in examining patients with polycystic kidney disease who have hematuria and are suspected of having a renal malignancy. CT can readily distinguish a mass with a high attenuation value from the multiple renal cysts, which have an attenuation value close to that of water. However, the presence of a mass with a high attenuation value does not necessarily imply the presence of a tumor. Hemorrhage or infection can increase the attenuation value of a cyst and thereby simulate a solid mass lesion (Fig. 15–22).[41] If a partial nephrectomy is planned as treatment for a solid renal mass, a contrast-enhanced CT scan helps estimate the amount and

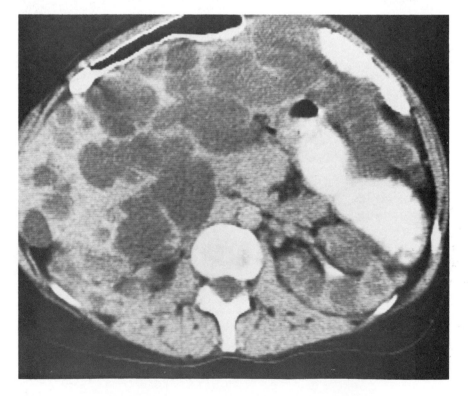

Figure 15–23. Polycystic kidney and liver disease. The kidneys contain multiple renal cysts but are not grossly enlarged. The liver is virtually replaced by multiple large hepatic cysts. The scan at a lower level demonstrated pancreatic cysts. Renal and hepatic functions were normal in this patient.

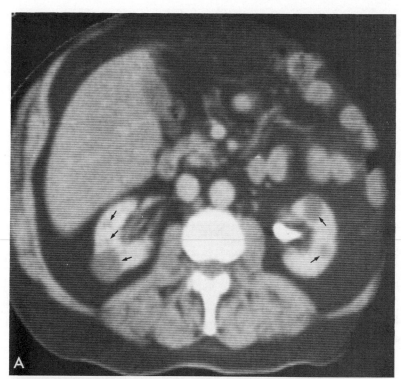

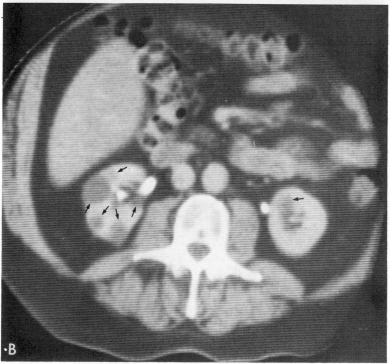

Figure 15–24. Multiple renal cysts. **A** Scan through level of midportion of both kidneys demonstrates multiple renal cysts (arrows) of varying size in each kidney. **B** Scan at lower level more clearly delineates multiple right renal cysts (arrows). The kidneys are not enlarged and function normally. No liver or pancreatic cysts are present.

location of functioning renal parenchyma before surgical excision.

MULTICYSTIC KIDNEY.   This is a dysplastic condition characterized by severe structural disorganization, incomplete corticomedullary differentiation, primitive ducts, and multiple cysts of various sizes.[37] Clinically, multicystic kidney is a frequent cause of an abdominal mass in an otherwise healthy infant or child.[37, 42] A plain abdominal film may show a flank mass, but excretory urography fails to reveal any renal function.[37, 42] CT shows that the entire kidney consists of numerous cystic masses that vary in size and have attenuation values similar to that of water. No function-

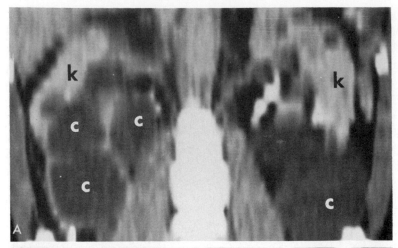

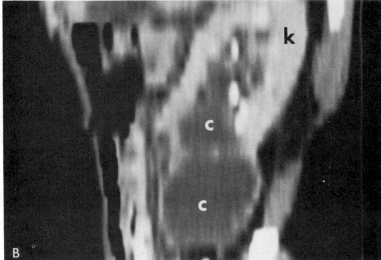

Figure 15–25. Multiple renal cysts. **A,B** Coronal **(A)** and right sagittal **(B)** reformatted scans through kidneys (k) containing multiple simple renal cysts (c). The relationships of the cysts to each other, to the renal collecting structures, and to the uninvolved renal parenchyma are clearly shown.

ing renal parenchyma is detectable after contrast administration, and the collecting structures cannot be distinguished from the mass. Multilocular cystic nephromas and unilateral polycystic disease may produce similar clinical findings but can be excluded if CT demonstrates the absence of functioning renal parenchyma.[42]

MULTILOCULAR RENAL CYSTS. This type of cyst is a "densely encapsulated solitary intrarenal mass composed of a myriad of noncommunicating cysts of varying size."[43] The multiple cysts have thick walls and septa that do not contain normal renal tissue. The external surface of the

mass is smooth, but the lack of normal renal tissue in the septa clearly distinguishes the multilocular cyst from contiguous benign renal cysts and most other congenital cystic diseases. Approximately 85 cases of multilocular renal cysts have been reported, half in children and half in adults.[43]

The etiology and pathogenesis of multilocular renal cysts are unclear.[43–45] In children, these cysts appear to be congenital; they are manifested as an abdominal mass under the age of 5 years (mean 17 months).[44] In adults, multilocular renal cysts are usually discovered as an incidental find-

Figure 15–26. Multilocular renal cyst. **A** Excretory urogram demonstrates distortion of the left collecting system by a lower pole renal mass (M). **B** CT scan shows a large cystic mass (C) that displaces (curved arrows) but does not invade adjacent functioning renal parenchyma. There are multiple septations (arrows) within the cystic mass, which has areas of different densities. **C** Renal angiogram reveals an avascular mass that stretches (arrows) the arteries supplying the left lower pole. No tumor vascularity is identified.

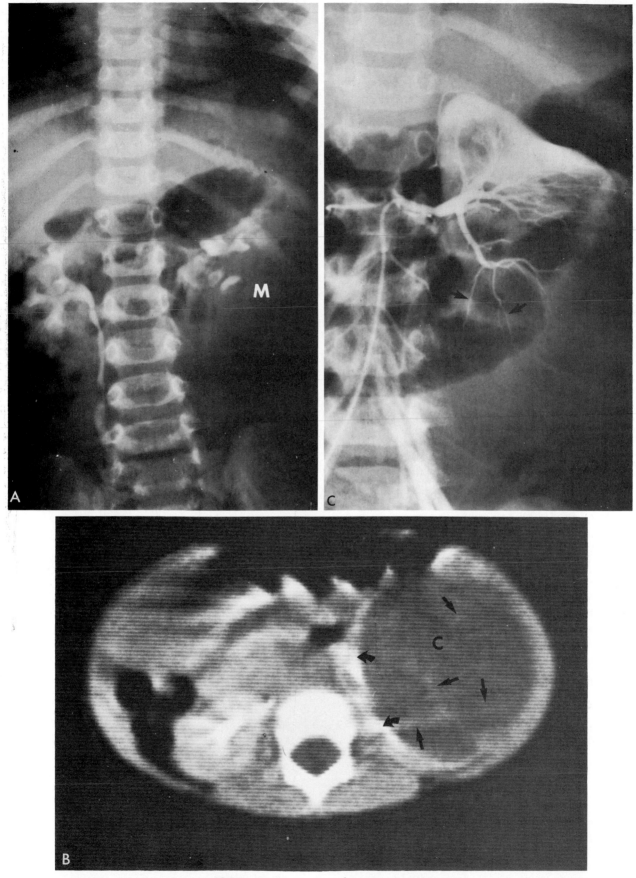

Figure 15–26. *See legend on opposite page*

ing during excretory urography in patients 40 to 70 years old.[43, 45] The lack of reported cases in the intervening years suggests acquired etiology in adult cases.

Because of the spectrum of histologic features and theories of its cause and pathogenesis, multi-locular renal cyst has been called by many names, including cystic adenoma, cystic lymphangioma, cystic hamartoma, cystadenoma, multilocular cystadenoma, cystic Wilms' tumor, polycystic nephroblastoma, cystic differentiated nephroblastoma, segmental polycystic kidney, segmental multicystic kidney, Perlmann tumor, multilocular cystic nephroma, and adenomatous polycystic kidney tumor.[43-45] The great variety of names has produced confusion as to the true incidence of these cysts.

CT demonstrates multiple fluid-filled cysts separated by thick septa and sharply demarcated from the normal renal parenchyma (Fig. 15–26).[43, 44] Peripheral or central calcification is present in 10 to 50 per cent of cases and may have a circular, stellate, flocculent, or granular pattern.[43] The attenuation values of multilocular cysts range from 2 to 40 H after contrast administration.[44] The sonographic appearance of multilocular renal cysts is that of multiple cystic masses separated by highly echogenic septa. Thus, the CT or ultrasonic features alone may be confusing, but the combined CT and ultrasonic features may suggest a preoperative diagnosis of multilocular renal cysts and permit a partial rather than a total nephrectomy to be performed.

Solid Renal Tumors

Solid renal masses can be benign or malignant; they are neoplastic, infectious, congenital, or traumatic in origin. The most common solid renal masses are malignant tumors arising from the renal parenchyma or from the epithelium of the renal pelvis.[46]

Various benign and malignant tumors originate in the kidney. Primary renal tumors may arise from the renal capsule, mature and immature renal parenchyma, renal mesenchymal derivatives, and the renal pelvis; various malignant lesions can secondarily involve the kidney. Malignant tumors of the kidney account for approximately 2 per cent of all neoplasms. Adenocarcinoma constitutes about 83 per cent of all renal malignancies; carcinoma of the renal pelvis, 8 per cent; nephroblastoma, 6 per cent; and other varieties, approximately 3 per cent.[46]

RENAL CELL CARCINOMA (ADENOCARCINOMA). Adenocarcinoma is the most common malignant renal tumor. It is three times more frequent in males than in females and is rare in children and young adults.[46] Gross hematuria occurs in approximately 60 per cent of patients, and about 50 per cent of patients have flank pain. However, less than 15 per cent of patients have the classic triad of renal carcinoma—gross hematuria, back pain, and flank mass.[46] Renal carcinoma occasionally produces hypertension and hyperparathyroidism. Familial occurrences are uncommon except in patients with von Hippel-Lindau disease, 12 to 83 per cent of whom develop adenocarcinoma.[46-49]

The characteristic CT appearance of a renal adenocarcinoma is a solid renal lesion that produces a mass or an abnormality of the renal contour (Figs. 15–27 and 15–28).[1-12, 29, 50] The tumor is frequently irregularly shaped and has a lobulated or ill-defined outer margin. In contrast to renal cysts, the demarcation between the tumor mass and normal renal parenchyma is usually ill defined. The attenuation value of the tumor on precontrast CT scans is often very close to that of normal renal parenchyma. Although the density of the tumor may be homogeneous, necrosis commonly causes the central part of the tumor to have a low, unhomogeneous CT density (Figs. 15–27 and 15–28). Recent intratumoral hemorrhage may cause areas of the tumor to have higher attenuation values than adjacent normal renal parenchyma. Central renal sinus fat is at least partially obliterated in approximately 50 per cent of cases (Figs. 15–28 and 15–29).[1, 11]

Administration of intravenous contrast medium accentuates the difference in CT density between normal parenchyma and tumor (Figs. 15–27B, 15–28B, and 15–29). The density of the normal renal parenchyma increases 80 to 120 H, whereas density of the tumor, which lacks functioning tubular elements, increases less and only in proportion to pooling of contrast medium in the tumor's vascular and extravascular compartments. Dynamic CT studies after a bolus injection of contrast medium may detect an early peak that corresponds to the early hypervascular phase on renal angiograms (Figs. 15–27 and 15–30).[2] Scans performed minutes after a bolus injection or an intravenous infusion of contrast medium will not detect the early hypervascular phase of renal cell carcinomas, but all postcontrast CT scans clearly demonstrate the interface between tumor and normal renal parenchyma.

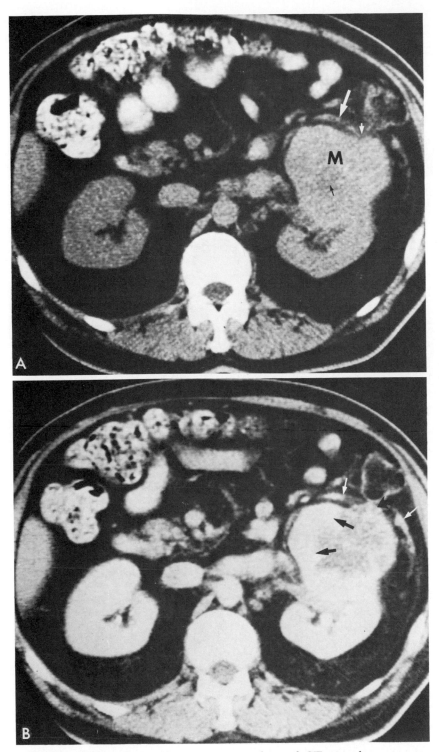

Figure 15–27. Renal cell carcinoma. **A** Noncontrast enhanced CT scan demonstrates a large solid mass (M) arising from the ventral surface of the left kidney. The outer contour is lobulated, and the demarcation from normal renal parenchyma is poorly defined. The center of the tumor (black arrow) has a slightly decreased attenuation compared with the periphery of the tumor. The tumor has extended into the perirenal space (small arrow) and has thickened the anterior renal fascia (large arrow). **B** CT scan after bolus injection of contrast material. The renal cell carcinoma shows areas of marked contrast enhancement (black arrows) and areas of lesser enhancement. The anterior renal fascia (white arrows) is thickened and enhances after contrast injection. Perirenal extension (curved arrow) is more clearly demonstrated.

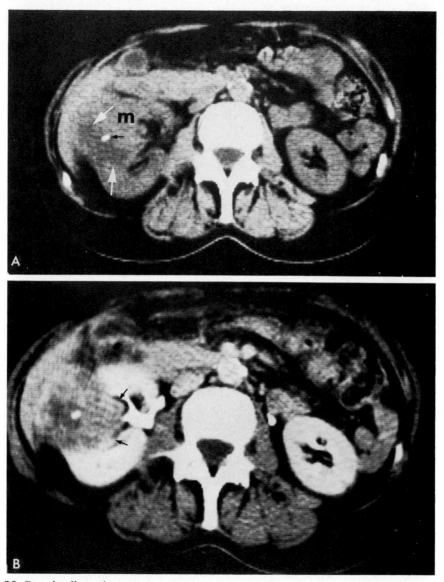

Figure 15–28. Renal cell carcinoma. **A**   Precontrast CT scan demonstrates a large mass (m) having an irregular outer margin, a focus of calcification (black arrow), areas of low density (white arrows), and a poor interface between tumor and normal kidney. **B**   Postcontrast injection, portions of the tumor enhance dramatically while others remain relatively unchanged. The tumor extends into the central renal sinus fat (arrows) and into the perirenal space.

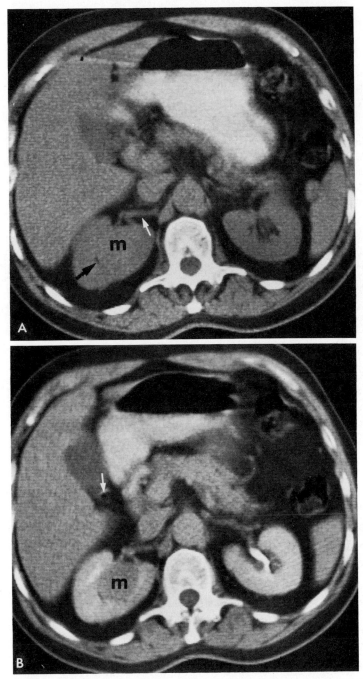

Figure 15–29. Central renal cell carcinoma. **A** Precontrast CT scan appears normal except for obliteration of the central renal sinus fat (arrow) by a mass (m) that has the same density as the adjacent kidney parenchyma. White arrow = Renal artery. **B** Postcontrast scan. The difference between the tumor mass (m) and the renal parenchyma is accentuated. The tumor has obliterated the renal sinus fat. White arrow = Low-density gallstone.

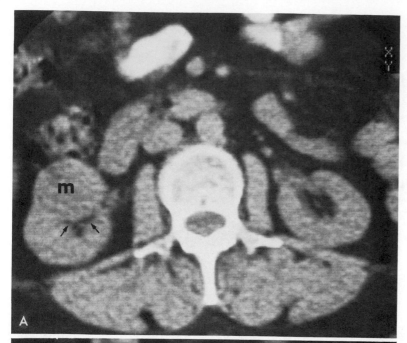

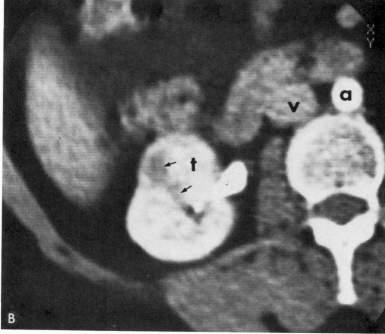

Figure 15–30. Hypervascular Stage I renal cell carcinoma—dynamic CT study. **A** Precontrast scan reveals small rounded mass (m) confined to renal parenchyma with a density similar to that of the normal kidney. The central renal fat (arrows) is preserved. **B** Scan during maximum arterial contrast. A portion of the tumor (t) greatly enhances, whereas other parts (arrows) are little enhanced. a = Aorta; v = inferior vena cava.

Illustration continued on opposite page

If the CT attenuation values of a renal lesion are between those of a simple renal cyst (0 to 15 H) and those of a solid mass lesion (30+ H), the mass is considered to be indeterminate, as it may represent a tumor (Fig. 15–31) or benign renal cyst (Figs. 15–18 and 15–20). Simple cysts may be septated, have higher attenuation values as a result of hemorrhage, inflammation, recent contrast administration, or calcification, and appear to have thick walls.[51] Calcification in renal cysts is peripheral (Fig. 15–18) and does not have a soft-tissue mass lateral to the calcification.

Solid renal masses may have lower CT atten-

uation values due to necrosis, hemorrhage, infection, or a high fat content in the lesion. Calcification in solid renal masses usually is central and associated with a soft-tissue mass, but the calcification may be peripheral.[46, 52] The presence of a low-density mass with central calcification or a higher-density mass with rim calcification is usually reason to classify a renal mass as indeterminate. However, the CT diagnosis of an indeterminate mass is made only after a thorough evaluation of all the morphologic features of the mass and adjacent structures on contrast-enhanced CT scans. When an indeterminate mass

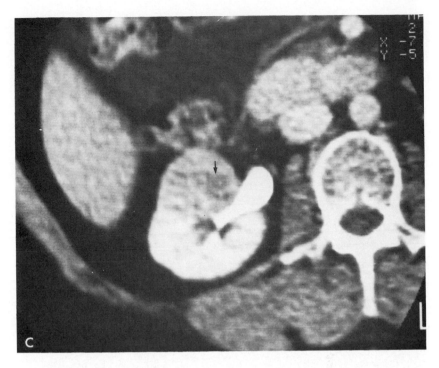

Figure 15–30. *Continued* **C**   Scan 45 seconds after injection. The central portion of the hypervascular tumor (arrow) now appears to be slightly lower in density than the remaining areas of tumor.

is diagnosed, additional studies, such as ultrasonography, angiography, nuclear imaging, and aspiration biopsy, are indicated to further clarify the nature of the renal mass. In our experience, the majority of indeterminate masses are benign but atypical malignancies are also encountered.

Pathologically, renal carcinoma can be divided into four stages.[2, 29, 53]

1. Stage I tumors are wholly confined within the renal parenchyma (Fig. 15–30).

2. Stage II tumors extend through the renal capsule and invade the perirenal fat but do not extend beyond Gerota's fascia (Figs. 15–27 and 15–31).

3. Stage III tumors involve the renal veins or lymph nodes (Figs. 15–32).

4. Stage IV tumors extend through Gerota's fascia and involve adjacent organs or have metastasized to distant organs (Fig. 15–33).

The overall prognosis is greatly affected by the

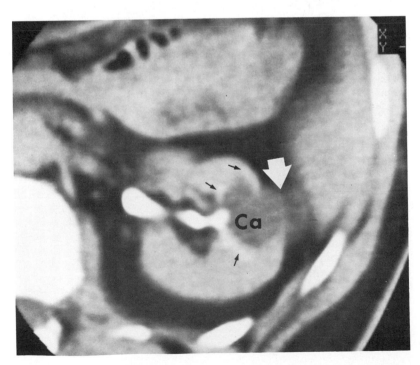

Figure 15–31. Stage II renal cell carcinoma. A cystic renal cell carcinoma (Ca) extends through the renal capsule into the perirenal space (large arrow). The density of the central portion of the carcinoma was 18 H, while the peripheral portion of the tumor demonstrated a higher-density rim (small arrows).

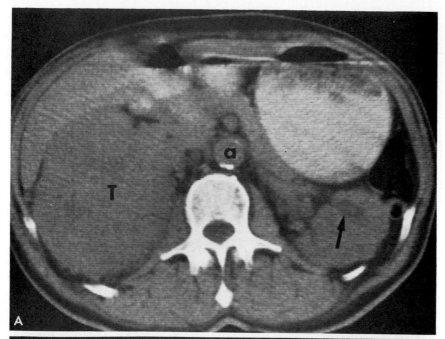

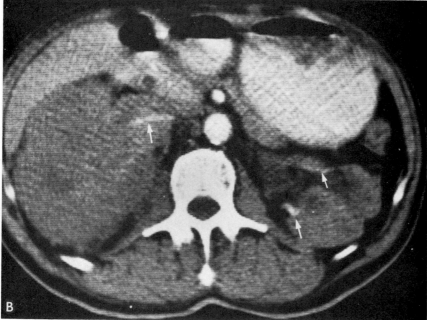

Figure 15–32. Stage III renal cell carcinoma—dynamic CT scan. **A** Precontrast CT scan. The right kidney is tremendously enlarged by a large tumor (T). The left kidney is small and has a dilated collecting system (arrow). The aorta (a) is seen, but the inferior vena cava is not identified. **B** Scan during peak aortic contrast enhancement reveals arterial flow to the right and left kidneys (arrows).

Illustration continued on opposite page

stage of the renal tumor at the time of diagnosis. The 10-year survival rate for Stage I and II adenocarcinomas is 60 to 67 per cent; Stage III lesions, only 38 per cent; and Stage IV tumors, less than a 5 per cent 5-year survival rate.[2, 29]

The surgical approach largely depends upon preoperative assessment of the tumor's stage. All Stage I tumors can be approached from the retroperitoneum, but radical nephrectomy and resection of Stage IV tumors require an abdominal approach. A thoracoabdominal incision is required if the tumor invades the inferior vena cava.[2] Rad-

ical nephrectomy increases the survival rate in patients with Stage II and III renal tumors. In this operation, the kidney and all of the perirenal fatty tissues are removed together, thereby reducing the chance of incomplete tumor resection or local seeding of tumor cells.

CT appears to be the best technique for detecting and staging renal cell carcinoma and can diagnose renal cell carcinoma with greater than 90 per cent accuracy.[1–12, 29, 50, 53–55] In addition, tumoral invasion of the inferior vena cava or main renal vein can be diagnosed with an 82 to 93 per

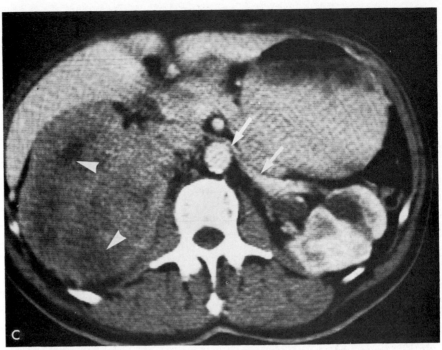

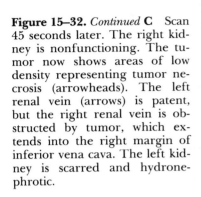

Figure 15–32. *Continued* **C** Scan 45 seconds later. The right kidney is nonfunctioning. The tumor now shows areas of low density representing tumor necrosis (arrowheads). The left renal vein (arrows) is patent, but the right renal vein is obstructed by tumor, which extends into the right margin of inferior vena cava. The left kidney is scarred and hydronephrotic.

cent accuracy.[29] Tumor extension produces hazy tumor margins, thickens the renal capsule, and obliterates the perinephric fat. Perinephric extension into adjacent organs can be detected in about 80 per cent of pathologically proved cases.[15, 29, 50, 52, 53] False-negative interpretations are usually due to microscopic invasion, and false-positive CT scans are caused by necrosis of perirenal fat or perinephric hematomas. Lymph node involvement is demonstrated by enlarged perirenal, para-aortic, paracaval, or retrocrural lymph nodes (Fig. 15–33). Perinephric extension, lymph node involvement, and metastatic disease are detected with greater accuracy by CT than by angiography, and renal vein or caval involvement is identified with equal or greater accuracy.[29, 50, 54, 56, 57] Preoperative angiography need not be performed in every patient with renal cell carcinoma. An-

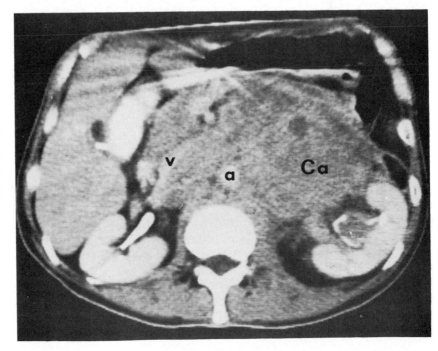

Figure 15–33. Stage IV renal cell carcinoma. Huge renal cell carcinoma (Ca) extends from the central portion of the left kidney through the renal fascia; surrounds the aorta (a) and inferior vena cava (v); and invades the adrenal gland, pancreas, and retroperitoneal lymph nodes.

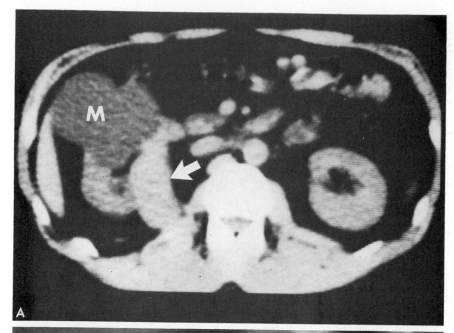

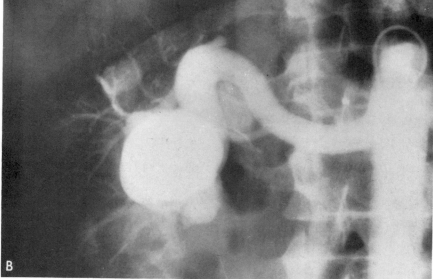

Figure 15–34. Renal cell carcinoma producing arteriovenous fistula. **A** Precontrast CT scan demonstrates large low-density mass (M) arising from right kidney and higher-density mass (arrow) medial to kidney, which has the same attenuation value as the aorta. **B** Aortogram reveals tremendously enlarged right renal artery feeding a large arteriovenous fistula.

giography is performed only in patients in whom the CT findings are uncertain or when the surgeon requires a complete depiction of renal vascular anatomy (Fig. 15–34).

VON HIPPEL-LINDAU SYNDROME. Patients with von Hippel-Lindau syndrome are at increased risk of developing renal cell carcinoma. In these patients, the carcinoma is frequently bilateral and multicentric (Fig. 15–35).[47–49] Multiple renal cysts and small benign adenomas are also frequently present (Fig. 15–36), making the diagnosis of small tumors difficult by urographic, angiographic and ultrasonic techniques.[58] Pancreatic cysts are commonly present (Fig. 15–36 and 15–37).

CT appears to be more accurate than ultrasonography in evaluating multiple renal masses[59] and has been able to detect and distinguish between renal cysts and small solid mass lesions in patients with von Hippel-Lindau syndrome (Fig. 15–37).[49] Solid mass lesions and cysts less than 2 cm in diameter are best evaluated by using finely collimated CT scans. Solid mass lesions larger than 3 cm are all classified as renal cell carcinomas, whereas solid lesions less than 3 cm are usually classified as benign "adenomas," although histologically they cannot be distinguished from renal cell carcinoma.

CT is recommended as the primary renal screening procedure in all patients suspected of

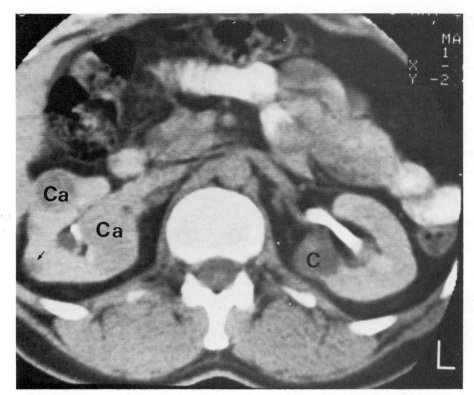

Figure 15–35. von Hippel-Lindau syndrome. There is a multicentric renal cell carcinoma (Ca) and a small adenoma (arrow) of the right kidney. A left renal cyst (C) is present.

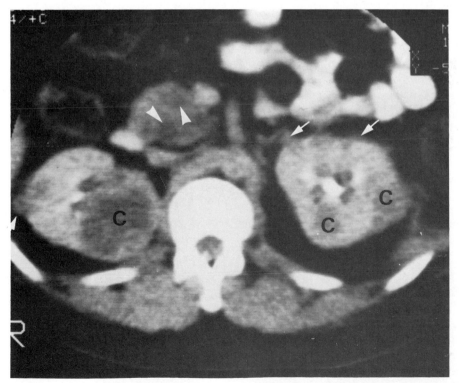

Figure 15–36. von Hippel-Lindau syndrome—postcontrast CT scan. Characteristic features demonstrated are multiple renal cysts (C), pancreatic cysts (arrowheads), and small solid adenomas (arrows).

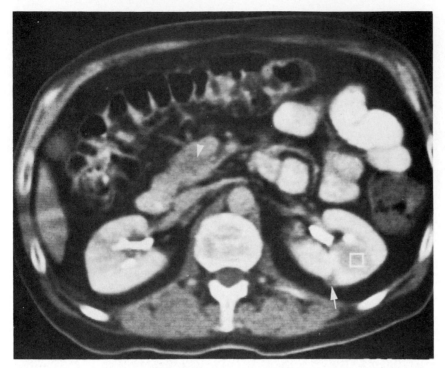

Figure 15–37. von Hippel-Lindau syndrome. The postcontrast CT scan findings demonstrated are a small peripheral left renal cyst (arrow), a central solid mass (box) measuring 56 H, proved to be a renal cell carcinoma, and a cyst in the head of the pancreas (arrowhead). Right renal cysts were present on lower CT scans.

having von Hippel-Lindau syndrome.[49] Relatives of patients with known von Hippel-Lindau syndrome should probably be studied. CT detection of a small, noninvasive tumor permits a wide local resection rather than a radical nephrectomy to be performed, thereby preserving renal function.[49]

NEPHROBLASTOMA (WILMS' TUMOR). This malignant tumor arises from immature renal parenchyma and occurs most frequently in children

1 to 5 years old.[46] It constitutes 6 per cent of all renal malignancies and is the most common abdominal malignant tumor in children (see Chapter 21). Approximately 25 per cent of Wilms' tumors occur in infants less than 1 year old; less than 5 per cent occur after the age of 6 years.[46] Bilateral involvement (1 to 13 per cent) occurs (Fig. 15–38) but is less frequent than in neuroblastoma.[46] Pathologically, nephroblastomas often

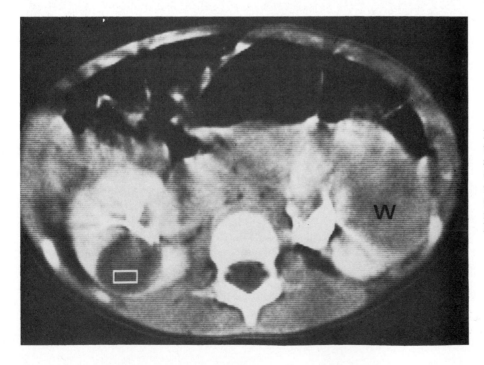

Figure 15–38. Bilateral Wilms' tumors. CT scan demonstrates a large left solid renal mass (W) and a smaller, more cystic-appearing right renal mass (box). At surgery the right tumor was found to contain a large amount of fatty tissue.

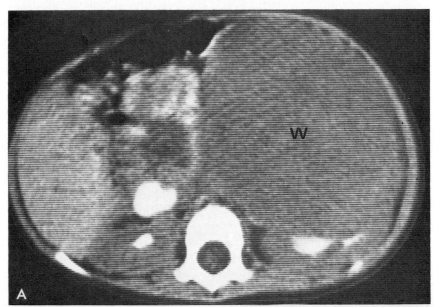

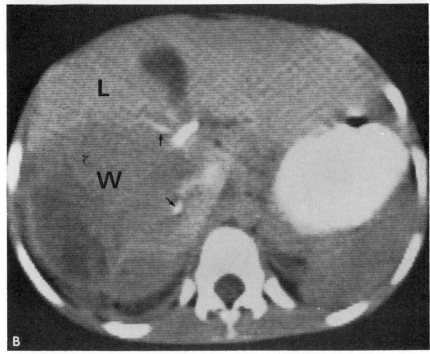

Figure 15–39. CT features of Wilms' tumor. **A** A large homogeneous, noncalcified mass (W) arising from the left kidney displaces but does not invade adjacent organs. **B** Inhomogeneous, noncalcified Wilms' tumor (W) of the right kidney is displacing the liver (L) and splaying the renal collecting structures (arrows).

show areas of necrosis or hemorrhage, and renal vein invasion is common (30 to 40 per cent).[46] Metastasis to lungs is frequent, but metastasis to bones, liver, and lymph nodes is uncommon.

Clinically, there is usually a palpable abdominal mass (60 per cent) and a low-grade fever (50 per cent). Hypertension is frequent, but hematuria is the presenting complaint in less than 20 per cent of cases.[46] The incidence of aniridia and hemihypertrophy is increased in patients with Wilms' tumor.

Nephroblastoma is most frequently demonstrated by CT to be a noncalcified (90 per cent), inhomogeneous solid mass lesion arising in the kidney (Figs. 15–38 and 15–39).[60, 61] Nephroblastoma usually cannot be differentiated from adult renal cell carcinoma based solely on the CT features.

ANGIOMYOLIPOMA.   The renal angiomyolipoma is an uncommon, benign renal tumor usually classified as a hamartoma, which is composed of various proportions of smooth muscle, blood vessels, and fat.[46] The term *angiomyolipoma* is used to describe the complete lesion; terms such as *angiomyoma* or *myolipoma* have been used when other tissues predominate.

Angiomyolipomas occur in two distinct groups of patients. In patients with tuberous sclerosis, 40 to 80 per cent have angiomyolipomas. The tumors in these patients are usually small, asymptomatic, bilateral, tend to occur in childhood or early adulthood, and are equally distributed between the sexes.[46] The majority of angiomyolipomas, however, are found in patients without tuberous sclerosis. The tumors in these patients are characteristically large, symptomatic, single, tend to occur in middle age, and have a 4:1 female predominance.[46]

Pathologically, the lesions are identical in the two groups. Angiomyolipomas are nonencapsulated, grow slowly, and tend to enlarge in an expansile fashion, replacing the renal parenchyma and distorting, but not destroying, the pelvicaliceal system. Some tumors may have a predominantly extrarenal growth pattern (25 per cent), which extends to, or even through, the renal capsule into the perirenal compartment.[62, 63] Because the prominent tumor vessels lack an internal elastic lining, intratumoral and perirenal hemorrhage is common, causing hematuria (40 per cent), flank pain (87 per cent), and a palpable mass (50 per cent).[62]

The CT findings in angiomyolipomas are often so distinctive that a histologic diagnosis may be suggested.[4, 11, 62–75] Single or multiple renal masses have zones of different density ranging from −150 (fat) to +150 H (calcification).[65] Because fat is present in most angiomyolipomas, there is usually at least one region with a CT density of at least −20 H (Fig. 15–40). However, in angiomyolipomas composed mainly of vascular tissue and muscle or in those in which recent hemorrhage has occurred, the majority of the tumor may have CT density values greater than 20H (Fig. 15–41).[64, 65, 73, 75, 76] Angiomyolipomas typically join the normal renal tissue at an acute angle, rarely obstruct the caliceal system, and are usually larger than 2 cm when detected.[62–72, 74, 75] After contrast medium injection, portions of the tumor may be enhanced, but fatty tissue and areas of necrosis do not increase in density. Dynamic CT may reveal an early hypervascular phase, which reflects the increased vascularity found at angiography. Even though angiomyolipomas may invade the perirenal compartment or adjacent structures such as the inferior vena cava,[77] CT detects no evidence of distant metastatic disease. The CT identification of fatty tissue within a renal mass usually permits an accurate diagnosis of renal angiomyolipoma.

Although the CT diagnosis of angiomyolipoma is highly specific, renal lipoma, liposarcoma, or retroperitoneal liposarcomas invading the kidney cannot be absolutely excluded. CT has also demonstrated fatty tissue in cases of Wilms' tumor (Fig. 15–38).[78] The diagnosis may be difficult in small lesions, as partial value averaging can erroneously elevate the measured CT density to that of water or solid tissue. The use of thinner CT scan sections helps avoid this potential pitfall. If

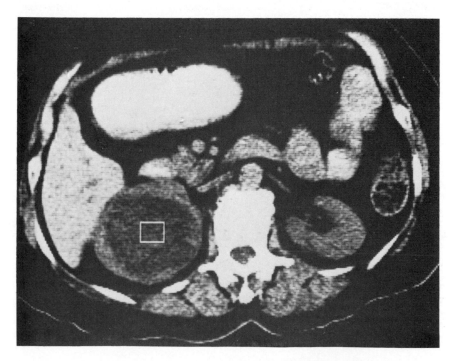

Figure 15–40. Renal angiomyolipoma. CT scan demonstrates large intrarenal mass (box) having a CT density ranging from −20 H to +20 H. Mean CT number in square = 6 H.

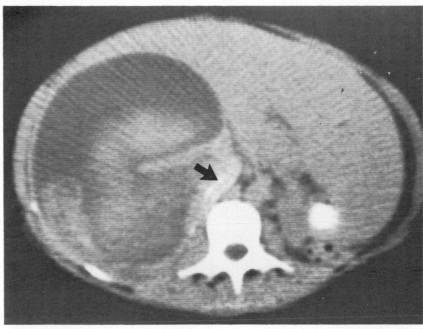

Figure 15–41. Angiomyolipoma with recent hemorrhage. CT scan demonstrates a large cystic-appearing right renal tumor, which is predominantly of low density but contains areas of higher attenuation value. The functioning renal parenchyma (arrow) is medially displaced. At surgery a large angiomyolipoma containing fat and recent hemorrhage was removed.

the diagnosis is still in doubt, ultrasonography can establish the diagnosis by demonstrating highly echogenic foci characteristic of fat rather than fluid or nonfatty solid tissue.[67, 68]

RENAL ONCOCYTOMA. These are rare, benign, solid renal tumors, always at least partially encapsulated, which are thought to originate from proximal tubular epithelial cells.[46, 79–81] Microscopically the oncocytes are large cells that have an eosinophilic, finely granular cytoplasm containing numerous mitochondria.[46, 79–81]

Oncocytomas are usually asymptomatic, may be single or multiple, and are often larger than 2 cm when discovered.[45, 79–81] Distinction from renal cell carcinoma is difficult by conventional radiologic

methods. Angiographically, a spoke wheel configuration of vessels, a homogeneous nephrogram, and a sharp interface with normal parenchyma have been described as characteristic of oncocytomas.[81]

The CT appearance of oncocytomas is that of a homogeneous solid renal mass that is only slightly less dense than the renal parenchyma after intravenous injection of contrast medium (Fig. 15–42).[81] The tumor mass is sharply separated from the normal cortex and does not invade the caliceal system or adjacent structures.[81] A diagnosis of oncocytomas should be considered whenever a solid, vascular renal mass is detected by CT, but distinction between oncocytoma, ade-

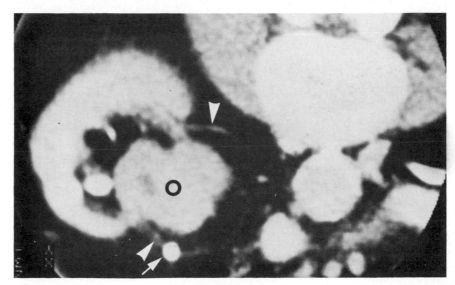

Figure 15–42. Oncocytoma. CT scan after injection of contrast material. A lobulated oncocytoma (o), seen as a homogeneous solid mass, is slightly less dense than functioning renal parenchyma. CT number of tumor was 70 H. The ureter (arrow) and renal vessels (arrowheads) are displaced by the tumor, but there is no evidence of obstruction of collecting structures, invasion of perirenal fat, or vascular occlusion. The tumor had been present for over 10 years.

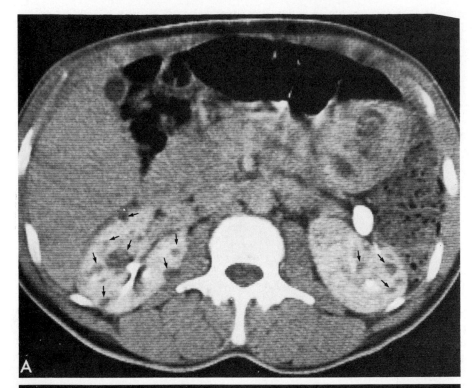

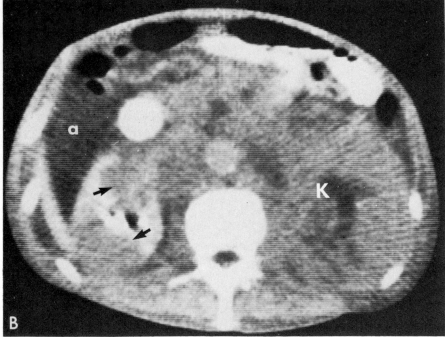

Figure 15–43. CT features of lymphoma involving the kidneys. **A** Multiple bilateral focal, nodular masses (arrows) of various sizes are seen scattered throughout the renal parenchyma in patient with Hodgkin's disease. **B** Two larger solid mass lesions (arrows) involving the right kidney and an enlarged nonfunctioning left kidney (K) due to lymphomatous infiltration are present. a = Ascites.

Illustration continued on opposite page

noma, and renal cell carcinoma by CT characteristics alone is usually not possible and requires additional diagnosing studies such as angiography or radionuclide imaging.[79–81]

UNUSUAL RENAL TUMORS. Tumors of the renal capsule, such as fibromas, leiomyomas, lipomas, and angiomas, are rare and can be benign or malignant.[46] Renal tumors arising from mesenchymal derivatives, muscle, and connective, adipose, or vascular tissue are also rare.[46, 82] Together, these rare tumors account for less than 1 per cent of renal tumors.[46] The CT findings of these tumors have not been reported, but it is unlikely that a specific CT diagnosis will be made except perhaps in cases of tumors of fatty tissue or the rare primary osteogenic sarcoma.

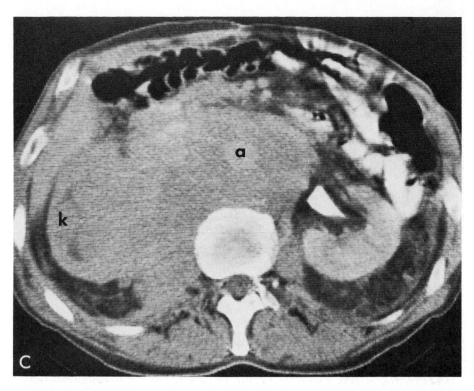

Figure 15–43. *Continued* **C** Nonfunction of the right kidney (k) due to invasion by a large retroperitoneal lymphomatous mass. a = Aorta.

Secondary Renal Tumors

RENAL LYMPHOMA. Renal involvement by lymphoma is commonly found at postmortem examination (30 to 50 per cent) but is seldom detected by conventional urographic studies.[46, 83–85] The most common manifestation of renal lymphoma is multiple parenchymal nodules (61 per cent). Invasion from perirenal disease (11 per cent), solitary nodules (7 per cent), large single lesions (6 per cent), and diffuse infiltration (6 per cent) are less frequent features.[83–86] Bilateral involvement is three times as common as unilateral involvement.[83, 86]

Urography may demonstrate diffuse or focal renal enlargement and indirectly detect extrarenal disease by ureteral obstruction or displacement.[87] However, Lalli and colleagues[84] reported that lymphomas produce lesions that are usually too small to be recognized by current roentgenographic methods.

CT manifestations of lymphomatous infiltration of the kidneys are varied and include:

1. Bilaterally enlarged kidneys without demonstrable masses.

2. Enlarged or normal kidneys with multiple, focal, nodular, solid masses of various sizes that have decreased density on postcontrast scans (Fig. 15–43A).

3. Focal, irregular, solitary, solid intrarenal mass lesions (Fig. 15–43B).

4. Perirenal disease that extends into the renal pelvis.

5. Dilatation of intrarenal collecting structures produced by diffuse interstitial infiltration of the kidneys.

6. Nonfunction (Fig. 15–43B,C).[83, 88, 89]

It may not be possible to distinguish among the various forms of lymphoma or to differentiate lymphoma from other solid intrarenal masses by CT. However, when CT reveals coexisting retroperitoneal adenopathy, splenomegaly, or mesenteric adenopathy, the possibility of renal lymphoma should be considered.

RENAL METASTASIS. Leukemic infiltration of the kidneys can produce bilateral renal enlargement and intrarenal masses.[46] Tumors from the lung (Fig. 15–44), breast, stomach, colon, cervix, and pancreas frequently metastasize to the kidneys but are rarely diagnosed.[46] Most metastases are small and do not produce renal failure, hydronephrosis, or hemorrhage. The CT appearance of a renal metastasis is that of a solid mass lesion that is indistinguishable from a primary renal malignancy.[1]

Tumors of the Renal Pelvis

Transitional cell carcinoma is the most common (82 per cent) epithelial tumor of the renal pelvis.[46] Transitional cell carcinoma is often multiple (42 per cent); similar tumors affect the bladder (10

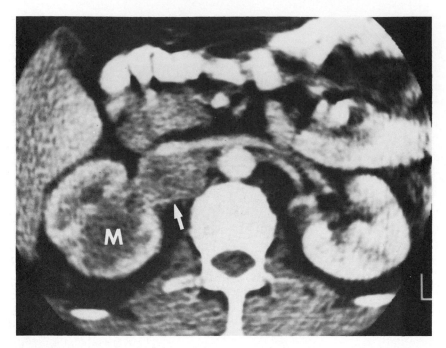

Figure 15–44. Metastatic carcinoma to the right kidney. A large, solid renal mass (M) and retrocaval nodal enlargement (arrow) resulting from metastatic lung carcinoma are seen. The metastasis was avascular and did not extend into the perirenal space.

per cent), ipsilateral ureter (17 per cent), or bladder and ureter (15 per cent). More than 85 per cent of transitional cell carcinomas are of the papillary type: low-grade malignancies that are slow to infiltrate and late to metastasize and follow a relatively benign course (50 per cent 5-year survival rate). The nonpapillary form of transitional cell carcinoma is a more aggressive malignancy; direct extension and metastasis occur early resulting in a 5-year survival rate of less than 10 per cent.[46] Transitional cell carcinoma is three to four times more common in males than in females, and more than 80 per cent of patients are 40 to 70 years old.

Squamous cell carcinoma constitutes 17 per cent of tumors of the renal pelvis and is frequently associated with chronic leukoplakia. Calculi are present in 50 per cent of cases, and extrarenal spread at the time of diagnosis is the rule rather than the exception. Hematuria and flank pain are common presenting symptoms, since the tumor is usually well advanced and has extended deeply into the adjacent tissues by the time the diagnosis has been made. There is no sex predilection, and the mean age of patients is greater than 60 years. The prognosis is very poor; the average survival is 1 to 1½ years, and there are almost no long-term survivors.[46]

The diagnosis of a pelvic tumor is usually suggested when an excretory urogram demonstrates hydronephrosis or a filling defect within the renal pelvis. Differentiation of renal pelvic tumors from filling defects due to nonopaque calculi, blood clots, polyps, aberrant or hypertrophied renal pa-

pillae, vascular impressions, prominent renal columns, or inflammatory conditions is frequently difficult by conventional urography and angiography.[90]

The CT appearance of renal pelvic tumors is varied. Small pelvic tumors that do not produce hydronephrosis or invade the peripelvic fat are usually not detected on precontrast CT scans.[90] After intravenous contrast injection, pelvic neoplasms are detected as pelvic filling defects that have a smooth, lobulated, or irregular margin (Fig. 15–45).[90] Tumor frequently prevents contrast from filling the dependent portion of the renal collection structures (Fig. 15–46). CT density values range from 30 to 40 H and do not dramatically increase after contrast medium administration. The peripelvic fat stripe is preserved when tumors are confined to the renal pelvis (Fig. 15–47) but obliterated when extrapelvic extension has occurred (Figs. 15–45 and 15–46). Larger tumors produce hydronephrosis, invade renal parenchymal or vascular structures, and are a cause of a nonfunctioning kidney.[90]

Distinguishing between transitional cell and squamous cell carcinoma by CT may not be possible except when the pelvic filling defect has a frondlike appearance (papillary transitional cell) or is associated with a pelvic calculus (squamous cell carcinoma). Nonopaque renal calculi have higher attenuation values than pelvic tumors,[90] and blood clots tend to be round, smooth, and dependently positioned within the renal pelvis, whereas tumors are frequently irregular, nondependent renal pelvic masses. Whenever a renal tumor is detected, the entire ureter and bladder should be examined to exclude uroepithelial tumors.

Tumors of the Ureter

The ureter has the same epithelium as the renal pelvis and bladder; ureteral tumors, therefore, are of cell types similar to those of the renal collecting system and bladder. Of all ureteral tumors, 75 to 80 per cent are malignant.[46] Transitional cell carcinoma occurs most frequently (85 per cent), but squamous cell carinoma accounts for 15 per cent of ureteral malignancies. Hematuria (80 per cent), pain (60 per cent), and flank mass (40 per cent) constitute the most frequent clinical presentation.[46] Urography reveals hydro-

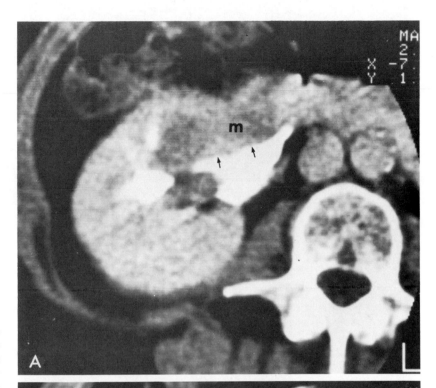

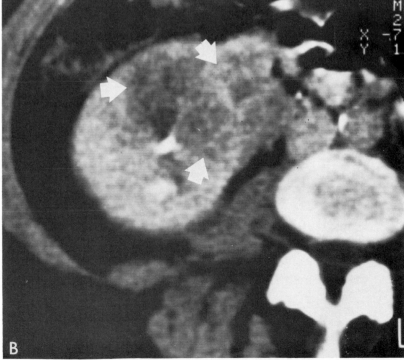

Figure 15–45. Transitional cell carcinoma of the renal pelvis. **A**   The carcinoma has produced a pelvic mass (m), which has a slightly irregular inferior margin (arrows). **B** CT scan at more caudal level demonstrates the mass to have invaded through the renal pelvis into the renal parenchyma (arrows).

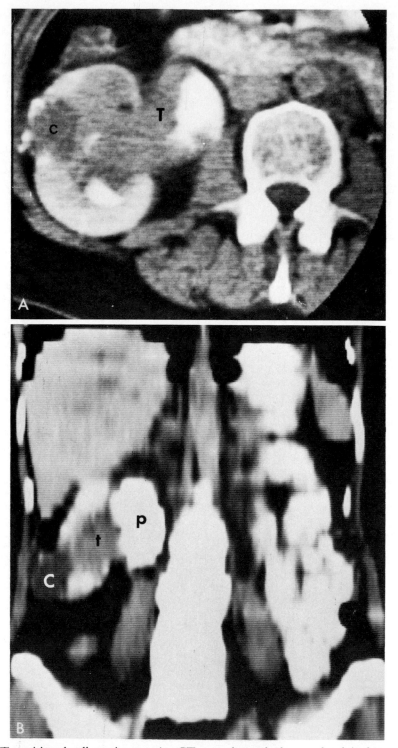

Figure 15–46. Transitional cell carcinoma. **A** CT scan through the renal pelvis demonstrates a large tumor (T), which partially fills the renal pelvis, preventing contrast material from filling the dependent portion of the collecting structure. The tumor has extended into the renal parenchyma, obliterating the peripelvic fat. c = Calcified renal cyst. **B** Sagittal reformation displays the relationship of the renal cyst (c), transitional cell tumor (t), and dilated renal pelvis (p).

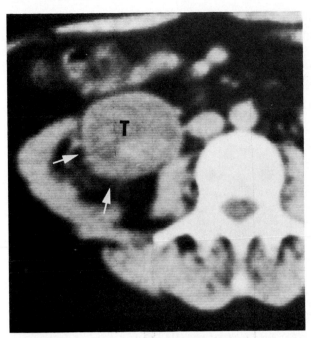

Figure 15–47. A large transitional cell carcinoma (T) causing marked enlargement of the extrarenal pelvis. The tumor is completely contained within the pelvis, and therefore the peripelvic fat planes (arrows) are preserved.

nephrosis, delayed renal excretion of contrast, and dilation of the ureter above a ureteral filling defect or stenosis.

In cases of ureteral tumor, CT typically demonstrates delayed renal excretion of contrast, hydronephrosis, and the obstructed ureter down to the level of the tumor. If a periureteral mass is present, CT usually cannot differentiate a primary ureteral neoplasm from obstruction because of direct ureteral involvement by metastasis from the cervix, rectum, bladder, prostate, ovary, or a distant site.[91, 92] However, ureteral obstruction resulting from calculi that are nonopaque by conventional radiography is possible, as nonopaque calculi have a CT density (50+ H) that permits easy identification.[90, 92, 95]

NON-NEOPLASTIC DISEASE

Renal and Ureteral Calculi

CT readily detects radiodense calculi in the ureters, renal pelvis, or caliceal collecting structures[92] and renal parenchymal calcifications also are frequently demonstrated during CT examinations performed for other clinical problems.[1–3, 5] Although it is not a primary diagnostic technique for evaluating urinary calculi, when employed, CT should be performed without intravenous

contrast injection because contrast material can obscure the diagnosis in more than 75 per cent of instances.[5]

Approximately 5 to 8 per cent of calculi are nonopaque, consisting mostly of uric acid, cystine, xanthine, struvite, calcium oxalate, and matrix calculi.[89, 93–97] Stones containing a mixture of components are also found.[93, 95–97] The usual appearance of a nonopaque calculus is a negative filling defect in the urinary collecting structures during excretory urography (Fig. 15–48A). Urographic differentiation is difficult because tumors, blood clots, papillomas, and nonopaque calculi produce similar urographic findings, and invasive diagnostic modalities such as ureteral biopsy, retrograde pyelography, and angiography are of limited value.

All reported nonopaque urinary calculi examined by CT have been of high density, 100 to 586 H (Fig. 15–48B).[90, 93, 94] Calculi in the renal collecting structures and ureter are readily identified as dense filling defects on nonenhanced scans. Differentiation between calculi of various compositions have not been possible by CT analysis because the CT densities of different calculi overlap.[95]

The increased CT density of nonopaque calculi is directly related to the increased physical density of the calculus,[94] and does not indicate calcium content.[95] Calculi exposed to urographic contrast material can have an increased density due to their absorption of contrast.[95] Thus, the detected CT density of calculi reflects a combination of inherent physical density and contrast effect on the calculi if the CT study is performed after administration of contrast medium.

CT can distinguish calculi from other nonopaque filling defects in almost every instance. Tumors of all types have soft-tissue attenuation values (30 to 60 H), and although blood clots may have a higher density than unopacified urine or renal parenchyma, they do not approach the density of urinary tract calculi.[90, 93, 95, 98] Contiguous thin CT sections (5 mm or less) through the region of the suspected calculi permit calculi as small as 2 to 3 mm to be detected and ensure that small calculi are not missed because of partial volume averaging or because the entire region of interest is not scanned.

Renal Trauma

CT findings can be used to diagnose and stage renal traumatic injuries.[99–105] Urography is a sen-

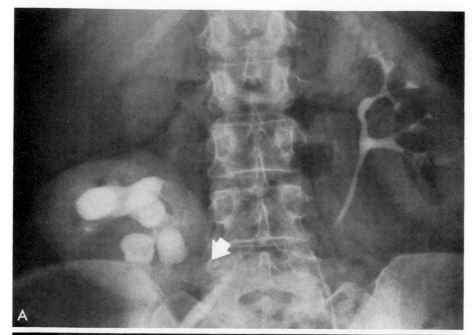

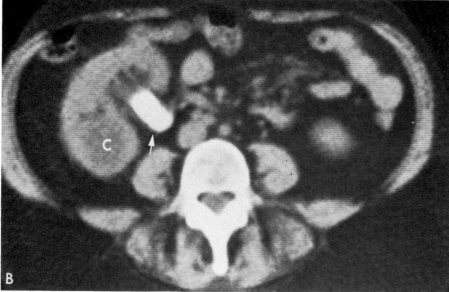

Figure 15–48. Uric acid calculus. **A** Excretory urogram. There is a hydronephrotic, distorted, and rotated right kidney. A nonopaque filling defect is present in the renal pelvis (arrow). **B** Noncontrast enhanced CT scan. A high-density calculus (arrow) fills the renal pelvis. A lower pole renal cyst (C) is present. The CT number of uric acid calculus was 150 + H.

sitive screening procedure, but it does not accurately reflect the type and extent of renal injury in 15 to 30 per cent of cases.[100] Based on CT findings, renal injuries have been grouped into various categories that can be used to guide therapy.[100, 101]

Subcapsular hematoma, the most frequent injury in most series,[100] is diagnosed when fluid is confined to the immediate extrarenal area and separated from Gerota's fascia by fat (Fig. 15–49).[100] The collection of fluid is frequently lenticular and the renal parenchyma is usually flattened.[99–104] Subcapsular hematomas can be caused by blunt or penetrating renal injuries and occur in 55 to

70 per cent of patients after percutaneous renal biopsy.[102–104] CT scans shortly after injury may show that the subcapsular hematoma has a higher density than the surrounding kidney because of fresh extravasation of blood (Fig. 15–49A); follow-up scans show that the hematoma diminishes in density as the hematoma liquifies.[103] CT scans after contrast medium administration demonstrate the hematoma as an area with a lower attenuation value than that of the functioning renal parenchyma (Fig. 15–49B). Isolated subcapsular hematomas are minor injuries that can be managed conservatively.[100–104]

Perirenal hematomas are larger fluid collections

extending to and confined by Gerota's fascia (Fig. 15–50).[99–103] A perirenal hematoma can be an isolated injury confined to the anterior or posterior perirenal space, but a subcapsular hematoma is frequently present.

Incomplete renal laceration and *intrarenal hematoma* are synonymous terms that indicate a focal renal parenchymal injury that prevents normal enhancement of the kidney after intravenous contrast administration (Fig. 15–51).[100] The nephrogram may be less dense than normal and the calices fill poorly, but no renal fracture is identified. Frequently, subcapsular and perirenal hematomas are also present. Conservative, nonsurgical management is usually sufficient in cases of intrarenal hematoma with or without subcapsular or perirenal hemorrhage.[100, 101]

Severe renal injury is diagnosed whenever there is a complete renal laceration, renal fracture, or shattered kidney.[100] The term *complete renal laceration* indicates a focal renal parenchymal injury that extends into the collecting system and results in extravasation of opacified urine. *Renal fracture* describes a single transection of the kidney into two poles accompanied by extravasation of urine; *shattered kidney* indicates the presence of multiple clefts.[100, 101] Surgery is indicated in cases of renal fracture, shattered kidney, or injuries to the vascular pedicle, but the role of surgery in complete renal laceration is controversial.[100] By accurately determining the extent of renal injury preoperatively, CT may reduce the number of exploratory laparotomies performed to evaluate kidney trauma.

Infection

Acute renal infection frequently produces fever, chills, flank pain, sepsis, nausea, and vomiting. Urinalysis reveals pyuria, and the white blood cell count is elevated. A clinical diagnosis of acute pyelonephritis is made, and excretory urography is performed to evaluate renal function and to detect renal calculi, abscesses, tumors, cysts, ureteral duplications, and congenital abnormalities. In acute pyelonephritis, the urographic findings are usually normal; minimal and nonspecific abnormalities are identified in only 24 to 28 per cent of patients.[106–108] Caliceal dilatation, diminished ureteral peristalsis, decreased density of the nephrogram, delayed caliceal appearance time, and generalized enlargement have been described in pyelonephritis.[107, 109–111] In rare instances, focal, patchy, or parenchymal opacification has been reported.[109, 112–114] When the acute infection is more severe, a focal mass demonstrated by excretory urography may represent a

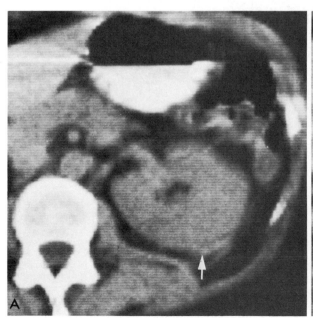 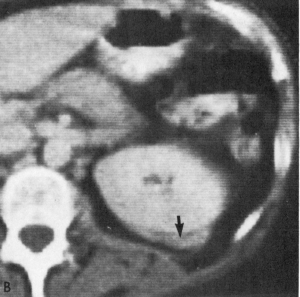

Figure 15–49. Subcapsular renal hematoma resulting from renal biopsy. **A** Precontrast CT scan. A slight irregularity posterior to the kidney is present (arrow). The hematoma has a slightly greater density than that of the kidney. **B** Postcontrast CT scan. The renal parenchyma increases greatly in attenuation value, whereas the hematoma does not. This permits the subcapsular hematoma (arrow) to be seen as a lenticular low-density mass confined to the immediate extrarenal area.

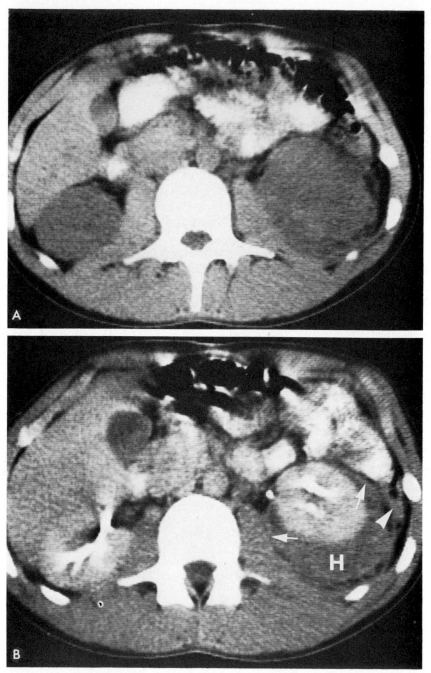

Figure 15–50. Perirenal hematoma due to renal biopsy. **A**   Precontrast CT scan. The left kidney cannot be clearly delineated from the soft-tissue mass in the left flank. The perirenal fat has been obliterated. **B**   Postcontrast CT scan. The left kidney, functioning normally, is now clearly identified. The perirenal hematoma (H) extends to the Gerota's fascia (arrows) and has produced thickening of the lateroconal fascia (arrowhead). The hematoma resolved on conservative therapy.

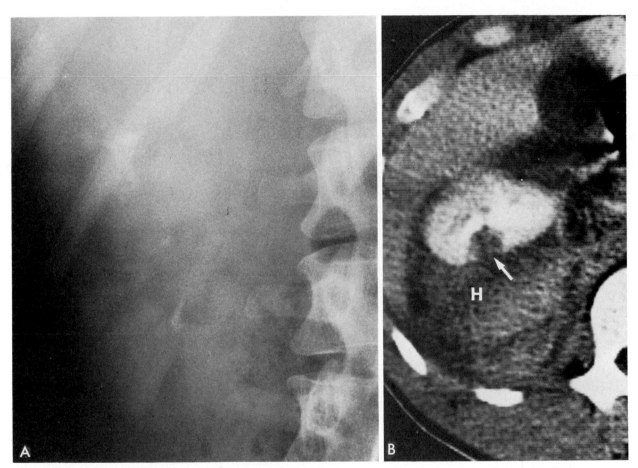

Figure 15–51. Incomplete renal laceration following blunt trauma. **A** Poor renal function is shown on the excretory urogram, but the extent of injury cannot be adequately assessed. **B** A focal laceration (arrow) resulting in a large perirenal hematoma (H) is present. The kidney is displaced but has good function. No extravasation of contrast material has occurred. The patient was successfully treated by conservative methods. (From Federle MP: CT of abdominal trauma. In Federle MP, Brant-Zawadski M (eds): Computed Tomography in the Evaluation of Trauma. Baltimore, Williams & Wilkins, 1982. Used with permission.)

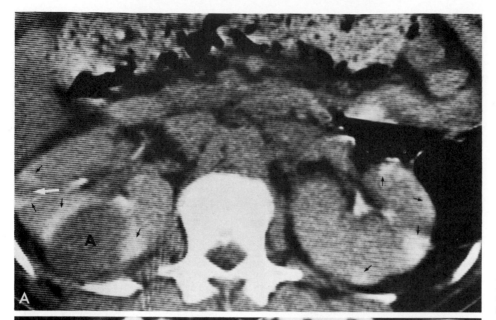

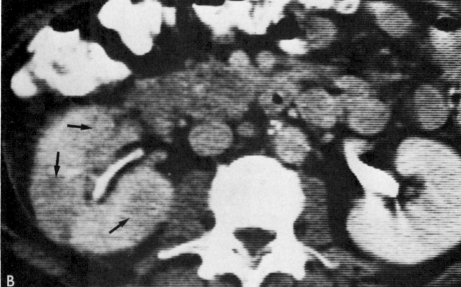

Figure 15–52. Acute bilateral pyelonephritis and renal abscess. **A** There are patchy, triangular areas of decreased renal function radiating into zones of normal renal function (black arrows). Some of the hypofunctioning areas of renal parenchyma appear as linear areas, which are radially oriented (white arrow). A focal renal abscess (A) is seen as a large, low-density mass in the right kidney. **B** CT scan following antibiotic therapy. The left kidney has returned to normal. There are still focal zones of diminished function (arrows) in the right kidney, but there has been marked improvement in its overall function.

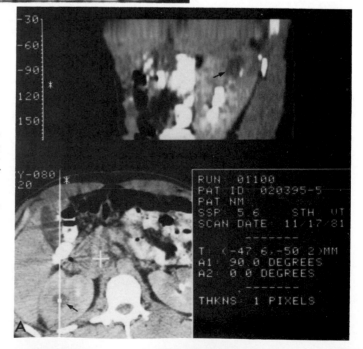

Figure 15–53. Acute pyelonephritis and renal abscess. **A** Axial and sagittal CT scans demonstrate low-density abscess (arrows) surrounded by a larger zone of decreased function in the upper pole of the right kidney.

Illustration continued on opposite page

frank abscess[115] or a mass without drainable pus (acute focal bacterial nephritis).[116]

The CT findings in acute pyelonephritis depend on the severity of the infection. In most cases, precontrast scans are normal[106] or reveal an area of slightly lower density in the renal parenchyma.[109, 112] Postcontrast CT scans demonstrate patchy, linear, radially oriented, low-density areas in the renal parenchyma (Fig. 15–52) that are absent on precontrast studies.[114, 116] These focal, striated abnormal zones of renal parenchymal en-

hancement correspond to similar findings or excretory urography and are thought to represent nonfunctioning nephrons resulting from obstruction or vascular compromise.[113, 114, 116–118]

More severe renal infection may extend into the perirenal space, produce a focal renal mass, or develop into a frank abscess (Fig. 15–53). Perirenal extension of infection causes increased density in the perirenal fat, thickens Gerota's fascia, and displaces the kidney. Gas-forming renal infections are readily identified by pelvocaliceal air,

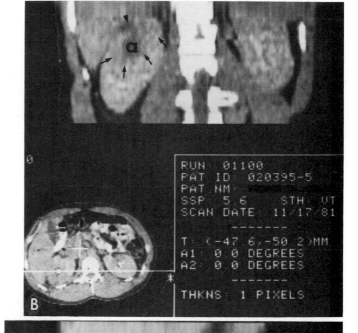

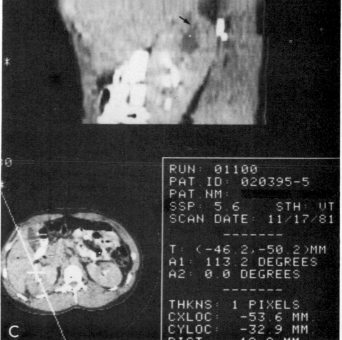

Figure 15–53. *Continued* **B** Coronal reformation showing abscess (a) extends to the renal cortical margin (arrowhead). A larger zone of poor function (arrows) is also seen. **C** Oblique reformation clearly demonstrates extension of the abscess to the renal margin (arrow).

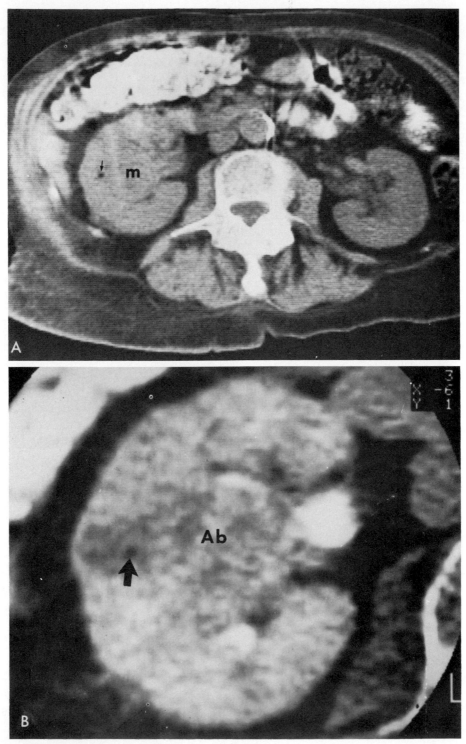

Figure 15–54. Gas-forming renal abscess. **A**   Precontrast CT scan. There is gross enlargement of the right kidney and a mass (m) obliterating the renal sinus fat, which contains a focus of gas (arrow). **B**   Postcontrast scan demonstrates renal abscess (Ab) containing gas (arrow), which has extended into the renal sinus, obliterating the fat planes.

air within a mass (Fig. 15–54), subcapsular gas (Fig. 15–55), or gas that has extended through the renal capsule into Gerota's fascia or the retroperitoneum.[119] However, renal gas must not be equated with infection in patients after embolization of renal tumors because intratumoral gas can occur in infarcted tissues without evidence of infection. The cause of gas formation is unclear, but similar occurrences in the adrenal gland and liver after embolization or vascular ligation have been reported.[120, 121]

The term *acute focal bacterial nephritis* is used to describe focal renal enlargement in the clinical setting of acute pyelonephritis.[116] Acute focal bacterial nephritis has also been called severe acute pyelonephritis,[110] focal or suppurative pyelonephritis,[27] acute lobar nephronia,[117] and acute bacterial nephritis.[109] Acute focal bacterial nephritis produces a solid renal mass with an attenuation value similar to or slightly lower than that of normal parenchyma on precontrast CT scans. The mass is enhanced in a patchy nonhomogeneous manner after contrast medium injection (Fig. 15–52). No capsule is demonstrated, and the margin with adjacent renal parenchyma is poorly defined. The adjacent renal fascia may be thickened, but paranephric extension is absent.[116]

Although difficult by clinical examination and urography, acute focal bacterial nephritis and renal abscess can usually be differentiated by CT. Renal abscesses frequently have a lower attenuation value than normal renal parenchyma on noncontrast scans and either fail to enhance or enhance in a patchy nonhomogeneous fashion after contrast medium administration. The abscess is often well delineated from the renal parenchyma and can have a thick, irregular wall or an ill-defined margin with adjacent parenchyma. The wall of the abscess may be enhanced after contrast medium injection, but the central part of the abscess is usually enhanced little, if at all. Perirenal extension, extension into the renal pelvis (Fig. 15–54), and thickening of the renal fascia are more common in renal abscess than in acute focal bacterial nephritis.[9]

Although CT distinction between abscess and acute focal bacterial nephritis is usually straightforward, the appearance of either is not pathognomonic. Benign and malignant tumors can have an identical appearance, although in the clinical setting of acute infection, differentiation from tumor is not difficult. Should confirmation be required, a needle aspiration for culture can be safely guided by ultrasound or CT.[122]

Renal infections are more frequent in diabetics and patients who have compromised immunologic systems.[114, 119, 123] In diabetic patients, the CT findings are those of acute pyelonephritis and, rarely, emphysematous pyelonephritis.[119] In patients with leukemia, we have noted a pattern of multiple small renal abscesses caused by fungal infections (Fig. 15–56).[123] These small abscesses are best demonstrated by enhanced CT scans and are associated with similar lesions in the liver and spleen. CT scans after treatment demonstrate resolution of the abscesses.

Aspergillosis[124] can produce pelvic filling defects; and tuberculosis,[125] xanthogranulomatous pyelonephritis,[1] and *Echinococcus*[126, 127] can produce renal mass lesions. Renal tuberculosis is often accompanied by renal calcifications or evidence of tuberculosis elsewhere in the chest or abdomen,[125] but absolute distinction from a solid tumor is often not possible by CT alone. CT in xanthogranulomatous pyelonephritis usually demonstrates poor or absent renal function, renal calculi, a mass with an attenuation value similar to that of the surrounding kidney, and extension into the perirenal fat (Fig. 15–57).[1] By CT criteria alone, xanthogranulomatous pyelonephritis usually cannot be absolutely distinguished from a renal malignancy.

Renal echinococcal infection occurs in 2 per cent of patients with systemic hydatid disease[127] and produces renal cystic lesions with calcification of the cyst wall, and daughter cysts of different density within the larger cysts.[126, 127] The fibroblastic wall of the cyst is enhanced after intravenous contrast administration, and the identification of daughter cysts distinguishes hydatid renal disease from simple renal cysts or polycystic renal disease. The most common symptom is a flank mass; pain and hydatiduria occur when a cyst ruptures into the renal collecting system. Associated findings may be liver and lung echinococcal disease.

Obstructive Uropathy

Obstructive uropathy can result in diminished or absent renal function on excretory urography.[128] Although an obstruction can usually be demonstrated by urography combined with conventional tomography even when there is renal failure, the site and cause of the obstruction often cannot be determined. Hydronephrosis is readily detected by CT because the dilated renal collectiong structures and ureter on nonenhanced scans are demonstrated as low-density structures with attenua-

Text continued on page 819

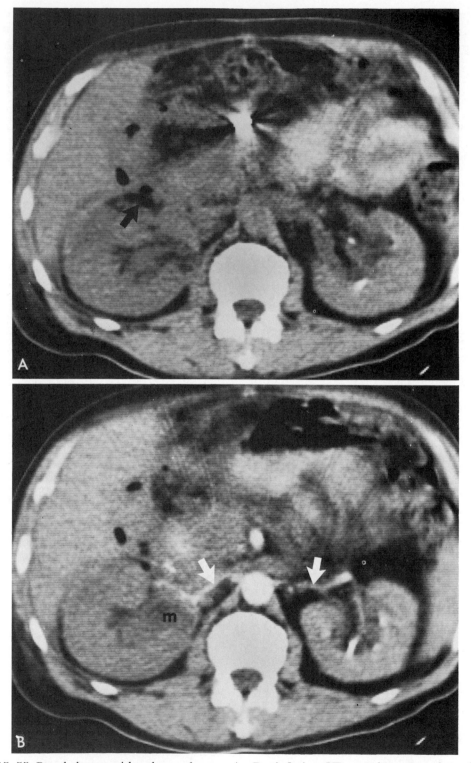

Figure 15–55. Renal abscess with subcapsular gas. **A** Postinfusion CT scan shows an enlarged, poorly functioning right kidney with a collection of gas (arrow) in the renal subcapsular space. **B** CT scan during bolus injection of contrast material demonstrates patency of both main renal arteries (arrows). A focal mass (m) is now apparent.

Illustration continued on opposite page

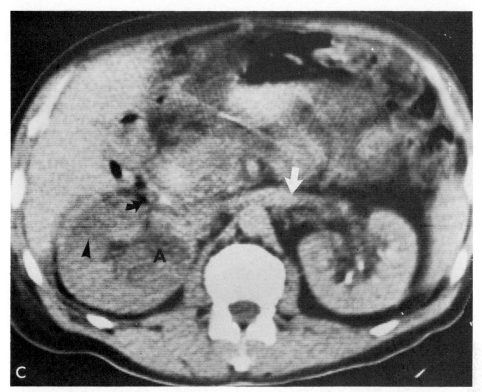

Figure 15–55. *Continued* **C**   CT scan during the venous phase. The left renal vein is patent (arrow), but the right renal vein is thrombosed. A renal abscess (A) and focal area of hypofunction (arrowhead) are seen. Subcapsular gas is present (curved arrow).

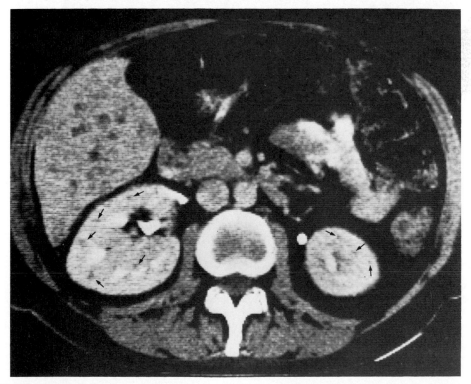

Figure 15–56. Fungal infection of the kidneys. Multiple small, rounded, low-density lesions (arrows) in both kidneys were proved to be fungal abscesses in an immunosuppressed patient with leukemia. Similar lesions were present in the liver.

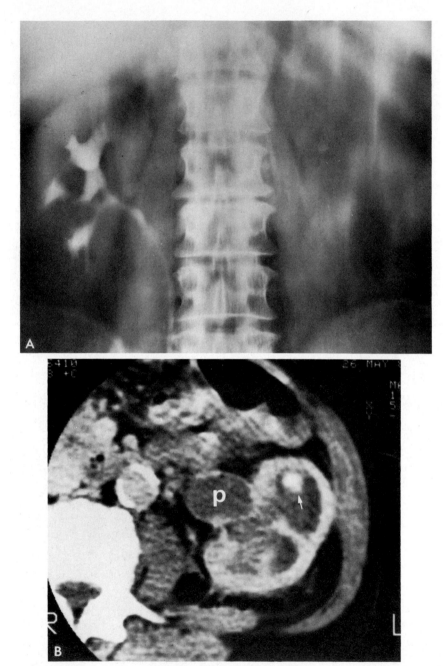

Figure 15–57. Xanthogranulomatous pyelonephritis. **A**   Excretory urogram demonstrates nonfunction of the left kidney. **B**   CT scan. There is prolonged opacification of the left renal cortex. The renal pelvis (p) is filled with pus, as are the intrarenal collecting structures. The high-density focus (arrow) is a renal calculus. At surgery xanthogranulomatous pyelonephritis with ureteral obstruction was found.

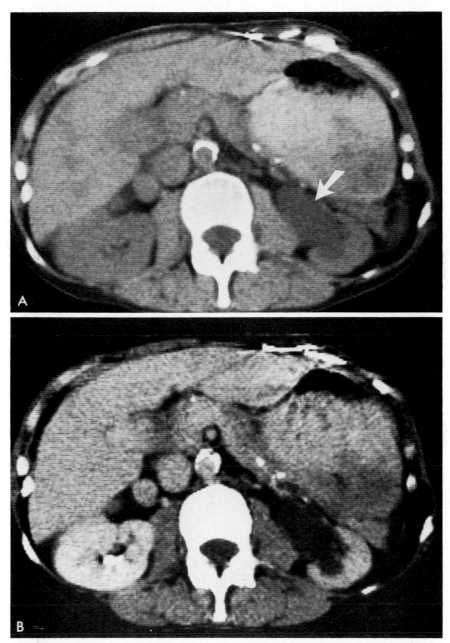

Figure 15–58. Hydronephrosis. **A** Precontrast CT scan reveals small left kidney and dilated renal pelvis (arrow), which has a CT density of 0 H. **B** Postcontrast scan demonstrates diminished function of the left kidney with no excretion of contrast material into the dilated renal pelvis.

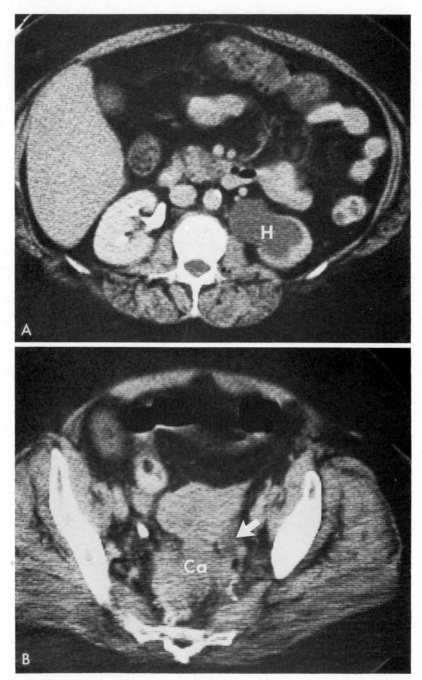

Figure 15–59. Chronic ureteral obstruction. **A** There is marked hydronephrosis (H) of the left kidney, which has resulted in atrophy of the kidney, manifested by cortical thinning, diminished function, and small size. **B** A dilated left ureter (arrow) is seen extending into the pelvis, where it was obstructed by a recurrent carcinoma of the colon (Ca).

tion values that approximate the density of water (Fig. 15–58A).[1, 4, 5, 128] After intravenous contrast medium is injected, the CT appearance of the collecting system depends on the degree of renal function remaining and the volume and concentration of contrast in the collecting system. Scans after contrast medium administration may show delayed function on the affected side and little excretion into the renal collecting structures (Figs. 15–58B and 15–59), or there may be an interface between urine and contrast medium, with the contrast medium layering in the dependent portions of the collecting structures (Fig. 15–60). The entire collecting system is usually opacified on delayed CT scans.

The obstruction is located by identifying a dilated collecting system down to the site of obstruction. Ureteropelvic junction obstructions result in dilated upper collecting systems and a normal-sized ureter, whereas distal ureteral obstructions result in a dilated ureter down to the obstructing lesion (Fig. 15–59). Nonopaque calculi, fibrosis, and retroperitoneal or pelvic tumors can be correctly diagnosed by CT as the cause of hydronephrosis (Figs. 15–59, 15–60).

As obstruction becomes chronic, the renal parenchyma atrophies, caliceal dilation progresses, and the kidney appears to be little more than a fluid-filled cyst with a thin rim of solid renal tissue (Fig. 15–61). At this stage, renal function is usually very poor or absent and cannot be restored.

CT detects hydronephrosis with a reported accuracy of virtually 100 per cent.[1, 3, 5, 88, 128] However, it may be difficult to detect very early hydronephrosis because no definite criteria for demonstrating slight degrees of caliceal dilatation have been established.[129]

Renal Failure

CHRONIC PYELONEPHRITIS. Renal failure resulting from chronic pyelonephritis is manifested by small, contracted kidneys that have broad-based inflammatory scars opposite a deformed calix and involve the entire thickness of the renal parenchyma. The scars cause the renal outline to be irregular but do not cause dilation of the collecting system (Fig. 15–62). Chronic pyelonephritis may affect one kidney predominantly and result in a small, marginally functioning kidney and a scarred cortex owing to severe focal parenchymal atrophy (Fig. 15–62).

RENAL FAILURE FROM MISCELLANEOUS ETIOLOGIES. Diffuse parenchymal atrophy, which uniformly involves the entire kidney, resulting in a small kidney, can occur as a result of renal artery stenosis, glomerulonephritis, or obstructive uropathy. The renal outline is smooth, and there is an apparent increase in the proportion of renal sinus and perinephric fat (Fig. 15–63).[4] The calices are normal in renal artery stenosis and glomerulonephritis but dilated in atrophy because of chronic obstruction (Figs. 15–58 and 15–59). Glomerulonephritis always involves both kidneys, but renal artery stenosis and obstructive uropathy can be unilateral or bilateral. Compensating hypertrophy of the uninvolved kidney frequently accompanies unilateral renal atrophy.

Differentiating renal agenesis from a small, nonfunctioning kidney, the result of pyelonephritis, is difficult by urographic techniques. Identification of renal vascular structures is vital (Fig. 15–63). In right renal agenesis, the right renal vein receives no tributaries and thus does not develop. Identifying the right renal vein by CT excludes a diagnosis of right renal agenesis. On the left side, the left renal vein receives inflow from the left adrenal and gonadal veins; therefore, in left renal agenesis, a small vein will always be demonstrated as it crosses in front of the aorta and enters the inferior vena cava.[88, 130]

Renal Ischemia

Renal ischemia resulting from renal parenchymal compression by a perirenal hematoma can cause mild hypertension. This clinical entity has been called the *Page kidney*[131] because Page demonstrated that hypertension could be produced in dogs by wrapping the kidney in cellophane.[132]

The perirenal hematoma usually results from biopsy, but infection, arterial diseases, blood disorders, and renal calculi have been implicated as etiologic factors.[131, 133–136] CT has demonstrated enlargement of the affected kidney and a surrounding perirenal mass of fluid or soft-tissue density.[131, 133] Postcontrast scans show decreased renal function and nonenhancement of a fibrotic band or crescent-shaped perirenal fluid collection. Extensive perirenal adhesions and concentric fibrosis extending to involve the contracted scarred kidney beneath the renal capsule are found at surgery.[133]

Regional renal infarction produced by segmental vascular ischemia produces wedge-shaped areas of decreased density in the renal cortex after contrast medium administration (Fig. 15–64 and 15–65).[137] The low attenuation values are due in part to nonperfusion of the infarcted tissue by con-

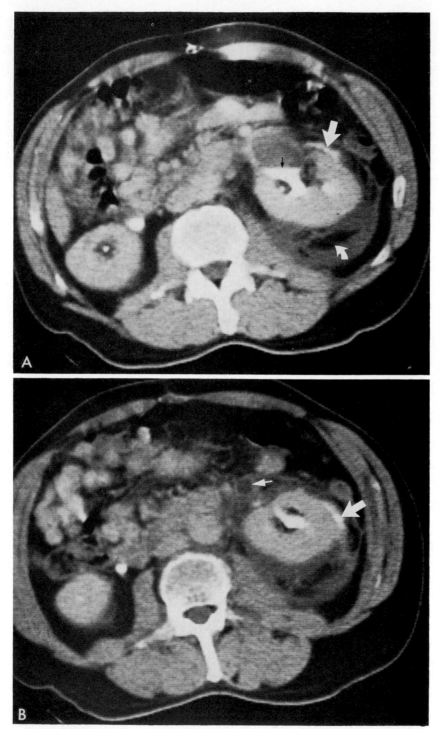

Figure 15–60. Hydronephrosis resulting from metastatic tumor. **A**   CT scan. The left renal pelvis is dilated and contains urine–contrast material (small arrow). A perirenal mass and urine extravasation (large arrow) are present. Areas of perirenal fat (curved arrow) are seen within the perirenal urinoma. **B**   Scan at slightly lower level than in **A**. The dilated ureter (small arrow) is filled with unopacified urine. Extravasation of opacified urine is again shown (large arrow).

Illustration continued on opposite page

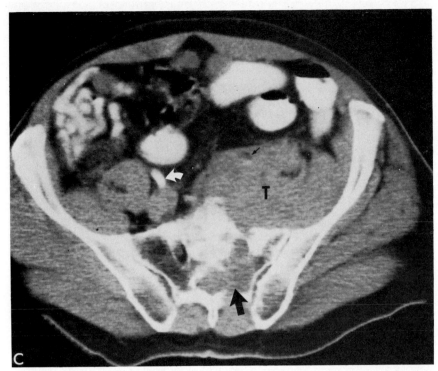

Figure 15–60. *Continued* **C**   Pelvic CT scan demonstrates a large tumor (T) encasing the left ureter (small arrow), which contains some contrast material. The tumor has partially destroyed the sacrum (large arrow). Curved arrow = normal right ureter. Biopsy revealed a liposarcoma of myxoid type.

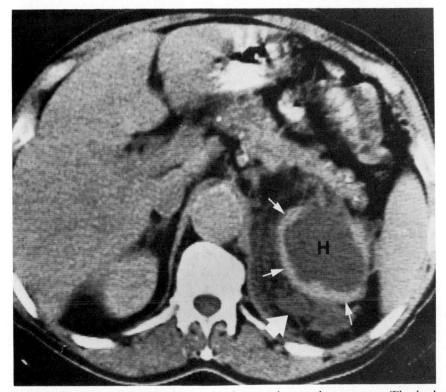

Figure 15–61. Chronic hydronephrosis, the result of an aortic pseudoaneurysm. The hydronephrotic, poorly functioning left kidney (H) appears as a large urine-filled sac surrounded by a thin rim of atrophied renal cortex (small arrows). There has been back-pressure rupture of the collecting system with leak of urine into the perirenal space (large arrow). At this stage, irreversible renal damage has occurred.

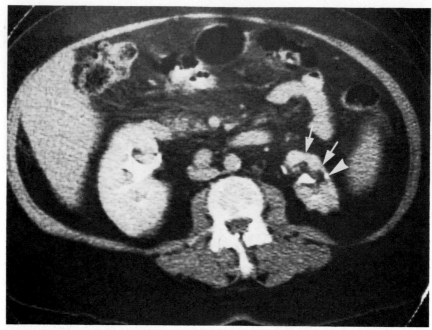

Figure 15–62. Chronic pyelonephritis. The left kidney is small, with marked cortical thinning (arrows). Renal function is poor, as evidenced by a diminished nephrogram compared with that for the right kidney. A focus of parenchymal calcification (arrowhead) is present in the region of maximal cortical atrophy. No hydronephrosis is noted. The pyelonephritis has been present long enough for the right kidney to hypertrophy.

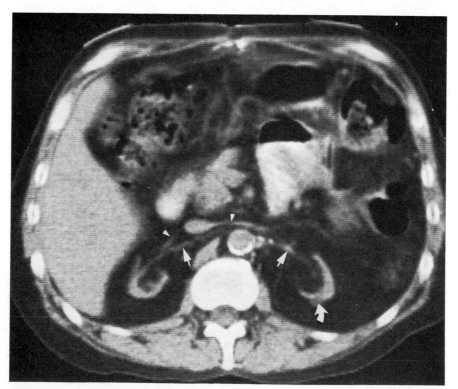

Figure 15–63. Glomerulonephritis. Bilateral small, poorly functioning kidneys with a smooth outline are seen; there is also an increase in renal sinus and perinephric fat. Renal arteries (arrows) and veins (arrowheads) are patent. There is no evidence of hydronephrosis. A small left renal cyst (curved arrow) is present.

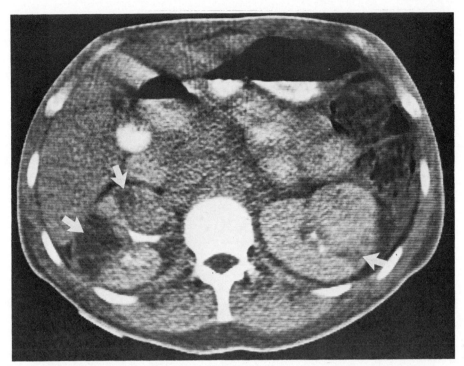

Figure 15–64. Segmented renal infarction. Wedge-shaped areas of decreased density (arrows) are present in both kidneys owing to renal infarction secondary to intravenous drug abuse. The infarcted areas did not enhance or demonstrate any function after contrast material injection.

trast-filled blood and in part to tissue edema. *Global renal infarction* indicates an entire kidney or region of a kidney is infarcted and is seen as a thin rim of high attenuation tissue surrounding a central zone of diminished density (Fig. 15–66). The high-density rim represents perfusion of the preserved outer rim of cortex by collateral vessels in the presence of renal artery occlusion.[138] Multiple areas of ischemia distal to intraparenchymal aneurysms in a patient with polyarteritis nodosa have been reported.[139] The CT features were identical with those of multiple focal areas of renal infarction.

Acute renal cortical necrosis is a rare cause of renal failure in which the renal medulla is spared but the renal cortex undergoes necrosis. Sepsis, shock, transfusion reactions, toxins, and severe dehydration are the usual clinical problems that produce renal cortical vasoconstriction, leading to necrosis of the renal cortex. CT demonstrates a thin rim of tissue with a low attenuation value between the thin capsule and adjacent medulla.[140] These CT findings correlate well with the pathologic features of the disease; thus, CT is valuable in confirming the clinical diagnosis and in determining the extent of involvement.

Renal vein obstruction can be produced by var-

ious neoplastic infectious or metabolic disorders.[141] In animals, acute renal vein thrombosis causes edema and hemorrhage, which produce an enlarged, poorly functioning or nonfunctioning kidney that on follow-up examinations shrinks and shows marked loss of parenchymal tissue.[114, 142] In patients, CT demonstrates an enlarged renal vein that contains a filling defect on enhanced CT scans (Fig. 15–67). The thrombosis may be the result of direct tumor extension or nontumorous causes of renal vein thrombosis.

Congenital Lesions

Congenital variation in the size, shape, and location of the kidneys is common. Pelvic kidney, (Fig. 15–68A)[143] "horseshoe" kidneys (Fig. 15–68B),[2] intrathoracic kidney,[144] and crossed, fused ectopia are readily detected by CT (Fig. 15–69). Pathologic enlargement of the left kidney can be simulated by splenic compression of the left kidney and by an ectopic pancreas. Unexpected motility of the kidneys[145] and alterations in the location of the colon, small bowel, and duodenum can result in malposition of the kidney, which simulates renal displacement by a mass lesion. We favor CT for evaluating the kidneys and retroperitoneum for suspected mass lesions that may cause

Text continued on page 828

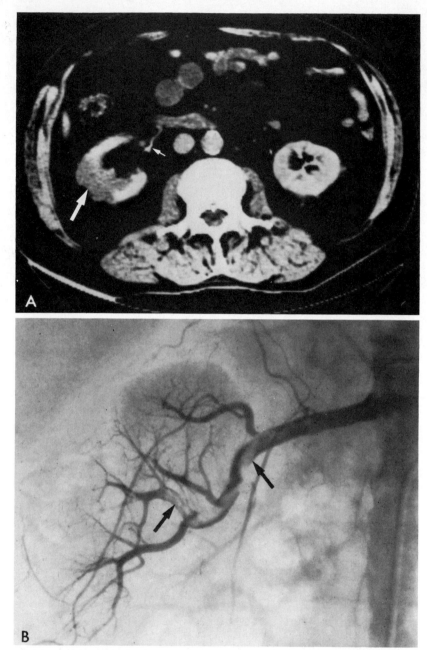

Figure 15–65. Renal artery thrombosis following coronary arteriography. **A** CT scan. A central area of the right kidney (large arrow) has no function, whereas other parts of the right kidney function normally. The kidney is not enlarged, the inferior vena cava is patent, and the renal artery (small arrow) is small. **B** Right renal arteriogram demonstrates multiple renal artery filling defects (arrows), which proved to be emboli at surgery.

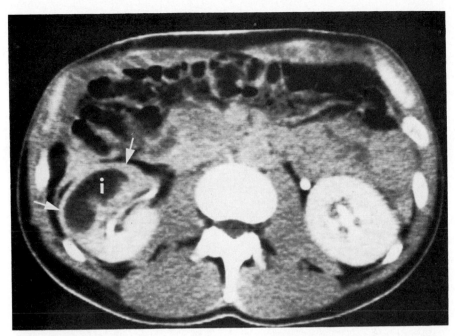

Figure 15–66. Global renal infarction. CT scan after contrast medium injection reveals a thin rim of high-attenuation tissue (arrows), which surrounds an infarcted area (i) of absent function having an attenuation value near that of water. The high-density rim is thought to be cortex preserved by capsular arteries and collateral vessels.

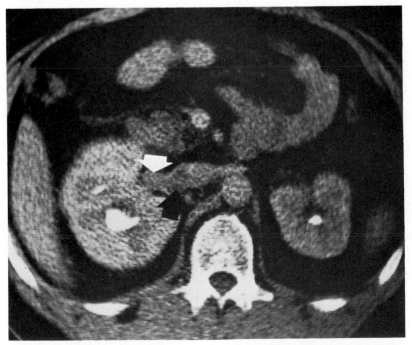

Figure 15–67. Renal vein thrombosis resulting from hypercoagulopathy. Dynamic CT scan after injection of contrast material shows thrombi in the right renal vein (white arrow) and inferior vena cava (black arrow). The kidney is markedly enlarged and there is delayed excretion of contrast material.

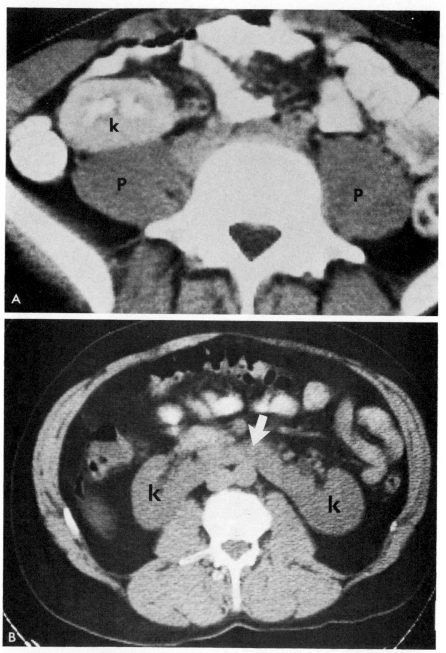

Figure 15–68. Common congenital variations in renal position or fusion. **A**   A normal functioning right pelvic kidney (k). P = psoas muscle. **B**   A horseshoe kidney (k) fusing anterior to the great vessels in a thin isthmus of renal parenchyma (arrow).

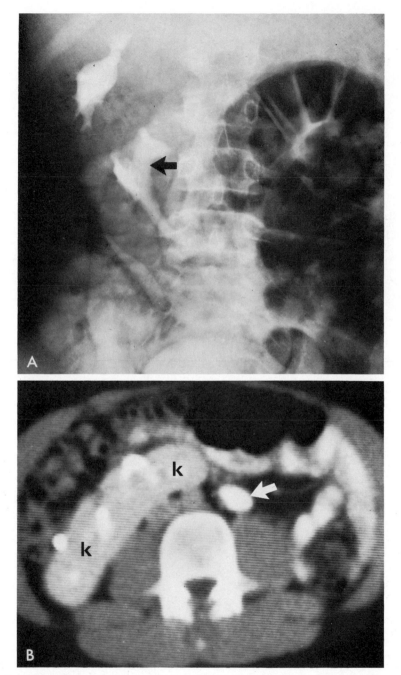

Figure 15–69. Crossed fused renal ectopia in a child with a palpable mass. **A** Excretory urogram showing the left kidney (arrow) to be positioned in the right abdomen. It is not possible to determine whether the left kidney is fused to the lower pole of the right kidney. **B** CT scan clearly shows the kidneys (k) to be fused. Despite the ectopic position of the left kidney, the left ureter (arrow) is in normal position.

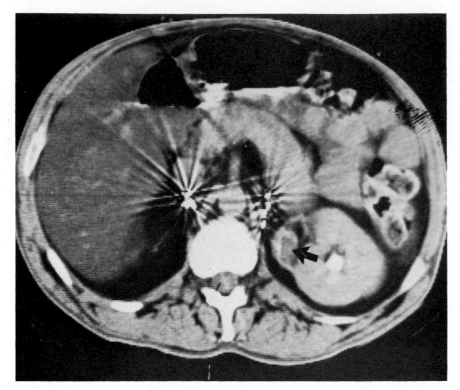

Figure 15–70. Duplicated ureter with obstructed upper pole collecting system. The obstructed collecting system is demonstrated as an oval, small, low-density mass (arrow) surrounded by cortical tissue. The nonobstructed portion of the kidney is shown lateral to the obstructed segment. A fatty liver is present. Clip artifacts are present from prior adrenalectomy.

deviation of the kidneys from their expected position. If CT does not demonstrate a mass lesion, no further evaluation is undertaken.

Fetal lobulation or compensatory hypertrophy of normal renal parenchyma can produce focal enlargement of the kidney, which simulates a tumor on excretory urography. If the "mass" is due to fetal lobulation or focal renal hypertrophy, however, enhanced CT scans show the "mass" to be functioning renal parenchyma. If a "renal mass" is due to peripelvic lipomatosis, CT demonstrates the fatty composition of the mass. If the peripelvic tissue contains enough fibrous tissue to raise the density above that of fat, differentiation from a solid peripelvic mass is difficult.

Unusual congenital variations of the ureter can be detected by CT scanning. The circumcaval ureter[146] is an anomaly in which the proximal right ureter courses medially behind and then ventral to the inferior vena cava, partially encircling it. Circumcaval ureter occurs in about one of every 1000 persons, and males are affected two to three times more frequently than females. Ureteral obstruction in varying degrees can be produced, but it is frequently an incidental autopsy finding. CT can demonstrate the retrocaval position of the ureter and the dilated proximal ureter without the need for retrograde urography or an inferior vena cavogram.[140]

CT is also useful in determining the cause of ureteral deviations, readily demonstrating those that are due to congenital variations in location, enlarged psoas muscles, tumors, retroperitoneal fibrosis, aortic aneurysms, lymphadenopathy, or retroperitoneal lipomatosis. Duplications of the ureter are identified as two high-density, rounded structures following contrast material injection. If one ureter is obstructed, the hydronephrotic part of the kidney (usually the upper pole) is readily apparent on CT (Fig. 15–70).

POSTSURGICAL EVALUATION

POSTNEPHRECTOMY

Interpretation of CT scans after nephrectomy demands a knowledge of postnephrectomy anatomy and the time-course of postoperative changes. Postoperative complications, such as hematoma or abscess (Fig. 15–71), must be diagnosed or excluded in the immediate postoperative period. After nephrectomy, small collections of retroperitoneal gas may be detected for a week or more without indicating abscess formation.[147] More important than the mere presence of retroperitoneal gas is whether the quantity of gas is increasing or decreasing. An increase in retroperitoneal gas is more indicative of abscess than the absolute volume of air or the time since surgery was performed.[147]

After right nephrectomy, the liver and colon shift to partially occupy the nephrectomy site; the second duodenum is located more posteriorly than usual and should not be mistaken for a paracaval tumor mass or recurrent renal neoplasm.[143, 148, 149] After left nephrectomy, the stomach and small bowel fill the renal bed and the tail of the pancreas falls posteriorly and medially to lie next to the left psoas muscle and aorta, giving the normal pancreas an inverted U-shape. Bowel in the empty renal fossa is common, and unopacified bowel must not be interpreted as an abscess.

Postoperatively, the psoas margins are usually symmetrical and are neither enlarged nor irregular.[148] Asymmetry, irregularity, or enlargement of the psoas muscle on the side of the nephrectomy is an important sign of recurrent or residual mass involvement. Postoperative scar tissue occurs in less than 10 per cent of patients who undergo radical nephrectomy.[149] Thus, a solid mass in the renal bed must be considered tumorous until proved otherwise. Local recurrence of renal cell or pelvic carcinoma is the most frequent[148, 149] and

produces a mass in the renal fossa, regional lymphadenopathy, or evidence of asymmetery of the psoas muscles (Fig. 15–72). When a mass is detected, fine-needle aspiration biopsy can be used to document or exclude recurrent neoplasm.

Although CT is the preferred procedure for evaluating the retroperitoneum after nephrectomy, by the time a patient becomes symptomatic, massive tumor recurrence is usually found.[149] CT examination of asymptomatic patients offers hope for early detection of recurrent tumor. Because the incidence of recurrence is related to the stage of carcinoma at nephrectomy, routine postoperative CT scans may be indicated in patients with Stage III or IV renal carcinoma or in patients with incomplete tumor resection.

RENAL TRANSPLANTS

Although potential complications of renal transplants are best evaluated initially by conventional urography, ultrasonography and radionuclide imaging techniques,[150] CT can provide additional information on possible causes of complications in certain patients. Urinoma, hematoma, lymphocele, and abscess can be diagnosed (Figs. 15–73 and 15–74), and the relationship of

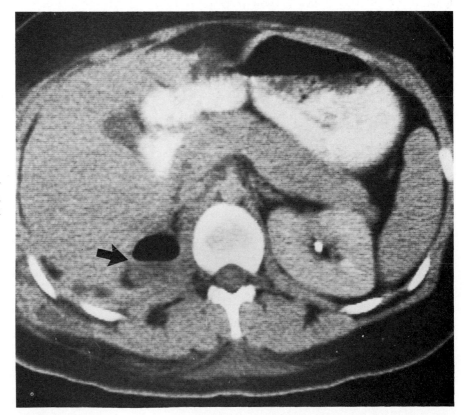

Figure 15–71. Postnephrectomy abscess (arrow) presents as a mass with an air-fluid level in the right renal fossa.

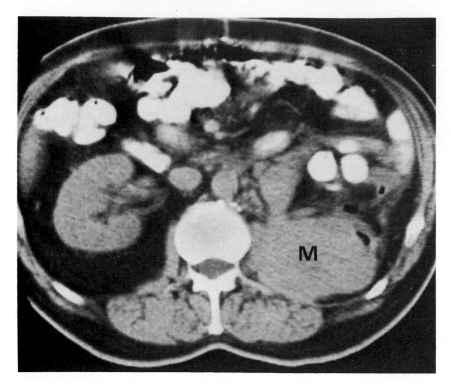

Figure 15–72. Recurrent left renal cell carcinoma producing a large, solid mass (M), which occupies the left renal fossa. Recurrence appeared 1 year after surgery. The preoperative CT scan for this patient shown as Figure 15–27.

the abnormality to the transplanted kidney can be depicted.[151] In cases of transplant dysfunction, after bolus injections of contrast medium, CT scans can be used to measure the renal cortical margin, demonstrate the vascular pedicle, and determine renal function (Figs. 15–75 and 15–76). CT can show the diagnosis of hydronephrosis, the size and position of the ureter, vascular occlusion (Figs. 15–75 and 15–76), the presence of calculi,[152] and the size of the transplanted kidney.[150] Renal size may increase abruptly when rejection is acute, but renal size decreases gradually in chronic rejection. A normal CT study virtually excludes any significant post-transplant abnormality.

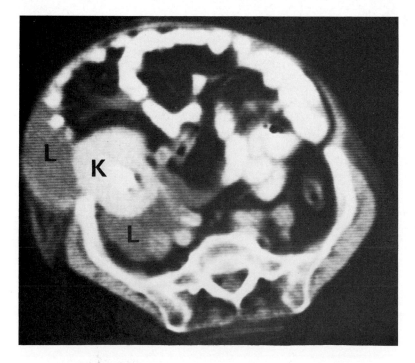

Figure 15–73. Post–renal transplant lymphocele. The CT scan demonstrates two lymphoceles (L) as homogeneous masses of water density surrounding a normally functioning transplanted kidney (K). The lateral lymphocele protrudes through the abdominal flank muscles.

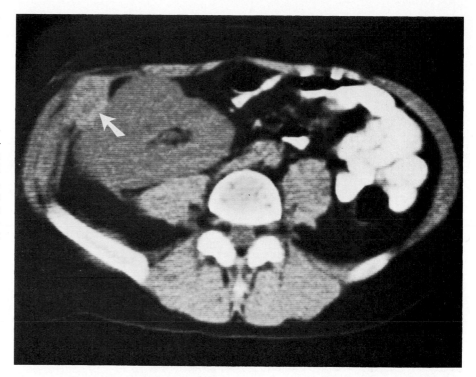

Figure 15–74. Hematoma following renal transplant. Non–contrast-enhanced CT scan shows a normal transplanted kidney in the right iliac fossa. A high-density mass (arrow) in the abdominal musculature proved to be a recent hematoma, which resolved without treatment.

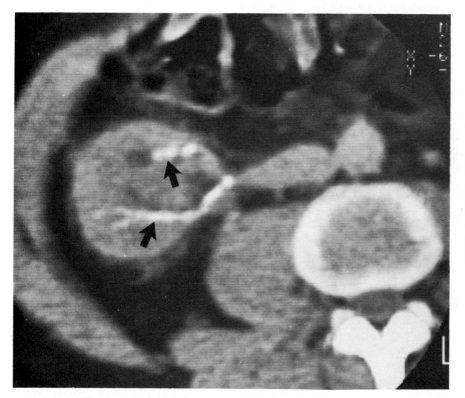

Figure 15–75. Long-standing renal transplant failure. CT scan following bolus injection of contrast material demonstrates no function of the right renal transplant. There is extensive calcification of the renal arteries (arrows).

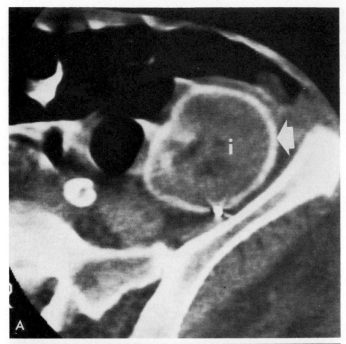

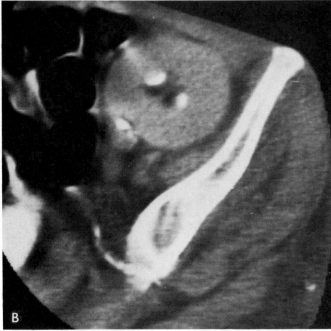

Figure 15–76. Regional infarction of transplanted kidney. **A** CT scan demonstrates thin rim of tissue having a high attenuation (arrow) value surrounding an area of renal infarction (i) which has a CT density of water in the upper pole of the transplanted kidney. **B** The lower pole of the transplant functions normally. Total occlusion of the arterial branch to the upper pole of the kidney was found at surgery.

REFERENCES

1. Sagel SS, Stanley RJ, Levitt RG, Geisse G: Computed tomography of the kidney. Radiology 124:359, 1977.
2. Love L, Reynes CJ, Churchill R, Moncada R: Third generation CT scanning in renal disease. Radiol Clin North Am 17:77, 1979.
3. Curtis JA, Brennan RE, Rubin C, Kurtz A, Goldberg BB: Computed tomography of the kidneys. Comput Tomogr 4:17, 1980.
4. Hattery RR, Williamson B, Stephens DH, Sheedy PF II, Hartman GW: Computed tomography of renal abnormalities. Radiol Clin North Am 15:401, 1977.
5. Engelstad BL, McClennan BL, Levitt RG, Stanley RJ, Sagel SS: The role of pre-contrast images in computed tomography of the kidney. Radiology 136:153, 1980.
6. Hattery RR, Williamson B Jr, Hartman GW: Urinary tract tomography. Radiol Clin North Am 14:23, 1976.
7. Haaga J, Reich NE: computed tomography of abdominal abnormalities. In Kidneys and Adrenal Glands. St Louis, CV Mosby, 1978, pp 177–211.
8. Williamson B, Hattery RR, Stephens DS, Sheedy PF: Computed tomography of the kidneys. Semin Roentgenol 13:249, 1978.
9. Magilner AD, Ostrum BJ: Computed tomography in

the diagnosis of renal masses. Radiology 126:715, 1978.

10. Havrilla TR, Reich NE, Seidelmann FE, Haaga JR: Computed tomography of the kidneys and retroperitoneum: Current status. CT 2:227, 1978.

11. Marchal G, Baert A, Wilms G: Value of computerized tomography and ultrasonography in the diagnosis of renal and adrenal space-occupying lesions. In Lohr E (ed): Renal and Adrenal Tumors: Pathology, Radiology, Ultrasonography, Therapy, Immunology. Springer-Verlag, 1979, pp 98–108.

12. Harris RD, Seat SG: Value of computerized tomography in evaluation of kidney. Urology 12:729, 1978.

13. Kim WS, Goldman SM, Gatewood OMB, Marshall FF, Siegelman SS: Computed tomography of calcified renal masses. J Comput Assist Tomogr 5:855, 1981.

14. Meyers MA: Dynamic Radiology of the Abdomen in Normal and Pathologic Anatomy. Heidelberg, Springer, 1976, pp 113–194.

15. Love L, Meyers MA, Churchill RJ, Reynes CJ, Moncada R, Gibson D: Computed tomography of extraperitoneal spaces. AJR 136:781, 1981.

16. Parienty RA, Pradel J, Picard JD, Ducellier R, Lubrano JM, Smolarski N: Visibility and thickening of the renal fascia on computed tomograms. Radiology 139:119, 1981.

17. Nicholson RL: Abnormalities of the perinephric fascia and fat in pancreatitis. Radiology 139:125, 1981.

18. Ritman EL, Kinsey JH, Robb RA, Gilbert BK, Harris LD, Wood EH: Three-dimensional imaging of the heart, lungs and circulation. Science 210:273, 1980.

19. Meyers MA, Whalen JP, Evans JA: Diagnosis of perirenal and subcapsular masses: Anatomic-Radiologic Correlation. AJR 121:523, 1974.

20. Siegelman SS, Copeland BE, Saba BE, Cameron JL, Sanders RC, Zerhouni EA: CT of fluid collections associated with pancreatitis. AJR 134:1121, 1980.

21. Somogyi J, Cohne WN, Omar MM, Makhuli Z: Communication of right and left perirenal spaces demonstrated by computed tomography. J Comput Assist Tomogr 3:270, 1979.

22. Mitchell GAG: Renal fascia. Br J Surg 37:257, 1950.

23. Gerota D: Beiträge zur Kenntniss des Befestigungsapparates der Niere. Arch f Anat u Entwicklungsgesch Leipz, 1895, 265–285.

24. Moss AA, Cann CE, Friedman MA, Brito AC: Determination of liver, kidney and spleen volumes by computed tomography: An experimental study in dogs. J Comput Assist Tomogr 5:12, 1981.

25. Buschi AJ, Harrison RB, Brenbridge ANAG, Williamson BRJ, Gentry RR, Cole R: Distended left renal vein: CT/sonographic normal variant. AJR 135:339, 1980.

26. Ishikawa I, Onouchi Z, Saito Y, Kitada H, Shinoda A, Ushitani K, Tabuchi M, Susuki M: Renal cortex visualization and analysis of dynamic CT curves of the kidney. J Comput Assist Tomogr 5:695, 1981.

27. Heinz ER, Dubois PJ, Drayer BP, Hill R: A preliminary investigation of the role of dynamic computed tomography in renovascular hypertension. J Comput Assist Tomogr 4:63, 1980.

28. Hammerschlag SB, Wolpert SM, Carter BL: Computed tomography of the spinal canal. Radiology 121:361, 1976.

29. Weyman PJ, McClennan BL, Stanley RJ, Levitt RG, Sa-

gel SS: Comparison of computed tomography and angiography in the evaluation of renal cell carcinoma. Radiology 137:417, 1980.

30. Turner RJ, Young SW, Castellino RA: Dynamic continuous computed tomography: Study of retroaortic left renal vein. J Comput Assist Tomogr 4:109, 1980.

31. Treugut H, Nyman U, Hildell J, Sequenz CT: Frühe Dichteveränderungen der gesunden Niere nach Kontrast mitt Elapplikation. Radiologie 20:558, 1980.

32. Brennan RE, Curtis JA, Pollack HM, Weinberg I: Sequential changes in the CT numbers of the normal canine kidney following intravenous contrast administration: II. The renal medulla. Invest Radiol 14:239, 1979

33. Hacker H, Becker H: Time controlled computed tomographic angiography. J Comput Assist Tomogr 1:405, 1977.

34. Boyd P, Gould RG, Quinn JR, Sparks R, Stanley JH, Hermannsfeldt WB: A proposed dynamic cardiac 3-D densitometer for early detection and evaluation of heart disease. IEEE Trans Nucl Sci NS-26:2724, 1979.

35. Ackerman LV, Rosai J: Surgical Pathology, 5th ed. St Louis, CV Mosby, 1974.

36. Kissane JM: The morphology of renal cystic disease. Perspect Nephrol Hypertension 4:31, 1976.

37. Elkin M: Renal cystic disease. In Elkin M (ed): Radiology of the Urinary System. Boston, Little, Brown & Company, 1980, pp 912–966.

38. McClennan BL, Stanley RJ, Nelson GL, Levitt RG, Sagel SS: CT of the renal cyst: Is cyst aspiration necessary? AJR 133:671, 1979.

39. Shanser JD, Hedgcock MW, Korobkin M: Transit of contrast material into renal cysts following urography or arteriography, abstract. AJR 130:584, 1978.

40. Ambos MA, Bosniak MA, Gordon R, Madayag MA: Replacement lipomatosis of the kidney. AJR 130:1087, 1978.

41. Foley WD: Polycystic kidney disease with hematuria. CT/T Clinical Symposium, vol 4, No 5. Milwaukee, General Electric Company, 1981.

42. Takao R, Amamoto Y, Matsunaga N, Tasaki T, Kakimoto S, Ito M, Fujii H, Futagawa S, Sekine I: Computed tomography of multicystic kidney. J Comput Assist Tomogr 4:548, 1980.

43. Banner MP, Pollack HM, Chatlen J, Witzleben C: Multilocular renal cysts: Radiologic-Pathologic Correlation. AJR 136:239, 1981.

44. Parienty RA, Pradel J, Imbert MC, Picard JD, Savart P: Computed tomography of multilocular cystic nephroma. Radiology 140:135, 1981.

45. Carlson DH, Carlson D, Simon H: Benign multilocal cystic nephroma AJR 131:621, 1978.

46. Elkin M: Tumors of the kidney. In Elkin M (ed): Radiology of the Urinary System. Boston, Little, Brown & Company, 1980, pp 296–397.

47. Horton WA, Wong V, Eldridge R: von Hippel-Lindau disease. Arch Intern Med 136:769, 1976.

48. Fill WL, Lamiell JM, Polk NO: The radiographic manifestations of von Hippel-Lindau disease. Radiology 133:289, 1979.

49. Levine E, Lee KR, Weigel JW, Farber B: Computed tomography in the diagnosis of renal carcinoma complicating von Hippel-Lindau syndrome. Radiology 130:703, 1979.

50. Levine E, Leek KR, Weigel J: Preoperative determina-

tion of abdominal extent of renal cell carcinoma by computed tomography. Radiology 132:395, 1979.

51. Segal AJ, Spitzer RM: Pseudo thick-walled renal cyst by CT. AJR 132:827, 1979.

52. Weymen PJ, McClennan BL, Lee JKT, Stanley RJ: CT of calcified renal masses. AJR 138:1095, 1982.

53. Love L, Churchill R, Reynes C: Computed tomography staging of renal carcinoma. Urol Radiol 1:3, 1979.

54. Marks WW, Korobkin M, Callen PW, Kaiser JA: CT diagnosis of tumor thrombosis of the renal vein and inferior vena cava. AJR 131:843, 1978.

55. Kothari K, Segal AJ, Spitzer RM, Peartree RJ: Preoperative radiographic evaluation of hypernephroma. J Comput Assist Tomogr 5:702, 1981.

56. Thomas JL, Bernardino ME: Neoplastic-induced renal vein enlargement: Sonographic detection. AJR 136:75, 1981.

57. Winfield AC, Gerlock AJ Jr, Shaff MI: Perirenal cobwebs: A CT sign of renal vein thrombosis. J Comput Assist Tomogr 5:705, 1981.

58. Lee KR, Wulfsberg E, Kepes JJ: Some important radiologic aspects of the kidney in Hippel-Lindau syndrome: The value of prospective study in an affected family. Radiology 122:649, 1977.

59. Levitt RG, Geisse GG, Sagel SS, Stanley RJ, Evens RG, Koehler RE, Jost RG: Complementary use of ultrasound and computed tomography in studies of the pancreas and kidney. Radiology 126:149, 1978.

60. Brasch RC, Korobkin M, Gooding CA: Computed body tomography in children: Evaluation of 45 patients. AJR 131:21, 1978.

61. Boldt DW, Reilly BJ: Computed tomography of abdominal mass lesions in children. Radiology 124:371, 1977.

62. Farrow GM, Harrison EG Jr, Utz DC, Jones DR: Renal angiomyolipomas: A clinical pathologic study of 32 cases. Cancer 22:564, 1968.

63. McCullough DL, Scott R Jr, Seybold HM: Renal angiomyolipoma (hamartoma): review of the literature and report of 7 cases. J Urol 105:32, 1971.

64. Hansen GC, Hoffman RB, Sample WF, Becker R: Computed tomography diagnosis of renal angiomyolipoma. Radiology 128:789, 1978.

65. Frija J, Larde D, Belloir C, Botto H, Martin N, Vasile N: Computed tomography diagnosis of renal angiomyolipoma. J Comput Assist Tomogr 4:843, 1980.

66. Hartman DS, Goldman SM, Friedman AC, Davis CJ, Madewell JE, Sherman JL: Angiomyolipoma: Ultrasonic-pathologic correlation. Radiology 139:451, 1981.

67. Kagan, RA, Steckel RJ (eds): Diagnostic oncology case study: Flank pain and hematuria in a child. AJR 136:597, 1981.

68. Totty WG, McClennan BL, Nelson GL, Patel R: Relative value of computed tomography and ultrasonography in the assessment of renal angiomyolipoma. J Comput Assist Tomogr 5:173, 1981.

69. Shawker TH, Horvath KL, Dunnick NR, Javadpoor N: Renal angiomyolipoma: Diagnosis by combined ultrasound and computerized tomography. J Urol 121:675, 1979.

70. Whittemore DM, Wendel RG: Bilateral involvement of renal hamartoma in 2 cases without tuberous sclerosis. J Urol 125:99, 1981.

71. Bush FM, Bark JC, Clyde HR: Benign renal angiomylipoma with regional lymph node involvement. J Urol 14:531, 1976.

72. Pitts WR Jr, Kazam E, Gray G, Vaughan ED Jr: Ultrasonography, computed transaxial tomography and pathology of angiomyolipoma of the kidney: Solution to diagnostic dilemma. J Urol 124:907, 1980.

73. Gentry LR, Gould HR, Alter AJ, Wegenke JD, Atwell DT: Hemorrhagic angiomyolipoma: Demonstration by computed tomography. J Comput Assist Tomogr 5:861, 1981.

74. Bagley D, Appell R, Pingoud E, McGuire EJ: Renal angiomyolipoma: Diagnosis and management. Urology 15:1, 1980.

75. Apitzsch DE, Wegener OH, Khalil M, Sorensen R: Advances in the diagnosis of renal angiomyolipoma. Acta Radiol (Diagn) (Stockh) 20:105, 1979.

76. Hattery RR, Williamson B Jr, Hartman GW: Computed tomography of the genitourinary tract and retroperitoneum. In Witten DM, Myers GH, Utz DC (eds): Emmett's Clinical Urography, 4th ed. Philadelphia, WB Saunders Company, 1977, p 362.

77. Kutcher R, Rosenblatt R, Mitsudo SM, Goldman M, Kogan S: Renal angiomyolipoma with sonographic demonstration of extension into the inferior vena cava. Radiology 143:755, 1982.

78. Parvey LS, Warner RM, Calliham TR, Magill HL: CT demonstration of fat tissue in malignant renal neoplasms: Atypical Wilms' tumors. J Comput Assist Tomogr 5:851, 1981.

79. Ambos MA, Bosniak MA, Valensi QJ, Madayag MA, Lefleur RS: Angiographic patterns in renal oncocytomas. Radiology 129:615, 1978.

80. Weiner SN, Bernstein RG: Renal oncocytoma: Angiographic features of two cases. Radiology 125:633, 1977.

81. Lautin FM, Gordon PM, Friedman AC, McCormick JF, Fromowitz FB, Goldman MJ, Sugarman LA: Radionuclide imaging and computed tomography in renal oncocytoma. Radiology 138:185, 1981.

82. Hartman DS, Lesar MSL, Madewell JE, Lichtenstein JE, Davis CJ Jr: Mesoblastic nephroma: Radiologic-pathologic correlation of 20 cases. AJR 136:69, 1981.

83. Rubin BE: Computed tomography in the evaluation of renal lymphoma. J Comput Assist Tomogr 3:759, 1979.

84. Lalli AF: Lymphoma and the urinary tract. Radiology 93:1051, 1969.

85. Martinez-Maldonado M, Ramirez de Arellano GA: Renal involvement in malignant lymphomas. J Urol 95:485, 1966.

86. Richmond J, Sherman RS, Diamond HD, Craver LF: Renal lesions associated with malignant lymphomas. Am J Med 32:184, 1962.

87. Kiely JM, Wagoner RD, Holley KE: Renal complications of lymphoma. Ann Intern Med 71:1159, 1969.

88. Forbes W St C, Isherwood I, Fawcitt RA: Computed tomography in the evaluation of the solitary or unilateral nonfunctioning kidney. J Comput Assist Tomogr 2:389, 1978.

89. Jafri SZH, Bree RL, Amendoke MA, Glazer GM, Schwab RE, Francis IR, Borlaza G: CT of renal and perirenal non-Hodgkin lymphoma. AJR 138:1101, 1982.

90. Pollack HM, Arger PH, Banner MP, Mulhern CB, Cole-

man BG: Computed tomography of renal pelvic filling defects. Radiology 138:645, 1981.

91. Mieza M, Rotstein JM, Geffen A: CT demonstration of periureteral fibrosis of malignant etiology. J Comput Assist Tomogr 6:290, 1982.

92. Bosniak MA, Megibow AJ, Ambos MA, Mitnick JS, Lefleur RS, Gordon R: Computed tomography of ureteral obstruction. AJR 138:1107, 1982.

93. Segal AJ, Spataro RF, Linke CA, Frank IN, Rabinowitz R: Diagnosis of nonopaque calculi by computed tomography. Radiology 129:447, 1978.

94. Brown RC, Loening SA, Ehrhardt JC, Hawtrey CE: Cystine calculi are radiopaque. AJR 135:565, 1980.

95. Federle MP, McAninch JW, Kaiser JA, Goodman PC, Roberts J, Mall JC: Computed tomography of urinary calculi. AJR 136:255, 1981.

96. Herring LC: Observations on the analysis of ten thousand urinary calculi. J Urol 88:545, 1962.

97. Prien EL: The analysis of urinary calculi. Urol Clin North Am 1:229, 1974.

98. Tessler AN, Ghazi MR: Case profile: Computerized tomographic assistance in diagnosis of radiolucent calculi. Urology 6:672, 1979.

99. Federle MP, Goldberg HI, Kaiser JA, Moss AA, Jeffrey RB Jr, Mall JC: Evaluation of abdominal trauma by computed tomography. Radiology 138:637, 1981.

100. Federle MP, Kaiser JA, McAninch JW, Jeffrey RB, Mall JC: The role of computed tomography in renal trauma. Radiology 141:455, 1981.

101. Sandler CM, Toombs BD: Computed tomographic evaluation of blunt renal injuries. Radiology 141:461, 1981.

102. Alter AJ, Zimmerman S, Kirachaiwanich C: Computerized tomographic assessment of retroperitoneal hemorrhage after percutaneous biopsy. Arch Intern Med 140:1323, 1980.

103. Schaner EG, Balow JE, Doppman JL: Computed tomography in the diagnosis of subcapsular and perirenal hematoma. AJR 129:83, 1977.

104. Rosenbaum R, Hoffsten PE, Stanley RJ, Klahr S: Use of computerized tomography to diagnose complications of percutaneous renal biopsy. Kidney Int 14:87, 1978.

105. Sagel SS, Siegel MJ, Stanley RJ, Jost RG: Detection of retroperitoneal hemorrhage by computed tomography. AJR 129:403, 1977.

106. Evans JA, Meyers MA, Bosniak MA: Acute renal and perirenal infections. Semin Roentgenol 6:274, 1971.

107. Little PJ, McPherson DR, de Wardener HE: The appearance of the intravenous pyelogram during and after acute pyelonephritis. Lancet 1:1186, 1965.

108. Shopfner CE: Urinary tract pathology with sepsis. AJR 108:632, 1970.

109. Davidson AJ, Talner LB: Urographic and angiographic abnormalities in adult-onset of acute bacterial nephritis. Radiology 106:249, 1973.

110. Silver TM, Kass EJ, Thornbury JR, Konnak JW, Wolfman MG: The radiological spectrum of acute pyelonephritis in adults and adolescents. Radiology 118:65, 1976.

111. Rauschkolb EN, Sandler CM, Patel S, Childs TL: Computed tomography of renal inflammatory disease. J Comput Assist Tomogr 6:502, 1982.

112. Bigongiari LR, Patel SK, Appelman H, Thornbury JR: Medullary rays: Visualization during excretory urography. AJR 125:795, 1975.

113. Wicks JD, Thornbury JR: Acute renal infection in adults: Radiol Clin North Am 17:245, 1979.

114. Hoffman EP, Mindelzun RE, Anderson RU: Computed tomography in acute pyelonephritis associated with diabetes. Radiology 135:691, 1980.

115. Kressel HY, McLean GK, Troupin RH: Correlative imaging conference: Hospital of the University of Pennsylvania: II. Lower abdominal pain and fever. AJR 135:1305, 1980.

116. Lee JKT, McClennan BL, Nelson GL, Stanley RJ: Acute focal bacterial nephritis: Emphasis on gray scale sonography and computed tomography. AJR 135:87, 1980.

117. Rosenfield AT, Glickman MG, Taylor KJW, Crade M, Hodson J: Acute focal bacterial nephritis (acute lobar nephronia). Radiology 132:553, 1979.

118. Lillienfeld RM, Lande A: Acute adult onset bacterial nephritis: Long-term urographic and angiographic follow-up. J Urol 114:14, 1975.

119. Kim DS, Woesner ME, Howard TF, Oson LK: Emphysematous pyelonephritis demonstrated by computed tomography. AJR 132:287, 1979.

120. Wilms G, Baert AL, Marchal G, Bruneel M: CT demonstration of gas formation after renal tumor embolization. J Comput Assist Tomogr 3:838, 1979.

121. Marks WM, Filly RA: Computed tomographic demonstration of intra-arterial air following hepatic artery ligation. Radiology 132:665, 1979.

122. Schneider M, Becker JA, Staiano S, Campos E: Sonographic-radiographic correlation of renal and perirenal infections. AJR 127:1007, 1976.

123. Callen PW, Filly RA, Marcus FS: Ultrasonography and computed tomography in the evaluation of hepatic microabscesses in the immunosuppressed patient. Radiology 136:433, 1980.

124. Flechner SM, McAninch JW: Aspergillosis of the urinary tract: Ascending route of infection and evolving patterns of disease. J Urol 125:598, 1981.

125. Elkin ME: Radiology of the urinary system. In Elkin M (ed): Computed Tomography of the Urinary Tract. Boston, Little, Brown & Company, 1980, pp 1114–1139.

126. Petrillo G, Tomaselli S, Greco S: Renal ecchinococcus. J Comput Assist Tomogr 5:912, 1981.

127. Gilzanz V, Lozano F, Jimenez J: Renal hydatid cysts: Communicating with collecting system. AJR 135:357, 1980.

128. Karasick SR, Herring W: Computed tomography evaluation of the poorly or nonvisualized kidney. Comput Tomogr 4:39, 1980.

129. Amis ES, Cronan JJ, Pfister RC: Pseudohydronephrosis on noncontrast computed tomography. J Comput Assist Tomogr 6:511, 1982.

130. Pozzo GD, Bozza A, Martorana G: Use of computed tomography in kidney agenesis. XTract 5:27, 1979.

131. Chamorro HA, Forbes TW, Padkowsky GO, Wholey MH: Multiimaging approach to the diagnosis of Page kidney. AJR 136:620, 1981.

132. Page IH: The production of persistent arterial hypertension by cellophane perinephritis. JAMA 113:2046, 1939.

133. Takahaski M, Tamakawa Y, Shibata A, Fukushima Y: Computed tomography of "Page" kidney. J Comput Assist Tomogr 1:344, 1977.

134. Hayward WG: Renal surgery as a cause for renal ischemia. J Urol 51:486, 1944.

135. Hellebusch AA, Simmons JL, Holland N: Renal ischemia and hypertension from a constrictive perirenal hematoma. JAMA 214:757, 1970.

136. McKay A, Proctor LD, Roome NW: Hypertension after removal of renal calculus. Can Med Assoc J 50:328, 1944.

137. Haaga JR, Morrison SC: CT appearance of renal infarct. J Comput Assist Tomogr 4:246, 1980.

138. Glazer GM, London SS: CT appearance of global renal infarction. J Comput Assist Tomogr 5:847, 1981.

139. Pope TL Jr, Buschi AJ, Moore TS, Williamson BRJ, Brenbridge ANAG: CT features of polyarteritis nodosa. AJR 136:986, 1981.

140. Goergen TG, Lindstrom RR, Tan H, Lille Y: CT appearance of acute renal cortical necrosis. AJR 137:176, 1981.

141. Rosenfield AT, Zeman RK, Cronan JJ, Taylor KJW: Ultrasound in experimental and clinical renal vein thrombosis. Radiology 137:735, 1980.

142. Hricak H, Sandler MA, Madrozo BL, Eyler WR, Sy GS: Sonographic manifestations of acute renal vein thrombosis: An experimental study. Invest Radiol 16:30, 1981.

143. Savolaine ER, Christoforidis AJ: Evaluation of pelvic mass: Bilateral pelvic kidneys disclosed by CT. CT/T Clinical Symposium, vol 2, No 9. Milwaukee, General Electric Company, 1979.

144. Nishitani H, Nakata H, Kowo J: Intrathoracic kidney. J Comput Assist Tomogr 3:409, 1979.

145. Sandler CM, Conley SB, Fogel SR, Brewer ED: Splenic compression of the left kidney simulating pathologic unilateral renal enlargement. J Comput Assist Tomogr 4:248, 1980.

146. Gefter WB, Arger PH, Mulhern CB, Pollack HM, Wein AJ: Computed tomography of circumcaval ureter. AJR 131:1086, 1978.

147. McDonald JE, Lee JKT, McClennan BL, Melzer JS, Sicard GA, Etheredge EE, Anderson CB: Natural history of extraperitoneal gas after renal transplantation CT demonstration. J Comput Assist Tomogr 6:507, 1982.

148. Bernardino ME, de Santos LA, Johnson DE, Bracken RB: Computed tomography in the evaluation of postnephrectomy patients. Radiology 130:183, 1979.

149. Alter AJ, Vehling DT, Zwiebel WJ: Computed tomography of the retroperitoneum following nephrectomy. Radiology 133:663, 1979.

150. Kittredge RD, Brensilver J, Pierce JC: Computed tomography in renal transplants. Radiology 127:165, 1978.

151. Nakstad P, Kilmannskog F, Kolbenstvedt A, Sodal G: Computed tomography in surgical complications following renal transplant. J Comput Assist Tomogr 6:286, 1982.

152. Nicholson RL: Renal transplant with secondary hyperparathyroidism. CT/T Clinical Symposium, vol 2, No 12. Milwaukee, General Electric Company, 1979.

16 COMPUTED TOMOGRAPHY OF THE ADRENAL GLANDS

Albert A. Moss

Conventional radiologic diagnostic examinations of the adrenal glands are frequently difficult and often unsuccessful. Plain abdominal roentgenography can detect adrenal calcification and large noncalcified adrenal neoplasms but has proved to be an insensitive method of demonstrating the majority of adrenal abnormalities.[1] Excretory urography is useful only when the adrenal gland becomes enlarged enough to displace the kidney[2] and even when excretory urography is combined with nephrotomography, adrenal masses less than 2.5 cm in diameter are usually undetectable.[3, 4] Conventional radiographic examinations are less than 70 per cent accurate in locating adrenal neoplasms,[4] and even when an adrenal mass is detected, its nature, extent, and relationship to surrounding organs usually cannot be characterized.

Radiologic techniques such as retroperitoneal pneumography,[5] adrenal angiography, and venography[6–8] are too invasive to be used as screening procedures. In addition, the technical difficulty, cost, and potential risk of adrenal hemorrhage or infarction are significant limitations.[9, 10]

Adrenal scintigraphy with ^{131}I-labeled iodocholesterol or [6B-^{131}I] iodomethyl-19-norcholes-5-(10)-en-3B-ol (NP-59) is useful for localizing functioning adrenal cortical neoplasms, but the examination takes up to 3 weeks to complete and requires a relatively high radiation exposure.[11–13] The isotopic method is further limited by the availability of radiopharmaceuticals and poor spatial resolution resulting from the limitations in dose required to avoid exposing the patient to excess radiation. Gray scale ultrasonography can delineate some normal-sized adrenal glands and most adrenal masses larger than 2 cm in diameter,[14–17] but obtaining and interpreting the ultrasonograms requires a high degree of technical proficiency.

Computed tomography (CT) can accurately display normal adrenal glands and adrenal pathology.[18–28] Normal-sized adrenal glands can be delineated in 85 to 99 per cent of patients.[18, 19, 21] Most adrenal tumors larger than 1.0 cm in diameter, and some as small as 0.5 cm, can be detected.[3, 22, 25, 26] In a comparison of CT and ultrasound for adrenal imaging, overall CT sensitivity

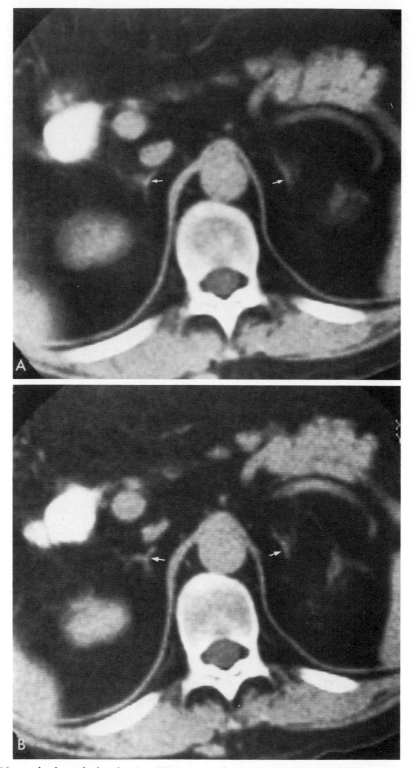

Figure 16–1. Normal adrenal glands. **A**   CT scan performed with 10-mm thick section clearly displays both adrenal glands (arrows). **B**   A 5-mm thick section at the same level gives slightly improved resolution. The margins of the adrenal glands are sharper, and individual limbs of the adrenal glands more clearly delineated (arrows). Both images are magnified 1.8 times.

was 84 per cent, specificity 98 per cent, and accuracy 90 per cent, compared with an ultrasound sensitivity of 79 per cent, specificity of 61 per cent, and accuracy of 70 per cent. Because of its greater overall accuracy in many centers, CT is the imaging procedure of choice for evaluating patients with suspected adrenal abnormalities.

TECHNIQUES OF EXAMINATION

The diagnostic accuracy of adrenal CT scanning is highest when meticulous attention to CT technique is coupled with a thorough understanding of the tomographic appearance of the normal adrenal glands and the alterations produced by adrenal pathology.

All adult patients are given 480 to 750 ml of a 1 to 2 per cent solution of sodium diatrizoate 30 minutes before CT scanning and another 240 ml of the same solution 5 minutes before scanning. This regimen identifies both the small bowel and duodenum and thus permits the adrenal glands to be easily differentiated from adjacent bowel. Pediatric patients are given a volume of 1 to 2 per cent sodium diatrizoate solution commensurate with their age and weight. If the CT scanner has a scan time greater than 6 seconds, a hypotonic agent should be administered to reduce artifacts caused by intestinal motility. Glucagon (0.5 mg) administered intravenously produces a marked hypotonic effect with low toxicity. Its duration action (5 to 10 minutes) is long enough to enable the study to be completed but brief enough to avoid the complications of longer-acting hypotonic agents. If bowel paralysis is required in patients with a suspected pheochromocytoma, propantheline bromide should be used because glucagon can precipitate a hypertensive crisis.

CT scans of the adrenal glands are performed using the small or medium calibration fields with the patient supine and the CT gantry at 0° angulation. Technical factors are chosen to ensure maximal spatial resolution without excessive radiation exposure. Spatial resolution with 3- to 5-mm-thick CT sections is slightly superior to those with sections 8 to 10 mm thick (Fig. 16–1). Contiguous nonoverlapping CT scans are usually sufficient, but the distance between scans should not be greater than 1 cm, even if the slice thickness is more than 1 cm. To ensure that the entire adrenal gland has been imaged, CT scans should encompass at least 1 cm above and below each adrenal gland.

The majority of patients can be scanned satisfactorily without intravenous administration of contrast material. Occasionally, in patients with a paucity of retroperitoneal fat, the CT scan may have to be repeated after intravenous administration of contrast material to distinguish the adrenal gland from adjacent vessels, the upper pole of the kidney, the liver, and/or pancreas.[29] A rapid infusion of 150 ml of 30 to 60 per cent meglumine diatrizoate usually allows the adrenal gland to be clearly delineated from adjacent structures. An intravenous bolus of 50 to 80 ml of 60 per cent meglumine diatrizoate is sometimes useful for opacifying adjacent vessels (Fig. 16–2).

Reformatting the axial CT images into coronal, sagittal, or oblique configurations gives additional anatomic information (Fig. 16–3) but is helpful only in a small percentage of patients. In certain patients, ultrathin CT sections (1.5 to 2 mm thick) can delineate subtle adrenal abnormalities, but routine use of ultrathin sections has not proved necessary.

Adrenal images are displayed at a moderately wide window (300 to 400 Hounsfield Units [H]) and an appropriate soft-tissue level (40 to 80 H). A 1.2- to 2-fold magnification makes it easier to view the adrenal glands and to determine contour abnormalities (Fig. 16–4). Scanning the adrenal glands using a limited field of reconstruction permits enlarged adrenal images to be obtained without sacrifice of spatial resolution.

ANATOMY

Each adrenal gland lies within Gerota's fascia in the perinephric space, embedded in adipose tissue and surrounded by a tough fibroelastic tissue capsule that penetrates the cortex and divides the gland into distinct columns.[30] Each adrenal gland has a thick cortex and a medulla of chromaffin tissue. The overall cortical/medulla ratio is 9:1 but varies from 5:1 in the head, to 15:1 in the body, to infinity in the tail.[31] The upper pole of each adrenal gland is firmly anchored to the top portion of Gerota's fascia by fibrous bands.

LOCATION
Right Adrenal Gland

The right adrenal gland is located just dorsal to the inferior vena cava at the level of its intra- and extrahepatic portions (Fig. 16–5A). The body of the gland extends dorsally and slightly laterally for several millimeters along its long axis. The right adrenal vein is very short and drains directly into the inferior vena cava. Laterally, the gland is separated from the posteromedial portion of the right lobe of the liver only by a variable amount of retroperitoneal fat. Medially, the crus of the

right diaphragm runs a course roughly parallel to the medial border of the gland.

Most right adrenal glands are positioned cephalad to the upper pole of the right kidney; the most caudal extent of the right adrenal gland is always cephalad to the renal vessels. The gland is usually 0 to 0.5 cm lateral to the vertebral body and between 0.5 cm posterior and 1 cm anterior

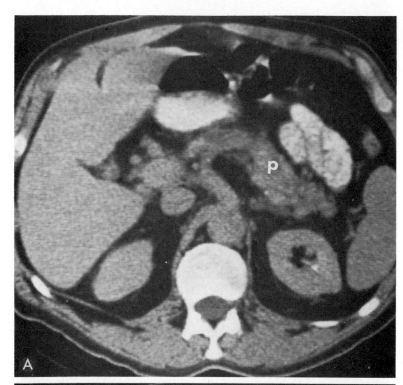

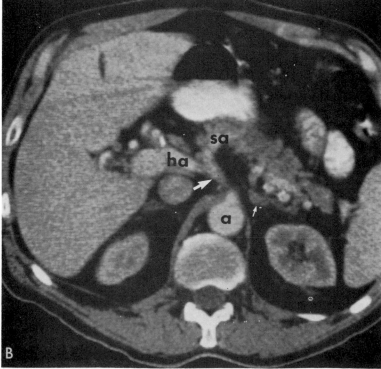

Figure 16–2. A CT scan performed after a contrast infusion demonstrates the tail of the pancreas (p), but the left adrenal cannot be absolutely separated from splenic vessels. **B** CT scan after bolus injection of contrast material showing opacified aorta (a), celiac axis (large arrow), hepatic artery (ha), and splenic artery (sa). The left adrenal (small arrow) is now clearly identified dorsal to the splenic vessels.

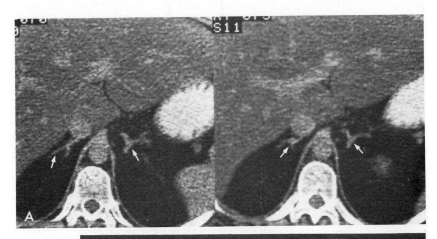

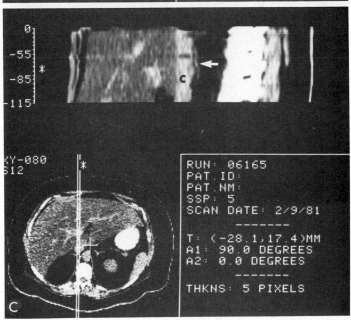

Figure 16–3. Normal adrenal glands. **A** Axial CT scans through level of both adrenal glands (arrows). Scans are 5 mm apart. **B,C** Plane of reformation of axial scan into coronal **B** or sagittal **C** images is indicated by parallel lines. Both limbs of each adrenal gland (arrows) are shown on the coronal reformation; on the sagittal reformation the right adrenal gland (arrow) is shown as a linear structure just dorsal to the inferior vena cava (c).

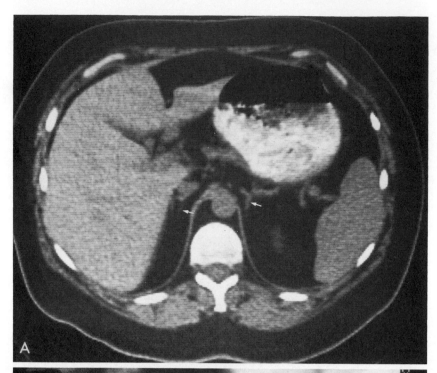

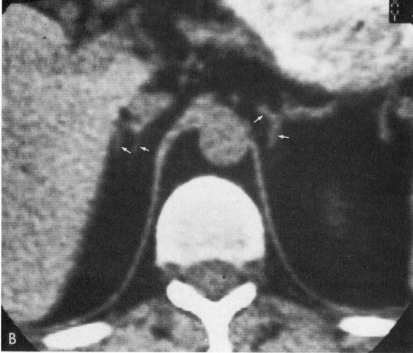

Figure 16–4. Normal adrenal glands. **A** Nonmagnified 5-mm-thick CT scan demonstrates both the right and left adrenal glands (arrows). **B** Same CT section magnified two-fold permits easier viewing of the adrenals and allows the contour of the individual adrenal limbs (arrows) to be better appreciated.

to the anterior vertebral body tangent.[18] Either limb of the right adrenal gland can extend to the dorsal margin of the vertebral body.

Left Adrenal Gland

The medial portion of the left adrenal gland is lateral to the crus of the left diaphragm, but its course may not be as parallel to the diaphragm as the medial limb of the right adrenal gland. Ninety-four per cent of left adrenal glands are anterior to the anterior vertebral margin (Fig. 16–5), and virtually all are posterior to the anterior aortic tangent.[18] The lower portion of the left adrenal gland and the superior pole of the left kidney are usually seen on the same CT section (Fig. 16–5A) because the base of the left adrenal touches the left kidney.[30] The upper margin of

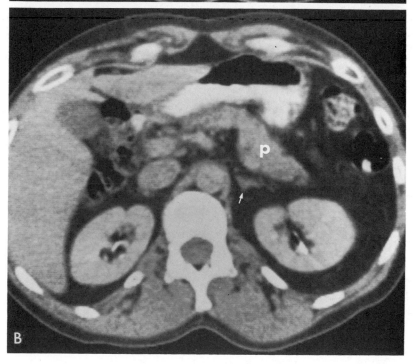

Figure 16.5. Normal position of adrenal glands. **A** Normal location of right adrenal gland (arrow) is just dorsal to the inferior vena cava (c). Retroperitoneal fat separates the medial margin of the liver from the right adrenal gland. The right adrenal gland lies above the upper pole of the right kidney and courses parallel to the crus of the diaphragm (curved arrow). The left adrenal gland (arrow) is usually seen on the same section as the upper pole of the left kidney (k) and is closely related to the dorsal margin of the stomach. **B** The left adrenal gland (arrow) is positioned just dorsal to the tail of the pancreas (p).

the right adrenal is cephalad to (34 per cent), at the same level (51 per cent) or lower than (15 per cent) the upper pole of the left adrenal.[19] The lower pole of the left gland is also cephalad to the renal vessels, but because the left adrenal arteries are shorter than the right, it is closer than the right adrenal to the aorta and renal vascular pedicle.

The tail of the pancreas is located anterior and/ or slightly lateral to the left adrenal gland (Fig. 16–5B). The tail of the pancreas is seen on at least one section with the left adrenal gland in more than 95 per cent of patients[18] and serves as a good marker for identification of the left gland. The splenic vessels are just dorsal to the lateral limb of the left adrenal (Fig. 16–2). The most cephalad

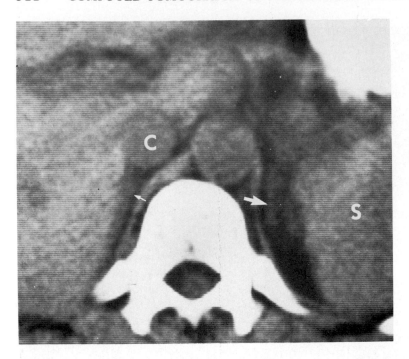

Figure 16–6. CT scan in patient with congenitally absent left kidney reveals the left adrenal gland to be in its normal position and to have normal shape (large arrow). The spleen (S), inferior vena cava (C), and right adrenal gland (small arrow) are in normal position.

portion of the left adrenal is related to the dorsal border of the stomach (Fig. 16–5A).[30]

The location of the adrenal glands is constant. Adrenal ectopia is extremely rare, and even in patients with renal ectopia or other congenital renal abnormalities, the adrenal glands are found in their expected positions (Fig. 16–6).[31]

MORPHOLOGY

Right Adrenal Gland

The right adrenal gland has a variety of cross-sectional configurations (Figs. 16–7 and 16–8). CT usually depicts the right adrenal as linear, with a course parallel to the diaphragmatic crura.

High-resolution CT scanners often show the body of the right adrenal split into medial and lateral limbs, giving it an inverted V shape. The lateral limb is frequently shorter than the medial limb; it usually courses parallel to the medial limb but may be directed laterally at a right angle from the body of the adrenal gland. The right adrenal gland can also appear as a horizontal linear structure or have a K-shaped configuration.

Left Adrenal Gland

The shape of the left adrenal also varies considerably (Figs. 16–7 and 16–8). Most frequently, it has an inverted V or Y shape but can appear lin-

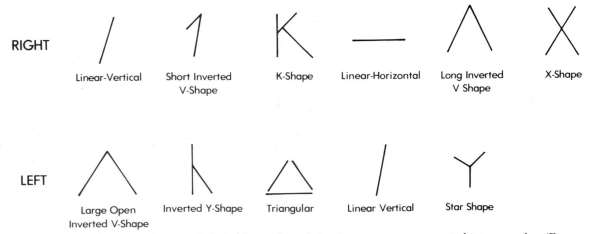

Figure 16–7. Diagram of some of the various adrenal shapes as seen on computed tomography. (From Moss AA: CT of the adrenal glands. In Ney C, Friedenberg RM (eds): Radiographic Altas of the Genitourinary System. Philadelphia, JB Lippincott, 1981.)

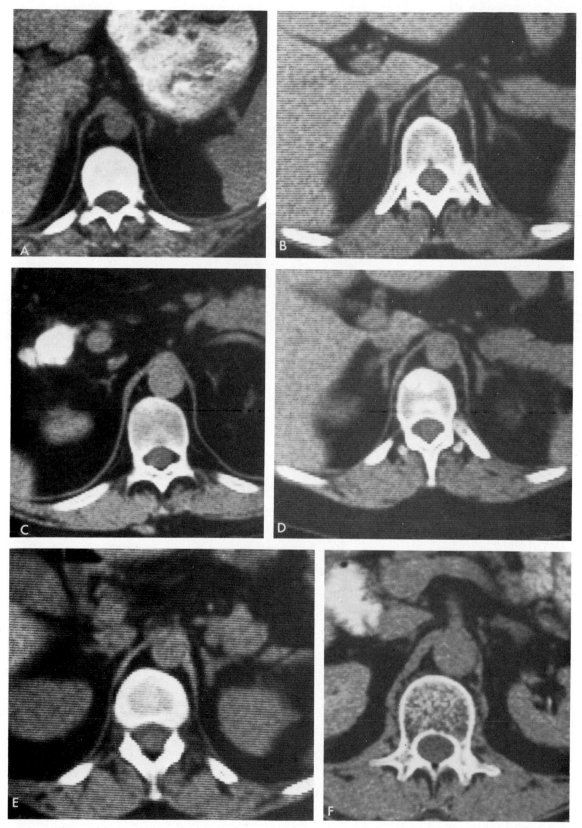

Figure 16–8. A–F   A range of different shapes of the adrenal glands demonstrated in different patients by computed tomography.

ear, triangular, crescentic, or V-shaped. The body of the left adrenal usually splits at an acute angle into medial and lateral limbs of equal length. When the limbs are of unequal length, the lateral limb is usually longer.

Because of the polymorphic shape of the adrenal glands and the differences in rotation about the longitudinal or transverse axis, the CT appearance of each adrenal gland varies, depending on the level of the CT section (Fig. 16–9).[21] When either kidney is congenitally absent, the adrenal gland on the affected side may be more rounded.[31] The margins of almost all normal adrenal glands are smooth, although accessory cortical bodies[18] can give a normal gland a slightly nodular configuration.

SIZE

Adrenal length, width, and thickness can be measured according to the method of Montagne and colleagues.[19] The length of each gland is determined by counting the number of contiguous

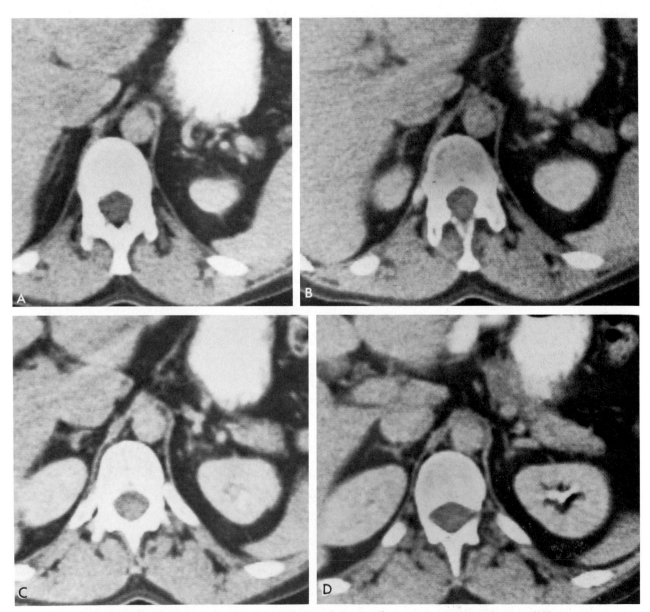

Figure 16–9. A–E   Variation in the shape of the adrenal glands in the same patient at different scan levels. Each scan is 5 mm caudal to the prior scan. The right adrenal gland goes through a dramatic configuration change, from a long inverted V shape with a very long medial limb **(A)** to a horizontal branching structure **(D)** and then to a horizontal linear shape **(E)**. The left adrenal changes from a horizontal linear configuration **(A)** to a star **(C)** and then seagull shape **(E)**.

Illustration continued on opposite page

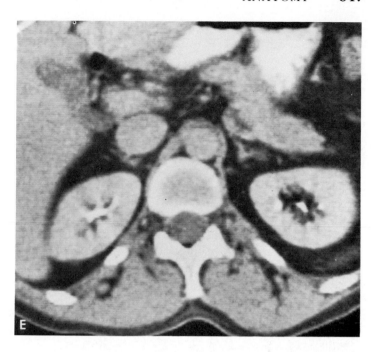

Figure 16–9. *Continued*

CT scans in which the gland is identified. The thickness of the adrenal gland is the greatest dimension perpendicular to the long axis of the gland or one of its limbs (Fig. 16–10A). The greatest thickness is usually at the junction of the adrenal body with its medial and lateral limbs. The width is measured by determining the greatest ventral-dorsal dimension of the gland (Fig. 16–10B).

Montagne and colleagues[10] found that 92 per cent of right and 96 per cent of left adrenal glands were 2 to 3.5 cm long. However, length measurements should be considered approximate because the length of the adrenal glands is difficult to measure accurately, since the cephalad and caudal extent of each gland is affected by partial volume averaging. Although 75 per cent of right and 80 per cent of left adrenal glands are 2.0 to 2.5 cm wide, great variations exist from patient to patient, and adrenal glands greater than 3 cm can be normal.[19]

Except for triangular left adrenal glands, the

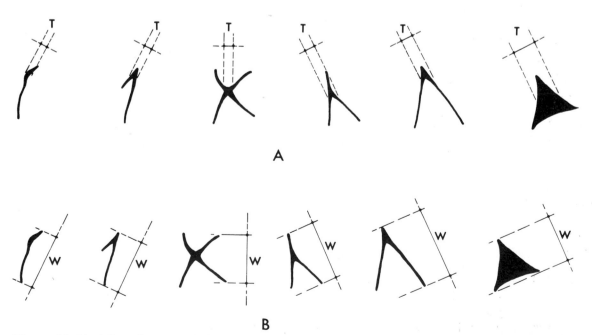

Figure 16–10. A,B   Diagrams of the method of measuring adrenal thickness (**A**) and width (**B**).

Table 16–1. CORRELATION OF ADRENAL CT MEASUREMENTS WITH PATHOLOGIC SPECIMENS

Author	Method	Adrenal Measurements		
		Length	Width	Thickness
Montagne et al.[19]	CT	2–4 cm	1–3 cm	0.5–1.0 cm
Meschan et al.[30]	Pathology	3–5 cm	3 cm	1.0–2.0 cm
Herbut et al.[32]	Pathology	3–5 cm	2–4 cm	0.4–0.6 cm
Soffer et al.[33]	Pathology	4–6 cm	2–3 cm	0.2–0.8 cm

thickness of each adrenal gland is usually 1.0 cm or less, with the left adrenal gland frequently being slightly thicker than the right. Measurement of adrenal thickness is frequently difficult. However, the thickness of the adrenal glands can be readily compared with the thickness of the diaphragmatic crus. In most instances, the adrenal gland will be no thicker than the maximal thickness of the crura at the same level on the side of the gland being evaluated (Figs. 16–1, 16–3, 16–5, 16–8, and 16–9).

The measurements of the adrenal gland size determined by CT are in agreement with measurements of pathologic specimens[19, 30, 32, 33] (Table 16–1) and indicate that CT is an accurate method of quantitating adrenal size and volume.

PATHOLOGY

CORTICAL ABNORMALITIES

Cushing's Syndrome

Patients with Cushing's syndrome have a constellation of symptoms and physical findings produced by continued exposure to elevated plasma corticosteroid levels. Patients have truncal and facial obesity with thin extremities (centripetal obesity), hypertension, purple striae, oligomenorrhea or amenorrhea, easy bruisability, acne, and weakness.[33] Biochemical studies confirm the diagnosis by documenting an absence of corticosteroid response to insulin-induced hypoglycemia, loss of normal corticosteroid circadian rhythm, and resistance to corticosteroid suppression by a low dose of dexamethasone.[34] Cushing's syndrome is three to four times more common in females than in males and occurs most frequently between the ages of 25 and 35 years.[35]

Cushing's syndrome can be produced by adrenocortical hyperplasia as a result of excessive pituitary adrenocorticotropic hormone (ACTH) or excess ACTH from ectopic nonendocrine tumors, adrenal neoplasm, nodular hyperplasia, or as a result of administration of ACTH or glucocorticoid medication. It is essential to separate patients with Cushing's syndrome that is the result of an adrenal neoplasm from those in whom it is due to an excessive ACTH production. Biochemical studies can be used to make this distinction, but the results can be equivocal.

A benign adrenal cortical adenoma is found in 10 to 15 per cent of patients with Cushing's syndrome (Figs. 16–11 and 16–12) and adrenal carcinoma in approximately 5 per cent (Fig. 16–13).[36] In less than 10 per cent of patients, the adenoma is bilateral. On CT scans the majority of functioning adrenal neoplasms appear as solid mass lesions ranging from 2 to 10 cm in diameter. The distinction between an adrenal adenoma and a carcinoma may not be possible unless metastatic disease or vascular extension of the neoplasm is demonstrated.[37] Intravenous administration of contrast material does not help distinguish benign from malignant adrenal neoplasia. The usual CT attenuation range of adrenal lesions is 30 to 50 H, but some adrenal cortical adenomas have lower attenuation values that are due to a high lipid content (Fig. 16–14),[3, 23, 38] and calcification has been demonstrated in both adrenal adenoma and carcinoma.[35]

In patients with Cushing's syndrome resulting from an overproduction of ACTH, the most frequent CT finding has been normal adrenal glands.[22] Diffuse, bilateral adrenal enlargement with preservation of shape is the second most frequently encountered finding of ACTH-dependent Cushing's syndrome (Fig. 16–15).[22] A nodular form of bilateral adrenal hyperplasia can be detected by identifying a nodule or nodules in a diffusely enlarged gland (Fig. 16–16A).[22, 39]

Pathologic studies have shown that some patients with ACTH-dependent Cushing's syndrome have adrenal glands that are grossly and histologically normal.[8, 40] This would explain the CT finding of "normal" adrenal glands in some patients with proven ACTH-dependent Cushing's syndrome. Although CT can never exclude a diagnosis of ACTH-dependent Cushing's disease, it can differentiate ACTH-dependent Cushing's syndrome from that due to an adrenal neoplasm in more than 90 per cent of cases.[3, 22, 23, 26, 27, 37, 39, 41–45]

Two associated CT findings in patients with

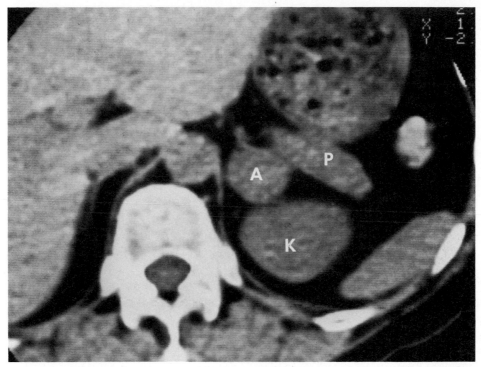

Figure 16–11. Cushing's syndrome. The CT scan demonstrates a solid left adrenal adenoma (A) 2 × 3 cm in size. The relationship of the adenoma to the kidney (K), pancreas (P), and aorta is clearly shown.

Cushing's syndrome are an abnormally low attenuation value of the liver resulting from hepatic fat deposition[43] and an increase in retroperitoneal and subcutaneous fat (Fig. 16–16A). CT usually does not demonstrate contralateral adrenal atrophy in patients with unilateral functioning adrenal neoplasms, but it can show the return of diffusely enlarged adrenal glands after pituitary surgery (Fig. 16–16B).

Primary Aldosteronism (Conn's Syndrome)

This condition results from excessive autonomous production of aldosterone[46] and is characterized by mild hypertension, hypokalemia, headache, sodium retention, and reduced or absent plasma renin.[25, 36] Primary aldosteronism is the cause of hypertension in approximately 1 per cent of patients with elevated blood pressure. Males are affected twice as frequently as females, and the patient's age at onset is usually between 30 and 50 years.[36]

Approximately 70 to 80 per cent of patients have a unilateral adrenal cortical adenoma, located twice as frequently on the right, which rarely exceeds 4 cm in diameter and is often less than 2 cm in greatest dimension.[25, 36, 47] Most of the remaining adult patients have idiopathic hy-

peraldosteronism that is due to nodular bilateral adrenocortical hyperplasia. In these patients, the adrenal glands may be slightly nodular and thickened or normal in size and shape.[40] In pediatric patients with primary aldosteronism, bilateral adrenocortical nodular hyperplasia is more common than functioning adenomas.[36] Carcinoma very rarely cause primary aldosternoism.[36]

The diagnosis of primary aldosteronism can be confirmed by an elevated rate of aldosterone secretion and a clinical response to spirolactone therapy. Patients with an adrenal adenoma tend to have higher urinary and plasma aldosterone levels, but biochemical distinction between adenoma and bilateral hyperplasia is often unclear.[25] Distinguishing patients who have an aldosterone-producing adenoma from those who have idiopathic hyperaldosteronism has important therapeutic implications. Resection of a solitary adenoma will restore normal aldosterone production and cure the patient's hypertension, but adrenal surgery, even bilateral adrenalectomy, may fail to affect the hypertension in patients with idiopathic hyperaldosteronism.[23, 26, 48]

The presence and location of an adenoma can be confirmed by arteriography,[6, 7, 49] venography,[8, 10, 49] adrenal venous sampling,[50] and adrenal

Text continued on page 856

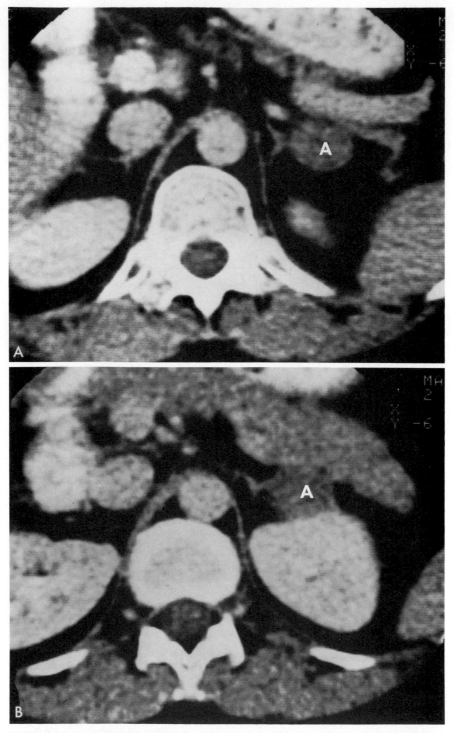

Figure 16–12. Cushing's syndrome—left adrenal adenoma. **A**   An adenoma (A) 2 × 3 cm in size arises from one limb of the left adrenal gland. **B**   On a scan at a lower level, the adenoma (A) cannot be separated from the pancreas or kidney.

Illustration continued on opposite page

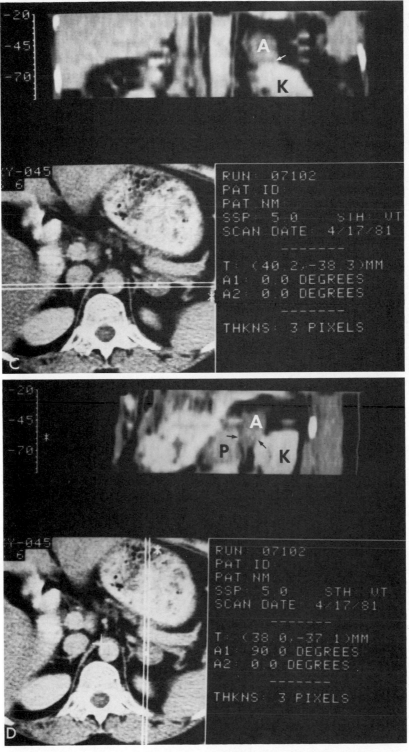

Figure 16–12. *Continued* **C,D**   Coronal (**C**) and sagittal (**D**) reformations show that a fat plane (arrows) separates the adenoma (A) from the upper pole of the kidney (K) and pancreas (P).

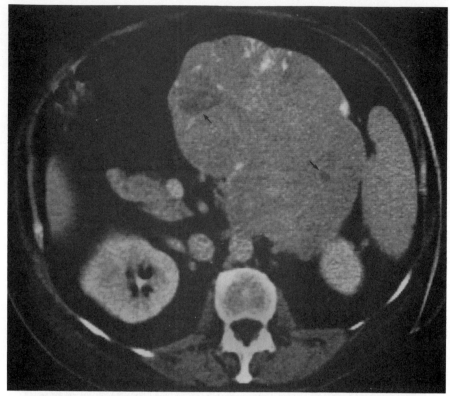

Figure 16–13. Cushing's syndrome from large adrenal carcinoma, which contains foci of calcification and areas of necrosis (arrows). (From Moss AA: CT of the adrenal glands. In Ney C, Friedenberg RM (eds): Radiographic Atlas of the Genitourinary System. Philadelphia, JB Lippincott, 1981.)

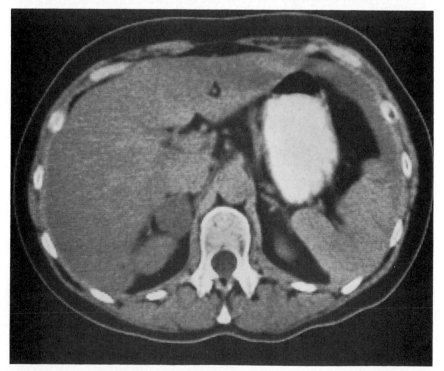

Figure 16–14. Solid right adrenal adenoma having an attenuation value of 18H due to a high fat content. Compare density of adenoma with that of the normal left adrenal gland, spleen, liver, and kidney. (From Moss AA: CT of the adrenal glands. In Ney C, Friedenberg RM (eds): Radiographic Atlas of the Genitourinary System. Philadelphia, JB Lippincott, 1981.)

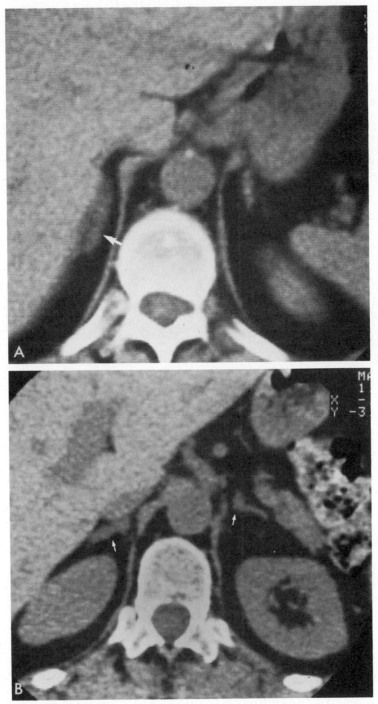

Figure 16–15. Cushing's syndrome secondary to overproduction of adrenocorticotropic hormone (ACTH). **A** CT scan at the level of the right adrenal gland. The right adrenal gland (arrow) is thickened but maintains a normal shape. Note the difference in size between the adrenal gland and diaphragmatic crus. **B** CT scan at a lower level shows both adrenal glands (arrows) to be diffusely enlarged.

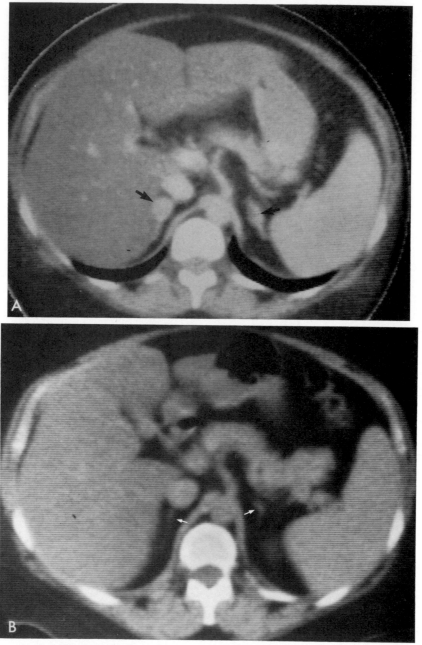

Figure 16–16. Cushing's disease from nodular adrenal gland hyperplasia. **A**   CT scan shows nodular masses (arrows) superimposed on enlarged adrenal glands. There is a excess of fat in the liver, permitting the hepatic vessels to be seen without contrast material. An excess of subcutaneous fat is also present. **B**   A CT scan 7 months after pituitary surgery reveals normal-sized adrenal glands (arrows) and less subcutaneous and hepatic fat.

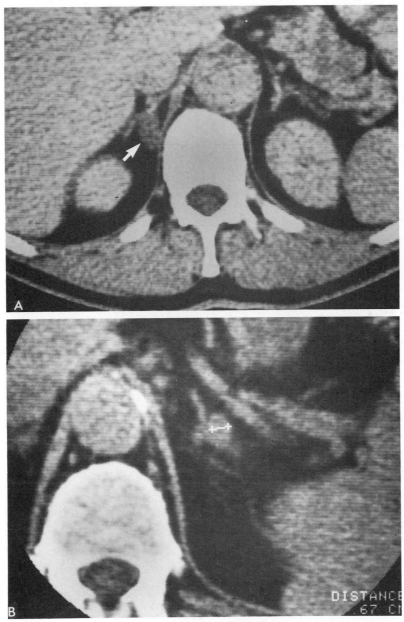

Figure 16–17. Aldosterone-producing adenomas. **A**   Small adenoma (arrow) arising from medial limb of right adrenal gland. **B**   An adenoma 0.67 cm in width arising from the lateral limb of left adrenal gland.

scintigraphy.[11–13] The angiographic procedures require technical expertise and all have some risk. Adrenal scintigraphy requires 4 to 20 days to complete, gives higher radiation exposure to the adrenal glands, and is limited by availability of the isotope.[11–13, 25, 51]

The risks and limitations of angiographic and radionuclide techniques have made CT the preferred initial imaging procedure in patients with hyperaldosteronism. CT usually shows a small, solid mass arising from one limb of the adrenal gland (Fig. 16–17). Adenomas as small as 0.5 cm in diameter can be identified with more than 83 per cent accuracy.[3, 22, 23, 25, 26, 32, 41–43, 47, 52] The size of adenomas measured by CT correlated well with measurements of surgical specimens.[25]

Because they contain as much as 5.1 per cent fat, aldosteronomas can have CT attenuation values significantly lower than those of adjacent organs (Fig. 16–18A),[23] whereas some aldosteronomas contain calcium and have higher attenuation values (Fig. 16–18B).[24] Intravenous administra-

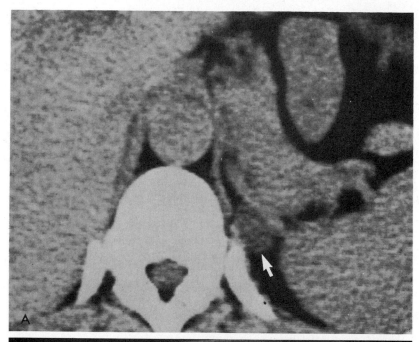

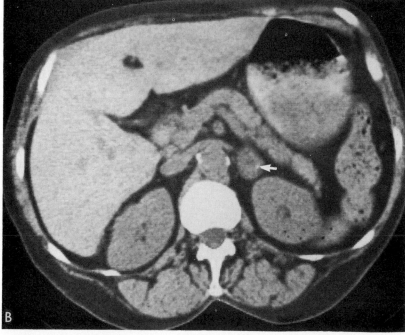

Figure 16–18. Variation in density of aldosteronomas. **A** Low-density left aldosteronoma (arrow) having high fat content. **B** High-density left aldosteronoma containing a focus of calcification (arrow).

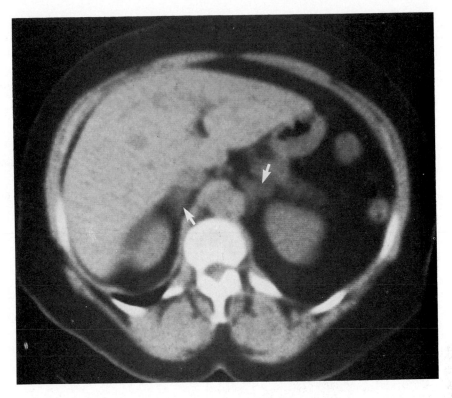

Figure 16–19. Bilaterally diffusely enlarged adrenal glands (arrows) in a patient with idiopathic hyperaldosteronism.

tion of contrast material usually does not greatly increase the attenuation value of the adenoma. Patients with idiopathic hyperaldosteronism have either diffusely thickened, slightly nodular, or normal adrenal glands (Fig. 16–19).[25] In more than 90 per cent of cases, CT can distinguish an aldosterone-producing adenoma from hyperplasia and thus determine the most effective mode of therapy.[25]

NONFUNCTIONING ADRENAL ADENOMA AND CARCINOMA

These are usually detected by CT as unilateral or bilateral solid mass lesions (Fig. 16–20). The adenoma is usually unilateral and less than 3 cm in diameter, whereas carcinomas are more frequently bilateral and larger. Adrenal carcinomas and adenomas usually grow slowly and can become extremely large before producing symptoms. Calcification is more common in carcinoma,[53] but adenomas can also contain calcium (Fig. 16–21). Frequently the CT features alone cannot distinguish whether a solid adrenal mass is benign or malignant unless there is evidence of metastatic disease or direct tumor extension into adjacent organs (Fig. 16–22).[37] Adrenal adenomas occur in 12 to 15 per cent of patients with renal cell carcinoma, compared with less than 2 to 3 per cent of the general population.[54]

It is usually not difficult to confirm whether a

mass is adrenal in origin by CT. However, when a right adrenal mass becomes very large, it may be difficult to determine from the axial CT scans alone whether the mass is hepatic, renal, or adrenal in origin. Reformatting the axial CT images into the coronal or sagittal plane may permit such a distinction to be made more easily (Fig. 16–23).

CT is useful in detecting recurrence of adrenal carcinoma after resection. In order not to confuse postoperative fibrosis and scarring with recurrent disease, CT scans are recommended 3 to 6 months after surgery as a baseline with which future CT scans may be compared.

MYELOLIPOMA AND ADENOLIPOMA

Myelolipomas are rare tumors (present in 0.8 per cent of autopsies)[55] of the adrenal cortex that contain varying proportions of bone marrow elements and fat.[13, 26, 27, 38, 55–58] Calcification occurs in approximately 20 per cent of cases.[39, 57] Adenolipomas are even rarer adrenal tumors composed predominantly of adipose tissue in which varying stages of degeneration, hemorrhage, fibrosis, and calcification are found.[44] Myelolipomas and adenolipomas seldom produce symptoms unless they become very large or undergo abrupt internal hemorrhage.

Myelolipomas and adenolipomas are readily detected by CT as well-circumscribed adrenal mass lesions that have attenuation values in the range

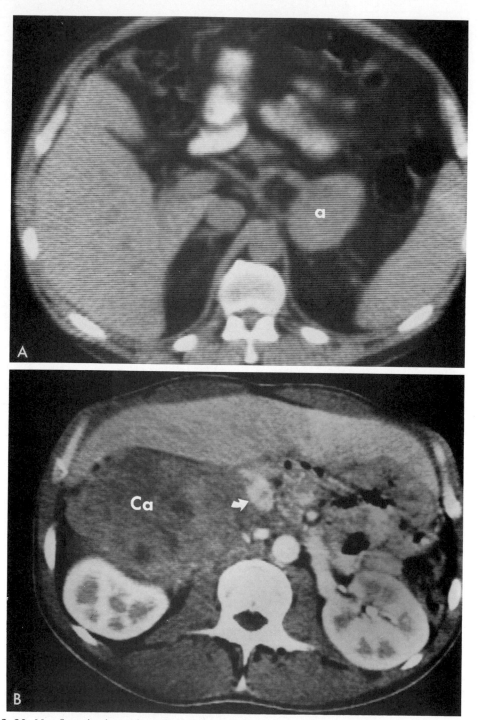

Figure 16–20. Nonfunctioning adrenal tumors. **A**   An asymptomatic left adrenal adenoma (a) measuring 5 × 6 cm. **B**   An enormous right adrenal carcinoma (Ca) displacing the right kidney, inferior vena cava (arrow), and liver. Scan was performed after bolus injection of contrast material. (From Moss AA: CT of the adrenal glands. In Ney C, Friedenberg (eds): Radiographic Atlas of the Genitourinary System. Philadelphia, JB Lippincott, 1981.)

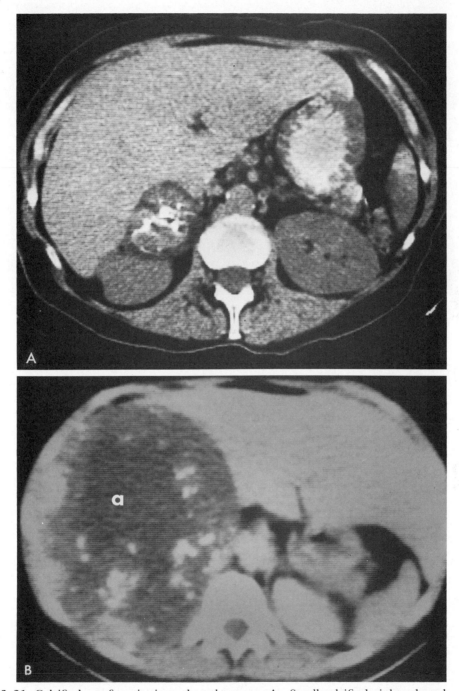

Figure 16–21. Calcified nonfunctioning adrenal tumors. **A** Small calcified right adrenal carcinoma. **B** Enormous, partially calcified right adrenal adenoma (a). (From Moss AA: CT of the adrenal glands. In Ney C, Friedenberg (eds): Radiographic Atlas of the Genitourinary System. Philadelphia, JB Lippincott, 1981.)

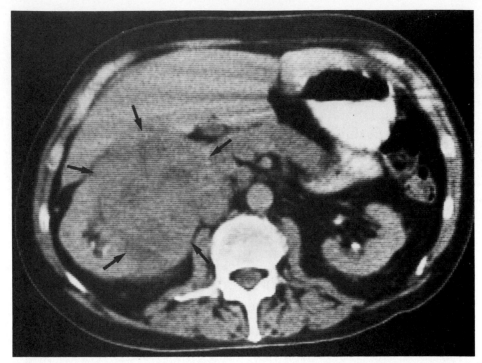

Figure 16–22. CT scan demonstrates a right adrenal carcinoma (arrows) which has invaded the right kidney.

of fat and frequently contain areas of calcification (Fig. 16–24). CT permits a specific diagnosis of a fat-containing adrenal tumor; however, this finding is not pathognomonic of a myolipoma or adenolipoma, as cortical adenomas and aldosteronomas can have low attenuation values as a result of their high fat content.[23, 44]

MEDULLARY ABNORMALITIES

Pheochromocytoma

Pheochromocytomas are tumors capable of secreting abnormal amounts of catecholamines. They are derived from chromaffin cell nests anywhere along the autonomic ganglia chain or from chromaffin bodies such as the adrenal medulla and organ of Zuckerkandl.[35, 36, 59–66] Paroxysmal attacks characterized by hypertension, diaphoresis, tachycardia, and anxiety are the most frequent clinical manifestations.[59] Pheochromocytomas are located in the adrenal glands in 90 per cent of cases but can arise anywhere along the axial skeleton from the base of the skull to the lower rectum.[61, 66, 67] Most pheochromocytomas are solitary and have a predilection for the right adrenal, but approximately 10 per cent are bilateral and 10 per cent are ectopic.[43, 60–63] In children, the right-to-left predominance increases to 2:1 and 20 per

cent are bilateral; multiple and ectopic locations are also much more common.[43] In patients with a suspected pheochromocytoma, CT usually rapidly and accurately confirms or excludes the diagnosis.

In 91 cases of proven pheochromocytoma evaluated by CT, the overall accuracy rate was 96 per cent.[3, 20, 22, 26, 31–43, 61–63, 65, 66, 68, 69] Most frequently, CT identified a unilateral adrenal mass with an attenuation of 16 to 70 H and a normal contralateral gland (Fig. 16–25). Pheochromocytomas are usually larger than 2 cm in diameter and may be entirely solid lesions, may contain both cystic and solid components, or may be almost entirely cystic; calcification is not common but does occur. Gross pathologic inspection of pheochromocytomas frequently reveals cystic areas, necrosis, and hemorrhage. Intravenous injection of contrast medium makes the nonhomogeneity of some pheochromocytomas more apparent and helps differentiate between a tumor and the inferior vena cava or kidney.

If the adrenal glands are normal despite strong clinical suspicion of pheochromocytoma, the rest of the abdomen and pelvis should be examined. The examination may be expanded to the neck and chest if the abdomen and pelvis are normal. The most common extra-adrenal location of a pheochromocytoma is in the organ of Zucker-

Text continued on page 865

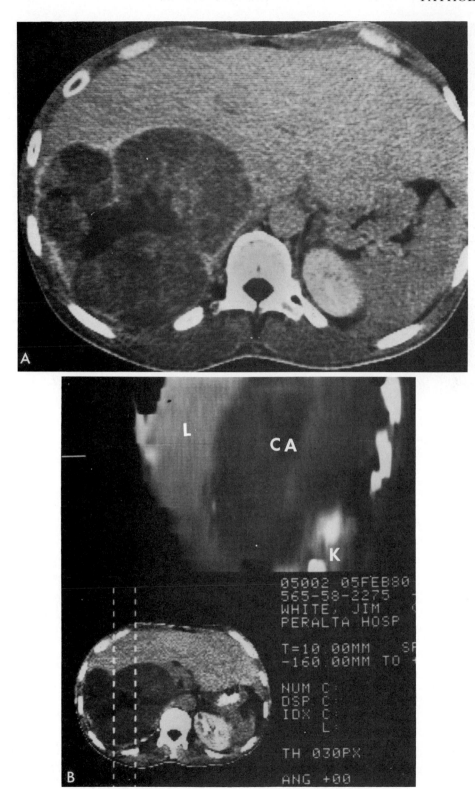

Figure 16–23. A Use of sagittal reformation to determine adrenal origin of a mass. An axial CT image reveals a large mass but it is difficult to determine whether the mass originates from the liver, adrenal gland, or kidney. **B** Sagittal reformation reveals the liver (L) to be displaced anteriorly by a large tumor mass (CA), which is anterior to the kidney (K) and extends up to the diaphragm. Adrenal carcinoma was found at surgery.

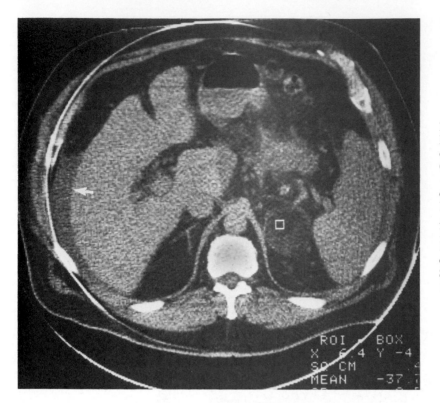

Figure 16–24. Myelolipoma of the left adrenal gland. A region-of-interest square reveals the mass to have a CT density of −37.7 H on a +500 to −500 H scale, indicating that considerable fat is present within the tumor. Note the normal right adrenal gland. Ascites is also present (arrow). (From Moss AA: CT of the adrenal glands. In Ney C, Friedenberg RM (eds): Radiographic Atlas of the Genitourinary System. Philadelphia, JB Lippincott, 1981.)

Figure 16–25. Right adrenal pheochromocytoma. **A** Nonhomogeneous pheochromocytoma (P), which had central necrosis at surgery.

Illustration continued on opposite page

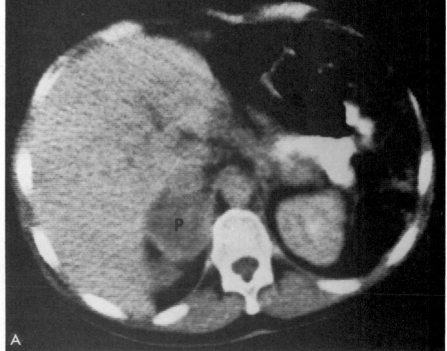

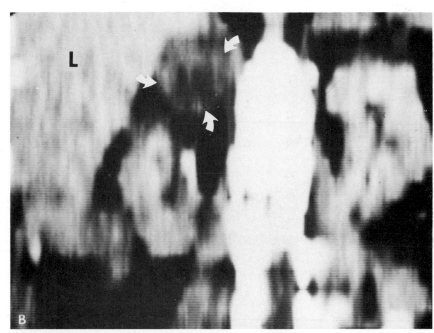

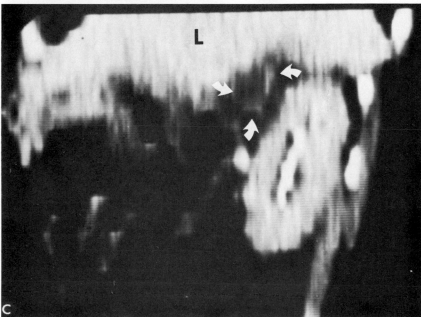

Figure 16–25. *Continued* Coronal **(B)** and sagittal **(C)** reformations of the same tumor show the pheochromocytoma (curved arrows) to be separate from the kidney and positioned just beneath the liver (L).

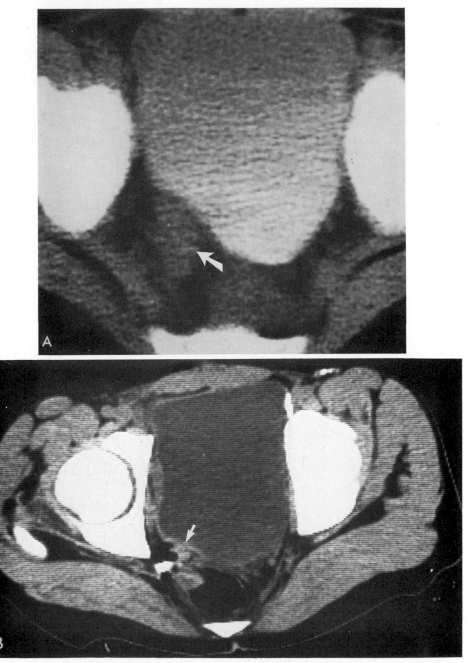

Figure 16–26. A Pheochromocytoma (arrow) arising in wall of bladder. (From Moss AA: CT of the adrenal glands. In Ney C, Friedenberg RM (eds): Radiographic Atlas of the Genitourinary System. Philadelphia, JB Lippincott, 1981.) **B** Repeat CT scan after surgery reveals a small residual pheochromocytoma (arrow) in the posterior portion of right bladder wall.

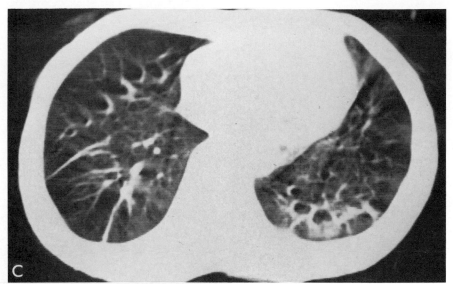

Figure 16–28 *Continued* **C** Diffuse pulmonary interstitial disease with bulla formation characteristic of neurofibromatosis is shown on the CT study of the lungs.

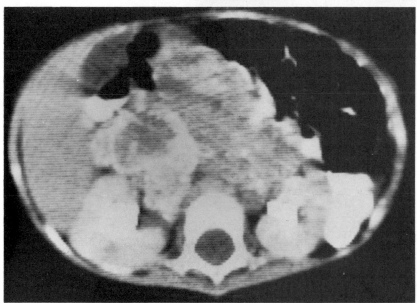

Figure 16–29. Neuroblastoma arising in right adrenal gland containing confluent as well as ringlike calcification.

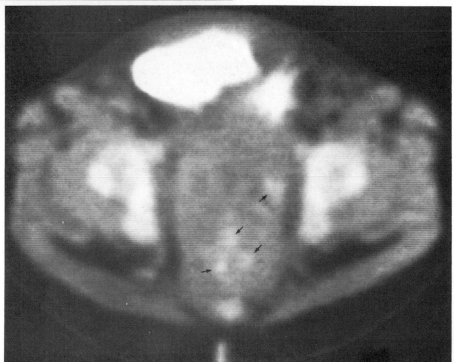

Figure 16–30. Pelvic neuroblastoma containing scattered areas of calcification (arrows). (Magnification 3×.)

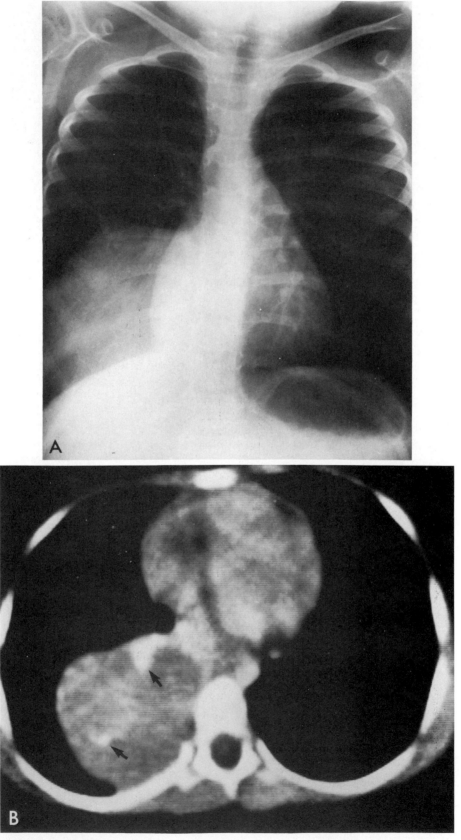

Figure 16–31. Supradiaphragmatic neuroblastoma. **A**   A chest radiograph shows a large, right-sided, noncalcified mass of undetermined etiology. **B**   An axial CT scan through the chest reveals the mass to contain areas of calcification (arrows), making neuroblastoma the most likely diagnosis.

Illustration continued on opposite page

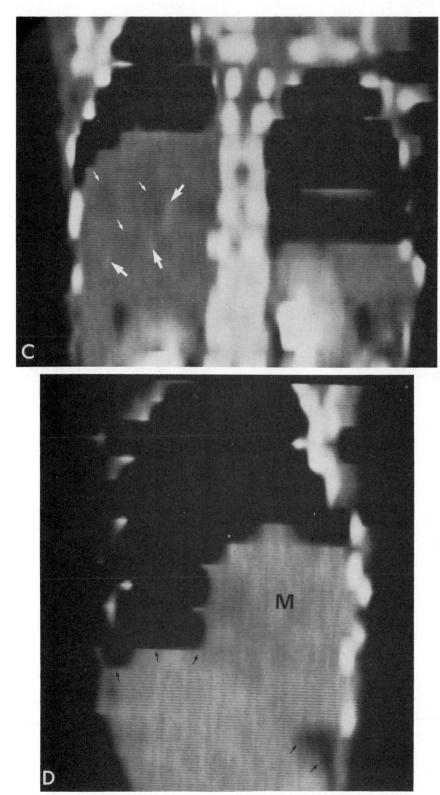

Figure 16–31. *Continued* **C**   Coronal reformation through the neuroblastoma demonstrates the mass to have calcified portions (large arrows) and areas of lower density (small arrows). **D**   Sagittal reformation confirms that the entire mass (M) is located above the diaphragm (arrows).

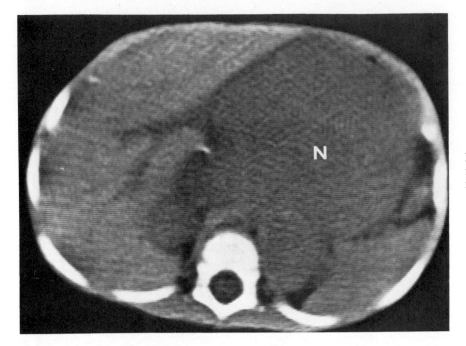

Figure 16–32. Large noncalcified neuroblastoma (N) displacing the liver.

and 60 to 75 per cent of patients have metastasis when initially seen.[71, 72] Skeletal, lymph node, and hepatic metastases are most common; pulmonary metastasis is present in only 11 per cent of patients at the initial diagnosis.[71] Plain abdominal radiography demonstrates a mass that has stippled, spiculated, solid, ringlike, or confluent calcification in only 50 per cent of neuroblastomas.[35, 72] CT readily detects calcification that is not readily apparent on conventional radiography (Fig. 16–31B,C).[72a] Neuroblastomas can also appear as solid, noncalcified masses of soft tissue or fatty density with or without cystic components (Figs. 16–32 and 16–33). Hepatic, skeletal, and pulmonary metastases are readily detected permitting CT to accurately stage primary neuroblastomas[72a] and detect recurrent disease (see Chapter 21).[72b, c]

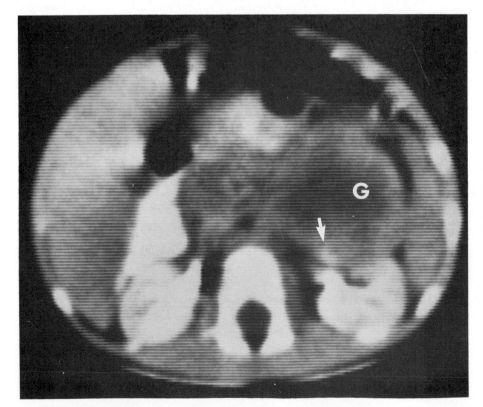

Figure 16–33. A ganglioneuroma (G) in a 5-year-old child has a central area of necrosis, a rim of higher density, and one focus (arrow) of calcification.

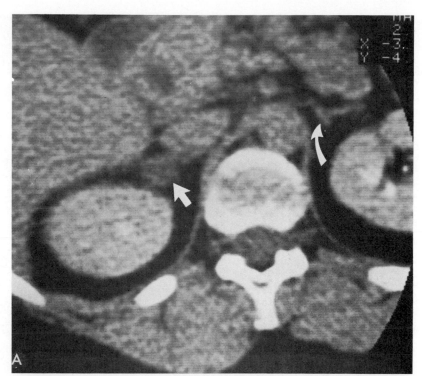

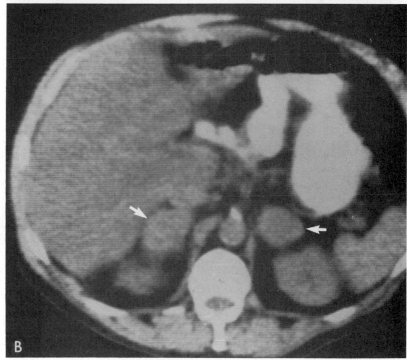

Figure 16–34. Adrenal metastases. **A** Unilateral right adrenal metastasis (arrow) from gastrin-producing tumor. Curved arrow = normal left adrenal gland. **B** Bilateral adrenal metastases (arrows) from primary lung carcinoma.

SECONDARY TUMORS

The adrenal glands are the fourth most frequent site of bloodborne metastatic disease. Metastasis from carcinoma of the lung is the most common, followed by carcinoma of the breast, thyroid, colon, and melanoma.[43, 53] Metastases produce circumscribed mass lesions in the adrenal gland that alter the gland's contour.[22, 27, 43, 53, 73, 74]

Metastases usually begin in the adrenal medulla and may be unilateral (Fig. 16–34A) but most often are bilateral (Fig. 16–34B). Metastases are usually relatively small (Fig. 16–34) but may reach enormous size (Fig. 16–35). The attenuation coefficient of the metastasis usually is close to or identical to that of the normal adrenal gland, but if tumor necrosis has occurred, the lesion may be nonhomogeneous or even cystic. Adrenal metas-

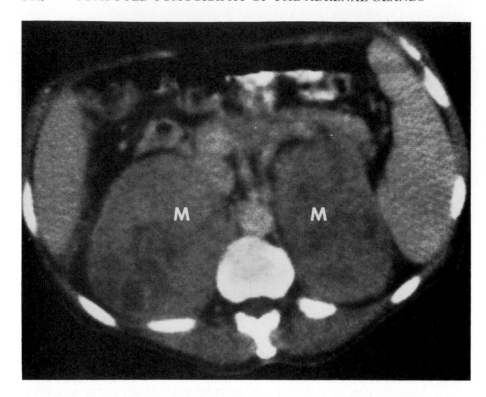

Figure 16–35. Enormous bilateral adrenal metastases (M) from a primary malignant melanoma. Areas of necrosis are scattered throughout both metastatic deposits. (From Moss AA: CT of the adrenal glands. In Ney C, Friedenberg RM (eds): Radiographic Atlas of the Genitourinary System. Philadelphia, JB Lippincott, 1981.)

tasis cannot be distinguished from nonfunctioning adrenal tumors by CT features alone. A CT-directed aspiration biopsy (Fig. 16–36) or a follow-up CT study in 3 to 6 months is recommended if it is critical to determine whether the adrenal mass is metastatic.[75]

Frequently, metastases to the liver, lungs, or bones will be present when adrenal metastasis has occurred. Adrenal metastases usually produce no symptoms and most adrenal metastases are detected when CT is performed to assess another clinical problem.[75a] However, rarely a clinical pic-

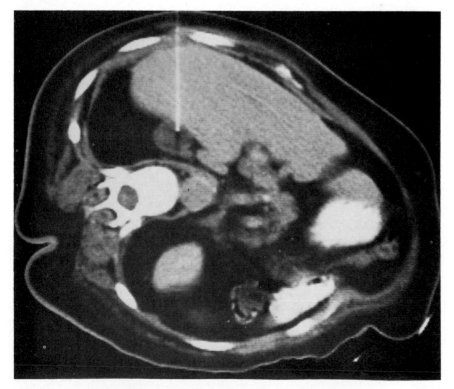

Figure 16–36. A CT-directed aspiration needle biopsy of a right adrenal mass which proved to be metastatic vulvar carcinoma. The patient was placed in the decubitus position, and the 22-gauge needle was passed through the liver to avoid traversing the pleura.

ture of hypoadrenalism will be produced by adrenal metastasis, usually by carcinoma of the lung.[43] It is important to evaluate all patients with idiopathic hypoadrenalism to exclude metastatic disease as the etiologic factor. Retroperitoneal and lymphomatous tumors can directly infiltrate the adrenal glands by local extension. When this occurs, it may be difficult to identify the origin of the primary tumor.

UNUSUAL PRIMARY TUMORS

Tumors can originate from any of the cellular components of the adrenal gland. Benign tumors such as lymphangiomas, hemangiomas, fibromas, neurofibromas, myomas, and hamartomas, as well as malignant degeneration of these tumors, can occur.[27, 35, 36, 43, 76] The CT appearance of these lesions has not been described since they all are extremely rare, and most are discovered incidentally at autopsy.

ADRENAL CYSTS

Adrenal cysts can be classified as parasitic, epithelial, endothelial (lymphangiectatic, angiomatous, and hamartomatous), and pseudocystic, resulting from degenerative necrosis and hemorrhage into an adrenal mass.[27, 35] Pseudocysts and lymphangiectatic cysts are the most common. Cysts range from small to very large, are usually unilat-

eral (85 per cent), and produce few symptoms. Adrenal cysts typically produce a rounded, low density mass within the adrenal gland; a rim of calcification is present in 15 per cent of cases (Fig. 16–37).[77, 78] The diagnosis of an adrenal cyst can be confirmed by surgery or by cyst puncture and aspiration under CT guidance.

MISCELLANEOUS ABNORMALITIES

Hypoadrenalism

Hypoadrenalism has not been widely investigated by CT. Small to normal-sized adrenal glands can be seen by CT in patients with hypoadrenalism secondary to pituitary irradiation or long-term steroid therapy.[22] In patients with acute hypoadrenalism secondary to adrenal hemorrhage, CT has demonstrated bilaterally enlarged adrenal glands that have a normal shape (Fig. 16–38).[79]

Infections

Various infections can affect the adrenal glands.[27, 35] Tuberculosis,[80] histoplasmosis, meningococcus, and infection caused by *Echinococcus* are the most frequent. Infection may result in adrenal calcification (Fig. 16–39), solid enlargement, or cystic masses. The CT findings are nonspecific, and the final diagnosis depends on biopsy or correlation with clinical course.

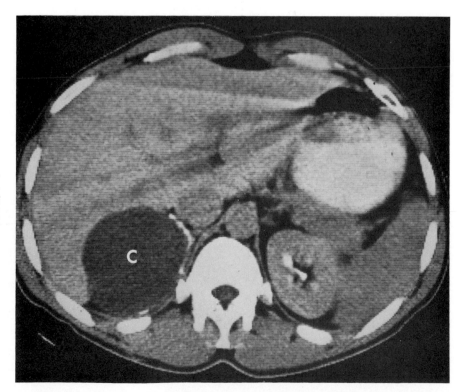

Figure 16–37. A large right adrenal cyst (C). The cyst has a uniform density close to that of water and a partially calcified rim.

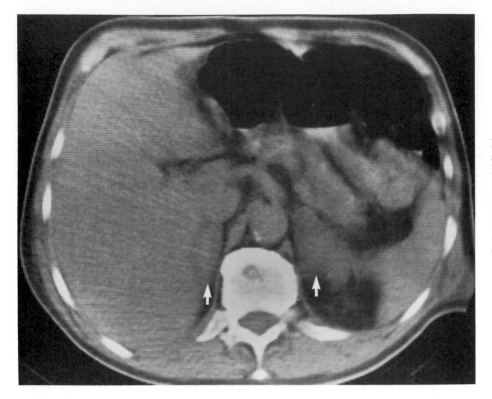

Figure 16–38. Acute hypoadrenalism secondary to bilateral adrenal hemorrhage in a patient with a hematologic disorder. Both adrenal glands (arrows) are diffusely enlarged but maintain a relatively normal linear configuration.

Acromegaly

The adrenal glands in acromegalic patients are larger than normal, but their shape and function are normal.

Hemochromatosis

The adrenal glands are frequently involved in hemochromatosis. The excessive deposition of iron in the adrenal glands is seldom seen by CT,

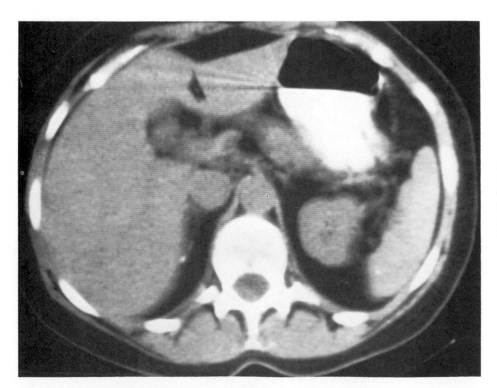

Figure 16–39. Histoplasmosis producing linear calcification in the right adrenal gland. A calcified granuloma is also present in the spleen.

but in patients with severe hemochromatosis the adrenal gland attenuation value may be greater than normal. The attenuation value of the liver and spleen will also be increased.

REFERENCES

1. McAlister WH, Lester PD: Diseases of the adrenal. Med Radiogr Photogr 47:62, 1971.
2. Lang EK: Roentgenographic diagnosis of suprarenal masses. Radiology 87:35, 1966.
3. Karstaedt N, Sagel SS, Stanley RJ, Melson GL, Levitt RG: Computed tomography of the adrenal gland. Radiology 129:723, 1978.
4. Pickering RS, Hartman GW, Week RE, Sheps SG, Hattery RR: Excretory urographic localization of adrenal cortical tumors and pheochromocytomas. Radiology 114:345, 1975.
5. Steinbach HL, Smith KL: Extraperitoneal pneumography in diagnosis of retroperitoneal tumors. Arch Surg 70:161, 1955.
6. Kahn PC, Nickrosz LV: Selective angiography of the adrenal glands. AJR 101:739, 1967.
7. Alfidi RJ, Gili WM Jr, Klein HJ: Arteriography of adrenal neoplasms AJR 106:635, 1969.
8. Mitty HA, Nicolis GL, Gabrilove JL: Adrenal venography: Clinical roentgenographic correlation in 80 patients. AJR 119:564, 1973.
9. Gold RE, Wisinger BM, Geraci AR, Heinz LM: Hypertensive crisis as a result of venography in a patient with pheochromocytoma. Radiology 102:579, 1972.
10. Bookstein JJ, Conn J, Reuter SR: Intraadrenal hemorrhage as a complication of adrenal venography in primary adosteronism. Radiology 90:778, 1968.
11. Troncone L, Galli G, Salvo D, Barbareno A, Bonoma L: Radioisotopic study of the adrenal glands using ^{131}I-19 iodocholesterol. Br J Radiol 50:340, 1977.
12. Hogan MJ, McRae J, Scharmbelan M, Biglieri EG: Location of aldosterone producing adenomas with ^{131}I-19 iodocholesterol. N Engl J Med 294:410, 1976.
13. Miles IM, Wahner HW, Carpenter PC, Salassa RM, Northcutt RC: Adrenal scintiscanning with NP-59, a new radioiodinated cholesterol agent. Mayo Clin Proc 54:321, 1979.
14. Yeh HC, Mitty HA, Rose J, Wolf BS, Gabrilove JL: Ultrasonography of adrenal masses: Unusual manifestations. Radiology 127:475, 1978.
15. Sample WF: A new technique for the evaluation of the adrenal gland with Gray scale ultrasonography. Radiology 124:463, 1977.
16. Bernardino ME, Goldstein HM, Green B: Gray scale ultrasonography of adrenal neoplasms. AJR 130:741, 1978.
17. Yeh H-C: Sonography of the adrenal glands: Normal glands and small masses. AJR 135:1167, 1980.
18. Brownlie K, Kreel L: Computer-assisted tomography of normal suprarenal glands. J Comput Assist Tomogr 2:1, 1978.
19. Montagne J-P, Kressel HY, Korobkin M, Moss AA: Computed tomography of the normal adrenal glands. AJR 130:963, 1978.
20. Sample WF, Sarti D: Computed tomography and Gray scale ultrasonography of the adrenal gland: A comparative study. Radiology 128:377, 1978.
21. Wilms G., Baert A, Marchal G, Goddeeris P: Computed tomography of the normal adrenal glands: Correlative study with autopsy specimens. J Comput Assist Tomogr 3:467, 1979.
22. Korobkin M, White EA, Kressel HY, Moss AA, Montagne J-P: Computed tomography in the diagnosis of adrenal disease. AJR 132:231, 1979.
23. Schaner EG, Dunnick NR, Doppman JL, Strott CA, Gill JR Jr, Javadpour N: Adrenal cortical tumors with low attenuation coefficients: A pitfall in computed tomography diagnosis. J Comput Assist Tomogr 2:11, 1978.
24. Epstein AJ, Patel SK, Petasnick JP: Computerized tomography of the adrenal gland. JAMA 242:2791, 1979.
25. White EA, Schambelan M, Rost CR, Biglieri EG, Moss AA, Korobkin M: Use of computed tomography in diagnosing the cause of primary adosteronism. N Engl J Med 303:1503, 1980.
26. Eghrari M, McLoughlin MJ, Rosen IE, St. Louis EL, Wilson SR, Wise DJ, Yeung HPH: The role of computed tomography in assessment of tumoral pathology of the adrenal glands. J Comput Assist Tomogr 4;71, 1980.
27. Hauser H, Battikba JG, Wettstein P: Pathology of the adrenal glands: Common and uncommon feelings on computed tomography. Europ J Radiol 1:215, 1981.
28. Abrams HL, Siegelman SS, Adams DF, Sanders R, Finkerg HJ, Hessel SJ, McNeil BJ: Computed tomography versus ultrasound of the adrenal gland: A prospective study. Radiology 143:121, 1982.
29. Pillari G, Mandon V, Cruz V, Chen M: Foot vein contrast medium infusion useful in computed tomography of the right adrenal gland. J Comput Assist Tomogr 6:169, 1982.
30. Meschan I: Synopsis of Radiologic Anatomy with Computed Tomography. Philadelphia, WB Saunders Company, 1978, pp. 534–538.
31. Symington T: Functional Pathology of the Human Adrenal Gland. Edinburg, E & S Livingstone Ltd, 1969, pp 13–16.
32. Herbut PA: Urologic Pathology, vol 2. Philadelphia, Lea & Febiger, 1952, pp 693–696.
33. Soffer LS: Diseases of the Endocrine Glands. Philadelphia, Lea & Febiger, 1951, pp 163–164.
34. Besser GM, Edwards CRW: Cushing's syndrome. Clin Endocrinol Metab 1:451, 1972.
35. McAlister WH, Koehler PR: Diseases of the adrenal. Radiol Clin North Am 2:205, 1967.
36. Bethune JE: The Adrenal Cortex. Kalamazoo, Mich, Upjohn Company, 1974.
37. Dunnick NR, Doppman JL, Geelhoed GW: Intravenous extension of endocrine tumors. AJR 135:471, 1980.
38. Behan M, Martin EC, Muecke EC, Kazam E: Myelolipoma of the adrenal: Two cases with ultrasound and CT findings. AJR 129:993, 1977.
39. Federle MP, Moss AA: Adrenal Abnormalities. CT/T Clinical Symposium, vol 1, No 4. Milwaukee, General Electric Company, 1979.
40. Neville AM, MacKay AM: The structure of the human adrenal cortex in health and disease. Clin Endocrinol Metab 1:361, 1972.
41. Ganguly A, Prott JH, Yune HY, Grim CE, Weinberger MH: Detection of adrenal tumors by computerized tomographic scan in endocrine hypertension. Arch Intern Med 139:589, 1979.
42. Dunnick NR, Schancer EG, Doppman JL, Strott CA, Gill JR, Javadpour N: Computed tomography in adrenal tumors. AJR 132:43, 1979.

43. Reynes CJ, Churchill R, Moncada R, Love L: Computed tomography of adrenal glands. Radiol Clin of North Am 17:91, 1979.

44. Costello P, Clouse ME, Kane RA, Paris A: Problems in the diagnosis of adrenal tumors. Radiology 125:335, 1977.

45. Curtis JA, Brennan RE, Kurtz AB: Evaluation of adrenal disease by computed tomography. Comput Tomogr 4:165, 1980.

46. Conn JW, Cohen EL, Rouner DR: Suppression of plasma activity in primary adosteronism: Distinguishing primary from secondary aldosteronism in hypertensive disease. JAMA 190:213, 1964.

47. Linde R, Coulam C, Battino R, Rhamy R, Gerlock J, Hollifield J: Localization of aldosterone-producing adenoma by computed tomography. J Clin Endocrinol Metab 49:642, 1979.

48. Biglieri EG, Schambelan M, Brust N, Chang B, Hogan M: Plasma aldosterone concentration: Further characterization of aldosterone producing adenomas. Circ Res 34 (suppl I):I-183, 1974.

49. Kahn PC, Killeher MD, Egdahl RH, Melby JC: Adrenal arteriography and venography in primary aldosteronism. Radiology 101:71, 1971.

50. Melby JC, Spark RF, Dale SL, Egdahl RH, Kahn PC: Diagnosis and localization of aldosterone-producing adenomas by adrenal-vein catheterization. N Engl J Med 277:1050, 1967.

51. Conn JW, Morita R, Cohen EL, Beierwaltes WH, MacDonald WJ, Herwig KG: Primary aldosteronism photo scanning of tumor after administration of ^{131}I-iodocholesterol. Arch Intern Med 129:417, 1972.

52. Prosser PR, Sutherland CM, Scullin DR: Localization of adrenal aldosterone adenoma by computed tomography. N Engl J Med 300:1278, 1979.

53. Bosniak MA, Siegelman SS, Evans JA: The adrenal, retroperitoneum and lower urinary tract. In Hodes PJ (ed): Atlas of Tumor Radiology, Chicago, Year Book Medical Publishers, 1976.

54. Ambos MA, Bosniak MA, Lefleur RS, Mitty HA: Adrenal adenoma associated with renal cell carcinoma. AJR 136:81, 1981.

55. Olsson CA, Krane RJ, Klugo RC, Selikowitz SM: Adrenal myelolipoma. Surgery 73:665, 1973.

56. Dykman J, Freidman D: Myelolipoma of the adrenal with clinical features and surgical excision. J Mt Sinai Hosp NY 24:793, 1957.

57. Fink DW, Wurtzebach LR: Symptomatic myelolipoma of the adrenal: Report of a case with computed tomographic evaluation. Radiology 134:451, 1980.

58. Liebman R, Srikantaswamy S: Adrenal myelolipoma demonstrated by computed tomography. J Comput Assist Tomogr 5:262, 1981.

59. Engleman K: Phaeochromocytoma. Clin Endocrinol Metab 6:709, 1977.

60. Thomas JL, Bernardino ME: Pheochromocytoma in multiple endocrine adenomatosis: Efficacy of computed tomography. JAMA 245:1467, 1981.

61. Thomas JL, Bernardino ME, Samaan VA, Hickey RC: CT of pheochromocytoma. AJR 135:477, 1980.

62. Tisnado J, Amendola MA, Konerding KF, Shirazik K, Beachley MC: Computed tomography versus angiography in the localization of pheochromocytoma. J Comput Assist Tomogr 4:853, 1980.

63. Laursen K, Damgaard-Pedersen K: CT for pheochromocytoma diagnosis. AJR 134:277, 1980.

64. Stewart BH, Bravo EL, Haaga J, Meaney T, Tarazi R: Localization of pheochromocytoma by computed tomography. N Engl J Med 299:460, 1978.

65. Hahn LC, Nadel NS, Bernstein NM, Satya KL: Localization of pheochromocytoma by computerized axial tomography. J Urol 120:349, 1978.

66. Foley WD: Ectopic pheochromocytmoa. CT/T Clinical Symposium, vol 3, no 10. Milwaukee, General Electric Company, 1980.

67. Zelch JV, Meany TF, Belhobek GH: Radiographic approach to the patient with suspected pheochromocytoma. Radiology 111:279, 1974.

68. Chok J, Freier DT, McCormick TL, Nishiyama RH, Forrest ME, Kaufman A, Borlaza GS: Adrenal medullary disease in multiple endocrine neoplasia type II. AJR 134:23, 1980.

69. Stewart GH, Bravo EL, Haaga J, Meany TF, Tarazi R: Localization of pheochromocytoma by computed tomography. N Engl J Med 299:460, 1978.

70. McLaughlin JE, Urich H: Maturing neuroblastoma and ganglion neuroblastoma: A study of four cases with long survival. J Pathol 121:19, 1977.

71. Dominick HC, Bachmann KD: Neuroblastoma. In Löhr E (ed): Renal and Adrenal Tumors. Berlin, Springer-Verlag, 1979, pp. 302–310.

72. Brasch RC, Korobkin M, Gooding CA: Computed body tomography in children: Evaluation of 45 patients. AJR 131:21, 1978.

72a. Stark DD, Moss AA, Brasch RC, deLorimier AA, Ablin AR, London DA, Gooding CA: Neuroblastoma: Diagnostic imaging and staging. Radiology 148:101, 1983.

72b. Stark DD, Brasch RC, Moss AA, deLorimier AA, Ablin AR, London DA, Gooding CA: Recurrent neuroblastoma: The role of CT and alternative imaging tests. Radiology 148:107, 1983.

72c. Podrasky AE, Stark DD, Hattner RS, Gooding CA, Moss AA: Radionuclide bone scanning in neuroblastoma: Skeletal metastases and primary tumor localization of ^{99m}TCMDP. AJR (in press).

73. Sheedy PF, Hattery RR: Adrenal glands. Computed Tomography of the Adrenal Gland. St Louis, CV Mosby, 1977, p 143.

74. Haaga J, Reich NE: Adrenal glands. Computed Tomography of Abdominal Abnormalities. St Louis, CV Mosby, 1978, pp 211–217.

75. Heaston DK, Handel DB, Ashton PR, Korobkin M: Narrow gauge needle aspiration of solid adrenal masses. AJR 138:1143, 1982.

75a. Gross BH, Goldberg HI, Moss AA, Harter LP: CT demonstration and guided aspiration of unusual adrenal metastases. J Comput Assist Tomogr 7:98, 1983.

76. Lee WJ, Weinreb J, Kumari S, Phillips G, Pochaczeusky R, Pillari G: Adrenal hemangioma. J Comput Assist Tomogr 6:392, 1982.

77. Palubinskas AJ, Christensen WR, Harrison JH, Sosman MC: Calcified adrenal cyst. AJR 82:853, 1959.

78. Daffener RH: Evaluation of suprarenal mass. CT/T Clinical Symposium, vol 1, no 3. Milwaukee, General Electric Company, 1979.

79. Albert SG, Wolverson MK, Johnson FE: Bilateral adrenal hemorrhage in an adult: Demonstration by computed tomography. JAMA 247:1737, 1982.

80. Wilms GE, Baert AL, Kint EJ, Pringot JH, Goddeeris PG: Computed tomographic findings in bilateral adrenal tuberculosis. Radiology 146:729, 1983.

17 COMPUTED TOMOGRAPHY OF THE SPLEEN

Michael P. Federle

The spleen is not often the primary organ of interest when abdominal CT scans are obtained. However, a wide variety of splenic variations and abnormalities may be detected on abdominal scans designed to evaluate the liver, pancreas, or retroperitoneum.[1]

TECHNIQUES OF EXAMINATION

In most instances, the spleen will be evaluated as part of a scan of the upper abdomen, and in only a few instances will a directed CT study of the spleen be requested. CT scans 1 cm thick taken at 1- or 2-cm intervals are usually adequate to evaluate the spleen. Precontrast CT scans add little information, and routine splenic CT studies are thus usually performed only after an intravenous infusion of contrast material.

SELECTIVE SPLENIC ENHANCEMENT

Uncommonly, it may be difficult to separate the spleen from contiguous structures such as kidney or pancreas on CT scans, and in such cases, renal or pancreatic tumors may be simulated. Experimental studies using intravenous liposoluble contrast material have demonstrated preferential increase in the attenuation of liver and spleen parenchyma (Fig. 17–1).[2–6] An alternative experimental contrast material has been produced using phospholiposomes carrying standard diatrizoic acid salts.[7] Such agents may prove clinically useful in a variety of hepatic and splenic pathologic processes, including evaluation of space-occupying lesions and separation of spleen from contiguous organs or masses.[6] However, these agents are still classified as investigational and have not yet been approved for general clinical use.

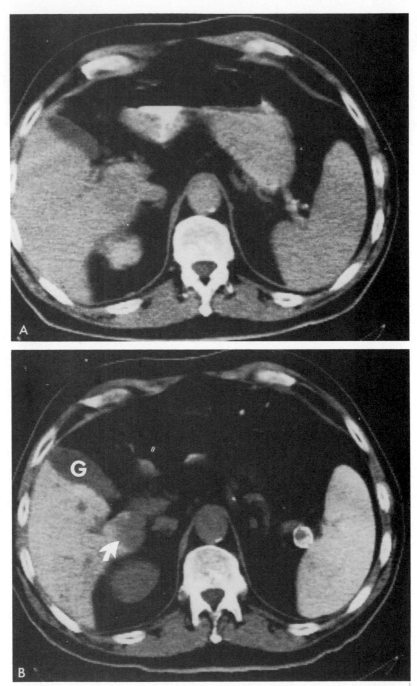

Figure 17–1. Liposoluble contrast material. **A**   CT scan through the liver and spleen following an intravenous infusion of Renografin 60 reveals a questionable lesion in the caudate lobe. **B**   Following intravenous infusion of iodinated oil, areas of normal reticuloendothelial cells in the liver and spleen become densely opacified. The questionable metastasis in the caudate lobe (arrow) is now obvious. G = Gallbladder. (Case courtesy of M.E. Bernardino, M.D., Atlanta, Ga.)

DYNAMIC CT SCANNING

Dynamic CT scanning following an intravenous bolus of 50 to 80 ml of meglumine diatrizoate is useful in assessing splenic vasculature and para-splenic masses. The splenic artery is clearly shown, and delayed CT scans are capable of determining patency of the splenic vein (Fig. 17–2). Dynamic CT studies are helpful for separating the spleen from adjacent organs and demonstrating abnormal vascular structures such as gastroesophageal varices, collateral vessels, and splenic artery aneurysms.

However, dynamic CT scanning of the spleen has not been as useful as dynamic scans of other solid parenchymal organs such as the liver or kidney. This is primarily due to the inhomogeneous pattern of contrast enchancement seen in many normal spleens (Fig. 17–2). The inhomogeneous contrast enhancement is most likely due to the variable rates of blood flow through the cords of the red pulp of the spleen.[7] Since the normal spleen often appears mottled on dynamic CT scans, dynamic splenic CT has not proven useful for detection of small intrasplenic masses, although it has been helpful in evaluating structures in or near the splenic hilum.

ANATOMY

SHAPE

The lateral border of the spleen along the abdominal wall and diaphragm has a smooth, convex margin. The visceral surface is usually lobulated, having a variety of notches, indentations, and ridges in its contour (Fig. 17–3). On axial CT sections, the appearance of the spleen varies, depending on the level of the CT scan (Figs. 17–3 and 17–4). An indentation or fossa is usually formed by the left kidney, and there may also be a less discrete fossa for the gastric fundus. Occasionally, a prominent notch appears as a complete transection through the splenic parenchyma and simulates a splenic laceration (Fig. 17–5).

A prominent ridge or bulge is commonly seen along the visceral surface[1] or occasionally appears as a discrete lobulation between the tail of the pancreas and the left kidney (Figs. 17–4B and 17–6). This variant may simulate a pancreatic mass on ultrasonography[8] or a pararenal mass on excretory urography,[9, 10] but it is easily recognized as a splenic variation by CT. It is more common with splenomegaly but can occur with normal-sized spleens. Sometimes an enlarged spleen almost encircles the kidney, displacing it anteriorly, posteriorly, or inferiorly (Fig. 17–7).[11]

SIZE

The spleen varies considerably in size among individuals and even within the same person according to age, state of nutrition, and body habits. The average adult spleen weighs about 150 gm (range: 100 to 250 gm with occasional extremes of 50 to 400 gm) and measures about 12 cm in length, 7 cm in breadth, and 3 to 4 cm in thickness.[12] Because of the variable size of the normal spleen, splenomegaly must be diagnosed with some reservation. From a practical standpoint, most experienced observers are able to judge splenic volume as smaller or larger than "normal" by a simple review of the CT scans. In general, the length of the normal spleen is less than 15 cm and the splenic tip does not extend caudally as far as the tip of the right lobe of the liver. The anterior edge of the spleen usually does not extend beyond the mid-axillary line, although thin crescentic spleens may do so.

When indicated, CT can be used to accurately measure splenic volume. Contiguous scans are obtained through the spleen, and the area occupied by the spleen on each CT section is calculated using a computer program and a track-ball system available on most CT scanners (Fig. 17–8). Since each CT section is of known thickness, the volume of the organ is determined by simple addition of the volumes displayed on each section. In experimental studies, splenic volume determination by CT has been found to be accurate to plus or minus 5 per cent of the organ volume measured by water displacement.[13–15] CT changes in spleen volume following distal splenorenal shunt surgery have been quantitated and correlated with shunt patency. Reduction in size of up to 23 per cent has been found in patients with patent shunts, but failure of the spleen to shrink, particularly early after surgery, does not indicate that the shunt is occluded.[16]

CT DENSITY

The absolute attenuation value of the spleen is variable within any patient population, although it is stable and reproducible within an individual. Piekarski and colleagues[17] reported a mean CT number of 42.2 Hounsfield Units (H) (range 29.8 to 68.6 H) with a standard deviation of 8.2 H.

Text continued on page 885

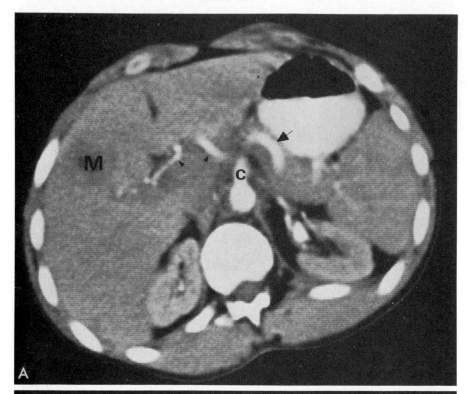

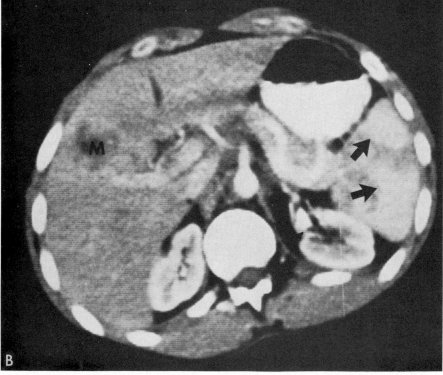

Figure 17–2. Dynamic CT section of normal spleen following intravenous bolus of contrast medium. **A** Early arterial phase. The splenic artery (arrow) arises from the celiac trunk (c). Arrowheads = Hepatic artery. **B** Capillary phase. There are areas of high density (arrows) separated by low-density clefts. The spleen enhances in a mottled pattern as a result of variable rates of blood flow in the red pulp of the spleen.

Illustration continued on opposite page

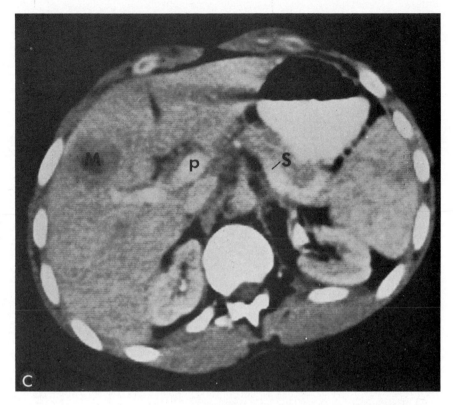

Figure 17–2. *Continued* **C** Venous phase. Splenic parenchyma gradually becomes more homogeneous. The splenic (S) and portal (p) veins are patent. M = hepatic metastasis. (From Federle MP, Moss AA: Computed tomography of the spleen CRC Crit Rev Diagn Imaging 19:1, 1983.)

VISCERAL SURFACE OF THE SPLEEN

CT APPEARANCE OF SPLEEN AT DIFFERENT LEVELS

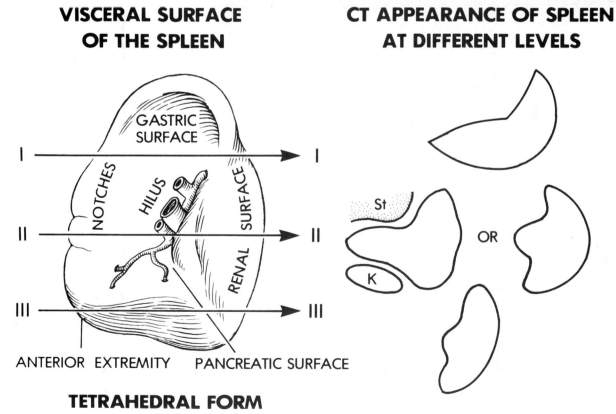

TETRAHEDRAL FORM

Figure 17–3. Diagram of the visceral surface of the spleen (tetrahedral form) with the corresponding axial CT appearance. Note the variable appearance at the level of the hilum, where a prominent ridge or lobulation is frequently seen. St = Stomach; K = kidney. (From Piekarski J, Federle MP, Moss AA, London SS: Computed tomography of the spleen. Radiology 135:683, 1980. Reprinted by permission.)

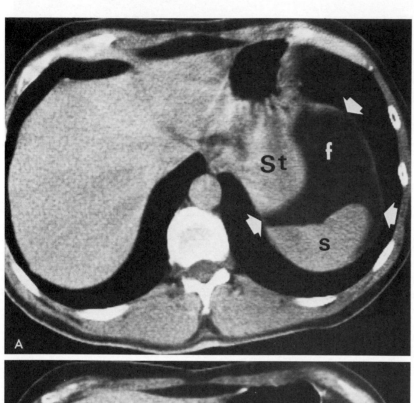

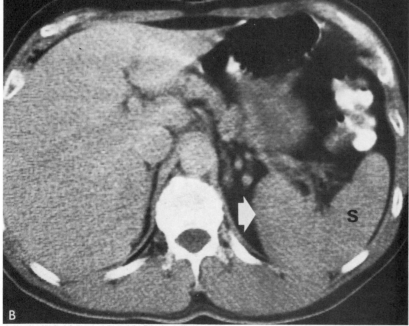

Figure 17–4. Variation in shape of normal spleen at different levels in the same patient. **A** The upper portion of the spleen (s) is semilunar in shape, surrounded by fat (f), and closely related to the diaphragm (arrows) and stomach (St). **B** The midportion of the spleen (s) has a prominent medial bulge (arrow), which should not be interpreted as a splenic mass.

Illustration continued on opposite page

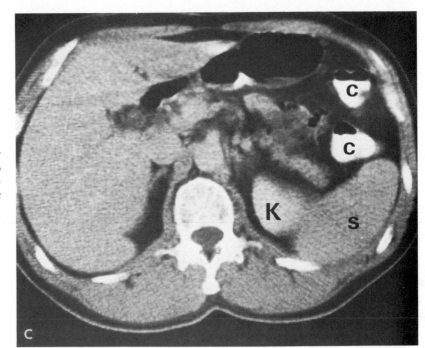

Figure 17–4. *Continued* **C** The lower portion of the spleen (s) is related to the left kidney (K) and the splenic flexure of the colon (c), and it has a more vertical, elongated shape.

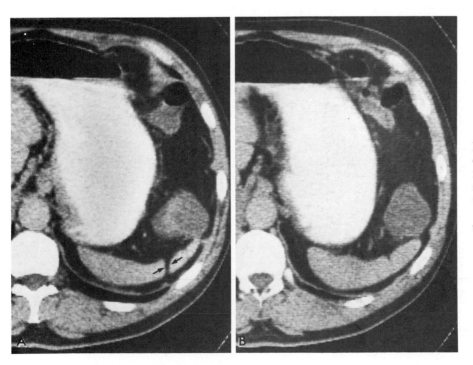

Figure 17–5. Pseudofracture of the spleen. **A** A prominent splenic notch (arrows) simulates a complete transsection of the spleen. **B** CT scan 1 cm lower demonstrates continuity of the spleen.

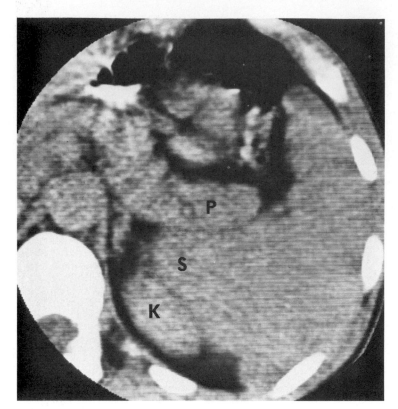

Figure 17–6. Prominent splenic lobulation (S) interposed between the pancreas (P) and the left kidney (K). (From Federle MP, Moss AA: Computed tomography of the spleen. CRC Crit Rev Diagn Imaging 19:1, 1983.)

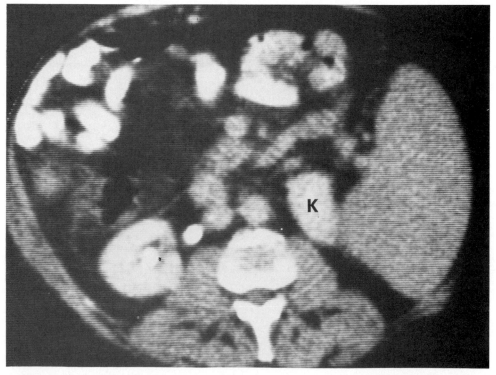

Figure 17–7. Splenomegaly displacing the left kidney (K) anteriorly and inferiorly.

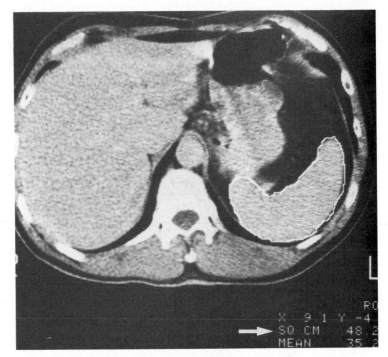

Figure 17–8. Splenic volume measurement. An electronic cursor was used to trace the outline of the spleen. Enclosed area is 48.2 cm² (arrow). As the CT slice is 1 cm thick, a volume of 48.2 cm³ is displayed. Volumes measured on contiguous 1-cm sections through spleen are then added to determine the total splenic volume.

Other authors,[18, 19] using different CT scanners, have reported a somewhat different range of attenuation values. The wide range of CT numbers is largely due to technical factors, such as beam-hardening artifacts, patient size and shape, varying kilovolt peak (kVp) of the anode, and intermittent software revisions in scanner systems. However, in the normal patient, the liver and spleen maintain a concordant relationship in attenuation values with the liver almost always slightly more dense than the spleen (Fig. 17–9)[17] Since the spleen is relatively inactive metabolically, large fluctuations of chemical content do not usually occur. Therefore, alterations in the concordant relationship between the liver and spleen CT numbers are usually due to changes in

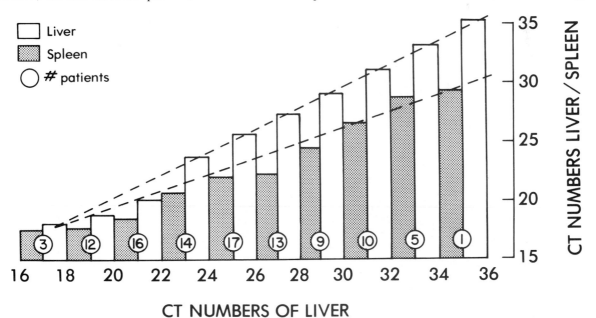

Figure 17–9. Relationship of liver CT number to spleen CT number in 100 adults, relating liver-spleen differences at specific liver CT numbers. Scale, +500 to −500 H. (From Piekarski J, Goldberg HI, Royal SA, Axel L, Moss AA: Difference between liver and spleen CT numbers in the normal adult: Its usefulness in predicting the presence of diffuse liver disease. Radiology 137:727, 1980. Reprinted by permission.)

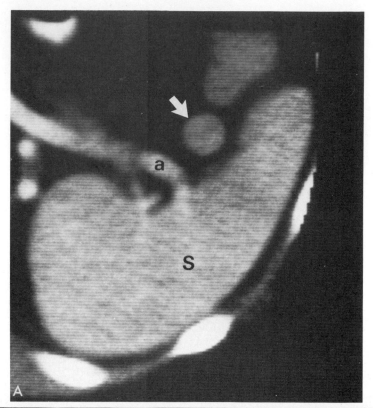

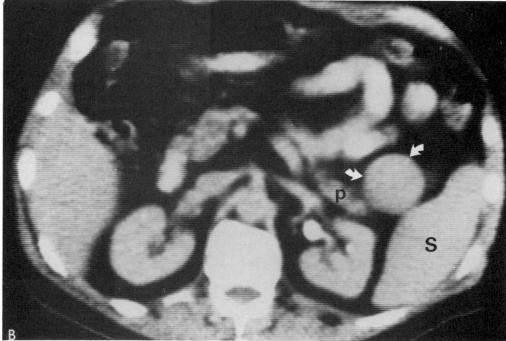

Figure 17–10. Accessory spleens. **A** A CT scan reveals a small, round accessory spleen (arrow) located in a typical position in the hilum of the spleen. S = Spleen; a = splenic artery. **B** Larger accessory spleen (curved arrows) in the hilum of the spleen, which displaces the tail of the pancreas (p). Despite the larger size of this accessory spleen it maintains a round shape and has the same density as the spleen (S). From Piekarski J, Federle MP, Moss AA, London SS: Computed tomography of the spleen. Radiology 135:683, 1980. Used with permission.)

liver composition (e.g., fat, glycogen, or iron deposition) rather than to changes in the attenuation value of the spleen. The spleen, however, may demonstrate increased attenuation as a result of hemosiderin deposition in beta-thalassemic patients after multiple blood transfusions,[20] but the spleen is usually of normal density in primary hemochromatosis.

CONGENITAL VARIATIONS

ACCESSORY SPLEEN

Accessory spleens are found in 10 to 30 per cent of unselected autopsy cases.[21, 22] They consist of nodules of normal splenic tissue and vary from a few millimeters to several centimeters in diameter. They occur most frequently in the hilar region and may be completely isolated from the spleen or connected to it by thin bands of tissue (Fig. 17–10). Most are small and of no clinical significance, going undetected on routine radiographic studies. However, occasionally they are sufficiently large or atypical in location to resemble a tumor on ultrasonography or excretory urography.[9, 10, 23] Following splenectomy, the accessory spleen may enlarge dramatically, sometimes presenting as a left upper-quadrant mass or causing recurrence of clinical problems in pa-

tients who have had splenectomy for hematologic or other disorders (Fig. 17–11).[24]

CT is an accurate method of diagnosing both symptomatic and asymptomatic accessory spleens.[1, 4, 25, 26] A round to oval mass in or near the hilum, having the same attenuation as a normal spleen both before and after intravenous contrast material, is virtually pathognomonic. If the CT diagnosis is still in doubt, technetium[99m] sulphur colloid images of the liver and spleen may be obtained.

POLYSPLENIA, ASPLENIA

The syndrome of polysplenia consists of multiple ectopic spleens associated with cardiovascular and visceral anomalies.[27–29] The multiple spleens are usually right-sided but may be bilateral. The syndrome differs from an accessory spleen in which there is a normal-sized spleen in normal position and one or more smaller accessory spleens. Asplenia and polysplenia may occur as isolated anomalies but are frequently associated with various cardiovascular abnormalities, partial or total failure of rotation of the intestinal tract, a midline mesentery, and occasional absence of the gallbladder. The right and left lobes of the liver are of equal size, and there is absence or hypoplasia[30] of the hepatic segment of the inferior vena cava and continuity of the cava with the azygos and hemiazygos veins (Fig. 17–12). CT provides a nonin-

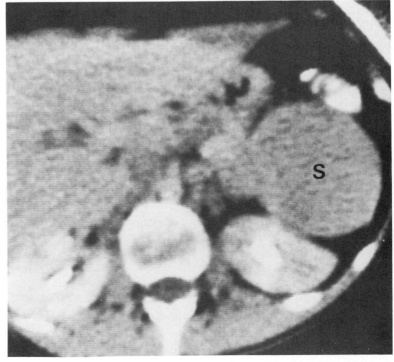

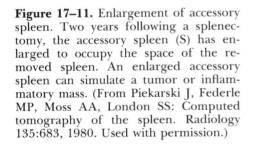

Figure 17–11. Enlargement of accessory spleen. Two years following a splenectomy, the accessory spleen (S) has enlarged to occupy the space of the removed spleen. An enlarged accessory spleen can simulate a tumor or inflammatory mass. (From Piekarski J, Federle MP, Moss AA, London SS: Computed tomography of the spleen. Radiology 135:683, 1980. Used with permission.)

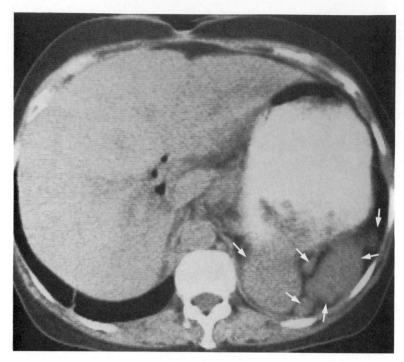

Figure 17–12. Polysplenia. CT scan showing multiple spleens (arrows) in a patient with azygous continuation of the inferior vena cava.

vasive means of evaluating several components of these syndromes.[29] Clearly seen are the multiple spleens, situs inversus, hepatic size anomalies, absence of the suprarenal vena cava, and enlarged azygos and hemiazygos veins adjacent to the aorta.

PATHOLOGY

TRAUMA

The spleen is the intraperitoneal organ that is most frequently injured in blunt abdominal trauma.[31] Abdominal injury can cause a frank splenic laceration or can result in a hematoma that is limited by the splenic capsule.[32-36] Most splenic subcapsular hematomas have a rather typical CT appearance of a crescentic peripheral low-density lesion along the lateral margin of the spleen, which flattens or indents the normally convex lateral margin of the spleen (Fig. 17–13). The size and limits of a subcapsular hematoma are best appreciated after administration of intravenous contrast material. If a CT scan is obtained very shortly after splenic trauma without intravenous contrast administration, subcapsular or intrasplenic hematomas may appear isodense or even slightly hyperdense when compared with the normal spleen (Fig. 17–14A,B). However, following intravenous contrast injection, the normal spleen increases in density; the subcapsular and intrasplenic hematomas do not enhance unless

there is continuing ongoing hemorrhage (Fig. 17–14C,D). The capsule of the spleen also can enhance and is seen as a thin rim surrounding the subcapsular hematoma (Fig. 17–13B,C).

As a splenic subcapsular hematoma matures, the density of the hematoma decreases (Fig. 17–15) as a result of a decrease in hemoglobin and increase in water content of the hematoma (Fig. 17–16).[37] Although the natural history of splenic subcapsular hematomas is not completely known, splenic subcapsular hematomas have been followed for months without change in size or delayed rupture.[34] Thus it appears when an isolated, well-defined subcapsular hematoma is demonstrated by CT that immediate surgery may not be required. This is especially important in patients who are poor surgical risks or with children in whom loss of the immunologic function of the spleen and risk of infection make splenectomy a less attractive procedure.[38]

Splenic lacerations can be diagnosed by CT, although the findings are more subtle and variable than those found in subcapsular hematoma. Splenic lacerations typically produce indistinct margins of the spleen and irregular low-density bands or clefts through the splenic parenchyma (Fig. 17–17). Lacerations virtually always involve part of the lateral contour of the spleen and are associated with perisplenic and free intraperitoneal blood in either the left paracolic gutter or Morrison's pouch (Fig. 17–17). Congenital splenic clefts may be differentiated from lacerations by a thin

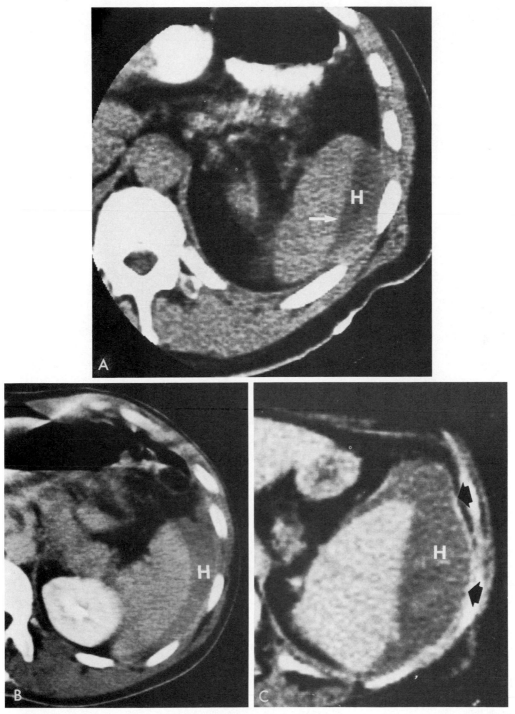

Figure 17–13. Variation in shape of subcapsular splenic hematoma. **A**   Crescentic low-density hematoma (H) indents the lateral margin of the spleen (arrow). **B**   Semilunar-shaped hematoma (H) displaces but does not flatten the lateral margin of the spleen. The density of this hematoma is mixed, indicating it is recent and has undergone only partial hemolysis of the blood clot. **C**   Subcapsular hematoma (H) flattening the spleen and surrounded by a thickened, hypervascular capsule (arrows).

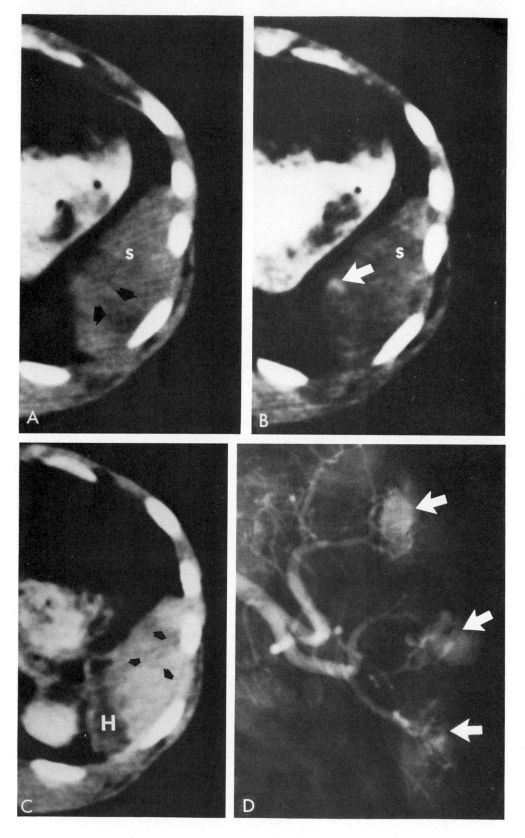

Figure 17–14. *See legend on opposite page*

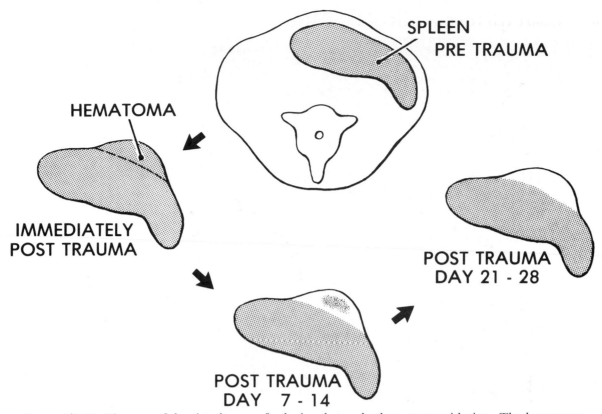

Figure 17–15. Diagram of density change of splenic subcapsular hematoma with time. The hematoma is initially isodense with the normal splenic tissue, then gradually becomes a low-density mass. (From Moss AA, Korobkin M, Price D, Brito AC: Computed tomography of splenic subcapsular hematomas: An experimental study in dogs. Invest Radiol 14:60, 1979. Used with permission.)

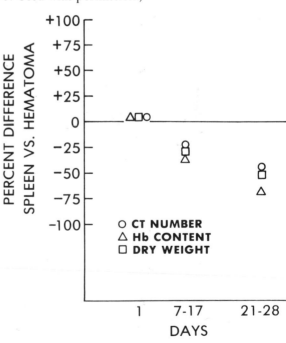

Figure 17–16. Graph of change in CT number, hemoglobin (Hb), and dry weight with time in experimentally produced splenic subcapsular hematomas. There is a linear decrease in hemoglobin content and a decrease in dry weight content of the hematoma, which correlates with the decrease in density over time of splenic subcapsular hematomas. (From Moss AA, Korobkin M, Price D, Brito AC: Computed tomography of splenic subcapsular hematomas: An experimental study in dogs. Invest Radiol 14:60, 1979. Used with permission.)

Figure 17–14. Traumatic intrasplenic hemorrhage and subcapsular hematoma. **A,B** Before contrast medium infusion, the spleen (s) has a mottled appearance with some areas of abnormally low attenuation (black arrows) and at other levels areas of high attenuation (white arrow). **C** Scan taken during bolus injection of contrast material shows areas of marked enhancement (black arrows), which proved to be areas of ongoing hemorrhage. The subcapsular hematoma (H) remains of low density. (From Piekarski J, Federle MP, Moss AA, London SS: Computed tomography of the spleen. Radiology 135:683, 1980. Used with permission.) **D** Splenic angiogram confirms multiple sites of ongoing intrasplenic hemorrhage (arrows).

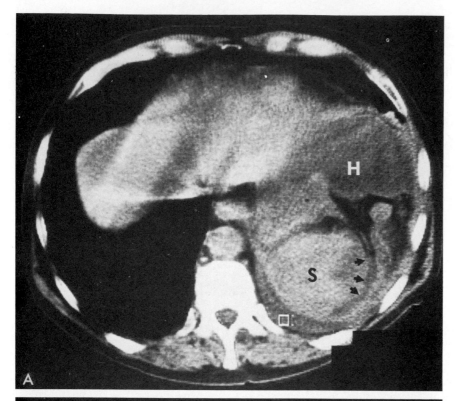

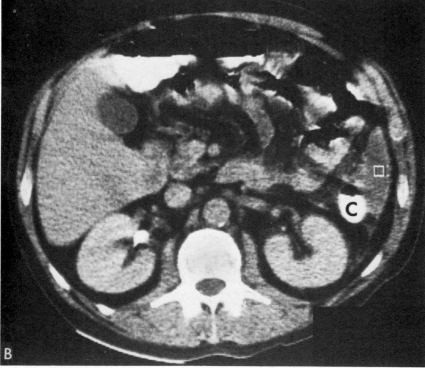

Figure 17–17. Splenic laceration. **A** Curvilinear laceration (arrows) through the upper pole of the spleen (S). Subphrenic blood collections (H and cursor box) are present. **B** Intraperitoneal blood (cursor box) is seen in the gutter lateral to the descending colon (C). From Federle MP: Abdominal trauma: The role and impact of computed tomography Invest Radiol 16:260, 1981. Used with permission.)

sharp linear margin along the medial contour of the spleen and lack of free or perisplenic blood (Fig. 17–5). A prominent left lobe of the liver extending across the midline to a point near the spleen must not be mistaken for a splenic laceration.

   To date, CT has proved to be extremely accu-rate in detecting splenic injury following blunt abdominal trauma.[32–36] An accuracy rate of 96 per cent was found in a prospective study of 50 patients suffering abdominal trauma.[36] CT correctly diagnosed 21 of 22 surgically proven traumatic lesions of the spleen and accurately distinguished between splenic lacerations and subcapsular hematomas. Because of the high accuracy, lack of morbidity, ease of performance and interpretation, CT has largely replaced arteriography and radionuclide scintigraphy in the evaluation of splenic trauma at some institutions.[39]

INFECTION

Splenic abscesses have been found in 0.2 to 0.7 per cent of autopsy reviews. Although patients have fever, leukocytosis, and frequently a mass or tenderness in the left upper quadrant,[40] the clinical diagnosis of splenic abscess is often extremely difficult, and a missed diagnosis can have fatal consequences. Most splenic abscesses (75 per cent) are associated with a hematogenous spread of infection, 15 per cent are associated with trauma, and 10 per cent with splenic infarction; only rarely is a splenic abscess secondary to contiguous spread of infection.[41, 42]

Splenic abscesses occur as multiple or solitary lesions. The majority of splenic abscesses are multiple, occurring most often in patients with immune deficiencies. Solitary splenic abscesses are more frequently related to direct extension or intravenous drug abuse.[42]

CT has proven to be an accurate means of early diagnosis of both isolated and multiple splenic abscesses[1, 43–45] and has been shown to be extremely valuable in the search for possible abscesses in the immune-compromised host.[43] In these patients, CT demonstrates multiple, small, rounded hypodense or cystic lesions that may have a central core of high density within the spleen (Fig. 17–18). The abscesses lack a well-defined wall and do not enhance following intravenous contrast administration, and the spleen is usually enlarged as a result of an underlying neoplastic disease. Similar small abscesses are frequently identified in the liver and kidneys. Although gram-negative bacilli have been reported to be the most frequent infectious agents in splenic abscesses in general,[42] fungal infections have been found in all immunosuppressed patients studied at our institution. A CT-guided aspiration and fungal stain of the contents can quickly determine whether or not fungi are responsible for a splenic abscess.

Certain viral and bacterial illnesses, such as mononucleosis, typhoid fever, and bacterial endocarditis, can produce mild to marked splenomegaly without frank abscess formation. CT in such cases usually reveals only nonspecific splenomegaly.[1] Occasionally, there may be intrasplenic hemorrhages or associated findings of enlarged retroperitoneal lymph nodes.[46]

INFARCTION

Acute and chronic forms of splenic infarction are both detectable by CT. Acute splenic infarction usually appears as a wedge-shaped area of decreased attenuation extending to the capsule of

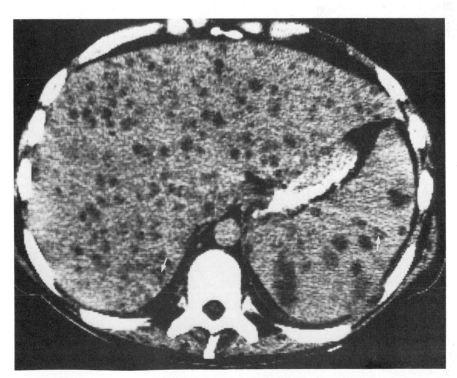

Figure 17–18. Fungal abscesses. Multiple splenic and hepatic fungal abscesses in a young man with acute myelogenous leukemia. Several of the abscesses have a central core of higher density (arrow), giving the abscesses a target appearance. (From Piekarski J, Federle MP, Moss AA, London SS: Computed tomography of the spleen. Radiology 135:683, 1980. Reprinted by permission.)

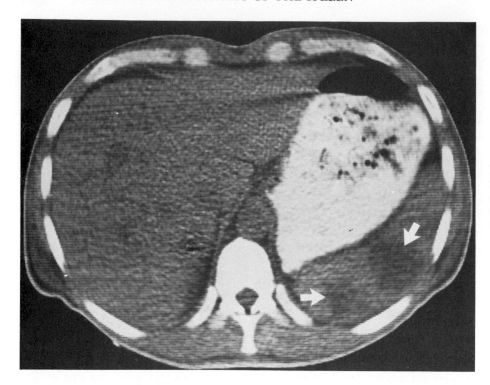

Figure 17–19. Acute splenic infarction in an intravenous drug abuser. Wedge-shaped defects (arrows) point toward splenic hilum.

the spleen (Figs. 17–19 through 17–21), which does not enhance after administration of intravenous contrast medium (Fig. 17–20) or liposoluble contrast (Fig. 17–21). The CT diagnosis of splenic infarction is usually straightforward, but care must be taken not to interpret the nonhomogeneous areas of contrast enhancement during a dynamic CT scan of the spleen as being due to infarcted tissue. Chronic splenic infarction, as seen in sickle cell anemia, frequently produces a spleen with areas of calcification (Fig. 17–22).

NON-NEOPLASTIC MASSES

Splenic cysts have been regarded as rare but are being recognized more frequently as ultrasound and CT have come into greater use.[47, 48] Non-neoplastic cystic splenic masses may be parasitic, congenital, or traumatic in origin. They are

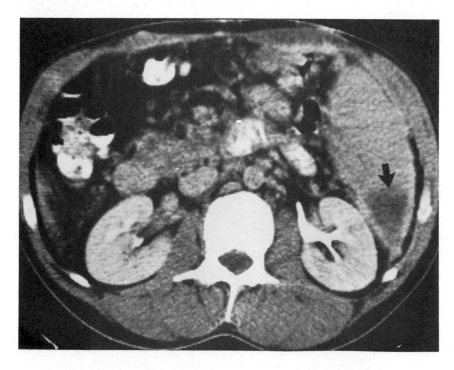

Figure 17–20. Acute splenic infarct. Wedge-shaped splenic infarct (arrow) due to splenic vein thrombosis, which does not increase in attenuation value after intravenous contrast administration. Marked splenomegaly is also present.

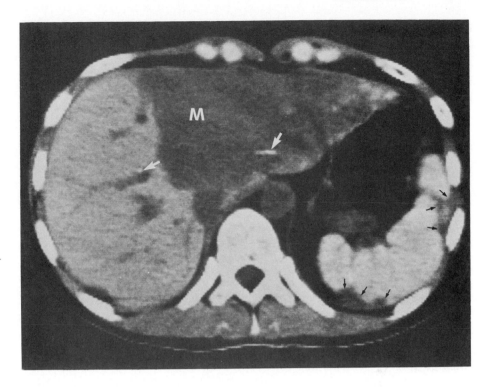

Figure 17–21. Acute splenic infarction: Following intravenous infusion of liposoluble contrast material, areas of normal reticuloendothelial cells in liver and spleen become densely opacified. The large, low-density mass (M) in the liver is metastatic carcinoma. High-density particles in the liver (white arrows) are embolic particles used as part of tumor therapy. The wedge-shaped defects (black arrows) in the spleen are infarcts caused by inadvertent iatrogenic embolization. (Case courtesy of M.E. Bernardino, M.D., Atlanta, Ga.) (From Federle MP, Moss AA: Computed tomography of the spleen. CRC Crit Rev Diagn Imaging 19:1, 1983. Used with permission.)

usually asymptomatic but may cause pain or an enlarging left upper-quadrant mass.

Parasitic Cysts

Parasitic splenic cysts are almost always due to *T. echinococcus.* The most common organism is *E. granulosus,* which tends to produce a round to oval mass of near-water density, having sharp margins (Fig. 17–23). CT reveals a nonhomogeneous mass, with sharp edges that may have foci of calcification (Fig. 17–23). The cyst wall may or may not contain foci of calcification. Noncalcified portions of the cyst wall enhance after contrast injection, and daughter cysts budding from the

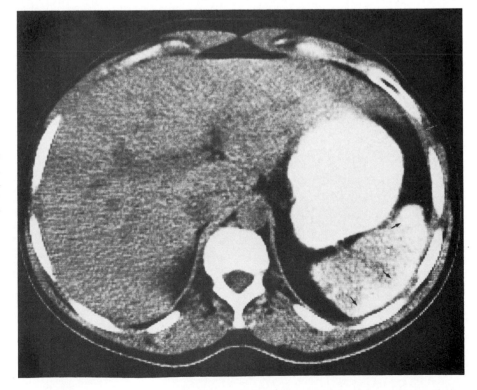

Figure 17–22. Chronic splenic infarction in a patient with sickle cell anemia (noncontrast scan). There is diffuse calcification of the spleen, which is most prominent in the subcapsular region (arrows).

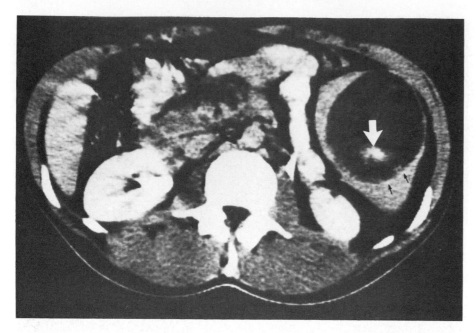

Figure 17–23. Echinococcal cyst of the spleen presenting as an intrasplenic rounded mass having an attenuation value of 0 H, an area of intracyst calcification (large arrow), pencil-sharp margins, and a rim (small arrows) that enhances after contrast injection. (From Piekarski J, Federle MP, Moss AA, London SS: Computed tomography of the spleen. Radiology 135:683, 1980. Used with permission.)

outer cyst wall often give a multiloculated appearance to the cyst.

Nonparasitic Cysts

Nonparasitic splenic cysts are usually either congenital or traumatic in origin. True cysts have a secreting epithelial lining—which implies a developmental origin. False cysts, which account for 80 per cent of splenic cysts, lack an epithelial lining and are the result of cystic degeneration of infarcts or hematomas.

True and false splenic cysts appear identical on CT. Both are characteristically unilocular, homo-

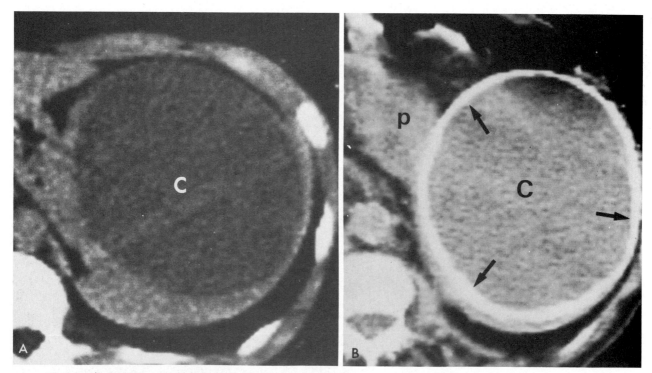

Figure 17–24. Nonparasitic splenic cysts. **A** Surgically proved epithelial cyst (c) had an attenuation value of 0 H before and after contrast infusion. The margins are pencil-sharp. **B** Post-traumatic intrasplenic cyst (c) with a completely calcified wall (arrows). The density of the cyst is near that of the pancreas (p). Thick material with a high hemoglobin content was removed at surgery.

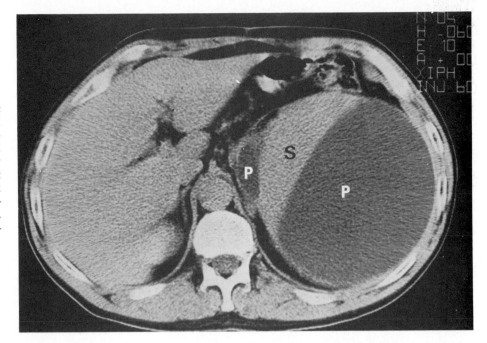

Figure 17–25. Intrasplenic pseudocysts. The normal spleen (S) is sandwiched between two well-defined fluid collections of water density proved to be intrasplenic pseudocysts (P) in a patient with a history of pancreatitis. (Courtesy of Pierre A. Schnyder, Lausanne, Switzerland.)

geneous, water-density lesions having pencil-thin margins that do not enhance after contrast medium administration (Fig. 17–24A). Although calcification in the wall of a splenic cyst is suggestive of *Echinococcus*, it also occurs in post-traumatic splenic cysts (Fig. 17–24B). However, often the history of trauma is minimal or nonexistent, and it is only after pathologic examination demonstrates the lack of a cellular epithelial lining and *Echinococcus* that a diagnosis of a traumatic, par-

tially calcified splenic cyst can be made with certainty.

A rare cause of a nonparasitic splenic cyst is pancreatitis. In these patients, dissection of enzymes into the spleen results in an intrasplenic pseudocyst (Fig. 17–25).[49] In the absence of other CT criteria to indicate pancreatitis, it may be difficult or impossible to differentiate an intrasplenic pseudocyst from a congenital or traumatic splenic cyst.

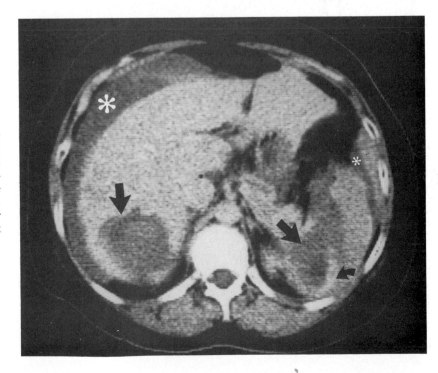

Figure 17–26. Angiosarcoma of the spleen and liver. There are masses in the spleen and liver (straight arrows) as well as fluid (asterisks) in the abdomen as a result of hemorrhage from rupture of one of the tumors. The periphery of the splenic tumor (curved arrow) shows enhancement following contrast infusion.

NEOPLASTIC MASSES

Benign Tumors

Benign splenic neoplasms, such as cystic lymphangiomas,[50, 51] hemangiomas, hamartomas, or desmoids,[42] can produce lesions of the spleen that are predominantly cystic in nature. Although CT appearance of these tumors has not been described, CT will probably be able to detect these benign splenic tumors; however, it is likely that differentiation between benign neoplasms will be difficult.

Malignant Tumors

PRIMARY NEOPLASMS. Although the spleen is a rare site of primary cancer, malignant tumors can arise within the spleen. Splenic angiosarcoma can present with fever, malaise, ascites, hepatosple-

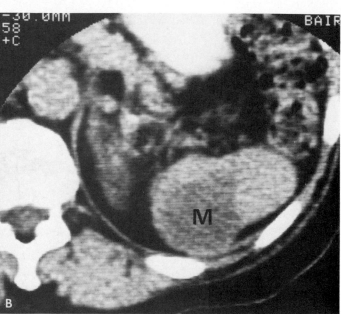

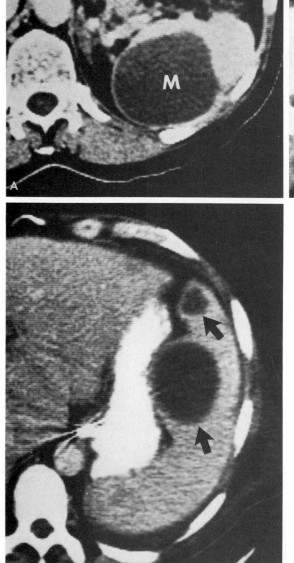

Figure 17–27. Splenic metastasis. **A** Sharply defined mass of water density (M) in the spleen proved to be endometrial carcinoma. CT number = 5 H. **B** Ill-defined splenic mass (M) having a CT number (20 H) higher than that of a simple cyst. Diagnosis: Metastatic endometrial carcinoma. **C** Multiple unilocular cystic metastasis (arrows) in an enlarged spleen resulting from ovarian carcinoma. CT number = 4 H.

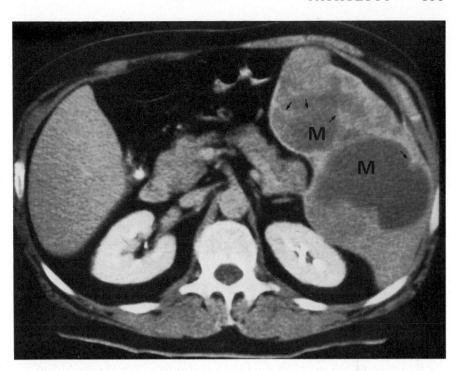

Figure 17–28. Metastatic malignant melanoma. CT scan shows multiple, irregularly shaped cystic masses (M). Internal septations are present (arrows).

nomegaly, and hematologic abnormalities, such as anemia, leukopenia, and thrombocytopenia.[52] These tumors grow rapidly and metastasize early. The CT pattern is that of a nonhomogeneous, complex mass of cystic and solid components which has a variable degree of tumor vascularity following contrast medium injection (Fig. 17–26).

METASTATIC NEOPLASMS.   The spleen is a relatively uncommon site of metastases in spite of its large mass of lymphoid tissue and its filtration of systemic blood flow. When present, splenic metastases are grossly visible at autopsy in only 67 per cent of cases but are detected by microscopic examination in the remaining 33 per cent.[53, 54] Thus, although CT can be expected to detect some cases of splenic metastases, a normal spleen CT examination can never be used to exclude metastatic disease to the spleen.

CT demonstrates splenic metastasis as ill-defined hypodense areas or well-delineated cystic lesions (Figs. 17–27 and 17–28).[55–56] The spleen may or may not be enlarged and the metastasis may appear unilocular (Fig. 17–27) or contain multiple septations (Fig. 17–28). Splenic metastases have been encountered from primary ovarian, pancreatic, and colonic tumors as well as from malignant melanoma, endometrial carcinoma, chondrosarcoma, and gastric lymphoma. In our experience, ovarian carcinoma has been the most frequent primary malignancy to metastasize to the spleen.[1] Differentiation of a cystic

splenic metastasis from a benign cystic lesion of the spleen is often difficult. The CT density and other CT features of cystic splenic metastasis can be identical to those of a benign cyst, and therefore the use of cyst puncture should be employed to document the nature of suspicious cystic lesions of the spleen.

Although splenic metastases usually have been believed to occur only in the setting of widespread tumor dissemination, CT has documented several instances of isolated splenic metastases.[1] In particular, CT has detected splenic lesions without any evidence of hepatic metastasis. Such findings may have important clinical implications, since CT detection of splenic involvement with tumor in the absence of other detectable metastatic foci may lead to initiation of focused therapy to the spleen rather than systemic therapy.

LYMPHOMA.   CT has been shown to play an important role in detecting para-aortic, paracaval, mesenteric, hilar, and mediastinal lymph node involvement in patients with lymphoma. However, in patients with Hodgkin's disease, the spleen is frequently the first and only site of abdominal involvement. Thus, if CT were a reliable method of documenting or excluding splenic involvement, many patients could be spared laparotomy and splenectomy for staging Hodgkin's disease. To date, however, CT has not proven to be an accurate method for determining splenic involvement with Hodgkin's disease or other lymphomas.

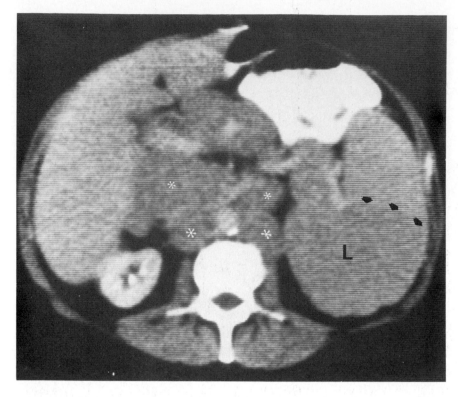

Figure 17–29. Non-Hodgkin's lymphoma demonstrated as splenomegaly containing a large nodule of low attenuation (L). The interphase between the lymphomatous nodule and the spleen is seen as a subtle change in density (arrows). There is also extensive adenopathy in the retroperitoneum and porta hepatis (asterisks). (From Piekarski J, Federle MP, Moss AA, London SS: Computed tomography of the spleen. Radiology 135:683, 1980. Reprinted by permission.)

Although CT is a reliable indicator of splenic size, splenic size alone is of limited diagnostic value in determining splenic involvement with lymphoma. If massive splenomegaly is detected in a patient with non-Hodgkin's lymphoma, there is a high probability of lymphomatous involvement. On the other hand, splenomegaly alone is not a reliable indicator of Hodgkin's disease because a third of such patients will not have pathologic splenic involvement; in addition, a third of the spleens in patients with Hodgkin's and non-Hodgkin's lymphoma will be normal in size but still harbor lymphoma.[57]

Occasionally, lymphoma may take the form of nodular implants in the spleen or liver. Since these nodules generally have a lower attenuation

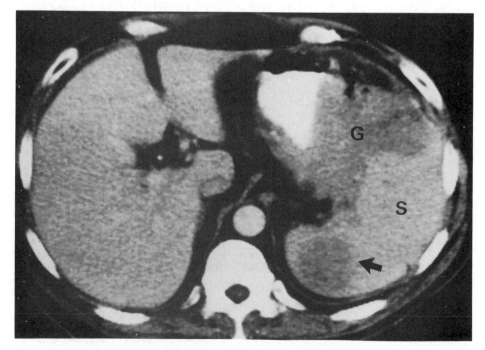

Figure 17–30. Gastric lymphoma (G) invading the spleen (S) and obliterating the fat plane between the spleen and the grater curvature of the stomach. A focus of lymphomatous tissue (arrow) is also noted in the tip of the spleen. (From Buy J-N, Moss AA: Computed tomography of gastric lymphoma. AJR 138:859, 1982. © 1982, American Roentgen Ray Society. Used with permission.)

value than the surrounding parenchyma, they can be detected by CT if they are greater than 1.0 to 1.5 cm in diameter (Fig. 17–29). However, only a minority of patients with splenic lymphoma have such a pattern, the usual pattern being a spleen with a completely homogeneous CT density. Splenic involvement can rarely occur from direct invasion by lymphoma originating in the stomach or colon (fig 17–30).

The use of water-soluble contrast agents has not aided in the detection of splenic lymphoma, but iodinated liposoluble contrast agents which selectively increase the attenuation of normal hepatic and splenic parenchyma will probably aid in

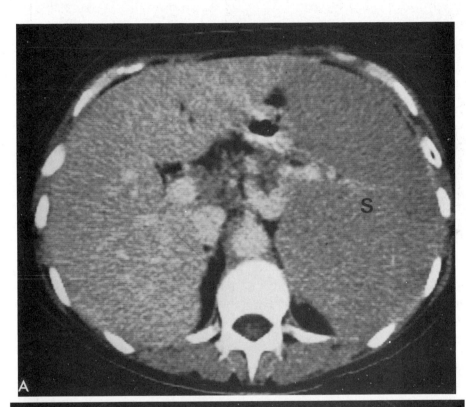

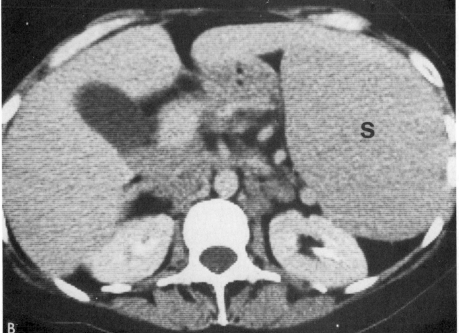

Figure 17–31. Splenic enlargement from leukemia. **A** Chronic lymphocytic leukemia producing marked splenomegaly without focal areas of decreased density. **B** Chronic myelogenous leukemia with identical appearance. S = Spleen.

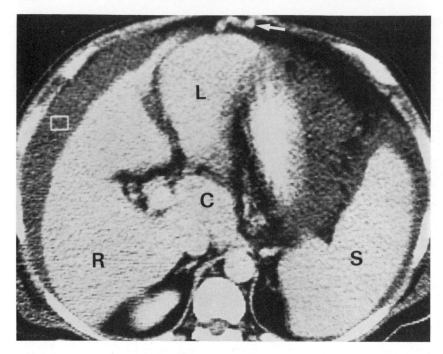

Figure 17–32. Splenomegaly from portal hypertension. Typical morphologic changes of Laennec's cirrhosis are present, including small right lobe of the liver (R), with enlarged left (L) and caudate lobes (C). Cursor (box) marks the presence of ascites. Splenomegaly (S) and a recanalized umbilical vein (arrow) indicate portal hypertension. (From Federle MP, Moss AA: Computed tomography of the spleen. CRC Crit Rev Diagn Imaging 19:1, 1983. Used with permission.)

the detection of subtle nodular implants of lymphoma.[2, 57] However, the common pattern of microscopic infiltrates will still escape CT detection and thus CT probably will not become the ultimate method of detecting splenic lymphoma.

SPLENOMEGALY

The diagnosis of splenomegaly is usually made by physical examination, radionuclide imaging, or plain abdominal radiography. However, the etiology of this condition is only rarely determined by these methods, and often splenomegaly is not appreciated until a CT scan is obtained. By virtue of its ability to accurately determine splenic volume, CT can detect splenomegaly; and although CT cannot provide a specific etiology in all instances, there frequently are indirect indicators of the underlying disease state.

Leukemia

The spleen in patients with leukemia can be markedly enlarged but it usually maintains a ho-

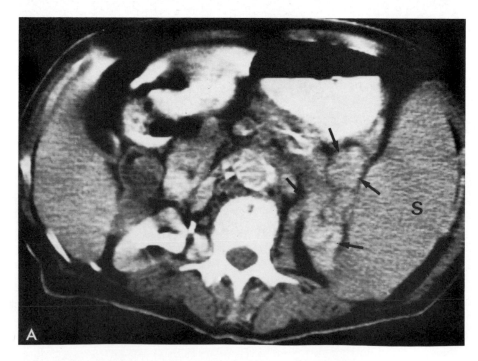

Figure 17–33. Portal hypertension with gastroesophageal varices and perisplenic collateral vessels. **A** CT scan demonstrating splenomegaly (S) and large vascular collaterals in splenic hilum (arrows).

Illustration continued on opposite page

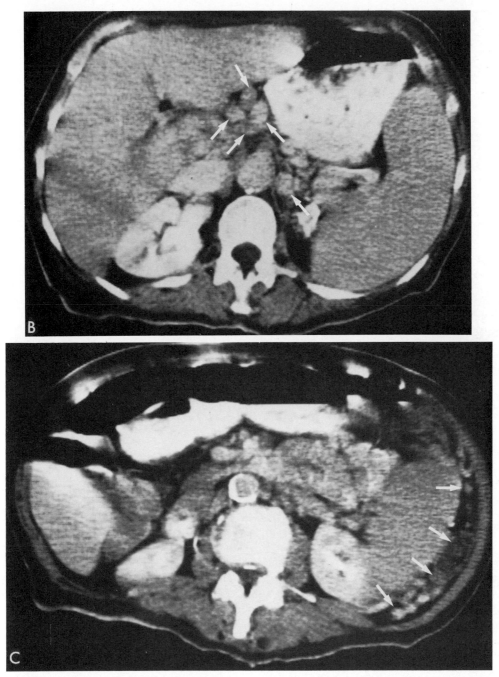

Figure 17–33. *Continued* **B**   Scan at slightly higher level reveals collateral vessels (arrows) along lesser curvature of the stomach, which represent dilated coronary veins. **C**   Scan 1 cm below scan **A**   reveals perisplenic collateral channels (arrows).

mogeneous, normal CT attenuation value (Fig. 17–31); often there is evidence of lymphadenopathy elsewhere. No difference in the CT appearance of the spleen has been noted between the various forms of leukemia.

Portal Hypertension

Portal hypertension is a frequent cause of splenomegaly. Associated CT findings commonly in-

clude a nodular liver, ascites, collateral vascular channels, and a prominent caudate lobe (Fig. 17–32). The demonstration of gastroesophageal varies and collateral vascular channels about the spleen is best demonstrated by dynamic CT scanning techniques (Fig. 17–33). Dynamic CT scanning can also demonstrate splenic vein thrombosis (Fig. 17–34), and in many patients it can suggest the underlying cause (e.g., pancreatitis, pancreatic carcinoma).

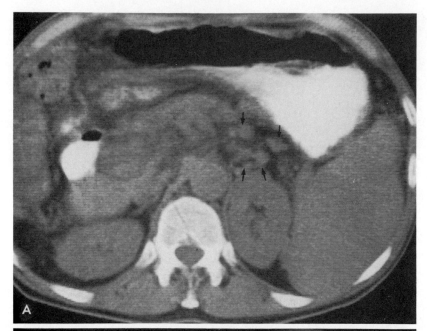

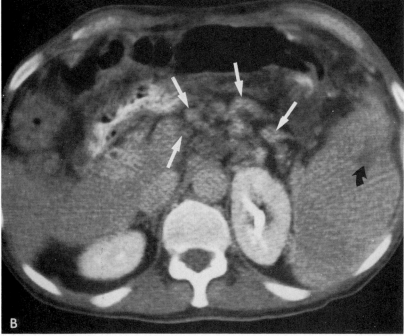

Figure 17–34. Splenic vein thrombosis with collateral flow. **A** Precontrast scan reveals splenomegaly and multiple rounded densities in the splenic hilum (arrows). **B** Scan following contrast injection reveals a network of collateral venous channels (arrows) but no definite splenic vein. An area of splenic infarction (curved arrow) is present.

REFERENCES

1. Piekarski J, Federle MP, Moss AA, London SS: Computed tomography of the spleen. Radiology 135:683, 1980.
2. Vermess M, Doppman JL, Sugarbaker P, Fisher RI, Chatterji DC, Luetzeler J, Grimes G, Girton M, Adamson PH: Clinical trial with a new intravenous liposoluble contrast material for computed tomography of the liver and spleen. Radiology 137:217, 1980.
3. Vermess M, Javadpour N, Blayney DW: Post-splenectomy demonstration of splenic tissue by computed tomography with liposoluble contrast material. J Comput Assist Tomogr 5:106, 1981.
4. Vermess M, Doppman JL, Sugarbaker PH, Fisher RI, O'Leary TJ, Chatterji DC, Grimes G, Adamson RH, Willis M, Edwards BK: Computed tomography of the liver and spleen with intravenous lipoid contrast material: Review of 60 examinations. AJR 138:1063, 1982.
5. Hauron A, Seltzer SE, Davis MA, Shulkin P: Radiopaque liposomes: A promising new contrast material for computed tomography of the spleen. Radiology 140:507, 1981.
6. Vermess M, Inscoe S, Sugarbaker P: Use of liposoluble contrast material to separate left renal and splenic parenchyma on computed tomography. J Comput Assist Tomogr 4:540, 1980.
7. Glazer G, Axel L, Goldberg HI, Moss AA: Dynamic CT of the normal spleen. AJR 137:343, 1981.

8. Gooding GAW: The ultrasonic and computed tomographic appearance of splenic lobulations: A consideration on the ultrasonic differential of masses adjacent to the left kidney. Radiology 126:719, 1978.

9. Madayag M, Bosniak MA, Beranbaum E, Becker J: Renal and suprarenal pseudotumors caused by variations of the spleen. Radiology 105:43, 1972.

10. Roa AKR, Silver TM: Normal pancreas and splenic variants simulating suprerenal and renal tumors. AJR 126:530, 1976.

11. Requard CK: Retroperitoneal spleen mimicking suprarenal mass in association with malpositioned left kidney: Embryologic theory. J Comput Assist Tomogr 5:443, 1981.

12. Gray H: Gray's Anatomy of the Human Body. In Goss, CM (ed): Philadelphia, Lea & Febiger, 28th ed. 1966, p 772.

13. Moss AA, Friedman MA, Brito AC: Determination of liver, kidney and spleen volumes by computed tomography: An experimental study in dogs. J Comput Assist Tomogr 5:12, 1981.

14. Brieman RS, Beck JW, Korobkin M, Glenny R, Akwari OE, Heaston DK, Moore AV, Ram PC: Volume determinations by computed tomography. AJR 138:329, 1982.

15. Heymsfield SB, Fulenwider T, Nordlinger B, Barlow R, Sones P, Kutner M: Accurate measurement of liver, kidney, and spleen volume and mass by computerized axial tomography. Ann Intern Med 90:185, 1979.

16. Hendersen JM, Heymsfield SB, Horowitz J, Kutner MH: Measurement of liver and spleen volume by computed tomography. Radiology 141:525, 1981.

17. Piekarski J, Goldberg HI, Royal SA, Axel L, Moss AA: Difference between liver and spleen CT numbers in the normal adult: Its usefulness in predicting the presence of diffuse liver disease. Radiology 137:727, 1980.

18. Ritchings RT, Pullan BR, Lucas SB, Fawcitt RA, Best JJK, Isherwood I, Morris AI: An analysis of the spatial distribution of attenuation values in computed tomographic scans of liver and spleen. J Comput Assist Tomogr 3:36, 1979.

19. Mategrano VC, Petasnick J, Clark J, Bin AC, Weinstein R: Attenuation values in computed tomography of the abdomen. Radiology 125:135, 1977.

20. Long JA, Doppman JL, Nienhus AW, Mills SR: Computed tomographic analysis of beta-thalassemic syndromes with hemochromatosis: Pathologic findings with clinical and laboratory correlation. J Comput Assist Tomogr 4:159, 1980.

21. Michaels NA: The variational anatomy of the spleen and splenic artery. AM J Anat 70:21, 1942.

22. Halpert B, Gyorkey F: Lesions observed in accessory spleens of 311 patients. Am J Clin Pathol 332:165, 1959.

23. Rosenkranz W, Kahmi B, Horowitz M: Retroperitoneal accessory spleen simulating a suprarenal mass. Br J Radiol 42:939, 1969.

24. Appel MF, Bart JB: The surgical and hematologic significance of accessory spleens. Surg Gynecol Obstet 143:191, 1976.

25. Stiris MG: Accessory spleen versus left adrenal tumor: Computed tomographic and abdominal angiographic evaluation. J Comput Assist Tomogr 4:543, 1980.

26. Beahrs JR, Stephens DH: Enlarged accessory spleens: CT appearance in post-splenectomy patients. AJR 135:483, 1980.

27. Vaughan T, Hawkins J, Elliot L: Diagnosis of polysplenia syndrome. Diagn Radiol 101:511, 1971.

28. Rose V, Izuhawa T, Moes CAF: Syndromes of asplenia and polysplenia. Br Heart J 37:840, 1975.

29. De Maeyer P, Wilms G, Baert AL: Polysplenia. J Comput Assist Tomogr 5:104, 1981.

30. Shadle CA, Scott ME, Ritchie DJ, Seliger G: Spontaneous splenic infarction in polysplenia syndrome. J Comput Assist Tomogr 6:177, 1982.

31. Stivelman RL, Glaubitz JP, Crampton RS: Laceration of the spleen due to nonpenetrating trauma: One hundred cases. Am J Surg 106:888, 1963.

32. Federle MP, Goldberg HI, Kaiser JA, Moss AA, Jeffrey RB Jr, Mall JC: Evaluation of abdominal trauma by computed tomography. Radiology 138:637, 1981.

33. Mall JC, Kaiser JA: CT diagnosis of splenic laceration. AJR 134:265, 1980.

34. Korobkin M, Moss AA, Callen PW, De Martini WJ, Kaiser JA: Computed tomography of subcapsular splenic hematoma. Clinical and experimental studies. Radiology 129:441, 1978.

35. Berger PE, Kahn JP: CT of blunt abdominal trauma in childhood. AJR 136:105, 1981.

36. Jeffrey RB, Laing FC, Federle MP, Goodman PC: Computed tomography of splenic trauma. Radiology 141:729, 1981.

37. Moss AA, Korobkin M, Price D, Brito AC: Computed tomography of splenic subcapsular hematomas: An experimental study in dogs. Invest Radiol 14:60, 1979.

38. Ein SH, Shandling B, Simpson JS, Stephens CA: Nonoperative management of traumatized spleen in children: How and why. J Pediatr Surg 13:117, 1978.

39. Federle MP: Abdominal trauma: The role and impact of computed tomography. Invest Radiol 16:260, 1981.

40. Rice LJ, Rosenstein R, Swikert NC. Splenic abscess: Review of the literature and report of case. J Ky Med Assoc 75:375, 1977.

41. Lawhorne TW Jr, Zuidema GO: Splenic abscess. Surgery 79:686, 1976.

42. Faer MJ, Lynch RD, Lichtenstein JE, Feigin DS: Traumatic splenic cyst RPC from the AFIP. Radiology 134:371, 1980.

43. Callen PW, Filly RA, Marcus FS: Ultrasonography and computed tomography in the evaluation of hepatic microabscesses in the immunosuppressed patient. Radiology 136:433, 1980.

44. Grant E, Mertens MA, Mascatello VJ: Splenic abscess: Comparison of four imaging methods. AJR 132:465, 1979.

45. Moss ML, Kirschner LP, Peereboom G, Ferris RA: CT demonstration of a splenic abscess not evident at surgery. AJR 135:159, 1980.

46. Federle MP, Moss AA: Computed tomography of the spleen. CRC Crit Rev Diagn Imaging 19:1, 1983.

47. Graves JW, Tayiem AK: Splenic cysts. J Kansas Med Soc 74:332, 1973.

48. Ghimji SD, Sooperberg PL, Naiman S, Morrison RT, Shergill P: Ultrasound diagnosis of splenic cysts. Radiology 122:787, 1977.

49. Vick CW, Simeone JF, Ferrucci JT Jr, Wittenberg J, Mueller PR. Pancreatitis-associated fluid collections, in-

volving the spleen: Sonographic and computed tomographic appearance. Gastrointest Radiol 6:247, 1981.

50. Pyatt RS, Williams ED, Clark M, Gasking R: CT diagnosis of splenic cystic lymphangiomatosis. J Comput Assist Tomogr 5:446, 1981.

51. Cornaglia-Ferraris P, Perlino GF, Barabino A, Soave F, Oliva L: A pediatric case of cystic lymphagnioma of the spleen. J Comput Assist Tomogr 5:449, 1981.

52. Mahony B, Jeffrey RB, Federle MP: Spontaneous rupture of hepatic and splenic angiosarcoma demonstrated by CT. AJR 138:965, 1982.

53. Marymont JG Jr, Gross S: Patterns of metastatic cancer in the spleen. Am J Clin Pathol 40:58, 1963.

54. Warren S, Davis AH: Studies on tumor metastasis: The metastases of carcinoma to the spleen. Am J Cancer 21:517, 1981.

55. Federle MP, Filly RA, Moss AA: Cystic hepatic neoplasms: Complementary roles of CT and sonography. AJR 136:345, 1981.

56. Newmark H III: Breast cancer metastasizing to the spleen: Seminar on computerized tomography. Comput Radiol 6:53, 1982.

57. Vermess M, Bernardino ME, Doppman JL, Fisher RI, Thomas JL, Velasquez WS, Fuller LM, Russo A: Use of intravenous liposoluble contrast material for the examination of the liver and spleen in lymphoma. J Comput Assist Tomogr 5:709, 1981.

18 COMPUTED TOMOGRAPHY OF LYMPHOVASCULAR STRUCTURES AND RETROPERITONEAL SOFT TISSUES

R. Brooke Jeffrey

Lymphatic Structures

A major contribution of computed tomography (CT) has been the noninvasive imaging of abdominal and pelvic lymph nodes. CT is well tolerated, simple to perform, and capable of directly imaging nodal areas not routinely visualized during bipedal lymphangiography. The CT demonstration of pelvic or retroperitoneal adenopathy (particularly when cytologically confirmed by directed biopsy), may obviate the need for more invasive procedures such as lymphangiography or lymph node dissection.

It is important to realize that CT does not evaluate intranodal architecture. Lymph node enlargement is the only CT criterion of lymph node abnormality and therefore metastasis to normal size nodes will escape detection (Fig. 18–1). Moreover, in patients with lymphadenopathy that is due to reactive hyperplasia or benign disease, CT will be unable to exclude malignancy as a cause for lymph node enlargement. Thus, while CT has become the initial screening procedure in patients with suspected primary or metastatic disease involving the lymph nodes, lymphangiography because of its ability to display intranodal architec-

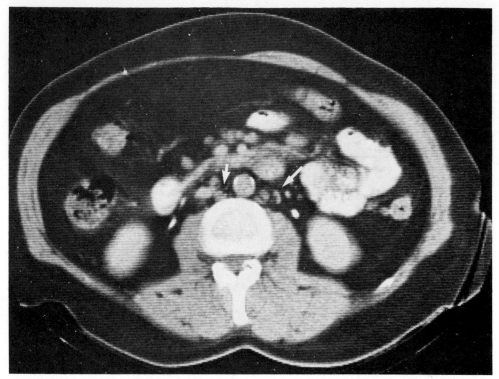

Figure 18–1. CT scan demonstrating a cluster of para-aortic lymph nodes (arrows), all less than 1 cm in diameter, which contained foci of metastatic prostatic carcinoma.

ture will continue to remain an important diagnostic procedure.

CT scans have proved quite accurate in the detection of lymphadenopathy in lymphoma and testicular neoplasms which characteristically produce bulky nodal enlargement.[1–14] CT has been less accurate in detecting focal nodal metastasis from pelvic malignancies such as carcinoma of the prostate, bladder, or cervix.[15–22] However, the improved resolution of new-generation scanners and a better understanding of the size and location of normal retroperitoneal and pelvic lymph nodes have resulted in a CT accuracy that is close to that achieved by lymphangiography.[20]

ANATOMY

Pelvic and retroperitoneal lymph nodes can be identified on CT by their relationship to normal abdominal and pelvic vascular structures, such as the external and common iliac vessels, abdominal aorta, and inferior vena cava (Fig. 18–2). Within the pelvis, the external iliac nodes may be subdivided into three separate nodal chains.[15] The ex-

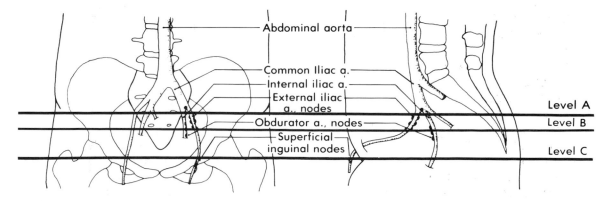

A

Figure 18–2. A Diagram of frontal and lateral projections displaying relationships of pelvic lymph notes to pelvic vascular structures.

Illustration continued on opposite page

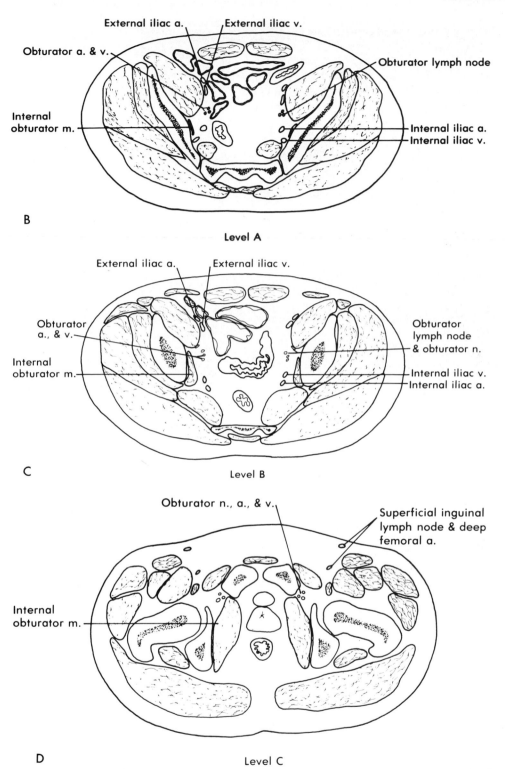

External iliac a. External iliac v.

Obturator a. & v.

Obturator lymph node

Internal obturator m.

Internal iliac a.
Internal iliac v.

B

Level A

External iliac a. External iliac v.

Obturator a., & v.

Obturator lymph node & obturator n.

Internal obturator m.

Internal iliac v.
Internal iliac a.

C

Level B

Obturator n., a., & v.

Superficial inguinal lymph node & deep femoral a.

Internal obturator m.

D

Level C

Figure 18–. *Continued* **B–D** Cross-sectional diagrams depicting anatomic relationships at levels A, B, and C. (Modified from Walsh JW, Amendola MA, Konerding KF, Tinsnado J, Hazra TA: Computed tomographic detection of pelvic and inguinal lymph node metastases from primary and recurrent pelvic malignant disease. Radiology 137:157, 1980.)

ternal (lateral), internal (medial), and middle chains are designated by their relationship to the external iliac artery or vein and are all well delineated by lymphangiography (Figs. 18–2 and 18–

3). The external group is composed of three to four nodes along the lateral aspect of the external iliac artery (Fig. 18–3A). The middle chain is related to the anterior and medial surface of the ex-

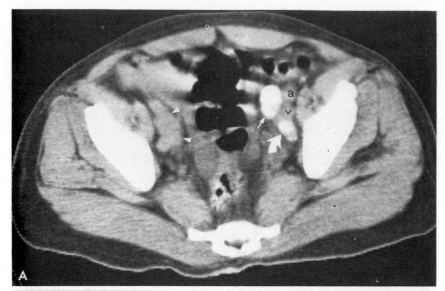

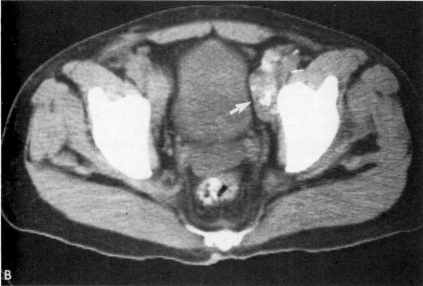

Figure 18–3. CT scan following lymphangiogram in a patient with lymphoma. **A** Enlarged external (lateral) (straight arrow) and middle (obturator) (curved arrow) nodes of the external iliac nodal group filled with lymphangiographic contrast material from left foot injection. Enlarged nonopacified external and obturator nodes (arrowheads) are present on the right side. Internal iliac nodes are also enlarged bilaterally. a = External iliac artery; v = external iliac vein. **B** Middle chain (large arrow) of external iliac nodes enlarged and partially filled with contrast material. Small arrow = External iliac vein.

ternal iliac vein (Fig. 18–3A,B). Lymph nodes in the middle chain are often referred to as the obturator nodes and are located along the lateral pelvic side walls medial to the obturator internus muscle and inferior to the external iliac vein. Obturator nodes are frequently the first to be involved in carcinomas of the cervix, bladder, or prostate (Fig. 18–4). Internal iliac nodes are related to the hypogastric artery dorsal to the obturator nodes (Fig. 18–2 and 18–3).

Inguinal nodes are located at the upper part of the femoral triangle and are usually divided into superficial and subinguinal groups.[15] The superficial nodes are immediately anterior to the femoral vessels (Fig. 18–5). The lumbar lymph nodes are also commonly divided into three separate nodal chains. These include nodes that are anterior, posterior, and lateral to the aorta (para-aortic); similar nodes positioned adjacent to the inferior

vena cava (paracaval); and nodes between the aorta and the cava (aortocaval) (Fig. 18–6). In the lumbar region, lymphadenopathy characteristically obscures the fat planes between the aorta and cava. When lymphadenopathy is massive, all three nodal chains merge to form a mantle of lymphadenopathy (Fig. 18–7). Lesser degrees of lymphadenopathy can cause asymmetry of contours of muscles or vascular structures.[16]

Retrocrural nodes (Fig. 18–8) are located beneath the reflections of the diaphragmatic crura. They can be differentiated from vascular structures (the azygos or hemiazygos veins) by their lack of enhancement with intravenous contrast material.

Pancreatic, celiac, and superior mesenteric lymph nodes are usually not identified with confidence unless enlarged or imaged against a background of a fatty mesentery (Fig. 18–8). The anatomy

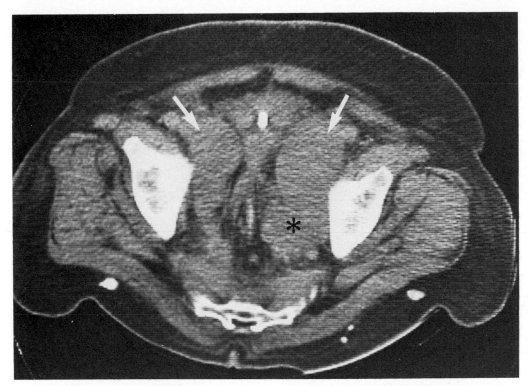

Figure 18–4. Bulky nodal metastases to obturator (middle) (asterisk) and external (lateral) iliac nodes (arrows) from prostatic carcinoma.

and pathology of mesenteric nodes are discussed in Chapter 19.

At present, it is difficult to designate precise size criteria for normal pelvic or retroperitoneal lymph nodes using CT. In general, pelvic or para-aortic nodes measuring 2 cm or greater are considered abnormal[15] and retrocrural nodes are

considered abnormal if larger than 6 mm in diameter (Fig. 18–8).[23] However, the size criteria for normal pelvic lymph nodes vary among investigators. Some authors state that only pelvic nodes greater than 2 cm are definitely abnormal,[15] whereas others suggest obturator nodes should be considered abnormal if greater than 1.2 cm and

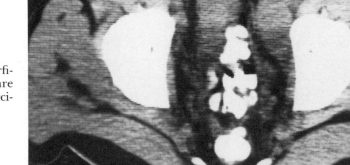

Figure 18–5. Enlarged superficial inguinal nodes (arrow) are due to metastatic adenocarcinoma of the colon.

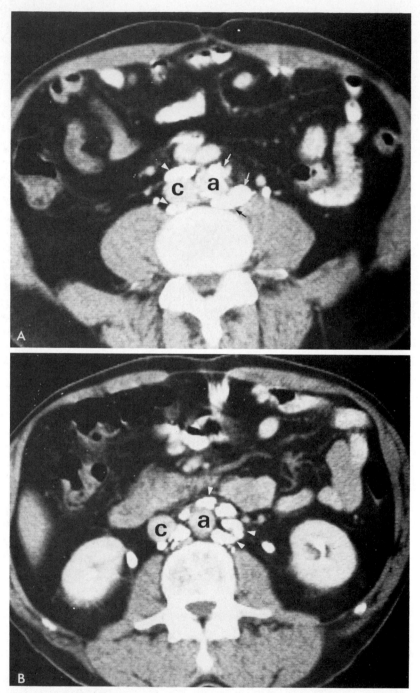

Figure 18–6. Anatomy of lumbar lymph nodes in patient with poorly differentiated nodular lymphoma. **A** Lymph nodes in the para-aortic (arrows) and paracaval nodal chains (arrowheads) are slightly enlarged and contain lymphangiographic contrast material. a = Aorta; c = inferior vena cava. **B** Scan at higher level demonstrates enlarged aortocaval (arrows) and para-aortic nodes (arrowheads). a = Aorta; c = inferior vena cava.

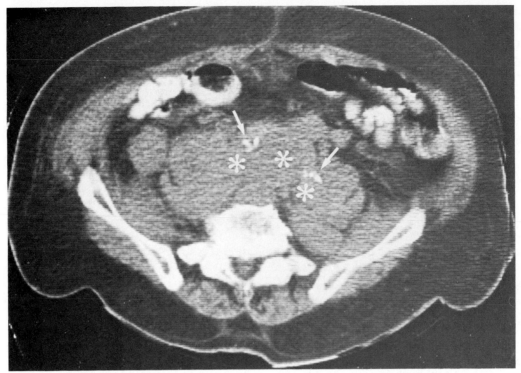

Figure 18–7. Massive adenopathy (asterisks) forming a mantle of tissue encasing and displacing calci-fied common iliac arteries (arrows).

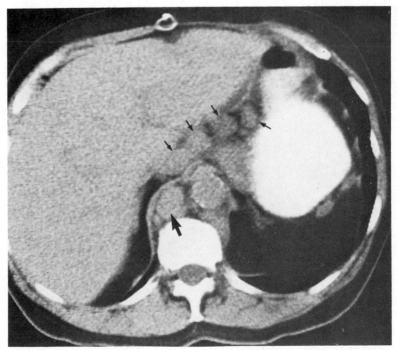

Figure 18–8. Retrocrural (large arrow) and celiac (small arrows) lymphadenopathy in a patient with non-Hodgkin's lymphoma.

the remainder of the external iliac chain abnormal if greater than 1.5 cm in diameter.[20] More detailed clinical and pathologic correlations are needed before strict size criteria can be applied to interpretation of retroperitoneal and pelvic nodes.

TECHNIQUES OF EXAMINATION

The accurate CT diagnosis of pelvic and retroperitoneal adenopathy depends upon both anatomic and technical factors. Lymph node enlargement is most readily identified in patients with ample pelvic and retroperitoneal fat and the preservation of fat planes surrounding the periaortic and pelvic vessels is an important CT finding in excluding lymphadenopathy. The detection of nodal enlargement in children and thin adults is often considerably more difficult because of a lack of perivascular fat.

Because fluid-filled loops of bowel can mimic adenopathy, it is essential to adequately opacify the small bowel with dilute oral contrast medium prior to the CT study. Administration of 480 ml of a 1 to 2 per cent meglumine diatrizoate (Gastrografin) solution 30 to 45 minutes prior to the

study followed by an additional 250 ml of 1 per cent Gastrografin just prior to the examination is usually sufficient to opacify both the proximal and distal small bowel. If the pelvis is to be scanned, a 300- to 400-ml enema of 1 per cent diatrizoate meglumine and diatrizoate sodium (Hypaque) is also administered. In selected patients having either slow or very rapid transit of contrast material, additional oral contrast and delayed scans may be required to avoid diagnostic errors.

In patients with ample pelvic and retroperitoneal fat, intravenous contrast injection is not crucial to detect lymphadenopathy. The normal ureter does not generally cause difficulty in interpretation, and hydronephrosis can be detected by CT without urographic contrast administration. In patients with a paucity of retroperitoneal fat, however, intravenous contrast injection given as a bolus of 70 to 80 ml, followed by a rapid intravenous infusion, is helpful to identify the retroperitoneal and pelvic vascular structures. On occasion, tortuous iliac vessels and normal variants such as a prominent left gonadal vein or duplicated inferior vena cava may simulate lymphadenopathy. Bolus scans of intravenous contrast medium are particularly helpful in diagnos-

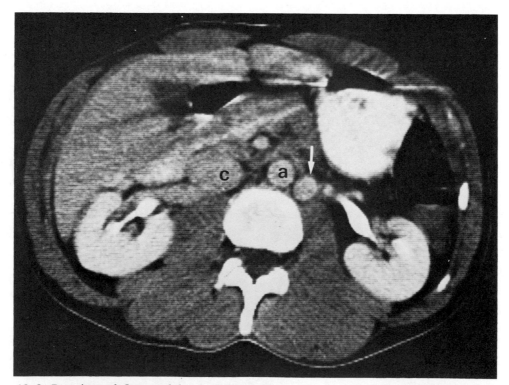

Figure 18–9. Prominent left gonadal vein (arrow) demonstrated by bolus injection enhances to the same degree as the aorta (a) and inferior vena cava (c). On nonenhanced scans, the unopacified gonadal vein can mimic an enlarged lymph node.

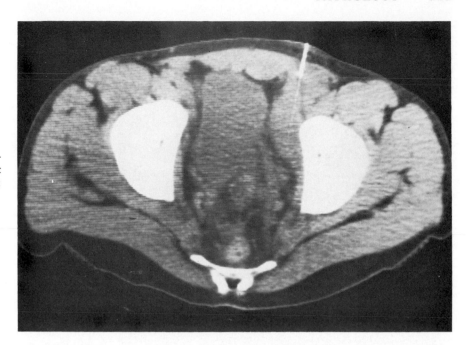

Figure 18–10. CT-guided biopsy of enlarged external iliac nodal mass. Final diagnosis: non-Hodgkin's lymphoma.

ing these vascular structures and in excluding lymphadenopathy (Fig. 18–9).

In the evaluation of lymphoma or testicular neoplasms, patients can be scanned throughout the abdomen at 2-cm intervals without loss of diagnostic accuracy.[24] Patients with pelvic carcinomas are optimally studied throughout the pelvis at 1-cm intervals because there may be only minimal nodal enlargement, but the remainder of the periaortic areas and abdomen is surveyed at 2-cm intervals. Reformatting of axial images into coronal or sagittal planes has not contributed substantially to the CT diagnosis of lymphadenopathy. However, CT-guided fine-needle aspiration of enlarged lymph nodes has proved an important adjunct to routine CT scanning (Fig. 18–10).

PATHOLOGY

LYMPHOMA

Accurate staging in both Hodgkin's and non-Hodgkin's lymphoma is vital in determining appropriate therapy and prognosis. Patients usually undergo a rigorous diagnostic evaluation, including bipedal lymphography and, frequently, a staging laparotomy.[8] Lymphangiography has been in clinical use for years, and in prospective studies it has an 85 to 90 per cent accuracy in staging of lymphoma.[25, 26] However, it is an invasive, time-consuming procedure requiring considerable skill to perform and interpret. Lymphography also is unable to evaluate mesenteric, high para-aortic, and internal iliac nodal chains.

When compared with the results of lymphography and staging laparotomies, CT has proved to be an accurate noninvasive method of detecting abdominal lymphadenopathy with overall accuracy rates ranging from 72 to 90 per cent.[1–8, 11, 25–27] Although CT does not provide any information concerning intranodal architecture, it can evaluate lymph nodes in the areas not visualized by lymphangiography. CT routinely detects retrocrural, mesenteric, and peripancreatic adenopathy (Figs. 18–8, 18–11, and 18–12) and enlarged nodes involving the splenic, renal, and hepatic hilum. In patients with lymphatic obstruction, lymphangiography may underestimate the extent of disease beyond the point of obstruction. In these patients, CT, which does not depend upon lymph node opacification, may better reflect the true degree of nodal involvement and permit more accurate planning of radiation therapy. At times, computed tomography may demonstrate lymphomatous involvement of solid organs such as the liver, spleen, or kidneys that is unsuspected. (Fig. 18–13).[28–30]

The precise role of computed tomography and lymphangiography in the staging and follow-up of lymphomas varies among institutions. At some oncologic centers, the initial screening examination is performed using CT. This is particularly true of patients with non-Hodgkin's lymphoma, a situation in which more than 50 per cent of patients have mesenteric nodal involvement that cannot be demonstrated by bipedal lymphangiography. Other centers consider the studies com-

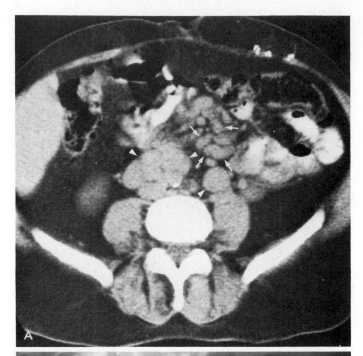

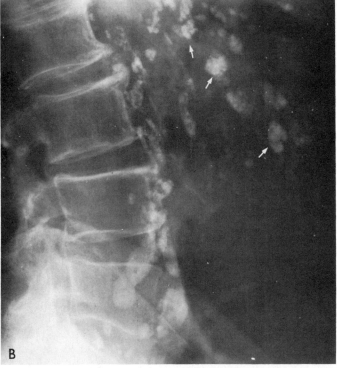

Figure 18–11. A Mesenteric adenopathy (arrows) demonstrated as multiple, small, rounded or oval densities. Para-aortic, paracaval, and aortocaval nodal enlargement (arrowheads) is also present. Diagnosis: non-Hodgkin's lymphoma. **B** Another patient. Enlarged mesenteric lymph nodes (arrows) filled with lymphangiographic contrast material.

Illustration continued on opposite page

plementary and routinely perform both CT and lymphography.[8]

Our current approach is to evaluate patients with newly diagnosed lymphoma initially by computed tomography. If widespread lymphadenopathy is present, no further staging procedures are performed. Lymphography is performed in patients with negative or equivocal CT studies. A CT-directed biopsy is performed whenever an

isolated lymph node is enlarged or when the lymphangiographic findings are equivocal.

Following the initial diagnosis, plain abdominal films or CT scans have been advocated for following the effect of therapy and for detecting recurrent disease. Abdominal radiographs are useful for following periaortic nodes as long as they contain sufficient lymphangiographic contrast material. However, approximately 50 per cent of clin-

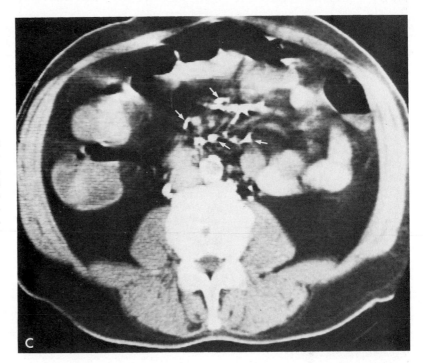

Figure 18–11. *Continued* **C** CT scan demonstrates the contrast-filled mesenteric lymph nodes (arrows). Normally, mesenteric lymph nodes do not fill at lymphangiography, but these did because the patient had obstructed cisternal chyli owing to non-Hodgkin's lymphoma.

ical relapses in lymphoma occur between 1-1/2 to 5 years and few patients retain adequate lymphographic contrast material for that period of time. Lee and co-workers[11] compared postlymphangiogram plain films with CT in patients with lymphoma. In 16 per cent of patients with apparent adequate residual contrast medium, plain films failed to demonstrate the extent of disease adequately. For this reason and because plain films cannot detect disease appearing in areas not opacified by lymphography (Fig. 18–14), we follow the majority of patients with lymphoma by computed tomography rather than by abdominal and pelvic radiography.

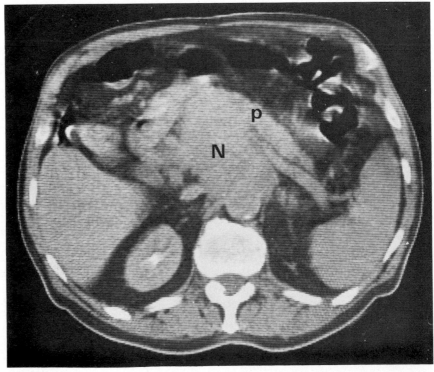

Figure 18–12. Enlarged peripancreatic lymph nodes (N), the result of non-Hodgkin's lymphoma, are displacing the pancreas (p) anteriorly, obliterating the peripancreatic and aortic fat planes, and mimicking a pancreatic neoplasm.

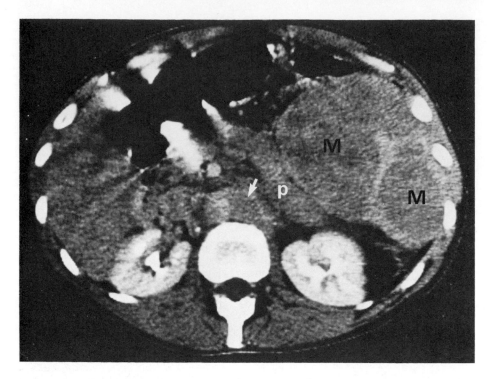

Figure 18–13. Parenchymal splenic metastasis (M) and para-aortic adenopathy (arrow) resulting from non-Hodgkin's lymphoma. p = Pancreas.

TESTICULAR NEOPLASMS

Testicular tumors account for 1 to 2 per cent of malignancies in males and are the most common cause of death from cancer in men between the ages of 25 to 35 years.[9, 10, 31] Histologically, testicular neoplasms are grouped into seminomatous and nonseminomatous categories. Nonseminomatous tumors are classified as embryonal, teratomatous, choriocarcinomatous, or mixed-element tumors on the basis of the predominant cellular component. The histologic nature of a testicular tumor directly relates to the rate of cure. Greater than 80 per cent of patients with seminoma will be free of disease 3 years after therapy but a similar disease-free period is only 62 per cent for teratoma, 55 per cent for mixed tumors, 39 per cent for embryonal carcinoma, and 26 per cent for choriocarcinoma.[12]

The choice of therapy of testicular neoplasms

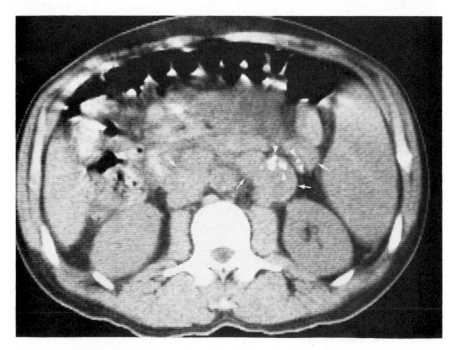

Figure 18–14. Recurrent lymphoma following therapy. A small amount of residual contrast material (arrowheads) is present in several "normal sized" para-aortic lymph nodes. The CT scan reveals extensive lymphadenopathy, which does not contain contrast material (arrows).

depends upon both histologic classification and the extent of tumor dissemination. Testicular tumors tend to spread by way of the lymphatics rather than by hematogenous routes; metastases from testicular neoplasms, therefore, tend to follow the lymphatic drainage of the involved testis. Testicular lymphatics drain into nodes located predominantly between T_{11} and L_4,[9, 12, 14] which are lateral to the para-aortic nodes usually opacified by lymphography. Spread to the lumbar para-aortic nodes that are filled by lymphography occurs only after involvement of nodes along the primary route of lymphatic drainage of the testis. This pattern of involvement accounts in part for the frequent finding of enlarged but nonopaci-

fied lymph nodes in patients with testicular neoplasms (Fig. 18–15A). The unopacified nodes tend to be lateral to the opacified nodes and displace the lumbar para-aortic nodes medially (Fig. 18–15B).

The drainage routes differs between the right and left testis as each follows the course of its gonadal vein. On the left side, the usual lymphatic drainage is to the lateral para-aortic nodes, just below the renal hilum and left renal vein at about the L_{1-2} level. On the right, the primary lymphatic channels flow more directly into paracaval nodes between the renal vein and aortic bifurcation at the L_{1-3} level (Fig. 18–16). However, crossover lymphatic channels are usually present,

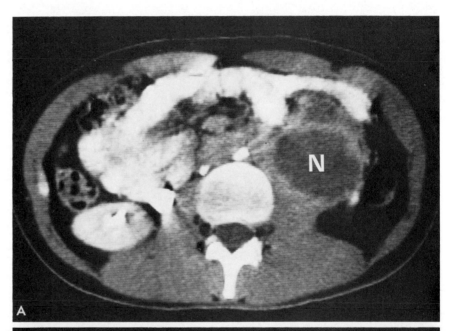

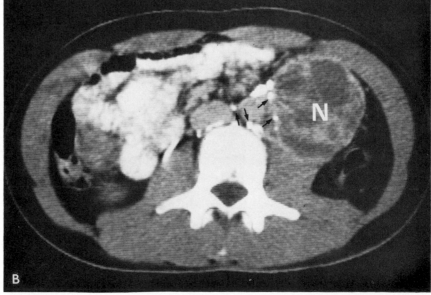

Figure 18–15. Metastatic seminoma. **A** CT scan demonstrating a huge, low-density, unopacified para-aortic nodal metastasis (N) from left testicular seminoma. **B** CT scan at lower level demonstrates multiple, normal-sized, opacified lymph nodes (arrows) medial to the large unopacified nodal metastasis (N).

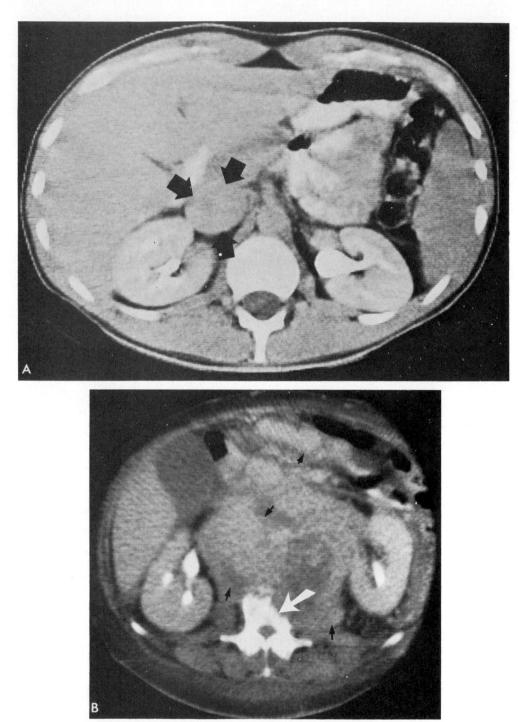

Figure 18–16. A   Right testicular carcinoma has metastasized to lymph nodes in the right renal hilum (arrows). The metastasis simulates the inferior vena cava but is three to four times the size of the normal inferior vena cava. At surgery the inferior vena cava was found to be severely compressed and crescent-shaped but not invaded. **B**   Right testicular seminoma producing massive paracaval, aorto-caval, para-aortic and mesenteric adenopathy (small arrows) as well as destruction of spine (large arrow). Crossover lymphatic drainage permits bilateral nodal enlargement.

particularly from the right to the left side, and account for bilateral nodal involvement from a unilateral testicular tumor (Fig. 18–16*B*). Involvement of pelvic, mesenteric, or femoral nodes is rare and usually occurs only with advanced disease or after primary routes of drainage have been altered by surgery or biopsy. Retrocrural nodal involvement occurs in only 7 to 14 per cent of patients with testicular neoplasms.[12, 14]

CT frequently demonstrates metastatic testicular tumors to have regions of low attenuation value (Fig. 18–15 and 18–16). CT density values close to those of a cyst—10 to 30 Hounsfield Units (H)—were found in 48 per cent of patients.[14] The exact cause of the low CT attenuation is unclear but is probably due to tumor degeneration or necrosis or both. However, there is little correlation between attenuation values and size or volume of nodes involved with metastatic testicular neoplasms.[14]

Several studies have compared the use of CT and lymphangiography in the staging of testicular neoplasms.[12, 14, 31] The accuracy of lymphography in detecting metastatic testicular carcinoma ranges from 62 to 89 per cent,[31] whereas CT has been found to be 66 to 90 per cent accurate.[9, 12, 27] Despite approximately equal overall accuracy rates, studies have documented the superiority of CT in delineating true extent of disease and in affecting the decision as to type of therapy to be employed.[12, 14] In the majority of patients, metastasis from testicular tumors produces large, bulky retroperitoneal lymphadenopathy that is easily detected by CT scans (Figs. 18–15 and 18–16) and not focal metastatic deposits in normal-sized nodes.

At the University of California, San Francisco, CT is employed as the initial staging modality in patients with newly diagnosed testicular carcinoma. If the CT study is positive, lymphography is not performed. However, if the CT scan is normal or equivocal, a lymphangiogram is obtained to take advantage of the lymphangiogram's ability to detect architectural abnormalities within nonenlarged nodes. Following diagnosis, CT can easily follow the effectiveness of therapy. However, caution must be exercised in interpreting residual retroperitoneal masses as representing a therapy failure. Residual fibrosis or necrosis after successful therapy can result in para-aortic masses that cannot be distinguished from recurrent or residual tumors.[13] In these patients, a fine-needle aspiration biopsy is a safe and accurate method of determining whether or not viable tumor is present.

PELVIC MALIGNANCIES

Studies evaluating the CT diagnosis of nodal metastasis from pelvic malignancies have revealed CT to be less accurate than in the staging of lymphoma or testicular neoplasms.[15–17, 21] This is primarily due to the inability of CT to detect metastasis to normal-size lymph nodes. Lee and associates reported a 73 per cent accuracy of CT when compared with staging laparotomy in a variety of pelvic malignancies,[17] and similar results were obtained by Walsh and colleagues, who noted a 77 per cent accuracy of CT in histologically confirmed cases.[18] However, only nodes larger than 2 cm were considered abnormal[18] and therefore the lower accuracy of CT in detecting pelvic lymphatic metastasis may in part be related to the size criteria of normal pelvic lymph nodes.

In a study by Levine and co-workers[20] comparing the accuracy of CT and lymphangiography in detecting metastasis from prostatic carcinoma, CT achieved an overall accuracy of 93 per cent. In this study, deep pelvic nodes (hypogastric or obturator nodes) were considered abnormal if they were greater than 1.2 cm. Koss and colleagues,[19] using 1.5 cm as the upper limit for normal pelvic lymph nodes, demonstrated 92 per cent accuracy for CT in bladder carcinoma.

In a comparison study of CT and lymphangiography in carcinoma of the cervix, Ginaldi and associates[16] emphasized the complementary role of CT and lymphography. CT has a greater diagnostic yield and more accurately reflects the true extent of disease in relatively advanced stages, whereas lymphangiography remains of considerable clinical value in detecting subtle changes in nodal architecture produced by early metastasis. We currently employ CT as the initial diagnostic procedure, followed by lymphangiography only if CT is negative or equivocal. CT guided-needle aspiration of nodes that are equivocally enlarged is likely to aid significantly in detecting pelvic metastasis.

Inferior Vena Cava
ANATOMY

Computed tomography can readily image the normal inferior vena cava (IVC) as well as its congenital variants.[32] The normal IVC lies to the right of the aorta and gradually tapers down to its bifurcation. The size of the normal IVC varies from a rounded structure 2 to 3 cm in diameter to a small slitlike structure that is barely detecta-

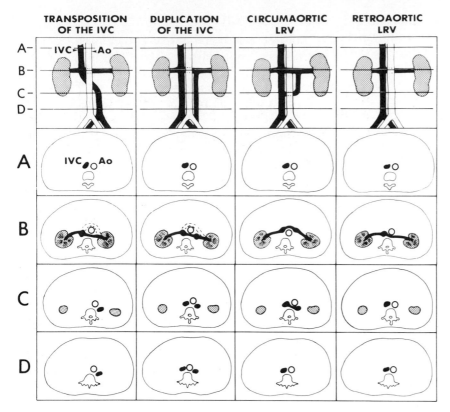

Figure 18–17. Diagram of inferior vena cava and left renal vein anomalies. **A–D** Axial CT appearance is diagrammed. (From Royal SA, Callen PW: CT evaluation of anomalies of the inferior vena cava and left renal vein. AJR 132:759, 1979. © 1979, American Roentgen Ray Society. Reprinted by permission.)

ble. The size is somewhat dependent on the phase of respiration and can vary from scan to scan within the same patient.

CONGENITAL ANOMALIES

Congenital anomalies that are demonstrable by computed tomography include caval duplication and transposition[32–34] and azygos continuation of the IVC (Fig. 18–17).[35–37] In caval transposition (incidence 0.2 to 0.5 per cent), there is a single IVC that is intially left-sided in the lower abdomen and crosses to the right side either anterior or posterior to the aorta at the level of the renal veins. On CT, a single venous structure is seen to the left of the aorta below the renal veins, which crosses to the right side at the level of the renal veins to continue on the right side above the renal veins (Fig. 18–18). In duplication (incidence 0.2 to 3 per cent) of the IVC, there is a second left-sided IVC that originates from the left common iliac vein and ascends to the level of the renal veins (Fig. 18–19). A variety of anomalous vascular communications link the left-sided IVC with the normally positioned vena cava at the level of the renal veins.

Computed tomography may also diagnose congenital anomalies of the left renal vein, including circumaortic (incidence 1.5 to 8.7 per cent) and

retroaortic left renal veins (incidence 1.8 to 2.4 per cent) (Fig. 18–20). In patients with a circumaortic left renal vein, there is a true vascular ring surrounding the aorta consisting of both preaortic and a retroaortic left renal veins. The preaortic left renal vein is seen in normal position, whereas the bridging retroaortic vein connects the normal vein to the IVC one to two vertebral bodies below the level of the preaortic vein. In patients with an isolated retroaortic left renal vein, there is a single left renal vein that courses posterior to the aorta either at the level of the normal left renal vein or courses obliquely caudad to enter the lower IVC.

Detection of azygos continuation (incidence 0.6 per cent) by CT depends on identification of an enlarged azygos (or hemiazygos) vein in the retrocrural space (Fig. 18–21).[35–37] The enlarged azygos vein appears as a tubular structure on multiple contiguous scans and enhances after injection of contrast material. When an enlarged retrocrural azygos vein is identified, obstruction of the superior IVC must be excluded before a diagnosis of azygos continuation is made. Congenital heart disease is present in 85 per cent of patients with azygos continuation.[37] Left pulmonary isomerism, polysplenia, dextrocardia, intracardiac defects, and transposed abdominal viscera are associated with azygos continuation.

Text continued on page 928

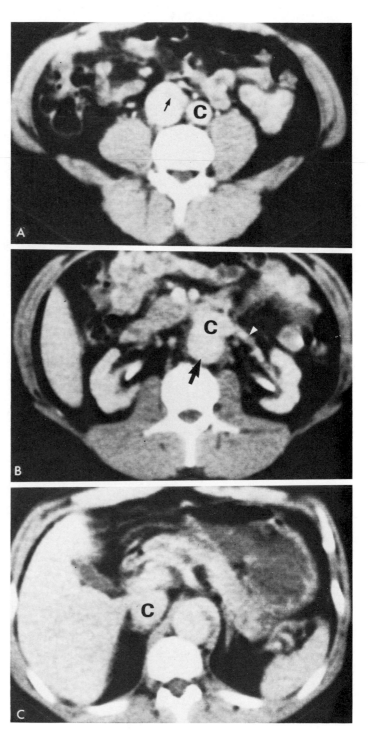

Figure 18–18. Transposition of the inferior vena cava. **A**   Scan below kidneys reveals left-sided inferior vena cava (C) and an aortic dissection (arrow). **B**   At level of the midportion of kidneys, the inferior vena cava (arrow) has moved to lie directly ventral to the aorta. The left renal vein (arrowhead) enters the inferior vena cava at this level. **C** CT scan above the kidneys demonstrates that the inferior vena cava (C) has crossed over to the right side of the abdomen.

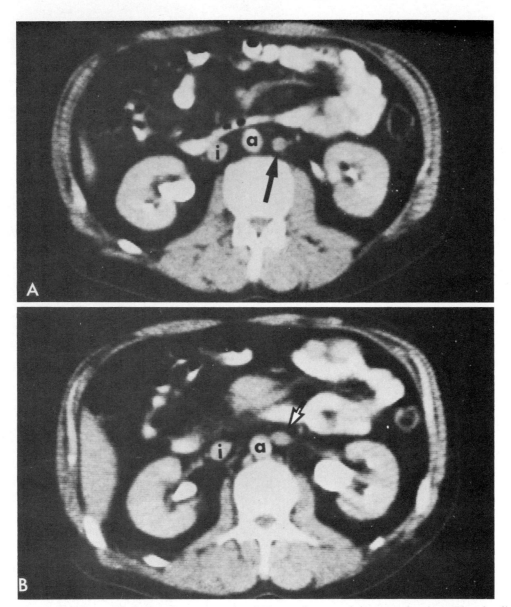

Figure 18–19. Duplicated inferior vena cava. **A**   CT scan just caudal to renal veins. The duplicated inferior vena cava (arrow) is a large vessel to the left of the aorta (a). **B**   At the level of the renal veins, the duplicated inferior vena cava (i) joins left renal vein, producing a focal dilatation (arrow) of the left renal vein.

Illustration continued on opposite page

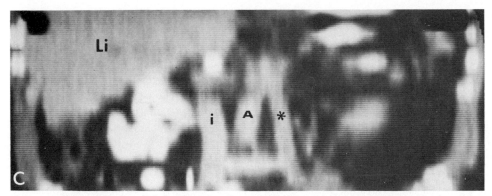

Figure 18–19. *Continued* **C**   Coronal reconstruction demonstrates the continuous nature of the duplicated inferior vena cava (asterisk), which runs from a level just cephalad to the iliac vein to its entrance into left renal vein. Li = Liver; A = aorta; i = normal right-sided inferior vena cava. (From Royal SA, Callen PW: CT evaluation of anomalies of the inferior vena cava and left renal vein. AJR 132:759, 1979. © 1979, American Roentgen Ray Society. Reprinted by permission.)

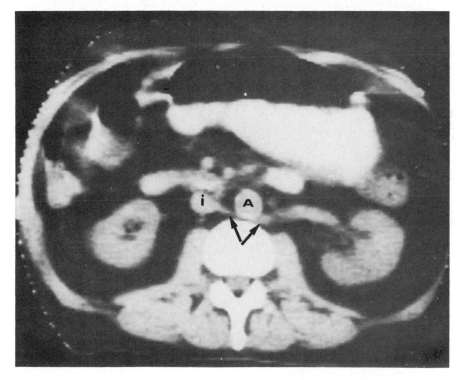

Figure 18–20. Retroaortic left renal vein. CT scan demonstrating the left renal vein (arrows) coursing dorsal to the aorta (A) to join the inferior vena cava (i). (From Royal SA, Callen PW: CT Evaluation of anomalies of the inferior vena cava and left renal vein. AJR 132:759, 1979. © 1979, American Roentgen Ray Society. Reprinted by permission.)

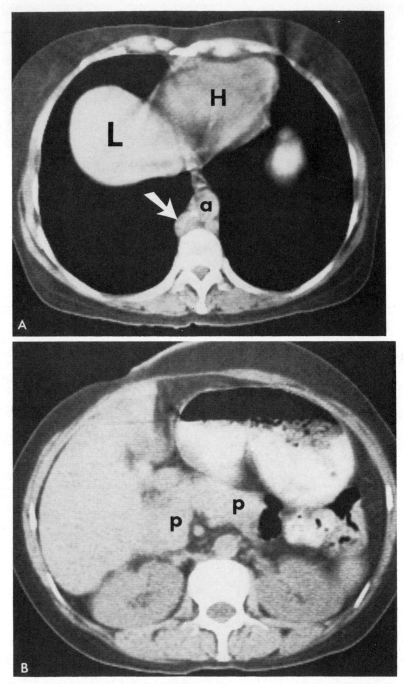

Figure 18–21. Azygos continuation of the inferior vena cava in a patient with polysplenia. **A**   CT scan at level of top of liver (L) and heart (H) demonstrates a dilated azygos vein (arrow) adjacent to descending aorta (a). There is no intrahepatic inferior vena cava. **B**   Scan through the abdomen demonstrates lack of a normal-sized inferior vena cava. p = Pancreas.

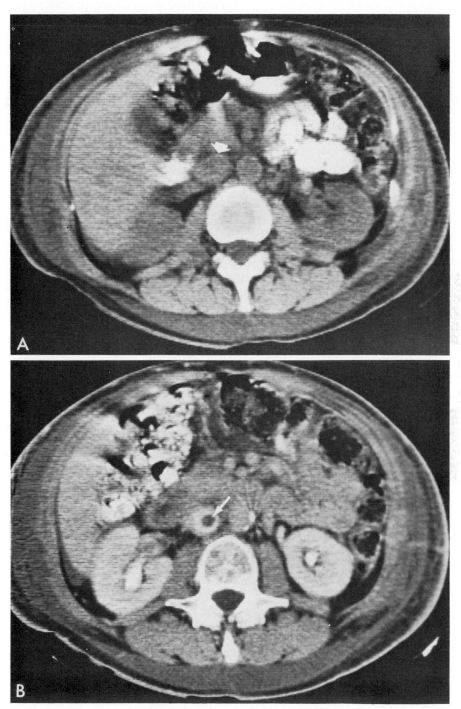

Figure 18–22. Inferior vena cava thrombus owing to thrombophlebitis. **A** Initial non-contrast scan demonstrates no definite abnormality of the inferior vena cava (arrow). **B** Scan after bolus injection of contrast material by way of a foot vein clearly outlines a thrombus (arrow) in the inferior vena cava.

TECHNIQUES OF EXAMINATION

The method of studying patients with suspected abnormalities of the IVC varies among investigators.[38–44] Infusion and bolus techniques have been used with contrast material being administered in both upper- and lower-extremity veins. A combination of a 50- to 70-ml bolus immediately followed by a rapid infusion of 60 per cent intravenous contrast material through a foot

vein consistently provides good opacification of the IVC. In patients with known or suspected IVC thrombosis, a bolus injection of 50 to 70 ml followed by a dynamic scan sequence at the level of suspected thrombosis usually will demonstrate caval patency or occlusion. However, laminar flow defects in the IVC can simulate a thrombosis after bolus injections into the lower extremities.[45] If the diagnosis of an IVC thrombosis is not clear, a repeated CT scan is obtained during a rapid intravenous infusion of contrast material into an upper-extremity vein.[45]

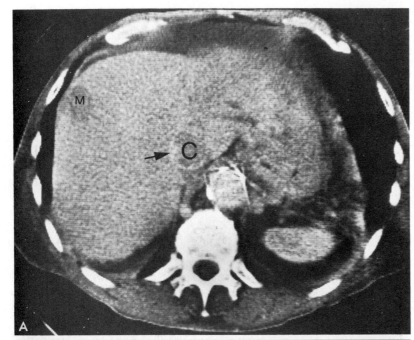

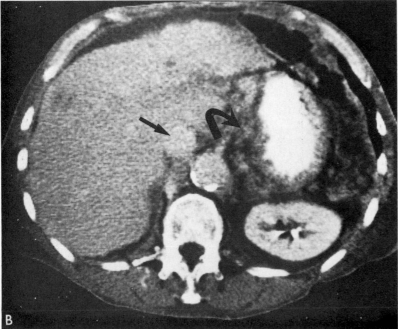

Figure 18–23. Thrombosis of inferior vena cava resulting from tumor. **A** CT scan through level of intrahepatic inferior vena cava (C) demonstrates the IVC to be enlarged and nonopacified except for a peripheral rim (arrow) of contrast enhancement. M = Metastasis. **B** CT scan at more caudal level demonstrates the inferior vena cava (arrow) to be patent. Large collateral vascular channels (curved arrow) are identified.

Illustration continued on opposite page

PATHOLOGY

THROMBOSIS

Both intrinsic and extrinsic lesions of the IVC are readily identified by computed tomography. Thrombus formation within the IVC may be the result of a bland or septic thrombosis or secondary to tumor extension.[37-46] The characteristic CT features of IVC thrombosis include caval enlargement due to intraluminal clot or neoplasm, a low-density intraluminal filling defect, and a rim of high density produced by contrast material surrounding the lower-density thrombus (Fig. 18–22).[37-46] Fresh thrombus within the IVC may be isodense with other vascular structures but will decrease in density with time. Although neoplastic invasion of the IVC often has a similar CT appearance similar to a bland thrombus (Fig. 18–23),[38-40] a specific diagnosis of a septic thrombus of the IVC can be made by identifying multiple gas bubbles within a low-attenuation intraluminal caval filling defect (Fig. 18–24).[46]

The CT demonstration of tumor extension into the IVC is an important prognostic sign in patients with primary carcinomas of the liver (Fig. 18–25), adrenal gland, or kidney.[41-43, 45, 47] Comparison studies of CT and angiography in patients with hypernephromas have demonstrated CT to be an accurate method of diagnosing tumor extension into the main renal vein and IVC.[41] A bolus injection of 80 to 100 ml of contrast material followed by a dynamic scan sequence will optimally demonstrate neoplastic involvement of the main renal veins. CT is less accurate in the diagnosis of intrarenal vein thrombosis; however, detection of isolated invasion of intrarenal veins is unlikely to alter surgical therapy and therefore has less prognostic significance.[41] In addition to demonstrating intrinsic involvement of the inferior vena cava, CT can also diagnose extrinsic displacement and compression of the IVC by primary hepatic or retroperitoneal masses (Fig. 18–26), such as lymphadenopathy, primary retroperitoneal tumors, abscesses, or hemorrhage. CT can also be used to evaluate the patency of portacaval and mesocaval shunts (Fig. 18–27). Documentation of contrast medium flowing through the shunt confirms patency, and the time course of filling provides information concerning the hemodynamics of the shunt.

Text continued on page 934

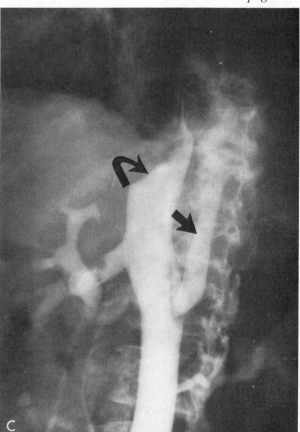

Figure 18–23. *Continued* **C** Inferior venacavogram showing total occlusion of the intrahepatic portion of the inferior vena cava (curved arrow) and an enlarged collateral venous channel (arrow).

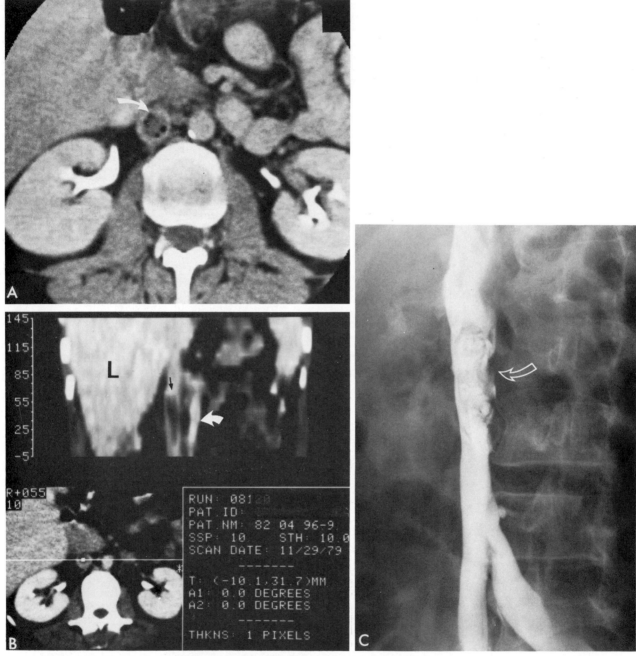

Figure 18–24. Septic thrombosis of inferior vena cava, the result of a toothpick perforating the duodenum and inferior vena cava. **A**   Axial CT scan demonstrates multiple gas bubbles within a caval thrombosis (arrow). **B**   Coronal reformation. Thrombus is present in the inferior vena cava (black arrow). White arrow = Aorta; L = liver. **C**   Inferior venacavogram confirms thrombus (arrow). (From Schmitz L, Jeffrey RB, Palubinskas AJ, Moss AA: CT demonstration of septic thrombosis of the inferior vena cava. J Comput Assist Tomogr 5:259, 1981. Reprinted by permission.)

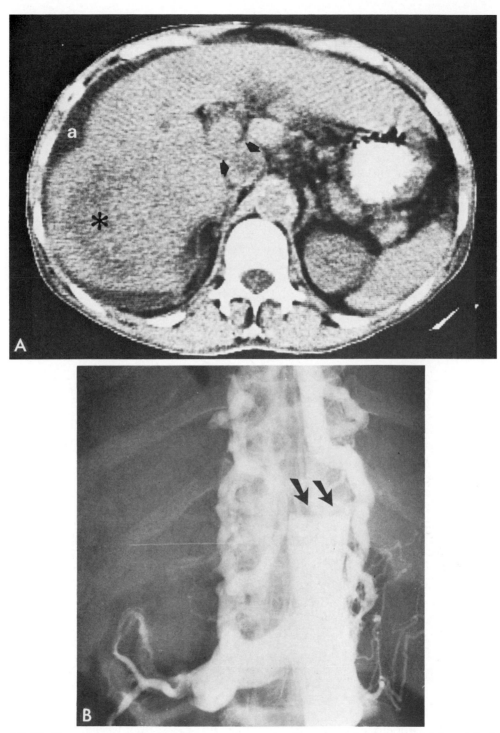

Figure 18–25. Hepatoma invading inferior vena cava. **A** Hepatoma (asterisk) involving right hepatic lobe. A low-attenuation filling defect is present in the intrahepatic segment of the inferior vena cava (arrows). a = Ascites. **B** Inferior venacavogram demonstrates total caval obstruction (arrows) with marked collateral flow.

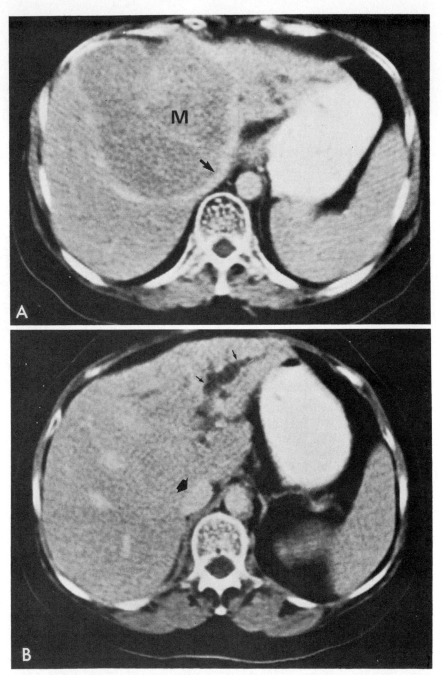

Figure 18–26. Extrinsic compression of intrahepatic portion of inferior vena cava by tumor. **A** CT scan reveals a hypodense mass (M) with an enhancing peripheral rim adjacent to the expected position of the intrahepatic portion of inferior vena cava (arrow). **B** Scan at lower level demonstrates a patent inferior vena cava (arrow). The left biliary system (small arrows) is obstructed.

Illustration continued on opposite page

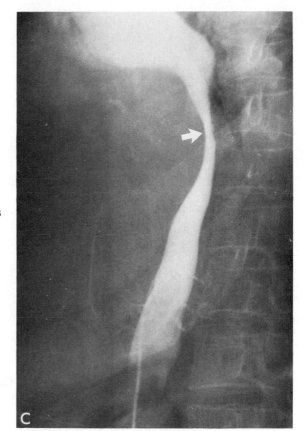

Figure 18–26. *Continued* **C** Inferior venacavogram outlines a compressed (arrow) but patent inferior vena cava.

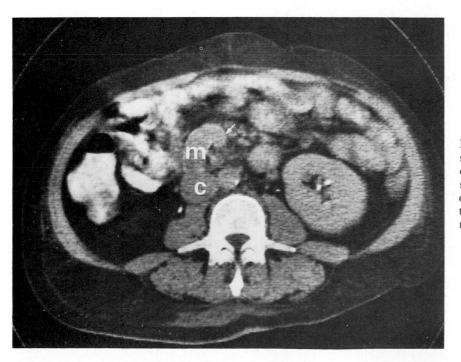

Figure 18–27. Patent mesocaval shunt. The shunt (m) is shown to connect a mesenteric venous vessel (arrow) with the inferior vena cava (c). Contrast material is seen to flow through the shunt, documenting patency.

Abdominal Aorta

ANATOMY

The normal abdominal aorta measures less than 3 cm in diameter and tapers gradually to its bifurcation at L_3-L_4. There is usually sufficient perivascular fat to outline the margin of the abdominal aorta and the origins of the renal arteries, celiac axis, and superior mesenteric artery (Fig. 18–28).[34] Common vascular variants such as multiple renal arteries and an anomalous hepatic artery (Fig. 18–28*B*) are routinely demonstrated.

TECHNIQUES OF EXAMINATION

In most patients, the abdominal aorta is well demonstrated by a rapid infusion of intravenous contrast medium via an 18-gauge needle in a peripheral vein. In patients suspected of having a

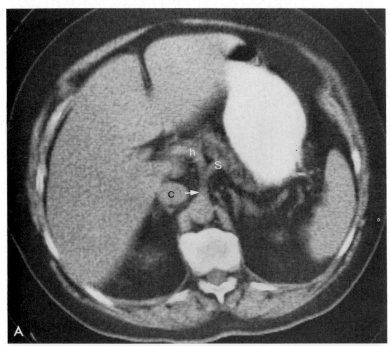

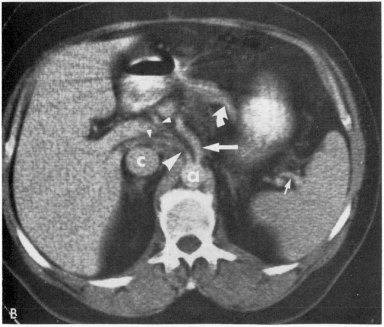

Figure 18–28. Normal aortic anatomy. **A** Celiac axis (arrow) branching into the splenic (s) and hepatic (h) arteries. The left gastric branch is not seen. c = Inferior vena cava. **B** Celiac artery and anomalous origin of hepatic artery. The celiac artery (large arrow) arises from the aorta (a) and divides into the left gastric (curved arrow) and splenic (small arrow) arteries. The proper hepatic artery (large arrowhead) originates directly from the aorta and divides into two branches (small arrowheads). c = Inferior vena cava.

Illustration continued on opposite page

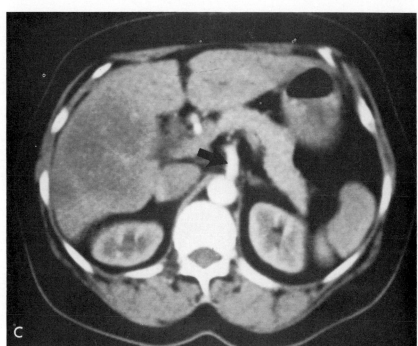

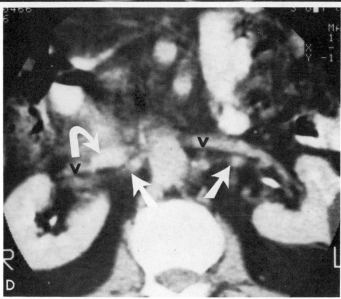

Figure 18–28. *Continued* **C** Superior mesenteric artery (arrow) arising from the aorta 1 cm below the celiac artery. **D** Scan through the level of the renal arteries (arrows) demonstrating typical position of the arteries dorsal to the renal veins (v). Curved arrow = Inferior vena cava.

dissecting abdominal aneurysm, a 50- to 80-ml bolus of contrast medium followed by rapid sequential scanning provides optimal delineation of the aortic lumen and detects intimal flaps better than the slow infusion of contrast medium. Relative flow through the true and false aortic lumen can be visually identified and calculated by computer programs that plot in graph form the changes in CT numbers with time. As with abnormalities of the IVC, both coronal and sagittal reformations are helpful in selected instances to better define anatomic relationships of the aorta to surrounding structures.

PATHOLOGY

AORTIC ANEURYSM

Currently, ultrasonography is the diagnostic method of choice in the initial screening of patients for suspected abdominal aortic aneurysms. However, if sonography is unsatisfactory, CT provides an alternative noninvasive method of detecting an aortic aneurysm, defining its extent and demonstrating its relationship to the major vascular structures (Fig. 18–29). The exact size of the aorta can be measured and the presence and extent of mural thrombus delineated.

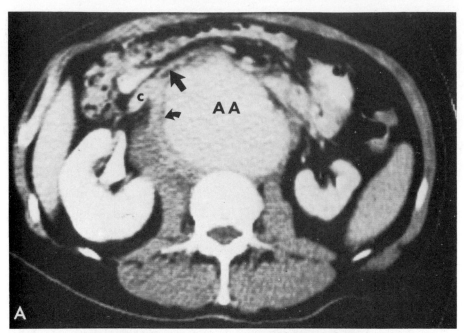

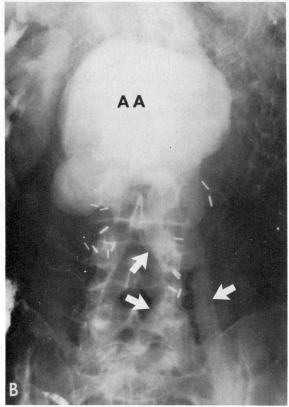

Figure 18–29. Abdominal aortic aneurysm. **A** Large saccular aneurysm of the abdominal aorta (AA) elevating the inferior vena cava (c) and stretching the left renal vein (arrow). Virtually the entire aneurysm fills with contrast material, only a small amount of mural thrombus being present (curved arrow). **B** Aortogram confirms the presence of a large saccular aortic aneurysm (AA), which fills with contrast material, as well as the patency of a distal aortic graft (arrows).

In patients with slowly leaking abdominal aortic aneurysms, the periaortic fat planes are obscured by a mass lesion representing a hematoma (Fig. 18–30A). The location and shape of the hematoma depend on the site and severity of the hemorrhage. Some hemorrhages tend to surround the aorta, forming a round mass; others dissect into the retroperitoneal space, producing an irregular mass that encases adjacent organs (Fig. 18–30B). The density of the hematoma depends on its age. A fresh hematoma can have a density higher than that of surrounding soft tissues, whereas a hematoma 2 to 4 weeks old will have a lower attenuation value. If a CT scan is done during active bleeding, the hematoma can have a very high density as a result of contrast material leaking from the aorta into the hematoma. A similar appearance is seen if a CT scan is performed shortly after a translumbar aortogram.[48, 49]

The presence of a circumferential mass surrounding an abdominal aneurysm does not always mean that an aortic leak has occurred. In asymptomatic patients with abdominal aortic aneurysms, CT may demonstrate a diffuse mantle of perianeurysmal fibrosis in the absence of hemorrhage. Although the exact etiology of this tissue is unknown, the lack of hemosiderin within the fibrotic mass suggests it is not related to hemorrhage.[50] Following contrast medium administration, this tissue may dramatically increase its attenuation value and simulate a periaortic hemorrhage. It is important to recognize this entity in order not to diagnose the intense perianeurysmal increase in CT density following a contrast injection as representing a life-threatening aortic hemorrhage. Perianeurysmal fibrosis can also simulate idiopathic retroperitoneal fibrosis by encasing the ureter and causing hydronephrosis.[50]

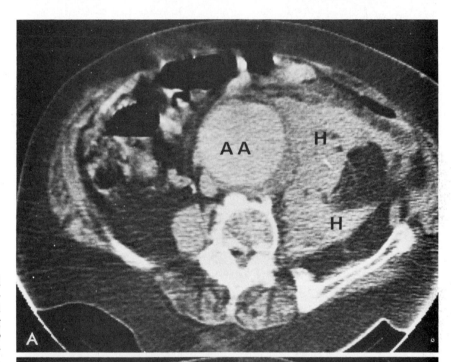

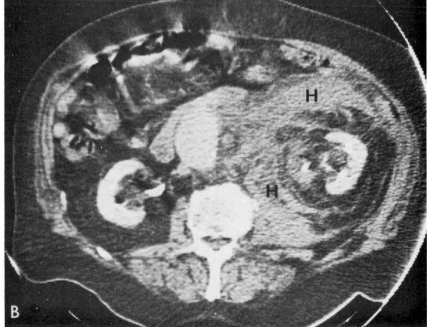

Figure 18–30. Leaking abdominal aortic aneurysm. **A** A large abdominal aortic aneurysm (AA) and a soft-tissue density representing hemorrhage (H), which extends to the left of the aneurysm and obscures the periaortic fat planes. **B** Scan at a higher level demonstrates the hematoma (H) to extend into the anterior and posterior pararenal spaces, encasing the left kidney.

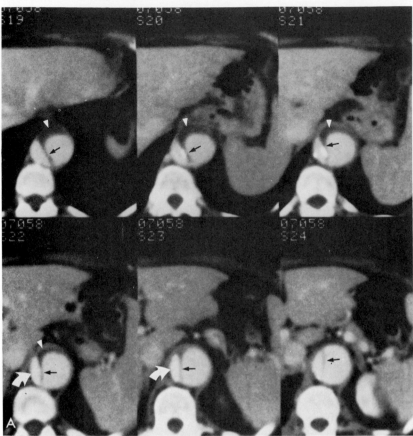

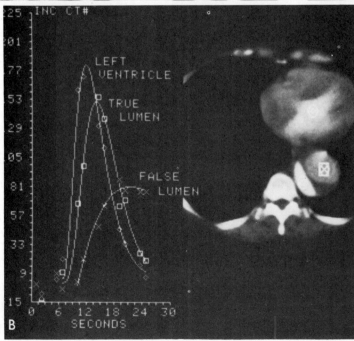

Figure 18–31. Dynamic CT scan of dissecting aneurysm of thoracic aorta extending into the abdomen. **A**   Six back-to-back CT scans following a 50-ml bolus injection of contrast material. There has been a 1-cm table incrementation during the interscan delay of 1.2 seconds. The intimal flap (black arrow) is readily demonstrated. The false lumen (curved arrow) is flattened by the patent true lumen, and a small clot (arrowhead) surrounds the true lumen. Calcification in the aortic wall is displaced inward. **B**   Time-density curve of contrast flow through the heart and true and false aortic lumens. The true lumen enhances maximally just after the left ventricle and rapidly decreases in density. The density of the false lumen rises more slowly to a lower peak, but the peak persists longer than that for the true lumen, indicating slow flow through the false lumen.

AORTIC DISSECTION

Dissection of the abdominal aorta as well as extension of thoracic dissections into the abdomen is readily demonstrated by CT (Fig. 18–31). Dynamic sequential scanning is helpful in diagnos-

ing differential opacification of the true and false lumen and in detecting the presence of intimal flaps (Fig. 18–31). The definitive CT finding is a contrast-filled double channel with an intervening intimal flap. If one channel is totally thrombosed, distinguishing a dissection from a fusiform aneurysm with an adherent clot can be difficult. Associated findings in dissection are inward displacement of intimal calcification, intraluminal thrombosis, dilatation of the aorta with compression of the true lumen, irregular contour of the contrast-filled part of the aorta, and differential flow to the kidneys (Fig. 18–31).

The accuracy of CT in detecting abdominal aortic dissections is high. At the University of California, San Francisco, no false-positive or negative diagnoses have been made in proven cases. As a result of the high accuracy and noninvasiveness, CT has largely replaced aortography as the initial diagnostic procedure except for patients in whom an immediate operation is warranted and in whom opacification of all aortic branch vessels is needed. Following treatment, CT is a noninva-

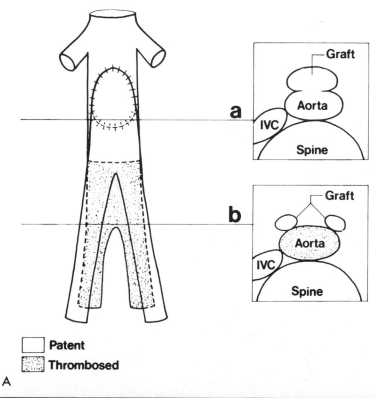

Figure 18–32. A Diagram of end-to-side aortic graft anastomosis. The graft is positioned ventral to the native aorta and usually bifurcates above the native bifurcation. Insets **(a,b)** demonstrate cross-sectional anatomy of the graft in relation to the native aorta. (From Mark A, Moss AA, Lusby R, Kaiser JA: CT Evaluation of complication of abdominal aortic surgery. Radiology 145:409, 1982. Used with permission.) **B** CT scan of a patent normal graft (arrow) located above the thrombosed native aorta (a).

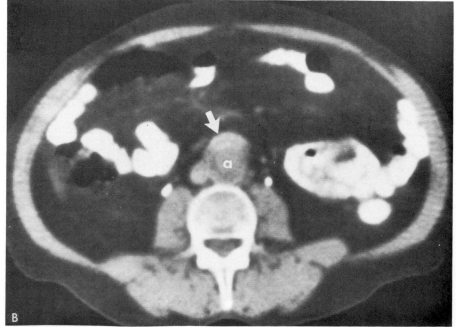

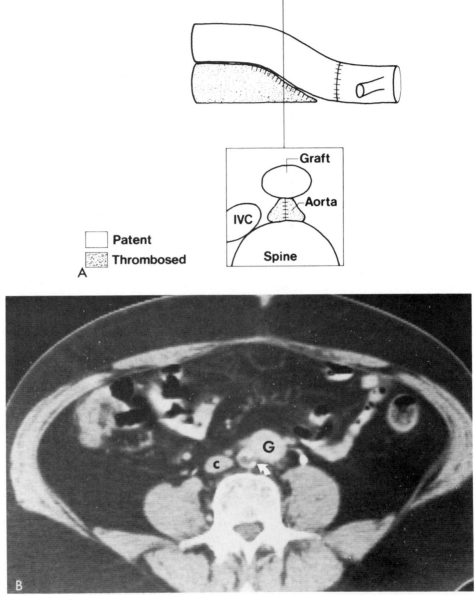

Figure 18–33. A Diagram of end-to-end aortic graft anastomosis (lateral and cross-sectional views). (From Mark A, Moss AA, Lusby R, Kaiser JA: CT Evaluation of complications of abdominal aortic surgery. Radiology 145:409, 1982. Used with permission.) **B** CT scan demonstrates a patent graft (G) and a small clotted native aorta between the graft and the spine. The native aorta is slightly more ventral than is usually seen. c = Inferior vena cava.

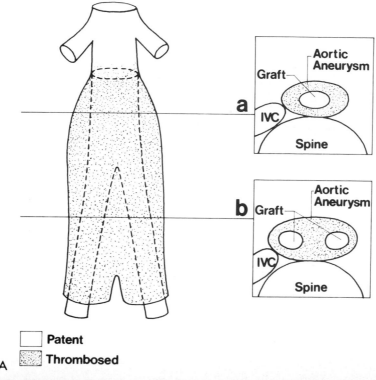

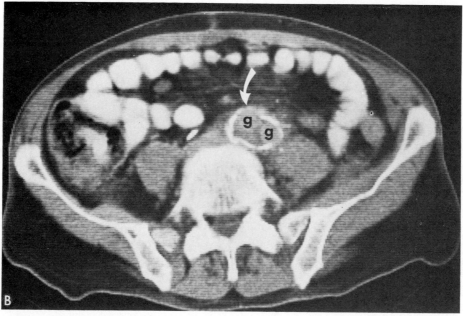

Figure 18–34. A   Diagram of graft and native aorta after aortic graft placement in a patient with aortic aneurysm. The graft is positioned within the aneurysm, which is sutured around the graft. Inserts **(a,b)** demonstrate cross-sectional anatomy of the graft in relation to the native aorta. (From Mark A, Moss AA, Lusby R, Kaiser JA: CT Evaluation of complications of abdominal aortic surgery. Radiology 145:409, 1982. Used with permission.) **B**   Scan through a lower level of the aneurysm reveals both limbs of the graft (g) surrounded by aneurysmal native aorta (curved arrow).

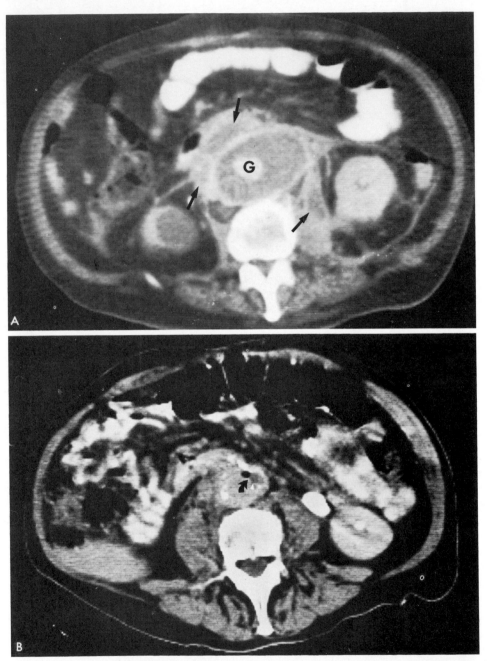

Figure 18–35. Perigraft infection following aortoiliac graft surgery. **A** Perigraft fluid collection (arrows), without gas, proved to be abscess. The patent graft (G) is wrapped by an aortic aneurysm and surrounded by a clot. **B** A small collection of gas (curved arrow) and fluid (arrowhead) adjacent to the graft indicates infection, an unsuspected aortoduodenal fistula, or both. Final diagnosis: Infection with aortoduodenal fistula.

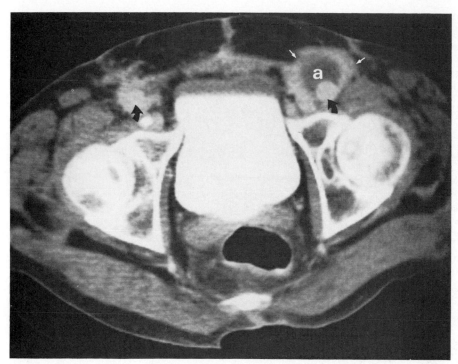

Figure 18–36. Localized perigraft abscess. A patent, well-incorporated right iliac graft (curved arrow) is surrounded by fibrosis but has no fluid collection. The patent left iliac graft (curved arrow) is partially surrounded by a fluid collection, proved to be a localized perigraft abscess (a). The abscess is surrounded by a thick, enhancing rim (arrows).

sive method of following patients who have had surgical or medical therapy for aortic dissection.

AORTIC SURGERY

Computed tomography has been shown capable of accurately displaying postsurgical anatomy (Figs. 18–32 through 18–34) and in diagnosing a variety of complications following aortoiliac surgery.[51–53] Common complications have included infection, hemorrhage, thrombosis, pseudoaneurysm, aortoduodenal fistula, and ureteral obstruction.[51, 52] In patients with infected grafts, CT usually demonstrates a periaortic fluid or gas collection (Fig. 18–35).[51, 52] A CT-guided aspiration can easily be performed to document the infection and obtains specimens for culture. Of particular value has been the capacity of CT to distinguish isolated groin infections that may be managed with local therapy (Fig. 18–36) from those that have spread to involve the abdominal graft and therefore require removal of the intra-abdominal graft.

Perigraft hemorrhage following aortoiliac surgery can also be diagnosed by CT. In a postoperative patient with a falling hematocrit, CT will demonstrate a perigraft mass that is usually ho-

mogeneous and related to either the abdominal or groin anastomosis. Pseudoaneurysms occur at the site of anastomosis and are shown by CT as mass lesions of fluid density, may contain septations and have rim enhancement after contrast injection (Fig. 18–37). Aortoduodenal fistulas are suggested by CT when there is presence of gas in the retroperitoneal region near the level of anastomosis, with or without a fluid collection being present (Figs. 18–35B and 18–38).

Ureteral obstruction is a well-known complication following aortoiliac surgery.[53] This generally results from the placement of the graft over the ureter with obstruction commonly occurring at the level of the pelvic inlet. On occasion, however, perigraft fibrosis may entrap the ureter, resulting in obstruction and hydronephrosis.

CT provides more information concerning the nature, extent, and location of complications following aortoiliac surgery than any other technique. Because of the high information content of aortic CT scans, CT is employed as the initial diagnostic procedure and arteriography is reserved for those patients requiring surgery and further delineation of vascular anatomy.

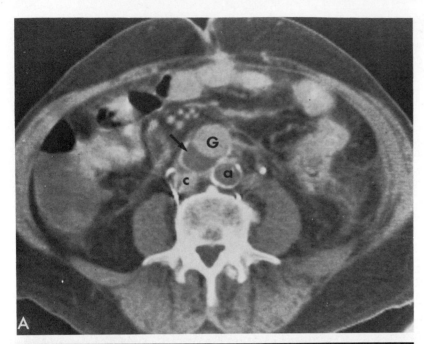

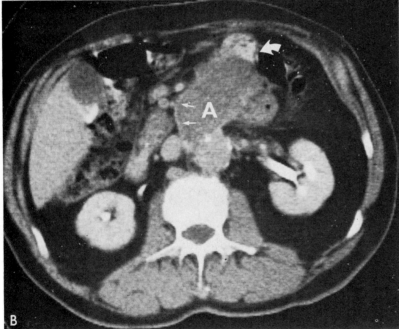

Figure 18–37. A Pseudoaneurysm following aortoiliac surgery. A patent end-to-side graft (G), clotted native aorta (a), normal inferior vena cava (c), and small pseudoaneurysm (arrow) are clearly shown. The pseudoaneurysm is clotted and has the same density as the aorta. **B** Large pseudoaneurysm (A) arising at the site of the anastomosis of the graft to the aorta and extending ventrally to displace the adjacent bowel (curved arrow). There is an enhancing rim (arrows) surrounding a portion of the pseudoaneurysm.

Retroperitoneum
PATHOLOGY

RETROPERITONEAL FIBROSIS

Retroperitoneal fibrosis occurs in patients aged 8 to 80 years with peak incidence in the fifth and sixth decades. Males are twice as frequently affected as females.[54] Patients with idiopathic retroperitoneal fibrosis develop a plaquelike mantle of fibrous tissue that encases the periaortic areas

(Fig. 18–39).[54–57] The fibrous mass can invade organs, but symptoms are usually due to constriction and compression of retroperitoneal structures. The ureters are the most common site of involvement, although the biliary tract, duodenum, inferior vena cava, aorta, pancreas and mesenteric vessels can also be affected.[54–56] Although the etiology of retroperitoneal fibrosis remains unknown, there is association with the drug methysergide, suggesting that in some cases the fibrosis represents a hypersensitivity reaction.[54]

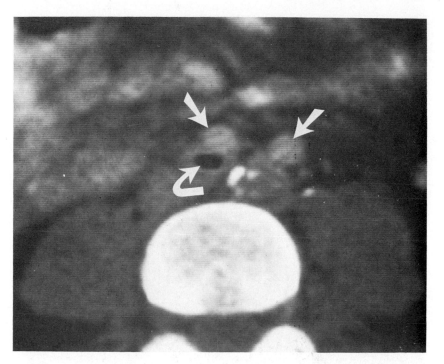

Figure 18–38. Aortoduodenal fistula seen as a focal pocket of gas (curved arrow) under the right limb of an aortic graft. Both limbs (arrows) of the graft are patent. (From Mark A, Moss AA, Lusby R, Kaiser JA: CT Evaluation of complications of abdominal aortic surgery. Radiology 145:409, 1982. Used with permission.)

Other patients with retroperitoneal fibrosis have either primary or metastatic neoplasms of the retroperitoneal space that apparently simulate a fibrotic reaction indistinguishable from the idiopathic form of the disease.[58]

The CT findings in retroperitoneal fibrosis are nonspecific. A similar CT appearance can be seen in patients with retroperitoneal hemorrhage, primary retroperitoneal sarcomas, and metastatic disease to the retroperitoneum.[54] A CT-guided biopsy is useful in distinguishing these entities. The CT findings are usually those of a solid mass

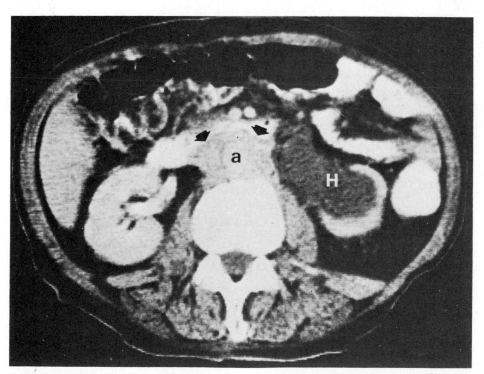

Figure 18–39. Idiopathic retroperitoneal fibrosis (arrows) surrounding the aorta (a) and obstructing the left ureter, producing hydronephrosis (H) of the left kidney.

located centrally and in the paravertebral regions. The mass tends to envelop and not displace adjacent structures such as the aorta, inferior vena cava, and ureters (Fig. 18–39). The anterior border of the fibrotic mass displaces the posterior peritoneum but does not break through into the peritoneal cavity. The anterior margin is usually sharply defined, the posterior margin poorly delineated. The CT density on noncontrast CT scans is in the range of muscle, but after contrast medium administration the mass may dramati-

cally increase in attenuation so that a vascular neoplasm is simulated. In a minority of patients with retroperitoneal fibrosis, no abnormalities will be detectable by CT.

HEMORRHAGE

Retroperitoneal hemorrhage may occur spontaneously or as a result of trauma, surgery, or excessive anticoagulation. Meyers[58] noted the most common site of retroperitoneal hemorrhage fol-

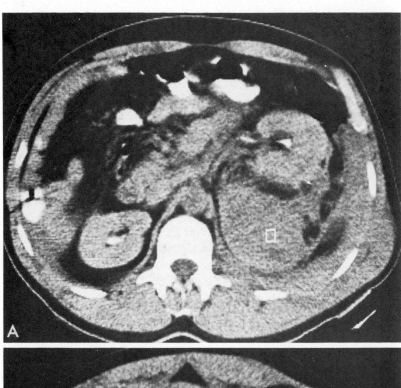

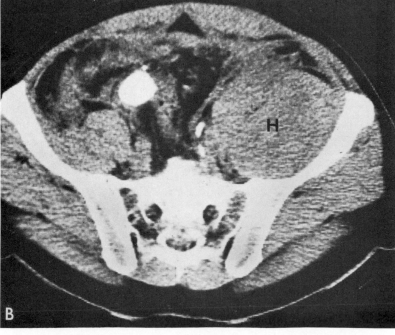

Figure 18–40. Spontaneous retroperitoneal hemorrhage secondary to anticoagulation therapy. **A** There is a mass extending primarily into the posterior pararenal space (box), which displaces the left kidney anteriorly. A small perirenal hematoma (arrow) is also present. **B** Scan at a lower level reveals that the hematoma (H) is dissecting into the left iliopsoas muscle group.

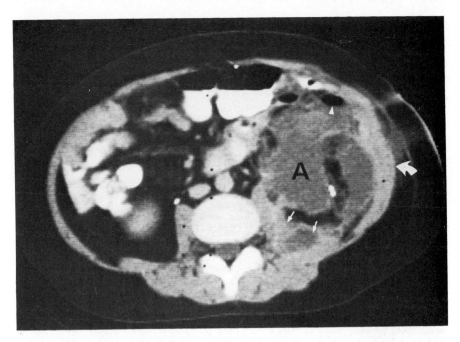

Figure 18–41. Multiloculated abscess (A) in left flank secondary to breakdown of primary colonic anastomosis. The abscess thickens the abdominal musculature (curved arrow), contains a foci of gas (arrowhead), and extends into the left psoas muscle (arrows).

lowing excessive anticoagulation to be the posterior pararenal space; we have had a similar experience (Fig. 18–40A). The clinical findings in patients with significant retroperitoneal hemorrhage are often distinctive, but in conjunction with the CT features of a relatively high-density mass lesion obliterating the periaortic fat planes, a confident diagnosis can be made.[59]

Retroperitoneal hemorrhage frequently is contained within well-defined muscle groups (Fig. 18–40B) and has a density that initially is higher than muscle but decreases to a low-density mass weeks after the hemorrhage.[59] Hemorrhage following translumbar aortography typically thickens the diaphragmatic crura and the left psoas muscle and obliterates the aortic outline.[48] Follow-up scans demonstrate that the hemorrhage usually resolves spontaneously over the course of several days.

ABSCESSES

The CT appearance of a retroperitoneal abscess is identical to the appearance of intraperitoneal abscesses (see Chapter 19). Typically, a well-defined mass of fluid density that may contain bubbles of gas is present (Fig. 18–41). Following contrast medium administration, the rim of the abscess enhances in 30 to 40 per cent of patients. The most frequent causes of retroperitoneal abscesses are colonic perforations, pancreatic abscesses, unsuspected duodenal perforations, or surgical contamination.

NEOPLASMS

Computed tomography is the imaging method of choice in the evaluation of primary retroperitoneal neoplasms.[60] The vast majority of primary retroperitoneal tumors are malignant with liposarcomas, leiomyosarcomas, fibrosarcomas, and malignant teratomas being the most frequently encountered. Metastatic retroperitoneal tumors are usually lymphomas or lymph node metastasis from pelvic, testicular, lung, or gastrointestinal neoplasms.

Liposarcomas are the most common primary retroperitoneal malignancy and have a variety of histologic subtypes relating to the anaplasia of the fat cells and the degree of admixture of fibrous or mucinous tissues.[60–62] As noted by Waligore and co-workers[61] liposarcomas may be classified histologically into lipogenic, myxoid, or pleomorphic varieties, with the myxoid subtype being the most common. Lipogenic liposarcomas contain primarily lipid elements (Fig. 18–42A), myxoid varieties have varying degrees of mucinous and fibrous tissues (Fig. 18–42B), and pleomorphic subtypes contain little mucin or lipid (Fig. 18–42C).

Friedman and associates[62] emphasized that liposarcomas had three distinct CT patterns: solid, mixed, and pseudocystic. In poorly differentiated liposarcomas, little fat is apparent and the lesion has a solid CT appearance with CT numbers greater than 20 H (Fig. 18–42C). Mixed lesions demonstrate focal fatty areas with attenuation values in the −40 to −20 H range (Fig. 18–42B). In the pseudocystic variety, there is a homogeneous

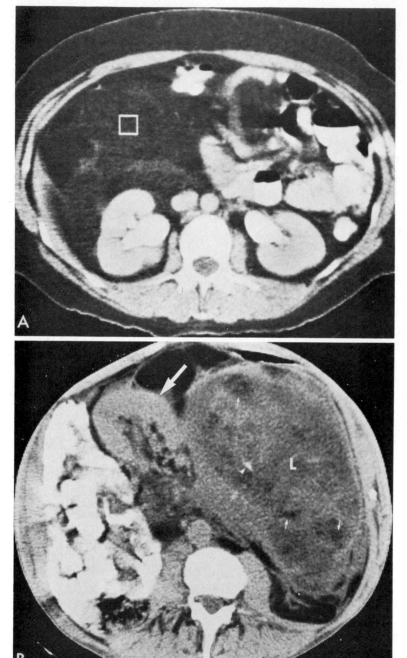

Figure 18–42. Various CT patterns of liposarcoma. **A** Lipogenic liposarcoma. A well-defined fatty mass (box) having a CT number only slightly higher than normal fat is displacing the bowel. **B** Myxoid liposarcoma (L) arising from the posterior pararenal space displaces the left kidney (large arrow) across the midline. The liposarcoma contains a mixture of low-density fatty elements (small arrows), high-density calcifications (arrowhead), and fibrous and mucinous tissue of intermediate density.

Illustration continued on opposite page

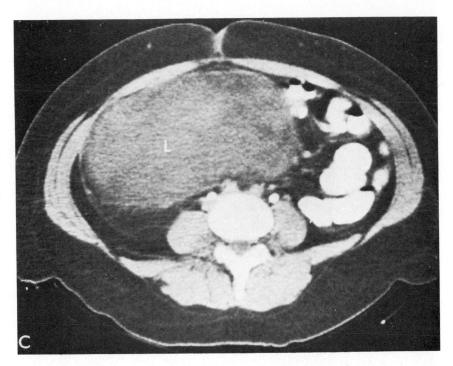

Figure 18–42. *Continued* **C** Pleomorphic liposarcoma (L) appearing as a mass having a density similar to that of soft tissue. The mass was composed mainly of fibrous and mucinous elements.

mass having a density close to that of water because partial volume averaging of fatty and solid elements creates a pseudocystic appearance. In general, even well-differentiated liposarcomas will demonstrate higher CT numbers than normal retroperitoneal fat, which ranges from −80 to −120 H. In evaluating a retroperitoneal mass, identification that even a small part of the mass has a CT density below zero is strong evidence that the mass is a liposarcoma (Fig. 18–43). Calcification may be present in a retroperitoneal liposarcoma (Fig. 18–42B), and when present it may not be possible to distinguish the liposarcoma from a malignant teratoma, which characteristically contains fat, bone, and calcium.

Leiomyosarcoma (Fig. 18–44), fibrosarcoma, fibrous histiocytoma, mesenchymal sarcoma, and malignant teratoma are other primary retroperitoneal tumors that may be indistinguishable by CT analysis. All of these tumors produce bulky, solid, retroperitoneal masses typically larger than 10 cm in diameter that have an attenuation value close to that of muscle (Fig. 18–44). Percutaneous biopsy is easily performed and readily distinguishes between the various entities. Metastatic retroperitoneal tumors are uncommon but do occur (Fig. 18–45) and appear identical to primary retroperitoneal malignancies.

UNDESCENDED TESTES

In patients with an impalpable testis, the usual standard diagnostic approach is to surgically explore the inguinal canal, and if no testis is located, to further explore the retroperitoneal space from the inguinal region along the course of the gonadal vein to the renal hilum. CT now permits accurate preoperative localization of the undescended testes and aids the surgeon in planning the operation so that in certain cases a more limited procedure can be performed.[63, 64]

Absence of palpable testes occurs in testicular agenesis, dysgenesis, and incomplete descent of a testis. The more normal the testis is in size (1.5 × 3 cm) and shape (oval), the more readily it is detected by CT. Atrophic and dysplastic testes appear as small foci of soft tissue similar in density to the adjacent abdominal wall or thigh musculature and are difficult to identify by CT.[63, 64]

Undescended testes are 12 to 40 times more likely to have foci of malignancy.[64] This is particularly true of testes that appear larger than normal by CT (Fig. 18–46A). The undescended testis is most frequently located in the superficial inguinal region or inguinal canal.[63, 64] An intra-abdominal testis is most often located near the internal inguinal ring adjacent to the iliac vessels (Fig. 18–46B).

Lee and co-workers[64] reported a 100 per cent accuracy in eight patients, and Wolversen's group[63] found only one incorrect localization in 15 impalpable testes. Accurate CT localization requires careful attention to pelvic anatomy, but it appears that CT should be performed routinely prior to surgery in every patient with an impalpable testis.

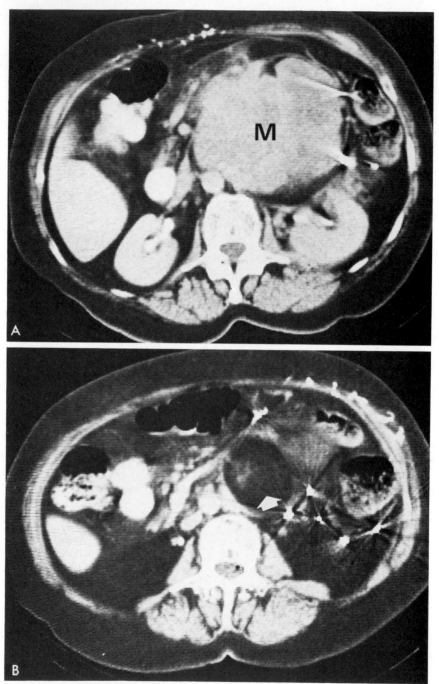

Figure 18–43. A   Liposarcoma appearing as a solid, rounded mass (M) having a soft-tissue density. At this level, a specific diagnosis cannot be made. **B**   Scan at a lower edge of the mass demonstrates that a portion of the mass contains fat (arrow), making a specific CT diagnosis of liposarcoma possible.

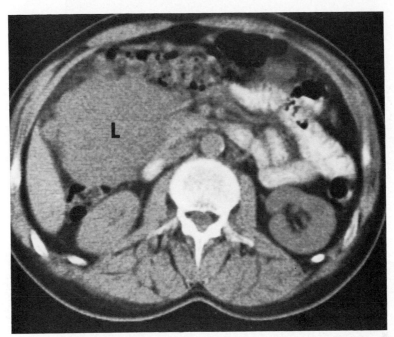

Figure 18–44. Leiomyosarcoma (L) appearing as a mass of homogeneous solid density displacing adjacent structures.

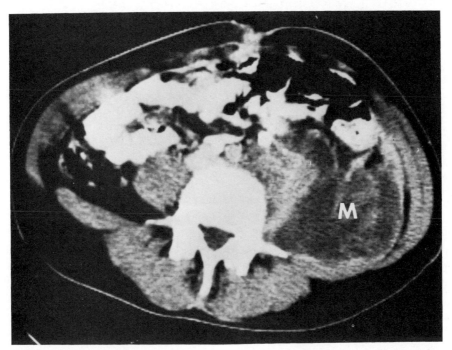

Figure 18–45. Carcinoma of the lung metastatic to the retroperitoneum, producing a large mass (M) of mixed density, which appears similar to a liposarcoma.

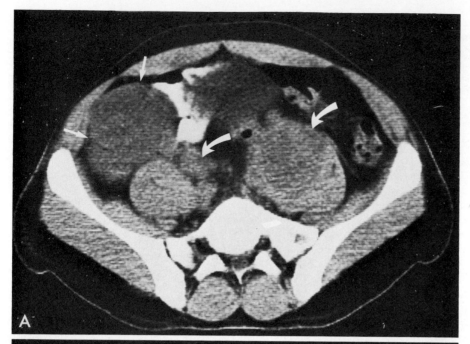

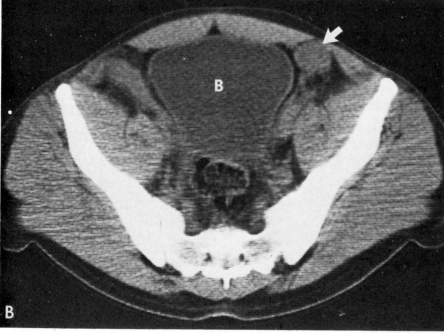

Figure 18–46. Bilateral undescended testes. **A** The undescended right testis is enlarged by a mass (arrows), which has proved to be an embryonal cell carcinoma. The tumor has metastasized to the lymph nodes (curved arrows), which are enlarged. **B** The nontumorous intra-abdominal left testis (arrow) is demonstrated as a smaller, rounded structure adjacent to the bladder (B).

REFERENCES

1. Ellert J, Kreel L: The role of computed tomography in the initial staging and subsequent management of the lymphomas. J Comput Assist Tomogr 4:368, 1980.
2. Lee JK, Stanley RJ, Sagel SS, Levitt RG: Accuracy of computed tomography in detecting intraabdominal and pelvic adenopathy in lymphoma. AJR 131:311, 1978.
3. Harell GS, Breiman RS, Glatstein EJ, Marshall WH, Castellino RA: Computed tomography of the abdomen in malignant lymphoma. Radiol Clin North Am 15:391, 1977.
4. Jones SE, Tobias DA, Waldman RS: Computed tomographic scanning in patients with lymphoma. Cancer 41:480, 1978.
5. Redman HC, Glatstein E, Castellino RA, Federal WA: Computed tomography as an adjunct in the staging of Hodgkin's disease and non-Hodgkin's lymphomas. Radiology 124:381, 1977.
6. Schaner EG, Head GL, Doppman JL, Young RC: Computed tomography in the diagnosis, staging and management of abdominal lymphomas. J Comput Assist Tomogr 1:176, 1977.
7. Alcorn FS, Mategran VC, Petrasnick JP, Clark JW: Contributions of computed tomography in the staging and management of malignant lymphomas. Radiology 125:717, 1977.

8. Breiman RS, Castellino RA, Harell GS, Marshall WH, Glatstein E, Kaplan HS: CT-pathologic correlations in Hodgkin's diseases and non-Hodgkin's lymphomas. Radiology 126:159, 1978.

9. Lee JK, McClennan BL, Stanley RJ, Sagel SS: Computed tomography in the staging of testicular neoplasms. Radiology 130:387, 1979.

10. Burney BT, Klatt EC: Ultrasound and computed tomography of the abdomen in the staging and management of testicular carcinoma. Radiology 132:415, 1979.

11. Lee JK, Stanley RJ, Sagel SS, Melson GL, Koehler RE: Limitations of the post-lymphangiogram plain abdominal radiograph as an indicator of recurrent lymphoma: Comparison to computed tomography. Radiology 134:155, 1980.

12. Thomas JS, Bernardino VWF, Bracken RB: Staging of testicular carcinoma: Comparison of CT and lymphangiography. AJR 137:991, 1981.

13. Soo CS, Bernardino ME, Chuang VP, Ordonez N: Pitfalls of CT findings in post-therapy testicular carcinoma. J Comput Assist Tomogr 5:39, 1981.

14. Husband JE, Peckham MJ, MacDonald JS: The role of abdominal computed tomography in the management of testicular tumors. Comput Tomogr 4:1, 1980.

15. Walsh JW, Amendola MA, Konerding KF, Tisnado J, Hazra TA: Computed tomographic detection of pelvic and inguinal lymph node metastasis from primary and recurrent pelvic malignant disease. Radiology 137:157, 1980.

16. Ginaldi S, Wallace S, Jing BS, Bernardino ME: Carcinoma of the cervix: Lymphangiography and computed tomography. AJR 136:1087, 1981.

17. Lee JK, Stanley RJ, Sagel SS, McClennan BL: Accuracy of CT in detecting intraabdominal and pelvic lymph node metastases from pelvic cancers. AJR 131:675, 1978.

18. Walsh JW, Amendola MA, Hall DJ, Tisnado J, Goplerud DR: Recurrent carcinoma of the cervix: CT diagnosis. AJR 136:117, 1981.

19. Koss JC, Arger PH, Coleman BG, Mulhern CB, Pollock HM, Wein AJ: CT staging of bladder carcinoma. AJR 137:359, 1981.

20. Levine MS, Arger PH, Coleman BG, Mulhern CB, Pollock HM, Wein AJ: Detecting lymphatic metastases from prostatic carcinoma: Superiority of CT. AJR 137:207, 1981.

21. Walsh JW, Goplerud DR: Prospective comparison between clinical and CT staging in primary cervical carcinoma. AJR 137:997, 1981.

22. Hamlin DJ, Burgener FA, Beecham JB: CT of intramural endometrial carcinoma: Contrast enhancement is essential. AJR 137:551, 1981.

23. Callen PW, Korobkin M, Isherwood I: Computed tomographic evaluation of the retrocrural prevertebral space. AJR 129:907, 1977.

24. Glazer GM, Goldberg HI, Moss AA, Axel L: Computed tomographic detection of retroperitoneal adenopathy. Radiology 143:147, 1982.

25. Castellino RA, Billingham M, Dorfman RF: Lymphographic accuracy in Hodgkin's disease and malignant lymphoma with a note on the "reactive" lymph node as a cause of most false-positive lymphograms. Invest Radiol 9:155, 1974.

26. Margolin S, Castellino R: Lymphographic accuracy in 632 consecutive previously untreated cases of Hodgkin's disease and non-Hodgkin's lymphoma. Radiology 140:351, 1981.

27. Best JJK, Blackledge G, Forbes WS, Todd IDH, Eddleston B, Crowther D, Isherwood I: Computed tomography of the abdomen in staging and clinical management of lymphoma. Br Med J 2:1675, 1978.

28. Zornoza J, Ginaldi S: Computed tomography in hepatic lymphoma. Radiology 138:405, 1981.

29. Burgener FA, Hamlin DJ: Histiocytic lymphoma of the abdomen: Radiographic spectrum. AJR 137:337, 1981.

30. Pierkarski J, Federle MP, Moss AA, London SS: Computed tomography of the spleen. Radiology 135:683, 1980.

31. Dunnick NR, Javadpour N: Value of CT and lymphography: Distinguishing retroperitoneal metastasis from nonseminomatous testicular tumors. AJR 136:1092, 1981.

32. Royal SA, Callen PW: CT evaluation of anomalies of the inferior vena cava and left renal vein. AJR 132:759, 1979.

33. Faer MJ, Lynch RD, Evans HO, Chin FK: Inferior vena cava duplication: Demonstrated by computed tomography. Radiology 130:707, 1979.

34. Korobkin M, Godwin JD: Computed tomography of the aorta and vena cava. In Goldberg HI (ed): International Radiology and Diagnostic Imaging Modalities. University of California, San Francisco, 1982, p 293–301.

35. Breckenridge JW, Kinlaw WB: Azygos continuation of inferior vena cava: CT appearance. J Comput Assist Tomogr 4:392, 1980.

36. Ginaldi S, Chuang VP, Wallace S: Absence of hepatic segment of the inferior vena cava with azygos continuation. J Comput Assist Tomogr 4:112, 1980.

37. Churchill RJ, Wesby G III, Marsan RE, Moncada R, Reynes CJ, Love L: Computed tomographic demonstration of anomalous inferior vena cava with azygos continuation. J Comput Assist Tomogr 4:398, 1980

38. Zerhouni EA, Barth KH, Siegelman SS: Demonstration of venous thrombosis by computed tomography. AJR 134:753, 1980.

39. Steele JR, Sones PJ, Heffner LT: The detection of inferior vena caval thrombosis with computed tomography Radiology 128:385, 1978.

40. Marks WM, Korobkin M, Callen PW, Kaiser JA: CT diagnosis of tumor thrombosis of the renal vein and inferior vena cava. AJR 131:843, 1978.

41. Weyman PJ, McClennan BL, Stanley RJ, Levitt GR, Sagel SS: Comparison of computed tomography and angiography in the evaluation of renal cell carcinoma. Radiology 137:417, 1980.

42. Van Breda A, Rubin VE, Dray EM: Detection of inferior vena cava abnormalities by computed tomography. J Comput Assist Tomogr 3:164, 1979.

43. Ferris RA, Kirschner LP, Mero JH, McCabe DJ, Moss ML: Computed tomography in the evaluation of inferior vena caval obstruction. Radiology 130:710, 1979.

44. Vujic I, Stanley J, Tyminski LJ: Computed tomography of suspected caval thrombosis secondary to proximal extension of phlebitis from the leg. Radiology 140:437, 1981.

45. Glazer GM, Callen PW, Parker JJ: CT diagnosis of tumor thrombus in the inferior vena cava: Avoiding false-positive diagnosis. AJR 137:1265, 1981.

46. Schmitz L, Jeffrey RB, Palubinskas AJ, Moss AA: CT demonstration of septic thrombosis of the inferior vena cava. J Comput Assist Tomogr 5:259, 1981.

47. Kunstlinger F, Federle MP, Moss AA, Marks W: Computed tomography of hepatocellular carcinoma. AJR 134:431, 1980.

48. Amendola MA, Tisnado J, Fields WR, Beachley MC, Vines FS, Cho S-R, Turner MA, Konerding KP: Evaluation of retroperitoneal hemorrhage by computed tomography before and after translumbar aortography. Radiology 133:401, 1979.

49. Bergman AB, Neiman HL: Computed tomography in the detection of retroperitoneal hemorrhage after translumbar aortography. AJR 131:831, 1978.

50. Vinton VC, Usselman JA, Warmath MA, Dilley RB: Aortic perianeurysmal fibrosis: CT density enhancement and ureteral obstruction. AJR 134:577, 1980.

51. Mark A, Moss AA, Lusby R, Kaiser JA: CT evaluation of the complications of abdominal aortic surgery. Radiology 145:409, 1982.

52. Haaga JR, Baldwin GN, Reich NB, Beven E, Kramer A, Weinstein A, Havrilla TR, Seidelmann FE, Namba AH, Parrish CM: CT detection of infected synthetic grafts: Preliminary report of a new sign. AJR 131:317, 1978.

53. Tracy DA, Eisenberg RL, Hedgcock M: Ureteral obstruction following aortoiliac bypass graft surgery. AJR 132:415, 1979.

54. Fagan CJ, Larrieu AJ, Amparo EG: Retroperitoneal fibrosis: Ultrasound and CT features. AJR 133:239, 1979.

55. Renner IG, Ponto GC, Savage WT II, Boswell WD: Idiopathic retroperitoneal fibrosis producing common bile duct and pancreatic duct obstruction. Gastroenterology 79:348, 1980.

56. Raper FP: Idiopathic retroperitoneal fibrosis involving the ureters. Br J Urol 28:436, 1956.

57. Brun B, Laursen K, Sorensen IN, Lorentzen JE, Kristensen JK: CT in retroperitoneal fibrosis. AJR 137:535, 1981.

58. Myers MA: Dynamic Radiology of the Abdomen: Normal and Pathologic Anatomy. Heidelberg, Springer 1976, p 174.

59. Sagel SS, Siegel MJ, Stanley RJ, Jost RG: Detection of retroperitoneal hemorrhage by computed tomography. AJR 129:403, 1977.

60. Stephens DH, Sheedy PF, Hattery RR, Williamson B: Diagnosis and evaluation of retroperitoneal tumors by computed tomography. AJR 129:395, 1977.

61. Waligore MP, Stephens DH, Soule EH, McLeod RA: Lipomatous tumors of the abdominal cavity: CT appearance and pathologic correlation. AJR 137:539, 1981.

62. Friedman AC, Hartman DS, Sherman J, Lautin EM, Goldman M: Computed tomography of abdominal fatty masses. Radiology 139:415, 1981.

63. Wolverson MK, Jagannadharao B, Sundaram M, Riaz MA, Nalesnik WJ, Houttuin E: CT in localization of impalpable cryptorchid testes. AJR 134:725, 1980.

64. Lee JK, McClennan BL, Stanley RJ, Sagel SS: Utility of computed tomography in the localization of the undescended testis. Radiology 135:121, 1980.

19 COMPUTED TOMOGRAPHY OF THE PERITONEAL CAVITY AND MESENTERY

R. Brooke Jeffrey

Peritoneal Cavity

ANATOMY

Much of our recent understanding of the radiologic anatomy of the peritoneal cavity and the spread of intraperitoneal disease processes comes from the anatomic-radiologic correlations pioneered by Meyers.[1-4] The peritoneal cavity may be divided into the pelvis, upper abdomen, and the lesser peritoneal sac (Figs. 19–1 and 19–2). The pelvic cul de sac is the most dependent portion of the peritoneal cavity (Fig. 19–3) and often is the initial location of intraperitoneal fluid collections, such as abscesses, hematomas, or ascites. Extending from the midline cul de sac, the paravesical fossae are in direct continuity with both the right and left paracolic gutters. Pelvic fluid collections preferentially extend into the upper abdomen by way of the right paracolic gutter, which is broader and deeper than the left and also because of the anatomic barrier created by the phrenicocolic ligament (Fig. 19–4). Upon examination by computed tomography (CT), fluid in the paracolic gutters is seen to displace the colon medially (Fig. 19–5); however, the extraperitoneal attachment along the posterior aspect of the ascending and descending colon is preserved.

In the upper abdomen, the transverse mesocolon divides the peritoneal cavity into supramesocolic and inframesocolic compartments (Fig. 19–6). In the right upper quadrant, the peritoneum reflects over the diaphragm and liver to create a right subphrenic and a right subhepatic space (Fig. 19–7). The right subphrenic space extends beneath the dome of the diaphragm to the edge of the coronary ligament, which suspends the right lobe of the liver from the diaphragm posteriorly. On CT scans, subphrenic fluid may be distinguished from a pleural effusion by its location anterior to the diaphragm (Fig. 19–8A). On occasion, it may be difficult to differentiate subphrenic from an intrahepatic fluid collection in

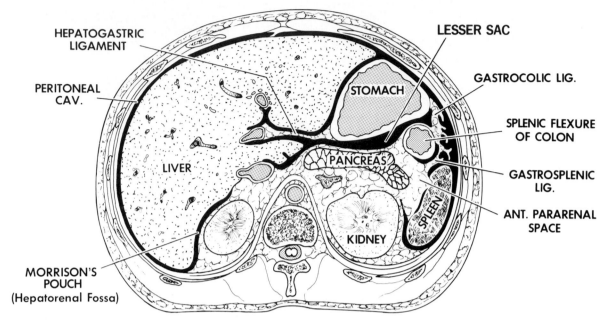

Figure 19–1. Diagram of transverse section of upper abdomen, demonstrating peritoneal cavity, Morrison's pouch, and the lesser sac. The relationships of the lesser sac, pancreas, colon, stomach, and liver are shown. The upper abdominal portion of the peritoneal cavity surrounds the liver, spleen, and lateral portion of the splenic flexure of the colon.

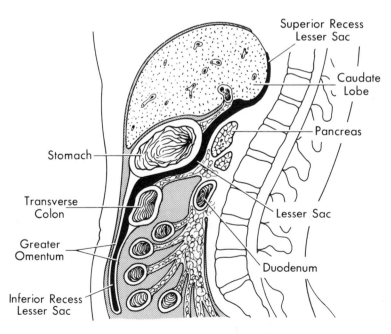

Figure 19–2. Sagittal section of upper abdomen through the region of the lesser sac. The drawing demonstrates that in some patients a well-defined inferior recess is present between the reflections of the greater omentum. In most patients, the caudal extent of the lesser sac is at the level of the transverse mesocolon. (From Jeffrey RB, Federle MP, Goodman PC: Computed tomography of the lesser peritoneal sac. Radiology 141:117, 1981.)

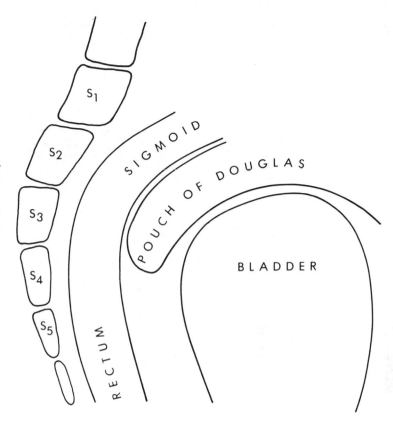

Figure 19–3. Sagittal section through the pelvis depicting the relationship of the pouch of Douglas to the rectum, sigmoid colon, and urinary bladder. The pouch of Douglas extends to the top of S_4 at the junction of the rectum and sigmoid colon. (Modified from Meyers MA: Dynamic Radiology of the Abdomen: Normal and Pathologic Anatomy. New York, Springer-Verlag, 1976.)

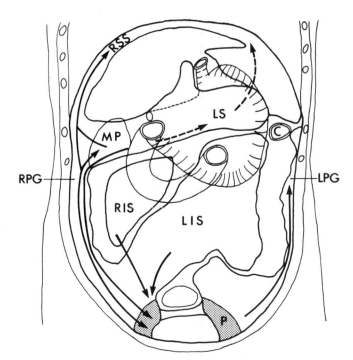

Figure 19–4. Diagram of flow patterns of intraperitoneal fluid. Dashed arrows indicate spread anterior to the stomach into the left subphrenic area. RPG = Right paracolic gutter; LPG = left paracolic gutter; MP = Morrison's pouch; LS = lesser sac; RSS = right subphrenic space; RIS = right infracolic space; LIS = left intracolic space; P = pelvic cul de sac; C = colon. (Modified from Meyers MA: Dynamic Radiology of the Abdomen: Normal and Pathologic Anatomy. New York, Spring-Verlag, 1976.)

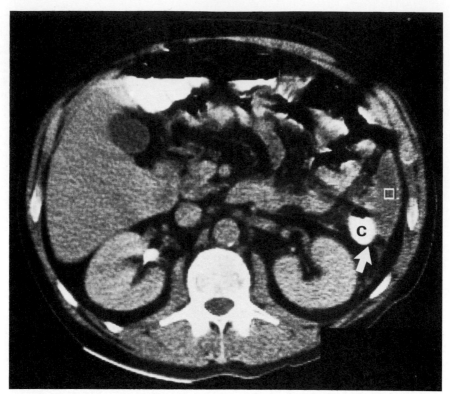

Figure 19–5. Free intraperitoneal fluid (box) displaces the contrast-filled colon (c) medially. The extraperitoneal attachment of the colon in the anterior pararenal space is preserved (arrow).

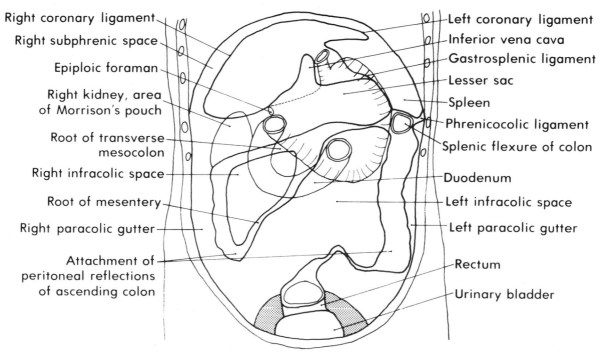

Right coronary ligament
Right subphrenic space
Epiploic foramen
Right kidney, area of Morrison's pouch
Root of transverse mesocolon
Right infracolic space
Root of mesentery
Right paracolic gutter
Attachment of peritoneal reflections of ascending colon

Left coronary ligament
Inferior vena cava
Gastrosplenic ligament
Lesser sac
Spleen
Phrenicocolic ligament
Splenic flexure of colon
Duodenum
Left infracolic space
Left paracolic gutter
Rectum
Urinary bladder

Figure 19–6. Diagram of posterior peritoneal reflections and recesses dividing the retroperitoneum into supramesocolic and inframesocolic compartments. (Modified from Meyers MA: Dynamic Radiology of the Abdomen: Normal and Pathologic Anatomy. New York, Springer-Verlag, 1976.)

Figure 19–7. Right parasagittal section. The right subphrenic space extends beneath the dome of the diaphragm to the superior edge of the coronary ligament. The right subhepatic space has both an anterior and posterior (Morrison's pouch) compartment and is contiguous with the right subphrenic space. The bare area of the liver lies between the reflections of the coronary ligament. (Modified from Meyers MA: Dynamic Radiology of the Abdomen: Normal and Pathologic Anatomy. New York, Springer-Verlag, 1976.)

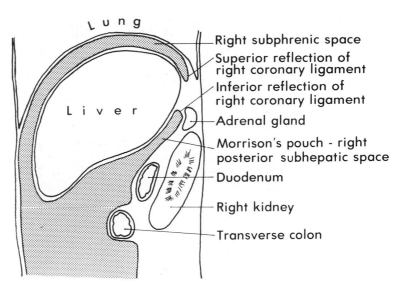

Lung

Liver

Right subphrenic space
Superior reflection of right coronary ligament
Inferior reflection of right coronary ligament
Adrenal gland
Morrison's pouch - right posterior subhepatic space
Duodenum
Right kidney
Transverse colon

the transverse plane. Sagittal and coronal reformations are often helpful in clarifying the location of fluid collections near the dome of the diaphragm (Fig. 19–8B,C).

The peritoneal reflections of the undersurface of the liver form an anterior and posterior subhepatic space roughly separated by the origin of the transverse mesocolon. The posterior subhepatic space, or Morrison's pouch (Figs. 19–1 and 19–7), is bounded by the peritoneal reflections between the posterior aspect of the right lobe of the liver and the right kidney. Morrison's pouch is the most dependent portion of the peritoneal cavity in the right upper quadrant and is frequently the site of postoperative abdominal abscesses. As stressed by Meyers,[2] intraperitoneal fluid extending from the pelvis up the right paracolic gutter initially localizes into the posterior subhepatic space (Figs. 19–4 and 19–9). With increasing volumes, intraperitoneal fluid extends from Morrison's pouch to the lateral peritoneal surface of the liver and finally into the subphrenic spaces. In patients with cirrhosis and other forms of hepatocellular disease, it is not unusual to identify varying amounts of ascitic fluid around the lateral aspect of the liver (Fig. 19–9). In addition, the lateral peritoneal surface is an important site for the diagnosis of peritoneal implants in patients with abdominal malignancies.

The falciform ligament separates the right and left subphrenic spaces. Both the right and left subphrenic space as well as the subhepatic space communicate freely along the edges of the falciform ligament. The left coronary ligament attaches more anteriorly than the right coronary ligament, and the left subphrenic space, therefore, does not extend as far posterior as the right (Fig. 19–10).

The lesser sac lies behind the lesser omentum, stomach, duodenum, and gastric ligament and communicates with the peritoneal cavity by way of the foramen of Winslow. Superiorly, the lesser sac extends to the diaphragm. The reflection of the parietal peritoneum off the gastrophrenic ligament extends to the gastric fundus and is contiguous inferiorly with the gastrosplenic ligament and the splenorenal ligament, which form the left lateral boundary of the lesser sac. The right lateral border of the lesser sac is the peritoneal reflection over the caudate lobe of the liver. In most individuals, the transverse mesocolon is the caudal extent of the lesser sac. However, in some patients there is a well-developed inferior recess of the lesser sac between the reflections of the greater omentum (Fig. 19–2). The anterior boundary of the lesser sac is formed by the posterior aspect of the stomach, the lesser omentum (hepatogastric ligament), and the anterior reflection of the greater omentum. Posteriorly, the lesser sac is bounded by the peritoneal reflection over the pancreas and left adrenal. In the anterior margin of the lesser sac, there is often a prominent fold created by the reflection of the peritoneum over the common hepatic and left gastric arteries.[5] Inflammatory lesions of the lesser sac may create adhesions along the plane of this fold, thus separating the lesser sac into two distinct compartments.

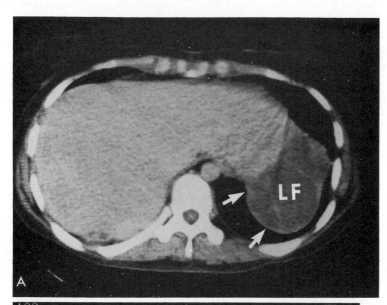

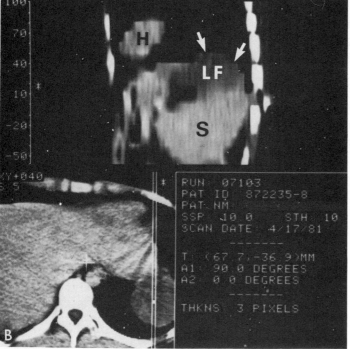

Figure 19–8. Bilateral subphrenic abscesses. **A** Transverse CT scan reveals fluid collection (LF) in left subphrenic space above the diaphragm (arrows). **B** Sagittal reformation more clearly demonstrates the relationship of left subphrenic fluid (LF) to diaphragm (arrows) and spleen (S). H = Heart.

Illustration continued on opposite page

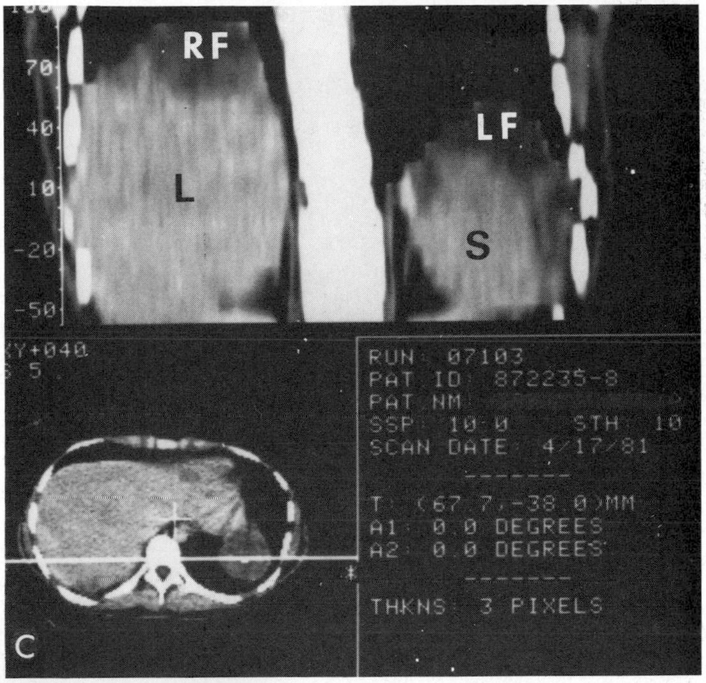

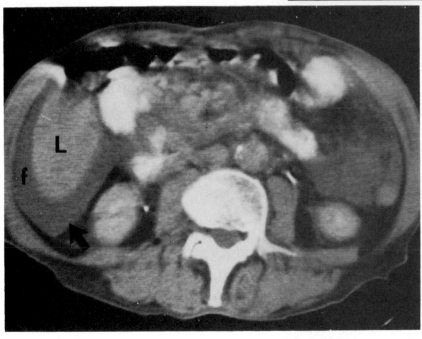

Figure 19–8. *Continued* **C** Coronal reformation reveals left (LF) and right (RF) subphrenic fluid collections. L = Liver; S = spleen.

Figure 19–9. Fluid (f) located lateral to the liver (L) and in Morrison's pouch (arrow). Small amounts of intraperitoneal fluid are often detectable in the right subhepatic space.

Figure 19–10. Parasagittal section through the left lobe of the liver. The coronary ligament attaches more anteriorly than the right and limits the posterior extent of the left subphrenic space. At this level, the perihepatic spaces are freely continuous. The lesser sac remains a separate space. (Modified from Meyers MA: Dynamic Radiology of the Abdomen: Normal and Pathologic Anatomy. New York, Springer-Verlag, 1976.)

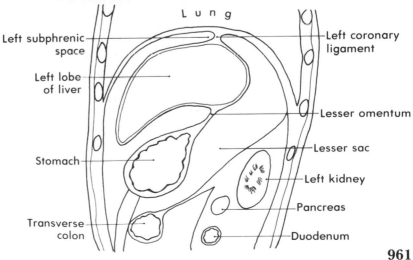

TECHNIQUES OF EXAMINATION

Scanning techniques used in evaluating suspected abnormalities of the peritoneal cavity must be individualized according to the clinical setting. Patients with possible intraperitoneal or pelvic abscesses are usually studied at 2-cm intervals from diaphragm to pelvis following oral and during an intravenous contrast medium infusion of contrast material. In the evaluation of pelvic fluid collections or masses, rectal contrast material is also given to help clarify the relationship of the mass to the colon. In patients evaluated for ascites and abdominal malignancies, scans are most frequently obtained at 2-cm intervals. However, in patients with known or suspected malignancies that may produce peritoneal implants or hepatic metastases, the liver and upper abdomen are scanned at 1-cm intervals and the lower abdomen and pelvis at 2-cm intervals.

Dunnick and colleagues[6] performed CT scans following injection of dilute contrast media through intraperitoneal catheters. They found the technique to be of value in selected cases of peritoneal metastasis, in demonstrating the distribution of intraperitoneal fluid, and in diagnosing the presence of adhesions. However, because of the invasiveness of the procedure, it has not gained wide acceptance and has not been utilized at our insti-

tution. Image reformation is not routinely performed but has proved helpful in distinguishing subphrenic from intrahepatic fluid collections (Fig. 19–8B,C).

PATHOLOGY

INTRAPERITONEAL FLUID

Intraperitoneal fluid collections may occur as either a primary or secondary manifestation of a variety of pathologic disorders, including peritonitis, trauma, metastatic disease, and cardiac, hepatic, or renal failure. CT can accurately diagnose and precisely delineate the location of very small quantities of intraperitoneal fluid and can distinguish between intraperitoneal and extraperitoneal fluid.[1, 2] Fluid in the supramesocolic compartment of the peritoneal cavity often initially collects in Morrison's pouch or in the posterior hepatorenal fossa, and is demonstrated as a rim of water density around the posterior edge of the right lobe of the liver (Fig. 19–9). In the inframesocolic compartment, fluid initially collects in the cul de sac and then extends from the paravesical fossae into the paracolic gutters. Intraperitoneal fluid in the paracolic gutters may be readily distinguished from extraperitoneal fluid by the preservation of the extraperitoneal fat posterior to the colon in the anterior pararenal space (Fig. 19–5). Extraperitoneal inflammatory processes such as pan-

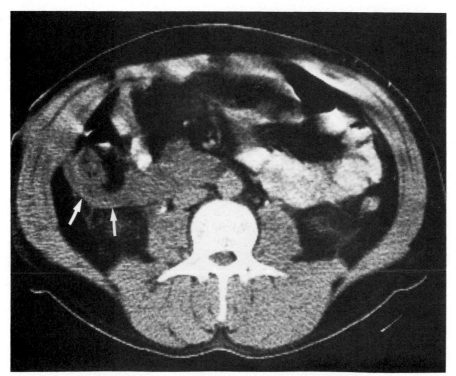

Figure 19–11. Extraperitoneal effusion in acute pancreatitis. An inflammatory reaction in the right anterior pararenal space (arrows) obliterates the extraperitoneal fat planes posterior to the ascending colon.

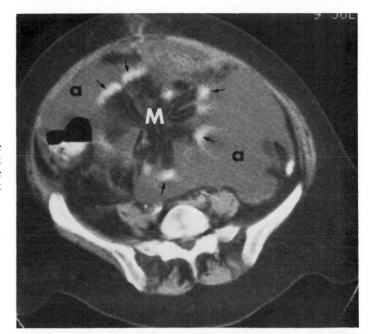

Figure 19–12. Massive ascites (a) causing the small bowel (arrows) and mesentery (M) to float in the central abdomen. The fat content of the mesentery is particularly well delineated against the background of ascitic fluid.

creatitis often obliterate the fat plane posterior to the colon in the anterior pararenal space (Fig. 19–11).

In patients with significant amounts of free ascites, the bowel loops are centrally positioned in the abdomen and the mesentery is clearly delineated (Fig. 19–12). Cystic masses can usually be distinguished from free intraperitoneal fluid by the presence of a mass effect, which displaces adjacent bowel loops in a focal manner. However, differentiation of a cystic mass from loculated ascites can be difficult at times and in patients with very tense ascites, bowel loops can be displaced from the central portion of the abdomen in the absence of an intraperitoneal mass.[7]

Loculated ascites is an important CT finding that indicates the presence of benign or malignant adhesions secondary to prior surgery, peri-

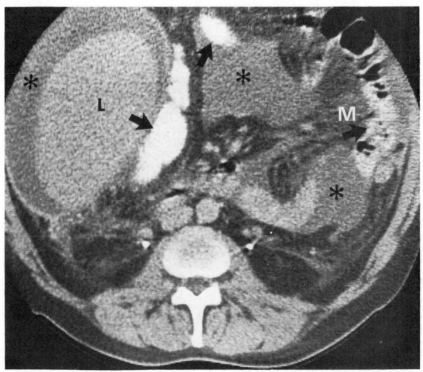

Figure 19–13. Loculated ascites (asterisk) in a patient with peritonitis resulting from tuberculosis. The bowel loops (arrows) and mesentery (M) are displaced by the loculated ascitic fluid and do not float freely in the central abdomen. The liver (L) is medially displaced.

tonitis or metastatic seeding in the peritoneum. The bowel loops in patients with loculated ascites do not float in the central abdomen but are displaced by the loculated ascitic fluid (Fig. 19–13).

The CT attenuation value of benign and malignant ascites has not proved sufficiently different to permit differentiation. However, the distribution of ascitic fluid can be a clue as to whether the ascitic fluid is benign or malignant. Gore and colleagues[8] found that benign ascites was found free within the intraperitoneal compartment, usually did not enter the lesser sac, and when present in the lesser sac, occurred in relatively small amounts (Fig. 19–14A). Malignant ascites resulting from peritoneal seeding was usually present in the lesser sac to as great a degree as in the peritoneal cavity (Fig. 19–14B). Fluid confined only to the lesser sac indicated a local etiologic factor, such as pancreatitis, lesser sac abscesses, or pancreatic carcinoma (Fig. 19–14C). The separation between benign and malignant ascites on the basis of distribution was not perfect, but it was sufficiently

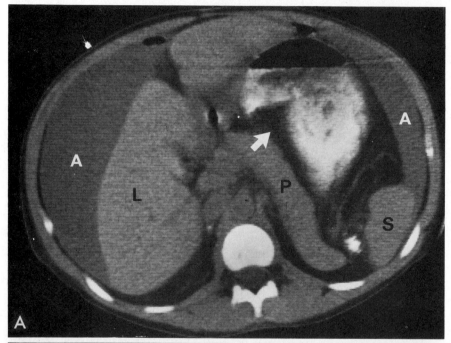

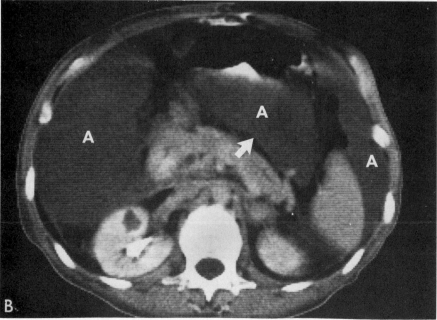

Figure 19–14. Patterns of ascites in benign and malignant disease. **A** Benign ascites (A) in the peritoneal cavity displaces the liver (L) and extends anterior to the spleen (S) but does not enter the lesser sac (arrow). P = pancreas. **B** Malignant ascites (A) secondary to ovarian carcinoma is distributed equally in the peritoneal cavity and lesser sac (arrow).

Illustration continued on opposite page

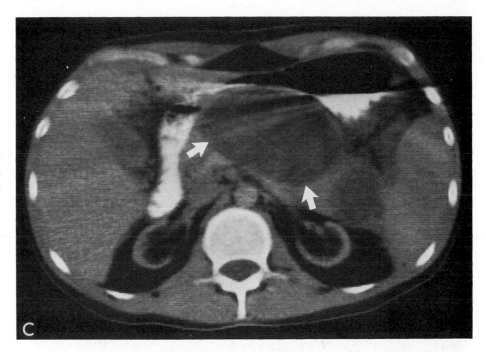

Figure 19–14. *Continued* **C** Fluid (arrows) confined to the lesser sac in a patient with acute pancreatitis.

accurate to warrant careful evaluation of the distribution of ascitic fluid in every patient with ascites.

Intraperitoneal hemorrhage most frequently is due to blunt abdominal trauma, which injures the liver or spleen. The presence of free intraperitoneal fluid (blood) is an important CT finding in the evaluation of blunt abdominal trauma because it indicates a laceration or fracture of the liver or spleen (Fig. 19–15).[9] In addition, intraperitoneal hemorrhage may occur following excessive anticoagulation[10] or from spontaneous rupture of various neoplasms, including hepatic adenomas, cavernous hemangiomas, and angiosarcomas (Fig. 19–16). The CT number of acute intraperitoneal hemorrhage is often greater than that of water, but

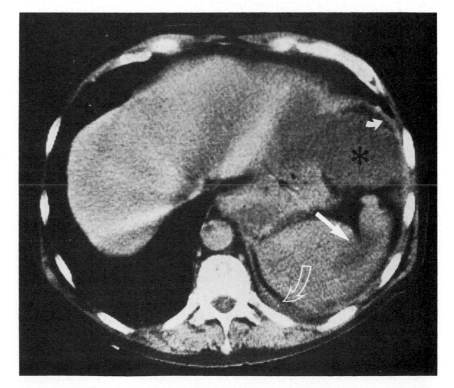

Figure 19–15. Intraperitoneal blood following splenic trauma. A left pleural effusion is shown posterior to the left diaphragm (curved open arrow). An intrasplenic hematoma (solid arrow) is evident, and free intraperitoneal blood (asterisk) is identified beneath the anterior aspect of the left hemidiaphragm (curved solid arrow).

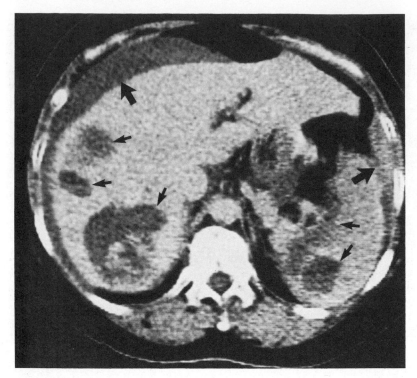

Figure 19–16. Spontaneous rupture of hepatic and splenic angiosarcoma. Free intraperitoneal blood (large arrows) is noted lateral to the liver and spleen. Multiple hepatic and splenic tumors (small arrows) are identified, but the site of extravasation is not identified. (From Mahony B, Jeffrey RB, Federle MP: Spontaneous rupture of hepatic and splenic angiosarcoma demonstrated by CT. AJR 138:965, 1982. © 1982, American Roentgen Ray Society. Used with permission.)

it may be difficult to differentiate exudative ascites from blood without a diagnostic needle aspiration.

Pseudomyxoma peritonei is an uncommon disorder characterized by intraperitoneal accumulations of gelatinous material. It is most often secondary to rupture of a mucinous cystadenocarcinoma of either the ovary or appendix or to rupture of a metastatic cystic mucin-producing implant in the peritoneum. The CT features of pseudomyxoma peritonei are a scalloping of the lateral contour of the liver produced by the gelatinous masses and the presence of septations extending from the liver margin to the lateral peritoneal surface.[11, 12] At times, pseudomyxoma peritonei produces a CT appearance indistinguishable from loculated ascites. Chronic pseudomyxoma peritonei may calcify (Fig. 19–17).

INTRAPERITONEAL ABSCESSES

In recent decades, the epidemiology of abdominal abscesses has changed so that postoperative abscesses rather than intestinal perforations are now the most common cause. Despite improved antibiotic and supportive therapies, abdominal

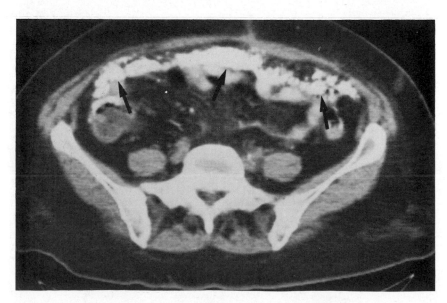

Figure 19–17. Pseudomyxoma peritonei producing a dense band of calcification (arrows) in the peritoneal cavity, which simulates a barium-filled colon.

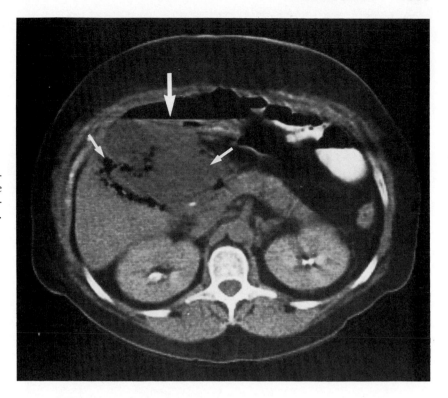

Figure 19–18. Gas-forming subhepatic abscess (small arrows) and free air (large arrow) following anastomotic leak from a gastrojejunostomy.

abscesses continue to be a major source of morbidity and mortality.[13, 14] Even with surgical drainage, there is a 30 per cent mortality in upper abdominal abscesses.[13] One of the major contributing factors to this continuing morbidity has been delay in diagnosis.

Plain films of the abdomen in patients with suspected abscesses are often helpful in demonstrating ectopic gas or fluid collections. However, if

the abdominal film is nondiagnostic, an additional imaging procedure should be employed. In our institution, computed tomography has become one of the primary diagnostic modalities in detecting abdominal abscesses.[15] The advantages of CT are its noninvasive quality, its high degree of accuracy, and its capability of imaging the entire abdomen in severely ill patients. In addition, CT can be used to guide diagnostic needle aspiration

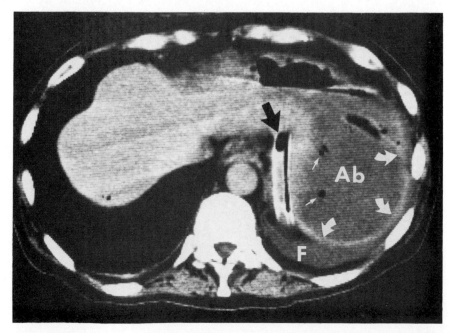

Figure 19–19. Left subphrenic abscess (Ab) following splenectomy, containing small gas bubbles (small arrows). A surgically placed drainage tube (large arrow) is seen to be medial to the abscess. A small amount of free intraperitoneal fluid (F) is present. The rim of the abscess (curved arrows) enhances after administration of contrast material.

for obtaining bacteriologic specimens as well as for directing percutaneous abscess drainage for definitive therapy.[16, 17] (See Chapter 22.)

The CT appearance of intra-abdominal and pelvic abscesses is varied. The most specific CT feature of an intra-abdominal or pelvic abscess is the presence of extraluminal gas (Figs. 19–18 and 19–19).[18, 19] Gas is found in slightly more than one third of abscesses[18] and may be present as multiple small bubbles of gas (Figs. 19–18 and 19–19) or a larger gas collection having an air-fluid inter-face (Fig. 19–20). When a large air-fluid level is identified, special attention must be given to the possibility of a perforated viscus or an intestinal fistula. Often, abscesses appear as rounded, oval, or biconvex, rather homogeneous, low-density masses having density values between 15 and 35 H.[18, 19] A definable wall and low-density center are seen in about a third of abscesses and are signs of a mature, drainable chronic abscess. The wall or rim of an abscess is frequently more clearly identified after intravenous contrast me-

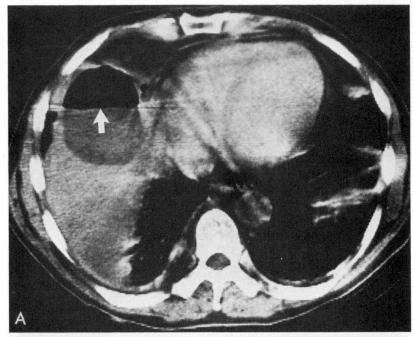

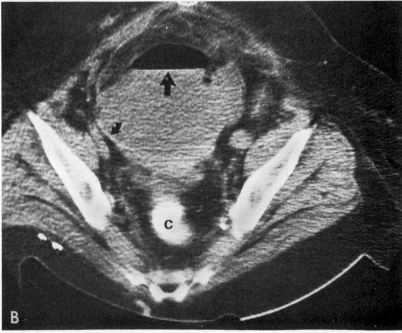

Figure 19–20. Abscesses with air fluid levels. **A** Subphrenic abscess with an air-fluid level (arrow). Note that it is difficult to distinguish whether an abscess is intrahepatic or subphrenic on a single transverse scan. Sagittal reformations are most helpful in these cases. **B** Large pelvic abscess with air-fluid level (arrow) following gynecologic surgery. A hypervascular rim (curved arrow) is seen around part of the abscess. There is contrast material in the rectosigmoid colon (c).

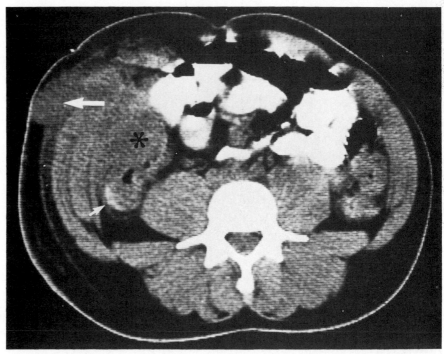

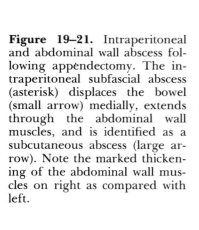

Figure 19–21. Intraperitoneal and abdominal wall abscess following appendectomy. The intraperitoneal subfascial abscess (asterisk) displaces the bowel (small arrow) medially, extends through the abdominal wall muscles, and is identified as a subcutaneous abscess (large arrow). Note the marked thickening of the abdominal wall muscles on right as compared with left.

dium administration because of the highly vascularized connective tissue that makes up the wall of the abscess.

Abscesses commonly produce obliteration of extraperitoneal fat, thickening of adjacent muscles, fascial planes, mesentery, or bowel wall (Figs. 19–21 and 19–22). On occasion, the CT characteristics of an abscess will provide a clue to its etiology. Identification of a high-density object within a postoperative abscess should suggest a diagnosis of a sponge abscess (Fig. 19–23); a calcific density within a right lower-quadrant abscess is evidence of a periappendiceal abscess (Fig. 19–24); and gas in the lesser sac in a patient with pancreatitis and fever is virtually diagnostic of a pancreatic abscess (Fig. 19–25). Commonly en-

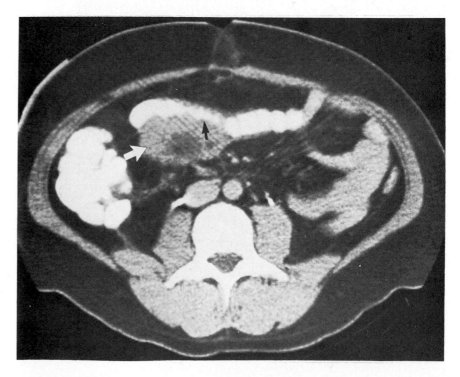

Figure 19–22. Abscess (large arrow) in mesentery of transverse colon following pancreatitis. There is marked thickening of the folds of the transverse colon with narrowing of the lumen (small arrow).

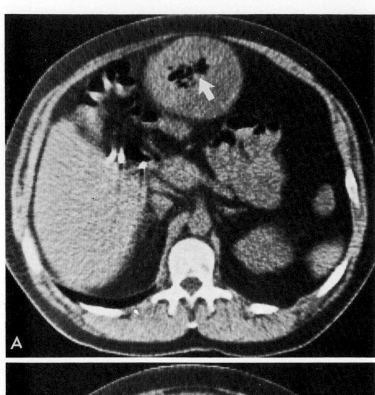

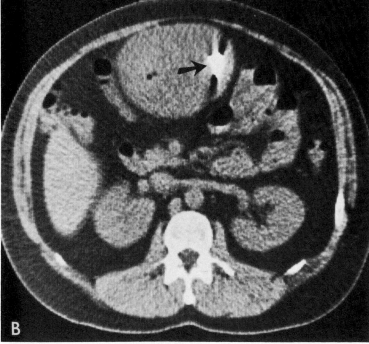

Figure 19–23. Sponge abscess. **A** A soft-tissue mass containing gas (arrow) is present in the peritoneal cavity. **B** At lower level, CT scan demonstrates a high-density object (arrow), proven to be a retained sponge.

countered associated findings in patients with abdominal or pelvic abscesses are ascites and pleural effusion or infiltrate.

Although almost all abscesses will be detected on a well-performed CT examination, the CT features may be nonspecific. Low-density abdominal masses can be produced by hematomas, bile collections, peritoneal implants (Fig. 19–26), pseudocysts, necrotic tumors, loculated ascites,

lymphocysts, and benign simple cysts. The CT features of abscesses overlap with these pathologic processes. The presence of gas may be found in a necrotic but noninfected tumor, and following intravenous contrast, hypervascular rims may be identified in tumors, hematomas, and pseudocysts (Fig. 19–26). However, in the proper clinical setting, the finding of an intra-abdominal or pelvic mass having the CT criteria of an ab-

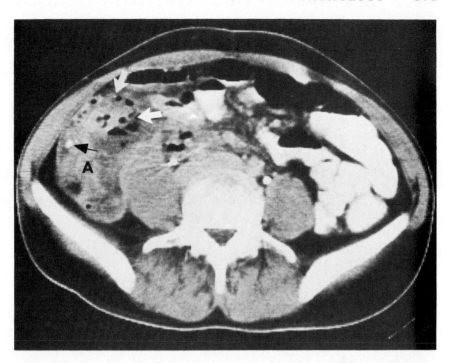

Figure 19–24. Periappendiceal abscess (A) fluid containing multiple gas bubbles (white arrows) and a high-density appendicolith (black arrow).

scess usually means an abscess is present. Should any doubt exist, diagnostic needle aspiration has proved to be a reliable, safe, and accurate method of providing a definitive diagnosis (Fig. 19–27).

The question of which imaging modality should be employed to diagnose abdominal and pelvic abscesses is still being debated. In a prospective study comparing computed tomography, ultra-

sound, and gallium imaging, McNeil noted that all three modalities had similar sensitivities (greater than 90 per cent) in the detection of abscesses.[21] The overall diagnostic yield could be increased slightly by combining two of the studies.[21] In a retrospective study of 170 patients with possible abscesses, a comparison of CT, ultrasound and indium-labeled leukocyte scans demonstrated that

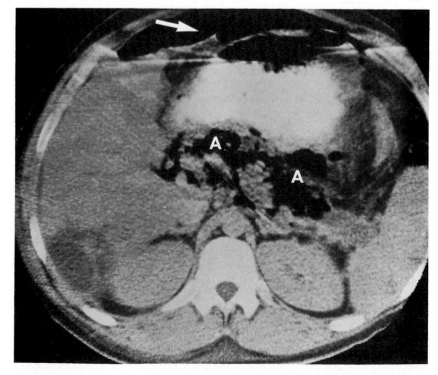

Figure 19–25. Extensive gas-forming pancreatic abscess (A) extending into the lesser sac. Free intraperitoneal air (arrow) results from escape of lesser sac gas by way of the foramen of Winslow.

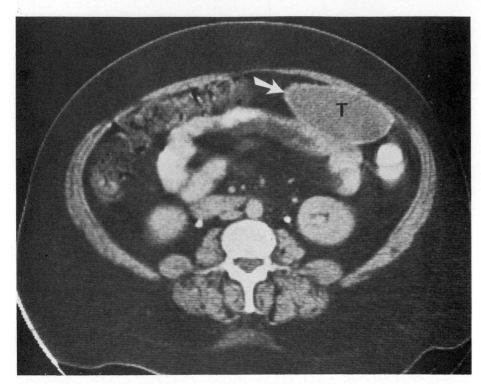

Figure 19–26. Cystic peritoneal tumor implant (T) from carcinoma of the ovary, which simulates a peritoneal abscess. The center of the implant has a density approaching that of water, and there is a well-defined rim (arrow) that enhances after contrast medium administration.

CT had a diagnostic accuracy of 96 per cent, ultrasound 90 per cent, and indium-labeled leukocyte scans 92 per cent.[9] Koehler and Moss[20] found CT to be 93 per cent accurate with a sensitivity of 99 per cent in 110 patients evaluated for possible abscesses. A number of other reports have documented CT accuracy rates for abscess detection to be above 90 per cent.[18, 19, 22–27]

Currently, patients who are not critically ill and have no focal signs of an abscess are initially imaged by an indium-labeled leukocyte scan. However, in critically ill patients, CT and ultrasound afford a more rapid and specific diagnosis. Because intestinal ileus, surgical wounds, drainage tubes, and ostomy appliances can restrict the usefulness of ultrasound in the postoperative patient, CT is usually selected for studying these patients. The relationship of an abscess to surrounding structures is best displayed by CT. Largely because of this factor, CT is becoming the imaging procedure of choice to evaluate patients with possible abscesses. If an abscess is detected, CT permits planning of the most appropriate route for percutaneous or surgical drainage.

PERITONEAL MASSES

The majority of solid peritoneal masses are secondary to metastatic implants from abdominal or pelvic malignancies. Peritoneal metastases occur in a variety of abdominal malignancies with carcinomas of the ovary, pancreas, stomach, and colon being the most common primary lesions. The CT demonstration of peritoneal metastasis may be the only evidence of recurrent disease, and the detection of a peritoneal nodule can help distinguish benign from malignant ascites.[28]

On CT scans, peritoneal implants appear as nodular (Fig. 19–28A) plaquelike (Fig. 19–28B), or sheetlike masses (Fig. 19–28C) of soft-tissue density along the peritoneal surface often outlined by ascites.[28] Occasionally, a peritoneal implant will have a cystic appearance (Fig. 19–26) and simulate an intra-abdominal abscess, pseudocyst or mesenteric cyst. One of the easiest sites for detecting peritoneal implants is along the lateral peritoneal surface of the liver (Fig. 19–28A), where the identification of neoplastic nodules is not hampered by loops of small intestine. In patients with known malignancies that characteristically seed via the peritoneum, this area, as well as all peritoneal surfaces, should be carefully scrutinized for the presence of peritoneal nodules. Because nonopacified loops of small bowel may mimic peritoneal implants, in order to avoid misdiagnosis, it is important to opacify the entire small bowel with dilute oral contrast material. Because of the superficial location of many peritoneal nodules, CT-directed aspiration biopsies to confirm recurrent malignancy are easily and safely performed.

The overall sensitivity of CT in detecting peritoneal implants is not known. However, because of the small size of most metastatic implants and the extensive surface of the peritoneum, it is probable that CT will prove to be relatively insensitive compared with endoscopic techniques, which directly visualize the peritoneal surface. In a comparison of laparoscopy and CT, small peritoneal implants not detected by CT were easily seen by laparoscopic methods.[29]

FREE INTRAPERITONEAL AIR

Although plain abdominal radiographs are the preferred method of diagnosing free air, on occasion the diagnosis of a perforated viscus is not suspected clinically and a patient is referred for CT scanning. Large amounts of free air can be distinguished by CT from gas with a segment of dilated bowel as a result of its lack of haustral or small bowel folds. In supine patients, free intraperitoneal air collects anteriorly beneath the abdominal musculature in the midabdomen (Fig. 19–29). Small amounts of free intraperitoneal air may be noted by CT up to 7 days after surgery and should not be interpreted as anastomotic breakdown or abdominal infection. However, loculated gas within a fluid or solid mass is almost always indicative of an abdominal abscess.

LESSER SAC ABNORMALITIES

Computed tomography is an extremely useful method in evaluating suspected lesser sac abnormalities.[30] Conventional radiologic studies, such as plain abdominal films and upper-gastrointestinal

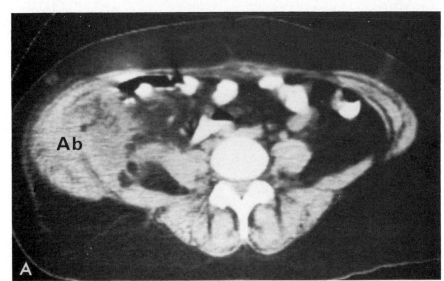

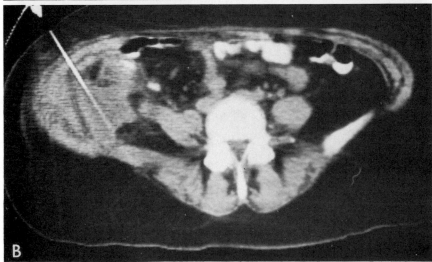

Figure 19–27. Needle aspiration to confirm abscess. **A** Right flank abscess (Ab) after nephrectomy causing marked thickening of the flank muscles. **B** Needle aspiration confirms presence of drainable pus.

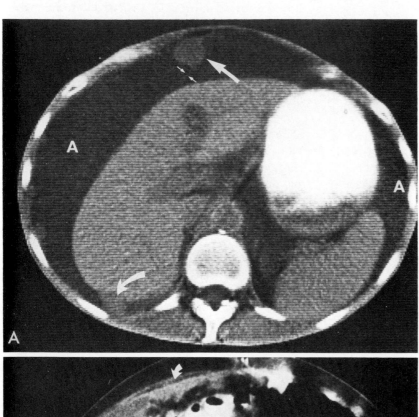

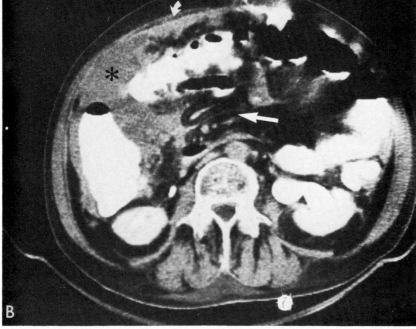

Figure 19–28. Varied CT appearance of peritoneal implants. **A** Nodular implants (large straight arrow) due to ovarian carcinoma are located adjacent to the falciform ligament (small arrows) and along lateral peritoneal surface of the liver (curved arrow). Massive ascites (A) is present in the peritoneal cavity, but only a small amount is present in the lesser sac. **B** Plaquelike peritoneal implant (curved arrow) is the result of ovarian carcinoma. Adjacent ascites (asterisk), marked angulation, and kinking of the mesentery (straight arrow) by serosal adhesions are shown.

Illustration continued on opposite page

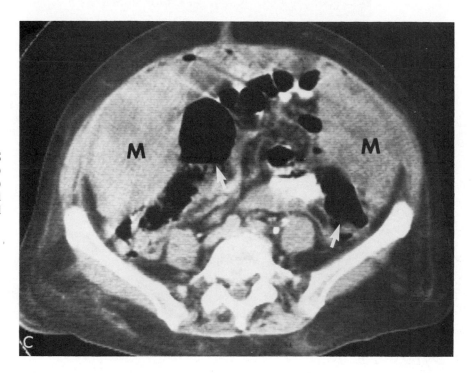

Figure 19–28. *Continued* **C** Sheetlike peritoneal masses (M) displacing the bowel (arrows) centrally are due to peritoneal metastasis from endometrial carcinoma.

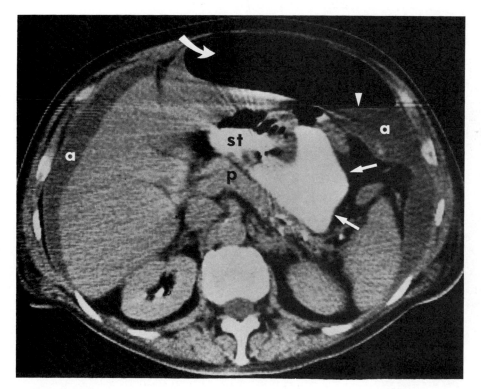

Figure 19–29. A large amount of free air (curved arrow) is seen to collect anteriorly following perforation of a gastric ulcer. Note air-fluid level (arrowhead). Oral contrast material has extravasated from the stomach (st) to outline the lesser sac (straight arrows) just anterior to the pancreas (p). a = Ascites. (From Jeffrey RB, Federle MP, Goodman PC: Computed tomography of the lesser peritoneal sac. Radiology 141:117, 1981.)

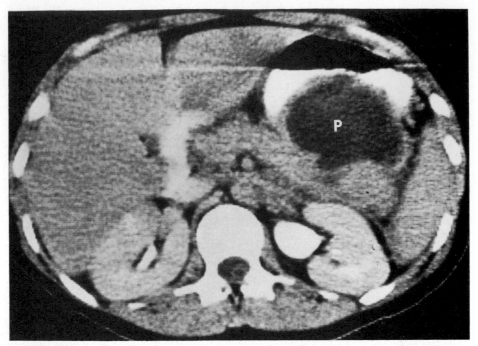

Figure 19–30. Lesser sac pseudocyst. A typical pancreatic pseudocyst (P) following acute pancreatitis is located in the lesser sac and displaces the stomach anteriorly.

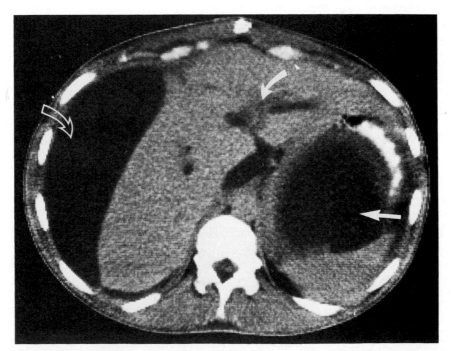

Figure 19–31. Post-traumatic lesser sac biloma following a gunshot wound to the porta hepatis that lacerated the common hepatic duct. Biliary dilatation (curved solid arrow) and subcapsular biloma of the liver (curved open arrow) are shown. A biloma (straight arrow) is present in the lesser sac and displaces the stomach anteriorly to the left. (From Jeffrey RB, Federle MP, Goodman PC: Computed tomography of the lesser peritoneal sac. Radiology 141:117, 1981.)

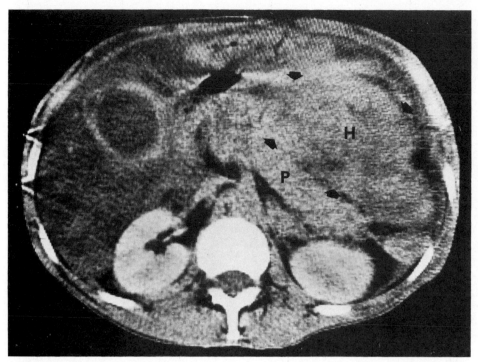

Figure 19–32. Hemorrhagic pancreatitis producing a hematoma (H), which is confined to the lesser sac (arrows). The hematoma contains both high- and low-density material, representing various stages in its evolution. The pancreas (P) appears grossly normal. (From Jeffrey RB, Federle MP, Goodman PC: Computed tomography of the lesser peritoneal sac. Radiology 141:117, 1981.)

tract examinations, can demonstrate only indirect signs of lesser sac pathology. CT directly images the lesser sac and readily distinguishes primary lesions of the lesser sac from pancreatic, adrenal, or retroperitoneal masses.

In axial projection, lesions of the lesser sac are usually diagnosed by their characteristic position between the stomach and body of the pancreas and spleen (Figs. 19–14B,C, 19–25, and 19–29 through 19–32).[30] On occasion, loops of small bowel or the splenic flexure of the colon may appear to be interposed between the stomach and pancreas without evidence of an internal hernia. The exact reason for this appearance is not certain, but may be secondary to variations of the origin of the transverse colon or small-bowel mesentery and degrees of gastric distention.

In most CT series, lesser sac abnormalities are most often pancreatic pseudocysts[30, 31] but abscesses, hematomas, perforated ulcers, and neoplastic invasion also involve the lesser sac. The CT findings, in conjunction with the clinical setting, must be considered in differentiating between these entities. Should the diagnosis still be in doubt, a CT-guided diagnostic needle aspiration or biopsy can be performed to distinguish infected from noninfected fluid collections or to diagnose neoplastic disease.

The Mesentery

Although barium examinations of the stomach, small intestine, and colon are capable of diagnosing mucosal abnormalities, they provide only an indirect image of the outer bowel wall and mesentery. In contrast, the outer wall of the bowel and the small- and large-bowel mesentery are directly imaged by computed tomography. By demonstrating mesenteric involvement, CT is capable of demonstrating the true extent of extramural neoplasms and inflammatory processes more accurately than conventional radiographic methods.

ANATOMY

The mesentery of the small bowel is formed by a "reflection of the posterior parietal peritoneum which connects the jejunum and ileum to the posterior wall of the abdomen" and thus acts as a suspensory ligament.[32] The root of the mesentery extends from the right sacroiliac joint across the origin of the superior mesenteric artery and vein to the left upper lumbar spine. At the intestinal margin, the peritoneum divides into two layers or leaves, which encase the small bowel and sur-

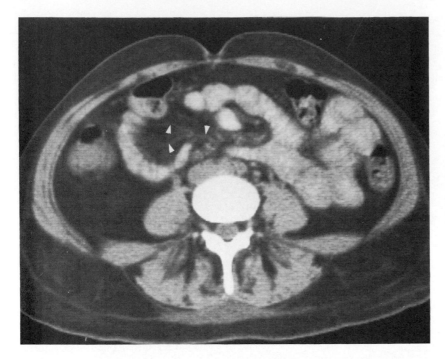

Figure 19–33. Mesenteric anatomy. Normal mesentery appears as a structure containing fat and vessels (arrowheads). Occasionally, a few normal-sized lymph nodes can be detected.

round the superior mesenteric artery, lymph nodes, and adjacent fat.[32] Thus, the small-bowel mesentery is a compartment that contains mainly fat but through which are scattered vascular and lymphatic channels and numerous mesenteric lymph nodes. The transverse mesocolon appears as a similar fatty structure containing lymphatic channels and vessels along the posterior medial aspect of the colon.

In patients with abundant fat, the mesentery is seen on CT as a structure having a density closely approximating abdominal and subcutaneous adipose tissue. Normal mesenteric lymph nodes measuring less than 1 cm in diameter can be identified, but usually only two or three are clearly demonstrated on any one CT section (Fig. 19–33).

TECHNIQUES OF EXAMINATION

Detection of mesenteric abnormalities is made easier by the presence of ample mesenteric fat and by complete opacification of both the large

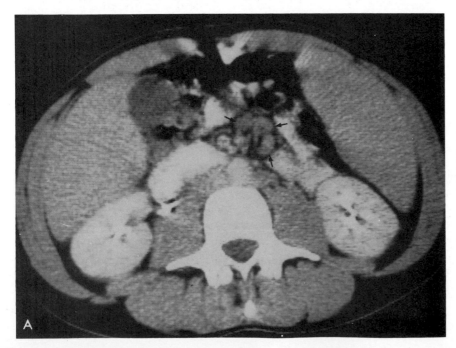

Figure 19–34. Patterns of mesenteric lymphadenopathy. **A** Multiple, small, rounded lymph nodes (arrows).

Illustration continued on opposite page

and small bowel with contrast material. At least 480 ml of oral contrast material—1 per cent meglumine diatrizoate (Gastrografin) or barium—is given 30 to 45 minutes before and another 250 to 300 ml just prior to the CT examination. The colon is filled with an enema of the same material.

Screening CT examinations are performed at 2-cm intervals, but in patients with conventional studies suggesting a mesenteric abnormality, CT scans at 1-cm intervals are taken through the area of interest. Intravenous contrast is not routinely given but a bolus injection or rapid intravenous

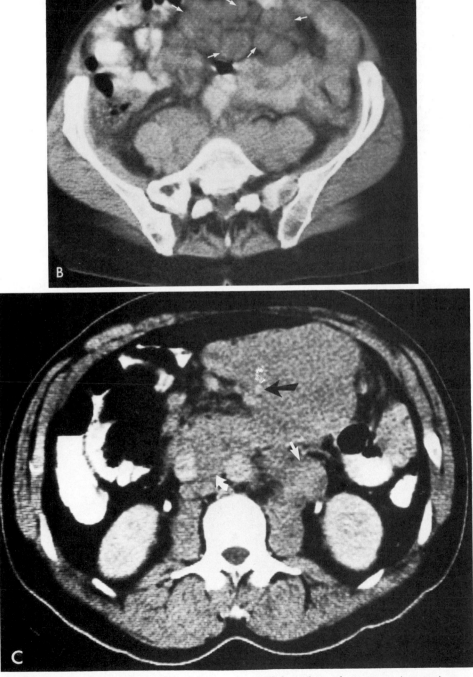

Figure 19–34. *Continued* **B** Groups of larger, rounded lymph node masses (arrows) are present. **(C)** Bulky mesenteric masses encase the mesenteric vessels (large arrow). Para-aortic (small arrow) and aortocaval nodes (curved arrow) are also enlarged.

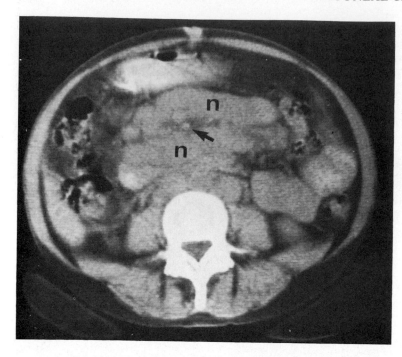

Figure 19–35. Advanced mesenteric adenopathy (n) resulting from lymphosarcoma surrounding the superior mesenteric artery (arrow); this produces the "sandwich sign" discussed by Mueller and others (Radiology 134:467, 1980).[32]

infusion is helpful in identifying the mesenteric vessels when a mesenteric mass is detected.

PATHOLOGY

LYMPHADENOPATHY—NEOPLASMS

Computed tomography can detect a variety of lesions involving the mesentery, including ade-nopathy, hematomas, abscesses, cysts, and in-flammatory thickening.[32–38] Mesenteric lymphade-nopathy is not demonstrated by pedal lymph-angiography but is readily detected by CT. The CT appearance of mesenteric lymphadenopathy varies from multiple, small, round soft-tissue densities to large, irregular, bulky masses (Fig. 19–34).[32–38] Advanced mesenteric adenopathy produces a characteristic CT appearance in which

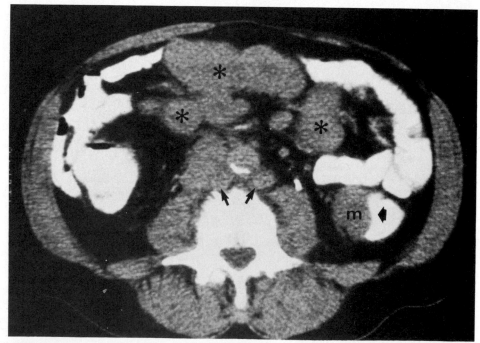

Figure 19–36. Melanoma metastatic to para-aortic (arrows) and mesenteric (asterisks) nodes. A mural metastasis (m) is seen along the medial margin (arrow) of a loop of small intestine.

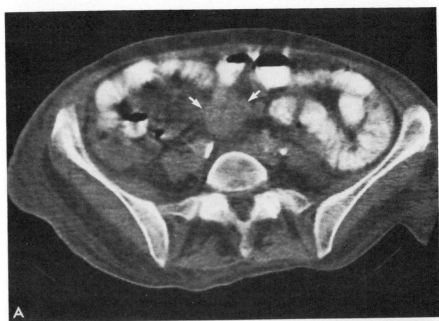

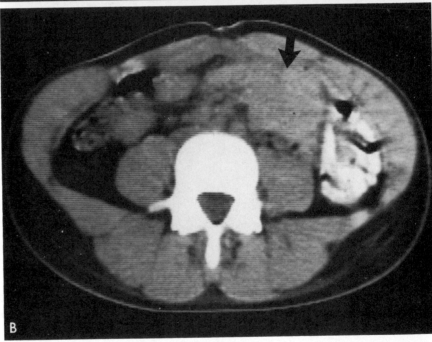

Figure 19–37. Nonlymphomatous mesenteric masses. **A** Carcinoid tumor involving the mesentery (arrows), resulting in a mesenteric mass. **B** Mesenteric desmoid tumor (arrow) in a patient with Gardner's syndrome, presenting as a solid mesenteric mass.

enlarged nodes between the dorsal and ventral leaves of the mesentery encase the superior mesenteric vessels producing a "sandwichlike" appearance (Fig. 19–35).[32]

The "sandwich" sign most frequently occurs in lymphoma; is often present in non-Hodgkin's lymphoma, a condition in which more than 50 per cent of patients have mesenteric nodal involvement at the time of the initial diagnosis (Fig. 19–35).[32] The ability to diagnose mesenteric adenopathy is an important contribution of CT in the evaluation of lymphomas[36–38] because mesenteric lymphadenopathy cannot be detected by

lymphangiography; the discovery of mesenteric involvement has important therapeutic and prognostic implications in all forms of lymphoma.

In addition to lymphoma, CT may demonstrate mesenteric involvement in other neoplastic disorders including carcinoid tumors, leukemia, and metastatic disease (Fig. 19–36).[34, 35] Carcinoid and desmoid tumors may produce mesenteric masses as well as an intense desmoplastic infiltration resulting in tethering and kinking of the mesentery (Fig. 19–37). Similar findings can be seen in other lesions that produce a dense fibroblastic infiltration of the mesentery, such as retractile mesenter-

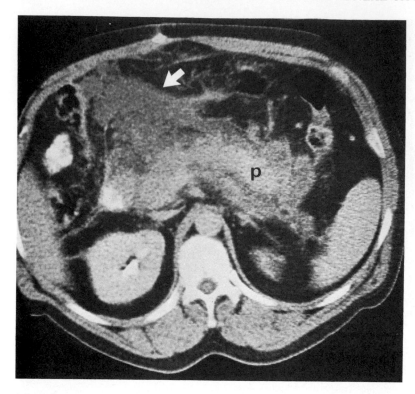

Figure 19–38. Acute pancreatitis. An inflammatory exudate encases the pancreas (p) and extends into the transverse mesocolon (arrow).

itis or metastatic carcinoma of the breast or pancreas.[35]

INFLAMMATORY DISEASE

In addition to diagnosing neoplastic lesions, CT can also diagnose a variety of benign lesions of the mesentery. In patients with necrotizing pancreatitis, the inflammatory reaction may extend directly down the transverse mesocolon (Fig. 19–38). This is the mechanism for the often associated ileus of the transverse colon or the "colon cut-off" sign. Pancreatic pseudocysts and abscesses may also dissect down the transverse mesocolon (Fig. 19–22) and may result in perforation of the colon and peritonitis.

In the later stages of Crohn's disease, there is often secondary inflammation of the mesentery adjacent to diseased loops of small bowel or colon.

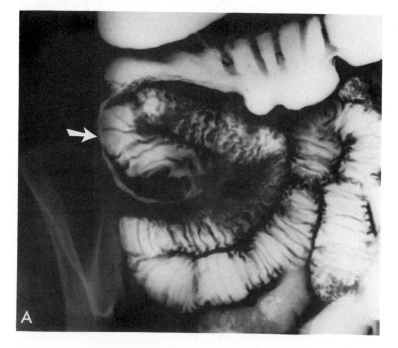

Figure 19–39. Recurrent Crohn's disease with fibrofatty thickening of the adjacent mesentery. **A** Barium enema demonstrates stenosis (arrow) of the small bowel following ileocolostomy for Crohn's disease.

Illustration continued on opposite page

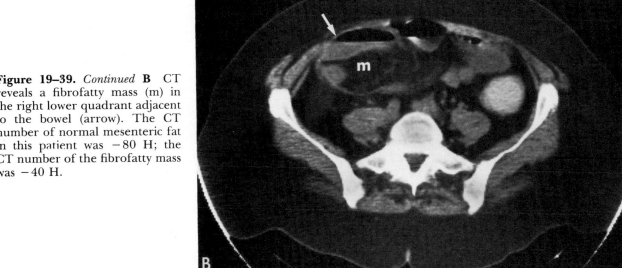

Figure 19–39. *Continued* **B** CT reveals a fibrofatty mass (m) in the right lower quadrant adjacent to the bowel (arrow). The CT number of normal mesenteric fat in this patient was −80 H; the CT number of the fibrofatty mass was −40 H.

The mesenteric thickening may be the result of sinus tracts which extend into the mesentery forming microabscesses or direct extension of the transmural inflammatory process. Mesenteric lymphatic obstruction by adjacent granulomatous reaction also occurs, contributing to thickening of the small bowel folds in Crohn's disease. The CT appearance is that of a fibrofatty mass surrounding the affected bowel and an increase in density of the adjacent mesenteric fat (Fig. 19–39). Infectious processes such as tuberculosis may cause mesenteric nodes to calcify. These nodes are readily identified by CT as high-density, rounded structures in the mesentery (Fig. 19–40).

TRAUMA

Blunt trauma to the abdomen, excessive anticoagulation or postoperative bleeding may cause mesenteric hematomas (Fig. 19–41). A specific diagnosis of mesenteric hematoma may be made when CT demonstrates a mass having the relatively high attenuation coefficient of fresh blood within the mesentery. Although most mesenteric hematomas do not require surgical evacuation,

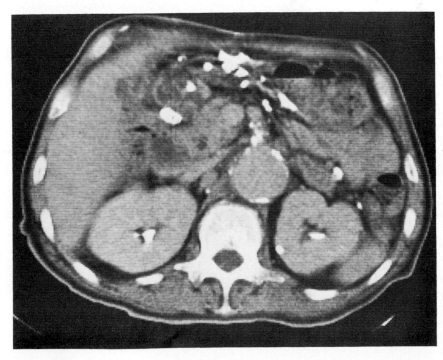

Figure 19–40. Multiple calcified mesenteric nodes resulting from tuberculosis are readily detected by computed tomography.

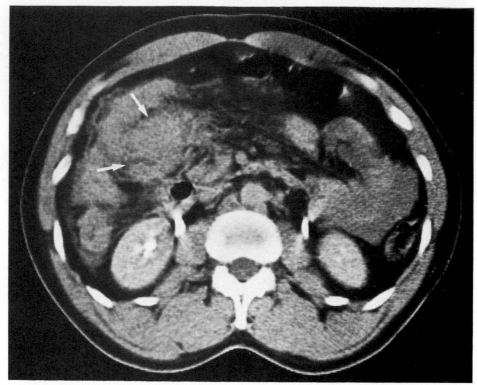

Figure 19–41. A mesenteric hematoma (arrows) secondary to blunt abdominal trauma is located adjacent to the ascending colon. The hematoma has a high attenuation value, indicating recent hemorrhage.

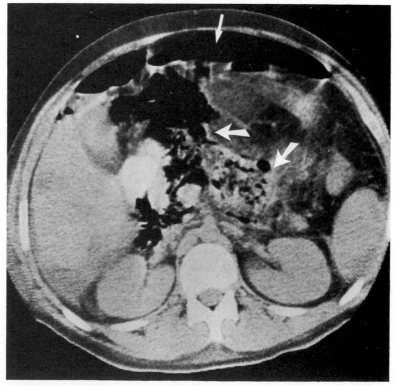

Figure 19–42. A pancreatic gas-forming abscess has extended into the root of the mesentery (large arrows). Free air is noted anteriorly (small arrow) from passage of gas through the foramen of Winslow.

they are an important finding and indicate possible injury to the bowel wall, which may result in delayed stenosis or perforation.[39]

ABSCESSES

Mesenteric abscesses can occur following pancreatitis, Crohn's disease, surgery, or penetrating injuries (Figs. 19–22 and 19–42). Mesenteric abscesses have a similar CT appearance to other abscesses and range from ill-defined areas of low density to well-encapsulated fluid collections with or without gas. As with mesenteric pseudocysts, abscesses may extend into the bowel wall, causing perforation.

Abscesses may also point to the skin and result in an abdominal sinus being formed. CT can delineate the sinus tract and determine its relationship to adjacent mesenteric and peritoneal structures.[40, 41] CT provides three-demensional information concerning the extent of a fistula or a sinus tract, which is complementary to information obtained from conventional sinograms or fistulograms.[40, 41]

REFERENCES

1. Meyers MA: Roentgen significance of the phrenicocolic ligament. Radiology 95:539, 1970.
2. Meyers MA: The spread and localization of acute intraperitoneal effusions. Radiology 95:547, 1970.
3. Meyers MA: Peritoneography: Normal and pathologic anatomy. AJR 123:67, 1975.
4. Meyers MA: Dynamic Radiology of the Abdomen. Normal and Pathologic Anatomy. New York, Springer-Verlag, 1976.
5. Walker LA, Weens HS: Radiological observations of the lesser peritoneal sac. Radiology 80:727, 1963.
6. Dunnick NR, Jones RB, Doppman JL, Speyer J, Myers CE: Intraperitoneal contrast infusion for assessment of intraperitoneal fluid dynamics. AJR 133:221, 1979.
7. Jolles H, Coulam CM: CT of ascites: Differential diagnosis. AJR 135:315, 1980.
8. Gore RM, Callen PW, Filly RA: The incidence and significance of lesser sac fluid in general peritoneal ascites. AJR 139:71, 1982.
9. Federle MP, Goldberg HI, Kaiser JA, Moss AA, Jeffrey RB, Mall JC: Evaluation of abdominal trauma by computed tomography. Radiology 138:637, 1981.
10. Lewin JR, Patterson EA: Recognition of spontaneous intraperitoneal hemorrhage complicating anticoagulant therapy. AJR 134:1271, 1980.
11. Seshal MB, Coulam CM: Pseudomyxoma peritonei: Computed tomography and sonography. AJR 136:803, 1981.
12. Mayes GB, Chuang VP, Fisher RG: CT of pseudomyxoma peritonei. AJR 136:807, 1981.
13. Connell TR, Stephens DH, Carlson HC, Brown ML: Upper abdominal abscess: A continuing and deadly problem. AJR 134:759, 1980.
14. Ariel IM, Kazarian KK: Diagnosis and treatment of abdominal abscesses. Baltimore, Williams & Wilkins, 1971, pp 174–206.
15. Wolverson MK, Jagannadharao B, Sundaram M, Joyce PF, Riaz MA, Shields JB: CT as a primary diagnostic method in evaluating intraabdominal abscess. AJR 133:1089, 1979.
16. Haaga JR, Weinstein AJ: CT guided percutaneous aspiration and drainage of abscesses. AJR 135:1187, 1980.
17. Harter LP, Moss AA, Goldberg HI: Computed tomographic guided fine needle aspirations for neoplastic and inflammatory disease. AJR 140:363, 1983.
18. Callen PW: Computed tomographic evaluation of abdominal and pelvic abscesses. Radiology 131:171, 1979.
19. Knochel JQ, Koehler PR, Lee TG, Welch DM: Diagnosis of abdominal abscesses with computed tomography, ultrasound and indium-111 leukocyte scans. Radiology 137:425, 1980.
20. Koehler PR, Moss AA: Diagnosis of intra-abdominal and pelvic abscesses by computerized tomography. JAMA 244:49, 1980.
21. McNeil BJ, Sanders R, Alderson PO, Hessel SJ, Fenberg H, Siegelman SS, Adams DF, Abrams HS: A prospective study of computed tomography, ultrasound and gallium imaging in patients with fever. Radiology 139:647, 1981.
22. Schneekloth G, Terrier F, Fuchs WA: Computed tomography of intraperitoneal abscesses. Gastrointest Radiol 7:35, 1982.
23. Rubinson KA, Isikoff MB, Hill MC: Diagnostic imaging of hepatic abscesses: A retrospective analysis. AJR 135:735, 1980.
24. Korobkin M, Callen PW, Filly RA, Hoffer PB, Shimshak RR, Kressel HY: Comparison of computed tomography, ultrasonography, and gallium-67 scanning in the evaluation of suspected abdominal abscess. Radiology 129:89, 1978.
25. Aronberg DJ, Stanley RJ, Levitt RG, Sagel SS: The evaluation of abdominal abscesses with computed tomography. J Comput Assist Tomogr 2:384, 1978.
26. Wolverson MK, Jagannadharao B, Sundaram M, Joyce PF, Riaz MA, Shields JB: CT as a primary diagnosis method in evaluating intra-abdominal abscess. AJR 133:1089, 1979.
27. Halber MD, Daffner RH, Morgan CL, Trought WS, Thompson WM, Rice RP, Korobkin M: Intraabdominal abscess: Current concepts in radiologic evaluation. AJR 133:9, 1979.
28. Jeffrey RB: CT demonstration of peritoneal implants. AJR 135:323, 1980.
29. Barth RA, Jeffrey RB Jr, Moss AA, Liberman MS: A comparison study of computed tomography and laparoscopy in the staging of abdominal neoplasms. Dig Dis Sci 26:253, 1981.
30. Jeffrey RB, Federle MP, Goodman PC: Computed tomography of the lesser peritoneal sac. Radiology 141:117, 1981.
31. Siegelman SS, Copeland BE, Sabe GB, Cameron JR, Sanders RC, Zerhouni BA: CT of fluid collections associated with pancreatitis. AJR 134:1121, 1980.
32. Mueller PR, Ferrucci JT, Harbin WP, Kirkpatrick RH, Simeone JF, Wittenberg J: Appearance of lymphomatous involvement of the mesentery of ultrasonography

and body computed tomography: The "sandwich sign." Radiology 134:467, 1980.

33. Levitt RG, Sagel SS, Stanley RJ: Detection of neoplastic involvement of the omentum by computed tomography. AJR 131:835, 1978.

34. Bernardino ME, Jing BS, Wallace S: Computed tomography diagnosis of mesenteric masses, AJR 132:33, 1979.

35. Siegel RS, Kuhns LR, Borlaza GS, McCormick TL, Simmons JR: Computed tomography and angiography in ileal carcinoid tumor and retractile mesenterits. Radiology 134:437, 1980.

36. Ellert J, Kreel L. The role of computed tomography in the initial staging and subsequent management of the lymphomas. J Comput Assist Tomogr 4:368, 1980.

37. Harell GS, Breiman RS, Glatstein EJ, Marshall WH, Castellino RA: Computed tomography of the abdomen in the malignant lymphomas. Radiol Clin North Am 15:391, 1977.

38. Lee JK, Stanley RJ, Sagel SS, Levitt RG: Accuracy of computed tomography in detecting intraabdominal and pelvic adenopathy in lymphoma. AJR 131:311, 1978.

39. Shuck JM, Lowe RG: Intestinal disruption due to blunt abdominal trauma. Am J Surg 136:668, 1978.

40. Frick MP, Feinberg SB, Stenlund RR, Gedgaudas E: Evaluation of abdominal fistulas with computed body tomography. Comput Radiol 16:17, 1982.

41. Alexander ES, Weinberg S, Clark RA, Belkin RD: Fistulas and sinus tracts: Radiologic evaluation, management and outcome. Gastrointest Radiol 7:135, 1982.

20 COMPUTED TOMOGRAPHY OF THE PELVIS

Ruedi F. Thoeni

The use of computed tomography (CT) in examination of the pelvis has become an important tool in the radiographic armamentarium for evaluating patients with suspected pelvic disease. The widespread use of CT is largely related to the excellent anatomic detail this technique provides. The ability of CT to display axial, coronal, and sagittal views of the pelvis ensures optimal display of normal and abnormal anatomy and enables extension of tumor into surrounding tissue (e.g. prostate, bladder, rectum, or sigmoid colon) to be determined with a high degree of accuracy. Thus,

CT scanning of the ovary, prostate, seminal vesicles, bladder uterus, and cervix has become important for both diagnosis and treatment planning.

TECHNIQUES OF EXAMINATION

Optimal CT scanning of the pelvis requires that all intestinal structures be well filled with contrast material at the time of the examination. To ensure that the distal small bowel and colon are opacified, each patient is asked to drink 500 ml of 1 per cent diatrizoate meglumine (Gastrografin or Gastroview) the evening before the examination. If possible patients who are not in the hospital are given 10 ml of Gastrografin in a small bottle at the time of scheduling and are instructed to mix the contrast material with 480 ml of water and to drink the mixture the evening before the examination. In addition, all patients are given 350 to 500 ml of 1 per cent diatrizoate meglumine to drink 45 minutes before the CT study. This method of administering oral contrast material ensures good filling of the distal small bowel and proximal colon and helps eliminates the diagnostic dilemma produced by nonopacified small-bowel loops that project deeply into the pelvis and simulate soft-tissue masses. To ensure better definition of the rectum and distal colon, approximately 300 ml of a 1 per cent solution of a soluble contrast material, such as diatrizoate sodium (Hypaque) is administered by way of the rectum just prior to the examination. In selected instances, 1 mg of glucagon is injected to paralyze the small bowel and to distend the colon. In female patients, vaginal tampons are used to mark the exact position of the vagina and cervix.

Intravenous contrast material is not routinely administered, but in some instances an infusion of contrast material or a bolus injection of 70 to 100 ml of contrast material is given to define the ureters or to distinguish vessels from enlarged lymph nodes.

When the bladder is being evaluated for a primary tumor or for determining whether invasion of the bladder wall is present, a single- or double-contrast examination of the bladder may be performed. For a single-contrast examination of the urinary bladder, 150 ml of contrast material is administered by rapid infusion before scanning and 150 ml as continuous intravenous infusion during the examination.[1, 2] For a double-contrast examination of the urinary bladder, a Foley catheter is inserted into the bladder and 100 ml of air or carbon dioxide and 100 ml of dilated contrast material (30 per cent diatrizoate meglumine) are instilled for better definition of the bladder wall. The double-contrast technique has been shown to be particularly helpful for evaluation of the anterior portion of the bladder dome[3] and most accurately demonstrates intraluminal and intramural tumor extension. Following air and contrast instillation, patients are scanned in the supine, decubitus, and prone positions. Disadvantages of the double-contrast examination of the urinary bladder are that the technique is time consuming and uncomfortable.

A scout view or digital radiograph of the pelvis permits localization of the bladder, prostate, inguinal canal, intrauterine contraceptive devices, ischial spines, and, occasionally, pelvic masses prior to performing positioning of transverse scans. In general, the initial scan of the pelvis is performed without intravenous contrast material in patients with suspected bladder or prostate pathology. In patients with suspected intramural endometrial carcinoma, the CT study is performed following an injection of contrast material.[4]

The routine CT examination of the pelvis is performed using contiguous sections 10 mm thick from the iliac crest to the symphysis during shallow breathing or suspended expiration. For staging of prostate, ovarian, uterine or bladder tumors, scans of 5 mm thickness at 5-mm intervals are employed. When searching for undescended testes, contiguous scan sections 5 mm thick are taken from the pubic symphysis to the anterior superior iliac spine, and if the testis is not identified, scans through the lower abdomen at 10-mm intervals up to the lower pole of the kidney are obtained. In patients being evaluated for superficial rectal tumors that are to be treated by endocavitary irradiation, 1 mg of glucagon is injected to ensure maximum colonic distention and scanning is initiated at the level of the symphysis. For tumor staging, the initial scans of the pelvis then are followed by contiguous sections 1 to 1.5 cm thick through the abdomen starting from the dome of the liver in order to identify metastases to liver, adrenals, spine, and mesenteric or retroperitoneal lymph nodes.

Maximum resolution will be obtained by performing scans using the smallest field of view that will include the entire pelvis. However, care must be taken to avoid the selection of too small a field in a large patient. Reformation of transverse CT images into sagittal and coronal sections is not routinely performed but has proven useful in determining tumor extension into the bladder or prostate.[5] Direct coronal or sagittal computed tomography of the pelvis has been described and offers improved image quality by avoiding partial volume averaging and patient motion disturbance.[6, 7] For coronal examination of the pelvis, a special seat is needed which connects to the patient support for automatic section indexing.[6] For direct sagittal CT sections of the pelvis, an accessory table at a 90 per cent angle to the regular table is required.[7]

Measurement of the volume of an organ (e.g. prostate, uterus, bladder) can be readily calculated by tracing the organ of interest with an electronic computer cursor and summating the surface area measurements obtained on the individual scans. This area is then multiplied by the slice thickness (usually 0.5 or 1 cm) to determine the segmental volume. The total volume of the organ to be measured is computed by the addition of all segmental volumes.

ANATOMY

At the level of the sacral promontory, the right colon is usually located anterior to the right psoas major and iliacus muscles, and the descending colon is positioned similarly on the left side. Ileal loops are located anteriorly, immediately below the rectus abdominis muscle and anterior to the sigmoid colon. The ileal loops are separated by the mesentery from the jejunal loops, which are located on the left side anterior to the psoas and iliacus (Fig. 20–1). In the midpelvis the sigmoid colon is identified by the one or two loops it forms prior to its joining the descending colon in its retroperitoneal location (Fig. 20–2). Distally, the rectum occupies a midline position surrounded by fat, just ventral to the sacrum (Fig. 20–3).

The urinary bladder is a homogeneous midline structure of water density whose size and configuration varies greatly depending on the amount of urine present. The outer margin of the bladder wall is smooth and usually well delineated by perivesical fat (Fig. 20–2). The bladder wall (2 to 5 mm) appears as a rim of soft tissue whose inner margins are better identified if the bladder contains only urine, or if air, carbon dioxide, or oil has been instilled into the bladder.

The ureters are best seen after intravenous administration of iodinated contrast material. At the level of the sacral promontory, the ureters are located anteromedial to the psoas major and anterior to the common iliac artery or lateral to the external iliac artery (Fig. 20–1). The ureters then course medially and posteriorly to the external iliac arteries until they reach the midportion of the internal obturator muscle. At this level, they course anteromedially to reach the trigonum of the bladder.

The pelvic muscles (psoas, iliacus, obturator in-

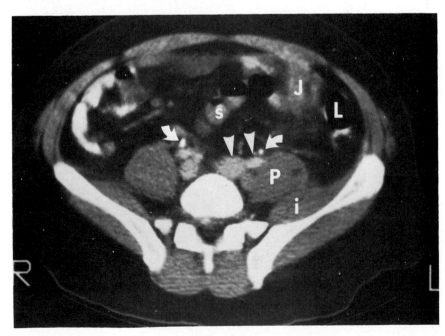

Figure 20–1. CT section at level of sacral promontory shows the common iliac arteries and veins (arrowheads) anteromedial to the psoas muscle (P). The ureters (curved arrows) are located anterior to the vessels. L=Left colon; J=jejunal loops; s=sigmoid colon; i=iliacus muscle.

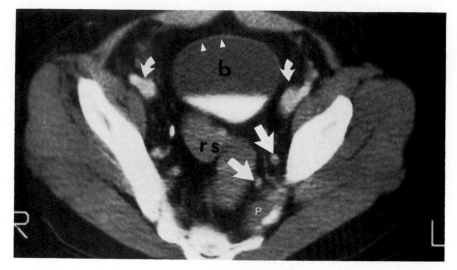

Figure 20–2. CT scan through midpelvis. A bolus of contrast material shows the location of internal (straight arrows) and external (curved arrows) iliac arteries and veins. Nodes accompanying the vessels are not identified in this normal patient. Rectosigmoid (rs) and bladder (b) also are well demonstrated. The bladder wall (arrowheads) is thin and has a smooth outer margin. The piriformis muscle (P) is seen on the left side, but not on the right, because of a slight tilt of the pelvis in the gantry.

Figure 20–3. CT scan through distal pelvis. A bolus of contrast material outlines the femoral artery (large solid arrow) and vein (curved arrow). Seminal vesicles (open arrows) are well delineated as oval structures between the bladder (b) and rectum (r), which is midline in position just anterior to the sacrum (arrowhead). Small arrows = Coccygeal muscle; i = internal obturator muscle; g = gluteus maximus muscle; ig = inferior gemellus muscle.

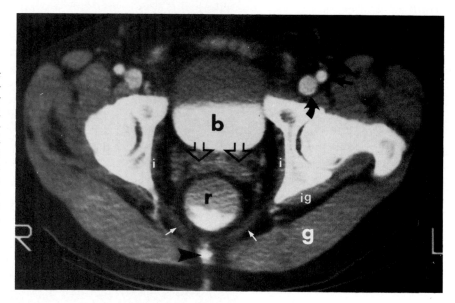

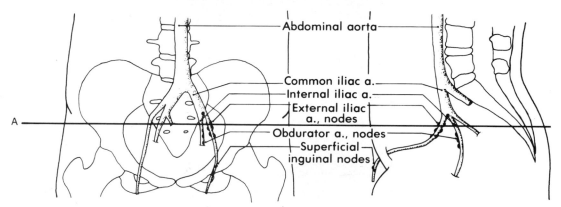

Figure 20–4. Diagram demonstrating the relationship of pelvic lymph nodes to pelvic arterial supply. Line A = level of CT scan shown in Figure 20–2. (Modified from Walsh JW, Amendola MA, Konerding KF, Tisnado J, Dazra TA: Computed tomographic detection of pelvic and inguinal lymph node metastases from primary and recurrent pelvic malignant disease. Radiology 137:157, 1980.)

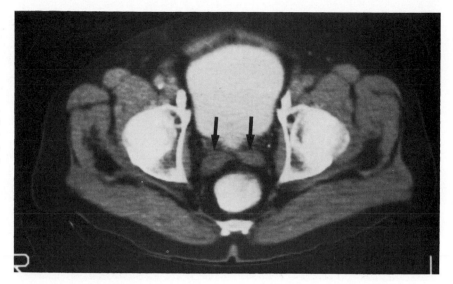

Figure 20–5. Normal male pelvis. The seminal vesicles are seen as oval to elliptical masses of soft-tissue density (arrows) posterior to the bladder and anterior to the rectum.

ternus, piriformis, and levator ani) are well outlined on cross sections of the pelvis and are symmetrical in the normal patient (Fig. 20–3). Pelvic lymph nodes accompany the common iliac, external iliac, internal iliac, and obturator vessels (Fig. 20–4), and although normal-sized pelvic lymph nodes often cannot be identified on CT scans (Fig. 20–2), if pelvic lymph nodes are enlarged, calcified, or contain ethiodized oil (Ethiodol), they are readily identified.

In the male pelvis, the seminal vesicles are seen dorsal to the bladder and anterior to the rectum (Figs. 20–3 and 20–5). They are oval- to tear-shaped structures and are clearly displayed as a result of the abundance of perirectal and perivesical fat. The position of the seminal vesicles is not fixed in the pelvis and their location and configuration change slightly, depending on the patient's position. The prostate is a homogeneous round structure of soft-tissue density, 2 to 4 cm in length, located just beneath the symphysis pubis immediately anterior to the rectum (Fig. 20–6). The spermatic cord with the vas deferens and testicular artery and vein can be recognized on lower cross sections of the pelvis. The spermatic cord appears as a circular or oval mass of soft-tissue density (Fig. 20–7A) or as a thin-walled, ringlike structure, containing a small dot or linear streak of soft-tissue density representing the vas deferens and the spermatic vessels (Fig. 20–7B). The

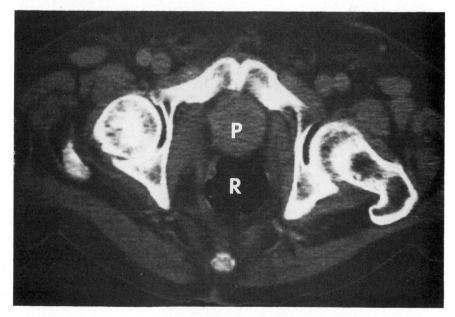

Figure 20–6. Male pelvis. A slightly enlarged prostate (P) is seen as a round soft-tissue density posterior to the symphysis and anterior to the rectum (R). At higher levels, the prostate is related to the base of the bladder.

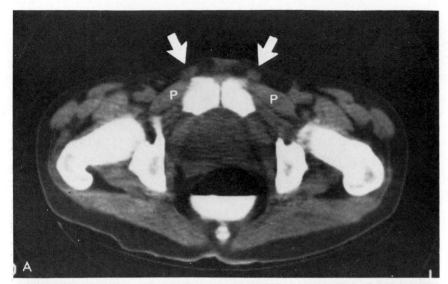

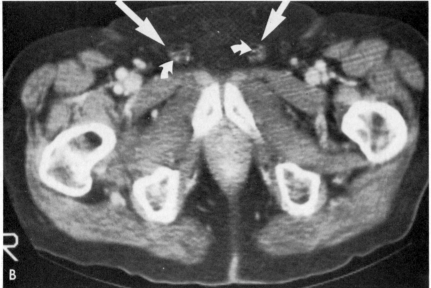

Figure 20–7. Male pelvis. **A**   The normal spermatic cords are shown as oval densities (arrows) anterior to the pectineal muscles (P). **B**   In an individual with sufficient fat, following intravenous administration of contrast medium the spermatic vessels (curved arrows) can be seen as small dots of high density within the spermatic cords (straight arrows).

normal testes appear as oval structures measuring 1 to 3 cm in anteroposterior diameter and 4 to 5 cm in length. The parenchyma of the testes is of low attenuation and is surrounded by the denser tunica albuginea.

The differences between the bony pelvis of the male and female are readily demonstrated by axial CT images. In females the pelvic inlet is larger; the iliac wings flare laterally, the sacrum is less curved and wider, and the ischial tuberosity and anterior iliac spines are more widely separated. On the cross sections of the female pelvis, three compartments can be recognized: an anterior sector containing ileal loops; a middle sector with the uterus, cervix, venous plexus, internal obturator muscle, and urinary bladder; and a posterior sector housing the rectum and sacrum.

The uterus is seen as a round, homogeneous, oval, or triangular soft-tissue mass located dorsal to the bladder, which may contain a central area of low attenuation (Fig. 20–8A–C). CT clearly demonstrates the pouch of Douglas as a recess between the uterus and rectum (Fig. 20–8A). Generally, the ovaries are not identified as discrete structures unless they are enlarged, and the oviducts are seen only if markedly abnormal in size, such as is found in an ectopic pregnancy. The demarcations between the vagina, cervix, and uterus are not clearly shown by CT scans. However, insertion of a vaginal tampon permits the vagina to be identified, demonstrates the close relationship between the wall of the vagina, urinary bladder, and rectum (Fig. 20–9), and permits delineation of the cervix and uterus.

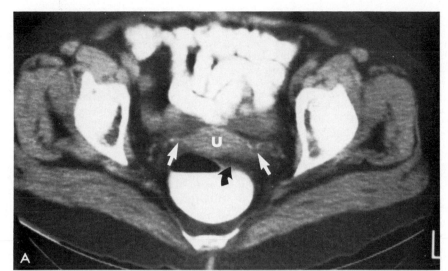

Figure 20–8. Normal female pelvis. **A** The normal uterus (u) is identified as an oval structure with deltoid extensions (arrows) on either side representing the adnexal structures. Pouch of Douglas is represented by a curved arrow. **B** At a higher level, CT scan shows the uterine cavity as an area of low attenuation (arrow). Broad ligaments (curved arrows) extend from the body of the uterus.

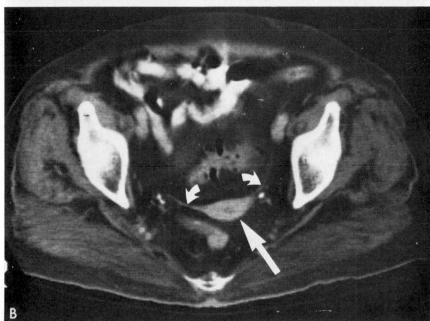

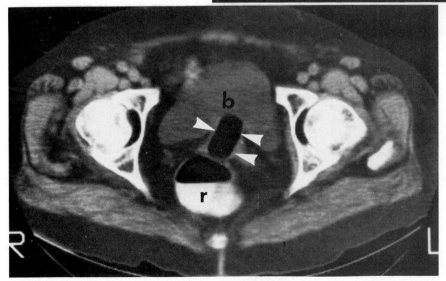

Figure 20–9. A tampon (arrowheads) outlines the vagina between rectum (r) and bladder (b).

Urinary Bladder
PATHOLOGY

BENIGN DISEASE

Masses seen on intravenous urography impressing, compressing, or displacing the bladder are readily evaluated by CT. True masses are easily distinguished from bladder impressions produced by loops of bowel present in the pelvis if the bowel loops are adequately filled with contrast material. Alterations in the shape of the bladder can be produced by retroperitoneal fibrosis, pelvic lipomatosis, hematoma, lymphoceles, or inferior vena caval thrombosis.[8-11] In these benign conditions, CT reveals elevation and narrowing of the bladder in such a way that the bladder appears pear-shaped. The cause of the pear-shaped bladder often can be determined by pelvic CT examinations. Large amounts of low-density fat are present surrounding the pelvic organs in pelvic lipomatosis (Fig. 20–10). Lymphoceles are cystic masses that compress the bladder, have sharp borders, and a CT density close to that of water. Acute hematomas have a density greater than that of surrounding muscles, and contrast-enhancing paravesical collateral vessels together with a filling defect in the inferior vena cava confirm a diagnosis of an inferior vena caval occlusion. If a mass has an irregular shape, obliterates perivesical fat planes, or appears to invade adjacent pelvic organs in the presence of a pear-shaped bladder, the most likely underlying cause is a pelvic malignancy.[12]

Extravesical inflammatory processes may extend to involve the bladder. Inflammatory bowel disease and diverticulitis can produce a localized thickening of the bladder wall that can be difficult to differentiate from tumorous thickening, and on rare occasions, localized irregular wall thickening may be caused by endometriosis of the urinary bladder.[13] In cases of endometriosis, ultrasound or CT—together with a history of classic cyclicity (seen in approximately 25 per cent of cases) and cystoscopy with biopsy—usually leads to the correct diagnosis. In addition, care must be taken not to confuse thickening of the bladder wall related to incomplete distention, trabeculation due to urinary outflow obstruction, radiation enema, or fibrosis (Fig. 20–11A), with thickening of the bladder wall related to a malignancy.

Nonmalignant bladder tumors are rare, but bladder fibromas, pheochromocytomas (Fig. 20–11B), and angiomas appear as smooth intravesical filling defects. Distinguishing these from a noncalcified bladder calculus or intravesical blood clot is usually easy because calculi have a high CT attenuation and blood clots change position as the patient is scanned in the prone or decubitus position.

MALIGNANT DISEASE

Bladder Carcinoma

The standard methods of examining patients with suspected primary or secondary bladder tumors are cystoscopy, biopsy using a transurethral approach, excretory urography, cystography, lymphangiography, arteriography, and bimanual

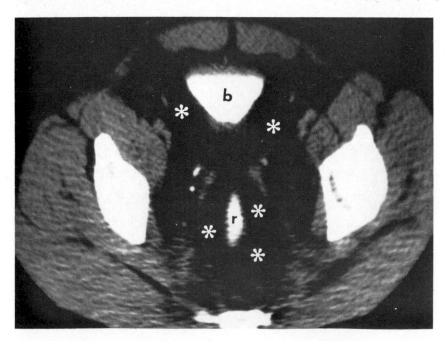

Figure 20–10. Pelvic lipomatosis. CT demonstrates excessive pelvic fat (asterisks) compressing the rectum (r) and bladder (b).

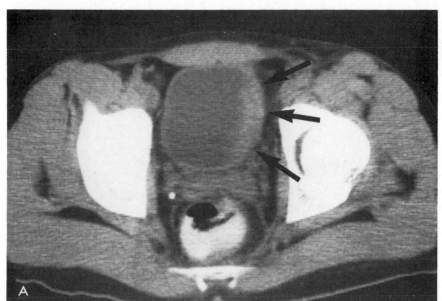

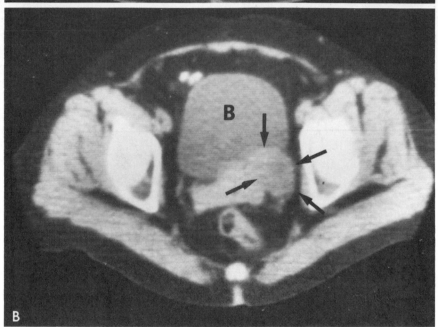

Figure 20–11. Benign bladder abnormalities.   **A** Irregular thickening of the left lateral wall of the bladder (arrows) is due to radiation cystitis but mimics a tumor. The clinical history is necessary for correct intepretation of bladder wall thickening. **B** A soft mass (arrows) representing a pheochromocytoma arising in the posterior wall of the bladder (B). The histologic nature of this mass cannot be determined by CT without biopsy or without confirming clinical evidence of a pheochromocytoma.

Table 20–1.   STAGING OF BLADDER TUMORS (JEWETT-MARSHALL SYSTEM)

Stage	Description
O	Confined to mucosa
A	Infiltration of submucosa
B_1	Infiltration of superficial muscle
B_2	Infiltration of deep muscle
C	Perivesical infiltration
D_1	Infiltration of adjacent organs and pelvic lymph nodes
D_2	Distant metastases to nodes above aortic bifurcation

examination under anesthesia.[14] The Jewett-Marshall system, generally used in the United States for staging bladder tumors (Table 20–1)[15] is based on results obtained from using standard methodology. Although there is extensive experience with this system, Kenny and associates[16] reported an accuracy rate of only 56 per cent for preoperative staging of bladder tumors using standard methods. Superficial tumors (Stages O and A) and tumors infiltrating the wall without extension beyond the margin of the bladder wall (Stages B_1 and B_2) generally were diagnosed accurately, but extension of tumor beyond the bladder wall

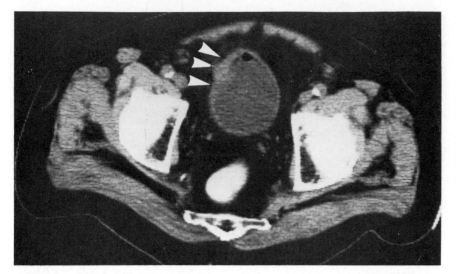

Figure 20–12. Bladder carcinoma. Focal thickening of the wall of the urinary bladder (arrowheads) from a stage B₂ transitional cell carcinoma. Air in the bladder was introduced during cystoscopy.

(Stages C, D₁ and D₂) was not adequately determined using conventional modalities.

Improvement in staging of bladder carcinoma has been obtained by the use of both ultrasound and computed tomography. Ultrasonographic examination of the bladder by means of an intravesical transducer is highly accurate,[17–19] but extensive infiltration into surrounding pelvic structures cannot be determined because of the limited depth penetration of the intraluminal transducer. Transabdominal ultrasonography of the bladder is accurate (80 per cent), but tumors in the bladder outlet or in the anterior wall near the outlet are difficult to evaluate by transabdominal ultrasonography.[17] Accurate evaluation of the extension of tumor into seminal vesicles or the prostate requires transrectal ultrasonographic scanning.[20, 21] Other drawbacks are that ultrasound of the pelvis requires a skilled operator, transvesical ultrasonography in men usually requires spinal or general anesthesia, and transrectal scanning is uncomfortable.

Compared with ultrasound, CT of the pelvis is easy to perform, is noninvasive, and can accurately detect mucosal or mural abnormalities. In general, CT cannot distinguish between Stage A, B₁, and B₂ bladder carcinomas[22] because CT cannot differentiate the various layers of the wall of the urinary bladder. However, CT is highly accurate in determining extension of tumor outside

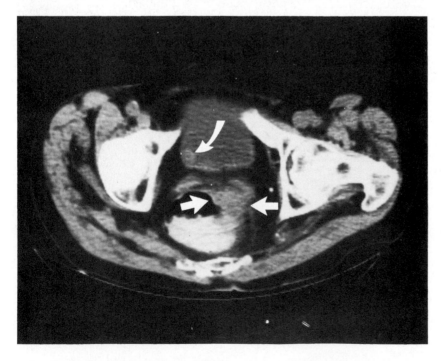

Figure 20–13. Stage B₁ transitional cell carcinoma of the bladder is seen as a localized nodule of soft-tissue density in the posterolateral aspect of the bladder (curved arrows). The tissue planes between the bladder and rectum are preserved. The patient also had a primary tumor of the rectum (straight arrows).

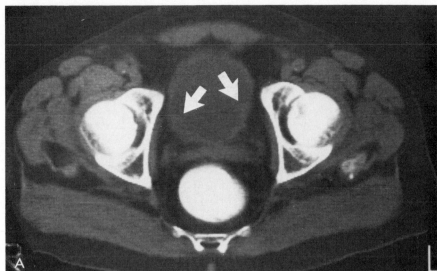

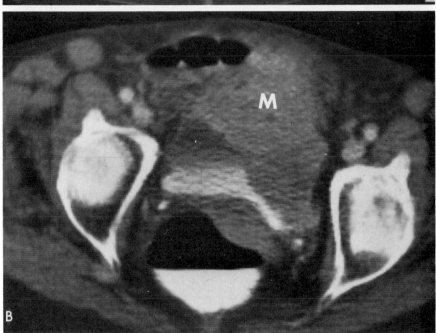

Figure 20–14. A Stage B_1 bladder carcinoma producing a thickening of the bladder wall (arrows), which extends to involve a large portion of the bladder wall. There is no extension of tumor into surrounding tissue. **B** A large mass (M) is seen to protrude into the lumen of the urinary bladder in a patient with transitional cell carcinoma Stage B_2.

the bladder to neighboring structures, pelvic side walls, lymph nodes and/or distant sites.[22, 23] Tumor confined to the bladder wall appears as thickening of the bladder wall with sharp borders. The tumor may produce localized bladder wall thickening (Fig. 20–12), a papillary projection into the lumen (Fig. 20–13), or involve a large portion of the bladder wall (Fig. 20–14). Bladder wall thickening is usually due to malignant disease, but inflammatory or radiation changes may mimic malignant wall thickening (Fig. 20–11).

Poor definition of the borders of the urinary bladder with loss of distinctness of the surrounding fat suggests perivesical tumor extension of disease (Fig. 20–15). If CT demonstrates a loss of

tissue planes and a tumor mass that clearly extends into the perivesical fat or involves neighboring structures such as seminal vesicles or obturator muscles, a diagnosis of Stage D_1 carcinoma can be made (Fig. 20–16). Hydronephrosis frequently is seen in Stage D_1 malignancies, but distinction by CT between an advanced Stage C and a D_1 tumor may not be possible. Stage D_2 is characterized by metastatic disease, usually in the form of retroperitoneal adenopathy or metastases to the liver or lungs (Fig. 20–17).

The reported accuracy rate for staging bladder tumors by CT has ranged from 64 to 90 per cent.[24–30] CT has proven superior to intravenous urography and to cystography for detecting ex-

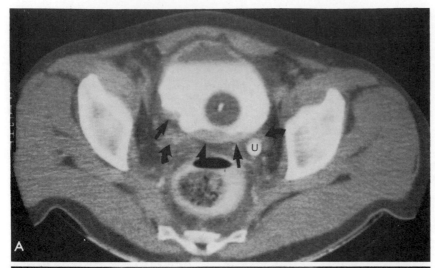

Figure 20–15. Stage C transitional cell carcinoma. **A** CT scan shows irregular thickening of the wall of the bladder (straight arrows) and extension of the tumor into surrounding tissues (curved arrows). The left ureter (U) is partially obstructed, and the right ureter is not identified. **B** CT scan through level of kidneys demonstrates hydronephrosis of the left kidney and a hydronephrotic nonfunctioning right kidney.

tension of a tumor mass beyond the bladder wall and often is more accurate for evaluation of anterior or posterior bladder wall lesions.[25] Axial CT scans accurately detect posterior spread of tumor into the seminal vesicles, but extension of carcinoma into the prostate is only rarely demon-

strated by CT. Sagittal and coronal image reconstruction is helpful for evaluating craniocaudad extension of tumor, for determination of the relationship of the tumor mass to seminal vesicles and prostate gland,[5] and in identifying lesions located in the dome and base of the urinary blad-

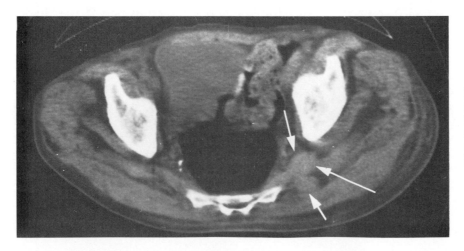

Figure 20–16. Stage D₁ transitional cell carcinoma of the bladder. Metastases from bladder carcinoma (arrows) adjacent to and invading the left piriformis muscle.

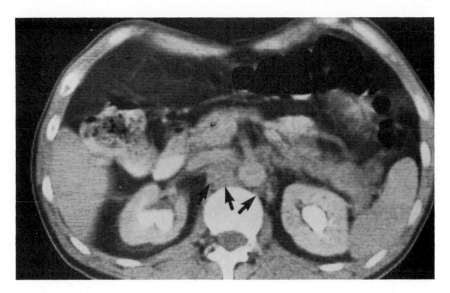

Figure 20–17. Stage D_2 bladder carcinoma producing retrocrural adenopathy (arrows).

der.[22] Kellet and co-workers found that in untreated patients, CT tended to reveal a higher stage than clinical examination.[26] This was particularly true among obese patients in whom increased fat facilitated CT differentiation of pelvic organs.

Although CT is a useful method for staging bladder carcinoma, it cannot reliably predict microscopic invasion of either the serosal surface of the bladder by pelvic malignancies or microscopic invasion of perivesical fat by intrinsic bladder tumor.[20, 27] In one study, 8 per cent of bladder tumors were understaged by CT; microscopic invasion of tumor to surrounding structures was present, and CT overstaging of bladder tumors can occur if insufficient body fat makes delineation of tissue planes impossible.

Following radiotherapy, CT has been utilized in an attempt to distinguish direct extension of recurrent tumor to the pelvic walls from simple radiation fibrosis with anchorage of the bladder to abdominal wall.[25] The recognition of fibrosis is important because patients with recurrent tumor not extending to the pelvic walls can undergo curative cystectomy.[31]

The major methods of evaluating patients with suspected lymph node metastases from bladder carcinoma are lymphangiography, CT, and lymphadenectomy. Although ultrasound is employed for screening of abdominal or pelvic adenopathy in some institutions, this method, despite reported accuracy rates of 78 per cent (sensitivity 73 per cent and specificity 89 per cent),[32] remains limited in its use because of the operator skill involved and the poor results achieved in patients with gas-distended abdomens.

The reported accuracy rates of lymphangiography in detecting lymph node metastasis from bladder tumors ranges between 90 and 94 per cent,[33, 34] while histologically confirmed CT accuracy rates have ranged from 73 to 77 per cent for evaluation of lymph node metastases from pelvic tumors and for evaluation of pelvic lymph nodes in patients with bladder carcinoma.[35, 36] CT routinely demonstrates enlarged celiac, renal pelvic, iliac, and obturator nodes that are not usually filled during lymphangiography. Lymph nodes are considered abnormal if they are larger than 1.5 or 2 cm in diameter,[35, 37] but CT cannot distinguish between benign and malignant lymphadenopathy without a histologic sample. Lymphangiography detects smaller metastasis, distinguishes between benign and malignant lymphadenopathy, and thus is more accurate than CT in diagnosing pelvic lymph node metastases.[36] However, lymphangiography is limited because it cannot detect microscopic metastases and it fails to fill certain groups of nodes in which metastases often are found.

Currently, a CT scan is initially obtained. If abnormal lymph nodes are demonstrated by CT, no further evaluation is performed unless histologic confirmation is required prior to institution of therapy. In such cases, a CT-guided percutaneous needle biopsy is performed to obtain tissue from the abnormal nodes. If CT is negative, lymphangiography may be performed.

EVALUATION OF THERAPY. Several reports have documented the value of CT in planning external beam radiation portals in patients with tumors of the bladder.[22, 38, 39] The use of computerized radiotherapy planning programs, coupled with anatomic and densitometric CT data, has increased the accuracy of portal planning and permitted the use of computerized dosimetry.[22] Often, based on CT results, treatment plans are changed, radiation ports adjusted, and dosages modified.

CT is also useful in following the effectiveness of radiation therapy. A CT scan obtained during or immediately following a course of radiotherapy usually will not demonstrate any significant change in the volume of the bladder tumor but will act as a baseline for assessment of tumor regression 6 months after irradiation. Following radiation therapy, fibrosis may occur; this can limit bladder mobility and simulate recurrent malignancy (Fig. 20–11A). Distinction between fibrosis and tumor is usually possible because fibrosis does not obscure organ margins[25] and tissue planes are preserved and often highlighted by increased perirectal and perivesical fat.[40]

A major role of CT in bladder tumors is to determine in which patients radical surgery should be avoided. CT also can detect early recurrence in patients following radiation therapy or resection. More data with larger series and longer follow-up periods are necessary to establish whether the additional information provided by CT will produce an overall improved survival rate because of earlier recognition of recurrence.

Carcinoma of the Urachus

This is a rare malignancy that arises from the intra- or juxtavesical segment (90 per cent), the middle (6 per cent), or from the umbilical end (4 per cent) of the urachus.[41] It accounts for less than 1 per cent of bladder carcinomas. Of urachal carcinomas, 75 to 80 per cent occur in males, typically between 40 and 70 years of age. Although most tumors are adenocarcinoma (94 per cent), transitional, squamous, and anaplastic carcinomas are found.[38] Patients with carcinoma of the urachus most commonly present with hematuria (78 per cent), with passage of mucoid material in the urine (10 per cent), discharge of blood or mucus from the umbilicus, dysuria, and abdominal pain being less frequent clinical manifestations. A suprapubic mass may be palpable, but plain radiography detects calcifications in less than 5 per cent of tumors. Urachal tumors can deform the bladder outline, cause lateral displacement of the ureters, or produce no abnormality. Urachal carcinoma is usually treated with radiation and partial cystectomy, but prognosis is poor, the 5-year survival rates ranging from 6.5 to 15 per cent.[41]

On CT scans, urachal carcinoma is seen as a soft-tissue mass that may contain calcium; it is located anterior to the bladder, extending toward the anterior abdominal wall. CT also provides information concerning extent of tumor spread, resectability, and local recurrence, which, unfortunately, occurs in 30 per cent of patients following partial cystectomy.

CT FOLLOWING CYSTECTOMY. The present practice of preoperative radiation and radical cystectomy consisting of a total cystectomy, pelvic lymphadenectomy, prostatectomy, and removal of seminal vesicles in men and total abdominal hysterectomy and bilateral salpingo-oophorectomy in women has reduced the rate of recurrence of bladder tumors. However, postoperative complications following such extensive surgery are not uncommon. Abscesses and urinary leaks at the anastomotic site are common immediately,[42–44] and CT has proved to be the best means for detecting these postcystectomy complications.[45] CT scans are not hampered by drains or surgical packing and can be performed with intravenous and oral contrast media to permit distinction of bowel from abscess and urine leak from hematoma or lymphocyst.

After radical cystectomy, axial CT scans of the abdomen demonstrate absence of bladder, prostate, and seminal vesicles in men, and bladder, uterus, and fallopian tubes in women. The space of the resected organs is occupied by small-bowel loops and occasionally a loop of sigmoid colon. Pelvic musculature remains symmetrical, but perivesical fat planes are often disrupted after cystectomy.

RECURRENT BLADDER TUMORS. Recurrent tumor appears as a soft-tissue mass with or without central necrosis; if the recurrent tumor is large, invasion of adjacent structures may be present. In general, any pelvic mass detected more than 3 months after cystectomy usually represents a tumor recurrence. However, a percutaneous biopsy may be necessary to differentiate tumor from postoperative fibrosis.

Prostate

The prostate is well visualized by CT in almost every male patient, and as a result of the clear delineation of the prostate, prostatic size and volume can be accurately measured. In men 30 years old and younger, the average craniocaudad diameter measures 3 cm, the anteroposterior diameter 2.3 cm, and the lateral diameter 3.1 cm. In the 60- to 70-year-old age group, these average measurements increase to 5 cm for the craniocaudad, 4.3 cm for the anteroposterior diameter, and 4.8 cm for the lateral diameter.[46] However, precise distinction is difficult between the apex of the gland and the levator ani and between the prostate and distal rectum. Therefore, the AP and lateral diameters of the prostate often are slightly overestimated because of inclusion of surrounding structures.

PATHOLOGY

As a general rule, the prostate is not enlarged if a scan 1 cm above the symphysis does not visualize the prostate.[46] However, prostatic enlargement can be diagnosed unequivocally only if the prostate is seen 2 to 3 cm or more above the symphysis, in which instances it is usually surrounded by the bladder (Fig. 20–18A). The actual volume of prostatic tissue can be calculated by summating prostatic volumes on sequential CT scans (Fig. 20–18B). The size of the prostate needs to be correlated with symptoms of the patient and the amount of residual urine in order to determine the clinical relevance of increase in prostatic size.

Prostatic calcifications are detected by CT more frequently with increasing age, reaching 60 per cent in the 50- to 70-year-old age group.[46] The calcifications usually appear as punctate, scattered, rounded densities that may not be identified on plain radiographs (Fig. 20–19). Large foci of calcification with irregular margins also are demonstrable.

BENIGN DISEASE

Despite the high density and spatial resolution of CT images, the margins of different prostatic lobes cannot be identified and prostatic gland tissue cannot be differentiated from the prostatic capsule. CT is a reliable indicator of prostatic disease only when the prostate is enlarged because benign prostatic tissue has a CT attenuation value similar to that of malignant tissue. In the presence of an enlarged prostate with sharp, smooth borders, it is impossible to distinguish between prostatic hypertrophy and a small focal adenocar-

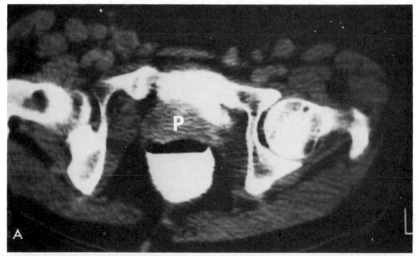

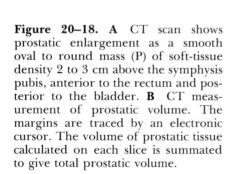

Figure 20–18. A CT scan shows prostatic enlargement as a smooth oval to round mass (P) of soft-tissue density 2 to 3 cm above the symphysis pubis, anterior to the rectum and posterior to the bladder. **B** CT measurement of prostatic volume. The margins are traced by an electronic cursor. The volume of prostatic tissue calculated on each slice is summated to give total prostatic volume.

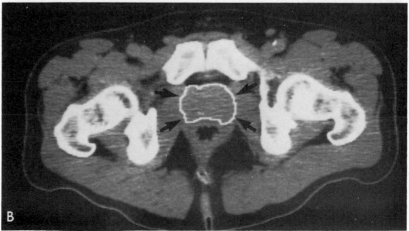

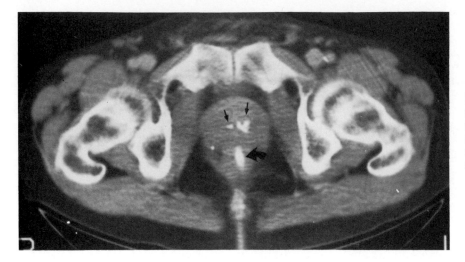

Figure 20–19. Calcifications (arrows) are demonstrated within the prostate gland. The rectum (curved arrows) contains contrast material and cannot be clearly separated from the prostate.

cinoma of the prostate (Figs. 20–18*A* and 20–20).

Sonographically benign hypertrophy presents as symmetrical enlargement having a homogeneous texture and sharp margination.[47–49] The accuracy of the transrectal ultrasonography in detecting benign prostatic hypertrophy ranges from 91 to 97 per cent and is 89 per cent in detecting prostatitis.[50, 51] Although the value of ultrasound in differentiating among benign diseases of the prostate is still unclear, it appears that currently ultrasonography is more specific than CT in evaluating benign prostatic disease.

MALIGNANT DISEASE

Prostatic Carcinoma

The diagnosis of prostatic carcinoma usually is made by physical examination and biopsy. Depending upon the clinical and surgical findings, prostatic carcinoma is placed in one of four stages (Table 20–2):

1. Stage A carcinoma is not clinically detectable.
2. Stage B malignancy produces a palpable mass that is confined to the prostate and causes no symptoms or abnormal laboratory tests.
3. Stage C tumor extends beyond the prostatic capsule or, if confined to the prostate, is associated with symptoms of prostatism and/or elevation of serum acid phosphatase.
4. Patients with Stage D prostatic cancer have distant metastatic disease. Elevated serum acid phosphatase levels are present in two thirds of patients with Stage D disease, and when elevated, lymph node metastases are present in 35 to 85 per cent of patients.[52, 53]

The major role of CT in prostatic carcinoma is not diagnosis but staging and evaluation of therapy. CT can neither diagnose Stage A disease nor detect Stage B carcinoma unless the tumor mass

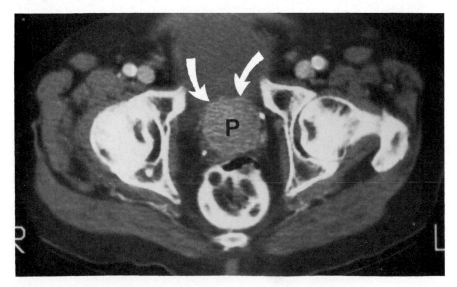

Figure 20–20. Stage B prostatic carcinoma producing symmetric enlargement of the prostate (P). The margins (arrows) are smooth, and there is no evidence of extension of tumor beyond the prostate. Distinction between benign prostatic hypertrophy and carcinoma is not possible.

Table 20–2. STAGING OF PROSTATE CARCINOMA

Stage	Extent of Carcinoma
A	Occult cancer, focus or foci of carcinoma
B	Cancer nodule confined within prostatic capsule
C	Cancer with extracapsular extension into surrounding structures or confined within capsule with elevation of serum acid phosphatase; pelvic nodes may be involved
D	Demonstrated bone or extrapelvic involvement

alters the contour of the prostate gland (Fig. 20–20). Based on the attenuation coefficient, a carcinoma confined within the capsule cannot be distinguished from a normal prostate gland.[22] A nodular contour or focally altered margin sug-

gests the presence of a carcinoma and a smooth contour in an enlarged gland benign prostatic hypertrophy, but the separation is imprecise. A smooth outer prostatic margin does not exclude a small, confined carcinoma, nor is an irregular margin pathognomonic of prostatic malignancy.

Extraprostatic extension of prostatic carcinoma (Stage C or D) is accurately diagnosed by computed tomography. Extension of prostatic carcinoma most frequently involves the seminal vesicles, producing loss of tissue fat planes and enlargement of the seminal vesicles (Fig. 20–21). Invasion of the seminal vesicles is found in 17 per cent of patients with newly diagnosed prostatic carcinoma,[54] while bladder and rectal invasion occurs less frequently (Fig. 20–21).

Stage D prostatic carcinoma is diagnosed when CT demonstrates metastatic lesions in the pelvis,

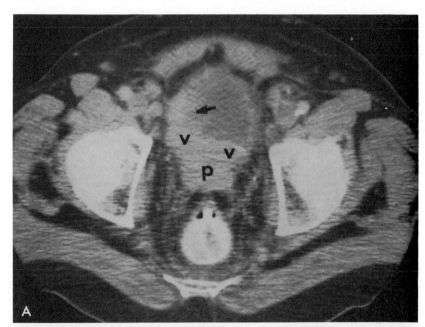

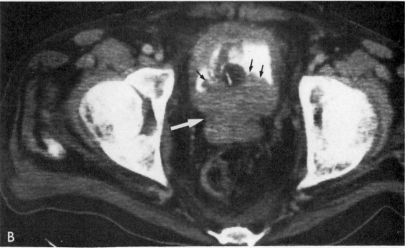

Figure 20–21. Prostatic carcinoma: **A** Stage C prostatic carcinoma (p) invading the wall of the bladder (arrow) and seminal vesicles (v). **B** Stage D prostatic carcinoma invading the bladder (black arrows) and seminal vesicles. The sharp angle between seminal vesicles and prostate is lost (white arrow).

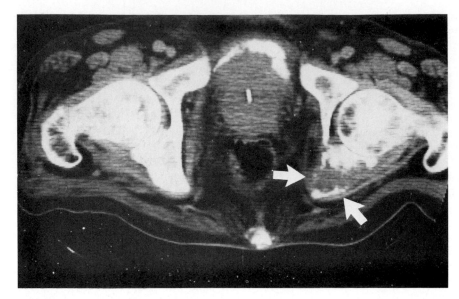

Figure 20–22. Stage D prostatic carcinoma. There is an irregular tumor mass invading the bladder and an expansile lytic lesion of the posterior portion of acetabulum (arrows).

spine, long bones, liver, lung, or retroperitoneal lymph nodes (Figs. 20–22 through 20–24). Bone metastases occur most frequently in the bony pelvis, lumbar vertebrae, and proximal femur,[55] appearing as osteoblastic (80 per cent), mixed osteolytic-osteoblastic (10 to 15 per cent), or osteolytic (5 per cent) lesions[22] (Figs. 20–22 and 20–23). Although CT can detect bone metastasis from prostatic carcinoma, CT is not used to screen for bone metastasis because radionuclide bone scintigraphy examines the entire skeleton and is a cheaper and more accurate method of detecting bone metastasis.

Evaluation of pelvic and retroperitoneal lymph nodes for metastatic prostatic carcinoma can be done by lymphangiographic or CT methods. Lymphangiographic accurancy ranges from 48 to 80 per cent[22, 56–58] with false-negative lymphangiograms usually due to nonfilling of internal iliac, obturator, or sacral lymph nodes that contain metastatic foci of prostatic carcinoma. Improvement in lymphangiographic accuracy is unlikely because the earliest lymphatic spread of prostatic carcinoma occurs by way of the obturator and internal iliac nodes,[56, 59, 60] and in 30 per cent of patients with lymphatic metastasis, these are the only lymph nodes involved with metastatic disease.

The reported accuracy of CT in detecting pelvic and retroperitoneal nodal metastasis from

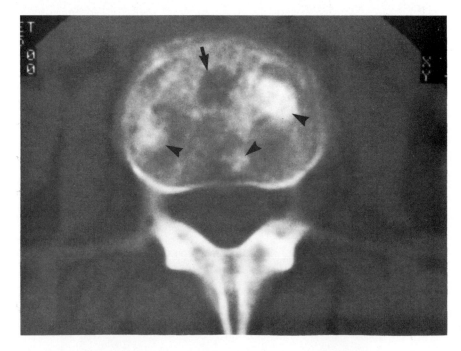

Figure 20–23. Stage D prostatic carcinoma producing lytic (arrow) and blastic (arrowheads) metastases in the vertebral body of the lumbar spine.

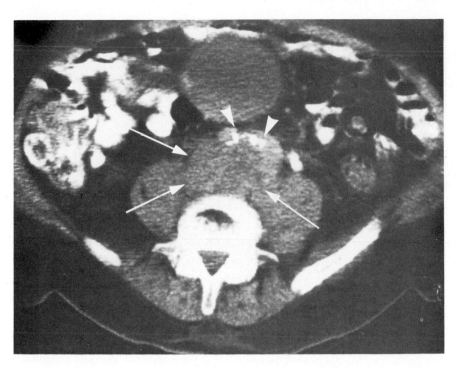

Figure 20–24. Stage D prostatic carcinoma with massive adenopathy (arrows) anteriorly displacing the calcified common iliac arteries (arrowheads).

prostatic carcinoma ranges from 33 to 93 per cent[22, 61] (Fig. 20–25). In a recent study, Levine and colleagues found CT to be more accurate (93 per cent versus 55 per cent) than lymphangiography in detecting lymph node metastasis from prostatic carcinoma[61] and attributed the greater accuracy of CT to its ability to demonstrate metastases to internal iliac and obturator nodes. However, despite high accuracy rates, CT detects nodal metastases solely on the basis of nodal enlargement and thus metastatic deposits that

do not produce lymphadenopathy go undetected. Therefore, a negative CT examination does not exclude lymph node metastasis, and pelvic lymphadenectomy must be performed if optimal staging of prostatic carcinoma is required.[61–63]

Percutaneous needle biopsy is recommended for documenting metastasis in patients with abnormal or suspicious lymph nodes seen on lymphangiography or CT.[62, 63] Preoperative staging by CT, coupled with percutaneous fine-needle biopsy, permits separation of patients with localized

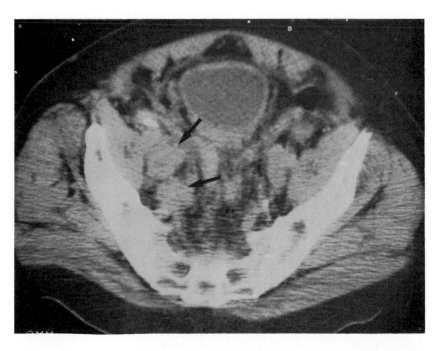

Figure 20–25. Metastatic prostatic carcinoma. CT scan demonstrates adenopathy in the external iliac lymph nodes (arrows) of the same patient with prostatic carcinoma, Stage C, as seen in Figure 20–21A.

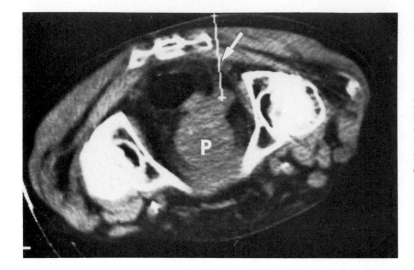

Figure 20–26. Prone CT scan demonstrating a Stage C prostatic carcinoma (P) extending beyond the capsule into surrounding tissue. A cursor line (arrow) indicates the proposed path for placement of a biopsy needle.

cancer (Stages A, B, and C) having relatively good prognosis from those with distant metastases and poor prognosis[64] (Fig. 20–26).

The overall accuracy of CT for staging prostatic carcinoma is approximately 75 per cent.[22] Most errors are due to the inability of CT to recognize depth of tumor within the gland and to detect microscopic invasion of surrounding fatty tissues or metastatic foci in normal-sized lymph nodes.

POSTOPERATIVE COMPLICATIONS. Following prostatic surgery, CT is useful for evaluating the pelvis for postoperative changes (Fig. 20–27) and for a variety of complications such as pelvic lymphoceles, hematomas, and/or abscesses that may follow pelvic lymphadenectomy.[65] Lymphoceles occur in the early postoperative period, usually within the first 10 postoperative days. They are usually located anterolaterally to the bladder and within 3 cm of the anterior abdominal wall.

Spring and colleagues[65] found lymphoceles in 27 per cent of 22 prospectively studied patients undergoing surgical staging of prostatic carcinoma and noted that lymphoceles appeared as sharply delineated cystic mass having an attenuation value close to water. Internal septations may or may not be present. Small lymphoceles without septations tend to resolve spontaneously, whereas large (greater than 30 cm³) nonseptated lymphoceles and lymphoceles with septations often require surgical intervention.

EVALUATION OF THERAPY. CT has proven to be a useful method for assessing the adequacy of portals for external beam radiation and for calculating the volume and average dimensions of the prostate for correct dosimetry of ^{125}I seeds (Figs. 20–18B, and 20–28).[22, 25, 54, 66, 67] Based upon CT results, error rates of 18 to 25 per cent were found in clinical estimation of treatment volume, thus requiring an adjustment in field size to

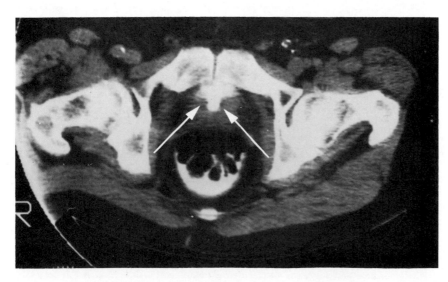

Figure 20–27. CT scan demonstrates the typical appearance of a widened bladder neck (arrows) following a transurethral resection of the prostate.

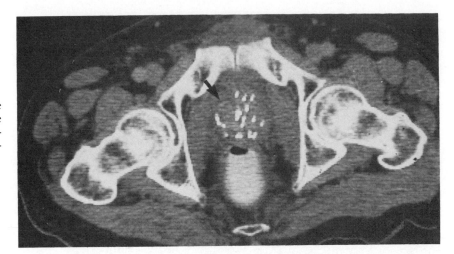

Figure 20–28. CT scan shows the distribution of ^{125}I seeds within the prostate. The right anterior portion of the prostate (arrow) demonstrates a lack of ^{125}I seeds.

ensure optimum external beam radiation therapy.[22, 25, 44, 67] Pilepich and others[54] found that in 23 per cent of patients the radiation portal was changed and in 11 per cent the field size had to be increased when compared with clinical findings. Our current approach to external radiation therapy is first to establish the isocenter and treatment volume using conventional simulation and then to adjust treatment portals based on information obtained by CT.

Recently localized carcinoma of the prostate (Stages A and B) has been shown to be effectively treated by prostatic implantation of ^{125}I seeds.[68–70] A significant advantage of this procedure is the reduced incidence of impotence or incontinence, complications that frequently occur following radical prostatectomy or external beam radiation. Because of the limited depth of irradiation capable using radioactive seeds, any extension of disease beyond the prostatic capsule precludes its use. In general, depending on tumor volume, 30 to 80 seeds containing 0.5 to 0.6 mCi of ^{125}I are surgically implanted by means of a suprapubic extraperitoneal approach. The seeds are placed at 5-mm intervals within and immediately around any palpable tumor nodules and at 10-mm intervals in the remaining prostatic tissue. The low-energy (27keV) emission and the short half-value layer (2 cm) of the ^{125}I radiation permits a dose of between 18,000 and 28,000 rads to be delivered to the tumor without causing cystitis or proctitis. Optimal therapy is given when there is even distribution of the seeds, but it is difficult to determine seed position accurately by conventional radiographic methods.

CT has proven capable of precisely assessing the distribution of seeds within the prostate and of determining whether extraprostatic radioactive

seeds have been placed (Fig. 20–28). In one study, CT detected inhomogeneous seed distribution (usually involving the cephalic portion of the prostate and/or extraprostatic seeds in 85 per cent of the patients examined.[66] Depending on clinical and CT findings, external radiation may be directed to areas that are not adequately treated by the ^{125}I seeds.[69, 71]

Testes

PATHOLOGY

UNDESCENDED TESTES

The absence of a palpable testis may be related to agenesis, dysgenesis, acquired atrophy, or incomplete descent. It is important to identify an undescended testis, or cryptorchidism, because there is a loss of fertility if the testis remains undescended and there is a 12 to 40-fold increased incidence of neoplasm, particularly in those testes located in the abdominal cavity.[72] In the prepubertal patient, generally an undescended testis is brought into the scrotum to assure fertility, to avoid repeated injury to the inguinal testis, and to preserve the patient's self-image. In the postpubertal patient, orchidectomy is usually performed because of the high incidence of malignancy in cryptic testes in older males.

Bilateral anorchidism is diagnosed readily by endocrinologic tests in patients under the age of 35 years, and no exploratory surgery or radiologic examination is needed. In patients over the age of 35 years, endocrinologic tests are unreliable because even if testes are present, their prolonged intra-abdominal position results in severe atrophy, which prevents a response to hormonal

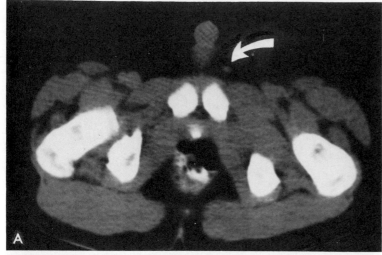

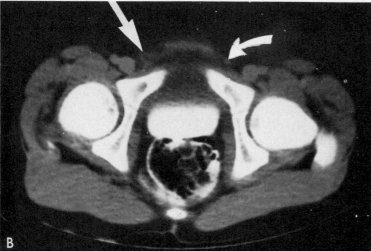

Figure 20–29. Undescended right testis in a 10-year-old boy. **A** CT scan at base of scrotum demonstrates a spermatic cord on the left side (curved arrow) but no spermatic cord on the right. A palpable testis was present on the left side but not on the right. **B** At a higher level, CT scan reveals an oval area of soft-tissue density in the right inguinal canal (straight arrow) that is larger than the normal spermatic cord (curved arrow) identified in the left inguinal canal. Right inguinal testis found at surgery.

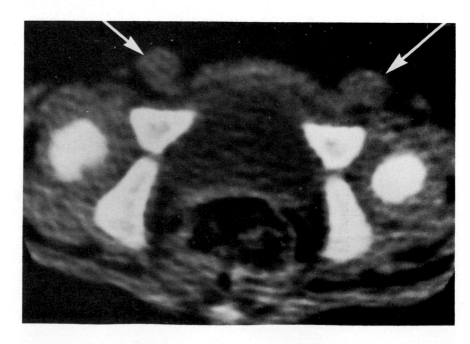

Figure 20–30. Bilateral oval soft-tissue masses (arrows) representing undescended testes are demonstrated in the inguinal canals.

stimulation. If only one testis is absent, endocrinologic tests are normal and the distinction between unilateral agenesis of the testis and a cryptorchidism must be made by other means.

The testis develops from an elongated embryonic gonad located ventral to the mesonephric ridge. During the descent of the gonad from its abdominal position, the vascular structures, nerve supply, and ductal connections are brought down into the inguinal canal and scrotum. The external descent, with migration of the testes through the inguinal canal into the scrotum, begins at about the 36th week of gestation.[73] This process, although usually completed at birth, may continue for approximately 4 to 6 weeks after birth in a full-term infant and for up to 12 weeks in a premature infant. The incidence of undescended testes is less than 1 per cent at 1 year of age.

Arrest of the migration of the testis may occur anywhere along the developmental pathway from the lower pole of the kidney to the external inguinal ring. In 80 per cent of the cases with undescended testes, the testis is palpable in the superficial inguinal region.[74–76] In approximately 20 per cent of cases, the testis is impalpable; this may be related to an absent testis or to a very small atrophic or dysplastic gland. Most impalpable undescended testes lie near the external ring located in the superficial inguinal pouch or at the neck of the scrotum. In some cases, the testis lies just above the internal inguinal ring, deep below the muscle layer of the anterior abdominal wall and close to the iliac vessels. In rare instances, a cryptic testis is located higher on the posterior abdominal wall.[77]

The standard approach to nonpalpable testes is complete surgical exploration of the inguinal canal followed by further exploration along the course of the gonadal veins if the initial search is negative. Because of the length of time involved in such a surgical procedure and because surgery may miss a small undescended testis, preoperative localization by other methods must be attempted. For this purpose, testicular venography, spermatic arteriography, ultrasonography and, more recently, CT have been used.[74–80]

Detection of undescended testes by CT is based upon recognition of an oval-shaped, soft-tissue mass along the course of the testicular descent (Figs. 20–29 and 20–30). CT scan sections must be carefully examined for the presence or absence of a cryptic testis between the internal inguinal ring, which lies approximately 5 to 6 cm caudad to the anterior superior iliac spine, and the external ring, which is located just cephalad to

the pubic ramus. The maldescended testis may be located in the lower abdomen, superficial inguinal pouch, inguinal canal, or scrotal neck. Because the normal structures in the inguinal area and lower pelvis are symmetrical, even a small, extra soft-tissue mass can be detected easily by CT. Detection of testes located higher in the pelvis or in the abdomen by CT is more difficult because the testis may be confused with bowel loops, vascular structures, or lymph nodes.[79]

Lymph nodes in the inguinal region can be distinguished from testicular tissue by their location; inferior to the inguinal ligament; or adjacent to femoral and iliac vessels, deep and lateral to the inguinal canal. In equivocal cases, a bolus injection of contrast material will permit separation of vascular structures from nonvascular soft-tissue masses.

Initial experience using CT to detect undescended testes has demonstrated the method to be highly accurate.[78, 80] In 20 patients with cryptorchidism, 22 undescended and one absent testes were identified. In only one patient with a small presacral testis was an erroneous diagnosis of an inguinal canal testis made.

Compared with other methods of localizing the undescended testis, CT has both advantages and disadvantages. The advantages are the excellent anatomic detail, ability to employ intravenous and gastrointestinal contrast, and ease of performance. The major disadvantages are a small irradiation risk (0.65 to 0.83 rad) and the need for sedation in young children.

Localization of undescended testes is also possible by testicular arteriography, venography, and ultrasonography. Both testicular arteriography and venography are accurate if they are technically successful,[74–78] but testicular angiography is invasive, and selective catheterization and injection into the spermatic artery is painful and technically difficult. Testicular venography is less traumatic and slightly less difficult to perform, but it is associated with a high radiation dose and some morbidity.

Ultrasonography can easily detect an undescended testis that is located in the inguinal canal.[77, 81] The sonographic diagnosis of an undescended testis is based upon recognition of an oval mass with medium-level echoes along the course of the testicular descent (Fig. 20–31). However, ultrasound is less useful in detecting undescended testes located in the lower abdomen and presents difficulty when there is an inguinal hernia present.

Our approach to examining patients with an

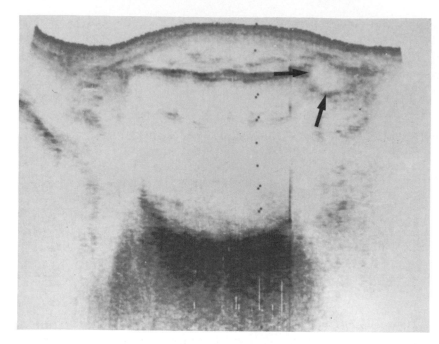

Figure 20–31. Ultrasonography of the inguinal canal shows an oval mass with medium-level echoes representing an impalpable testis (arrows). (Courtesy Dr. H. Hricak, University of California, San Francisco.)

impalpable testis is to initially perform an ultrasonographic study. Because over 70 per cent of undescended testes are located in the inguinal canal, ultrasonography will detect the vast majority of ectopic testes. If the ultrasound examination is equivocal or negative, CT is performed. When spermatic cord structures but no testes are identified or when the testes cannot be localized unequivocally by CT, testicular venography or arteriography is used for further evaluation.

BENIGN TESTICULAR DISEASE

There has been only limited experience using CT to examine the scrotum and testes because CT carries some radiation risk, whereas ultrasound is highly accurate and completely risk-free.[81–89] In addition, testicular lesions that do not cause testicular enlargement are not detected by

CT unless the testicular margin has become irregular. Extratesticular lesions such as hernias, hydroceles, varicoceles, or spermatoceles are readily demonstrated by CT (Figs. 20–32 and 20–33), but it may be difficult to distinguish between testicular and extratesticular masses with CT if there is insufficient peritesticular fat.

MALIGNANT TESTICULAR NEOPLASMS

The yearly incidence of testicular carcinoma in the United States for Caucasian males is 2.5 to 3.7 per 100,000 men.[90] Although testicular tumors account for only 2 per cent of all malignancies in men, they are the most common cause of death in men between the ages of 24 and 35 years. The most common malignant testicular tumor is seminoma, closely followed by embryonal carcinoma

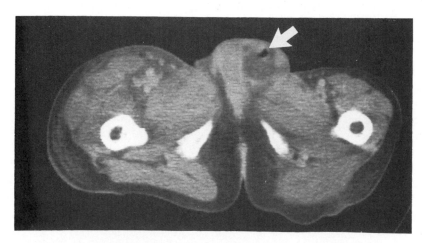

Figure 20–32. A left inguinal hernia descending into the scrotum is seen in a low-density area containing air (arrow).

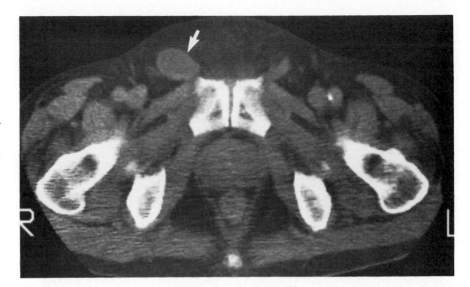

Figure 20–33. An oval mass of water density in the right inguinal canal (arrow) proved to be a hydrocele.

and teratoma.[91] The rarest primary tumor of the testes is choriocarcinoma.

Localized pain in the testes is the most common presenting symptom, but many patients present with symptoms related to tumor spread at the time of diagnosis. Testicular tumors commonly metastasize by way of the lymphangitic route to the iliac, para-aortic, mediastinal, and supraclavicular lymph nodes. If hematogenous spread occurs and if it is the predominant early route in choriocarcinoma of the testes, metastases can involve any organ, but the lungs, liver, and kidney are the most frequent sites.

Prognosis and treatment of testicular malignancy depend on the stage of the disease when it is first diagnosed (Table 20–3).[92] Because testicular tumors commonly metastasize by way of the lymphatic system, clinical staging has been heavily dependent upon lymphangiographic findings. Lymphangiography is 62 to 89 per cent accurate, 50 to 90 per cent sensitive, and 67 to 100 per cent specific in demonstrating lymphatic spread of testicular neoplasms.[93–99] Metastases may be missed because of the microscopic size of the metastatic focus or because involved nodes are not visualized on bipedal lymphangiography. Lymph nodes in or near the renal hilum, which receive lymphatic drainage directly from the testes, are often insufficiently opacified.[100, 101] False-positive lymphangiographic interpretations are due to fibrosis, fatty replacement, or inflammatory disease,[99] which produce areas of incomplete lymph node filling.

Both CT and ultrasound can be used to stage testicular tumors.[102–104] Reported accuracies of CT in demonstrating lymph node metastases range from 74 to 87 per cent, ultrasound accuracies from 75 to 81 per cent.[105, 106] Although the overall accuracy rates are comparable with those achieved with lymphangiography, lymphangiography is slightly more accurate as it detects metastases in nonenlarged nodes.[93] However, CT is superior for detecting abnormal nodes in the upper retroperitoneum and inferior mediastinum and provides visualization of enlarged nodes in the mesentery and renal hilar areas[94, 107, 108] (Fig. 20–34). In addition, CT can evaluate extranodal tissue and demonstrate lesions in the liver, kidney, bone, and lungs during a single examination (Fig. 20–35). CT is also the most accurate of all methods for demonstrating the actual volume of the metastatic disease, which is important for planning surgical resection or for predicting the outcome of radiation treatment.

Table 20–3.   STAGING OF TESTICULAR TUMORS

Stage	Extent of Carcinoma
I	Tumor clinically limited to the testis and spermatic cord
II	Clinical or radiographic evidence of tumor spread beyond the testis and spermatic cord, but limited to the regional lymphatics below the diaphragm
II$_A$	Moderate-sized retroperitoneal metastasis
II$_B$	Massive retroperitoneal metastasis
III	Metastasis beyond the diaphragm
III$_A$	Extension beyond the diaphragm, but still confined to the mediastinum or supraclavicular lymphatics
III$_B$	Extranodal metastasis

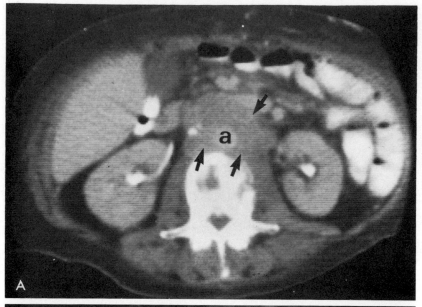

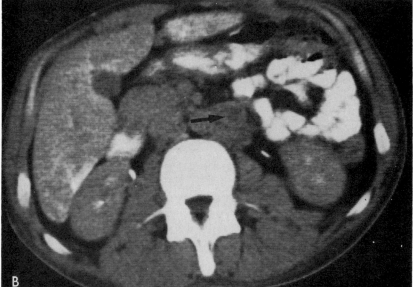

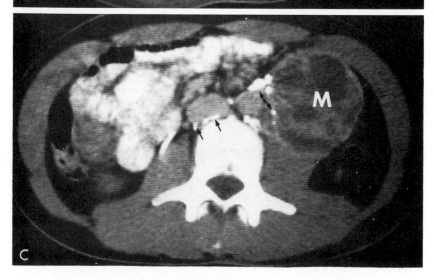

Figure 20–34. A Periaortic and pericaval adenopathy (arrows) is present in the retroperitoneum of a patient with metastatic seminoma. a = Aorta. **B** Para-aortic adenopathy of low density (arrow) in patient with Stage D testicular malignancy. **C** Massive lymph node metastases (M) from seminoma of the left testis. Normal-sized lymph nodes filled with lymphangiographic contrast material (arrows) are displaced by the nonopacified low-density, septated tumor mass.

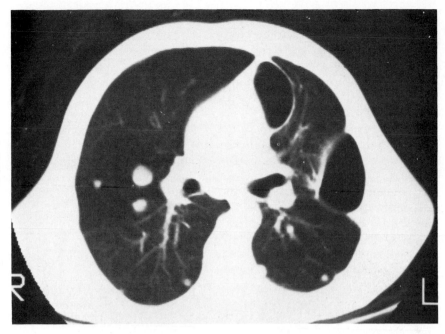

Figure 20–35. Multiple lung nodules and a localized pneumothorax with pleural thickening in a patient with testicular carcinoma treated with bleomycin.

Our current approach to a newly diagnosed testicular neoplasm is to perform a CT study as the initial staging procedure. We obtain lymphangiography only in patients having a normal CT examination and agree with other investigators that neither phlebography nor excretory urography is necessary for staging testicular tumors.[93, 105, 108]

EVALUATION OF THERAPY. CT findings in patients undergoing chemotherapy and/or cytoreductive therapy have correlated closely with clinical and surgical results and the level of serum tumor markers.[109] Because CT readily demonstrates changes in the attenuation value and size of nodal metastases, (Fig. 20–36) it is routinely used to evaluate the results of therapy and to follow patients after orchidectomy and during

chemotherapy.[102, 110–113] CT is also useful in following patients for development of metastatic lung disease[110] and in differentiating Bleomycin-induced pulmonary fibrosis from recurrent metastatic disease.[114]

Following therapy, measurement of mean CT numbers may provide useful information concerning changes in tumor composition.[113] Conversion of a solid to a cystic mass during therapy is strong evidence that no viable tumor remains or that a tumor such as an embryonal cell carcinoma has matured into a cystic teratoma.[111] Although lymph nodes with persistent active malignancy have higher CT attenuation values (32.7 ± 4.8 H versus 18.7 ± 7.8 H) than lymph nodes without tumor, a decrease in CT numbers during therapy suggests that a residual mass does not

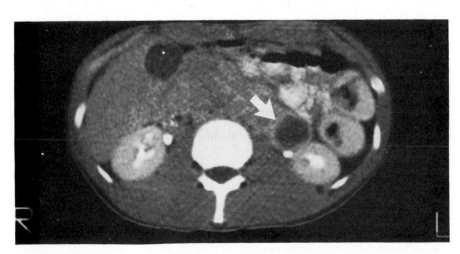

Figure 20–36. Teratocarcinoma. Marked adenopathy is present in the retroperitoneum of a patient with teratocarcinoma of the testis undergoing treatment. Most of the nodes have a soft-tissue density, but one large node on the left side shows cystic degeneration (arrow).

contain tumor irrespective of the final absolute CT number.[113] An overall increase in CT density during treatment strongly suggests viable malignant tissue. Measurement of CT numbers does not appear as useful in evaluating therapy for seminomas because they do not usually undergo cystic degeneration.[113]

Quantitative estimation of tumor volume following therapy provides additional information concerning viability of a tumor. In one study, residual masses less than 20 cm³ contained no active malignancy, whereas masses greater than 20 cm³ were either benign or malignant.[113] Currently a fine-needle biopsy is obtained to exclude viable tumor in lymph node masses that do not return to normal size or that decrease in attenuation value.

Pelvis

PATHOLOGY

PELVIC INADEQUACY

In many institutions, CT pelvimetry is employed whenever a vaginal delivery is being considered for a patient with breech presentation in order to avoid the high fetal morbidity that results from delivery of an after-coming unmolded head through an inadequate maternal pelvis. In addition, predelivery identification of a hyperextended fetal head permits avoidance of damage to the umbilical cord. Although both the inadequate pelvis and malpositioned fetal head can be detected with conventional pelvimetry, the radiographs are often underexposed, the lateral films are often not truly lateral, and portions of the pelvis can be cut off the films. Gonadal radiation dose to the fetus using conventional pelvimentry is estimated to be 885 mrad.[115] and technical failures necessitating additional radiographs often further increase the radiation dose to the mother and fetus.

Pelvimetry using digital radiography and a single CT scan at the level of the fovae of the femoral heads has replaced conventional pelvimetry at the University of California at San Francisco.[116] An anteroposterior digital radiograph of the abdomen and pelvis and a lateral digital radiograph of the pelvis are taken and pelvic measurements are made using the CT console (Fig. 20–37). The technique is rapid, positioning problems are avoided and radiation exposure is markedly reduced. The abdominal pelvic digital radiograph gives a maximum entrance skin dose of less than 10 mrad and an exit skin dose of approximately

22 mrads.[116] The CT scan (Fig. 20–38) taken at the level of the ischial spines, exposed with reduced factors of 80mA, 2.2 msec pulse width, and a 5.7-sec scan time, results in an average absorbed dose of 380 mrads.[116] In many instances, even lower radiation factors may be employed. Radiation exposure is further reduced by CT because the gonads of the fetus and mother are effectively shielded from scattered radiation as a result of the tight collimation of the CT scanner and the fact that the CT scan level is inferior to the fetus and level of the ovaries.

MEASUREMENTS.   The pelvic inlet or true conjugate is measured on the lateral scout view from the sacral promontory to the upper portion of the symphysis pubis (normal >11.0 cm) (Fig. 20–37A). The transverse diameter of the pelvis is measured on the anteroposterior scout view as the largest transverse diameter in the pelvis (normal >12.0 cm) (Fig. 20–37B). The interspinous distance (midpelvic diameter) is measured between two points connecting the ischial spines on a CT section obtained at the level of the fovae of the femoral heads (normal >10 cm) (Fig. 20–38). The measurements obtained with the electronic cursor do not require adjustments for magnification and are highly accurate.[116] Pelvimetry using digital radiography, therefore, offers the advantage of lower radiation exposure to fetus and mother and higher accuracy of measurements as compared with conventional pelvimetry.

Ovaries

PATHOLOGY

The ovaries generally are not identified on CT scans as separate structures unless they are enlarged as a result of ovarian cysts, benign tumors, tubo-ovarian abscesses, or malignant neoplasms. CT readily demonstrates most ovarian masses and can usually determine whether the mass is fluid-containing or hemorrhagic but often gives little information concerning the internal architecture of cystic ovarian masses. When very large ovarian masses are present, it is often difficult to identify the ovary as the origin of the mass because of the marked distortion of the relationship of the intrapelvic organs to one another produced by the mass.

BENIGN OVARIAN TUMORS

Teratomas account for approximately 10 to 15 per cent of all ovarian neoplasms and typically occur in women during their reproductive years, being rare before puberty and not developing

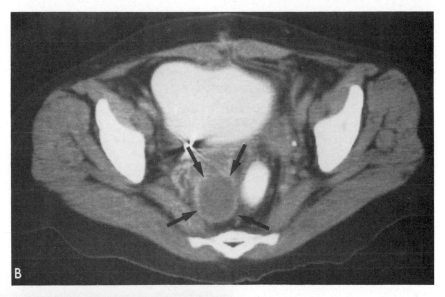

Figure 20–44. *Continued* **B** Tubo-ovarian abscess producing a well-defined oval mass having a low attenuation center surrounded by a thin rim (arrows). On CT scanning, differentiation of a tubo-ovarian abscess from a simple ovarian cyst or cystadenoma cannot be made unless septations or gas is present.

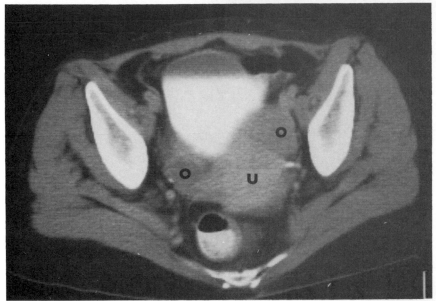

Figure 20–45. Bilateral tubo-ovarian abscesses (o) are identified as ill-defined areas of low density on each side of the uterus (u).

Figure 20–46. Pelvic inflammatory disease. An irregular mass with areas of low attenuation (arrowheads) is seen in the pelvis slightly to the right of the midline. Surgery revealed pelvic inflammatory disease, but a malignant tumor of the ovary or uterus cannot be excluded based on the CT images alone.

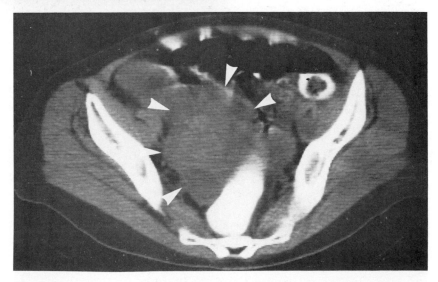

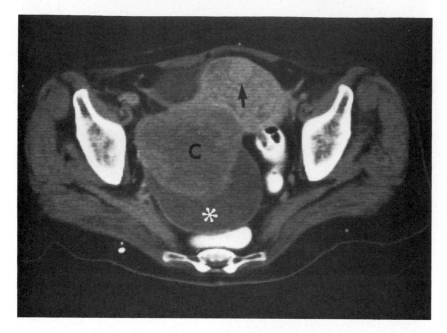

Figure 20–47. Adenocarcinoma of the ovary. CT scan demonstrates a poorly differentiated adenocarcinoma of the ovary (C) producing an inhomogeneous pelvic mass containing cystic (asterisk), solid (arrow), and mixed solid cystic components.

MALIGNANT OVARIAN TUMORS

Ovarian cancer ranks sixth among all cancers in women. Approximately one of every seven newborn females is expected to develop cancer of the ovary at some time in her life.[124, 125] The prognosis is poor, the overall 5 year survival rate for all stages and grades of ovarian cancer being only 20 to 25 per cent. The poor prognosis is related to the fact that 60 to 70 per cent of patients with ovarian cancer present initially with Stage III or IV disease. The delay in detection of ovarian cancer is primarily due to the absence of early symptoms and the nonspecific nature of many of the symptoms.[126]

The most common primary malignant ovarian tumors are adenocarcinoma (Fig. 20–47) (papillary or undifferentiated), serous or mucinous cystadenocarcinoma (Fig. 20–48), and endometroid carcinoma. Less frequently encountered are malignant teratoma, endodermal sinus tumor, mixed müllerian tumor (Fig. 20–49), malignant thecoma and dysgerminoma (Fig. 20–50). A frequent ovarian tumor, the so-called ovarian Krukenberg tumor (Fig. 20–51) is actually a metastatic tumor to the ovary from the gastrointestinal tract.

The most generally accepted classification of ovarian carcinoma is the one proposed by the International Federation of Gynecologists and Ob-

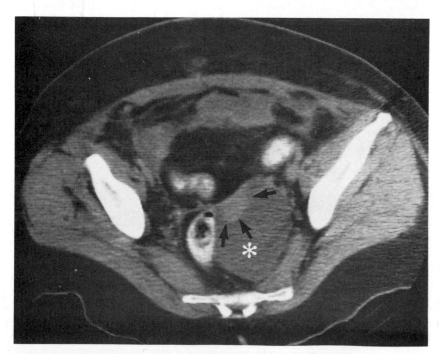

Figure 20–48. Papillary serous cystadenocarcinoma of the ovary. CT reveals the tumor as a predominantly cystic mass (asterisk) having irregular margins and a soft-tissue component (arrows) projecting into the low-density portion of the tumor.

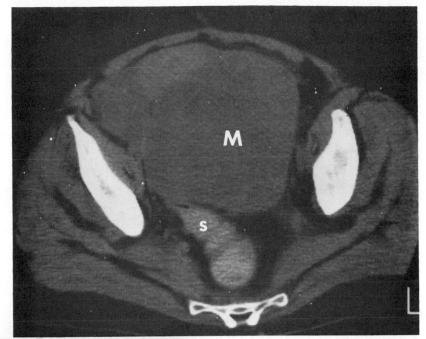

Figure 20–49. A malignant mixed-müllerian tumor of the ovary (M) producing a large, inhomogeneous pelvic mass that displaces the sigmoid colon (s) and extends to but does not invade the pelvic side walls.

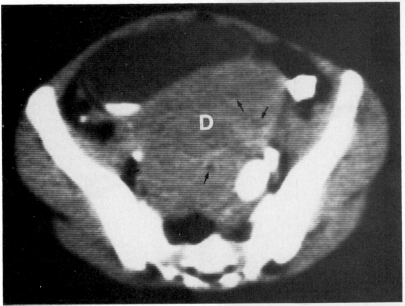

Figure 20–50. Ovarian dysgerminoma: CT scan shows an ovarian dysgerminoma (D) as a predominantly solid pelvic mass containing only a few areas of lower attenuation (arrows).

Figure 20–51. Bilateral Krukenberg tumors (K) due to metastasis from a colonic carcinoma. The ovarian metastases have a mixed cysticsolid appearance. U = Uterus.

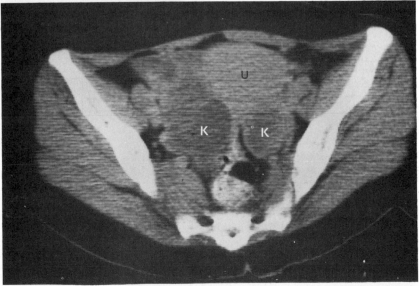

Table 20–4. STAGING OF OVARIAN CARCINOMA

Stage	Extent of Tumor
I	Tumor limited to ovary
II	Tumor with pelvic extension with or without ascites
III	Tumor with widespread intraperitoneal metastases outside pelvis with or without ascites and/or positive retroperitoneal nodes
IV	Tumor with spread to distant sites includes liver parenchyma and/or outside peritoneal cavity with or without ascites

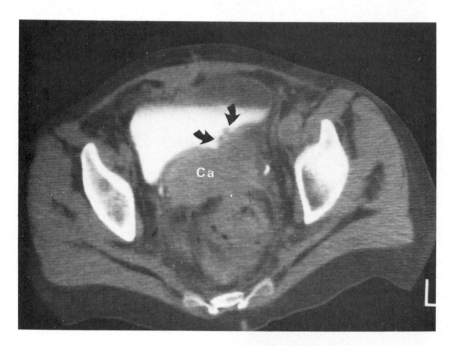

Figure 20–52. Cystadenoma of the ovary (Ca) presenting as a large solid cul-de-sac mass. Invasion of the bladder (curved arrows) is clearly demonstrated.

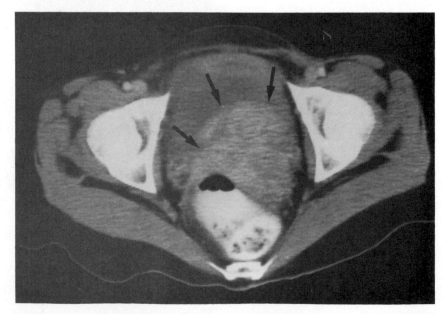

Figure 20–53. Ovarian metastases. A large inhomogeneous mass (arrows), located in the pouch of Douglas, was the result of melanoma metastasizing to both ovaries. Tissue planes are not preserved, indicating infiltration of the bladder and possibly the rectum.

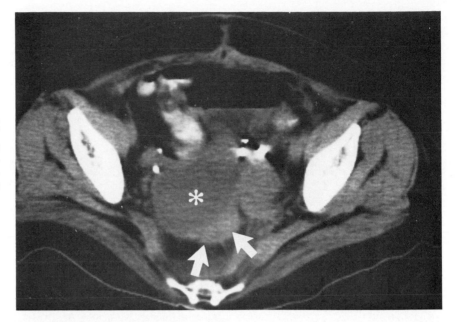

Figure 20–54. Papillary cystadenocarcinoma of the ovary. CT scan reveals a large cystic mass (asterisk) having slightly irregular margins and a solid component (arrows) projecting into the cystic portion of the tumor.

stetricians (FIGO).[127] However, recently the FIGO staging has been simplified for use in classifying ovarian tumors using CT scanning (Table 20–4). The main difference between the two classifications is the elimination of subgroups in Stage I and II disease.

On CT sections, primary and metastatic ovarian tumors can appear as abdominal or pelvic masses (Figs. 20–49 and 20–50), as cul-de-sac lesions (Figs. 20–52 and 20–53), or as uni- or bilateral adnexal masses (Figs. 20–48 and 20–51). Cystadenocarcinomas usually appear on CT as large predominantly cystic tumors having CT attenuation values ranging from 10 to 20 H. The margins of

the tumor are irregular, and often there are soft-tissue components within the cystic central portion of the tumor (Figs. 20–48, 20–54, and 20–55). These features usually permit differentiation between simple cysts and cystadenocarcinomas. Amorphous calcifications and internal septations commonly found in benign cystadenomas are less frequently present in cystadenocarcinomas.

Other ovarian tumors present as mixed solid-cystic (Figs. 20–47, 20–49, 20–51) or predominantly solid masses (Figs. 20–50 and 20–56) with density readings of 40 to 50 H.[128] CT distinction between histologic types of solid or mixed cystic-solid ovarian tumors is usually not possible, and

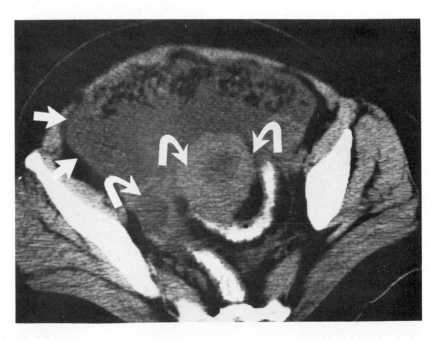

Figure 20–55. Bilateral papillary serous cystadenocarcinomas of the ovary. CT scan reveals noncalcified ovarian masses (curved arrows) with low-density centers and shaggy margins. A large amount of ascites (straight arrows) is present in the pelvis.

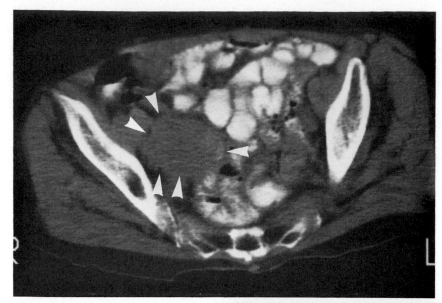

Figure 20–56. Leiomyosarcoma of the ovary (arrowheads), producing a homogeneous soft-tissue mass in the right pelvis.

Figure 20–57. A cystadenocarcinoma (C) of the ovary, producing a large pelvic mass of mixed density. The origin of the mass cannot be determined by axial CT scans.

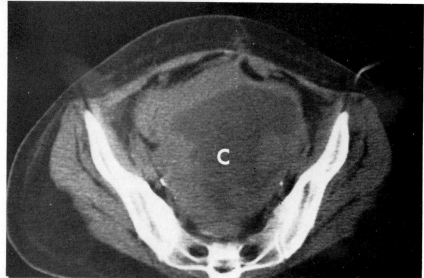

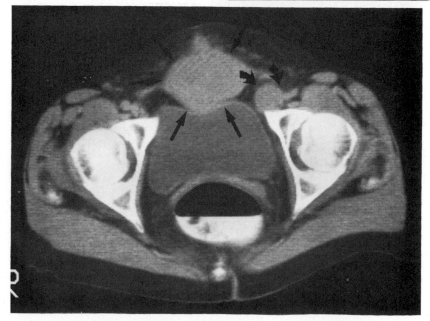

Figure 20–58. A large abdominal wall mass (straight arrows) and an enlarged superficial inguinal node (curved arrows) are produced by recurrent ovarian carcinoma.

at times even determining whether a tumor originates from the ovary is impossible (Figs. 20–49, 20–50, 20–52, and 20–57). Invasion of the bladder (Figs. 20–52 and 20–53), small bowel, or colon (Fig. 20–53) can be suggested when there is a loss of adjacent soft-tissue planes, but caution must be taken in order to avoid false-positive diagnoses in thin patients and in situations when a tumor is touching but not invading an adjacent organ. The presence of even small amounts of ascites can be diagnosed accurately by CT[129] (Fig. 20–55) and indicates at least Stage II disease. Peritoneal implants and retroperitoneal adenopathy can frequently be detected by CT,[128] and tumor invasion of the pelvic side walls produces asymmetry of the pelvic musculature.[130] When recurrent ovarian tumor is present, CT identifies abdominal masses, retroperitoneal or inguinal adenopathy (Fig. 20–58), ascites and/or soft tissue masses in the pelvis or cul-de-sac.

Staging

Ultrasonography has been found to be highly accurate (97 per cent) in detecting both solid and cystic ovarian tumors.[134] Because it is safe and inexpensive, ultrasonography is widely employed as the initial study in evaluating suspected ovarian tumors.[128, 132, 133] However, despite high detection rates, in one report, accurate sonographic staging was achieved in only 48 per cent of patients with malignant ovarian tumors.[131] Small amounts of ascites may be missed; bladder and bowel involvement are not easily demonstrated; lymph node metastases are often missed; and small omental and peritoneal implants are not detectable in up to 55 per cent of patients with ovarian tumors.[131]

Lymphangiography is helpful in staging ovarian tumors, but contrary to the situation found with other pelvic tumors, a preferential site of nodal involvement cannot be predicted, as lymphatic spread of ovarian tumors has an unpredictable distribution.[134] False-negative results are often related to microscopic metastasis, but when lymphangiography is compared with results from needle biopsy or surgical resection, it is evident that in every stage of ovarian cancer, lymphatic spread is more extensive than demonstrated on the bipedal lymphangiogram.[135]

CT appears superior in staging, following the effects of therapy and as an aid to radiation therapy. CT better defines the extent of tumor invasion into bone, muscle, mesentery, lymph nodes, bowel, and bladder and has been shown to give accurate assessment of the response to cytotoxic therapy.[136] CT is not limited by bowel adhering in the pelvis following surgery or radiation therapy. For these reasons, CT is assuming a dominant role in staging and in the post-therapy follow-up of patients with ovarian carcinoma.

Uterus
PATHOLOGY

BENIGN ABNORMALITIES

A variety of benign conditions affecting the uterus are best evaluated by a combination of bimanual pelvic examination and ultrasonography. Ultrasound has become the primary method of locating intrauterine contraceptive devices (IUDs)[137–139], examining suspected molar pregnancy[140, 141] endometrial fluid collections unassociated with pregnancy,[142] hydrocolpos and hydrometrocolpos,[143] the persistently retroverted gravid uterus,[144] the gravid uterus for gestational age or suspected abnormal pregnancy,[145–148] ectopic pregnancy,[149–150] endouterine abnormalities,[151, 152] endometriosis, myomas, and fetal anomalies. In many of these abnormalities CT has proven a valuable secondary method for studying the uterus when ultrasound results are equivocal.

Dislocation of Intrauterine Devices

Ultrasonography has been the method of choice for locating IUDs because Lippes loop, Copper-7, Gravigards, Safety Coils, and Dalkon shields can be readily identified. However, sonographic differentiation between various types of IUDs is accurate only for the Lippes loop (78 to 94 per cent),[137, 138] and the Copper-7 device (81 per cent), and precise sonographic localization of extrauterine devices can be difficult.[137–139] Therefore, whenever the ultrasonographic findings are equivocal, when an IUD is thought to be extrauterine in position, or when the type of device must be confirmed, CT is used to determine the type of device and to identify an intra- or extrauterine location of an IUD (Figs. 20–59 and 20–60).[153] CT is fast, easy to perform, and less invasive than hysterosalpingography and achieves a high degree of accuracy.

In order to reduce radiation exposure to an absolute minimum, a preliminary digital scout radiograph is used to locate the position of the IUD within the pelvis, thus reducing the number of CT scans necessary to locate and characterize the IUD. The calculated radiation dose delivered to the patient in a single CT section is less than 2

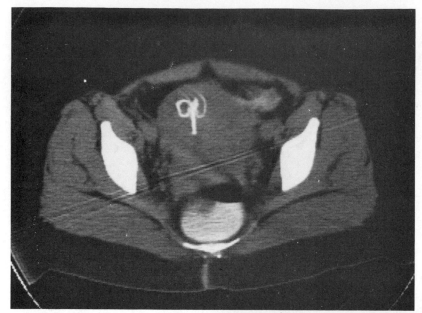

Figure 20–59. CT scan demonstrates a double-coil IUD in an anteverted uterus.

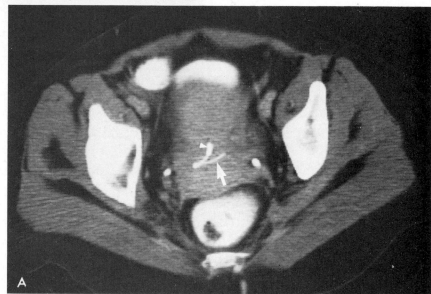

Figure 20–60. CT documentation of intrauterine position of two intrauterine devices (IUDs). **A** CT cross-section reveals a Copper-7 (arrow) and Lippes loop (arrowhead) IUD within the intrauterine lumen. The uterus contains multiple leiomyomas. **B** The Lippes loop is better demonstrated on a CT scan obtained at a higher level.

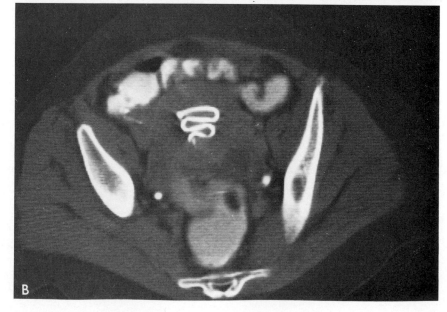

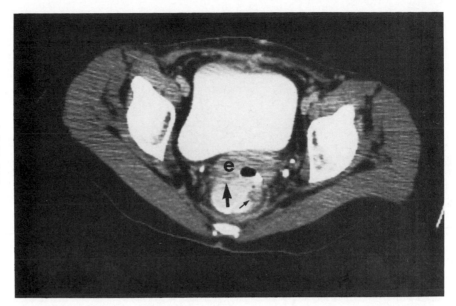

Figure 20–61. Endometriosis (e) located in the cul-de-sac, producing irregularities in the anterior rectal wall (large arrow). A small focus of endometriosis (small arrow) involves the left lateral wall of the rectum.

rads skin dose and about a 0.2 rad gonadal dose.[153] Further reduction is achieved by performing CT scans for IUD localization at the lowest possible exposure factors.

Endometriosis

Endometriosis is a common disease among women, having an incidence ranging from 8 to 30 per cent in women undergoing gynecologic surgery.[154, 155] Endometriosis usually produces sharply delineated spherical lesions, most frequently located in the cul-de-sac, which sonographically appear as cystic or predominantly cystic adnexal masses. Scattered echoes are confined to the pe-

riphery or dependent portion of the mass.[156] Even when typical sonographic findings are present, a specific diagnosis of endometriosis can be suggested by ultrasound only if strongly supported by clinical history because similar sonographic features are seen in a variety of gynecologic abnormalities.

The CT findings in endometriosis are varied. There may be a thickening of the tissues adjacent to the ovaries or uterus, involvement of the bladder, rectum (Fig. 20–61), or small bowel by single or multiple solid masses or fluid-filled cysts (Fig. 20–62). The cul-de-sac of the pelvis is the most common site for endometriosis (Fig. 20–61); how-

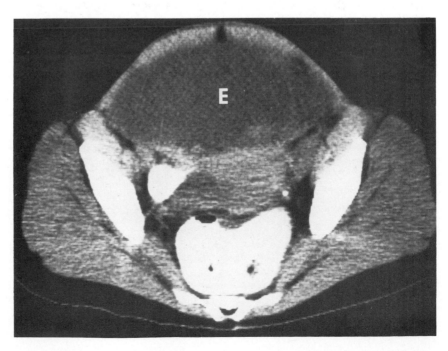

Figure 20–62. A large fluid-filled structure proved to be cystic endometriosis (E). A typical clinical history was available, permitting a specific diagnosis to be made.

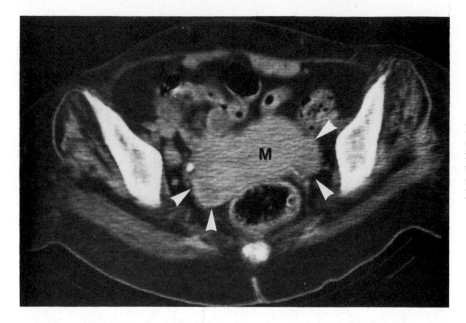

Figure 20–63. Uterine myoma (M), producing a lobulated uterine mass. The mass obliterates the uterine cavity, and has two rounded protrusions (arrowheads) with low-density centers.

ever, even when endometriosis is present, a definitive CT diagnosis cannot be made without a typical clinical history (Fig. 20–62). If extensive or chronic disease is present, a correct CT diagnosis is very difficult to make because the loss of tissue planes mimics a primary or metastatic pelvic malignancy. If the ovaries, fallopian tubes, uterus, rectosigmoid colon, or bladder is the primary site, a specific diagnosis is impossible without the characteristic clinical setting.

Uterine Myoma

The uterine myoma or fibroid is a common benign tumor in adult women, affecting approximately 20 per cent of women over 30 years of age. In general, the lobulated masses projecting from the outer surfaces of the uterus are subserous, the intracavitary masses are submucous, and the masses obliterating the uterine cavity are interstitial in location.[157]

Four major CT features suggest the diagnosis of a uterine myoma:

1. A focal solid mass causing a lobulation and/or protrusion from the outer margin of the uterus (Fig. 20–63).

2. Soft-tissue masses that distort or obliterate the uterine cavity (Fig. 20–63).

3. Areas of calcification within uterine masses (Figs. 20–64 and 20–65).

4. Irregular, low-density areas within the uter-

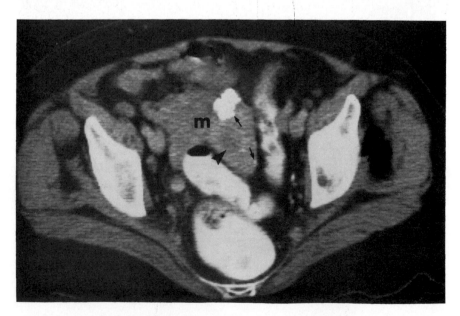

Figure 20–64. A uterine myoma (m) contains calcifications (arrows) and an area of low attenuation (arrowhead). The outer margins of the myoma are smooth, and the periuterine fat planes are preserved.

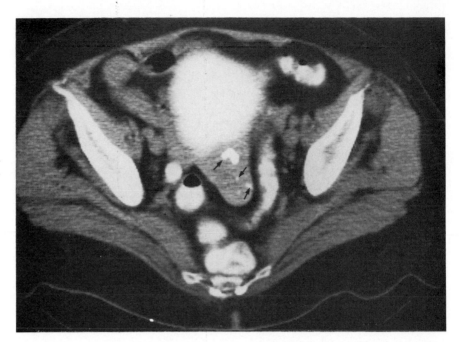

Figure 20–65. Typical calcifications (arrows) in a smoothly lobulated myoma of the uterus.

ine masses representing degeneration of the myoma (Figs. 20–63 through 20–66).[157]

Occasionally, myomas produce diffuse enlargement of the uterus. Solid noncalcified uterine myomas usually cannot be distinguished from other solid uterine masses, but occasionally a diagnosis of a uterine lipoleiomyoma can be made when CT demonstrates a well-encapsulated uterine mass that is predominantly the density of fat (-70 to -100 H).[158]

A bolus injection of contrast material enhances the attenuation value of the uterus, helping to outline the margins of the uterus and identify the uterine cavity. Separation of the uterus from adjacent adnexal tissue is improved when CT images are taken after administration of contrast material; but unless a definite tissue plane is seen around the uterus, a uterine mass may not be distinguished from ovarian masses that have invaded the uterus.

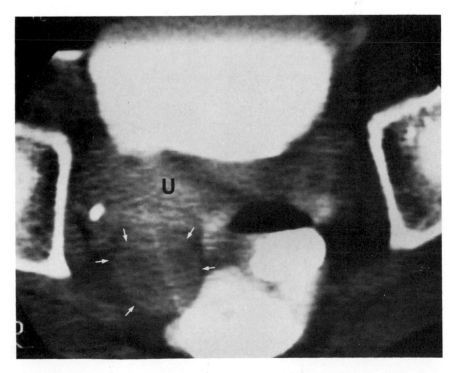

Figure 20–66. Pelvic CT scan (magnification 2.5×) demonstrates a lobulated mass (arrows) protruding from the right side of the uterus (U). The areas of low density within the myoma represent regions of degeneration.

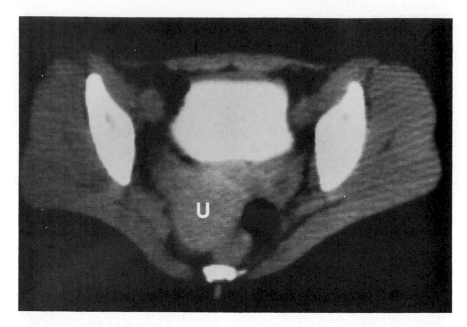

Figure 20–67. Postcontrast CT scan. A retroverted uterus (U) is seen as a high-density solid mass projecting posteriorly and to the right. As usual, the uterus has increased its attenuation value to a greater degree than that of surrounding muscle.

MISCELLANEOUS UTERINE ABNORMALITIES

Malposition of the Uterus

CT has proven useful in demonstrating abnormalities in position, such as a retroverted uterus (Fig. 20–67). The administration of intravenous contrast medium enhances normal uterine tissue to a greater degree than surrounding muscle and permits an abnormally positioned uterus to be distinguished from other pelvic masses. Reformation of axial images into coronal and sagittal planes is also useful in evaluation of the malpositioned uterus.

Abscess

Uterine abscesses following surgery (Fig. 20–68) and pyometrium (Fig. 20–69) from a variety of etiologies are readily demonstrated by CT. Gas within the wall of the uterus is indicative of an intrauterine abscess, especially if the inner margins of the uterus are irregular. Differentiating a pyometrium from other causes of uterine fluid

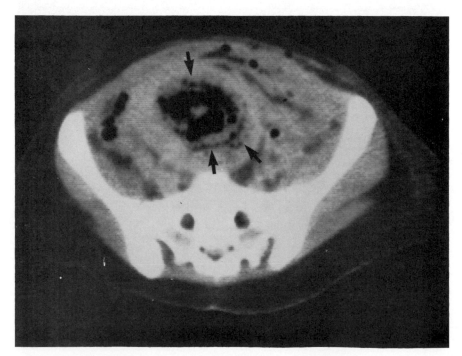

Figure 20–68. Intrauterine abscess. An enlarged thick-walled uterus is seen in a patient post partum and after cesarean section. The inner margins of the uterus are irregular, and air is seen in the wall of the uterus (arrows), indicating an intrauterine abscess.

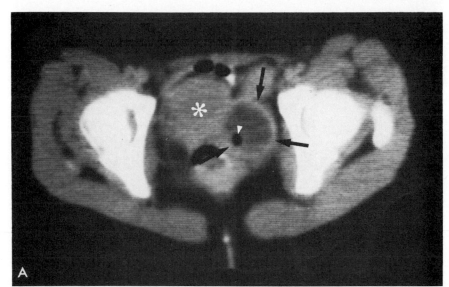

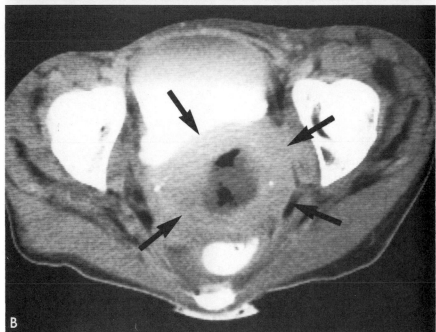

Figure 20–69. Pyometrium of the uterus. **A** An oval low-density mass (arrows) containing air (arrowhead) represents a pyometrium in a patient with a bicornuate uterus and an obstructed left horn. The unobstructed right horn (asterisk) has a normal soft-tissue density. **B** An enlarged thick-walled uterus (arrows) containing a central collection of fluid and air represents a hydrocolpos and pyometrium in a patient with cervical carcinoma obstructing the uterus.

collections is possible if gas is noted within the area of low density.

Gravid Uterus

CT is not usually used to study the gravid uterus, but occasionally a pelvic scan will be performed in a patient who does not know she is pregnant. In early pregnancies, CT demonstrates an enlarged, thick-walled uterus containing a fluid-filled gestational sac (Fig. 20–70). CT scans performed later in pregnancy will demonstrate the fetal skeleton and rarely detect fetal anomalies (Fig. 20–71). CT scans obtained shortly after delivery reveal an enlarged uterus with a dif-

fusely thickened wall and a central cavity (Fig. 20–72).

MALIGNANT UTERINE DISEASE

Endometrial Carcinoma

This is the most frequent invasive gynecologic malignancy, with 39,000 new cases and 3000 deaths estimated in 1982.[159] Most frequently occurring in women over 50 years of age, endometrial cancer usually presents with postmenopausal bleeding. Choice of treatment is dependent upon depth of myometrial invasion, histologic grade, and tumor stage (Table 20–5).[160] Simple curet-

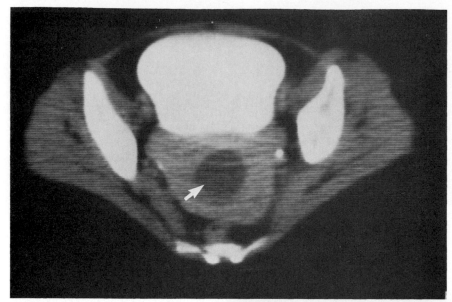

Figure 20–70. Early intrauterine pregnancy producing an enlarged thick-walled uterus. The uterus contains a fluid-filled gestational sac.

Figure 20–71. A CT scan following instillation of contrast material into the amniotic sac reveals a single intrauterine pregnancy and contrast-filled bowel (arrow) present within the left chest, resulting from the presence of a fetal diaphragmatic hernia.

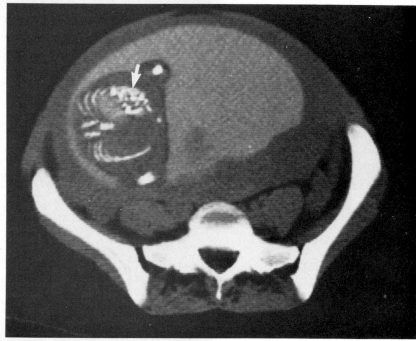

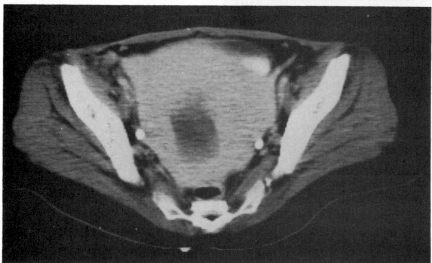

Figure 20–72. A CT scan shortly following delivery demonstrates a normally enlarged uterus with thick walls and a central fluid cavity. Compare with the postpartum abscess shown in Figure 20–68.

Table 20–5. STAGING OF ENDOMETRIAL CARCINOMA

Stage	Extent of Tumor
I	Carcinoma limited to corpus uteri
II	Carcinoma involving corpus uteri and cervix
III	Extension of carcinoma beyond uterus into surrounding tissue without involvement of bladder or rectum
IV	Extension of tumor into bladder and/or rectum or spread to distant sites

tage, hysterectomy, surgery with postsurgical radiotherapy, radiation, and subsequent hysterectomy or chemotherapy and/or external irradiation are used, depending on extent and histologic features of the tumor.[161–164]

Assessment of tumor extent has historically relied upon findings obtained by cystoscopy, lymphangiography, sigmoidoscopy, chest radiography, barium enema, excretory urography, and bimanual pelvic examination under anesthesia. More recently, CT and ultrasonography have been utilized in an attempt to decrease the number of

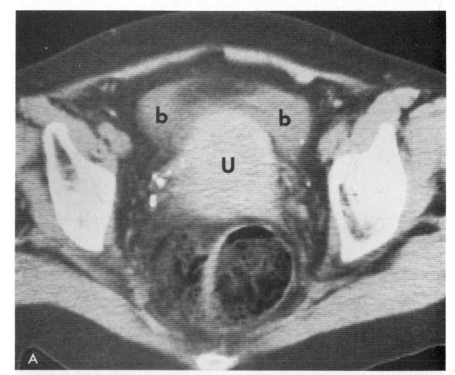

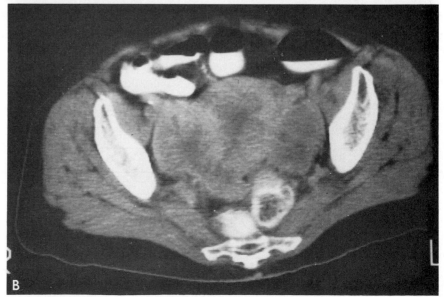

Figure 20–73. Endometrial carcinoma producing focal enlargement of the uterus (U). In this patient, the carcinoma has a uniform solid appearance. There is preservation of the fat planes between the uterus and rectum and uterus and bladder (b), indicating lack of direct tumor spread. **B** Global enlargement of the uterus. There are multiple areas of tumor necrosis, and the tumor fills the entire pelvis.

treatment failures stemming from inaccurate detection of extrauterine extension of tumor.

Ultrasonography has been evaluated as a method of detecting and staging endometrial carcinomas by several investigators.[121, 132, 165–168] Requard and colleagues[165] found a statistically significant difference between the echo pattern of Stage I and II disease compared with Stage III and IV disease and suggested that ultrasonographic features could distinguish between Stage II and III endometrial carcinoma, even though the distinction is clinically difficult. However, overall results to date indicate that ultrasonography does not have a major role in detecting Stage I or II endometrial

carcinomas; cannot be used to exclude a tumor; is insensitive for detecting bowel, mesentery, omental, lymphatic, bone and peritoneal involvement; and thus has a limited role in staging endometrial carcinoma. However, by accurately assessing uterine size, shape, and position relative to the bladder and rectum, ultrasonography has proved to be of value in planning treatment by endocavitary irradiation.[169, 170]

CT has been widely employed to detect, stage, and follow the effects of therapy in patients with endometrial carcinoma.[4, 167, 170–173] Endometrial carcinoma in a normal-sized uterus cannot be detected on precontrast CT scans because the atten-

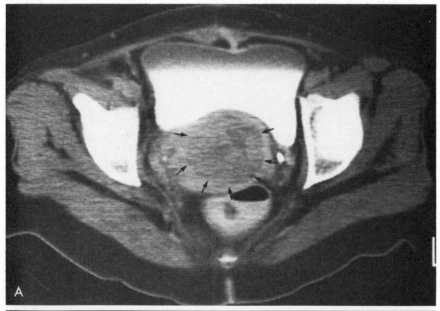

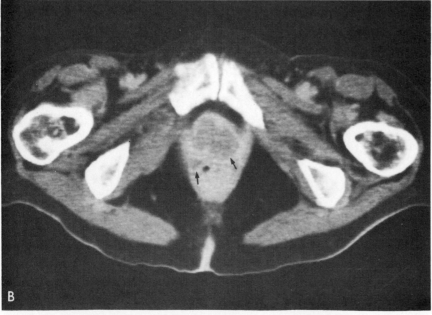

Figure 20–74. Endometrial carcinoma. **A** CT scan following intravenous infusion of contrast material demonstrates a hypodense lesion (arrows), representing necrotic tumor, sharply demarcated from normal endometrium. **B** Postcontrast CT study demonstrates uterine tissue to enhance more than foci of endometrial carcinoma (arrows).

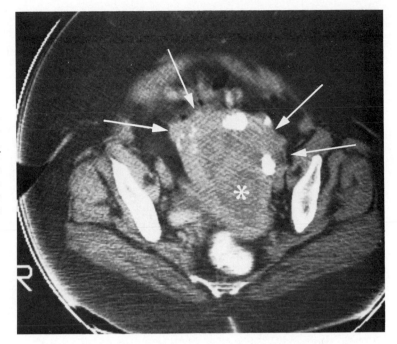

Figure 20–75. Uterine sarcoma is manifested as a large mass with irregular margins (arrows). The tumor has a central area of necrosis (asterisk) and foci of benign-appearing calcifications. In this case, the presence of calcifications erroneously led to a diagnosis of a uterine myoma. The irregular margins give a clue as to the true nature of the mass.

uation coefficient of the normal myometrium and that of endometrial carcinoma are similar. However, if the tumor involves at least a third of the uterine wall,[4] it can be detected as a hypodense lesion surrounded by densely opacified normal endometrium following a rapid infusion of contrast material (Fig. 20–73). The hypodense area seen on contrast scans represents necrotic tumor; less necrotic tumor contains regions of central contrast enhancement within a hypodense mass. On CT sections, submucous leiomyomas, particularly if they undergo cystic changes, cannot be differentiated from endometrial carcinoma. However, only 5 per cent of leiomyomas occur in a submucous location, and they tend to regress after menopause, reducing the likelihood of confusion with endometrial carcinoma.

On axial CT images, carcinoma of the endometrium is usually manifest by focal or global enlargement of the uterine body (Fig. 20–73). The attenuation values of endometrial carcinoma on precontrast CT scans can be indistinguishable from those found in myomas of the uterus (Fig. 20–73A). Bolus injections or rapid contrast infusion usually enhances normal uterine tissue and benign myomas more than endometrial carcinoma, thus permitting separation of normal from abnormal and benign from malignant uterine tumors (Fig. 20–74). The presence of calcification and/or fatty degeneration within a uterine mass is strong evidence the mass is a benign myoma (Figs. 20–64 and 20–65), but rarely a malignancy

will be present in a uterus containing benign-appearing calcifications (Fig. 20–75).

Adnexal spread of tumor is seen as a lobulated, triangular-shaped mass extending from the central neoplasm (Fig. 20–76). Extrauterine extension is manifest by obliteration of normal parametrial and paravaginal fat planes (Figs. 20–77 and 20–78). However, caution should be employed in interpreting fat plane loss without an associated tumor mass invading into an adjacent structure as unequivocal evidence of extrauterine extension. Invasion of bladder, pelvic side wall, or rectum may be simulated by a tumor that is continuous with but not invading an adjacent structure. Therefore, a confident diagnosis is made only where there is unequivocal evidence of asymmetrical thickening of the wall of the rectum, bladder, or pelvic musculature (Figs. 20–77 and 20–78). The presence of normal pelvic fat planes excludes direct gross extension into an adjacent organ (Fig. 20–74A), but does not exclude microscopic foci of tumor being present in pelvic fat adjacent to a malignant tumor.

Endometrial carcinoma occludes the internal cervical os and results in a hydrometra, hematometra, or pyometra.[166] In these conditions, CT demonstrates a symmetrically enlarged uterus containing a central water-density mass but cannot distinguish hydrometra from pyometra unless gas is present.

The incidence of lymph node metastasis from endometrial carcinoma varies with the clinical

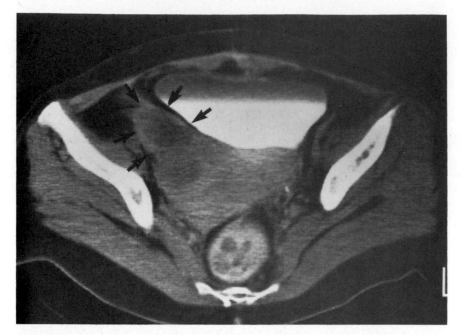

Figure 20–76. Endometrial carcinoma. Extension of tumor (arrows) into the right adnexal structures seen as a triangular-shaped mass containing areas of necrosis.

stage. Initial metastases occur in the external and internal iliac lymph node groups with the obturator group, a part of the medial subgroup of the external iliac chain being most frequently involved.[174]

The sensitivity of CT for detecting lymph node metastasis in the pelvis ranges between 73 and 80 per cent, with a specificity of 92 per cent.[173, 175, 176] This compares with reported lymphangiographic sensitivities ranging from 75 to 90 per cent with specificities varying between 57 and 87 per cent.[177–180] Lymphangiography has the advantage of detecting small foci of metastasis in normal-sized nodes and in directing needle biopsies to suspicious areas in normal-sized nodes.[181] An additional advantage of lymphangiography is that reactive hyperplasia and lymph node metastasis can often be distinguished because of the internal nodal architecture displayed by lymphangiography. As a result of different capabilities, CT and lymphangiography are largely complementary in the evaluation of patients with endometrial carcinoma. CT is performed initially, and in advanced disease it is usually sufficient. However, if nodes

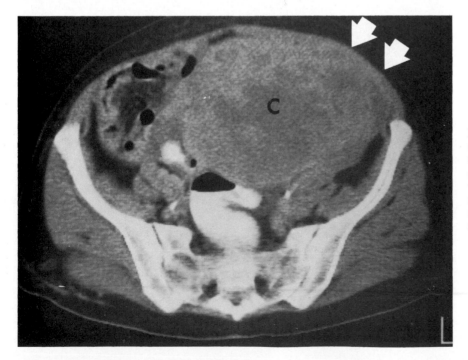

Figure 20–77. A very large endometrial carcinoma (C) containing multiple areas of tumor necrosis. The tumor has invaded the abdominal wall (arrows), resulting in loss of normal fat planes and thickening of the abdominal wall musculature.

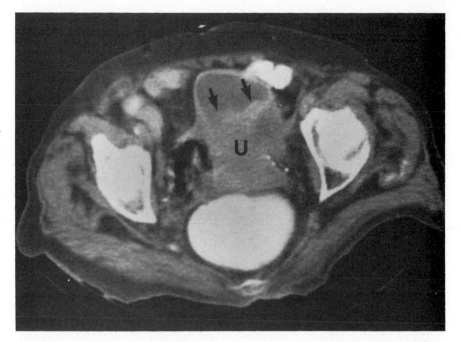

Figure 20–78. Endometrial carcinoma. Irregularity of posterior bladder wall (arrows) and loss of tissue planes between the bladder and uterus (U) indicates direct invasion of the bladder by endometrial carcinoma. Based on the CT images alone, a transitional cell carcinoma with extension into uterus cannot be excluded.

are normal or only slightly enlarged, lymphangiography is performed because lymph node size alone can lead to false-positive results.[182]

CT should not be performed in patients with Stage I disease because it adds little information to that obtained by dilation and curettage. However, CT is recommended in all patients with infiltrative endometrial carcinoma to evaluate pelvic and retroperitoneal extension of tumor. If lymphadenopathy is present, a percutaneous biopsy is performed; if the biopsy is positive, it terminates the presurgical workup. Lymphangiography is performed if CT shows no contraindications for surgery. Additional studies such as excretory urography, barium enema examination, liver/spleen scan, and cystoscopy are not done unless there is clinical evidence (i.e., hematuria, gastrointestinal bleeding) of abnormalities involving the kidneys, colon, ureters, or bladder.

CT is useful in planning intracavitary irradiation by providing measurements of the uterus and cervix as well as three-dimensional anatomic information that enables selection of the appropriate applicator for proper implantation of radioactive sources.[183] CT accurately determines the relationship of the applicator to adjacent structures, and based on CT, radiation treatment can be individualized in regard to total radiation dose and the number and spatial distribution of radioactive sources.[170]

RECURRENT ENDOMETRIAL CARCINOMA. Recurrent disease most frequently is confined to the pelvis, producing symptoms of low back or sciatic pain, leg edema, or obstructive uropathy. Because bimanual pelvic examinations are difficult to perform and interpret in patients with suspected recurrent tumor due to pelvic adhesions or radiation fibrosis, we employ CT as the primary technique for assessing the pelvis for recurrent endometrial carcinoma. Data obtained by CT regarding the presence or absence of a tumor mass (Fig. 20–79A), extension of tumor to the pelvic side walls, inguinal (Fig. 20–79B), para-aortic or pelvic lymph nodes, bladder, rectum, bone, or ureters (Fig. 20–79C), complements the physical examination and facilitates appropriate therapeutic decisions.

In our experience, CT can detect recurrent uterine carcinoma with greater than 90 per cent accuracy. Most false-positive examinations are related to radiation changes that simulate recurrent tumor. False-negative results are often due to small superficial tumor deposits in the perineum or vagina. False-positive interpretations are minimized if baseline CT scans of patients with Stage II or III lesions are obtained after initial radiation therapy.

Sarcoma

Although sarcomas are rare uterine tumors, accounting for only 3 per cent of malignant uterine neoplasms, they are the most lethal of all uterine malignancies.[159] Leiomyosarcoma is the most common uterine sarcoma and is believed to arise in pre-existing leiomyomas,[159] although malignant degeneration must be extremely rare, considering prevalence of benign myomas. CT most fre-

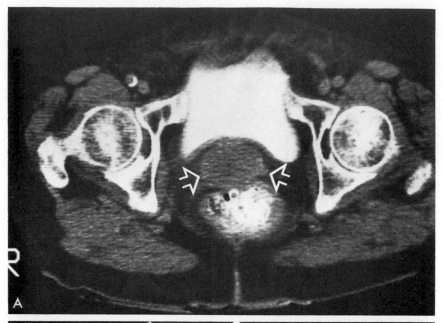

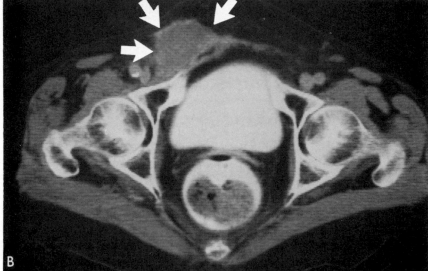

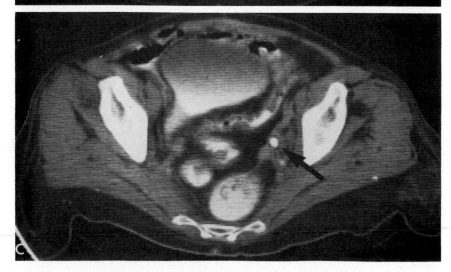

Figure 20–79. Patterns of recurrent endometrial carcinoma. **A** A solid pelvic mass (arrows) following total hysterectomy. **B** Invasion of the abdominal wall (arrows) by a large necrotic tumor mass. **C** Endometrial carcinoma encasing the left ureter (arrow).

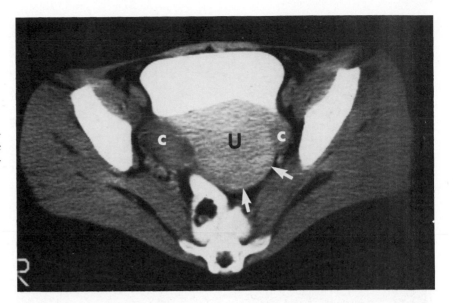

Figure 20–80. Gestational tropho-blastic disease producing a uterine mass (U) having sharp margins (arrows). c = Corpus luteum cysts.

quently demonstrates uterine enlargement with inhomogeneity and zones of low attenuation. Foci of calcification may be present (Fig. 20–75). Although detection of uterine sarcomas is usually straightforward, the CT features are identical to those of endometrial carcinoma and do not permit a preoperative diagnosis of uterine sarcoma to be made.

Gestational Trophoblastic Disease

This condition refers to a spectrum of prolif-erative abnormalities of trophoblasts ranging from hydatidiform mole to choriocarcinoma.[140, 141, 152] Treatment varies according to the degree of invasion or presence of metastases, and thus accurate assessment of extent of disease is critical. Currently, plain chest radiography, whole lung tomography, and abdominopelvic ultrasound are used to determine extent of disease, although these techniques are less sensitive than CT in detecting pulmonary and retroperitoneal disease. Recently, we have substituted a CT scan of the chest, abdomen, and pelvis for conventional radiographic techniques to detect both local extension of disease and distant metastasis in patients with gestational trophoblastic disease. CT most often demonstrates an enlarged inhomogeneous uterus containing a central area of low attenuation (Fig. 20–80), but an enlarged homogeneous uterus may also be demonstrated. An associated finding is the presence of multiple enlarged ovaries containing multiple corpus luteum cysts (Figs. 20–80 and 20–81). Following therapy, CT is employed to document response of both the enlarged uterus and areas of tumor extension or metastasis.

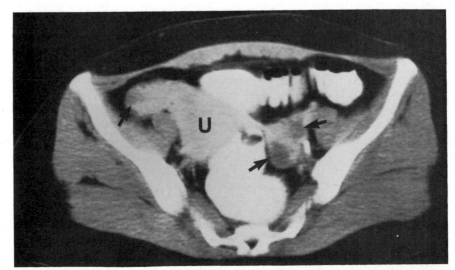

Figure 20–81. Gestational tro-phoblastic disease. CT scan demonstrates a solid uterine mass (U) and enlarged ovaries containing multiple corpus luteum cysts (arrows).

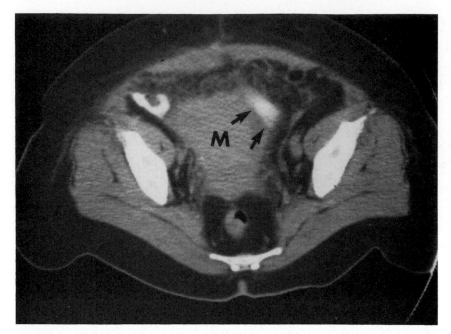

Figure 20–82. A large solid uterine mass (M) produced by metastatic breast carcinoma. The tumor cannot be separated from the small bowel (arrows). At surgery, infiltration of the small bowel was found.

Metastasis

Uterine metastases most commonly arise from tumors originating in the ovary, whereas extrapelvic neoplasms that metastasize to the uterus most frequently arise in the breast and gastrointestinal tract. Metastatic tumors produce lobular, homogeneous soft-tissue masses that are nonspecific in appearance and indistinguishable from benign or malignant primary uterine neoplasms (Fig. 20–82).

Cervical Carcinoma

Cervical carcinoma is the most frequent gynecologic malignancy, with 61,000 new cases and 7200 deaths occurring yearly.[159] Approximately 75 per cent of new cases will be detected as carcinoma in situ by a cervical smear cytologic examination while the patient is asymptomatic. Peak incidence of invasive cervical carcinoma occurs in women younger than 50 years of age; 95 per cent are squamous cell carcinomas arising in the external surface of the cervix and vagina and 4.5 per cent are adenocarcinomas arising from endocervical epithelium.[159]

Accurate staging of cervical carcinoma is vital in selecting optimal therapy because therapeutic failures are often due to undetected tumor involvement of regional lymph nodes in the pelvic and para-aortic chains. Although bimanual pelvic examinations, cystoscopy, excretory urography, sigmoidoscopy, and lymphangiography are used to evaluate extent of disease in patients with invasive cervical carcinoma, when compared with surgical findings, these methods have been found to have error rates ranging from 35 to 39 per cent.[167]

The overall accuracy of CT in staging patients with cervical carcinoma is reported as ranging between 66 and 80 per cent,[175, 184] with a sensitivity as high as 93 per cent.[175] In one study, CT gave more accurate results than clinical and postsurgical staging but was slightly less accurate than a combination of clinical and cytoscopic techniques.[176] CT is more accurate than clinical staging in the detection of local spread with parametrial involvement (Stage II) or pelvic side wall disease (Stage III) and more reliably demonstrates Stage IVB disease (metastasis to pelvic and para-aortic lymph nodes; liver or other organs) than any other modality.

The CT appearance of a normal cervix varies, depending on the shape and position of the uterus. However, in all instances the outer cervical margins are smooth and sharply delineated by paravaginal fat, and overall size is usually less than 3 cm in diameter. Invasive carcinoma of the cervix typically produces a mass of soft-tissue density that is confined to the cervix or extends into the uterus and parametrium (Fig. 20–83). In 50 per cent of the tumors, areas of tumor necrosis are seen as foci of decreased attenuation within the tumor (Fig. 20–83).[176] Extension of tumor to the parametrium results in an irregular, lobulated or triangular extension from the central tumor, and obliteration of tissue fat planes between the mass and pelvic side walls is considered evidence of fixation of tumor to the side wall (Fig. 20–84). Spread of cervical carcinoma to involve the blad-

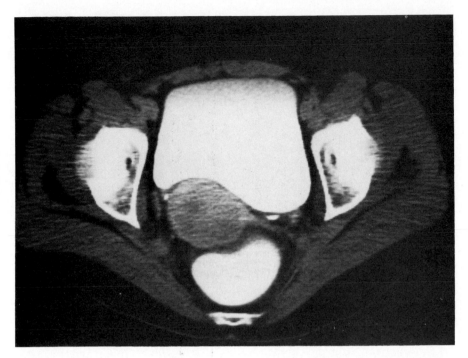

Figure 20–83. Cervical carcinoma, producing a rounded inhomogeneous mass. The mass is well demarcated from the bladder and rectum.

der, rectum, lymph nodes, pelvic musculature, or distant organs is diagnosed as described for uterine carcinoma (Fig. 20–85).

The sensitivity of CT in detecting lymph node metastasis in cervical carcinoma has ranged from 70 to 80 per cent, with up to 30 per cent false-negative and 22 per cent false-positive interpretations.[173, 175, 177, 184] Lymphangiographic sensitivity rates approach 90 per cent,[177, 180–182] and thus a negative CT examination does not exclude lymph node spread of cervical carcinoma. Our current

approach is to perform a CT scan as the initial study for detecting lymphatic metastases and to proceed with lymphangiography and/or biopsy if the CT study is normal or suspicious.

As in carcinoma of the uterus, CT has applications in the radiotherapy of cervical carcinoma. Calculation of tumor volume and determination of extent is useful for the planning of radiation portals and CT after insertion of radiation applicator (Fig. 20–86) permits accurate dosimetric calculations[170, 183] and may detect unsuspected uter-

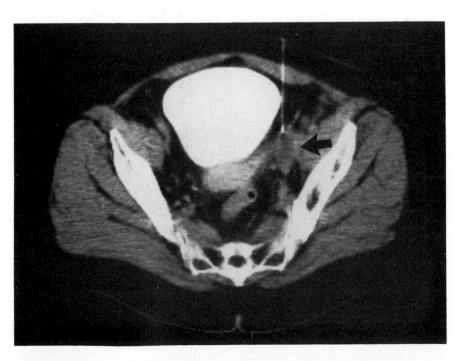

Figure 20–84. Needle biopsy of cervical carcinoma. Extension of cervical carcinoma into the left parametrium (arrow), proven by CT-guided biopsy.

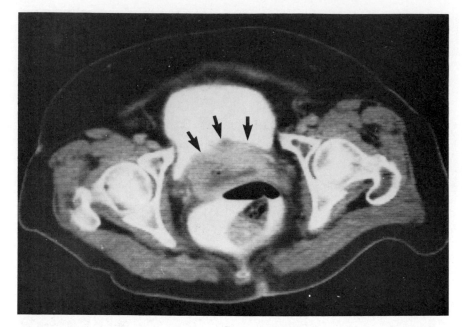

Figure 20–85. Cervical carcinoma has invaded the base of the bladder (arrows) and extends dorsally to involve the anterior wall of the rectum.

ine perforation. Results of therapy can be monitored by follow-up CT studies.

RECURRENT CERVICAL CARCINOMA. Carcinoma of the cervix most frequently recurs within 2 years after treatment, with approximately 50 per cent of patients having pelvic recurrences and 50 per cent having distant metastases.[176] Computed tomography offers the advantage of being able to evaluate the pelvis, chest, and abdomen with a single examination and thus has become the procedure of choice for screening patients with suspected recurrent tumor.

Recurrent tumor typically produces an irregular pelvic mass larger than 4 cm in diameter. The mass can be either uniformly solid or have an area of central necrosis. Pelvic side wall extension is commonly present and produces either irregular linear soft-tissue strands extending to the internal obturator muscle or a solid tumor mass that invades muscle and obliterates the pelvic fat planes (Fig. 20–87). Recurrent tumor can also be detected by demonstrating lymphadenopathy, rectal or bladder invasion, or liver or bone metastasis.

The sensitivity of CT in detecting recurrent tumor is greater than 90 per cent.[176] The main disadvantage of CT is its difficulty in distinguishing between radiation fibrosis and recurrent tumor.

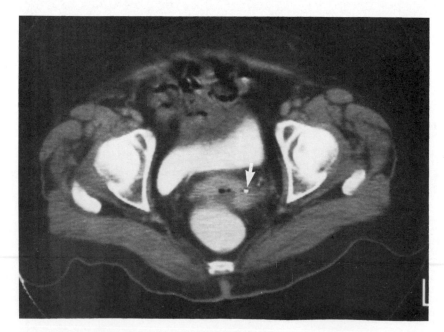

Figure 20–86. A cesium applicator (arrow) inserted for cervical carcinoma is identified. Computed tomography is useful for calculating doses to critical organs, such as the rectum and small bowel, and for measuring the tumor volume to be irradiated.

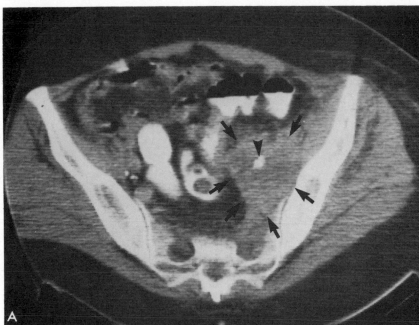

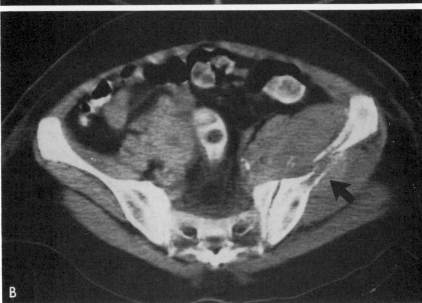

Figure 20–87. Recurrent cervical carcinoma. **A** A large recurrent cervical carcinoma (arrows) invades the left pelvic side wall and encases the left ureter (arrowhead). **B** Recurrent cervical carcinoma invading the left iliacus muscle and destroying the left iliac wing (arrow).

Performance of a baseline CT study after initial radiation therapy of advanced tumors is recommended as a method of decreasing false-positive or equivocal CT studies. The use of CT-guided percutaneous needle biopsies is advocated whenever a CT study is equivocal.

Vagina

PATHOLOGY

SQUAMOUS CELL CARCINOMA

Squamous cell carcinoma accounts for over 90 per cent of the relatively rare primary vaginal neoplasms. Although the tumor is readily diagnosed by clinical examination, CT gives additional information regarding local extension, nodal metastasis, or bladder and/or rectal invasion. On CT scans, carcinoma of the vagina typically produces a mass caudal to the uterus which contains areas of low attenuation representing necrotic tumor (Fig. 20–88).

RHABDOMYOSARCOMA (SARCOMA BOTRYOIDES)

This is a rare vaginal tumor usually occurring in children under the age of 5. It is highly malignant despite a relatively innocuous microscopic appearance. CT reveals a large solid pelvic mass

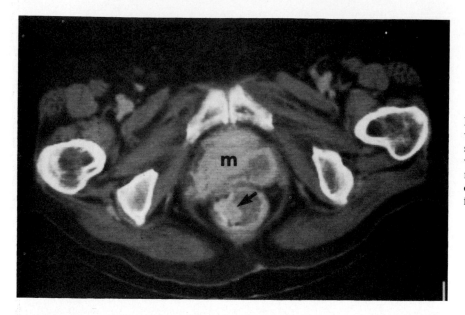

Figure 20–88. Carcinoma of the vagina. CT scan, in a patient with squamous cell carcinoma of the vagina, demonstrates a soft-tissue mass (m) with areas of decreased density. The rectum is partially filled with tumor (arrow).

having multiple zones of decreased attenuation. The mass is often so large and local invasion so extensive that it can be difficult to identify the organ of origin.

CT FINDINGS FOLLOWING RADIATION THERAPY OF THE PELVIS

External and intracavitary irradiation for gynecologic malignancies may damage the rectum, sigmoid colon, distal small bowel, vagina, and bladder.[185] The most common changes demonstrated by CT after pelvic irradiation are widening of the presacral space, an increase in perirectal fat, thickening of the perirectal fibrous tissue and bladder wall, and fibrotic connection between the sacrum and rectum (Fig. 20–89).[40]

In contrast to changes found with recurrent tumor, postirradiation changes usually are symmetrical. Increased pelvic fat secondary to irradiation can be distinguished from pelvic lipomatosis by demonstration of the presence of fibrosis in the fatty tissue. Sacral-rectal fibrosis appears to occur more frequently after radiation therapy for cervical carcinoma than for bladder tumors. The reasons for this are unclear, but they may be related to the different radiation doses and techniques used in these two groups of patients.

Soft Tissue

In addition to displaying pathologic changes in the pelvic organs, CT is valuable in detecting a variety of primary tumors of pelvic soft-tissue and osseous structures (Figs. 20–90 and 20–91). Among the more common pelvic soft-tissue masses are

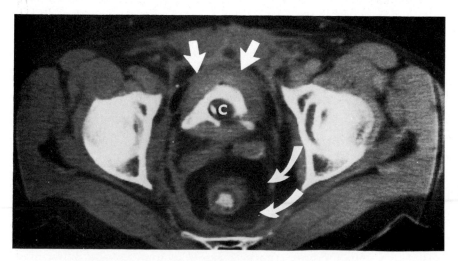

Figure 20–89. Postradiation changes. The bladder wall (straight arrows) is markedly thickened because of radiation cystitis. Increased fat surrounds the rectum (curved arrows). There is thickening of the perirectal tissue and narrowing of the rectum as a result of pelvic irradiation. A catheter (c) is present in the bladder.

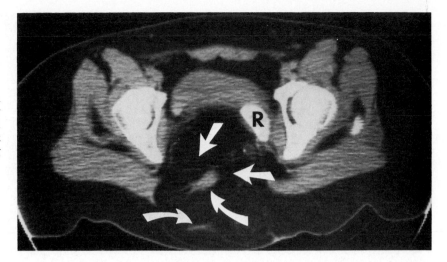

Figure 20–90. Pelvic liposarcoma. A pelvic mass is shown to have fatty (straight arrows) and solid (curved arrows) components in a patient with a large liposarcoma, displacing the rectum (R).

the anterior meningocele, the lumbosacral lipoma, and the hemophilic pseudotumor.

PATHOLOGY

ANTERIOR MENINGOCELE

The anterior sacral meningocele usually herniates through a ventral defect in the sacrum or through an enlarged intervertebral or sciatic foramen.[186] Therefore, it can present as a soft-tissue mass either anterior to the sacrum or in the gluteal region. Commonly identified is an anterior sacral bony defect which is smooth and well demarcated. The tip of the sacrum and coccyx is seen to hook under the meningocele, producing a scimitar appearance.

The diagnosis of an anterior sacral meningocele is made from plain radiography of the sacrum, excretory urography, and/or myelography, whereas ultrasound is useful in defining the meningocele as a transsonic cystic mass. CT usually is not necessary for diagnosis but can determine the relationship of the meningocele to the intrapelvic organs and, in equivocal cases, can exclude other tumors. On CT, a sacral meningocele appears as a smooth, well-defined mass of low attenuation that lies just anterior to the sacrum and is associated with sacral defects. The differential diagnosis includes chordoma, dermoid cyst, teratoma, lipoma, chondroma, and neurogenic tumor.

LIPOMA

Lumbosacral lipomas are rare benign tumors that are often associated with neural defects. Serious neurologic deficits may result from sever-

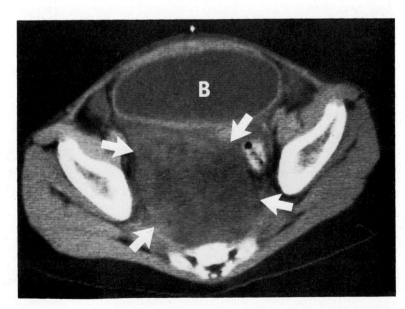

Figure 20–91. Rhabdomyosarcoma producing a large soft-tissue mass containing areas of low attenuation. The appearance of the rhabdomyosarcoma is similar to that of a large endometrial carcinoma. B = Bladder.

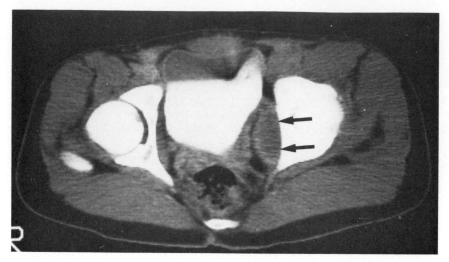

Figure 20–92. Hemophilic pseudotumor. A pelvic CT scan reveals enlargement of the left internal obturator muscle (arrows) in a hemophiliac boy. The low-density component of the mass represents a partially organized hematoma. Without the clinical history, a malignant mass could not be excluded based on the CT appearance.

ance of neural elements during surgery, nerve root traction, and increased thecal pressure produced by the tumor mass. The CT examination demonstrates the lipomatous nature of the tumor; defines the superior and inferior extent of the lesion; gives detailed information about extension into neighboring tissue; outlines the origin of the tumor; and identifies bony abnormalities in the sacrum and cartilaginous tissue within the lipoma.[187]

HEMOPHILIC PSEUDOTUMOR

Hemophilic pseudotumors are old hematomas surrounded by thick fibrous capsules and filled with coagulum. Hemophilic pseudotumors of the pelvis occur as rare complications of bleeding in 1 to 2 per cent of severe hemophiliacs. They may be contained exclusively within soft tissue or may originate in subperiosteal or intraosseous sites

(Fig. 20–92). In patients with bony involvement, CT of the pelvis demonstrates a large soft-tissue mass that destroys bone and often extends into the external oblique, iliopsoas, or the gluteus muscles.[188, 189] If only a soft-tissue pseudotumor is present, CT reveals a noncalcified pelvic mass containing regions of low or high density, suggesting fresh and old hemorrhage. (Fig. 20–93). Because CT accurately demonstrates the true extent of osseous destruction and extraosseous extension of hemophilic pseudotumors, CT is employed as a complementary procedure to plain film radiography whenever a complete evaluation of a pelvic hemophilic pseudotumor is warranted.

ILIOPSOAS BURSITIS

The iliopsoas bursa overlies the hip capsule, lies behind the iliopsoas muscle, and is lateral to the femoral vessels. A communication between the

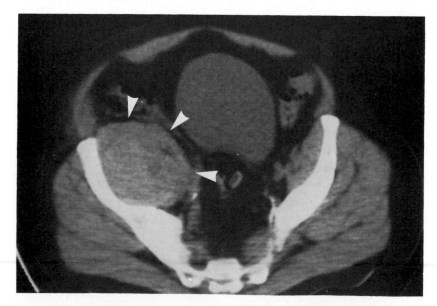

Figure 20–93. Iliopsoas hemorrhage. Markedly enlarged iliopsoas muscle (arrowheads). Regions of high attenuation value indicate recent hemorrhage into the iliopsoas muscle.

hip joint and bursa exists in 15 per cent of autopsies. Bursal enlargement may occur if the bursa is inflamed as a result of osteoarthritis, rheumatoid arthritis, pigmented villonodular synovitis, or synovial chondromatosis. If significant enlargement is present, CT demonstrates a mass of low attenuation, lateral to the femoral vessels, that displaces the iliopsoas muscle.[190] If bursal enlargement extends beneath the inguinal ligament, CT may reveal compression of the sigmoid colon, cecum, ureter, or bladder by the water-density mass.

Fluid Collections

Abnormal fluid collections within the pelvis may be caused by ascites, free blood, pelvic hematomas, abscesses, necrotic tumors, lymphoceles. Although it is not always possible to differentiate among various pelvic fluid collections, certain CT findings give clues as to the true nature of pelvic fluid.

PATHOLOGY

ASCITES

The most frequently observed pelvic fluid collection is ascites resulting from cirrhosis, neoplasm, inflammation, trauma, congestive heart failure, abnormal metabolism, or renal failure. In general, ascitic fluid has a CT density near to that of water but can have an attenuation value of 10 to 30 H, depending on the protein content of the fluid. Initially, ascites collects in the rectovesical or rectouterine (pouch of Douglas) recesses. Larger amounts fill the lateral paravesical recesses and extend up along the paracolic gutters to be contiguous with fluid in the perihepatic and perisplenic spaces.

The accuracy of CT in detecting ascites approaches 95 per cent,[191] with CT readily demonstrating even small amounts of intra-abdominal and pelvic fluid. Ascitic fluid conforms to surrounding structures, insinuating around and between organs.[192] Bowel loops tend to float out of the pelvis except when a tense ascites develops and they are displaced to one side. Distinction between benign and malignant ascites is not usually possible on the basis of the amount or attenuation value of the fluid. However, demonstration of peritoneal implants, liver metastasis, matted bowel loops in the pelvis, and lymphadenopathy are factors indicating that the ascitic fluid is malignant.

Differentiation between blood and ascitic fluid is possible only in the acute circumstance when fresh blood has a CT attenuation value significantly greater than water.[193]

HEMATOMA

Pelvic hematomas are usually due to trauma, excessive anticoagulation, hemophilia, surgical error, or neoplasia. The CT features of an acute hematoma consist of a soft-tissue mass of relatively high density (20 to 60 H) with sharp margins. As in hematomas elsewhere in the body, the attenuation value of the hematoma decreases with time as the hemoglobin content decreases and the water content increases. Hematomas 2 to 4 weeks old can be confused with other pelvic fluid collections, since they appear on CT as a cystic structure of low density. A necrotic- or cystic-appearing tumor such as cystic teratoma or an abscess may mimic an old hematoma, and clinical history and results from physical examination are needed for the correct diagnosis. In difficult cases, percutaneous needle aspiration permits a definitive diagnosis.

ABSCESS

Pelvic abscesses most often are related to inflammatory adnexal disease, appendicitis, or diverticulitis, but they are also commonly found to be secondary to Crohn's disease, pelvic surgery, carcinoma, trauma, or colonic perforation. Peripelvic abscesses are frequently due to needle contamination during parenteral administration of drugs into the buttocks. Gluteal abscesses may be due to infection of degenerated hematomas or seromas following trauma or surgery (particularly hip surgery), a necrotic neoplasm,[194] extension of an abscess along the iliacus,[194, 195] or they may be the result of a pelvic abscess spreading to the buttocks and hip through the greater and lesser sciatic foramen. This latter phenomenon is seen in postpartum patients and in patients with diabetes and inflammatory pelvic disease such as tubo-ovarian abscesses.

As in other areas of the body, CT has proved to be an accurate method for detecting and documenting the extent and size of pelvic abscesses.[196] On CT sections, an acute pelvic abscess usually appears as a low-density mass that has either a sharp or irregular outer margin (Fig. 20–94). The wall or rim of the abscess, which often is irregular, is best demonstrated following intravenous administration of contrast material. Chronic abscesses usually possess a rim that is better defined

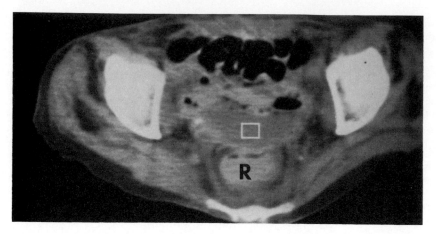

Figure 20–94. Acute pelvic abscess. A large oval area of low density (box) posterior to the small bowel and anterior to the rectum (R) is seen in a patient with a large abscess in the cul-de-sac resulting from perforation of the sigmoid colon. The abscess does not have well-defined walls.

than those found in acute abscesses, and their internal contents are generally of lower density. The fact that abscesses often obscure adjacent fat planes permits CT to exclude a cyst or seroma, both of which leave the tissue planes intact. If an abscess is caused by a gas-forming organism, air bubbles may be identified within the fluid collection. Without the presence of intraluminal gas, which was seen in 38 per cent in one series,[195] hematomas, noninfected inflammatory masses, and cystic or necrotic tumors cannot be excluded. Not all gas collections within a mass are due to infection, since gas within a mass also may be secondary to ischemia, and subsequent necrosis, or may be iatrogenically administered.

Although both ultrasound and CT can accurately diagnose pelvic abscesses, CT is superior in the postoperative patient because postoperative ileus, abdominal surgical dressing, and drains often prevent an adequate ultrasonographic examination.[196] In addition, CT is of greater help in demonstrating fistulous tracts and in guiding placement of percutaneous drainage catheters into pelvic abscesses. For these reasons, CT is employed as the initial imaging procedure in high-risk postoperative patients and in patients undergoing percutaneous drainage procedures. Ultrasonography is employed initially for most other patients suspected of a pelvic abscess with scintigraphy and/or CT utilized as complementary to ultrasonography.[197]

REFERENCES

1. Hamlin DJ, Cockett AT: Modification for computerized tomographic staging of infiltrative bladder carcinoma. J Urol 123:489, 1980.
2. Hamlin DJ, Burgener FA: Positive and negative contrast agents in CT evaluation of the abdomen and pelvis. J Comput Tomogr 5:82, 1981.
3. Seidelmann FE, Cohen WN, Bryan PJ, Temes SP, Kraus D, Schoenrock G: Accuracy of CT staging of bladder neoplasms using the gas-filled method: Report of 21 patients with surgical confirmation. AJR 130:735, 1978.
4. Hamlin DJ, Burgener FA, Beecham JB: CT of intramural endometrial carcinoma: Contrast enhancement is essential. AJR 137:551, 1981.
5. Hamlin DJ, Cockett AK, Burgener FA: Computed tomography of the pelvis: Sagittal and coronal image reconstruction in the evaluation of infiltrative bladder carcinoma. Comput Assist Tomogr 5:27, 1981.
6. van Waes PF, Zonnveld FW: Patient positioning for direct coronal computer tomography of the entire body. Radiology 142:531, 1982.
7. Osborn AG, Koehler PR, Gibbs FA, Leavitt DD, Anderson RE, Lee TG, Ferris DT: Direct sagittal computed tomographic scans in the radiographic evaluation of the pelvis. Radiology 134:255, 1980.
8. Church PA, Kazam E: Computed tomography and ultrasound in diagnosis of pelvic lipomatosis. Urology 14:631, 1979.
9. Harris RD, Bendon JA, Robinson CH, Seat SG, Herwig KR: Computed tomographic evaluation of pear-shaped bladder. Urology 14:528, 1979.
10. Schapira DV, Asbury RF, Wandtke JC, Macintosh PK: Hematuria secondary to perivesical tumors. NY State J Med 1:67, 1980.
11. Hueber F, De Faveri D, Franceschi L, Canciani L: Su di un caso di lipomatosi pelvica constrittiva: Rilievi con la TAC. Radiol Med (Torino) 66:277, 1980.
12. Brun B, Kristensen JK: Computed tomography in the evaluation of a pelvic tumor. J Comput Assist Tomogr 3:547, 1979.
13. Goodman, JD, Macchia RJ, Macasaet MA, Schneider M: Endometriosis of the urinary bladder: Sonographic findings. AJR 135:625, 1980.
14. Voelter D, Keller AJ: Diagnostik des Harnblasenkarzinoms. Aktuelle Diagnostik 105:746, 1980.
15. Marshall VF: The relation of the preoperative estimate to the pathologic demonstration of the extent of vesical neoplasms. J Urol 68:714, 1952.
16. Kenny GM, Hartoner GJ, Moore RM, Murphy GP: Current results from treatment of stage C & D bladder tumors at Roswell Park Memorial Institute. Urology 107:56, 1972.
17. Schueller J, Walther V, Staehler G, Schmiedt E, Bauer HW: Intravesikale Ultraschalltomographie zur Bestimmung der infiltrationstiefe von Blasentumoren. Muench med Wschr 122:1431, 1980.

18. Resnick MI, Willard JW, Boyce WH: Recent progress in ultrasonography of the bladder and prostate. J Urol 117:444, 1977.

19. Nakamura S, Nijima T: Staging of bladder cancer by ultrasonography: A new technique by transurethral intravesical scanning. J Urol 124:341, 1980.

20. Harada K, Igari D, Tanahashi Y, Watanabe H, Saiton M, Mishina T: Staging of bladder tumors by means of transrectal ultrasonography. J Clin Ultrasound 5:388, 1977.

21. Gammelgaard J, Hom HH: Transurethral and transrectal ultrasonic scanning in urology. J Urol 124:863, 1980.

22. Morgan CL, Calkins RF, Cavalcanti EJ: Computed tomography in the evaluation, staging, and therapy of carcinoma of the bladder and prostate. Radiology 140:751, 1981.

23. Froedin L, Hemmingsson A, Johannson A, Wicklund HL: Computed tomography in staging of bladder carcinoma. Acta Radiol (Diagn) 21:763, 1980.

24. Bruneton JN, Dilhuydy MH, Elie G, Calabet A, Le Treut A: Apport de la tomodensitometrie dans le bilan des tumeurs vesicales. J Radiol 61:343, 1980.

25. Asbell SO: CT scanning in the male genital tract and in recurrent rectal carcinoma: A review. CT: J Comput Tomogr 5:244, 1981.

26. Kellett MJ, Oliver RT, Husband JE, Fry IK: Computed tomography as an adjunct to bimanual examination for staging bladder tumors. Br J Urol 52:101, 1980.

27. Jeffrey RB, Palubinskas AJ, Federle MP: CT evaluation of invasive lesions of the bladder. J Comput Assist Tomogr 5:22, 1981.

28. Yu WS, Sagerman RH, King GA, Chung CT, Yu YW: The value of computed tomography in the management of bladder cancer. Int J Radiat Oncol Biol Phys 5:135, 1979.

29. Seidelman FE, Cohen WN, Bryan PJ: Computed tomography staging of bladder neoplasms. Radiol Clin North Am 15:419, 1977.

30. Koss JC, Arger PH, Coleman BG, Mulhern CH, Pollack HM, Wein AJ: CT staging of bladder carcinoma. AJR 137:359, 1981.

31. Wallace DM, Bloom HJG: The management of deeply infiltrating (T3) bladder cancer: Controlled trial of radical radiotherapy versus preoperative radiotherapy and radical cystectomy. Br J Urol 48:587, 1976.

32. Beyer D, Peters PE: Real-time ultrasonography—An efficient screening method for abdominal and pelvic lymphadenopathy. Lymphology 13:142, 1980.

33. Wajsman Z, Baumgartner G, Murphy GP, Merrin C: Evaluation of lymphangiography for clinical staging of bladder tumors. J Urol 114:712, 1975.

34. Johnson DE, Kaesler KE, Kaminsky S, Jing BS, Wallace S: Lymphangiography as an aid in staging bladder carcinoma. South Med J 69:28, 1976.

35. Walsh JW, Amendola MA, Konerding KF, Tisnado J, Dazra TA: Computed tomographic detection of pelvic and inguinal lymph node metastases from primary and recurrent pelvic malignant disease. Radiology 137:157, 1980.

36. Lee JK, Stanley RJ, Sagel SS, McClennan BL: Accuracy of CT in detecting intraabdominal and pelvic lymph node metastases from pelvic cancers. AJR 131:675, 1978.

37. Castellino RA, Marglin SI, Carroll BA, Young SW, Narell GS, Blank N: The radiographic evaluation of abdominal and pelvic lymph nodes in oncologic practice. Cancer Treat Rev 7:153, 1980.

38. Schlager B, Asbell SO, Baker AS, Aklaroff DM, Seydel MG, Ostrum BJ: The use of computerized tomography scanning in treatment planning for bladder carcinoma. Int J Radiol Oncol Biol Phys 5:99, 1979.

39. Brizel HE, Livingston PA, Grayson EV: Radiotherapeutic applications of pelvic computed tomography. J Comput Assist Tomogr 3:453, 1979.

40. Doubleday LC, Bernardino ME: CT findings in the perirectal area following radiation therapy. J Comput Assist Tomogr 4:634, 1980.

41. Kwok-Liu JP, Zikman JM, Cockshott WP: Carcinoma of the urachus: The role of computed tomography. Radiology 137:731, 1980.

42. Wajsman Z, Merrin C, Moore R, Murphy GP: Current results from treatment of bladder tumors with total cystectomy at Roswell Park Memorial Institute. J Urol 113:806, 1975.

43. Richie JP, Skinner DG, Kaufman JJ: Radical cystectomy for carcinoma of the bladder: 16 years of experience. J Urol 113:186, 1975.

44. Johnson DE, Lamy SM: Complications of a single stage radical cystectomy and ileal conduit diversion: Review of 214 cases. J Urol 117:171, 1975.

45. Lee JK, McClennan BL, Stanley RJ, Levitt RG, Sagel SS: Use of CT in evaluation of postcystectomy patients. AJR 136:483, 1981.

46. Van Engelshoven JM, Kreel L: Computed tomography of the prostate. J Comput Assist Tomogr 3:45, 1979.

47. Greenberg M, Neiman HL, Brandt TD, Falkowski W, Carter MF: Ultrasound of the prostate: Analysis of tissue texture and abnormalities. Radiology 141:757, 1981.

48. Watanabe H: Prostatic ultrasound. Clinics in Diagnostic Ultrasound 2:125, 1979.

49. Resnick MI: Ultrasound evaluation of the prostate and bladder. Seminars in Ultrasound 1:69, 1980.

50. Harada K, Igari D, Tanahashi Y: Gray scale transrectal ultrasonography of the prostate. J Clin Ultrasound 7:45, 1979.

51. Harada K, Tanahashi Y, Igari D, Numata I, Orikasa S: Clinical evaluation of inside echo patterns in gray scale prostatic echography. J Urol 124:216, 1980.

52. Murphy GP, Gaeta JF, Pickren J, Wajsman Z: Current status of classification and staging of prostate cancer. Cancer 45:1889, 1980.

53. Whitehead ED, Leiter E: Prostatic carcinoma: Clinical and surgical staging. NY State J Med 81:184, 1981.

54. Pilepich MV, Perez CA, Prasas S: Computed tomography in definitive radiotherapy of prostatic carcinoma. Int J Radiat Oncol Biol Phys 6:923, 1980.

55. Hovsepian JA, Byar DP: Quantitative radiology for staging and prognosis of patients with advanced prostatic cancer. Urology 14:145, 1979.

56. Loening SA, Schmidt JP, Brown RC, Hawtrey CE, Fallon B, Culp DA: A comparison between lymphangiography and pelvic node dissection in the staging of prostatic cancer. J Urol 117:752, 1977.

57. Spellman MC, Castellino RA, Ray GR, Pistenma DA, Bagshaw MA: An evaluation of lymphography in localized carcinoma of the prostate. Radiology 125:637, 1977.

58. Prando A, Wallace S, Von Eschenbach AC, Jing BS, Ro-

sengren JE, Hussey DM: Lymphangiography in staging of carcinoma of the prostate. Radiology 131:641, 1979.

59. McLaughlin AP, Saltzstein SL, McCullough DL, Gittes RF: Prostatic carcinoma: Incidence and location of unsuspected lymphatic metastases. J Urol 115:89, 1976.

60. Paulson DF: The impact of current staging procedures in assessing disease extent of prostatic adenocarcinoma. J Urol 121:300, 1979.

61. Levine MS, Arger PH, Coleman BG, Mulhern CB Jr, Pollack HM, Wein AJ: Detecting lymphatic metastases from prostatic carcinoma: Superiority of CT. AJR 137:207, 1981.

62. Efremidis SC, Dan SJ, Nieburgs H, Mitty MA: Carcinoma of the prostate: Lymph node aspiration for staging. AJR 136:489, 1981.

63. Goethlin JH, Hoiem L: Percutaneous fine-needle biopsy of radiographically normal lymph nodes in the staging of prostatic carcinoma. Radiology 141:351, 1981.

64. Klein LA: Prostatic carcinoma. N Engl J Med 300:824, 1979.

65. Spring DB, Schroeder D, Babu S, Agee R, Gooding GAW: Ultrasonic evaluation of lymphocele formation after staging lymphadenectomy for prostatic carcinoma. Radiology 141:479, 1981.

66. Gore RM, Moss AA: Value of computed tomography in interstitial I-125 brachytherapy of prostatic cancer. Radiology 146:453, 1983.

67. Lee DJ, Leibel S, Sheils R, Sanders R, Siegelman S, Order S: The value of ultrasonic imaging and CT scanning in planning the radiotherapy for prostatic carcinoma. Cancer 45:724, 1980.

68. Lytton B, Schiff M, Shonk CR: Treatment of early stage prostatic cancer by implantation of Iodine-125. Surg Clin North Am 60:1215, 1980.

69. Goffinet DR, Alvaro M, Freiha F, Toolers DM, Pistenma DA, Cumes D, Bagshaw MA: [125] Iodine prostate implants for recurrent carcinomas. Cancer 45:2717, 1980.

70. Ambrose SS: Transcoccygeal [125]Iodine prostatic implantation for adenocarcinoma. J Urology 125:365, 1981.

71. Elkon D, Kim JA, Constable WC: Anatomic localization of radioactive gold seeds of the prostate by computer-aided tomography. Comput Tomogr 5:89, 1980.

72. Pinch L, Aceto T JR, Meyer-Bahlburg HFL: Cryptorchidism: A pediatric review. Urol Clin North Am 1:573, 1974.

73. Scorer CG: The descent of the testis. Arch Dis Child 39:605, 1964.

74. Khademi M, Seebode JJ, Falla A: Selective spermatic arteriography for localization of an impalpable undescended testis. Diagnostic Radiology 136:627, 1980.

75. Diamond AB, Meng CH, Kodroff M, Goldman SM: Testicular venography in the nonpalpable testis. AJR 129:71, 1977.

76. Glickman MG, Weiss RM, Itzchak Y: Testicular venography for undescended testes. AJR 129:67, 1977.

77. Madrazo BL, Klugo RC, Parks JA, Diloretto R: Ultrasonographic demonstration of undescended testes. Radiology 113:181, 1979.

78. Weiss RM, Glickman MG, Lytton B: Clinical implications of gonadal venography in the management of the non-palpable undescended testes. Urol 121:745, 1978.

79. Lee JK, McClennan BL, Stanley RJ, Sagel SS: Utility of computed tomography in the localization of the undescended testis. Radiology 135:121, 1980.

80. Wolverson MK, Jagannadharao B, Sundaram M, Riaz MA, Nalesnik WJ, Houttuin E: CT in localization of impalpable cryptorchid testes. AJR 134:725, 1980.

81. Hricak H, Filly RA: Ultrasonography of the scrotum. AJR Invest Radiol 18:112, 1983.

82. Arger PH, Mulhern CB Jr, Coleman BG, Banner MP: Prospective analysis of the value of scrotal ultrasound. Radiology 141:763, 1981.

83. Leopold GR, Woo VL, Scheible W, Nachtsheim D, Gosink BB: High-resolution ultrasonography of scrotal pathology. Radiology 131:719, 1979.

84. Friedrich M, Claussen CD, Felix R: Immersion ultrasound of testicular pathology. Radiology 141:235, 1981.

85. Winston MA, Handler SJ, Pritchard JH: Ultrasonography of the testis—Correlation with radiotracer perfusion. J Nucl Med 19:615, 1978.

86. Claussen CD, Friedrich M, Kemper J: Diagnosis of scrotal lesions by means of new immersion ultrasound technique. ROEFO 133:465, 1980.

87. Black RE, Cox JA, Han B, Babcock DS: Abdominal hydrocele—Cause of abdominal mass in children. Pediatrics 67:420, 1981.

88. Phillips GN, Schneider M, Goodman JD, Macchia RJ: Ultrasonic evaluation of the scrotum. Urol Radiol 1:157, 1979.

89. Rodriguez DD, Rodriguez WC, Rivera JJ, Rodriguez S, Otero AA: Doppler ultrasound versus testicular scanning in the evaluation of the acute scrotum. J Urol 125:343, 1981.

90. Holder LE, Martire JR, Holmes ER, Wagner HN: Testicular radionuclide angiography and static imaging: Anatomy, scintigraphic interpretation, and clinical indications. Radiology 125:739, 1977.

91. Beard CM, Benson RC Jr, Kelalis PP, Elveback LR: Incidence of malignant testicular tumors in the population of Rochester, Minnesota, 1935 through 1974. Mayo Clin Proc 52:8, 1977.

92. Castro JR: Tumors of the testis. In Fletcher GH (ed): Textbook of Radiotherapy, 2nd ed. Philadelphia, Lea & Febiger, 1973, pp 737–751.

93. Dunnick NR, Janadpour N: Value of CT and lymphography: Distinguishing retroperitoneal metastases from nonseminomatous testicular tumors. AJR 136:1093, 1981.

94. Lackner, K, Weissbach L, Boldt I, Scherholz K, Brecht G: Computed tomographic demonstration of lymph node metastases in malignant tumors of the testicles: Comparison of results of lymphography and computed tomography. ROEFO 130:636, 1979.

95. Storm PB, Kern A, Leoning SA, Brown RC, Culp DA: Evaluation of pedal lymphangiography in staging non-seminomatous testicular carcinoma. J Urol 118:1000, 1977.

96. Maier JG, Schamber DT: The role of lymphangiography in the diagnosis and treatment of malignant testicular tumors. AJR 114:482, 1972.

97. Safer ML, Green JP, Crews QE, Hill DR: Lymphangiographic accuracy in the staging of testicular tumors. Cancer 35:1603, 1975.

98. Watson RC: Lymphography of testicular carcinoma. Semin Oncol 6:31, 1979.

99. Kademian M, Wirtanen G: Accuracy of bipedal lymphangiography in testicular tumors. Urology 9:218, 1977.

100. Chiappa S, Uslenghi C, Gonadonna G, Marano P, Ravasi G: Combined testicular and foot lymphangiography in testicular carcinomas. Surg Gynecol Obstet 123:10, 1966.

101. Zaubauer W, Kunz R, Lauppi R: Diagnostic reliability of lymphography in patients with malignant testicular tumors. Fortschr Roentgenstr 126:335, 1977.

102. Husband JE, Peckham MJ, MacDonald JS, Hendry WF: The role of computed tomography in the management of testicular teratoma. Clin Radiol 30:243, 1979.

103. Frick MP, Feinberg SE, Knight LC: Evaluation of retroperitoneum with computerized tomography and ultrasonography in patients with testicular tumors. Comput Tomogr 3:181, 1979.

104. Glazer HS, Lee JKT, Melson GL, McClennan BL: Sonographic detection of occult testicular neoplasms. AJR 138:673, 1982.

105. Burney BT, Klatte EC: Ultrasound and computed tomography of the abdomen in the staging and management of testicular carcinoma. Radiology 132:415, 1979.

106. Williams RD, Reinberg SB, Knight LC, Fraley EE: Abdominal staging of testicular tumors using ultrasonography and computed tomography. J Urol 123:872, 1980.

107. Lee JK, McClennan BL, Stanley RJ, Sagel SS: Computed tomography in the staging of testicular neoplasms. Radiology 130:387, 1978.

108. Lien HH, Kolbenstvedt A, Kolmannskog F, Liverud K, Aakhus T: Computer tomography, lymphography and phlebography in metastases from testicular tumors. Acta Radiologica Diagnosis 21:505, 1980.

109. Javadpour N, Doppman JL, Bergmann SM, Anderson T: Correlation of computed tomography and serum tumor markers in metastatic retroperitoneal testicular tumor. J Comput Assist Tomogr 2:176, 1978.

110. Husband JE, Barrett A, Peckham MJ: Evaluation of computed tomography in the management of testicular teratoma. Br J Urol 53:179, 1981.

111. Javadpour N, Anderson T, Doppman JL: Computed tomography in evaluation of testicular cancer during intensive chemotherapy. J Urol 122:565, 1979.

112. Soo CH, Bernardino ME, Chuang VP, Ordonez N: Pitfalls of CT findings in post-therapy testicular carcinoma. J Comput Assist Tomogr 5:39, 1981.

113. Husband JE, Hawkes DJ, Peckham MJ: CT estimations of mean attenuation values and volume in testicular tumors: A comparison with surgical and histologic findings. Radiology 144:553, 1982.

114. Nachman JB, Baum ES, White H, Chuang VP, Ordonez N: Bleomycin-induced pulmonary fibrosis mimicking recurrent metastatic disease in a patient with testicular carcinoma. Cancer 47:236, 1981.

115. Osborn SB: The implications of the reports of the Committee on Radiological Hazards to Patients (Adrian Committee). A symposium given at the Annual Congress of the British Institute of Radiology, April 27, 1962. I. Variations in the radiation dose received by the patient in diagnostic radiology. Br J Radiol 36:230, 1963.

116. Federle MP, Cohen HA, Rosenwein MF, Brant-Zawadzki MN, Cann CE: Pelvimetry by digital radiography, a low dose examination. Radiology 143:733, 1982.

117. Friedman AC, Pyatt RS, Hartman DS, Downey EF, Olson WB: CT of benign cystic teratomas. AJR 138:659, 1982.

118. Peterson WF, Prevost EC, Edmunds FT, Hundley MJ, Morris FK: Benign cystic teratomas of the ovary. Am J Obstet Gynecol 70:368, 1955

119. Sloan RD: Cystic teratoma (dermoid) of the ovary. Radiology 81:847, 1963.

120. Laing FC, Van Dalsem VF, Marks WM, Burton JL, Martinez DA: Dermoid cysts of the ovary: Their ultrasonographic appearances. Obstet Gynecol 57:99, 1981.

121. Walsh JW, Taylor KJ, Wasson JF, Schwartz PE, Rosenfeld AT: Gray-scale ultrasound in 204 proved gynecologic masses: Accuracy and specific diagnostic criteria. Radiology 130:391, 1979.

122. Sandler MA, Silver TM, Karo JJ: Gray-scale ultrasonic features of ovarian teratomas. Radiology 131:705, 1979.

123. Lindsay AN, Voorhess ML, MacGillivray MH: Multicystic ovaries detected by sonography in children with hypothyroidism. Am J Dis Child 134:588, 1980.

124. Wolff JP: Tumeurs ovariennes—ovariumtumoren, cancer de l'ovarie. Acta Chirurgica Belgica 79:227, 1980.

125. Silverberg BS: Gynecologic Cancer: Statistical and Epidemiological Information. American Cancer Society Professional Education Publication 6–8, 1975.

126. Watring WG, Edinger DD, Anderson B: Screening and diagnosis in ovarian cancer. Clin Obstet Gynecol 22:745, 1979.

127. Rutledge F, Boronow RC, Wharton JT: Gynecologic Oncology. New York, John Wiley & Sons, 1976, p 160.

128. Amendola MA, Walsh JW, Amendola BE, Tisnado J, Hall DJ, Goplerud DR: Computed tomography in the evaluation of carcinoma of the ovary. J Comput Assist Tomogr 5:179, 1981.

129. Haertell VM: Zur Computertomographie gynekologischer Karzinome. Fortschr Roentgenstr 132:652, 1980.

130. Photopulos GJ, McCartney WH, Walton LA, Staab EV: Computerized tomography applied to gynecologic oncology. Am J Obstet Gynecol 135:381, 1979.

131. Musumeci R, De Palo G, Kenda R, Tesoro-Tess JD, Di RE F, Petrillo R, Rilke F: Retroperitoneal metastases from ovarian carcinoma: Reassessment of 365 patients studied with lymphography. AJR 134:449, 1980.

132. Nash CH, Alberts DS, Suciu TN, Giles HR, Tobias DA, Waldman RS: Comparison of B-mode ultrasonography and computed tomography in gynecologic cancer. Gynecol Oncol 8:172, 1979.

133. Walsh JW, Rosenfield AT, Jaffe CC, Schwartz PE, Simeone J, Dembner AG, Taylor KJW: Prospective

comparison of ultrasound and computed tomography in the evaluation of gynecologic pelvic masses. AJR 131:955, 1978.

134. Requard CK, Mettler FA, Wicks JD: Preoperative sonography of malignant ovarian neoplasms. AJR 137:79, 1981.

135. Dunnick NR, Fisher RI, Chu EW, Young RC: Percutaneous aspiration of retroperitoneal lymph nodes in ovarian cancer. AJR 135:109, 1980.

136. Pickel H, Schreithofer H, Sager WD: Zur Anwendung der Computertomographie in der Gynekologischen Onkologie. Gerburtsh Frauenheilk 40:912, 1980.

137. Watt I, Watt E, Halliwell M, Ross GM: Sonographic demonstration of intrauterine contraceptive devices. J Clin Ultrasound 5:378, 1977.

138. Callen PW, Filly RA, Munyer TP: Intrauterine contraceptive devices: Evaluation by sonography. AJR 135:797, 1980.

139. Queenan JT, Kubarych SF, Douglas DL: Evaluation of diagnostic ultrasound in gynecology. Am J Obstet Gynecol 123:453, 1975.

140. Santos-Ramos R, Forney JP, Schwartz BE: Sonographic findings and clinical correlations in molar pregnancy. Obstet Gynecol 56:186, 1980.

141. Wittmann BK, Fulton L, Cooperberg PL, Lyons EA, Miller C, Shaw D: Molar pregnancy: Early diagnosis by ultrasound. J Clin Ultrasound 9:153, 1981.

142. Laing FC, Filly RA, Marks WM, Brown TW: Ultrasonic demonstration of endometrial fluid collections unassociated with pregnancy. Radiology 137:471, 1980.

143. Wilson DA, Stacy TM, Smith EI: Ultrasound diagnosis of hydrocolpos and hydrometrocolpos. Radiology 128:451, 1978.

144. Laing FC: Sonography of a persistently retroverted gravid uterus. AJR 136:413, 1981.

145. Callen PW, Filly RA: Placental-subplacental complex: Specific indicator of placental position on ultrasound. J Clin Ultrasound 8:21, 1980.

146. Chinn DH, Filly RA, Callen PW: Prediction of intrauterine growth retardation by sonographic estimation of total intrauterine volume. J Clin Ultrasound 9:125, 1981.

147. Wexler P, Gottesfield KR: Early diagnosis of placenta previa. Obstet Gynecol 54:231, 1979.

148. Carroll VA: Ultrasonic features of preeclampsia. J Clin Ultrasound 8:457, 1980.

149. Brown TW, Filly RA, Laing FC, Barton J: Analysis of ultrasonographic criteria in the evaluation for ectopic pregnancy. AJR 131:967, 1978.

150. Schoenbaum SW, Rosendorf L, Kappelman N, Rowan T: Gray scale ultrasound in tubal pregnancy. Radiology 127:757, 1978.

151. Shenker L, Brickman FE: Bicornuate uterus with incomplete vaginal septum and unilateral agenesis: Ultrasound demonstration in two patients. Radiology 133:455, 1979.

152. Reuter K, Michlewitz H, Kahn PC: Early appearance of hydatiform mole by ultrasound. AJR 134:588, 1980.

153. Richardson ML, Kinard RE, Watters DH: Location of intrauterine devices: Evaluation by computed tomography. Radiology 142:690, 1982.

154. Ranney B: The prevention, inhibition, palliation and treatment of endometriosis. Am J Obstet Gynecol 123:778, 1975.

155. William TJ, Pratt JH: Endometriosis in 1,000 consecutive celiotomies: Incidence and management. Am J Obstet Gynecol 129:245, 1977.

156. Coleman BG, Arger PH, Mulhern CH: Endometriosis: Clinical and ultrasonic correlation. AJR 132:747, 1979.

157. Tada S, Tsukioka M, Ishii C, Tanaka H, Mizunuma K: Computed tomographic features of uterine myoma. J Comput Assist Tomogr 5:866, 1981.

158. Oppenheimer DA, Carroll BA, Young SW: Lipoleiomyoma of the uterus. J Comput Assist Tomogr 6:640, 1982.

159. Kestner RW: Gynecology Principles and Practice, 3rd ed. Chicago, Year Book Medical Publishers, 1979, pp 255–276.

160. Staging as recommended by the Cancer Committee of the International Federation of Gynecology and Obstetrics. Gynecol Oncol 4:13, 1976.

161. De Saia PJ, Creasman WT: Clinical gynecologic oncology. St Louis, CV Mosby Company, 1981, pp 128–152.

162. Cox JD, Komaki R, Wilson JK, Greenber M: Locally advanced adenocarcinoma of the endometrium: Results of irradiation with and without subsequent hysterectomy. Cancer 45:715, 1980.

163. Jobson VW, Girtanner RE, Averette HE: Therapy and survival of early invasive carcinoma of the cervix uteri with metastases to the pelvic nodes. Surg Obstet Gynecol 151:27, 1980.

164. Baker HW, Makk L, Morrissey RW, Ockstein H: Stage I adenocarcinoma of the endometrium: A clinical and histopathological study of 65 cases treated with preoperative radium. Obstet Gynecol 54:146, 1979.

165. Requard CK, Wicks JD, Mettler FA: Ultrasonography in the staging of endometrial adenocarcinoma. Radiology 140:781, 1981.

166. Scott WW, Rosenheim NB, Seigelman SS, Sander RC: The obstructed uterus. Radiology 141:767, 1981.

167. Walsh JW, Rosenfield AT, Jaffe CC, Schwartz PE, Simeone J, Dembner AG, Taylor KJW: Prospective comparison of ultrasound and computed tomography in the evaluation of gynecologic pelvic masses. AJR 131:955, 1978.

168. Schlensker KH, Beckers H: The use of ultrasound in the diagnosis of pelvic pathology. Arch Gynecol 229:91, 1980.

169. Brascho DJ, Kim RY, Wilson EE: Use of ultrasonography in planning intracavitary radiotherapy of endometrial carcinoma. Radiology 129:163, 1978.

170. Lee KR, Mansfield CM, Dwyer SJ, Cox HL, Levine E, Templeton AW: CT for intracavitary radiotherapy planning. AJR 135:809, 1980.

171. Chen SS, Kumari S, Lee L: Contribution of abdominal computed tomography (CT) in the management of gynecologic cancer: Correlated study of CT image and gross surgical pathology. Gynecol Oncol 10:162, 1980.

172. Piana L, Rosello R, Boutiere JL, Padaut J, Roux, Clement R: Interet de la tomodensitometrie dans le traitement du cancer du col uterin. Bulletin Du Cancer 66:519, 1979.

173. Walsh JW, Amendola MA, Karsten FK, Tisnado J, Hazra TA: Computed tomographic detection of pelvic and inguinal lymph-node metastases from primary

and recurrent pelvic malignant disease. Radiology 137:157, 1980.

174. Liu W, Meigs JV: Radical hysterectomy and pelvic lymphadenectomy. Am J Obstet Gynecol 95:706, 1966.

175. Whitley NO, Brenner DE, Francis A, Villa Santa U, Aisner J, Wiernik PH, Whitley J: Computed tomographic evaluation of carcinoma of the cervix. Radiology 142:439, 1982.

176. Walsh JW, Amendola MA, Hall DJ, Tisnado J, Goplerud DR: Recurrent carcinoma of the cervix: CT diagnosis. AJR 136:117, 1981.

177. Ginaldi S, Wallace S, Jing BS, Bernardino ME: Carcinoma of the cervix: Lymphangiography and computed tomography. AJR 136:1087, 1981.

178. Wallace S, Jing BS, Zornoza J, Hammond JA, Hamberger A, Herson J, Freedman R, Wharton T: Is lymphangiography worthwhile? Int J Radiat Oncol Biol Phys 5:1873, 1979.

179. Musumeci R, de Palo G, Conti U, Kenda R, Mangioni C, Belloni C, Marzi M, Bandieramonte G: Are retroperitoneal lymph node metastases a major problem in endometrial adenocarcinoma? Cancer 46:1887, 1980.

180. Piver MS, Wallace S, Castro JR: The accuracy of lymphangiography in carcinoma of the uterine cervix. AJR 111:278, 1971.

181. Brown RC, Buchsbaum HJ, Tewfik HH, Platz CE: Accuracy of lymphangiography in the diagnosis of paraaortic lymph node metastases from carcinoma of the cervix. Obstet Gynecol 54:571, 1979.

182. Henrikson E: The lymphatic spread of carcinoma of the cervix and of the body of the uterus. Am J Obstet Gynecol 58:924, 1949.

183. Yu WS, Sagerman RH, Chung CT, King GA, Dalal PS, Bassano DA, Ames TE: Anatomical relationships in intracavitary irradiation demonstrated by computed tomography. Radiology 143:537, 1982.

184. Kilcheski, Arger PH, Mulhern CB, Coleman BG, Kressel HY, Mikuta JI: Role of computed tomography in the presurgical evaluation of carcinoma of the cervix.

J Comput Assist Tomogr 5:378, 1981.

185. Mayer JE: Review: Radiography of the distal colon and rectum after irradiation of carcinoma of the cervix. AJR 136:691, 1981.

186. De Klerk DJJ, McCusker I, Loubser JS: Anterior sacral meningoceles. S Afr Med J 54:361, 1978.

187. Carter BL, Hahn PC, Wolpert SM, Hammerschlag SB, Schwartz AM, Scott RM: Unusual pelvic masses: A comparison of computed tomographic scanning and ultrasonography. Radiology 121:383, 1976.

188. Osborn AG, Koehler PR, Gibbs FA, Leavitt DD, Anderson RE, Lee TG, Ferris DT: Direct sagittal computed tomographic scans in the radiographic evaluation of the pelvis. Radiology 134:255, 1980.

189. Sundaram M, Wolverson MK, Joist JH, Riaz MA, Rao BJ: Case Report 133. Skeletal Radiol 6:54, 1981.

190. Penkava RR: Iliopsoas bursitis demonstrated by computed tomography. AJR 135:175, 1980.

191. Jolles H, Coulam CM: CT of ascites: Differential diagnosis. AJR 135:315, 1980.

192. Doust BD, Quiroz F, Stewart JM: Ultrasonic distinction of abscesses from other intra-abdominal fluid collections. Radiology 125:213, 1977.

193. Edell SL, Gefter WB: Ultrasonic differentiation of types of ascitic fluid. AJR 133:111, 1979.

194. Wolverson, MK, Jagannadharoa B, Sundaram M, Heiberg E, Grider R: Computed tomography in the diagnosis of gluteal abscesses and other peripelvic fluid collections. J Comput Assist Tomogr 5:34, 1981.

195. Callen PW: Computed tomographic evaluation of abdominal and pelvic abscesses. Radiology 131:171, 1979.

196. Koehler PR, Moss AA: Diagnosis of intraabdominal and pelvic abscesses by computerized tomography. JAMA 244:49, 1980.

197. Filly RA: Detection of abdominal abscesses: A combined approach employing ultrasonography, computed tomography and gallium-67 scanning. Journal De L'Association Canadienne Des Radiologistes 30:202, 1979.

21 COMPUTED TOMOGRAPHY OF CHILDREN

Robert C. Brasch

The array of imaging techniques established for the diagnosis of pediatric diseases has expanded beyond conventional radiography to include ultrasonography, nuclear scintigraphy, and, more recently, computed tomography. Anticipated future additions are digital imaging and nuclear magnetic resonance imaging. Using the new imaging techniques, we are able to diagnose, stage, and follow the progress of disease more accurately than was possible a decade ago. Yet, the multiplicity of different techniques has placed an added responsibility to choose the most appropriate imaging modality for a specific diagnostic problem. The most efficacious examination should be performed; at the same time, the temptation to order excessive tests must be avoided.

Factors that influence the choice of imaging test may differ between adult and pediatric populations. Children are not "small adults" in several regards. In addition to the requirement for accurate, useful diagnostic information, the need to minimize radiation exposure has particular relevance for the younger patient. Frequently, diseases and their natural evolution differ between adults and children. For example, only children develop neuroblastoma, and juvenile myasthenia gravis is not associated with thymomas.[1] CT procedures and techniques must be specifically tailored for children to ensure that a diagnostic examination is obtained without jeopardizing the child's safety.

The increased use of CT in pediatric diagnosis has largely been due to the continued evolution and improvement of scanning equipment. The early body CT scanners gave relatively high radiation exposures and required 18 seconds or longer per scan, too long a period for young children to suspend respiration.[2] Streak artifacts were common, and radiation exposure was comparable with or above that given in conventional radiologic procedures.[2] Newer CT scanners, which complete a scan in as little as 2 seconds, have dramatically reduced the frequency of motion artifacts and now permit dynamic examinations. In addition, CT images can now be reformatted in virtually any plane, again increasing the diagnostic utility of this method. Engineering improve-

1055

ments have made the newer scanners more dose efficient, and superior resolution can be obtained with less absorbed dose.[3, 4]

PRACTICAL CONSIDERATIONS AND TECHNIQUES OF EXAMINATION

The CT examination of an infant or small child may pose a unique and often troublesome situation for the CT diagnostician. Some radiologists are reluctant to scan a very small child because they lack experience and confidence in performing pediatric CT studies. Using a rational management plan and paying meticulous attention to technique, however, professionals should be able to perform the pediatric examination smoothly and safely.

CT images of infants and young children tend to demonstrate anatomic detail less accurately compared with images of older children and adults. The greater difficulty in defining organs and tissue interfaces in small children can be attributed to multiple factors:

1. Small object size is one contributing factor but can be partially compensated by electronic image magnification, use of thinner sections and limited field of reconstruction software.

2. Patient motion, particularly respiratory motion, is a problem that can be partially overcome by using faster scanning times.

3. Additionally, small children have less of the perivisceral fat that normally permits the sharp delineation of organs seen in older, fatter patients.

Despite the summed negative effects of these several pediatric characteristics on CT image quality, experience demonstrates that the carefully performed CT examination can provide uniquely valuable diagnostic images, even for the tiny newborn infant (Fig. 21–1).

PREPARATION AND SEDATION

CT scanner rooms must be kept cool for untroubled operation of the computer, but newborn infants must be kept warm to prevent hypothermia. Complications of hypothermia include metabolic imbalances, disruption of coagulation (which may predispose to intracranial hemorrhage), and even death. Accordingly, maintenance of normal infant temperature must not be ignored and attention should be given toward maintenance of safe body temperatures when newborn infants are scanned. Two effective and safe techniques are to wrap the infant in a warm-water heating blanket (Fig. 21–2) or position the child within the beam of a thermaster-controlled radiant heating device. Both of these techniques can be used while the infant is being scanned; but regardless of which method is employed, the newborn infant's skin temperature should be electronically monitored to avoid the possibility of hyperthermia.

How to give safe and effective sedation to pediatric patients is often a perplexing problem for the CT specialist. Generally, no sedation is needed

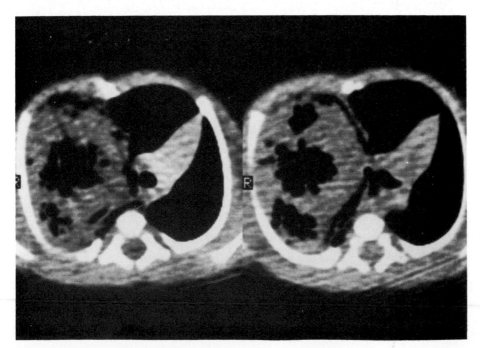

Figure 21–1. Cystic adenomatoid malformation. Two transverse CT sections through the chest of a 1-day-old infant with respiratory distress demonstrate a large mass in the right hemithorax with displacement of the mediastinal structures to the left. The combination of water-density and irregular air-density structures within the mass support the plain film impression of cystic adenomatoid malformation. The CT scan helps to identify the extent of the abnormality and to demonstrate which portions of the right lung were normally aerated and could be spared surgical resection.

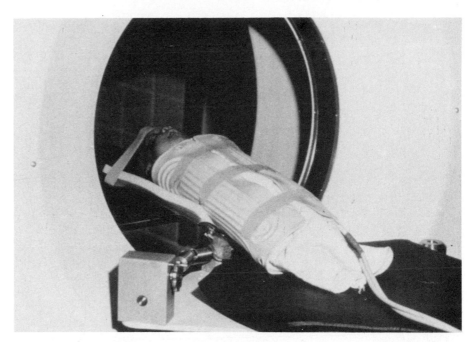

Figure 21–2. A warm-water heating blanket wrapped around a cotton sheet serves to prevent hypothermia in the temperature-sensitive newborn infant during the CT procedure. Wrapping the baby snugly also helps to limit motion and thus reduces artifacts on the CT images.

for babies less than 1 year old if they are snugly wrapped in blankets and restrained on wooden boards. However, children from 1 to 6 years old rarely lie still and usually require sedation. Our current procedure is to give pentobarbital in a dose of 5 mg per kg of body weight as an intramuscular injection 30 minutes prior to the CT examination. If adequate sedation is not achieved in 1 hour, a supplementary dose of 2 mg per kg can be administered. An alternative method of sedation is to use a combination of drugs frequently termed a "cardiac cocktail." Meperidine 2 mg per kg, promethazine 1 mg per kg, and chlorpromazine 1 mg per kg, can be administered intramuscularly 20 minutes prior to the CT study. Disadvantages of both of these drug regimens are that sedation may persist for several hours after completion of the CT examination and the children must be professionally monitored until they regain alertness. Children who are old enough to understand the CT procedure should be given kind words of explanation and assurance before the examination. Using patience, it is usually possible to gain patient cooperation in children 6 years of age or older and complete the CT examination without sedation.

CONTRAST MEDIUM ADMINISTRATION

Children are routinely fasted for 3 to 4 hours prior to the CT examination because of possible vomiting from contrast medium administration and the attendant risk of aspiration. If the child

is to have another radiologic procedure requiring barium and if the reason for scheduling the CT examination is not dependent upon the results of the barium study, the CT examination is performed first. Regardless of scanner speed, barium causes artifacts, and if a barium study has been performed prior to the CT scan, a scout radiograph should be obtained to check for retained barium before initiating the CT scan.

Virtually all children having an abdominal or pelvic CT scan receive dilute, oral iodinated contrast material prior to sedation. The only exception is when the CT scan is performed as part of a search for subtle abdominal calcifications (Fig. 21–3). Oral contrast material is given as a 1 to 2 per cent solution of diatrizoate in fruit juice with from 100 to 500 ml, depending on body weight, administered 45 minutes or longer before the CT study. For infants, contrast material may be mixed with formula. A dilute (1 per cent) barium suspension can be used as an alternative to diatrizoate.

For the uncooperative patient, a nasogastric tube may be necessary for contrast medium instillation. Immediately prior to obtaining the initial CT scan, another 50 to 250 ml of dilute contrast medium is administered to fill the proximal gastrointestinal tract if the child has not been sedated. Failure to opacify the intestine adequately often leads to major difficulties in interpretation because unopacified bowel can simulate an abdominal or retroperitoneal mass. When scans of the pelvis are performed, an enema with 50 to

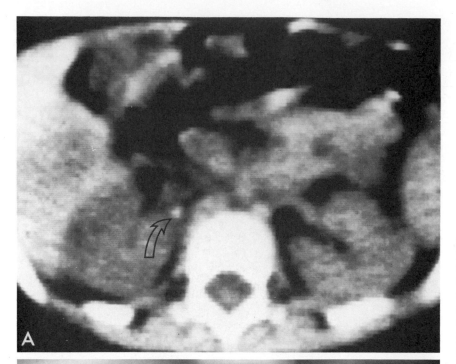

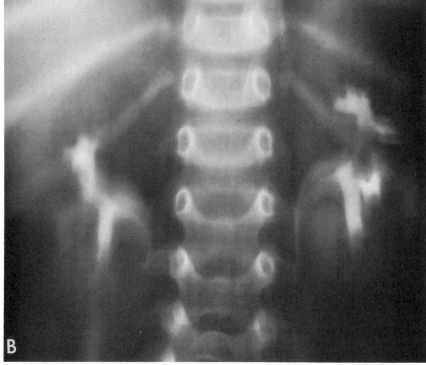

Figure 21–3. Occult neuroblastoma in a 2-year-old with opisclonus and myoclonus. **A** Noncontrast enhanced CT scan through the upper poles of the kidneys demonstrates a small mass anterior to the right kidney containing a tiny focus of calcium (arrow). The histologic diagnosis was ganglioneuroblastoma. All previous imaging studies including a plain film of the abdomen and nephrotomography after intravenous contrast medium administration **(B)** failed to demonstrate any calcification or mass. (From Hecht ST, Brasch RC, Styne D: CT localization of occult secretory tumors in children. Pediatr Radiol 12:67, 1982.)

200 ml of dilute contrast medium is administered (Fig. 21–4).

If possible, children are brought to the x-ray department with an intravenous line in place; patient agitation is reduced by having the venipuncture performed prior to administration of sedation and arrival in the CT suite. For most pediatric abdominal CT examinations, 2 ml per kg of a 50 to 60 per cent solution of contrast medium is administered intravenously. This is a dose similar to that used for pediatric urography and can be given safely to children with normal renal function.

The intravenous contrast material is administered in a bolus with scanning begun after half the bolus is injected. Usually no precontrast scans

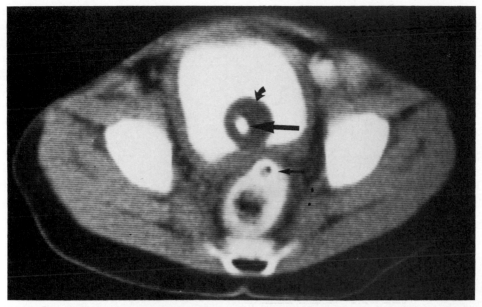

Figure 21–4. Prostatic rhabdomyosarcoma. The rectal administration of contrast material (small arrow points to rectal tube) and the instillation of contrast material through a Foley catheter (large arrow) help to define the extent of a mass in a 3-year-old boy with urinary retention. The central low-density filling defect within the bladder (curved arrow) was proved histologically to be a prostatic embryonal rhabdomyosarcoma.

are obtained, since post-contrast CT scans offer higher diagnostic yield and permit the study to be completed more rapidly and with less radiation exposure. Injection of contrast medium into a lower-extremity vein may be advantageous when pathology within the inferior vena cava is being sought, such as tumor thrombus in Wilms' tumor

(Fig. 21–5). An exception to the routine use of intravenous contrast medium is made when the liver is being scanned for possible primary or metastatic disease. In this case, the initial CT scan is performed without intravenous contrast material in order not to miss the rare lesion that becomes isodense after intravenous injection. Le-

Figure 21–5. Tumor thrombus in the inferior vena cava. Transverse CT section through the inferior vena cava after intravenous administration of radiographic contrast agent through a foot vein demonstrates a low-density filling defect (arrow) within the inferior vena cava at the level of the renal hilum. A rim of contrast material surrounds the thrombus. The CT diagnosis of Wilms' tumor (W) with venous tumor thrombus was confirmed surgically.

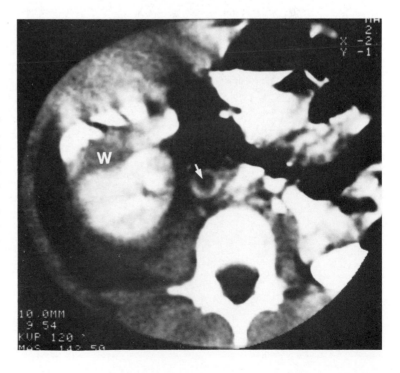

sions clearly identified on precontrast CT scans can be followed without a repeated injection of contrast material.

TECHNICAL FACTORS

A prescan scout radiograph is used to locate with precision the region to be scanned. Generally contiguous CT sections 1 cm thick are obtained through the area of interest. Exposure settings are tailored to the individual child but are selected to ensure minimum radiation exposure. Pediatric CT scans can be reconstructed using the infant or head CT reconstruction file and magni-

fied 1.3 to two times prior to filming. Improved pediatric CT scans can also be obtained by using a limited field reconstruction scan. This technique requires the child to be scanned in the medium or large adult body file and have the image reconstructed from the center portion of the larger file. This technique reconstructs the image using a smaller pixel size and produces an image magnified 1.3 to two times. These factors contribute to improved spatial resolution and sharper, larger images that are more easily interpreted (Fig. 21–6). Because no additional radiation is required to obtain these images, limited field reconstruction scans should be employed routinely for pediatric CT scanning.

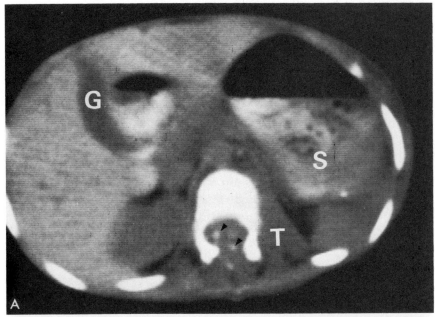

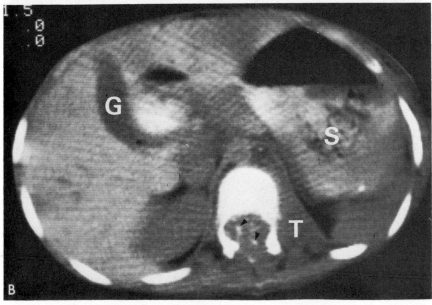

Figure 21–6. Pediatric CT using limited field reconstruction. **A** Conventional CT scan through liver and spine in patient with neuroblastoma (magnification 1.5×). The calcifications (arrowheads) in the tumor are visible, but they are not sharp. The remaining abdomen has an overall lack of sharpness. **B** CT scan using limited field reconstruction with factor of 1.5×. The margins of organs are sharp, and the calcifications (arrowheads) are more well delineated. G = Gallbladder; S = stomach; T = paraspinous tumor.

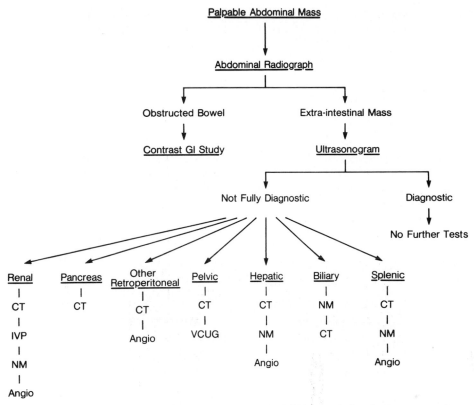

Figure 21–7. Diagnostic algorithm for the evaluation of childhood abdominal masses. Computed tomography is generally performed after the completion of plain film radiography and ultrasonography when significant diagnostic uncertainty remains.

CLINICAL INDICATIONS

Generally, the unique capabilities that include tomographic imaging in virtually any plane, quantification of data, and extraordinary density resolution dictate the utility of CT in children.[5] The clinical indications for CT scanning in adults in many instances can be extended to the pediatric population. However, there are certain specific and unique indications for pediatric CT scanning.

ABDOMINAL MASS LESIONS

The diagnostic evaluation of the infant or child with an abdominal mass can be a challenging problem requiring multiple examinations. The goal of the imaging evaluation is to determine the location, extent, and nature of the mass lesion using the most direct and accurate examinations but with the greatest possible safety to the child. The widespread availability of ultrasonography and computed tomography have significantly changed the traditional approach of the pediatric radiologist in diagnosing abdominal mass lesions.

A suggested algorithm for the evaluation of childhood abdominal masses is shown in Figure 21–7. This decision pattern is not meant to be inviolate and is frequently altered according to the circumstances of an individual patient. However, it serves as a general guide to the use of various imaging techniques.

In children with abdominal masses, the abdominal radiograph is recommended as the initial imaging examination. If the plain abdominal radiograph suggests a bowel obstruction, the appropriate fluoroscopic examination of the gastrointestinal tract is performed. If the abdominal radiograph suggests an extraintestinal mass, an ultrasonogram is usually the next imaging procedure.

In certain instances, the ultrasound examination will be diagnostic and eliminate the need for any further imaging procedures. The most frequent cause of an abdominal mass in newborns is hydronephrosis, which ultrasonography can accurately diagnose and usually indicate the severity, location, and cause of the urinary blockade.[6] CT is only rarely indicated in this clinical situation.

Ultrasound requires no radiation and can differentiate solid, cystic, and mixed-nature abdom-

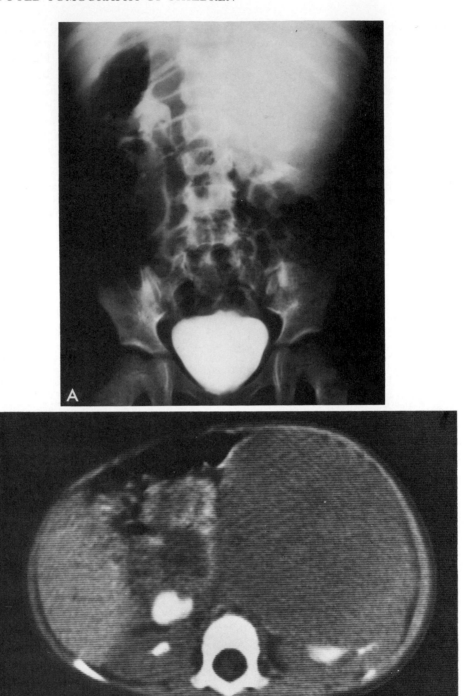

Figure 21–8. Wilms' tumor. **A**   Intravenous urogram in a 1-year-old with a palpable abdominal mass demonstrates displacement of contrast-filled intrarenal collecting structures. The urographic appearance could be attributable to either an intrarenal tumor, such as Wilms' tumor, or an extrarenal neuroblastoma **(B)**. The CT scan reveals a large mass arising from the left kidney. Renal origin of the mass is demonstrated by the continuity between the mass and the renal parenchyma. The homogeneous appearance of this tumor tends to exclude a large degree of tissue necrosis.

inal masses; it frequently can define the size and extent of the lesion. Compared with CT, ultrasonography is less expensive, requires no sedation or contrast medium, can be performed portably, and can readily produce anatomic sections in numerous planes. Disadvantages are that it is highly operator-dependent, provides only indirect data about organ function, and may be hindered by gas and bony structures. If ultrasonography is not fully diagnostic, a CT scan of the abdomen is usually performed as the next diagnostic procedure. A CT scan is also employed if pathologic calcification is sought, if both the lungs and abdomen need to be evaluated, or if an open wound or dressing hinders the ultrasound examination.

Pediatric abdominal ultrasonography and computed tomography have been shown to have similar sensitivities (87 per cent) and specificities (100 per cent).[7] However, differential diagnostic accuracy in abnormal cases was greater with CT (95 per cent) than with ultrasonography (71 per cent).[7] The highest diagnostic accuracy is achieved when the information from CT and ultrasonography is combined, indicating that these are more complementary than competitive procedures. However, it is neither necessary nor desirable to perform both examinations in every child but only when the results of the initial study leave significant diagnostic uncertainty. In these cases, the use of the complementary technique will usually provide sufficient additional information to permit an accurate diagnosis to be made.

WILMS' TUMOR

Wilms' tumor is the most common abdominal neoplasm in childhood accounting for greater than 20 per cent of all abdominal masses occurring after the newborn period.[8] Almost always arising from within the kidney, Wilms' tumors frequently metastasize to the lung and liver, making the examination of multiple organs and regions mandatory. Prior to institution of therapy, CT is particularly well suited to a multiple-region examination and has assumed an important role in the pretherapy and post-therapy evaluation of children with Wilms' tumor.

On CT scans Wilms' tumors appear as solid intrarenal masses that displace and distort intrarenal collecting structures (Figs. 21–8 and 21–9). Tumors arising in the upper poles may be difficult to differentiate from adrenal or hepatic tumors by urography alone (Fig. 21–8A),[9] but CT usually readily defines the tissue of origin (Fig. 21–8B). Calcifications are identified in less than 10 per cent of cases. Following intravenous contrast injection, tumor inhomogeneity is frequently shown to be present (Fig. 21–9).[10] Frequently, the most central portion of the tumor does not enhance after contrast medium administration (Fig. 21–9), indicating a certain measure of necrosis of the tumor core. Demonstration of metastasis to the liver (Fig. 21–10), lungs (Fig. 21–11), or other abdominal organs permits accurate pretherapy staging of Wilms' tumors.

With modern treatment for Wilms' tumor consisting of surgical resection, chemotherapy, and radiation, the prognosis is excellent with an overall survival of from 80 to 90 per cent.[11] Because of the excellent prognosis but the potential for late tumor recurrences, follow-up evaluations of Wilms' tumor patients have particular importance. When diagnostic accuracy, expense, exam-

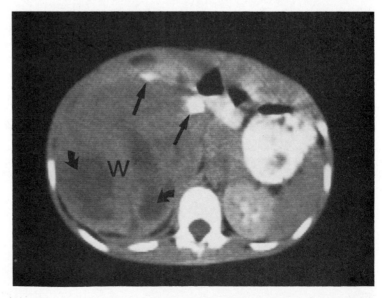

Figure 21–9. Necrotic Wilms' tumor. Transverse CT scan of a 4-year-old child with a right-sided abdominal mass demonstrates a large mass (W) containing irregular low-density areas which displace renal calices (arrows) anteromedially. The low-density regions (curved arrows) within this Wilms' tumor represented areas of tumor necrosis.

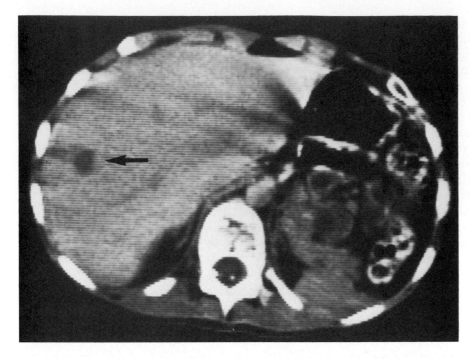

Figure 21–10. Wilms' tumor metastasis in the liver. A 1-cm metastatic lesion (arrow) is well defined on a CT image but was not evident, even in retrospect on liver scintigraph. (From Brasch RC, Randel SB, Gould RG: Follow-up of Wilms' tumor: Comparison of CT with other imaging procedures. AJR 137:1005, 1981. © 1981, American Roentgen Ray Society. Used with permission.)

ination time, and radiation exposure were compared for CT and a package of "routine" diagnostic imaging procedures (angiography, chest radiography, liver scintigraphy, ultrasonography) used for follow-up evaluations of patients with Wilms' tumors, CT was shown to be superior.[12]

Results indicated CT most accurately answered the pertinent diagnostic queries: the presence and extent of bilateral renal tumors, local recurrence, contralateral renal hypertrophy, and metastasis to liver and lungs. For diagnosing pulmonary metastases, CT was superior to conventional chest radiography both in sensitivity and specificity. In depiction of liver metastases, CT was superior to liver scintigraphy and the extent of bilateral Wilms' tumors was better defined by CT than by

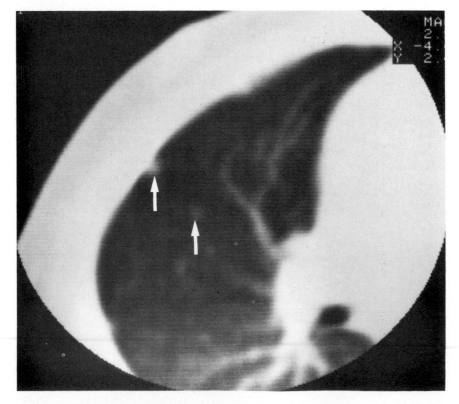

Figure 21–11. Lung metastases from Wilms' tumor. Two pulmonary metastases (arrows) are demonstrated on a CT scan of a 1-year-old with previously resected Wilms' tumor. These lesions, measuring less than 1 cm in diameter, were not identified on conventional chest radiographs.

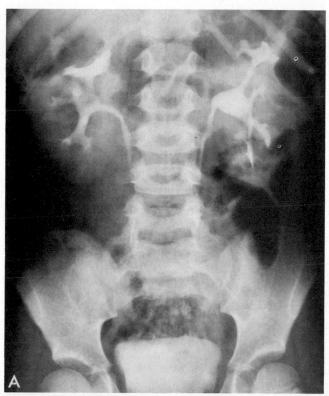

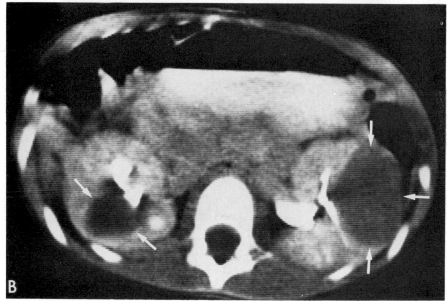

Figure 21–12. Bilateral Wilms' tumors in 5-year-old child after therapy with radiation and chemotherapy. **A** The degree of caliceal distortion on, the urogram suggests tumor growth in the left kidney. **B** The CT section at the midrenal level more clearly demonstrates tumor size and extent and revealed bilateral tumor enlargement (arrows), prompting surgical intervention. (From Brasch RC, Randel SB, Gould RG: Follow-up of Wilms' tumor: Comparison of CT with other imaging procedures. AJR 137:1005, 1981. © 1981, American Roentgen Ray Society. Used with permission.)

urography (Fig. 21–12). CT has also proved valuable in the examination of the surgically evacuated renal fossa for local tumor recurrence (Fig. 21–13).

In no instances were the alternative diagnostic studies more accurate than CT. The average cost for a CT examination ($344) was considerably less than the cost for a "routine" combination of other imaging studies ($594) (Table 21–1). Moreover, examination time and diagnostic radiation doses were also reduced when CT was employed. Pending larger comparison studies, CT is recommended as the primary diagnostic method of follow-up evaluation in all patients with Wilms' tumor.

MULTILOCULAR CYSTIC NEPHROMA

This is a rare benign intrarenal mass occurring in children that can mimic exactly the urographic appearance of Wilms' tumor (Fig. 21–14A).[13] Both

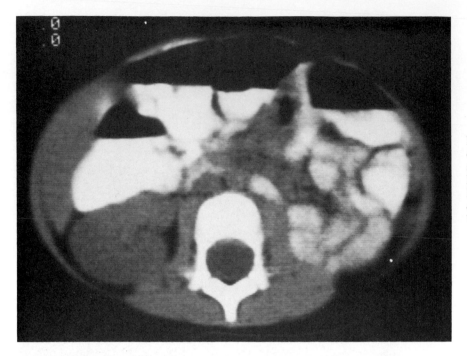

Figure 21–13. CT imaging of the evacuated renal fossa. Demonstration of contrast-filled bowel loops within the left renal fossa helps to exclude local tumor recurrence after nephrectomy for Wilms' tumor.

Table 21–1. COMPARISON OF AVERAGE COST* AND DURATION OF EXAMINATION FOR WILMS' TUMOR FOLLOW-UP

Follow-up Diagnostic Questions	Type of Procedure	Cost	Hours
Lung metastases?	Chest radiography, two views	$ 49	0.25
	Linear chest tomography	151	1.00
Liver metastases?	Liver scintigraphy	219	0.75
Local recurrence in renal fossa?	Abdominal ultrasonography (optional)	(136)	(0.85)
Contralateral renal tumor or hypertrophy?	Excretory urography with nephrotomography	175	1.25
	Arteriography (optional), three runs	(615)	(1.50)
	Total cost without options	594	3.25
	Total cost with options	($1345)	(5.60)
All questions above	Body CT (using contrast material)	$ 344	1.2

*1980 data from four medical referral centers for children.

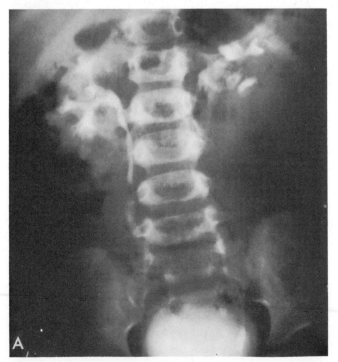

Figure 21–14. Multilocular cystic nephroma. **A** An excretory urogram in a 6-year-old girl shows a large intrarenal mass arising from the lower pole of the left kidney with displacement and distortion of caliceal structures. This appearance is indistinguishable from that of Wilms' tumor.

Illustration continued on opposite page

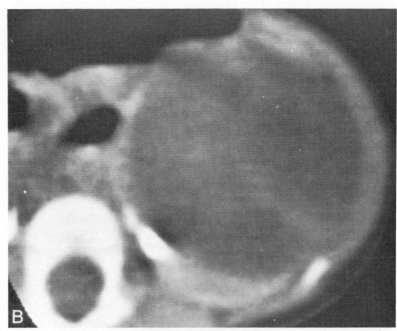

Figure 21–14. *Continued* **B** A contrast-enhanced CT scan reveals a large intrarenal mass. Within the mass are multiple rounded areas of decreased density. The attenuation coefficients differed between the multiple cystic areas, suggesting that the cysts did not communicate. The cystic nature of the renal lesion was confirmed by ultrasonography. On the basis of the CT and ultrasonic examinations, a preoperative diagnosis of multicystic nephroma was made; the lesion was locally excised without nephrectomy. **C** The pathologic appearance closely corresponds to the CT findings and confirmed the diagnosis of multilocular cystic nephroma.

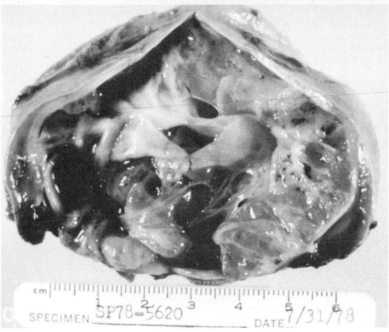

multilocular cystic nephroma and Wilms' tumor appear as nonfunctioning intrarenal masses. Prior to CT and ultrasound, the inability to diagnose these benign tumors preoperatively led to complete nephrectomies when local tumor excision could have provided definitive treatment.

CT reveals a renal mass containing multiple low-density cysts separated by curvilinear septae (Fig. 21–14B). The presence of varying CT densities within the multiple cysts gives evidence of the integrity of the individual cystic collections and strengthens the preoperative suspicion of multilocular cystic nephroma. Because of the diagnostic confidence afforded by CT and ultrasound, a preoperative diagnosis of a multilocular cystic nephroma may be suggested, leading to surgical resection of the tumor without nephrectomy. Pathologically, multilocular cystic nephromas are composed of multiple cysts separated by thin septa (Fig. 21–14C).

NEUROBLASTOMA

Neuroblastoma is the second most frequent malignant abdominal mass in childhood.[8, 14] Most

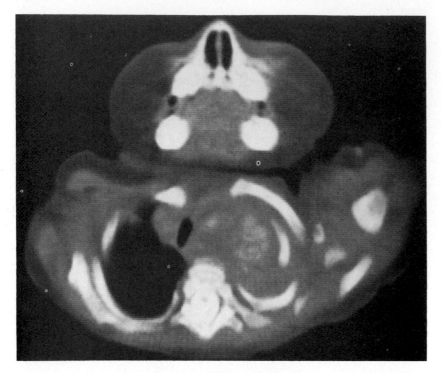

Figure 21–15. Primary neuroblastoma. CT scan through the upper thoracic region of a 2-year-old with respiratory distress demonstrates a mass containing diffuse calcifications displacing the trachea to the right. Although the chest radiograph also demonstrated a soft-tissue mass in this region, the calcifications could not be identified. The subarachnoid instillation of metrizamide helped to exclude intraspinous extension of this mediastinal tumor.

neuroblastomas arise from the adrenal glands, but primary tumors (Fig. 21–15) may originate anywhere along the sympathetic chain from the cervical region to the pelvis. These small, round cell tumors metastasize early; many patients have marrow, skeletal (Fig. 21–16), liver, lymph node (Fig. 21–17), or skin metastases at the time of clinical presentation, but lung metastases are rare and generally occur late in the course of disease.[15]

On plain film radiography, approximately 50

per cent of neuroblastomas contain calcification. Using CT, calcification is demonstrated in more than 85 per cent of primary neuroblastomas.[15a] Most frequently, the calcifications are scattered irregularly throughout the neuroblastoma (Fig. 21–18A) but large solid (Fig. 21–18B) and ring (Fig. 21–18C) calcifications surrounding areas of lower attenuation within the tumor are also identified. The exact nature of the regions of low attenuation within the neuroblastoma is unclear but probably represents areas of hemorrhage or ne-

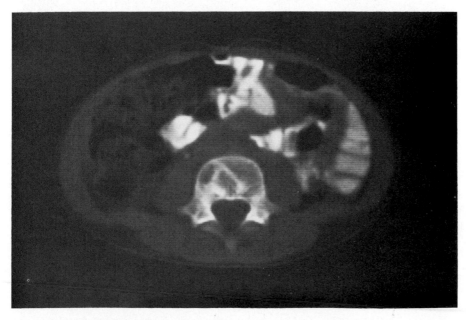

Figure 21–16. Metastatic neuroblastoma. A transverse CT scan of a 2-year-old child with proven neuroblastoma demonstrates a metastasis within the third lumbar vertebral body. A bone scintigram was positive in this region, but high-resolution magnification radiographs failed to demonstrate the abnormality.

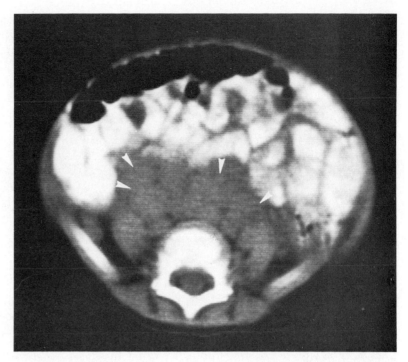

Figure 21–17. Metastatic neuroblastoma. A mantle of enlarged, retroperitoneal lymph nodes in a 2-year-old child with a primary adrenal neuroblastoma. CT demonstrates the nodal metastases as multiple, rounded masses (arrowheads) of soft-tissue density which can be easily differentiated from contrast-filled small bowel loops.

crosis. Detection of calcifications within a mass is of great diagnostic importance, since in most cases it permits differentiation of a neuroblastoma from Wilms' tumor or other renal or suprarenal masses (Figs. 21–3).[16]

The treatment for neuroblastoma varies considerably, depending on the stage of the tumor when diagnosed. Although a variety of imaging techniques can be employed, CT most accurately determines the nature and extent of the primary lesion and simultaneously defines nodal or liver metastasis, spread of tumor across the diaphragm, and bone destruction.[15a] CT is the most single accurate staging procedure but has not proved as accurate as bone scintigraphy or bone marrow aspirates in detecting spread of disease to bone prior to bone destruction. Bone scintigraphy, therefore, remains a valuable procedure in the staging of neuroblastoma.[16a] Following therapy, CT is valuable in monitoring the success of therapy and for detecting local recurrent disease or distant metastases.[16b] As in patients with Wilms' tumor, CT can substitute for a combination of imaging studies and thereby reduce hospital time, expense, and radiation exposure.

TERATOMAS

Teratomas are usually benign tumors that can arise anywhere in the retroperitoneum but are most common in the presacral region. Tissue from any of the three embryonic germ layers may

be predominant within a particular tumor. Subtle calcifications and areas of fat are frequently detected by CT, permitting the true nature of the mass to be determined preoperatively. CT can define tumor extent and relationships to surrounding structures precisely, thus aiding the surgeon in planning an adequate resection.

PANCREATIC LESIONS

Because of a lack of retroperitoneal fat, the pancreas is one of the most difficult organs to evaluate by CT in pediatric patients. In order to clearly identify the pancreas in infants and children, it is vital to completely opacify the small bowel, or the unopacified bowel will "appear" as large pancreatic mass. Fortunately, pancreatic mass lesions attributable to either pancreatitis or neoplasms are rare in children. Yet when a pancreatic abnormality is suggested clinically or by ultrasonography, CT is valuable in clarifying the presence, nature, and extent of disease.

CT detects pseudocysts (Fig. 21–19) as low-density, cystic masses in patients with familial or traumatic pancreatitis and is capable of detecting calcifications not seen on plain abdominal radiography. Pancreatic neoplasms in children are extremely rare and usually are suspected only when they are hormonally active. In these instances, CT can detect a solid focal pancreatic mass (Fig. 21–20) and confirm the location and extent of a functioning pancreatic tumor.

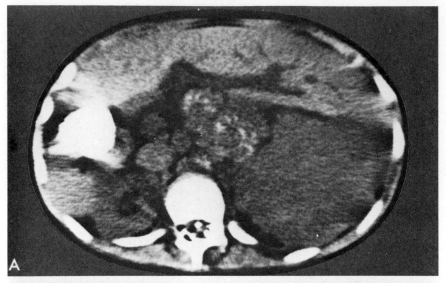

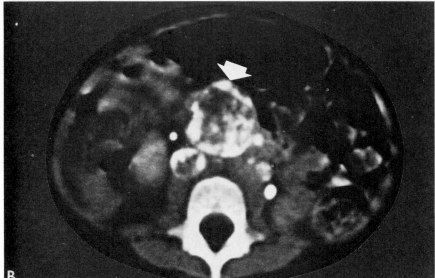

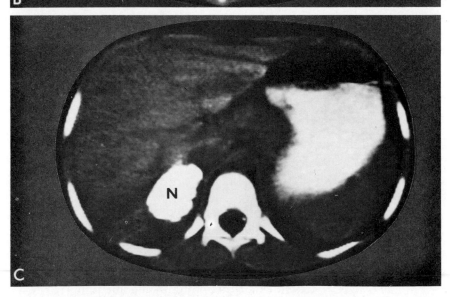

Figure 21–18. Patterns of calcification in neuroblastoma. **A** Scattered, punctate calcifications throughout a mass. **B** Ring or rim calcification (arrow) surrounding a low-density portion of a tumor. **C** Solid clumps of calcification in primary neuroblastoma (N).

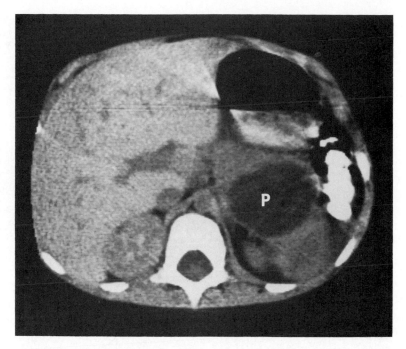

Figure 21–19. Pancreatic pseudocyst in a 4-year-old girl: CT demonstrates the pseudocyst (P) as a rounded, low-density mass within the pancreatic tail. The patient had a positive family history for pancreatitis.

RETROPERITONEAL MASSES

The differential diagnosis of retroperitoneal masses of childhood, in addition to Wilms' tumor, neuroblastoma, and teratomas, include rhabdomyosarcoma, lymphoma, lipoma, abscess, and occult secretory tumors such pheochromocytomas (Fig. 21–21), and adrenal adenomas.[13, 16] In all instances, CT readily detects the mass and localizes it to the retroperitoneal compartment. However, differentiation between solid masses is usually not possible without a biopsy unless calcification or fatty tissue is identified. Gas within a mass indicates infection[17] but does not exclude the presence of a tumor that has become infected. In staging retroperitoneal tumors, the entire abdomen and pelvis is scanned to detect lymphadenopathy and in cases where hematogenous spread of ma-

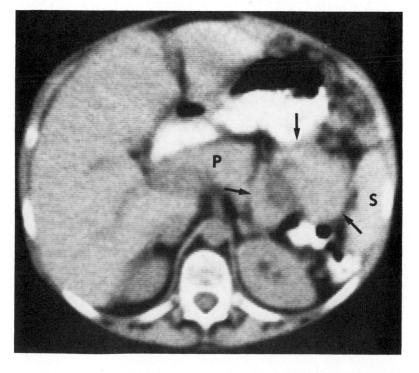

Figure 21–20. Islet cell carcinoma of the pancreas. Transverse CT scan through upper abdomen of a 9-year-old boy demonstrates a large exophytic mass (arrows) arising from the body and tail of the pancreas (P). The mass was delineated by contrast-filled loops of bowel and the spleen (S). Metastatic peritoneal implants were evident on other sections. (From Hecht ST, Brasch RC, Styne D: CT localization of occult secretory tumors in children. Pediatr Radiol 12:67, 1982.)

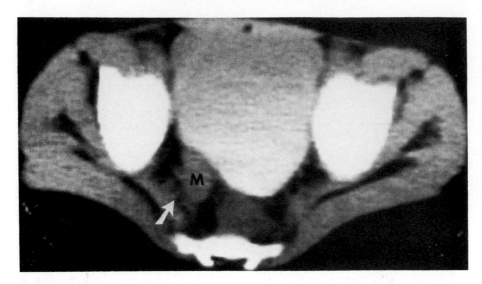

Figure 21–21. Pheochromocytoma. Transverse CT scan through the pelvis of a 10-year-old boy demonstrates a mass lesion (M) indenting the right posterolateral aspect of the contrast-filled bladder. The tumor also obscures the margin of the right piriform muscle, suggesting local invasion (arrow). (From Hecht ST, Brasch RC, Styne D: CT localization of occult secretory tumors in children. Pediatr Radiol 12:67, 1982.)

lignancy is common, the CT examination is routinely extended to include the chest.

LIVER TUMORS

The majority of primary pediatric hepatic tumors are malignant, with hepatoblastoma (34 per cent) and hepatoma (26 per cent) being the most commonly encountered.[18] Usually these tumors clinically present as palpable masses associated with anorexia and weight loss. The right hepatic lobe is involved more often than the left, but both lobes are affected in 30 to 45 per cent of cases.[18] Chemotherapy and radiation therapy have not proved curative, and complete surgical resection is thus the only method of ensuring a permanent cure.

Accurate localization of a hepatic tumor is required if the surgeon is to plan the most appropriate operation. Preoperative localization of the segmental extent of hepatic tumors can be uncertain with ultrasonography,[13] and angiography is an invasive procedure. However, CT can usually define hepatic segmental anatomy and thus accurately determine the location and extent of the malignant tumor. Because lung metastases occur with malignant hepatic tumors, the CT examination is routinely extended to include the thorax.

CT demonstrates hepatomas and hepatoblastomas as solid, hepatic mass lesions having attenuation values lower than those of surrounding normal liver (Fig. 21–22). Calcification (Fig. 21–22A) can be seen in both, and following contrast medium injection the tumors can dramatically enhance, reflecting the underlying hypervascularity of the lesions. Metastatic liver tumors appear similar to primary malignancies and usually cannot be absolutely differentiated from primary tumors without a biopsy.

The benign hypervascular liver tumors, hemangiomas, and hemangioendotheliomas are relatively more common in the newborn period. Diagnosis is usually made by ultrasound, dynamic nuclear scintigraphy, or angiography. Although focal lesions can be resected, diffuse lesions are treated conservatively with hope they will spontaneously regress.

Following a segmental surgical resection of the liver in a child, CT demonstrates the remaining liver to hypertrophy (Fig. 21–23). The density of the enlarged liver can be slightly greater than normally encountered, perhaps because of additional glycogen deposits within the remaining segment of liver. The appearance of recurrent tumor or metastatic disease can be easily monitored by follow-up CT scans.

BILIARY ABNORMALITIES

CT detects obstructed bile ducts as branching structures of low density within the liver in both children (Fig. 21–22A) and in adults. However, because the incidence of tumors causing obstruction in pediatric patients is low and because ultrasound can determine the status of the biliary system with as high a degree of accuracy, ultrasound is recommended to initially evaluate the liver of the jaundiced child.

Choledochal cysts are uncommon lesions classically presenting with abdominal pain, a palpable abdominal mass, and jaundice; however, the clinical diagnosis can be obscure because the complete classic clinical triad is present in only 10 per cent of patients. Usually ultrasonography and technetium-IDA scintigraphy will permit a diagnosis of choledochal cyst to be made and additional imaging with CT is not necessary. However, if the diagnosis remains in doubt, CT will readily demonstrate the choledochal cyst as a cystic mass in continuity with the biliary system and will confirm the diagnosis.

SUSPECTED ABDOMINAL ABSCESSES

The localization of abscesses in children with fever and abdominal pain can be difficult. Plain abdominal films are sometimes diagnostic but additional imaging studies such as [67]gallium scanning, indium-labeled white blood cell scanning, ultrasonography, and CT are frequently needed.[17] Radionuclide imaging is useful in detecting abscesses but requires time (hours or days) to be completed and the images are often difficult to interpret because of nonspecific accumulation of the isotope within the bowel. The ultrasonographic search for abdominal abscesses can be

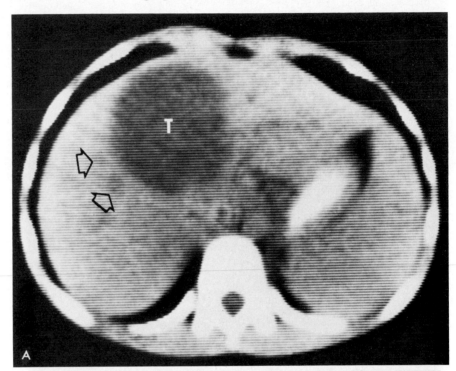

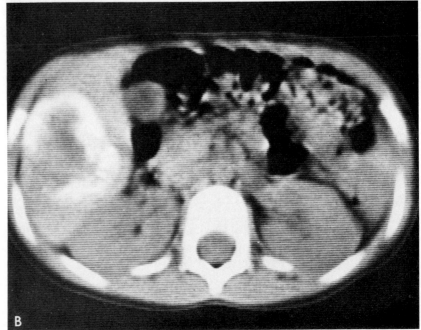

Figure 21–22. Two children with hepatoblastomas. range of CT appearances. **A** In one patient, the tumor (T) appeared as a rounded, low-density mass within the porta hepatis. Dilated bile ducts (open arrows) correlated well with clinical jaundice. Angiography was obtained preoperatively to better define the extent of this tumor. **B** In a second patient, the tumor is confined to the right lobe of the liver and is densely calcified. Because the tumor could be clearly localized to the right hepatic lobe, a hemihepatectomy was performed without preoperative angiography.

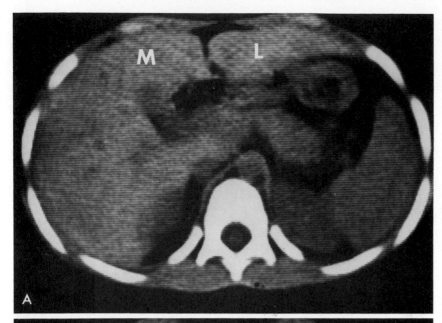

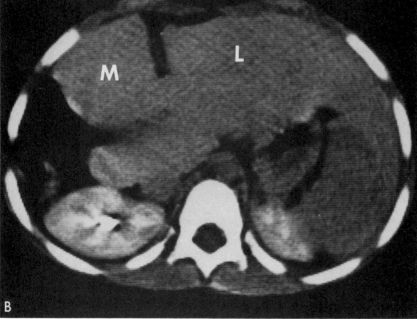

Figure 21–23. Hepatoblastoma. **A** CT scan demonstrates an ill-defined mass in the right hepatic lobe, but the medial (M) and lateral (L) segments of the left lobe are normal. **B** CT scan following right lobectomy reveals marked growth of the medial (M) and lateral (L) segments of the left lobe of the liver.

hindered by surgical dressings or by the presence of large amounts of gas (Fig. 21–24A). CT is rapid, noninvasive, accurate, and unaffected by dressings or gas and has become the most frequently employed imaging procedure for detection of abdominal abscesses (Fig. 21–24B).

The CT appearance of an abscess will depend in part on its location. Abscesses are often rounded, low-density mass lesions but may adapt to the shape of adjacent organs. Typically, the center of an abscess contains pus that does not enhance after contrast medium administration; however, the solid, inflammatory wall of the abscess fre-

quently does.[17] CT can detect gas within abscesses (Fig. 21–25), which is not clearly delineated by plain abdominal radiographs, and clearly determines the relationship of the abscess of adjacent structures. CT-guided aspiration of suspected abscesses can be safely performed to obtain a specimen for culture prior to treatment.

ABDOMINAL TRAUMA

The accuracy and ease of performance have made CT a primary imaging modality in cases of severe abdominal trauma to children. CT has been shown to be of value by accurately defining

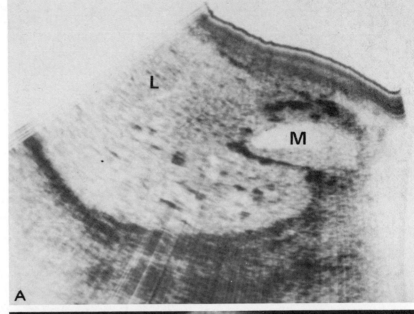

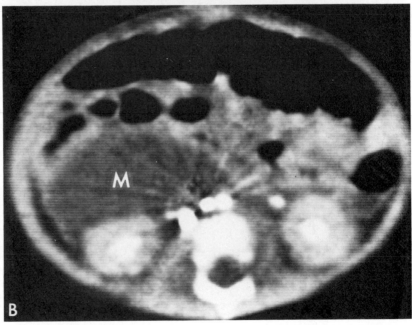

Figure 21–24. Postoperative abscess. **A** Right parasagittal ultrasonogram reveals a fluid collection (M) caudal to the liver (L). The mass contained high-amplitude margin echoes and was thought most likely to represent a loop of dilated right colon. **B** The corresponding transverse CT scan through the level of the kidneys shows a right upper-quadrant, low-density retroperitoneal mass (M) displacing the transverse colon. The CT diagnosis of abscess was confirmed surgically and attributed to dehiscence of appendectomy wound. (From Brasch RC, Abols IB, Gooding CA, Filly RA: Abdominal disease in children: A comparison of computed tomography and ultrasound. AJR 134:153, 1980. © 1980, American Roentgen Ray Society. Used with permission.)

the extent and severity of abdominal injury and by reducing the number of needed ancillary tests.[19] With CT, all abdominal viscera and compartments are imaged; unlike ultrasonography, CT does not require direct contact with the traumatized abdomen. Furthermore, contrast-enhanced CT enables vessel integrity, organ vascularity, and renal function to be evaluated. Ribs or a distended bowel pose no obstacle to the CT examination and compared with angiography, CT is less invasive, quicker, and easier to perform and interpret.

CT is employed as the initial imaging procedure in our center for the severely traumatized child whose vital signs are sufficiently stable to permit a safe CT examination. Unstable pediatric patients requiring operative intervention proceed directly to surgery without preliminary CT or other imaging examinations; the child who has signs or symptoms suggesting only a mild injury can be followed clinically, CT being performed only when the patient does not respond to conservative therapy or when there is sudden or marked deterioration.

The CT signs of renal trauma have been discussed extensively in Chapter 15. As in adults, ex-

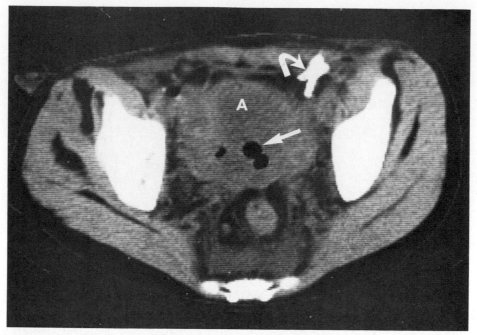

Figure 21–25. A pelvic abscess (A) containing gas (arrow) due to Crohn's disease. A surgical drain (curved arrow) does not communicate with the abscess.

perience with children indicates that CT is more accurate than urography in defining the extent of renal and perirenal injury (Fig. 21–26). The decision to treat conservatively or to operate can best be made after a CT examination.

Splenic (Fig. 21–27) and hepatic hematomas, either acute or subacute occult lesions, are clearly defined by CT. Subcapsular collections of fluid appear as low-density, homogeneous or mixed collections that can flatten or indent the splenic parenchyma. The treatment of a subcapsular splenic hematoma is becoming more conservative

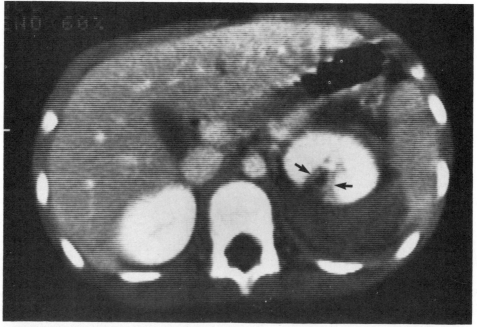

Figure 21–26. Perirenal hematoma and renal laceration. CT scan after intravenous administration in a child suffering a motor vehicle accident vividly depicts a large collection of blood posterior to the left kidney and a laceration (arrows) of the kidney extending from the surface to the center of the organ. The intravenous urogram of this patient underestimated the extent of the injury. (Courtesy of Dr. J. Kuhn, Buffalo Children's Hospital, Buffalo, N.Y.)

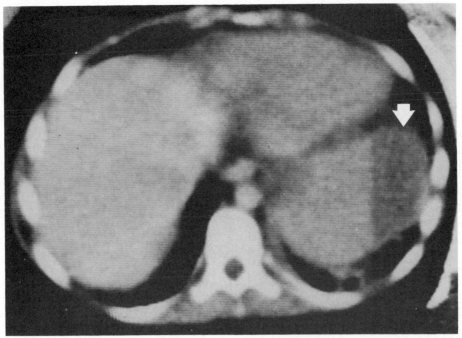

Figure 21–27. Splenic hematoma. Transverse CT scan through the upper abdomen of 12-year-old boy after contrast medium administration demonstrates area of low density (arrow) on the lateral aspect of the spleen. Note straight interface with medially compressed splenic tissue. (From Brasch RC, Korobkin M, Gooding CA: Computed body tomography in children: Evaluation of 45 patients. AJR 131:21, 1978. © 1978, American Roentgen Ray Society. Used with permission.)

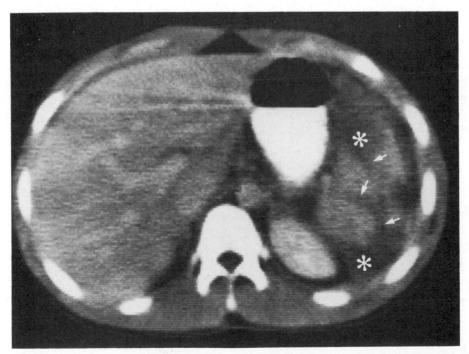

Figure 21–28. Fractured spleen. Transverse CT section through the upper abdomen of a child performed 1 hour after a severe motor vehicle accident demonstrates multiple low-density fracture planes (arrows) and blood (asterisks) surrounding the spleen.

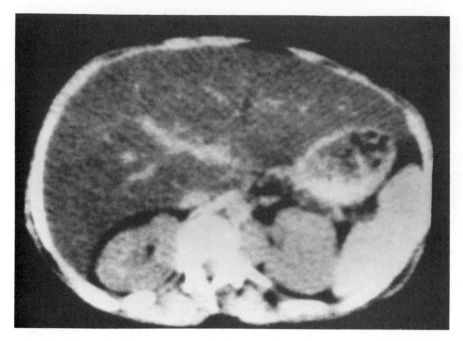

Figure 21–29. Fatty infiltration of the liver. CT section of an infant with lipoprotein-lipase deficiency demonstrates an overall decrease in attenuation of the liver attributable to fatty infiltration. The spleen and kidneys are uninvolved in this disorder and demonstrate normal attenuation values.

as the risks of splenectomy have become more appreciated, and repeated CT studies have shown that stable subcapsular hematomas do not enlarge or appear to be prone to rupture.

Splenic fractures appear on CT as irregular, linear low-density bands, separating solid parenchymal tissue (Fig. 21–28). Blood is identified in the paracolic gutter, or Morrison's pouch.

INFILTRATIVE DISEASES OF THE LIVER

The ability to measure the x-ray absorption of a tissue numerically is a unique feature of the CT method, which has amplified its diagnostic yield. For example, CT can measure the change in density of a lesion after intravenous contrast medium administration and thus gauge the vascularity of the lesion. The ability to measure density numerically has also been used to diagnose and precisely quantitate infiltration of the liver by a variety of substances.

Fatty infiltration of the liver occurs in a variety of diseases and is manifest on CT by a focal or diffuse decrease in hepatic density (Fig. 21–29). The decrease in hepatic attenuation value is directly proportional to the amount of fat present

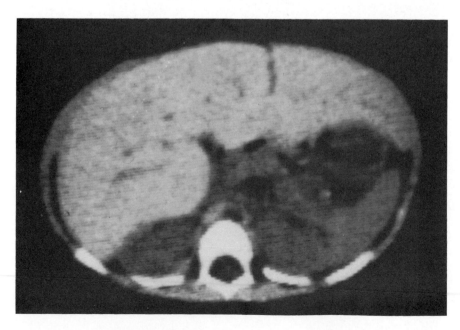

Figure 21–30. Glycogen storage disease manifest as a diffuse increase in hepatic density. The kidneys and spleen are of normal density in Type I glycogen storage disease.

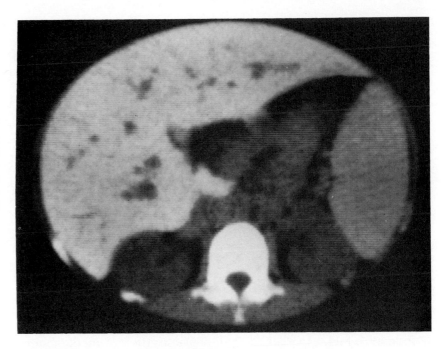

Figure 21–31. Hemochromatosis. CT section of a 15-year-old child with thalassemia treated with repeated blood transfusions. There is a dramatic increase in liver density as a result of iron deposition. The attenuation increase of the spleen is less prominent.

in the liver.[20] Conversely, glycogen infiltration of the liver, which occurs in newborn infants with glycogen storage disease and infants of diabetic mothers, can be manifest on CT as a diffuse (Fig. 21–30) or patchy increase in liver density.[21]

Iron deposition in hemachromatosis is similar to glycogen in that it also causes an increase in the liver density (Fig. 21–31). Using a dual-energy scanning technique, scanning the same region at 80 and 120 kVp, there is a linear relationship between the amount of iron deposition and the difference in the CT number observed at the two scanning energies.[20] In experimental animal studies, these investigators found a change of 24 Hounsfield Units (H) per gram per cent of iron within the liver. Dual-energy CT scanning thus can provide an accurate, noninvasive method for quantitating liver iron content. However, dual-energy CT techniques are not as precise for quantification of hepatic glycogen because the potassium edge of glycogen, unlike iron, is relatively close to the potassium edge for water. The CT density of glycogen thus changes less than iron when scanned at lower energies.[20] (A more complete discussion of the use of CT to quantitate hepatic iron, glycogen, and fat is presented in Chapter 23.)

As in adults, CT frequently does not detect hepatic density changes in children with hepatitis or cirrhosis. Portal hypertension is diagnosed only indirectly by demonstrating collateral vascular channels, and leukemia and lymphoma usually are manifest only by diffuse hepatomegaly.

THORACIC ABNORMALITIES

Computed tomography of the thorax of children is valuable in the evaluation of abnormalities involving the lungs, mediastinum, pleurae, and chest wall.[22–25] The use of CT scanners with scan times less than 5 seconds has sharply increased the number of diagnostic examinations by reducing the motion artifacts present in CT studies obtained with longer scan times. Reduction of scan times to 2 seconds or less promises to further increase the diagnostic yield of pediatric thoracic CT studies. Although a great variety of the pediatric thoracic abnormalities can be studied by CT, the two most common indications for thoracic CT are to search for pulmonary metastatic lesions and to evaluate mediastinal mass lesions.

PULMONARY METASTASES

The search for metastatic pulmonary lesions is the most frequent indication for pediatric chest CT. Small metastatic nodules that cannot be diagnosed by conventional chest radiography or linear tomography can be demonstrated by CT (Fig. 21–11). Conversely, the cross-sectional anatomic format of CT permits the exclusion of lesions that are suggested by conventional radiographic studies. In children with known primary extrathoracic tumors that frequently metastasize to the lungs, a chest scan is performed in concert with CT imaging of the primary extrathoracic tumor. Wilms' tumor, osteogenic sarcoma, rhabdomyosarcoma, and malignant teratoma are common pediatric tumors that frequently metastasize to the lung and warrant a thoracic CT examination. The thoracic CT examination is performed in lieu of full lung tomography and is always obtained prior to surgery to resect pulmonary metastasis.

Numerous studies have demonstrated the remarkable sensitivity of CT for the detection of pulmonary nodules.[25-26] Unfortunately, in adult patients the specificity of CT for the differentiation of benign and malignant pulmonary nodules is poor, with greater than 50 per cent of adult pulmonary nodules detected by CT being benign histologically.[26] However, in children benign subpleural lymph nodes or granulomas are considerably less common and the CT detection of a nodule in a child with malignancy is thus highly specific for metastases. After scanning of more than 100 children with neoplasms, in only one instance did a benign pulmonary nodule mimic a metastatic lesion. Demonstration of a pulmonary nodule in a child, especially if granulomatous disease of the lung is not endemic to the area, then, should be taken as evidence of metastatic disease until the nodule is proved to be benign.

MEDIASTINAL MASSES

The CT evaluation of mediastinal masses can provide accurate information concerning the anatomic compartment of origin, the relationships of the mass to adjacent structures, and tissue characteristics of the mass itself. Mediastinal CT is complementary to pain chest radiography and should be performed in all children with suspected or definite mediastinal masses. In a series of 23 children having mediastinal CT and plain chest radiography, CT provided information additional to that from chest radiographs in 82 per cent of cases and contributed to a substantial change in therapy in 65 per cent of patients.[23] Elimination of a planned thoracotomy was the most frequent change in therapy brought about by CT.

Frequent causes of mediastinal masses in children include neurogenic tumor, teratoma, lymphoma, foregut cysts, and thymus (Fig. 21–32). Masses of vascular origin, although relatively rare in children, can be readily differentiated by CT (Fig. 21–33). Pediatric CT metrizamide myelography is particularly useful in the evaluation of intraspinal extension of posterior mediastinal masses whether or not neurologic abnormalities are present.[27]

The thymic gland of children is highly variable in size and shape and prior to CT was a particularly difficult organ to examine radiographically.

However, both the normal and pathologic thymus gland is readily imaged by CT.[28, 29] Baron and colleagues identified the thymus by CT in 100 per cent of patients under 30 years of age and described the CT appearance of the normal and abnormal thymus.[28, 29]

The thymus is usually located in the anterior mediastinum between the brachiocephalic vessels superiorly and the base of the great vessels inferiorly. The thymus gland frequently appears as two separate lobes or as an arrowhead-shaped structure formed by the confluence of the two lobes (Fig. 21–32). In children, the thymus tends to be less fatty than in adults and has a correspondingly higher CT number that is equal to or greater than that of the chest wall musculature.

Thymic attenuation values progressively decrease in older patients, finally approaching those of fat.[28] The thickness of the normal thymus is less than 1.8 cm. When thicker glands are identified, abnormalities such as Hodgkin's disease, hyperplasia associated with myasthenia gravis, or Graves' disease, cystic teratoma, germ cell tumor,

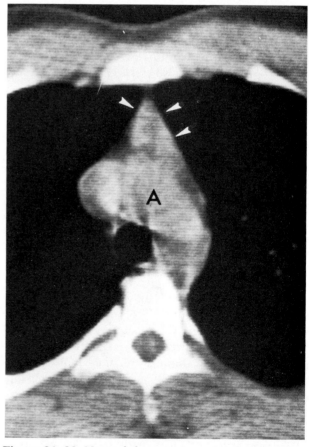

Figure 21–32. Normal thymus. Arrowhead-shaped thymus (arrowheads) lies anterior to the aorta (A). Density of the thymus is similar to that of the chest wall muscles.

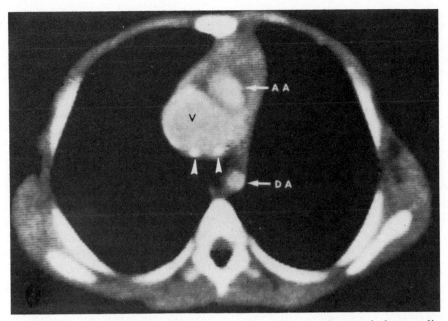

Figure 21–33. Thoracic aortic aneurysm. A 6-year-old boy with an abnormal chest radiograph demonstrating curvilinear mediastinal calcification. A CT scan with intravenous contrast enhancement, demonstrates that the calcification (arrowheads) proven to be an aortic aneurysm surrounded a markedly dilated vessel (v) is arising from the ascending aorta (AA). DA=Descending aorta. (From Skoildbrand CG, Brasch RC, Lipton MJ: Utility of computer tomography in the diagnosis of thoracic aneurysm in childhood. Cardiovasc Intervent Radiol 4:30, 1981.)

and benign cysts must be excluded. Focal thymic masses are produced by teratomas, germ cell tumors, and benign cysts. Either benign hyperplasia or malignant lymphoma can cause diffuse thymic enlargement. Compared with adult patients having myasthenia gravis, there is no need to examine the thymus of a child with myasthenia gravis in search for a thymoma because thymomas are not found in patients with juvenile myasthenia gravis.[1]

RISKS OF COMPUTED TOMOGRAPHY IN CHILDREN

Computed tomography is not a noninvasive procedure. Although CT scanning may be less invasive than certain diagnostic procedures such as angiography and exploratory surgery, there is still a potential for morbidity and even death. Potential complications may arise from sedation, hypothermia, the administration of radiographic contrast media, and radiation exposure. Although these risks associated with CT scanning appear relatively slight compared with the potential diagnostic benefit, only by considering the "down-

side" risks can we make intelligent decisions about when to employ CT or alternative diagnostic modalities.

The risk of contrast medium toxicity in children appears to be extremely low. The rate of fatal reactions in patients of all ages is approximately one in 40,000 exposures,[30] and a prospective toxicity study limited to children receiving intravenous contrast material indicates that reactions may be even less common in the pediatric age group.[31] Major reactions were observed in only five of 12,419 contrast medium administrations and none of these was fatal.[31]

Exposure to ionizing radiation is perhaps the major negative aspect of CT scanning and is of particular import for pediatric patients. Information on radiation exposure levels is essential for both the radiologist and the referring clinician if they are to make appropriate selection of patients for CT examinations.

A study by Brasch and Cann compared the radiation exposures and resolving capabilities of seven different late-model CT scanners.[4] Surface and internal radiation exposures for abdominal CT of children were measured using child- and infant-sized phantoms. High-contrast resolving power and low-contrast discrimination for each scanner were determined simultaneously with ra-

Table 21–2. SKIN DOSE AND RESOLVING POWER WITH 66 CM PHANTOM*

CT Model (year)	Average Quadrant Skin Dose		High-Contrast (12%) Resolving Power
	rad	(Gy)	mm
General Electric 8800 (1980)	0.5	(0.005)	1.25
EMI 7070 (1979)	1.0	(0.01)	1.00
Pfizer 0450 (1979)	4.6	(0.046)	1.50
Technicare Delta 2020 (1980)	2.2	(0.022)	1.25
Elscint Excel 905 (1980)	0.8	(0.008)	1.50–1.75
Picker Synerview 600 (1980)	1.0	(0.01)	1.25
Siemens Somatom 2 (1980)	0.6	(0.006)	1.50
Mean	1.5	(0.015)	1.38
General Electric CT/T7800 (1977)	0.5	(0.005)	2.25
EMI CT 500 (1977)	3.1	(0.031)	2.25
Pfizer 200FS (1977)	2.3	(0.023)	2.00
Ohio Nuclear Delta 2000 (1977)	2.5	(0.025)	1.75
Ohio Nuclear Delta 50FS (1977)	1.0	(0.01)	2.00
Ohio Nuclear Delta 50 (1977)	1.8	(0.018)	2.00
Varian CT (1977)	4.3	(0.043)	1.75
Mean	2.2	(0.022)	2.00

*From Basch RC, Cann CE: Computed tomographic scanning in children: II. An updated comparison of radiation dose and resolving power of commercial scanners. AJR 138:127, 1982. © 1982, American Roentgen Ray Society. Used with permission.

diation measurements, and the results were compared with those from a similar study conducted in 1977 with earlier CT models.[3] Because the two studies were performed in a similar fashion and using the same phantoms, it was possible to evaluate trends in radiation exposure and resolving power resulting from design alterations in CT equipment.

The average circumferential surface doses for simulated pediatric CT body examinations were 31 per cent lower in the later study compared with 1977 results with a mean of 1.5 rad (0.015 Gy) versus 2.2 rad (0.022 Gy), respectively (Table 21–2). At the same time, resolving power for high-contrast (12 per cent) improved by 31 per cent to a mean of 1.38 mm from 2.0 mm (Fig. 21–34) and all scanners of current vintage could resolve low-contrast differences of 0.25 per cent for a 5-mm object. Results of radiation dose determinations from the 66-mm phantom, designed to simulate the size of a 10-year-old abdomen, revealed a relative uniformity of radiation exposure throughout the cross sections (Fig. 21–35). In some cases, the central radiation measurement exceeds the maximum surface exposure.

The general improvement in CT dose efficiency can be attributed to several engineering modifications in the newer CT scan models. Early stationary-ring scanners had comparatively few

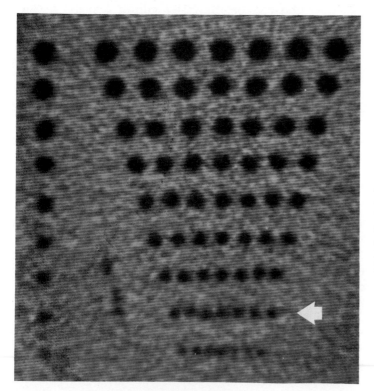

Figure 21–34. CT image of resolving power phantom. Holes in the eighth row (arrow), 1.25 mm in diameter, are seen as distinct and separate circles. Holes in the ninth row, 1.00 mm in diameter, are indistinct. Resolving power of this image is recorded as 1.25 mm. (From Brasch RC, Cann CE: Computed tomographic scanning in children: II. An updated comparison of radiation dose and resolving power of commercial scanners. AJR 138:127–133, 1982. © 1982, American Roentgen Ray Society. Used with permission.)

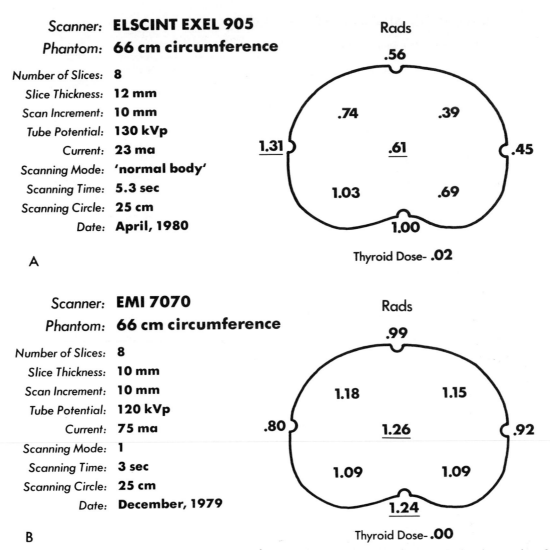

Scanner:	**ELSCINT EXEL 905**
Phantom:	**66 cm circumference**
Number of Slices:	**8**
Slice Thickness:	**12 mm**
Scan Increment:	**10 mm**
Tube Potential:	**130 kVp**
Current:	**23 ma**
Scanning Mode:	**'normal body'**
Scanning Time:	**5.3 sec**
Scanning Circle:	**25 cm**
Date:	**April, 1980**

A

Rads

.56

.74   .39

1.31   .61   .45

1.03   .69

1.00

Thyroid Dose- **.02**

Scanner:	**EMI 7070**
Phantom:	**66 cm circumference**
Number of Slices:	**8**
Slice Thickness:	**10 mm**
Scan Increment:	**10 mm**
Tube Potential:	**120 kVp**
Current:	**75 ma**
Scanning Mode:	**1**
Scanning Time:	**3 sec**
Scanning Circle:	**25 cm**
Date:	**December, 1979**

B

Rads

.99

1.18   1.15

.80   1.26   .92

1.09   1.09

1.24

Thyroid Dose- **.00**

Figure 21–35. A–F Pediatric radiation dosimetry. Results of radiation dose determinations using 66 cm diameter pediatric phantom and six commercially available CT scanners. All dose data except thyroid dose reflect radiation exposure in the central plane of eight CT sections. Midplane and maximum skin doses are underlined. International system of units: 1 rad = 0.01 Gy. (From Brasch RC, Cann CE: Computed tomographic scanning in children: II. An updated comparison of radiation dose and resolving power of commercial scanners. AJR 138:127, 1982. © 1982, American Roentgen Ray Society. Used with permission.)

Illustration continued on following page

detectors in the beam path with gaps between detectors, which resulted in underutilization of transmitted x-ray photons and higher patient dose. New configurations using closely packed detectors, more efficient scintillators, and more stable photodiodes have made the newer systems more dose efficient. Further, new x-ray tubes with high heat-load capabilities allow shorter scan times, reducing motion artifacts and the need for repeat scans. Another factor is the trend toward the use of small focus x-ray tubes and improvements in collimator design to reduce out-of-plane penumbra radiation.

Simultaneous to the technologic improvement in CT systems, radiologists have become more facile in the performance and interpretation of CT studies. Although future technologic advances may continue to increase CT dose efficiency, the radiologist and technologist have an important role in minimizing the patient radiation exposures by selecting the optimal technique factors for each patient and diagnostic problem. For example, a search for lung metastases (high contrast) can be done using lower exposure than the evaluation of the liver for low-contrast infiltrative or metastatic disease.

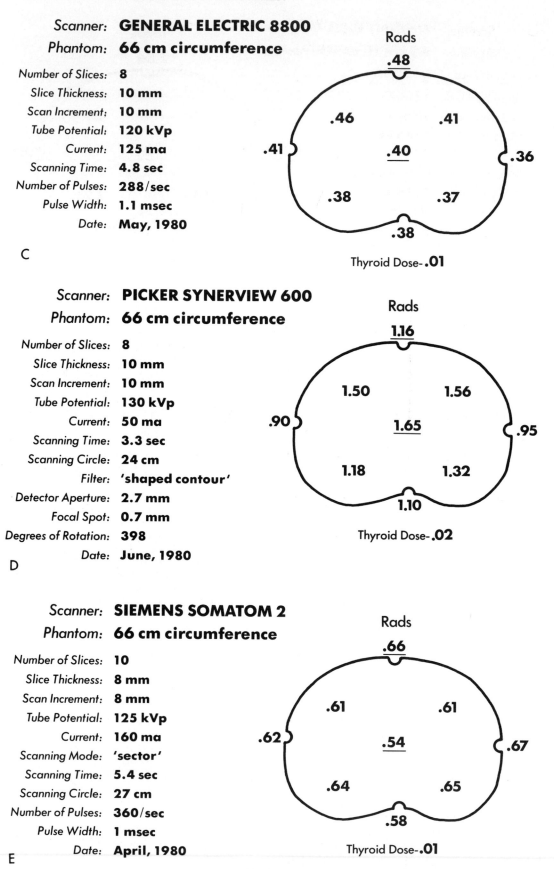

Scanner: **GENERAL ELECTRIC 8800**
Phantom: **66 cm circumference**

Number of Slices: **8**
Slice Thickness: **10 mm**
Scan Increment: **10 mm**
Tube Potential: **120 kVp**
Current: **125 ma**
Scanning Time: **4.8 sec**
Number of Pulses: **288/sec**
Pulse Width: **1.1 msec**
Date: **May, 1980**

C

Rads
.48
.46   .41
.41   .40   .36
.38   .37
.38
Thyroid Dose-**.01**

Scanner: **PICKER SYNERVIEW 600**
Phantom: **66 cm circumference**

Number of Slices: **8**
Slice Thickness: **10 mm**
Scan Increment: **10 mm**
Tube Potential: **130 kVp**
Current: **50 ma**
Scanning Time: **3.3 sec**
Scanning Circle: **24 cm**
Filter: **'shaped contour'**
Detector Aperture: **2.7 mm**
Focal Spot: **0.7 mm**
Degrees of Rotation: **398**
Date: **June, 1980**

D

Rads
1.16
1.50   1.56
.90   1.65   .95
1.18   1.32
1.10
Thyroid Dose-**.02**

Scanner: **SIEMENS SOMATOM 2**
Phantom: **66 cm circumference**

Number of Slices: **10**
Slice Thickness: **8 mm**
Scan Increment: **8 mm**
Tube Potential: **125 kVp**
Current: **160 ma**
Scanning Mode: **'sector'**
Scanning Time: **5.4 sec**
Scanning Circle: **27 cm**
Number of Pulses: **360/sec**
Pulse Width: **1 msec**
Date: **April, 1980**

E

Rads
.66
.61   .61
.62   .54   .67
.64   .65
.58
Thyroid Dose-**.01**

Figure 21–35. *Continued*

Illustration continued on opposite page

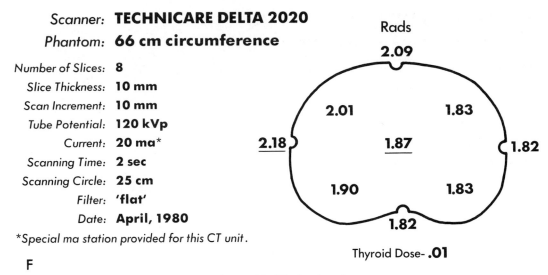

Figure 21–35. *Continued*

REFERENCES

1. Thurmond HS, Brasch RC: Radiologic evaluation of the thymus in juvenile myasthenia gravis. Pediatr Radiol 7:136, 1978.
2. Brasch RC, Korobkin M, Gooding CA: Computed body tomography in children: Evaluation of 45 patients. AJR 131:21, 1978.
3. Brasch RC, Boyd DP, Gooding CA: Computed tomographic scanning in children: Comparison of radiation dose and resolving power of commercial CT scanners. AJR 131:95, 1978.
4. Brasch RC, Cann CE: Computed tomographic scanning in children: II. An updated comparison of radiation dose and resolving power of commercial scanners. AJR 138:127, 1982.
5. Berger PE, Kuhn JP (eds): Pediatric Computed Tomography. Radiol Clin North Am, vol 19, No. 3, 1981, pp. 399–545.
6. Chopra II, Teele RL: Hydronephrosis in children: Narrowing the differential diagnosis with ultrasound. JCU 8:473, 1980.
7. Brasch RC, Abols IB, Gooding CA, Filly RA: Abdominal disease in children: A comparison of computed tomography and ultrasound. AJR 134:153, 1980.
8. Melicow MS, Urar AC: Palpable abdominal masses in infants and children: A reported based on a review of 653 cases. J Urol 81:705, 1959.
9. Shackelford GD, McAlister W: Errors in diagnosis of Wilms' tumor. CRC: Critical Rev Radiol Sci 3:171, 1972.
10. Brasch RC: Computed tomography in the evaluation of pediatric genitourinary disease. Urol Clin North Am 7:223, 1980.
11. Grossman H: Wilms tumor. In Parker and Castellino RA (eds): Pediatric Oncologic Radiology. St Louis, CV Mosby Co, 1977, pp 237–263.
12. Brasch RC, Randel SB, Gould RG: Follow-up of Wilms'
tumor: Comparison of CT with other imaging procedures. AJR 137:1005, 1981.
13. Kirks DR, Merten DF, Grossman A, Bowie JD: Diagnostic imaging of pediatric abdominal masses: An overview. Radiol Clin North Am 19:527, 1981.
14. Griscom NT: The roentgenology of neonatal abdominal masses. AJR 93:447, 1965.
15. Towbin R, Cruppo RA: Pulmonary metastases in neuroblastoma. AJR 138:75, 1982.
15a. Stark DD, Moss AA, Brasch RC, deLorimier AA, Ablin AR, London DA, Goading CA: Neuroblastoma: Diagnostic imaging and staging. Radiology 148:101, 1983.
16. Hecht ST, Brasch RC, Styne D: CT localization of occult secretory tumors in children. Pediatr Radiol 12:67, 1982.
16a. Podrasky AE, Stark DD, Hattner RS, Gooding CA, Moss AA: Radionuclide bone scanning in neuroblastoma: Skeletal metastases and primary tumor localization of 99m TCMDP. (in press).
16b. Stark DD, Brasch RC, Moss AA, deLorimier AA, Ablin AR, London DA, Gooding CA: Recurrent Neuroblastoma: The role of CT and alternative imaging tests. Radiology 148:107, 1983.
17. Afshani E: Computed tomography of abdominal abscesses in children. Radiol Clin North Am 19:515, 1981.
18. Exelby PR, Miller RM, Grosfeld JL: Liver tumors in children in the particular reference to hepatoblastoma and hepatocellular carcinoma. J Pediatr Surg 10:329, 1975.
19. Berger PE, Kuhn JP: CT of blunt abdominal trauma in childhood. AJR 136:105, 1981.
20. Goldberg HI, Cann CE, Moss AA, Ohto M, Brito A, Federle M: Non-invasive quantitation of liver iron in dogs with hemochromatosis using dual energy CT scanning. Invest Radiol 17:375, 1982.
21. Goldberg HI: CT scanning of diffuse parenchymal liver disease. In Moss AA, Goldberg HI (eds): Computed Tomography, Ultrasound and X-Ray: An Integrated

Approach 1980. Berkeley, University of California Press, 1980, pp 177–188.

22. Kirks DR, Korobkin M: Computed tomography of the chest wall, pleura, and pulmonary parenchyma in infants and children. Radiol Clin North Am 19:421, 1981.

23. Siegel JM, Sagel SS, Reed K: The value of computed tomography in diagnosis and management of pediatric mediastinal abnormalities. Radiology 142:149, 1982.

24. Skoildbrand CG, Brasch RC, Lipton MJ: Utility of computed tomography in the diagnosis of thoracic aneurysm in childhood. Cardiovasc Intervent Radiol 4:30, 1981.

25. Muhm JR, Brown LR, Crowe JK, Sheedy PF II, Hattery RR, Stephens DA: Comparison of computed and conventional whole lung tomography in detecting pulmonary nodules. AJR 131:981, 1978.

26. Siegelman SS, Zerhouni EA, Leo FP, Khouri NF, Titik FP: CT of the solitary pulmonary nodule. AJR 135:1, 1980.

27. Harwood-Nash DC: Computed tomography of the pediatric spine: A protocol for the 1980's. Radiol Clin North Am 19:479, 1981.

28. Baron RL, Lee JKT, Sagel SS, Peterson RL: Computed tomography of the normal thymus. Radiology 142: 121, 1982.

29. Baron RL, Lee JKT, Sagel SS, Peterson RL: Computed tomography of the abnormal thymus. Radiology 142:127, 1982.

30. Shehadi WH, Toniolo G: Adverse reactions to contrast media. Radiology 137:299, 1980.

31. Gooding CA, Berdon WE, Brodeur AE, Rowen M: Adverse reactions to intravenous pyelography in children. AJR 123:801, 1975.

22 INTERVENTIONAL COMPUTED TOMOGRAPHY

Albert A. Moss

Many imaging techniques, including fluoroscopy,[1–4] angiography,[5–6] endoscopic retrograde cholangiopancreatography (ERCP),[7] ultrasonography,[8–11] nuclear imaging,[12] and computed tomography (CT)[13–19] have been used to guide fine-needle interventional procedures. Each technique has advantages and limitations in guiding specific interventional procedures, and selection of the most appropriate technique demands the consideration of a variety of factors.

Since its introduction, CT has been used to guide percutaneous interventional procedures.[20] CT precisely defines the relationship of a needle to the surrounding tissues. Thus, if the needle tip is demonstrated by CT, its precise position is assured, limited only by the thickness of the CT section. In a CT section, 1 cm thick, the needle tip can be located within a 5-mm range on the z-axis, and because the spatial resolution of current CT scanners is less than 3 mm in the x-y plane,[21] the actual location of the needle is known within very narrow limits. Because CT can identify and localize lesions less than 1 cm in diameter, the size of the smallest lesion that can undergo biopsy depends more on the technical skill of the radiologist in placing the needle into a small mass rather than in detecting the lesion.

A major advantage of CT over other imaging techniques is its capacity to image materials ranging in density from air to metal. The capability of CT to image materials with high attenuation values permits the use of oral, rectal, and intravenous contrast material as diagnostic aids in CT scanning. An abscess can be readily distinguished from bowel when the bowel is filled with contrast medium. Intravenous contrast medium permits better definition of the relationship of a mass to nearby vascular structures, improves the detectability of certain mass lesions, and provides an assessment of tumor vascularity before biopsy. Injection of iodinated urographic contrast medium into cysts, abscesses, or fistulas delineates the true extent of the abnormal cavity, reveals any communicating tracts, and permits assessment of the inner margin of the cystic space. In addition, CT images are not significantly degraded by external dressings, open wounds, ostomy devices, or drainage catheters and low-density lesions can be imaged even if they are adjacent to high-density material.

The indications for percutaneous interventional procedures are rapidly evolving as new equipment is developed, experience is accumulated, and the risks and benefits of the procedures are more completely defined. Lesions readily demonstrated by conventional radiographic techniques are biopsied under fluoroscopic guidance and ultrasonography is employed whenever ultrasound clearly images a lesion and a safe approach can be assured.

CT is most frequently used to guide interventional procedures for:

1. Biopsy of lesions not easily demonstrated by other imaging techniques.

2. Masses less than 3 cm in diameter.

3. Lesions closely related to bone, blood vessels or bowel.

4. Deep lesions.

5. Mediastinal masses.

6. Pulmonary parenchymal lesions that cannot be biopsied fluoroscopically.

7. Intra-abdominal abscesses requiring catheter drainage.

8. Neurolysis.

9. Repeated biopsies when a biopsy has been unsuccessful by other methods.

CT-guided interventional procedures require expensive, often heavily used scanning instruments, and therefore, such procedures are more costly than those guided by fluoroscopy or ultrasound.

CT-GUIDED PERCUTANEOUS BIOPSIES

Whenever possible, a full diagnostic CT scan is performed before a CT-guided biopsy. The biopsy is scheduled only after review of the diag-nostic CT scan, history, physical findings, and laboratory results with the referring physician. Selection of the type of needle and technique to be used is based on the depth and location of the abnormality and its relationship to bone, vascular structures, bowel, or pleura.

PATIENT PREPARATION

Patients are given a clear liquid diet on the day of the biopsy to minimize the chance of aspiration

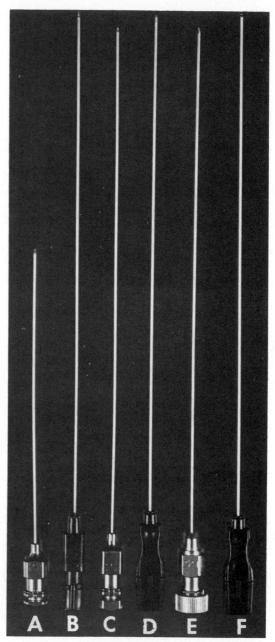

Figure 22–1. Various 22-gauge needles used for cytologic biopsies. A = Spinal needle; B = Green needle; C = Madayag needle; D = Turner needle; E = Franseen needle; F = Chiba needle.

DESIGN   GAUGES

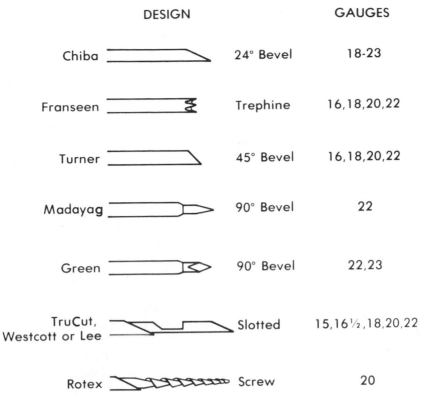

Chiba   24° Bevel   18-23

Franseen   Trephine   16,18,20,22

Turner   45° Bevel   16,18,20,22

Madayag   90° Bevel   22

Green   90° Bevel   22,23

TruCut,   Slotted   15,16½,18,20,22
Westcott or Lee

Rotex   Screw   20

Figure 22–2. Needles most frequently employed in CT-directed biopsies. (Modified from Lieberman RP, Hafez GR, Crummy AB: Histology from aspiration biopsy: Turner needle experience. AJR 138:561, 1982. © 1982, American Roentgen Ray Society. Used with permission.)

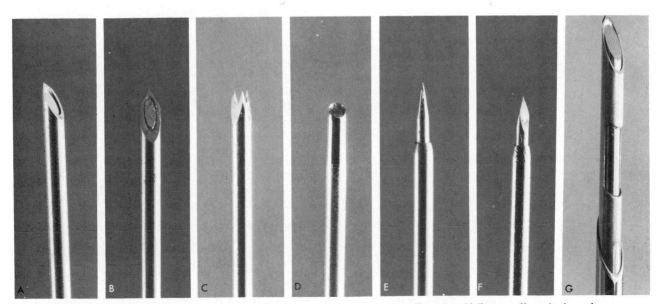

Figure 22–3. Close-up photographs of tips of various biopsy needles. **A** Chiba needle—tip has short (24°) noncutting bevel. **B** Spinal needle—tip has slightly longer, cutting bevel. **C** Franseen needle—trephine tip with three cutting teeth. **D** Turner needle—beveled tip (45°) with inner cutting edge. **E** Madayag needle—beveled tip (90°) with a conical stylet. **F** Green needle—beveled tip (90°) with a diamond-shaped stylet. **G** TruCut Lee, or Westcott needle—slotted, three pieces.

should emesis occur. Premedication is not routinely given except to pediatric patients. As a precaution, a prothrombin time and platelet count are obtained before performing a biopsy with a needle larger than 20 gauge. A low platelet count or a prothrombin time more than 50 per cent above normal are relative contraindications to a percutaneous biopsy; in these situations, we attempt to correct the abnormality before proceeding with the biopsy. If a bleeding tendency still persists after attempted correction, the indications for the biopsy should be carefully reassessed in view of the increased hazards of the procedure. Should a biopsy still be clinically indicated, the smallest needle possible should be used, and typed, cross-matched whole blood should be readily available. Using a 22-gauge thin needle, we

have performed biopsies without complications in patients with abnormal clotting factors.

MATERIALS

Needles for Cytologic Aspiration

Material for cytologic evaluation can be aspirated using a variety of fine-gauge needles (Figs. 22–1 and 22–2). Because each needle for cytologic aspiration has advantages and limitations, a complete selection should be available before the biopsy. We usually use a 22-gauge, thin-walled flexible Chiba needle. The original Chiba 22-gauge needle had an outer diameter of 0.028 inch and an inner diameter of 0.015 inch[22]; a more flexible needle with the same outer diameter and a larger inner diameter (0.020 inch) has since become available (Cook, Inc.).[22]

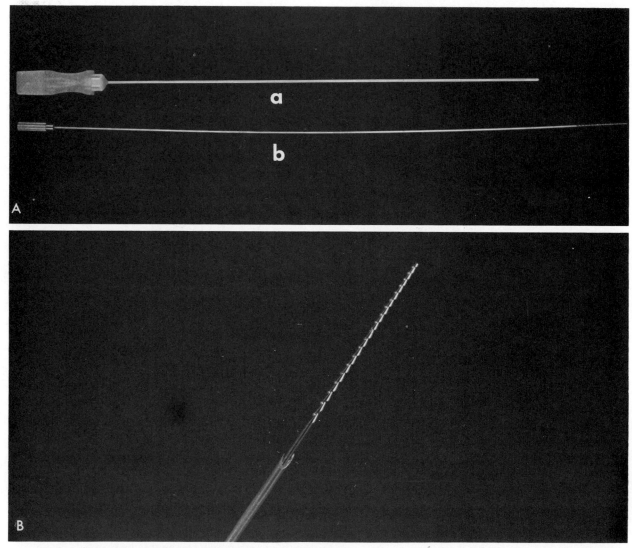

Figure 22–4. Rolex needle. **A** Components. a=Outer cannula; b=inner screw-shaped needle. **B** Tapered screw passing through outer cannula (magnified view).

The thinner-walled needle permits slightly more material to be obtained but is somewhat more difficult to direct. Both needles are made of flexible steel and have an inner stylet. The original Chiba needle had noncutting bevel of 30°,[22] which was modified to 24° to facilitate introduction of the needle and dislodgment of bits of tissue as the needle is rotated (Fig. 22–3A). Needles of the same design are available in 18- to 23-gauge sizes.

The 22-gauge needle is employed for cytologic aspiration because larger needles frequently permit aspiration of more blood but little additional tissue. Biopsies of deep-seated lesions or masses in obese patients are more easily performed using a larger-gauge needle, which provides improved direction control as it is passed through the abdomen, retroperitoneum, and subcutaneous tissue.

Cytologic aspiration can also be done with spinal needles of various lengths and gauges

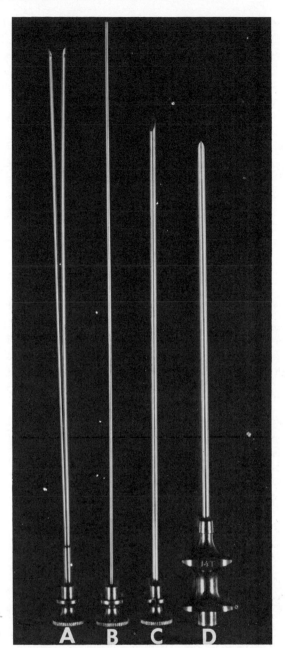

Figure 22–6. Vim-Silverman needle. A = 17-gauge inner split cutting cannula; B = blunt stylet for removing tissue from split cannula; C,D = 14-gauge outer beveled cannula with fitted stylet.

(Figs. 22–1A and 22–3B). Spinal needles are less flexible and easier to control than thinner-walled needles; their short length makes them ideal for biopsies of superficial lesions.

Needles for Histologic Sampling

Many needles with a cutting edge for obtaining tissue for histologic analysis are available. Some needles are designed for biopsy of a particular or-

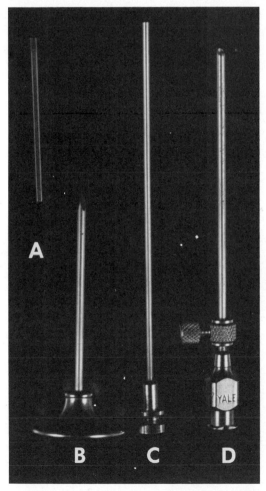

Figure 22–5. Menghini needle. A = Biopsy-retaining pin to prevent biopsy sample from extending up entire length of cannula or extruding into syringe; B = trocar for initial skin puncture; C = stylet to push biopsy specimen out of needle; D = thin-wall needle with bevel of 45° to 50° and sharpened edge (side stop can be adjusted to ensure biopsy at premeasured depth).

gan, such as liver or bone, while others are used as general-purpose biopsy needles.

Thin-walled needles designed to obtain tissue for histologic analysis are available in 22-, 20-, and 18-gauge sizes (Fig. 22–3). The Franseen needle (Cook, Inc.) has three cutting teeth that detach pieces of tissue when the needle is rotated (Fig. 22–3C). The Turner needle (Cook, Inc.) consists of a cutting cannula with a flat, 45° beveled cutting tip and a fitted obturator (Fig. 22–3D). The tip of the Turner needle occasionally makes entry difficult, but it cuts a core of tissue that remains in the needle when the needle is rotated. The Madayag needle (Johannah Medical Services, Inc.) has a 90° bevel and a conical stylet (Fig. 22–3E). The Green needle (Cook, Inc.) is identical except for its multifaceted diamond-shaped stylet (Fig. 22–3F).

Larger-gauge needles permit larger pieces of tissue to be obtained, and the tissue specimens can be fixed and stained in a conventional manner. The TruCut needle (Travenol Laboratories, Inc.) (Fig. 22–3G) has been used for biopsies of pleural, chest wall, and soft-tissue lesions.[4, 23] The

needle has an outer cutting cannula through which an inner component containing a 2-mm specimen slot is passed. After insertion of the needle, the cutting cannula is slid over the inner component, slicing the specimen and holding it for retrieval. The Lee and Westcott needles (Becton-Dickinson) are similar to the TruCut but have a smaller gauge.

The Rotex (Travenol Laboratories, Inc.) biopsy instrument is designed to collect tissue without significant dilution of the specimen by blood (Figs. 22–2 and 22–4). The instrument consists of two parts: a stainless steel needle 0.55 mm in diameter and 205 mm long with a distal end consisting of a 17-mm tapered screw, and a cannula 0.8 mm in diameter and 157 mm long. The needle is passed through the cannula and rotated into the mass by a small handle on the needle. The outer cannula slides over the screw, and the needle and cannula are removed together.

The Menghini needle (Fig. 22–5) is a cutting instrument used primarily for biopsy of the liver and solid avascular abdominal or pelvic masses. The needle is available in 15 to 19-gauge sizes in

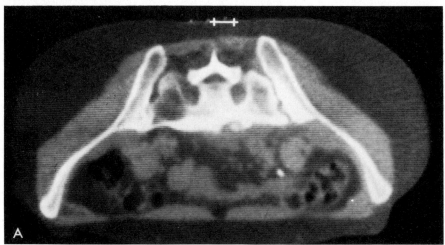

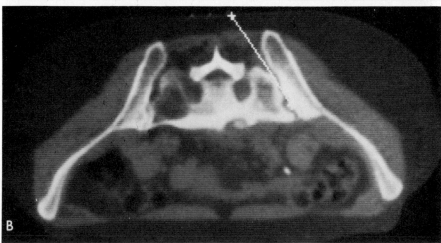

Figure 22–7. Method of CT-guided biopsy. **A** CT scan in prone position. There is sclerosis of the right sacroiliac joint with slight widening of the joint space. A distance of 1.6 cm was measured from the midline and selected as the site of needle entry. **B** Simulated placement of needle into joint space. CT console-measured depth was 8.3 cm at an angle of −55°.

Illustration continued on opposite page

lengths of 7 or 13 cm.[17] A mechanical stop on the side of the needle can be adjusted to the depth of the lesion. The needle is inserted to the premeasured depth and withdrawn in a single motion.

The Vim-Silverman (Fig. 22–6) is a 14-gauge cutting needle that provides a larger core of tissue and is used primarily for liver biopsies. However, because safer, more easily used biopsy needles are available, this needle is now rarely used.

Needles for biopsy of bone are large, pointed instruments consisting of an outer cannula, a pointed obturator, and a cutting inner cannula. The Turkel needle is a 10-gauge triephine instrument that has a slightly blunt obturator beveled to wedge into the bone. The inner cannula has three sharp teeth that are rotated by two hexagonal metal pieces that attach to the hub of the inner cannula and act as a handle.

The Craig needle has a serrate inner cannula and a very large bore (3.5 mm inner diameter). Blunt stylets are provided for all triephine needles to expel the biopsy material.

The Jamshide needle (Kormed Corp.) combines the features of cutting and triephine needles. It is available in 11- and 12-gauge sizes and consists of a cannula with a sharp, beveled tip and a flat obturator.

METHODS

The initial diagnostic CT scans are reviewed to select the biopsy site and to determine the position in which the patient will be placed for biopsy. We use an anterior transabdominal or transthoracic approach with the patient in the supine position, except for paravertebral and deep retroperitoneal masses. The supine position is easier for the patient to maintain without discomfort than the prone or decubitus position.

The abnormality to be biopsied is relocated on a series of scans at levels preselected from the initial diagnostic CT scans, and the level is marked

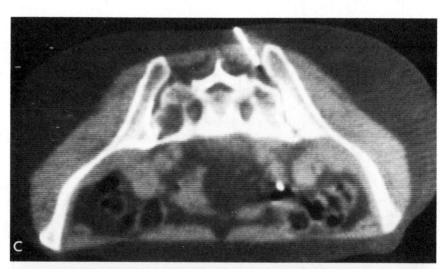
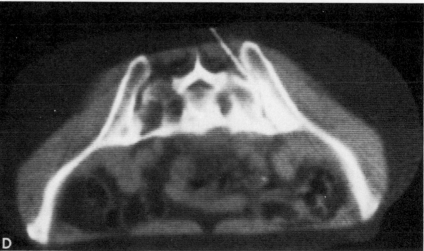

Figure 22–7. *Continued* **C** Anesthetic needle is confirmed to be in satisfactory position. **D** CT confirmation of satisfactory needle placement in sacroiliac joint. Diagnosis: Nonpyogenic sacroilitis.

on the skin with an ink marker. An alternative method is to tape a grid marker to the skin.[15, 17] A repeat scan ensures that the entry point is appropriate. Once a suitable entry site is chosen, the skin is cleansed with povidone-iodine (Betadine) and the area sterilely draped. The distance from the midabdominal or midthoracic line to the entry site, the depth from the skin to the anterior and posterior margins of the lesion, and the angle of insertion of the needle are measured from the CT scan (Fig. 22–7A,B). The depth from the skin to the lesion is indicated on the needle with sterile tape. The skin and subcutaneous tissues are anesthetized, and the 23-gauge needle used for anesthesia is left in position. A CT scan through the anesthetic needle (Fig. 22–7C) is obtained to verify that the entry site is still appropriate. If necessary, the needle is repositioned and CT scans are repeated until the anesthestic needle is properly oriented.

Cytologic Biopsy Techniques

Using the anesthetic needle as a guide, a thin-walled 22-gauge needle is inserted to the measured depth and its position is verified by a CT scan (Fig. 22–7D). CT scans are obtained until the needle tip is shown to be in the lesion. When included within the scan slice, the needle tip will appear square[13] and the needle with have a uniform density throughout its length. To minimize radiation exposure, CT scans for needle verification should be performed at the lowest possible exposure factors.

We have found it easier to place the biopsy needle accurately if the needle is inserted perpendicular to the lesion through the abdominal wall or chest (Fig. 22–8A,B). This usually can be accomplished in the abdomen, since a 22-gauge needle can be passed through bowel without complication.[24] When the needle is being passed, it is important to maintain it on a straight path because a slight deviation at skin level will produce a larger deviation within the body. The needle should be advanced in small increments with one hand stabilizing the needle at the skin margin. It is helpful for the x-ray technician to assume a position at the head or side of the patient to visually verify that the needle is being directed on a straight path at the proper angle. If the needle is directed incorrectly, its course cannot be corrected by altering the position of the needle hub; the entire needle must be removed and reintroduced. In obese patients, a short, 18-gauge, thin-walled needle can serve as a cannula through which a smaller needle can be passed, but direct passage of a 20- or 21-gauge needle also gives satisfactory results.

Once the needle tip is verified to be within the lesion, a second needle is passed parallel to the first needle into the mass (Figs. 22–8C and 22–9). The tandem needle technique, first described by Ferrucci and Wittenberg,[15] permits repositioning of biopsy needles after aspiration so accurately that a repeat CT scan to verify the position of additional needles is not needed. If there is doubt as to which tip belongs to which needle, injecting a small amount of contrast medium through one needle will resolve the problem.[19]

Increased resistance to passage of the needle is frequently felt as the mass is reached. When resistance is met, the needle should be advanced slightly into the lesion and rotated several times to dislodge cellular material from around the needle tip. After the stylet is removed, suction is applied by a 12-ml syringe as the needle is again rotated and moved 0.5 to 1 cm in the vertical plane.

After aspiration is completed, the suction is released and the pressure permitted to equalize before the needle is removed from the mass. Release of suction ensures the aspirated material will be retained in the needle and easily expelled onto a glass slide. Suction is discontinued if blood is aspirated because excessive blood makes interpretation of the specimen more difficult. The biopsy procedure is repeated until an adequate sample is obtained. Large lesions are routinely biopsied at several sites, and if a lesion is necrotic, samples are obtained from the periphery and central portion of the lesion.

When the pleura, lung, or a critical vascular structure intervenes between the lesion and a biopsy performed in the same plane, the needle can be angulated into the mass by simple triangulation (Fig. 22–10).[25, 26]

Preparation of Cytologic Specimens

The accuracy of diagnosis depends to a great degree upon the skill of the cytopathologist and the quality of the biopsy material. The cytopathologist is notified at the beginning of the biopsy and, if possible, is present during the biopsy to prepare the specimens. Specimens are immediately smeared on glass slides and wet fixed with 95 per cent ethanol or, if the aspirate is bloody, Carnoy's solution (ethyl alcohol and 5 per cent glacial acetic acid). Although specimens can first be placed in a preservative solution, then centrifuged, smeared on ground glass slides and postfixed in 95 per cent ethanol, rapid wet fixation better preserves the entire cell and prevents dis-

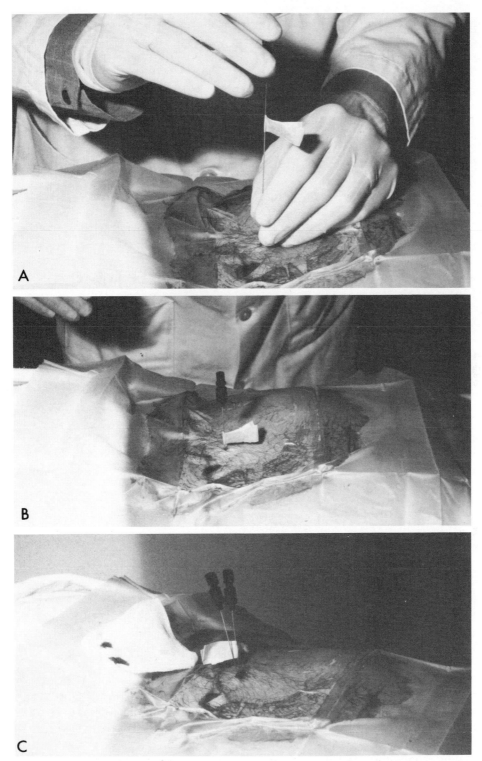

Figure 22–8. Fine-needle aspiration biopsy technique. **A** Placement of needle vertically through abdominal wall. Holding the needle close to the entry point helps stabilize the flexible needle. Tape placed around needle at desired depth. **B** Needle positioned vertically up to tape. **C** Second needle in place using first needle as guide.

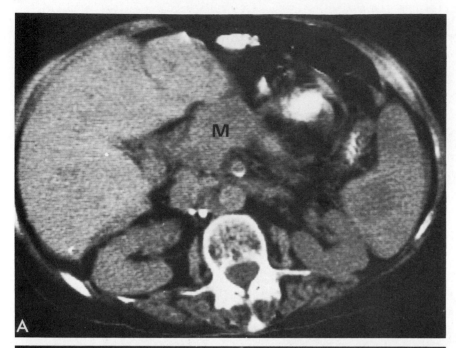

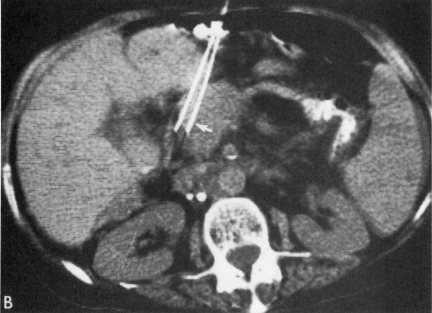

Figure 22–9. CT-guided pancreatic biopsy using tandem technique. **A** A small mass (M) is identified in the head of the pancreas. **B** Two needles are placed into pancreatic mass. The tip of one needle (arrow) appears to be just in the pancreas.

Illustration continued on opposite page

tortion, shrinkage, and swelling. Immediately after fixing the specimen, it is stained with toluidine blue and the cytopathologist views the specimen on the microscope to determine whether the sample is adequate (Fig. 22–11). This practice has virtually eliminated inadequate biopsies and frequently permits a preliminary diagnosis to be made while the patient is still in the CT suite. A final diagnosis is made after the aspirated material is permanently stained.

Knowledge of the expected diagnosis can influence the diagnostic approach. Because epithelial tumors such as adenocarcinomas and squamous cell carcinomas usually provide adequate cellular material, fine-needle cytologic aspiration biopsies are usually satisfactory.[19, 21] However, solid mesodermal tumors tend to have great cellular cohesiveness and may not yield good specimens unless histologic samples are obtained. Therefore, the radiologist and pathologist must be prepared to obtain and preserve histologic as well as cytologic tumor material.

Histologic Biopsy Techniques

Tissue core biopsies can be obtained with flexible 20- or 22-gauge needles as well as with large-

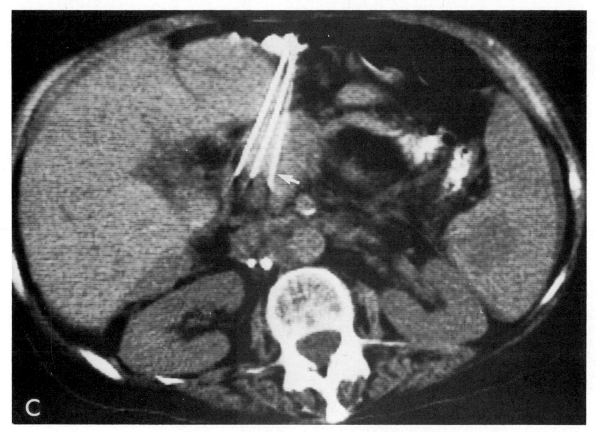

Figure 22–9. *Continued* **C**   Placement of another needle (arrow) into the pancreatic mass. Diagnosis: Carcinoma of the pancreas.

bore needles.[17, 27–29] The technique for obtaining histologic material depends largely on the organ to be biopsied and the needle used to obtain the material. Obtaining core biopsies with thin needles requires only a slight modification of the technique used for cytologic aspiration biopsies. Patient preparation is identical and no additional laboratory studies are obtained. Thin-needle core biopsies are often performed as outpatient procedures.

The 22-gauge flexible biopsy needles are placed into the lesion using the tandem needle technique. A syringe containing 1 to 2 ml of normal saline is attached to the needle, and suction is applied as the needle is slowly advanced and rotated. As soon as blood or bits of tissue are aspirated into the syringe, the needle and syringe are removed together and the contents of the syringe are injected into a sterile test tube. The tissue fragments are individually removed in the pathology laboratory and processed by the usual histologic techniques. The remaining portion of the supernatant may be filtered and processed for cytologic analysis.

Using this technique, both cytologic and histologic specimens can be obtained from a single aspiration biopsy. However, fine-needle core biopsy techniques provide a wet aspirate for cytologic review, in contrast to the dry aspirate obtained by cytologic biopsy. If the cytologist prefers a dry specimen for analysis or if rapid staining and interpretation are required, a separate cytologic biopsy must be performed.

Larger tissue samples can be obtained with various larger and less flexible needles.[30, 31] To avoid complication, vascular structures, bowel, and solid parenchymal organs should not be traversed. Solid, superficial masses without intervening lung or bowel can be safely biopsied. Prior to obtaining a biopsy, the vascularity of the lesion is determined by injecting a bolus of contrast material and performing a dynamic scan sequence by large-bore cutting needles (Fig. 22–12). If a lesion is hypervascular, a large-bore biopsy is not performed. Determination of the vascularity of hepatic lesions is particularly important prior to biopsy in order to avoid biopsy of a hepatic cavernous hemangioma.

Large-bore biopsies are performed only on hospitalized patients who are closely monitored for signs of hemorrhage.

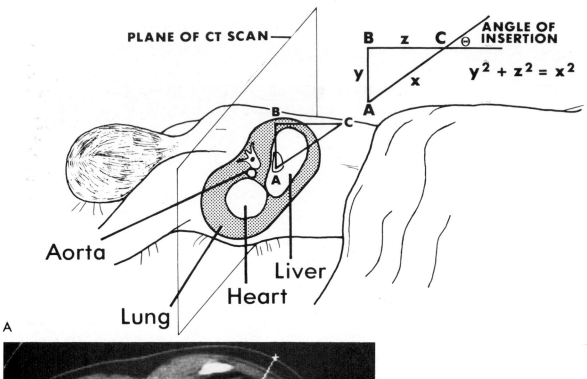

PLANE OF CT SCAN

ANGLE OF
INSERTION

$y^2 + z^2 = x^2$

Aorta

Liver

Heart

Lung

A

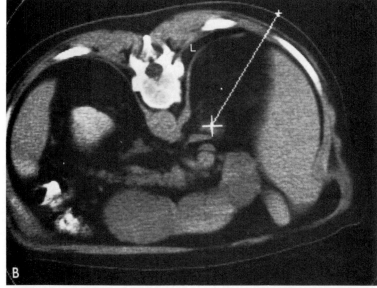

B

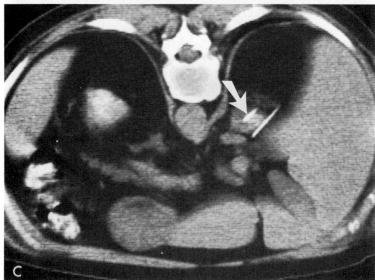

C

Figure 22–10. Triangulation method of CT guided biopsy. **A** Plane of CT scan passes through liver lesion (A) surrounded by lung. Entry point (C) selected caudad to diaphragm. Point B is directly above liver lesion (A). Triangle ABC (inset). Distance y measured from scan; z measured on skin; x calculated by Pythagorean theorem ($y^2 + z^2 = x^2$). Distance x is actual needle path. Entry/ angle = calculated by tangent y/z (opposite/ adjacent). (Modified from Gerzof SG: Triangulation: Indirect CT guidance for abscess drainage. AJR 137:1080, 1981. © 1981, American Roentgen Ray Society. Used with permission.) **B** Adrenal mass biopsy using triangulation method. Prone CT scan on entry site is chosen to avoid the lung (L). A distance of 12.3 cm is measured. **C** Tandem needle technique. Two needle tips are demonstrated; one (arrow) is in adrenal mass. Final diagnosis: Metastatic transitional cell carcinoma from the bladder.

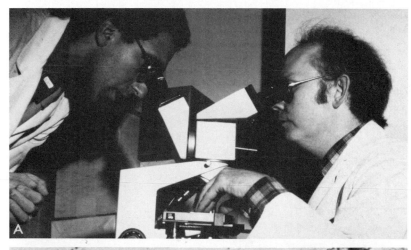

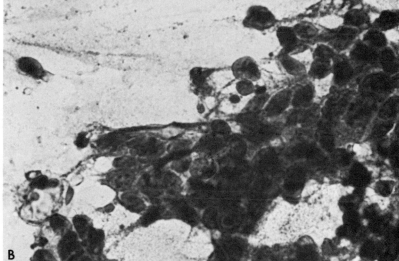

Figure 22–11. A Immediate viewing of cytologic specimen to determine whether sample is adequate for diagnosis. **B** Cytologic material from hepatic aspirate of metastatic carcinoma is stained with toluidine blue. Excellent preservation of cytologic characteristics permits a preliminary diagnosis and termination of the aspiration procedure. **C** The same aspirate stained with the final Papanicolaou stain. Cytologic detail is excellent and is not affected by prior toluidine blue stain.

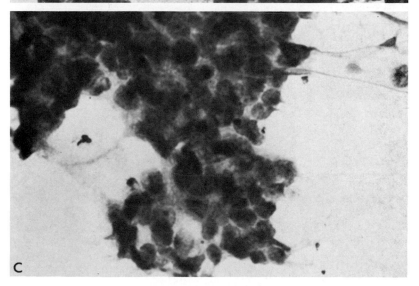

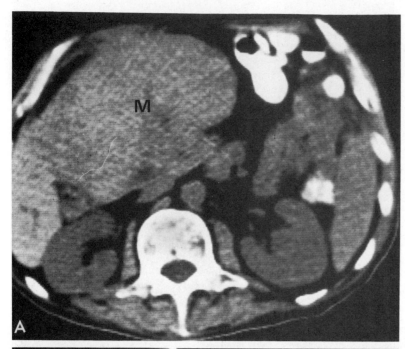

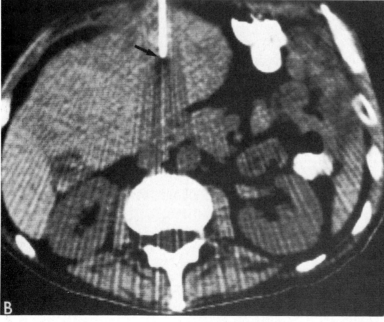

Figure 22–12. Large-bone biopsy of hepatic tumor. **A** A large hepatic mass (M) is demonstrated in the left lobe of the liver. The mass was not highly vascular on a dynamic CT scan series performed following a bolus injection of contrast. **B** Histologic biopsy using 18-gauge needle. The tip of the needle appears square (arrow). Streak artifacts are due to the hub of the needle. Diagnosis: Metastatic adenocarcinoma.

Larger histologic specimens can be obtained using a single-needle or double-needle technique. With the single-needle technique, the entry site, depth of biopsy, needle angulation, and anesthesia are accomplished in a manner identical to that in a cytologic aspiration biopsy. After verification that the anesthetic needle is in the correct plane and orientation, the larger needle is advanced into the mass parallel to the anesthetic needle and the position of the needle is verified by CT. A specimen is then obtained by a continuous inward and outward motion.

The double-needle technique involves placing a thin needle into the lesion and using it as a guide for inserting the cutting needle into the mass. A verifying CT scan is not performed, and the tissue sample is obtained immediately.

BIOPSY OF SPECIFIC ORGANS

Pancreas

The most frequent indication for a thin-needle pancreatic biopsy is to differentiate pancreatic carcinoma from chronic pancreatitis in a patient with abdominal pain, weight loss, and a pancreatic mass. This distinction remains difficult despite advances in ultrasonography, CT, en-

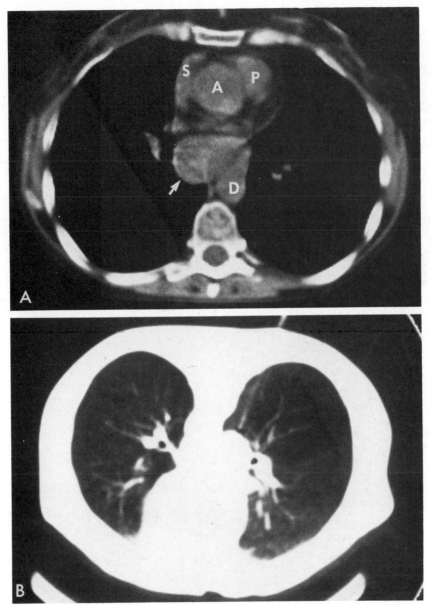

Figure 22–20. CT-directed biopsy of mediastinal mass. **A** CT scan demonstrating a rounded, predominantly right-sided mediastinal mass (arrow). A = Root of aorta; P = main pulmonary artery; S = superior vena cava; D = descending aorta. **B** Biopsy of mass performed in prone position using single-needle technique. Final diagnosis: Oat cell carcinoma.

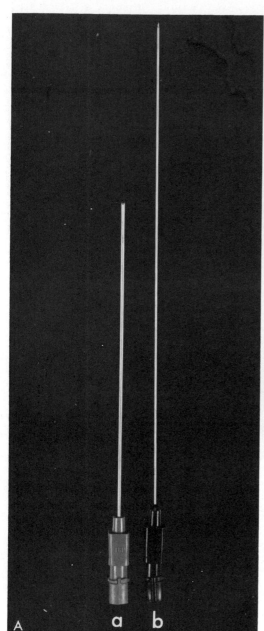

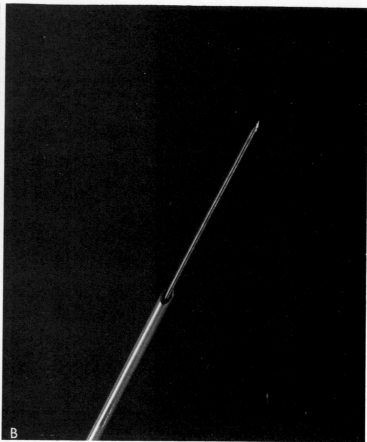

Figure 22–21. Green needle set used for double-needle method of lung biopsy. **A** Two needles are shown: a = 19-gauge guidance cannula with stylet; b = 22-gauge biopsy needle with diamond-shaped stylet. **B** Close-up photograph of biopsy needle projecting through guidance cannula.

Figure 22–22. Double-needle technique for CT-guided biopsy of pulmonary nodule. **A** CT scan demonstrates a small nodule (arrow) in the left lung.

Illustration continued on opposite page

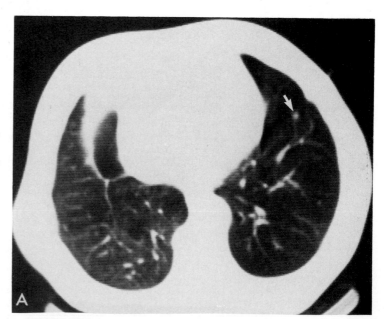

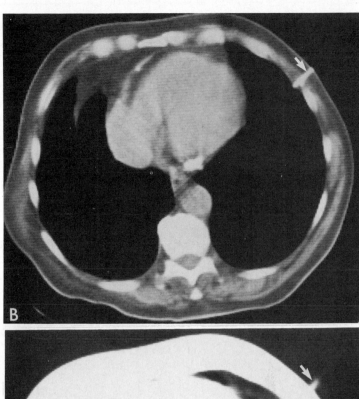

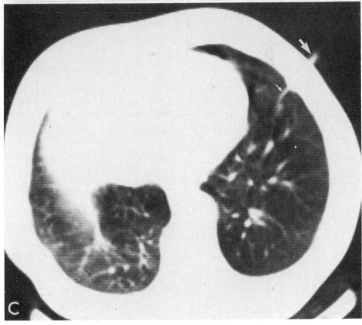

Figure 22–22. *Continued* **B** The short guidance cannula (arrow) is directed toward the lung nodule. **C** CT scan after placement of the thin biopsy needle (small arrow) through the guidance cannula (large arrow) into the pulmonary nodule. Final diagnosis: Metastatic adenocarcinoma.

Pneumothorax is the principal complication of CT-guided transthoracic biopsies. In our series, pneumothorax occurred in 52 per cent and 12 per cent required placement of a chest tube. This compares with a 31.2 per cent rate of pneumothorax reported for fluoroscopically guided transthoracic needle aspiration biopsies.[52] Most patients with pneumothorax require no therapy, but the means to treat a pneumothorax rapidly and effectively should be available whenever transthoracic biopsy is performed.

If a pneumothorax occurs during a CT-directed transthoracic biopsy, the biopsy is stopped.

Further needle punctures increase the hazard to the patient, and because of the changing position of the mass relative to the entry point, additional needle passages are unlikely to be successful. If the needle misses the lesion on the initial placement, the needle and stylet are left in position and a second attempt is made with another needle. Left in place, the needle serves as a guide for the next attempt and tends to prevent rapid formation of a pneumothorax. After the biopsy, 5 to 10 ml of clotted blood is injected through the guidance needle in an attempt to seal the needle track. The clotted blood produces a parenchymal

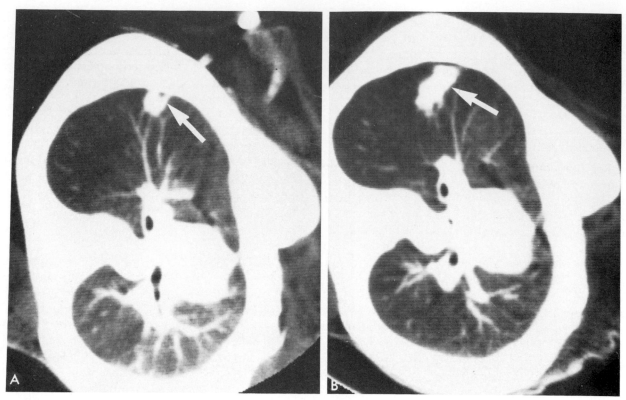

Figure 22–23. Blood patch technique to seal pleura after biopsy. **A** Left decubitus position. Biopsy needle (arrow) in right lung nodule. **B** Injection of 10 ml of clotted blood through guidance needle after biopsy. The blood patch (arrow) is seen in the right lung but no pneumothorax is present. Final diagnosis: Metastatic adenocarcinoma.

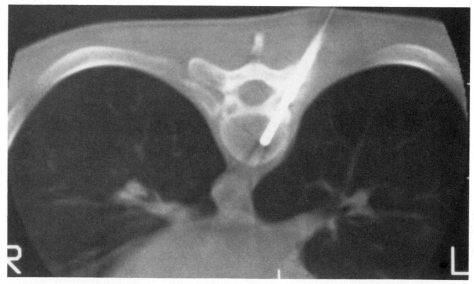

Figure 22–24. Large-bore biopsy of vertebral body. CT scan demonstrates the tip of a Craig needle in the center of the body of a thoracic vertebra. Despite the large bore needle, the use of the extended scale (-1000 to $+3000$ H) permits CT scans of nonmoving high-density objects to be obtained that are relatively free of artifacts. Final diagnosis: Compression fracture, no tumor or infection.

density (Fig. 22–23) that resolves quickly but tends to seal the needle track and reduces the likelihood of a major pneumothorax. After biopsy, an expiratory chest radiograph is obtained, and if a pneumothorax is present, the patient is closely monitored.

Skeletal System

Percutaneous bone biopsies are utilized to diagnose primary bone tumors, metastasis, or infection. Most investigators prefer to perform bone biopsies using fluoroscopic guidance because the technique is safe, convenient and familiar and has an accuracy rate of greater than 90 per cent.[28]

Despite the ease and accuracy of fluoroscopically guided skeletal biopsy, CT can provide information that permits more accurate prebiopsy planning. Hardy and colleagues[31] reported that among 19 patients referred for percutaneous bone biopsy, CT influenced the choice of needle, biopsy site, or needle path in seven and demonstrated that no biopsy should be performed in four. When a vertebral biopsy is indicated, CT can make a percutaneous large-bore biopsy of the spine (Fig. 22–24) safer[30] and in other instances CT may permit smaller, less invasive needles to be used. The use of CT for planning and guiding percutaneous bone biopsies will increase as more experience is obtained.

CT-GUIDED THERAPEUTIC PROCEDURES

ABSCESS ASPIRATION AND DRAINAGE

Computed tomography has contributed much to the diagnosis of intra-abdominal and pelvic abscesses. More than 90 per cent of abscesses are detected by CT, and in many centers CT is the preferred procedure for detecting abscess.[55–57] CT precisely localizes an abscess and defines its relationship to adjacent organs and peritoneal spaces. This information is vital in planning surgical procedures, aspirating abscesses for culture, and determining suitability for percutaneous drainage.

Patient Selection

CT-guided needle aspiration of a suspected abscess is indicated to confirm the diagnosis and to provide material for culture to aid in selecting an-

tibiotics. Fine-needle aspiration for culture can be performed in virtually any patient. Percutaneous drainage of a documented abscess is indicated when there is a well-defined abscess cavity, a safe drainage route and the surgeon and radiologist agree the procedure is warranted. In contrast to the technique of Gerzof and co-workers,[58, 59, 61] we frequently drain abscesses in patients who are poor operative risks. Infected phlegmons and multiple, extensive, or multiloculated abscesses are best treated with surgically placed drains. Occasionally, however, large, loculated abscesses can be successfully drained.[60, 61]

Techniques

Antibiotics are administered intravenously before a diagnostic aspiration or percutaneous drainage procedure. Subsequent antibiotic therapy is governed by the results of Gram stain and culture of aspirated material. The site of entry for diagnostic and drainage procedures is based on the size, location, and relationship of the abscess to surrounding organs.

Following a diagnostic CT scan, the shortest straight line from the skin to the abscess that does not traverse bowel or other organs is measured. The skin is marked, cleansed, and anesthesized as for a percutaneous needle biopsy. Whenever possible, an extraperitoneal approach is employed.

DIAGNOSTIC ASPIRATION. If the lesion has an accessible, safe aspiration route, a diagnostic aspiration can be performed using either a Teflon-sheathed (Fig. 22–25) or non-sheathed 18- to 20-gauge needle. If a sheathed needle is employed, a small incision made in the skin to facilitate entry. The needle is inserted into the abscess to the premeasured depth, the stylet is removed, and a small amount of abscess is aspirated for culture and Gram stain (Fig. 22–26).

Aspiration of small, deep, or critically positioned abscesses requiring needle passage through bowel or solid parenchymal organs is performed with a 22-gauge needle. The location of the needle should be verified by CT before aspiration (Fig. 22–27). Only thin, nonviscous material can be aspirated, through a 22-gauge needle, but often enough material is obtained for culture and smear. Thin-needle aspiration is useful for diagnostic purposes only, since the contents of an abscess can seldom be completely aspirated through a small-gauge needle.

THERAPEUTIC DRAINAGE. Abscesses can be drained using a pigtail angiographic catheter or

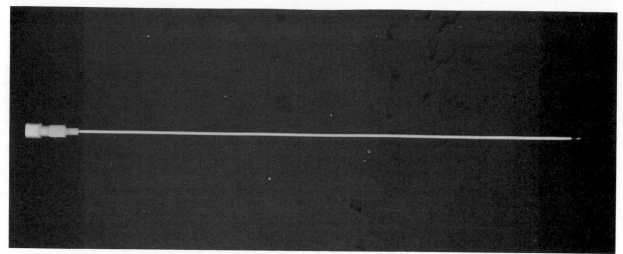

Figure 22–25. Ring catheter-stylet combination (Cook, Inc.). An inner trocar stylet and outer 5 French polyethylene catheter used for diagnostic aspiration of intra-abdominal or pelvic abscesses. If necessary, a guide wire can be passed through the sheath and a larger-gauge catheter placed into the abscess to aspirate pus that is too thick to be aspirated through the smaller Teflon sheath.

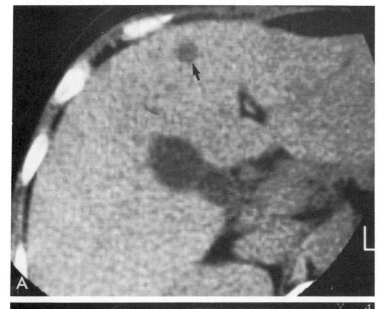

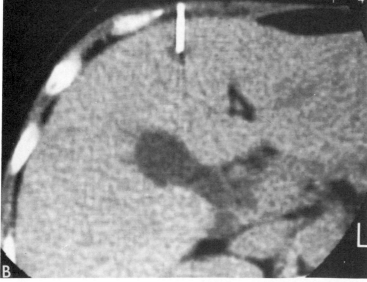

Figure 22–26. Diagnostic aspiration of small liver abscess. **A** CT scan reveals a 1 × 1 cm low-density mass (arrow) in the medial segment of the left hepatic lobe. **B** CT scan documenting placement of an 18-gauge needle into the liver mass. Note the square appearance to the tip of the needle. A small amount of fluid was aspirated. Final diagnosis: Fungal abscess resulting from *Candida albicans*.

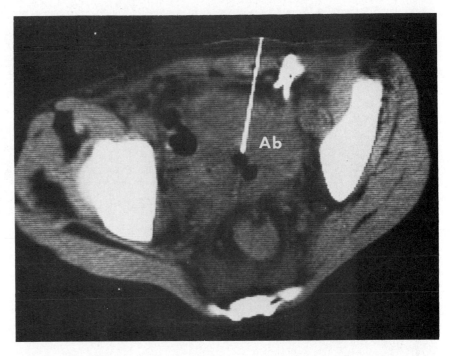

Figure 22–27. Diagnostic aspiration of pelvic abscess (Ab), resulting from Crohn's disease, with a 22-gauge needle. The thin needle was used because the abscess could not be clearly separated from bowel and the thin-gauged needle provided an extra margin of safety.

large trocar catheters (Figs. 22–28 and 22–29). The pigtail catheter is best suited for draining small, deep intraparenchymal abscesses or abscesses close to bowel or the diaphragm and is the more frequently used drainage technique.

The placement of a pigtail catheter entails a series of steps (Fig. 22–30). After the abscess is located and the needle path is planned, a diagnostic aspiration of the abscess is performed using a sheathed catheter. A J-shaped guide wire is passed through the sheath into the abscess and the sheath removed. The track is dilated with an 8 French (8F) angiographic dilator, and an 8.3F or 10F pigtail catheter (Cook, Inc.) is passed over the guide wire into the abscess. The position of the pigtail catheter is then documented by CT. The pigtail shape prevents perforation of the catheter through the wall of the abscess and protects against dislodgement. Continuous drainage

is promoted because the drainage holes are on the inner curve of the pigtail where they will not be occluded if the catheter lodges against the wall of the abscess.

The abscess is aspirated to dryness by manual suction. If abscess contents are viscous, 3 to 10 ml of 10 to 20 per cent acetylcysteine (Mucomyst, Mead-Johnson) is injected into the cavity. This frequently turns thick pus into thin readily drainable fluid. Repeated flushing with saline and acetylcysteine ensures complete drainage.[61a]

Water-soluble contrast material injected into the abscess cavity permits detection of undrained loculated portions of the abscess, outlines fistulous tracts, and documents catheter position (Figs. 22–30 and 22–31).

Abscesses can also be drained using a variety of large-bore (12F–16F) trocar catheters (Fig. 22–29). After diagnostic aspiration of the abscess, the

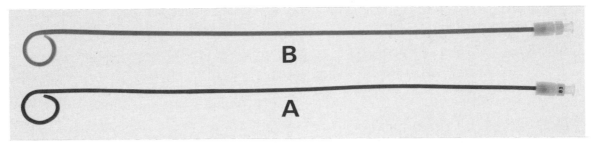

Figure 22–28. Photograph of pigtail catheters (Cook, Inc.) used for percutaneous drainage of abscesses. A = Black 8.3 French catheter; B = white 10.0 French catheter.

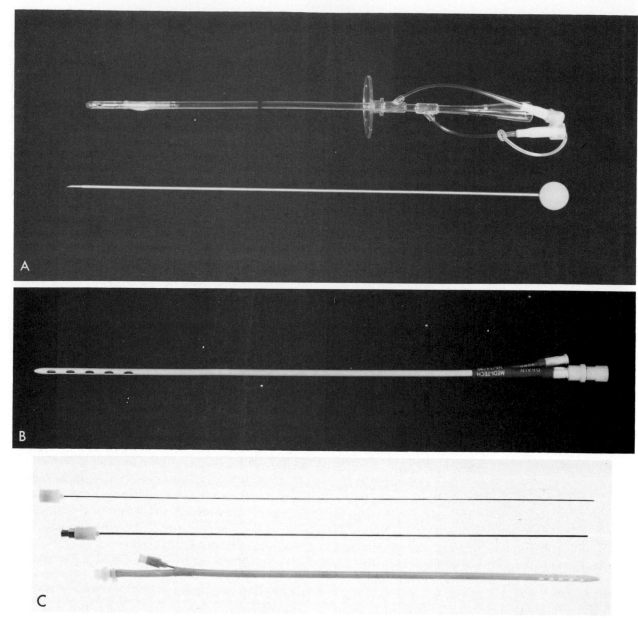

Figure 22–29. Large-bore catheters used for drainage of nonparenchymal abscesses. **A** Ingram trocar catheter (Sherwood Medical Co.). Special features include a very stiff metal stylet for introduction, a balloon tip to contain catheter in the abscess, a flange for anchoring the catheter to the skin, and a separate injection port. **B** Von Sonnenberg catheter (Medi-Tech, Inc.). Special features include a stiff metal stylet for introduction when used as a trocar catheter, a distal hole permitting passage over a guide wire, multiple large side holes, a separate injection port, long length, and extreme flexibility. **C** Ring-McLean abscess drainage catheter (Cook, Inc.). Special features include: true sump design; a pointed stylet that fits through a metal stiffening cannula for introduction when used as a trocar catheter; catheter and metal cannula with end hole for easy passage over a guide wire; multiple, large side holes; separate injection port; long length, and extreme flexibility.

large trocar catheter is passed into the abscess along the same path and to the same depth as the needle used for the diagnostic aspiration. During the passage of the trocar catheter, solid parenchymal organs, bowel, and the pleural space must be avoided. Once the catheter is advanced into the abscess, the stylet is removed and the contents of the abscess are totally drained. The initial position of the metal trocar is not verified by CT because the subcutaneous tissues usually cannot support the weight of the large metal stylet, and for safety it is important to remove the stylet immediately after the abscess is punctured.

After evacuation of the abscess, the catheter is securely fastened to the skin to prevent inadvertent dislodgment. A biliary drainage bag is attached to the catheter, and the system is left to drain by gravity or attached to continuous low-pressure suction. If the abscess contents are viscous, the drainage catheter is irrigated four times daily with sterile saline.

If a pigtail catheter has been used, after 3 to 4 days, the catheter is removed and a straight catheter is reinserted. The straight catheter is then slowly withdrawn and removed when there is cessation of drainage and evidence on a follow-up CT scan or abscessogram of complete resolution of the abscess cavity. Clinical response is frequently immediate and almost always occurs by 96 hours,[58-61] but it can take 15 to 30 days of drainage before all of the conditions for catheter removal are met.[59, 61] Patients who have an enteric communication usually require a longer period of drainage. Catheter drainage has been maintained for up to 120 days without complications.[61]

Results and Complications

Properly performed percutaneous catheter drainage is a safe and effective method of treating abdominal abscesses. Gerzof and colleagues[61] successfully drained 61 of (86 per cent) 71 abscesses. Haaga's group[60] obtained satisfactory specimens for culture in 33 of 36 abscesses (92 per cent) and successfully treated 28 of 33 abscesses (85 per cent) by CT-guided percutaneous catheter drainage. Other investigators report similar success rates.[62, 63] We have been successful in 85 per cent of abscesses aspirated for culture and catheter drainage.[38] Failure occurs most frequently in patients with very large, multiloculated, or multiple abscesses, infected tumors, pancreatic phelgmons, colonic or enteric fistulas, intrarenal abscesses, and abscesses containing material too thick to be drained by large-bore catheters.[58-61]

Complications occur in approximately 15 per cent of patients undergoing drainage procedures.[61] Sepsis is the most common, but empyema, hemorrhage, and fistula formation are also encountered.[60, 61] Gerzof[59] reported 4 per cent mortality secondary to inadequate drainage and a 1 per cent recurrence rate.[61] This is significantly lower than the 11 to 43 per cent mortality and 14 to 49 per cent recurrence rates after surgery.[64, 65] These results indicate that percutaneous drainage should be performed before surgical drainage in most accessible abscesses. No immediate catastrophic complications have occurred, and whenever percutaneous drainage proves inadequate, surgical intervention can be performed. In some cases, percutaneous catheter drainage can be used as an intermediate step; a patient who is a poor operative candidate can be made fit to undergo surgical drainage.

PANCREATIC PSEUDOCYST ASPIRATION AND DRAINAGE

Patient Selection

Conventional surgical management of pancreatic pseudocysts is internal drainage of a mature pseudocyst into an adjacent viscus.[66, 67] Surgical internal drainage is a safe, reliable method of treating pancreatic pseudocysts but requires a 6- to 8-week waiting period while the cyst wall matures sufficiently to permit a satisfactory enteric anastomosis.[66, 67] Although more than 10 per cent of pseudocysts resolve during the wait for cyst wall maturation,[66, 68] others can become infected, expand rapidly, and cause severe unrelenting pain, duodenal or biliary obstruction, or hemorrhage.[67] Surgical intervention before the cyst wall is mature is difficult and is associated with high morbidity and mortality.[69]

Although experience is still limited, the results indicate that percutaneous aspiration and drainage of pancreatic pseudocysts can safely and effectively relieve symptoms and treat sepsis in selected patients without serious complications.[61, 70-73]

Techniques

The technique is identical to that employed for diagnostic aspiration of abscesses. In nonseptic patients, a 22-gauge needle is inserted and the cyst is aspirated until it collapses (Fig. 22-32). Viscous fluid may require an 18- or 20-gauge needle,

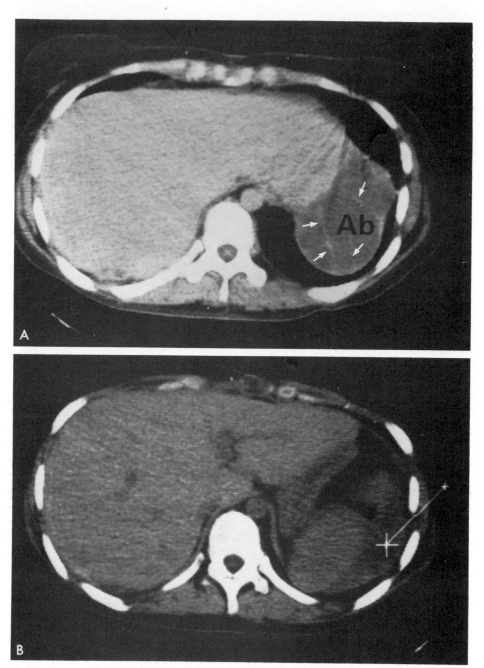

Figure 22–30. Percutaneous drainage of left subphrenic abscess using pigtail catheter. **A** A well-defined multiseptated (arrows) abscess (Ab) in the left subphrenic space. **B** CT scan at slightly lower level demonstrating projected path of drainage catheter chosen to avoid the pleural space. The distance from skin to abscess center is approximately 5.7 cm.

Illustration continued on opposite page

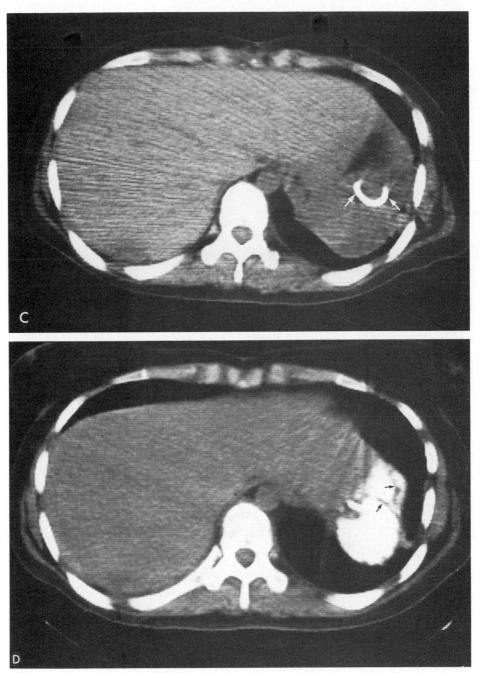

Figure 22–30. *Continued* **C** CT scan through curved tip of pigtail catheter (arrows) documents the catheter in the abscess. **D** Contrast medium injection into abscess cavity confirms catheter communication with abscess. Contrast material fills entire abscess despite presence of septations (arrows). No extravasation of contrast into the pleural space is noted.

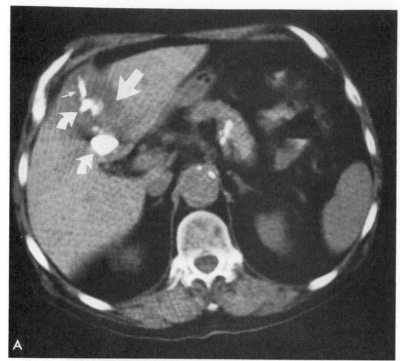

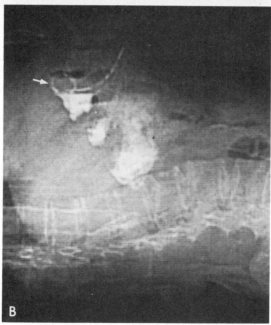

Figure 22–31. Catheter drainage of hepatic abscess. **A** CT scan through a hepatic abscess (large arrow) following injection of contrast material (curved arrows) through the drainage catheter. The contrast material is contained wholly within the abscess. **B** A lateral computerized radiograph demonstrates that pigtail catheter (arrow) is located in the most cephalad, anterior portion of the irregularly shaped hepatic abscess. A preferred catheter position would have been in the most dependent part of the abscess.

and multiple pseudocysts require separate punctures and aspirations (Fig. 22–33). Communication of a pseudocyst with the main pancreatic duct has been shown by injecting contrast material into a pseudocyst.[70]

Results and Complications

After drainage, pain is usually relieved immediately[71] and no serious complications have been reported.[70–73] The incidence of recurrence after percutaneous drainage is unknown; MacErlean's group[71] reported that effectively drained pseudocysts had not recurred for up to a year and Gerzof and associates[61] successfully treated nine patients without recurrence or complications.

Pseudocysts should be aspirated in patients who develop sepsis and who are not surgical candidates. If the fluid is purulent or Gram-stain positive, antibiotics and catheter drainage therapy are begun. Although experience has been limited,

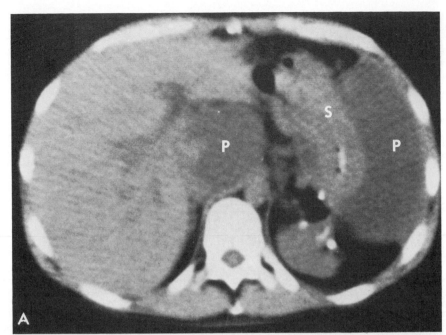

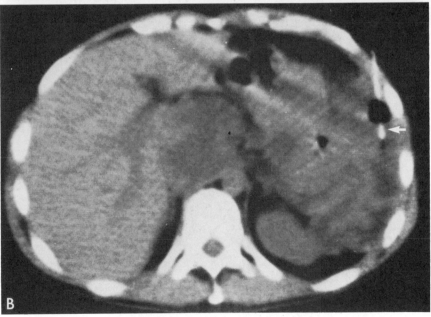

Figure 22–32. Percutaneous drainage of extrapancreatic pseudocysts. **A** Extrapancreatic pseudocysts (P) located in the lesser sac and lateral to the stomach (S). **B** CT scan following aspiration of 150 ml of fluid from the lateral pseudocyst through a 22-gauge needle (arrow). The pseudocyst was almost completely evacuated and did not recur after removal of the needle. A separate needle puncture successfully drained the pseudocyst in the lesser sac.

CT-guided aspiration and drainage of acute, complicated pancreatic pseudocysts will undoubtedly become a valuable therapeutic procedure.

MISCELLANEOUS ASPIRATION AND DRAINAGE PROCEDURES

Pancreatic Phlegmons

The role of CT-guided needle aspiration and drainage in nontumorous, semisolid, phlegmonous masses involving the pancreas is not well defined. Treating infected pancreatic phlegmons by percutaneous drainage has been successful in only 40 per cent of cases[61] because the solid components of an infected lesion are not adequately drained. However, injection of acetylcysteine into a pancreatic phlegmon may convert the semisolid mass into a drainable fluid collection.[61a]

Percutaneous diagnostic needle aspiration of noncystic pancreatic masses is a useful, accurate method of determining whether a pancreatic abscess is present. In patients with pancreatitis and a suspected pancreatic abscess, pancreatic aspirations with an 18- or 20-gauge needle are imme-

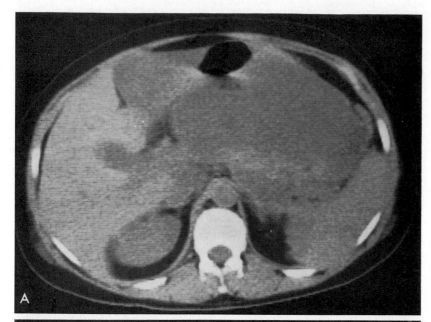

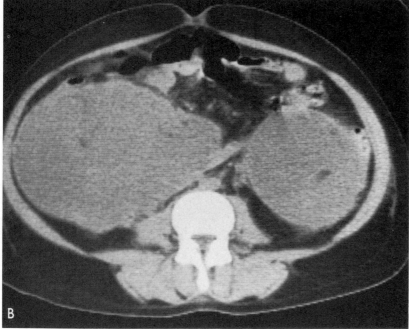

Figure 22–33. Percutaneous drainage of multiple extrapancreatic pseudocysts in a patient with congenital excess of serum triglycerides. **A** CT scan at level of pancreas demonstrates large extrapancreatic pseudocysts (P). **B** Pseudocysts extend down into the flanks.

Illustration continued on opposite page

diately stained and examined for bacteria. The aspirate is also cultured, but a culture can be positive in the absence of a frank pancreatic abscess. If the aspirate contains numerous bacteria, the patient is considered to have a pancreatic abscess and appropriate therapy is instituted.

Percutaneous Nephrostomy

This well-established procedure is usually performed under fluoroscopic or ultrasonic guidance. Although rarely used to place the drainage catheter,[37] CT can be used to guide percutaneous nephrostomies in patients in whom placement of catheters by fluoroscopy and ultrasound has failed. In patients with absent renal function, CT visualization of the renal collecting system without injection of contrast medium permits accurate placement of the drainage catheter. The use of CT also permits the nephrostomy catheter to be placed laterally, allowing the patient to lie more comfortably during drainage.

The technique of percutaneous nephrostomy is similar to that used in abscess puncture and drainage. A sheathed needle is inserted into the collecting system. A J-shaped guide wire is then passed through the sheath and the sheath is re-

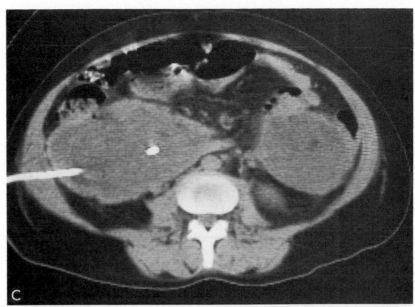

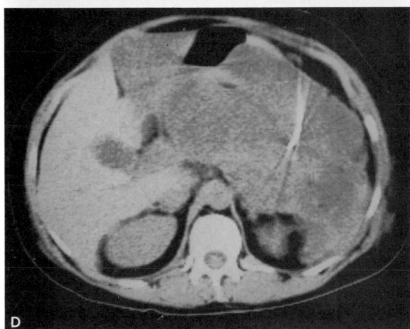

Figure 22–23 *Continued* **C** Drainage catheters placed into cyst located in the right flank and **(D)** left upper abdomen.

Illustration continued on following page

moved, leaving the wire in place. The needle track is dilated and an 8.3F or 10F pigtail catheter is inserted for drainage. A follow-up CT scan confirms the catheter's position. Haaga and coworkers[74] reported successful placement in 12 of 13 CT-guided percutaneous nephrostomies (93 per cent) without serious complications.

Biliary Decompression

CT has been used to guide the puncture of a dilated biliary radicle and to place a drainage catheter to effect biliary decompression.[75] However, because biliary decompression can almost al-

ways be performed under fluoroscopic guidance, CT is not often recommended to guide this procedure. CT can be used to guide drainage of a locally obstructed biliary system when drainage guided by fluoroscopy or ultrasound has failed.

Hematoma Evacuation

Chronic subcapsular and intrahepatic hematomas that have undergone liquefaction can be aspirated and evacuated using CT to guide catheter placement.[76] CT usually reveals a low-density mass lesion that can be completely evacuated (Fig.

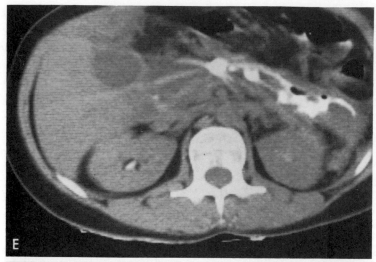

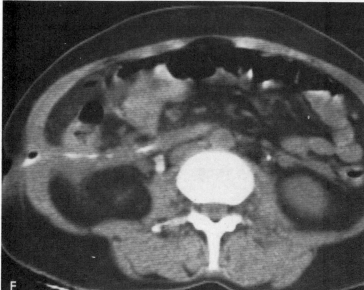

Figure 22–33. *Continued* **E,F** Five weeks after drainage was initiated, pseudocysts have almost resolved.

Illustration continued on opposite page

22–16). Even if the hematoma is not infected, it should be evacuated to decrease the mass effect on the liver and promote hepatic healing.[76]

NEUROLYSIS

Splanchnic nerve neurolysis in the management of upper abdominal pain was first described in 1919 by Kappis.[77] Only in the last decade, however, has splanchnic nerve and celiac ganglion neurolysis become an accepted form of therapy in patients with intractable back or upper-abdominal pain stemming from pancreatic carcinoma, abdominal malignancy, or pancreatitis.[78–82]

Fluoroscopy and bony landmarks have been used to direct the placement of needles prior to the alcohol injection. However, the relationship of the needle tips to surrounding structures and the spread of the neurolytic agent in the retroperitoneum cannot be accurately determined by conventional radiologic techniques. Thus, while using the fluoroscopic method, the overall complication rate is low (less than 5 per cent), there is a 1 per cent incidence of serious complications such as paralysis and peritonitis.[79, 81, 82]

Techniques

The celiac artery reliably indicates the position of the celiac ganglia.[83] The average distances of the ganglia below the celiac artery on the right and left sides are 0.6 and 0.4 cm, respectively,

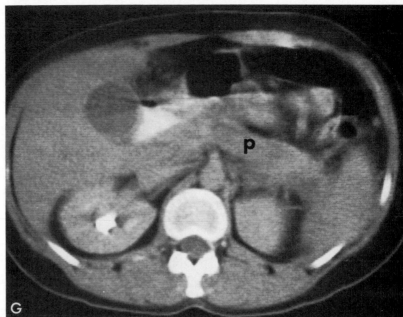

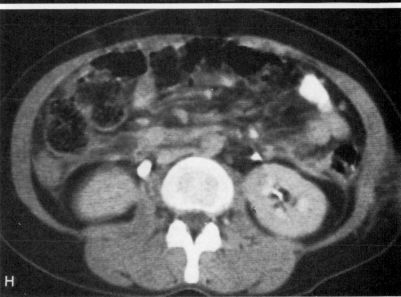

Figure 22–33. *Continued* **G,H** Three months after initiation of drainage, the abdomen is almost normal. p= Pancreas.

while the location of the ganglia relative to the spine varies from the middle of L_2 to the intervertebral disk between T_{12} and L_1.[83] Thus, reliance on bony landmarks is an imprecise way to ensure proper needle position. CT by displaying the aortic, celiac, and superior mesenteric arteries in almost every patient can provide reliable guidance for celiac ganglion neurolysis.[84] The splanchnic nerves are in a retrocrural location on either side of the aorta (Fig. 22–34). If a splanchnic block is to be performed, CT demonstration of the diaphragmatic crura permits accurate retrocrural needle placement.

CT-guided splanchnic nerve and celiac gan-

glion neurolysis has been described by several investigators.[37, 74, 84, 85] A computed radiograph of the upper abdomen is obtained with the patient prone. The level of T_{12} is identified, and CT scans at 1-cm intervals are obtained from the bottom of T_{11} until the celiac axis is clearly demonstrated.

Visceral sympathetic neurolysis may be accomplished by celiac plexus or splanchnic nerve ablation. Both techniques require accurate insertion of two 15-cm needles of 20 to 22 gauge. The needle tips can be positioned either retrocrurally (classic splanchnic nerve neurolysis) or transcrurally, with the needle tips located anterior and lateral to the aorta at the level of the celiac artery

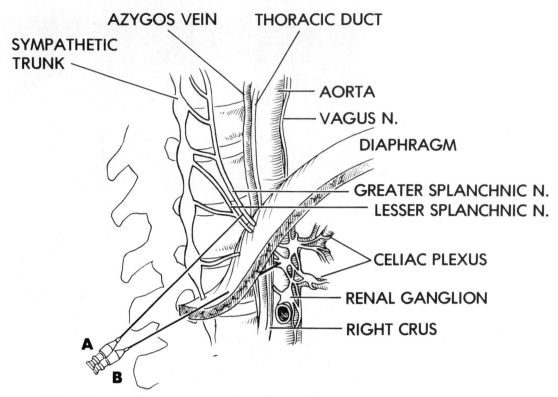

Figure 22–34. Diagram showing location of needle tips for retrocrural splanchnic nerve neurolysis (A) and transcrural celiac plexus neurolysis (B). (From Buy J-N, Moss AA, Singler RC: CT Guided celiac plexus and splanchnic nerve neurolysis. J Comput Assist Tomogr 6:315, 1982.)

(Fig. 22–34). The distances from the midline to the puncture site, the angle of needle entry, and the depth to the site of injection are measured directly from the CT scan with the scan cursor (Fig. 22–35). To avoid the kidneys and lungs, the needles are angled an average of 40° in a cephalocaudal direction. The location of the needle tips is verified by CT before the injection of the neurolytic agent (Fig. 22–36).

Neurolysis is accomplished by injecting 18 to 22 ml of absolute alcohol and 2 to 3 ml of iothalamate meglumine through each needle. After the

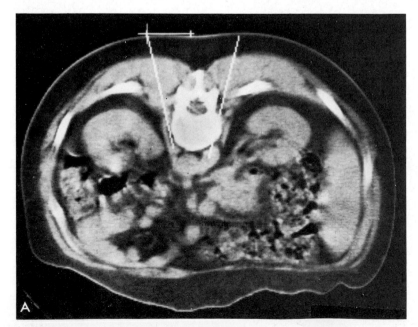

Figure 22–35. CT-guided retrocrural splanchnic neurolysis technique. **A** CT-measured distance from midline to puncture site is 4.3 cm. (From Buy J-N, Moss AA, Singler RC: CT Guided celiac plexus and splanchnic nerve neurolysis. J Comput Assist Tomogr 6:315, 1982.)

Illustration continued on opposite page

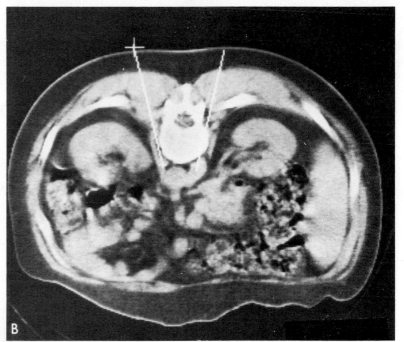

Figure 22–35. *Continued* **B** Distance from skin to just beneath aorta measures 11.96 cm. The angle of needle insertion is 77.1°.

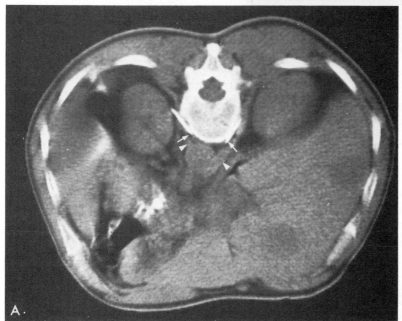

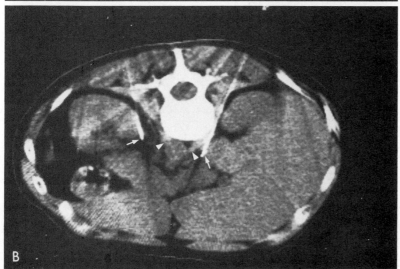

Figure 22–36. CT verification of **(A)** needle tips (arrows) in a retrocrural or **(B)** transcrural position. Diaphragmatic crura (arrowheads) are shown. (From Buy J-N, Moss AA, Singler RC: CT guided celiac plexus and splanchnic nerve neurolysis. J Comput Assist Tomogr 6:315, 1982.)

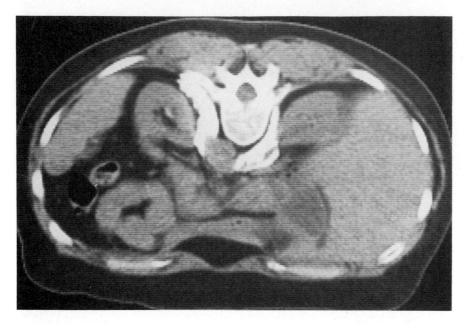

Figure 22–37. Alcohol spread following retrocrural injection for splanchnic neurolysis. Alcohol spreads into the retrocrural and retroaortic space. Diaphragmatic crura limit ventral extension of alcohol spread. (From Buy J-N, Moss AA, Singler RC: CT Guided celiac plexus and splanchnic nerve neurolysis. J Comput Assist Tomogr 6:315, 1982.)

injections, eight to ten CT scans are obtained at 1-cm intervals to assess the spread of alcohol around the celiac ganglia or splanchnic nerves. Retrocrural injection permits alcohol to spread into the retrocrural and retroaortic spaces from T_9 to L_2, but the diaphragmatic crura prevent alcohol from extending around the celiac ganglia (Fig. 22–37). Transcrural alcohol injection spreads around the celiac plexus and into the anterior pararenal, posterior pararenal, or perirenal space (Fig. 22–38).

Results and Complications

Success in relieving pain with percutaneous sympathetic nerve blocks has varied from 33 per cent[86] to 94 per cent.[81] In our experience, 12 of 14 CT-directed neurolytic procedures (86 per cent) relieved pain at least partially.[85] However, because pain relief is subjective, it is difficult to quantitate the degree of success in relieving abdominal and back pain with neurolytic techniques.[83, 85] The duration of pain relief has varied from total pain relief for 3 to 9 months to partial relief for 1 to 2 weeks.[85] It is unclear why some patients have excellent results and others experience poor results. The location and extent of alcohol spread may be critical factors in determining the degree and longevity of pain relief after neurolysis. The transcrural technique directly ablates the celiac plexus and appears to produce slightly longer pain relief.[85]

Serious complications of splanchnic blocks oc-

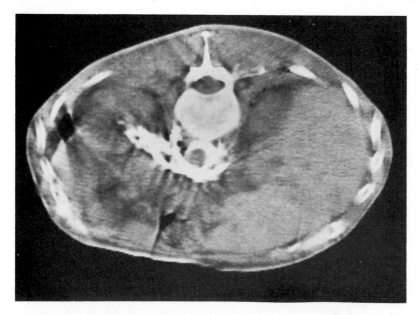

Figure 22–38. Alcohol spread after transcrural injection for celiac plexus neurolysis. Alcohol spreads anterior to aorta and into the left anterior pararenal and perirenal spaces. (From Buy J-N, Moss AA, Singler RC: CT Guided celiac plexus and splanchnic nerve neurolysis. J Comput Assist Tomogr 6:315, 1982.)

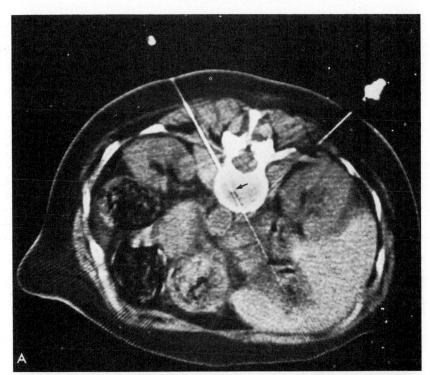

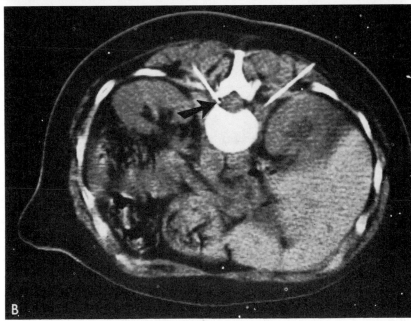

Figure 22–39. CT documentation of needle malpositions during neurolytic procedures. **A** Inadvertent placement of left needle tip (arrow) into intervertebral disc. **B** Placement of left needle tip (arrow) into spinal canal. Injection of alcohol in this position could have produced paralysis. (From Buy J-N, Moss AA, Singler RC: CT Guided celiac plexus and splanchnic nerve neurolysis. J Comput Assist Tomogr 6:315, 1982.)

cur in less than 1 per cent of patients.[81] When the needle tip is inadvertently placed into the peritoneal cavity, chemical peritonitis may follow the injection of alcohol and paralysis occurs after a direct subarachnoid injection or spread of alcohol along nerve roots into the subarachnoid space.[81] Back pain and moderate hypotension are common, minor complications that are usually transient.[79, 83] No serious complications have been reported after CT-guided neurolytic procedures.[74, 85] CT guidance and verification of needle position should detect needle malpositions (Fig. 22–39) and avoid inadvertent subarachnoid injections. Transcrural needle placement virtually eliminates the chance of alcohol flowing back along nerve roots into the spinal canal.

REFERENCES

1. Goldstein H, Zornoza J, Wallace S: Percutaneous fine needle aspiration biopsy of pancreatic and other abdominal masses. Radiology 123:319, 1977.
2. Göthlin JH: Post-lymphographic percutaneous fine needle

biopsy of lymph nodes guided by fluoroscopy. Radiology 120:205, 1976.

3. Pereiras RV, Meiers W, Kunhardt B, Troner M, Hutson D, Barkin JS, Viamonte M: Fluoroscopically guided thin needle aspiration biopsy of the abdomen and retroperitoneum. AJR 131:197, 1978.

4. Westcott JL: Direct percutaneous needle aspiration of localized pulmonary lesions: Results in 422 patients. Radiology 137:31, 1980.

5. Tylen U, Arnesjo B, Lindberg LG, Lunderquist A, Akerman M: Percutaneous biopsy of carcinoma of the pancreas guided by angiography. Surg Gynecol Obstet 142:737, 1976.

6. Oscarson J, Stormby N, Sundgren R: Selective angiography in fine needle aspiration cytodiagnosis of gastric and pancreatic tumors. Acta Radiol (Diag) 12:737, 1972.

7. Ho C-S, McLoughlin MJ, McHattie JD, Tao L-C: Percutaneous fine needle aspiration biopsy of the pancreas following endoscopic retrograde cholangiopancreatography. Radiology 125:351, 1977.

8. Hancke S, Holm HH, Koch F: Ultrasonically guided percutaneous fine needle biopsy of the pancreas. Surg Gynecol Obstet 140:361, 1975.

9. Holm HH, Pedersen JF, Kristensen JK, Rasmussen SN, Hancke S, Jensen E: Ultrasonically guided percutaneous puncture. Radiol Clin North Am 13:493, 1975.

10. Smith EH, Bartrum RJ Jr, Chang YC: Ultrasonically guided percutaneous aspiration biopsy of the pancreas. Radiology 112:737, 1974.

11. Bjork JT, Foley WD, Varma RR: Percutaneous liver biopsy in difficult cases simplified by CT or ultrasonic localization. Dig Dis Sci 26:146, 1981.

12. Johansen P, Svendsen KN: Scan-guided needle aspiration biopsy in malignant hepatic disease. Acta Cytol 22:292, 1978.

13. Haaga JR, Alfidi RJ: Precise biopsy localization by computed tomography. Radiology 118:603, 1976.

14. Haaga JR: New techniques for CT-guided biopsies. AJR 133:633, 1979.

15. Ferrucci JT Jr, Wittenberg J: CT biopsy of abdominal tumors: Aids for lesion localization. Radiology 129:739, 1978.

16. Ferrucci JT Jr, Wittenberg J, Mueller PR, Simeone JF, Harbin WP, Kirkpatrick RH, Taft PD: Diagnosis of abdominal malignancy by radiologic fine-needle aspiration biopsy. AJR 134:323, 1980.

17. Haaga JR, Vanek J: Computed tomographic guided liver biopsy using the Menghini needle. Radiology 133:405, 1979.

18. Jaques PF, Staab E, Richey W, Photopulos G, Swanton M: CT-assisted pelvic and abdominal aspiration biopsies in gynecological malignancy. Radiology 128:651, 1978.

19. Mueller PR, Wittenberg J, Ferrucci JT Jr: Fine-needle aspiration biopsy of abdominal masses. Semin Roentgenol 16:52, 1981.

20. Alfidi RJ, Haaga JR, Meaney TF, MacIntyre WJ, Gonzalez L, Tarar R, Zelch MG, Boller M, Cook SA, Jelden G: Computed tomography of the thorax and abdomen: A preliminary report. Radiology 117:257, 1975.

21. Boyd DP: Computed tomography. In Margulis AR, Burhenne HJ (eds): Alimentary Tract Radiology: Abdominal Imaging. St Louis, CV Mosby, 1979, pp 3–11.

22. Okuda K, Tanikawa K, Emura T, Kuratomi S, Jinnouchi S, Urabe K, Suminkoshi T, Kawada Y, Fukuyama Y, Musha H, Mori H, Shimokawa Y, Yakushiji F, Matsoura Y: Nonsurgical percutaneous transhepatic cholangiography—Diagnostic significance in medical problems of the liver. Am J Dig Dis 19:21, 1974.

23. Zornoza J: Abdomen. In Zornoza J (ed): Percutaneous Needle Biopsy. Baltimore, Williams & Wilkins, 1981, pp 102–140.

24. Coel MN, Niwayama G: Safety of percutaneous fine-needle pancreatic biopsy: A porcine model. Invest Radiol 13:547, 1978.

25. Gerzof SG: Triangulation: Indirect CT guidance for abscess drainage. AJR 137:1080, 1981.

26. Van Sonnenberg E, Wittenberg J, Ferrucci JT Jr, Mueller PR, Simeone JF: Triangulation method for percutaneous needle guidance: The angled approach to upper abdominal masses. AJR 137:757, 1981.

27. Lukeman JM: Cytological diagnosis and techniques. In Zornoza J (ed): Percutaneous Needle Biopsy. Baltimore, Williams & Wilkins, 1981, pp 1–12.

28. DeSantos LA, Zornoza J: Bone and soft tissue. In Zornoza J (ed): Percutaneous Needle Biopsy. Baltimore, Williams & Wilkins, 1981, pp 141–178.

29. Isler RJ, Ferrucci JT Jr, Wittenberg J, Simeone JF, Van Sonnenberg E, Hall DA: Tissue core biopsy of abdominal tumors with a 22 gauge cutting needle. AJR 136:725, 1981.

30. Adapon BD, Legada BD Jr, Lim EVA, Silao JV Jr, Cruz-Dalmacio A: CT guided closed biopsy of the spine. J Comput Assist Tomogr 5:73, 1981.

31. Hardy DC, Murphy WA, Gilula LA: Computed tomography in planning percutaneous bone biopsy. Radiology 134:447, 1980.

32. Anacker H: Efficiency and Limits of Radiologic Examination of the Pancreas. Publishing Sciences Group, Inc., Littleton, Mass, 1975, pp 273–276.

33. Arnesjo B, Stormby N, Akerman M: Cytodiagnosis of pancreatic lesions by means of fine-needle biopsy during operation. Acta Chir Scand 138:363, 1972.

34. Weiss VA, Koo AH, McClendon D: Percutaneous pancreatic aspiration biopsy. CT/T Clinical Symposium, vol 2, No 11. Milwaukee, General Electric Company, 1979.

35. Goldman ML, Naibz M, Galambos JT, Rude JC III, Oen K-T, Bradley EL III, Salam A, Gonzalez AC: Preoperative diagnosis of pancreatic carcinoma by percutaneous aspiration biopsy. Dig Dis Sci 22:1076, 1977.

36. Goldstein HM, Zornoza J: Percutaneous transperitoneal aspiration biopsy of pancreatic masses. Dig Dis Sci 23:840, 1978.

37. Haaga JR, Reich NE: CT-Guided needle procedures. In Haaga JR, Reich NE (eds): Computed Tomography of Abdominal Abnormalities. St Louis, CV Mosby, 1978, pp 315–354.

38. Harter LP, Moss AA, Goldberg HI: Computed tomographic guided fine needle aspirations for neoplastic and inflammatory diseases. AJR 140:363, 1983.

39. Ferrucci JT Jr, Wittenberg J, Margolies MN, Carey RW: Malignant seeding of the tract after thin-needle aspiration biopsy. Radiology 130:345, 1979.

40. Menghini G: One-second biopsy of the liver—Problems of its clinical application. N Engl J Med 283:582, 1970.

41. Ovlisen B, Baden H: Liver biopsy by the method of Menghini. Nord Med 83:297, 1970.

42. Conn HO, Yesner RA: A re-evaluation of needle biopsy in the diagnosis of metastatic cancer of the liver. Ann Intern Med 59:53, 1963.

43. Zamcheck N, Klausenstock O: Liver biopsy II. The rest of needle biopsy. N Engl J Med 249:1062, 1953.

44. Madden RE: Complications of needle biopsy of the liver. Arch Surg 83:778, 1961.

45. Zornoza J, Wallace S, Ordoncz N, Lukeman J: Fine-needle aspiration biopsy of the liver. AJR 134:331, 1980.

46. Zornoza J, Cabanillas FF, Altoff TM, Ordonez N, Cohen MA: Percutaneous needle biopsy in abdominal lymphoma. AJR 136:97, 1981.

47. Zornoza J, Wallace S, Goldstein HM, Lukeman JM, Jing B-S: Transperitoneal percutaneous retroperitoneal lymph node aspiration biopsy. Radiology 122:111, 1977.

48. Stephenson TF, Mehnert PJ, Marx AJ, Boger JN, Roth-Moyo L, Balaji MR, Nadaraja N: Evaluation of contrast markers for CT aspiration biopsy. AJR 133:1097, 1979.

49. Göthlin JH, Rupp N, Rothenberger KH, MacIntosh PK: Percutaneous biopsy of retroperitoneal lymph nodes: A multicentric study. Europ J Radiol 1:46, 1981.

50. Dunnick NR, Fisher RI, Chu EW, Young RC: Percutaneous aspiration of retroperitoneal lymph nodes in ovarian cancer. AJR 135:109, 1980.

51. Haaga J, Alfidi RJ: Computed tomography. In Margulis AR, Burhenne HJ (eds): Alimentary Tract Radiology: Abdominal Imaging. St Louis, CV Mosby, 1979, pp 623–640.

52. Thornbury JR, Burke DP, Naylor B: Transthoracic needle aspiration biopsy: Accuracy of cytologic typing of malignant neoplasms. AJR 136:719, 1981.

53. Lalli AF, McCormack LJ, Zelch M, Reich NE, Belouich D: Aspiration biopsies of chest lesions. Radiology 127:35, 1978.

54. Zornoza J: Lung and pleura. In Zornoza J (ed): Percutaneous Needle Biopsy. Baltimore, Williams & Wilkins, 1981, pp 52–77.

55. Koehler PR, Moss AA: Diagnosis of intraabdominal and pelvic abscesses by computed tomography. JAMA 244:49, 1980.

56. Haaga JR, Alfidi RJ, Havrilla TR, Cooperman AM, Seidelmann FE, Reich NE, Weinstein AJ, Meaney TF: CT detection and aspiration of abdominal abscesses. AJR 128:465, 1977.

57. Callen PW: Computed tomographic evaluation of abdominal and pelvic abscesses. Radiology 131:171, 1979.

58. Gerzof SG, Spira R, Robbins AH: Percutaneous abscess drainage. Semin Roentgenol 16:62, 1981.

59. Gerzof SG, Robbins AH, Birkett DH, Johnson WC, Pugatch RD, Vincent ME: Percutaneous catheter drainage of abdominal abscesses guided by ultrasound and computed tomography. AJR 133:1, 1979.

60. Haaga JR, Weinstein AJ: CT-guided percutaneous aspiration and drainage of abscesses. AJR 135:1187, 1980.

61. Gerzof SG, Robbins AH, Johnson WC, Birkett DH, Nabseth DC: Percutaneous catheter drainage of abdominal abscesses: A five year experience. N Engl J Med 305:653, 1981.

61a. van Waes PFGM: Management of loculated abscesses containing hardly drainable pus: A new approach. In Moss AA (ed): NMR, Interventional Radiology and Diagnostic Imaging Modalities. San Francisco, University of California Press, 1983, pp 347–360.

62. Martin EC, Karlson FB, Fankuchen E, Cooperman A, Casarella WJ: Percutaneous drainage in the management of hepatic abscesses. Surg Clin North Am 61:157, 1981.

63. von Sonnenberg E, Ferrucci JT Jr, Mueller PR, Wittenberg J, Simeone JF: Percutaneous drainage of abscesses and fluid collections: Technique, results and applications. Radiology 142:1, 1982.

64. De Cosse JJ, Poulin TL, Fox PS, Condon RE: Subphrenic abscess. Surg Gynecol Obstet 138:841, 1974.

65. Deck KB, Berne TV: Selective management of subphrenic abscesses. Arch Surg 114:1165, 1979.

66. Anderson MC: Management of pancreatic pseudocysts. Am J Surg 123:209, 1972.

67. Rosenberg IK, Kahn JA, Walt AJ: Surgical experience with pancreatic pseudocysts. Am J Surg 117:11, 1969.

68. Sankaran S, Walt AJ: The natural and unnatural history of pancreatic pseudocysts. Br J Surg 62:37, 1975.

69. Polk HC, Zeppa R, Warren WD: Surgical significance of differentiation between acute and chronic pancreatic collections. Ann Surg 169:444, 1969.

70. Haaga JR, Highman LM, Cooperman AV, Owens FJ: Percutaneous CT-guided pancreatography and pseudocystography. AJR 132:829, 1979.

71. MacErlean DP, Bryan DJ, Murphy JL: Pancreatic pseudocyst: Management by ultrasonically guided aspiration. Gastrointest Radiol 5:255, 1980.

72. Hancke S, Pedersen JF: Percutaneous puncture of pancreatic cysts guided by ultrasound. Surg Gynecol Obstet 142:551, 1976.

73. Andersen BN, Hancke S, Neilsen SAD: The diagnosis of pancreatic cyst by endoscopic retrograde pancreatography and ultrasonic scanning. Ann Surg 185:286, 1977.

74. Haaga JR, Reich NE, Havrilla TR, Alfidi RJ: Interventional CT scanning. Radiol Clin North Am 15:449, 1977.

75. Reich NE, Haaga JR, Havrilla TR, Cooperman A, Geiss A: Computed tomography—Guided percutaneous biliary drainage. Comput Axial Tomogr 1:111, 1977.

76. Bhatt G, Jason RS, Delany HM, Rudavsky AZ: Hepatic hematoma: Percutaneous drainage. AJR 135:1287, 1980.

77. Kappis M: Sensibilitat und lokale Anästhesie und chirugischen Gebiet der Bauchhole mit besonderer Berücksichtigung der Splanchnicus Anästhesis. Beitrage zur Klin Chirurgie 115:161, 1919.

78. Jones RR: A technic for injection of splanchnic nerves with alcohol. Anesth Analg 36:75, 1957.

79. Bridenbaugh LD, Moore DC, Campbell DD: Management of upper abdominal cancer pain. JAMA 190:877, 1964.

80. Bell SN, Cole R, Roberts-Thomson IC: Celiac plexus block for control of pain in chronic pancreatitis. Br Med J 281:1064, 1980.

81. Thompson GE, Moore DC, Bridenbaugh DL, Artin RY: Abdominal pain and alcohol celiac plexus nerve block. Anes Analges Current Res 56:1, 1977.

82. Boas RA: Sympathetic blocks in clinical practice. Int Anesthesiol Clin 16:149, 1978.

83. Ward EM, Rorie DK, Nauss LA, Bahn RC: The celiac ganglia in man: Normal anatomic variations. Anesth Analg 58:461, 1979.

84. Jackson SA, Jacobs JB, Epstein RA: Angiologic approach to celiac plexus block. Anesthesiology 31:373, 1969.

85. Buy J-N, Moss AA, Singler RC: CT Guided celiac plexus and splanchnic nerve neurolysis. J Comput Assist Tomogr 6:315, 1982.

86. Elmgilie RC, Slavotinek AH: Surgical objectives in unresected cancer of the head of the pancreas. Br J Surg 59:508, 1972.

23 QUANTITATIVE COMPUTED TOMOGRAPHY

Christopher E. Cann

Computed tomography (CT) as an imaging modality has in many ways revolutionized diagnostic radiology. The cross-sectional display of anatomy afforded by this technique has provided the means whereby an isolated region can be examined free from surrounding tissue that overlies the region of interest (ROI) in a conventional radiograph. However, the pictorial display of a CT image has also overshadowed the very basis of that image, in that the superb contrast resolution of CT enables visualization of organs by virtue of their differences in x-ray attenuation. The CT image is a pictorial map of x-ray attenuation values of a cross-sectional region of the body, and this map is stored in digital form in a computer memory and can be easily accessed. The use of this digital information, the CT numbers, to provide diagnostic information about a patient study can be referred to as quantitative computed tomography, or QCT.

Several investigators recognized the potential of QCT early after the introduction of the first commercial CT scanner, the EMI head scanner. The use of the CT numbers to characterize lesions in the brain[1] was a novel approach to the definition of pathology and may have aided in diagnosis because of the low spatial resolution of the early scanners, which made pictorial identification of the type and extent of many lesions difficult. The early scanners by virtue of their configuration—using a water bag to provide constant path length—provided relatively reproducible and accurate CT numbers that could be used with confidence. These scanners were also used by researchers in non-neurologic fields to begin quantification of tissue densities, particularly for bone.[2, 3] The development of whole body CT scanners that did not require a water bag[4] was a major step forward in imaging of both the head and body. However, by surrounding the irregularly shaped body with air rather than water, the equivalent soft-tissue path length of the x-ray beam could vary dramatically, depending upon the position of the source and detector relative to the object being scanned. This characteristic of whole body scanners introduced significant errors in the CT numbers, especially the accuracy with which they represented the true tissue attenuation coefficients. Errors of several per cent or up to 40 to 50 Hounsfield Units (H) resulting from object size and inhomogeneities were common. Factors such as dependence on object position within the scanning field and improper correction for the polychromatic nature of the x-ray source (beam hardening) are only now being corrected to any satisfactory extent. The accuracy of the CT numbers is finally being brought back to the level that was available with the water-bag systems and the level at which we can expect to be able to use the CT numbers on a routine basis to aid in diagnosis and evaluation of treatment.

THE BASIS OF QUANTITATIVE CT

The data that are displayed as the CT image are a representation of the x-ray attenuation coefficients of a series of volume elements (voxels), which are defined by their size and position within the reconstructed image. In a perfect CT scanner, the CT number of each voxel would be an accurate reflection of the true tissue attenuation coefficient in that element.

Current CT scanners have limitations because of volume averaging between adjacent voxels (spatial resolution) and statistical fluctuations in the value of the CT number calculated for each voxel as a result of limitations in detected photon flux. For homogeneous material such as a water phantom, the major contribution to CT number variation between voxels is the statistical variation based on limited photon transmission. In this case, we can define a distribution of CT numbers by a mean (equal to zero for water) and a standard deviation about this mean, which is determined primarily by the administered x-ray dose. The CT number variations are random in nature and are well represented by a symmetric function approaching a gaussian distribution when a large enough region is examined. Mixing a second material of slightly different density into the first will produce a distribution of materials rather than a homogeneous material and we are faced with two possibilities:

1. If the second material is composed of particulates larger than the nominal spatial resolution of the CT system, we would see a discrete separation between the two materials.

2. If the particulate size is smaller than the resolving element, we would have volume averaging between the two materials. In this case, we would have a material that looks homogeneous but has a wider distribution or standard deviation about a mean CT number than would be expected on the basis of purely dosimetric considerations.

These two factors that affect the CT number, statistical fluctuation because of limited photon transmission and physical inhomogeneities in a two-component system, are common to all densitometry studies using CT. Other factors, however, greatly affect the accuracy and reproducibility of specific types of QCT studies, often to the point of severely restricting or eliminating their usefulness. These factors can be inherent in scanner design or in the physiology or morphology of the system under study and can affect primarily accuracy, primarily reproducibility, or both.

ACCURACY

The largest inaccuracies in a CT number are due to suboptimal corrections for the polychromaticity and scatter of the x-ray beam. If a CT scanner source were monoenergetic, the attenuation of the beam along any projection would be truly exponential, dependent only upon the attenuation coefficients of the composite of materials through which the beam passed. A monoenergetic CT scan and subsequent reconstruction, exclusive of numerical reconstruction errors, would be an accurate representation of the map of attenuation coefficients in the scanned region. Unfortunately, all commercial CT scanners use a filtered bremsstrahlung x-ray source that provides an effective energy of 60 to 70 keV but with a range of x-ray energies from about 40 to the nominal peak voltage of 120 to 130 kVp.

As this spectrum of x-rays passes through tissue, the lower-energy photons are absorbed with a greater frequency than the high-energy photons because of the increased attenuation coefficient of matter (μ) at lower photon energies. At each successive point along the projection from source to detector, the mean x-ray energy of the remaining photons has become slightly higher, so that by the time the beam has passed through a thick part of the body or head, its mean energy has shifted, for example, from 60 to 80 keV. However, if the beam passes through a thin part of the body, its energy may shift from only 60 to 65 keV, and the average attenuation per unit path length (μ, cm^{-1}) will be higher, even if the object is of identical material along the two path lengths. This beam-hardening effect can be corrected empirically and accurately if the precise size and composition of the object being scanned are known, for example, a cylindrical water phantom. However, if the exact size and composition of most objects (i.e., patients) were known, there would be no need to scan them. Therefore, some assumptions must be made about the object if one attempts to correct for beam hardening inaccuracies in the CT numbers.

The first and most logical assumption is that a body is a cylinder of uniform density and known size and a head is a cylinder of uniform density contained within a thin shell of higher density. Proper implementation of this correction can eliminate most of the beam-hardening error in the abdomen or head, and CT numbers in these areas of the body have been shown to reflect tissue attenuation moderately well.[5, 6] However, the same correction applied to the chest (which contains mostly air) or the thigh (which contains large amounts of dense bone) will produce an inaccurate result. Special techniques such as postprocessing beam-hardening corrections[7] or preprocessed dual-energy CT[8, 9, 9a] must be used in these cases to eliminate the errors.

The accuracy of a CT number can be affected by technical factors other than x-ray polychromaticity. Older whole body CT scanners, especially some of the translate-rotate design, have reconstruction algorithms and x-ray beam compensa-

tors ("bowtie filters") that produce severe nonuniformities in CT number for identical objects placed at various positions in the scanning field. These errors must be corrected empirically (that is, by calibrating with an object similar in density and spatial characteristics as the patient) if these scanners are to be used for QCT. Unfortunately, some of these undesirable characteristics have carried over to some of the newer scanner designs as well, so that not all of the advanced CT scanners now on the market are suited to QCT applications.[10]

Another factor that may be less of a technical error than an error of interpretation of data is "volume averaging." Consider an ideal CT scanner in which the photon beam is monoenergetic and perfectly collimated (Fig. 23–1, top left). A scan of an object that is smaller in length than the slice thickness will always produce a CT number in the final image which corresponds to an average attenuation for the object and its surrounding medium in proportion to the contribution of each to the total μ. The only way to eliminate this effect is to reduce the slice thickness to the point where the object is totally contained within the beam profile. In this case we can then obtain a "true" CT number for the object in the ideal scanner.

Figure 23–1. Partial-volume errors may be caused by different factors. **Left** Object smaller than the slice thickness will be averaged with surrounding material to produce attenuation value smaller than expected. Reducing slice thickness eliminates volume averaging. **Right** Object not centered with respect to sensitive width of beam produces low-attenuation reading for source-detector position, higher attenuation with 180° position change. Reconstructed image will contain error from variable volume averaging in projections as a function of rotational angle. Plane of rotation about the isocenter is into or out of the page.

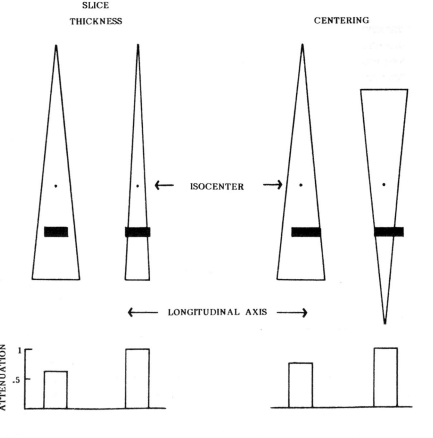

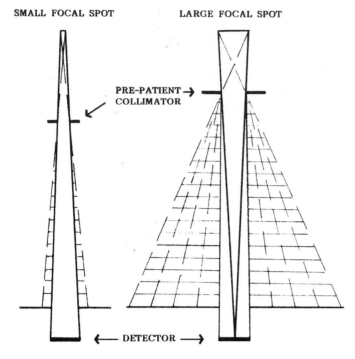

SMALL FOCAL SPOT   LARGE FOCAL SPOT

PRE–PATIENT → COLLIMATOR

← DETECTOR →

Figure 23–2. Shape of sensitivity profile of x-ray beam varies according to focal spot size, collimator and detector aperture, and source-collimator distance. **Left** Small focal spot, large source-collimator distance produces relatively uniform beam profile in longitudinal axis. **Right** Larger focal spot, shorter source-collimator distance can produce gaussian profile so that object in center of beam contributes more to intensity in reconstructed image than surrounding medium, causing artificially high or artificially low CT number.

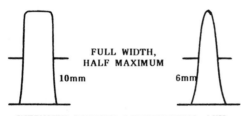

FULL WIDTH, HALF MAXIMUM

10mm   6mm

INTENSITY PROFILE, LONGITUDINAL AXIS

However, CT scanners are far from ideal, and several effects contribute to inaccuracies as a result of volume averaging.

One of the most important factors is the shape of the x-ray beam profile as it passes through the patient. For many commercial scanners, this profile is not square, as for an ideal scanner, but is weighted more heavily toward the center of the beam; that is, there is greater sensitivity at the center of the slice than at the edges. The exact profile depends on focal spot size and on prepatient and postpatient collimation and can vary from nearly square to nearly gaussian (Fig 23–2). For an object larger than the slice thickness and a properly calibrated scanner, the CT number of the object can usually be represented adequately for any beam profile. However, for the object thinner than the slice, a gaussian profile will weight the centered object more than its surrounding medium when the projection data are obtained and so may give an inaccurate representation of the x-ray attenuation of that scanned region. In addition, if the object is not centered in the scanning circle, the beam profile that it sees at different times during the scan will be different (Fig. 23–1, top right) and even postprocessing or preprocessing beam-hardening corrections may be suboptimal because of this partial volume effect.

On a practical basis, volume averaging due just to slice thickness too large for the object can be compensated by using a thinner slice.[11] However, the error caused by beam profile may not be completely correctable,[11] and it may be futile to try to extract quantitative information from a technically unsuitable scan. In most cases, the volume-averaging effect can be empirically corrected or taken into account, and this will be illustrated later with discussion of some clinically useful techniques for QCT.

Accurate measurement of the CT number, or x-ray attenuation, may not be adequate to provide

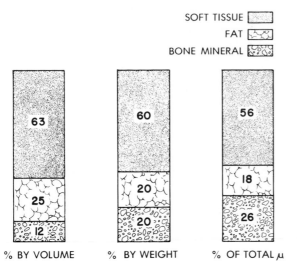

SOFT TISSUE
FAT
BONE MINERAL

% BY VOLUME   % BY WEIGHT   % OF TOTAL μ

Figure 23–3. Composition of the vertebral trabecular bone mixture of an older individual, showing the fraction of volume occupied by bone, red marrow, and fat. Presence of fat reduces the x-ray attenuation of the mixture relative to case with only red marrow and bone, and assumptions about marrow composition must be made to estimate bone mineral content.

the desired diagnostic information. The CT number represents total x-ray attenuation in a volume element, or voxel, in a CT scan, and is the sum of the attenuation of all the different materials contained in that voxel. If the voxel contains two components (such as fat mixed with soft tissue) and each component has a known attenuation coefficient the concentrations of these two components can be uniquely determined. However, when a third component of different attenuation is added to the mixture, determination of the composition is no longer unique. For example, the addition of 10 per cent fat with a CT number

about −100 H (density 0.92 gm cm^{-3}) to normal liver at 50 H (density 1.05 gm cm^{-3}) would produce a CT number of about 37 H. If a patient also stores several per cent glycogen (density about 1.2 gm cm^{-3}), this would raise the CT number back to normal, so that this three-component system would look like the initial single component.

A similar situation for the vertebral bone mixture is illustrated in Figure 23–3, wherein the three components are bone, marrow, and fat, and the primary component of interest, bone, cannot be measured independently of the other components if the fat content is high. If one of the components is sufficiently different from the others in terms of its x-ray attenuation properties, it may be uniquely distinguished (Fig. 23–4). This is true, for example, for calcium-containing stones or diffuse nephrocalcinosis, iron in liver, or bone mineral in the spine, which can be separated from soft tissue by scanning at two energies and attributing the differential absorption at high and low x-ray energies to the high atomic number component (calcium, iron, phosphorus). In this way the physiologic contribution to inaccuracy of measurement may be minimized. Proper assessment and correction for these physical and physiologic factors can provide not only an accurate CT number but also a relatively accurate determination of the component of interest.

REPRODUCIBILITY

Although many quantitative CT studies require only that a diagnosis be made on the basis of the CT number, and thus a separation from a normal population, perhaps the greatest use of QCT is in

Figure 23–4. X-ray attenuation coefficient (μ) as a function of energy for iron and muscle. At the energies normally used for CT scanning (55 to 70 keV), there is a dramatic change in μ for iron and a very slight change for muscle. By scanning a tissue containing iron at two energies, the measured change in μ will be due primarily to the iron content.

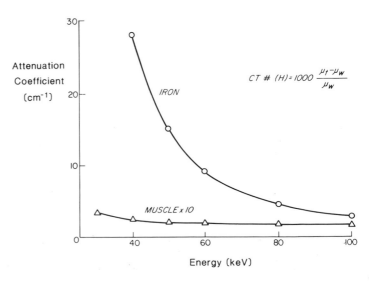

$$CT \ \# \ (H) = 1000 \ \frac{\mu_t - \mu_w}{\mu_w}$$

IRON

MUSCLE x 10

Attenuation Coefficient (cm^{-1})

Energy (keV)

serial studies for the management of patients. For this application, the most stringent requirement on any QCT technique is that it be reproducible, that is, multiple measurements of an unchanging quantity should be constant over the period of the study.

It is important to recognize that the quantity measured need not be the CT number. For densitometry studies, a relative measure of CT number, or x-ray attenuation, is often sufficient to provide the desired information. In the head, for example, the CT number of relatively constant CSF can be used as a reference in serial studies of brain density as long as one knows that CSF is not changing. Likewise, the relationship between liver and spleen CT number is known[12] and can be used to look at various hepatic disorders, and the CT number of blood in the aorta can be used in the chest. These internal references, however, are certainly not optimal because of variability between patients and changes with time in the same patient. For those scanners in which field uniformity is good and has been well documented, a reference standard of known composition can be scanned at the same time as the patient[13, 14]. In all cases, the reference material is used to improve the reliability of the relative CT number of the object of interest.

In an ideal CT scanner, a reference material would not be necessary because the CT number would be accurate. However, as discussed earlier, many factors can affect the accuracy of the CT numbers in the short term. In addition to these scan-to-scan effects, there are longer-term effects caused by x-ray tube aging, software and hard-ware changes, detector drifts, and other factors that cause the CT number of an object to change. Most scanners are calibrated on a day-to-day basis using air and water, so that the CT number changes for soft tissue are compensated.[14] However, because some scanners still do not correct the projection data for object size, there can be scan-to-scan variation in the CT number of a uniform object such as the liver. Thus, even for soft-tissue densitometry (low atomic number components), it is desirable to have a reference standard in the scanning field.

The situation for CT number stability for high-atomic-number (Z) components such as iron or calcium is more complex. The x-ray attenuation coefficient of these elements has a significant photoelectric component at the scanning energies normally used, and because photoelectric absorption varies approximately as Z^4 and is highly dependent on energy, a slight shift in the effective x-ray energy can be manifest as a significant change in CT number. Thus, as an x-ray tube gets older and tungsten plates out on the window, filtering and hardening the beam, the measured CT number decreases. Likewise, a high tube current may reduce the effective kVp and increase the CT number (Fig. 23–5).[15] Therefore, for measurement of bone mineral or other tissue calcium concentration, or for liver iron concentration, a standard containing the appropriate high-Z material must be scanned along with the patient.

The duration of any study and the desired reproducibility determine the necessity of a reference standard. A study of the vascularity of a tu-

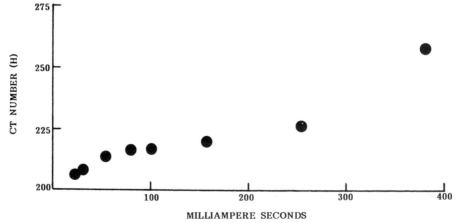

Figure 23–5. Effect of x-ray tube loading on effective kVp. Calculated CT number for mineral-equivalent solution containing potassium (Z = 19) and phosphorus (Z = 15) changes depending upon tube current (generator load). CT number of solution is measured in a phantom simulating the human abdomen, 30 cm in diameter, minimizing differences in beam hardening. The effect would be magnified if object were smaller or less homogeneous, for example, in the lung or peripheral skeleton.

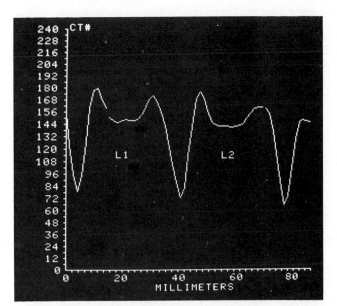

Figure 23–6. CT number profile along the longitudinal axis of the spine. High densities are vertebral endplates, low densities through the intervertebral discs. There is a relative plateau in the center of the vertebral body, 13 to 15 mm thick, allowing positioning of an 8- to 10-mm thick scanning volume within this plateau region. A positioning error of ± 1 to 2 mm will not significantly affect the measured CT number; an error of 3 to 4 mm may affect the CT value by 8 to 10 per cent.

mor by contrast enhancement over a period of minutes or hours may not require a reference other than a precontrast scan, whereas measurements of long-term degenerative liver changes or vertebral bone mineral changes must be calibrated to compensate for machine-related changes which occur between measurements.

A major factor that affects reproducibility in some types of studies is repositioning to the same volume for sequential analysis. This is particularly important when the CT number changes rapidly over a short distance, such as passing from vertebral trabecular bone into the compact bone or end plate (Fig. 23–6), or from a lung nodule into lung tissue.[16] Repositioning is less critical when the CT number change at a boundary is relatively slow and monotonic as in liver infiltrated by tumor.[17] The amount of volume averaging of a region of interest depends strongly on slice thickness, as discussed earlier, and it significantly affects the repositioning capabilities for small objects. Newer CT scanners provide computed radiographic localization systems for specification of one or more scanning planes. Proper utilization of these external localizers can provide positioning to 1 to 1.5 mm for relatively stationary objects like the spine, but other positioning methods

such as software reformatting or rapid-sequence scanning must be used for objects like lung nodules, which will move between the time a localizer scan and a CT scan are done. For larger objects, repositioning is not as critical, with errors due to volume averaging introduced only at the edges of the object. Thus, positioning requirements can be tailored to the exam, and adequate techniques are currently available that can be used or modified to fit almost any type of study.

The radiation dose necessary to provide quantitative information from CT scans depends upon the study to be done. High-contrast objects, such as bone, can be quantified using a low-dose, one tenth to one twentieth that used for imaging because edges are easily detected and a large ROI can be used to average statistical noise in the data and obtain the desired information.[15] In this case, the pixel standard deviation has little effect on the standard deviation of the mean CT number in a large ROI. The study of low-contrast objects such as edema in brain[18] necessitates a higher dose to better define the boundaries between edema and normal tissue (Fig. 23–7). A low-dose scan in this case may increase the pixel standard deviation significantly, so that measurement of edema based on CT number may be masked by the wide variation of CT number for normal tissue. In general, however, quantitative CT studies require significantly less radiation dose to the patient than a routine diagnostic imaging study. This is particularly important in the management of patients in whom serial studies are necessary.

The clinical utility of QCT relies on the development of techniques which have accuracy, reproducibility, and sensitivity *sufficient* to answer the diagnostic question. Methods and clinical results for specific applications in the liver, bone, and chest are discussed in the following sections to illustrate the diagnostic capabilities of QCT.

DENSITOMETRY AND VOLUME STUDIES OF THE LIVER
(with Albert A. Moss and Henry I. Goldberg)

The clinical application of QCT in the abdomen has found its greatest use in studies of diffuse liver disease of metabolic origins and metastatic disease. Densitometry provides quantitative information about fatty infiltration, glycogen storage, and iron storage.[19, 20, 20a] Volumetric analysis

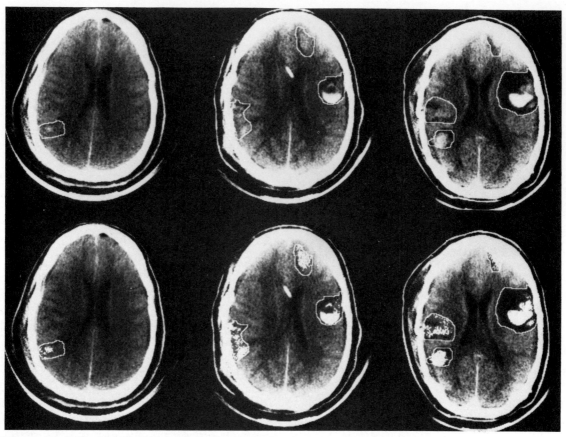

Figure 23–7. Evolution of hematomas in the brain, demonstrating necessity for high radiation dose to define low-contrast boundaries. **Top** First, second, and seventh day after traumatic injury, showing appearance and change in composition of lesions, including high-density, isodense, and edematous components. **Bottom** Volume of high-density component is determined using histogram-based region-of-interest analysis. Highlighted pixels define high-density regions within lesions.

can quantify the amount of tumor whether as a large lesion or distibuted small lesions.[17, 21] Both types of studies provide information useful in patient diagnosis and management.

Iron storage in the liver can be a complication of hemochromatosis or secondary to the congenital or chronic acquired anemia in patients who receive repeated blood transfusions. In both these disorders, it is desirable to have both a sensitive measure of iron content to detect iron overload and a reproducible method of monitoring iron changes during the treatment of patients by phlebotomy or desferroxamine or after transfusions. Serum ferritin levels are often used as an indirect assessment of iron stores but are subject to significant inaccuracies for prediction of total body iron.[22] Percutaneous needle biopsy of the skin or liver provides a tissue sample for pathologic analysis but is invasive and subject to sampling site errors because of the small biospies obtained. In addition, specialized techniques such as neutron activation analysis must be used to provide the sensitivity and reproducibility necessary for meas-

urement of the microgram amounts of iron present in these samples. Dual-energy CT can be used to measure liver iron quantitatively based on the differential attenuation of iron at two effective scanning energies which produces a linear relationship between the change in CT number and the concentration of iron present in the tissue (Figs. 23–8 and 23–9). Predictive accuracy for liver iron (dispersion about the regression) is 8 per cent, compared with iron concentration measurements made by neutron activation analysis of needle biopsies from dogs (Fig. 23–10).[20] Studies in patients have shown that liver iron can be detected with a sensitivity of about 2 mg of iron per gm of tissue when a patient is scanned with special calibrations (Fig. 23–8). Prediction of cardiac iron overload from liver iron content is desirable but may not be possible.[23]

Excessive glycogen deposition in the liver results in an increased x-ray attenuation which is proportional to the amount of glycogen in the liver cells. In contrast to iron deposition, which can be quantified with dual-energy CT, glycogen

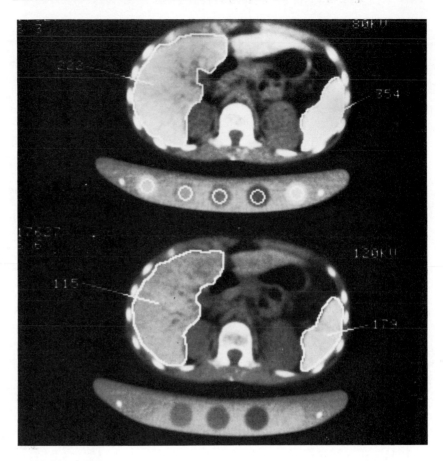

Figure 23–8. CT scans of a patient with iron storage disease at 80 and 120 kVp. CT number of muscle or kidney change about 50 H, similar to water and resulting from different attenuation of soft tissue at 80 versus 120 kVp. Change in CT number for liver or spleen is much greater, indicating high atomic number component to the tissue (iron). Calibration standard under patient contains solutions of iron-dextran as reference material to quantify tissue iron content accurately.

produces no unique tissue signature on CT and is quantified only by the increased attenuation over that of normal liver. In a similar manner, as described in Chapter 13, fatty infiltration of the liver causes a decrease in CT number proportional to the triglyceride content. Based on these relationships and the ability to estimate the normal CT value of the liver by measuring the attenuation value of the spleen,[12] quantification of hepatic fat or glycogen is possible. However, the

clinical usefulness of this technique may be limited if there is concomitant increase in liver fibrosis as occurs in cirrhosis.

In contrast to iron or glycogen storage, which is diffusely spread throughout the liver, metastatic disease can manifest as diffuse disease or isolated lesions. The clinician is faced with the diagnosis of metastases to the liver but also wishes to know the extent of liver involvement to correlate with liver function. A measure of response to treat-

Figure 23–9. Sensitivity of dual-energy CT for detection of iron. Change in CT number as a function of iron content produces a linear relationship used to calibrate measured difference in liver or spleen CT number. (From Goldberg HI, Cann CE, Moss AA, Ohto M, Brito A, Federle M: Noninvasive quantitation of liver iron in dogs with hemochromatosis using dual-energy CT scanning. Invest Radiol 17:375, 1982. Used with permission.)

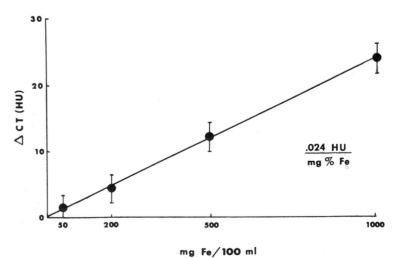

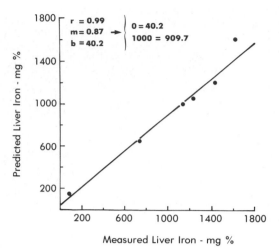

Figure 23–10. Correlation between iron concentration in liver measured by quantitative CT and by neutron activation analysis.[20] Dispersion about the regression line Sy/$\bar{y}$ is 8 per cent. Part of the dispersion is due to small size of biopsies used for neutron activation analysis (1 to 3 mg) reflecting possible inhomogeneity in liver iron content. *In vivo* accuracy with CT appears to be 3 to 5 per cent in humans, with a reproducibility for iron measurement better than 3 per cent. (From Goldberg HI, Cann CE, Moss AA, Ohto M, Brito A, Federle M: Non-invasive quantitation of liver iron in dogs with hemochromatosis using dual-energy CT scanning. Invest Radiol 17:375, 1982. Used with permission.)

ment or progression of disease is also useful. In many cases, the number of discreet lesions is very great (Fig. 23–11, top), and volumetric analysis of tumor is difficult if the size of individual lesions must be determined. A grading system for change may be used, but it is subjective and not quantitative.[21]

Most tumor in the liver is of low density and can be differentiated from normal liver parenchyma, and this provides the basis for tumor quantification using CT attenuation values. Normal liver tissue can be represented by a symmetric distribution of CT numbers (Fig. 23–11, bottom). The addition of tumor to this distribution adds a component to the low CT number side of the distribution, making it nonsymmetric. The total number of pixels or voxels below the mean CT value for normal liver is greater than that above the mean, and the difference in volume represents the volume of tumor in the liver. With measurement of total liver volume, the percentage of tumor can also be calculated. This method is simple, easily implemented, reproducible (± 10 per cent) and provides the clinician with a number which can be directly compared to previous studies to quantify patient response.[17, 21]

The use of dual-energy CT for measurement of liver iron and quantitative volumetric analysis

of hepatic tumors has so far been restricted because of the special procedures necessary to either obtain or analyze the data. Newer CT scanners provide multiple-energy scanning capabilities and more accurate CT values for tissue components. The software for data analysis is becoming more user-oriented as well. The combination of technical improvements and clinician demand will provide the impetus for implementation of these techniques in routine radiologic diagnosis and patient management.

QUANTITATIVE SPINAL BONE MINERAL ANALYSIS
(with Harry K. Genant)

The clinical evaluation of patients with metabolic bone disorders by quantitative bone mineral determination provides an important objective criterion of the progress of disease or response to therapy. Computed tomography has been used

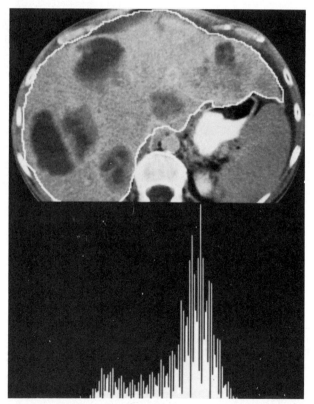

Figure 23–11. Top Liver infiltrated with tumor. Number of metastases is very large, precluding volumetric analysis by quantifying individual lesions. **Bottom** Histogram of CT numbers of region outlined in top figure. Gaussian distribution at right is distribution for normal liver, depending primarily on administered x-ray exposure (noise in image). Tumor component of liver is lower density (left of figure) and can be quantified using straightforward techniques.[17]

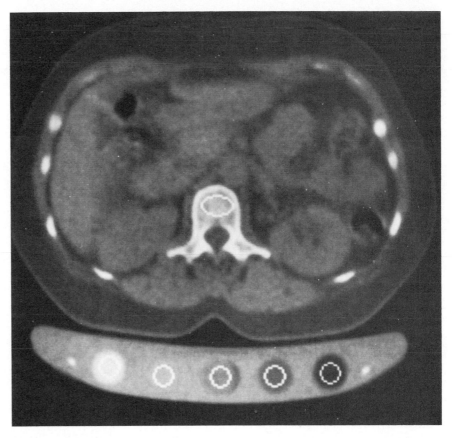

Figure 23–12. CT scan of patient at the level of the midportion of the first lumbar vertebra. Calibration phantom contains mineral and soft-tissue equivalent solutions for reference.

for mineral analysis in the radius[24, 25] and the spine.[26–30] Perhaps its greatest clinical potential lies in its ability to measure the content of purely trabecular bone in the spine and to make this measurement with high reproducibility and acceptable accuracy. This provides an assessment of mineral content at the site of earliest clinical involvement, the spine, and in bone, which has a high turnover rate and is most responsive to metabolic stimulus.

The technical requirements for QCT for spinal mineral analysis are strict and have been detailed previously.[13, 29] A standardized reference calibration phantom is used to correct for machine changes (Fig. 23–12), and vertebral mineral values are expressed in terms of mineral equivalent, referenced to this phantom. Positioning precisely to the center of the vertebral body may be accomplished either by software localization procedures[13] or by the use of the computed radiographic localization system available on most newer scanners. Reproducibility for measurement using the calibration phantom and software localization is 1.6 per cent in vivo at the University of California at San Francisco.[31] When the external localization method is used, reproducibility appears to be 3 to 3.5 per cent. Theoretical and phantom work[2] predicts inaccuracy of single-energy QCT of as much as 15 to 20 per cent if

large amounts, up to 50 per cent, of the vertebral marrow volume is replaced by fat. However, this appears only to be the case in the elderly population where hemopoetic marrow is replaced by yellow marrow, or in specific diseases such as steroid-induced osteoporosis. Dual-energy CT may reduce this error to 3 to 5 per cent[2, 9] but may not be necessary in the normal case, wherein biological variability about the normal mean for mineral content is 15 to 20 per cent (Fig. 23–13).

Two clinical areas in which QCT is useful for measurement of spinal trabecular mineral content are in diagnosis of osteoporosis or osteopenia (decrement of bone relative to normal) and in treatment of patients. For diagnosis, the ability to separate a patient from the normal population is of paramount importance, and the accuracy of a measurement must be adequate for this purpose. Patient management, on the other hand, requires a method that is very reproducible, so that measurements made serially with time will determine if bone mass is increasing or decreasing as a result of therapy or disease progression. QCT in the spine, when properly done, is adequate for both these purposes.

Cross-sectional studies of normal and osteoporotic men and women have been done to determine the capability of QCT to distinguish osteo-

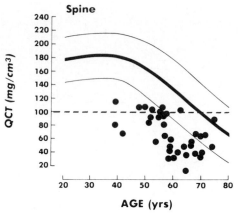

Figure 23–13. Mineral equivalent of the vertebral cancellous bone as a function of age in females. Solid lines are normal age-related changes. Closed circles represent patients with at least one vertebral fracture. A threshold level of bone mineral content exists at about 100 mg/cm³, above which patients do not experience fracture but below which a high probability of fracture appears to exist.

porotic patients from the normal population.[32] Figure 23–13 shows the normal range for 200 female controls, and the spinal mineral values for osteoporotic women (one or more vertebral crush fractures) superimposed upon this normal range; Figure 23–14 shows a similar curve for 120 normal males and 40 osteoporotics. It can be seen that below a threshold value of mineral content, about 100 mg/cm³, fractures occur in the spine. On the other hand, the number of patients with mineral content above this threshold and who have fractures is very small. Thus, it appears that

QCT may be a useful predictive index of fracture in osteoporotic or osteopenic patients.

Changes in bone mass with time as measured by QCT and compared with standard quantitative bone measurements can be illustrated with a group of women who were studied serially following oophorectomy.[27, 31, 33] Graded doses of conjugated estrogens (e.g., Premarin) were given to determine the minimum dose of estrogen that prevented bone loss. Bone mass was measured at 0, 6, 12, and 24 months in the spine using QCT, and in the cortical bone of the radius and the metacarpals using photon absorptiometry and radiogrammetry, respectively. At 24 months, the mean changes for the estrogen dose groups and the individual correlations between peripheral cortical bone and spinal trabecular bone were determined. Figure 23–15 shows the spinal bone loss, in per cent per year, in the patients receiving the different estrogen doses. It can be seen that only the dose of 0.625 mg/day prevents spinal loss. The correlation between peripheral cortical bone loss and spinal trabecular bone loss (Fig. 23–16) was weak, and the dispersion of the data precludes accurate prediction of vertebral mineral loss from peripheral measurements in individual patients. This figure also shows the much greater magnitude of spinal mineral loss than peripheral bone loss.

Measurements of spinal bone mass using QCT are still being refined, but the present state of the techniques is suitable for many applications. Continued improvements in CT hardware and software, such as multiple energy CT and better lo-

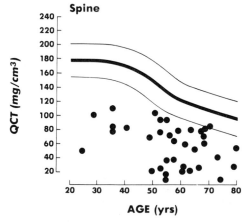

Figure 23–14. Age-related changes in normal males (solid lines) and vertebral trabecular mineral content in osteoporotic males (closed circles). As in Figure 23–13, a threshold level exists above which fractures do not occur. Note also an apparent age-related loss in the osteoporotics superimposed on the decrement of bone mass compared with normal condition.

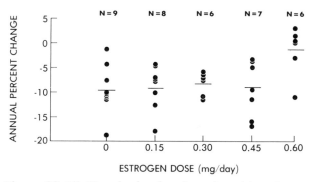

Figure 23–15. Vertebral trabecular mineral loss, in per cent per year, for oophorectomized women receiving graded doses of replacement estrogens. Only the equivalent of 0.6 mg/day of conjugated estrogens prevented vertebral mineral loss. (From Genant HK, Cann CE, Ettinger B, Gordan GS: Quantitative computed tomography of vertebral spongiosa: A sensitive method for detecting early bone loss after oophorectomy. Ann Intern Med 97:799, 1982. Used with permission.)

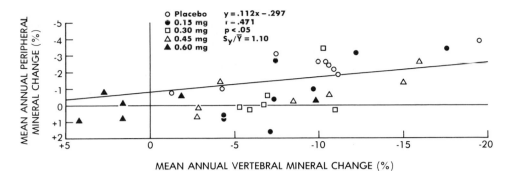

Figure 23–16. Comparison of peripheral cortical and vertebral trabecular bone loss in individual patients. The regression indicates a nine-fold greater loss from trabecular bone than peripheral cortical bone. In addition, the wide dispersion around the regression precludes prediction of spinal loss from a measurement of peripheral bone loss. (From Genant HK, Cann CE, Ettinger B, Gordan GS: Quantitative computed tomography of vertebral spongiosa: A sensitive method for detecting early bone loss after oophorectomy. Ann Intern Med 97:799, 1982. Used with permission.)

calization capabilities, will provide a method which can be accurate, reproducible, convenient, and inexpensive for routine use, and, when properly implemented, can have widespread clinical applicability in the assessment of metabolic bone disease.

EVALUATION OF PULMONARY NODULES AND PARENCHYMAL DENSITY
(with Gordon Gamsu)

Pulmonary density changes may reflect pathological conditions, and an accurate measurement of lung tissue density may be useful in diagnosis. In particular, the evaluation of solitary pulmonary nodules by QCT has been reported to provide information about the nature of the lesions.[34, 37] However, QCT densitometry of the chest, particularly for small isolated lesions, is one of the most technically difficult procedures to accomplish. Commercial scanners can provide relatively accurate CT numbers when the scanned field is homogeneous, such as in the abdomen or head. However, in the chest the changes in density over short distances are very large, going from rib or spine into lung or from the heart into the lung. In addition, the moving heart causes artifacts in the image and in the CT numbers. These anatomic discontinuities cause major problems for a reconstruction algorithm which is tailored to the abdomen, as are most commercial body routines. This problem, coupled with the volume averaging artifacts discussed earlier, makes measurement of absolute tissue densities in the lung very difficult.

These technical difficulties can be approached in two ways to make CT densitometry in the lung feasible. The first approach is to standardize the CT numbers to a reference scale so that they can be interpreted. This may be accomplished either by improvements in the reconstruction algorithms done by the manufacturer or by empirical corrections to the image done by the investigator. The latter requires the construction of phantoms to simulate the chest and extensive measurements of regional differences in CT number. The second approach, which we have investigated,[35, 36] uses dual-energy CT to measure CT number shifts and to correlate this with tissue characteristics such as calcification. This approach eliminates many of the positional and algorithm-related errors but can provide only a relative measure of tissue density. However, it can accurately quantify tissue calcification and thus may be clinically useful in the study of solitary pulmonary nodules.

Results for quantitative CT analysis of simulated pulmonary nodules are shown in Figure 23–17 for single-energy CT and Figure 23–18 for dual-energy CT. The dispersion about the regression is 3.82 per cent at 120 kVp on a GE CT/T 8800 and 1.48 per cent for dual energy at 80 and 120 kVp. The lower dispersion with the dual-energy method results from the elimination of positional and algorithm-related errors when the difference between two images is used. Limited patient studies with single- and dual-energy CT (Fig. 23–19) show a correlation between results obtained with the two methods. The wide dispersion may be due to errors in either the single- or dual-energy methods, although internal scan calibration with a reference phantom and rapid back-to-back dual-energy scanning to eliminate patient

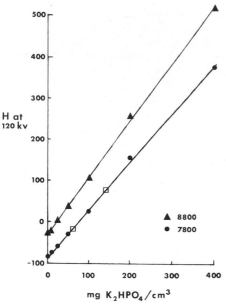

Figure 23–17. CT number versus mineral content for simulated pulmonary nodules in a lung phantom on two scanners from the same manufacturer. Relationship is linear on both machines; however, CT number for water (intercept of regression line) is -80 H on one scanner and -23 H on the other instead of 0 as expected. Absolute CT numbers in the lung can vary widely from scanner to scanner, especially among manufacturers, making it difficult to measure density of lung nodules. (From Cann CE, Gamsu G, Birnberg FA, Webb WR: Quantification of pulmonary calcification using single and dual energy CT. Radiology 145:493, 1982. Used with permission.)

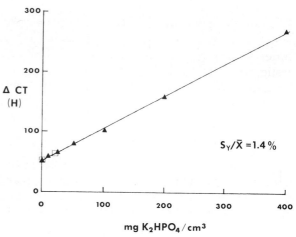

Figure 23–18. Change in CT number as a function of mineral content for simulated lung nodules. Mineral content can be predicted accurately using dual-energy CT, eliminating many of the inaccuracies in the single-energy method. (From Cann CE, Gamsu G, Birnberg FA, Webb WR: Quantification of pulmonary calcification using single and dual energy CT. Radiology 145:493, 1982. Used with permission.)

motion errors were done. Unfortunately, the patient population for this study was such that a wide range of CT values was seen but the CT range in which diffuse calcification in benign nodules was expected was not observed. We may look toward more use of QCT in the chest for characterization and quantification not only of nodules

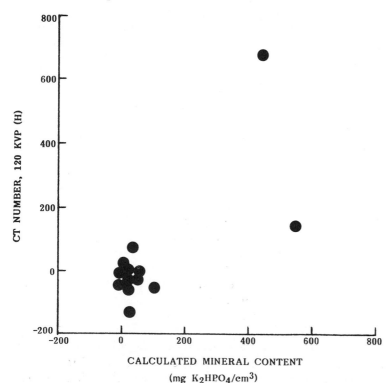

Figure 23–19. CT number of solitary pulmonary nodules in patients versus calculated mineral content from dual-energy measurement. Lack of data in the middle range of either CT number or mineral content precludes assessment of correlation.

but of pulmonary edema, fibrosis, and vascular changes as well. The recent improvements in scanner performance have opened these areas to investigation and may lead to considerably more information and clinically useful methods for pulmonary quantification.

CONCLUSION

Quantitative computed tomography can be defined as the use of the digital data in a CT scan, rather than the filmed image, to provide useful clinical information. Volume studies can be done to quantify the presence or change in the size of a lesion within an organ and to provide this result to the clinician. Computed tomographic densitometry utilizes the CT number as a reasonably accurate representation of tissue x-ray attenuation to extract clinically useful information. In its basic form, densitometry may be used to separate a renal cyst from parenchyma by virtue of its lower CT number or to characterize a tumor as a lipoma by noting a CT number close to that of fat.

With careful standardization and calibration techniques, QCT can be used for many tissue density studies. More advanced techniques such as dual-energy CT provide information about specific tissue components, especially high atomic number materials such as iron or calcium. Dual-energy CT is used to quantify liver and myocardial iron content in iron storage disease. Renal stones can be characterized as organic or calcium-containing based on dual-energy scans, as can pulmonary nodules. The measurement of bone mineral content in the spine is now an accepted technique that is useful in the diagnosis of bone disease and in the assessment of therapeutic response. Techniques to do studies such as these are available and can be implemented in a clinical radiology setting. It only remains for the clinician to understand the capabilities of the instrumentation well enough to request these studies and for the radiologist to do likewise to provide the results.

REFERENCES

1. New PFJ, Scott WR, Schnur JA, Davis KR, Taveras JM: Computerized axial tomography with the EMI scanner. Radiology 110:109, 1974.
2. Genant HK, Boyd DP: Quantitative bone mineral analysis using dual-energy computed tomography. Invest Radiol 12:545, 1977.
3. Isherwood I, Rutherford RA, Pullan BR, Adams PH: Bone mineral estimation by computer assisted transverse axial tomography. Lancet 1:712, 1976.
4. Ledley RS: Computerized transaxial x ray tomography of the human body. Science 186:207, 1974.
5. DiChiro G, Rieth KG, Klatzo I, Fujiwara K, Brooks RA: Comparison of CT attenuation and specific gravity in cerebral edema in the rhesus monkey. J Comput Asst Tomogr 3:860, 1979.
6. Heymsfield SB, Fulenwider T, Nordlinger B, Barlow R, Sones P, Kutner M: Accurate measurement of liver, kidney and spleen volume and mass by computerized axial tomography. Ann Intern Med 90:185, 1979.
7. Joseph PM, Spital RD: A method for correcting bone-induced artifacts in computed tomography scanners. J Comput Assist Tomogr 2:100, 1978.
8. Avrin DE, Macovski A, Zatz LM: Clinical application of compton and photoelectric reconstruction in computed tomography: Preliminary results. Invest Radiol 13:217, 1978.
9. Faul DD, Couch JL, Cann CE, Boyd DP, Genant HK: Composition-selective reconstruction for mineral content in the axial and appendicular skeleton. J Comput Assist Tomogr 6:202, 1982.
9a. Rutt B, Fenster A: Split-filter computed tomography: A simple technique for dual energy scanning. J Comput Assist Tomogr 4:501, 1980.
10. Cann CE, Rutt BK, Genant HK: Comparison of advanced CT scanners for vertebral mineral determination. 68th Scientific Assembly, Radiological Society of North America, Chicago, Ill., November 1982.
11. Glover GH, Pelc NJ: Nonlinear partial volume artifacts in x-ray computed tomography. Med Phys 7:238, 1980.
12. Piekarski J, Goldberg HI, Royal SA, Axel L, Moss AA: Difference between liver and spleen CT numbers in the normal adult: Its usefulness in predicting the presence of diffuse liver disease. Radiology 137:727, 1980.
13. Cann CE, Genant HK: Precise measurement of vertebral mineral content using computed tomography. J Comput Assist Tomogr 4:493, 1980.
14. Fike JR, Cann CE, Berninger WH: Quantitative evaluation of the canine brain using computed tomography. J Comput Assist Tomogr 6:325, 1982.
15. Cann CE: Low-dose CT scanning for quantitative spinal mineral analysis. Radiology 140:813, 1981.
16. Godwin JD, Fram EK, Cann CE, Gamsu G: CT densitometry of pulmonary nodules, a phantom study. J Comput Assist Tomogr 6:254, 1982.
17. Moss AA, Cann CE, Friedman MA, Marcus FS, Resser KJ, Berninger WH: Volumetric CT analysis of hepatic tumors. J Comput Assist Tomogr 5:714, 1981.
18. Cann CE, Fike JR, Brant-Zawadski MN, Pitts L: Quantitative evaluation of mass lesions in cerebral trauma by CT. AJR (in press).
19. Goldberg HI: Differential diagnosis of diffuse liver disease with use of dual energy CT. J Comput Assist Tomogr 3:858, 1979.
20. Goldberg HI, Cann CE, Moss AA, Ohto M, Brito A, Federle M: Non-invasive quantitation of liver iron in dogs with hemochromatosis using dual-energy CT scanning. Invest Radiol 17:375, 1982.
20a. Long JA, Doppman JL, Nieuhus AW, Mills SR: Computed tomographic analysis of beta-thalassemic syndrome with hemochromatosis: Pathologic findings with clinical and laboratory correlation. J Comput Assist Tomogr 4:159, 1980.
21. Friedman MA, Marcus FA, Resser KJ, Moss AA, Cann CE: Inaccuracy of routine interpretation of CT scans

for detecting volume changes in the liver—A volumetric analysis. Clin Res 29:548A, 1981.

22. Lipschitz DA, Cook JD, Finch CA: A clinical evaluation of serum ferritin as an index of iron stores. N Engl J Med 290:1213, 1974.

23. Lipton MJ, Cann CE, Goldberg HI, Carrera CJ, Boyd DP: Dual energy CT for quantitating myocardial iron levels in hemochromatosis. American Heart Association, 54th Scientific Sessions, Dallas, 1981.

24. Ruegsegger P, Niederer P, Anliker M: An extension of classical bone mineral measurements. Ann Biomed Engr 2:194, 1974.

25. Orphanoudakis S, Jensen P, Rauschkolb EN, Lang R, Rasmussen H: Bone mineral analysis using single energy computed tomography. Invest Radiol 14:122, 1979.

26. Bradley JG, Huang HK, Ledley RS: Evaluation of calcium concentration in bones from CT scans. Radiology 128:103, 1978.

27. Cann CE, Genant HK, Ettinger B, Gordan GS: Spinal mineral loss in oophorectomized women. Determination by quantitative computed tomography. JAMA 244:2056, 1980.

28. Cann CE, Genant HK, Young DR: Comparison of vertebral and peripheral mineral losses in disuse osteoporosis in monkeys. Radiology 134:525, 1980.

29. Genant HK, Cann CE: Vertebral mineral determination using quantitative computed tomography. In DeLuca HF, Frost HM, Jee WSS, Johnston CC, Parfitt AM (eds): Osteoporosis: Recent Advantages in Pathogenesis and Treatment. Baltimore, University Park Press, 1981, pp 37–47.

30. Laval-Jeantet M, Laval-Jeantet AM, Lamarque JL, Demoulin B: Evaluation de la minéralisation osseuse vértébrale par tomographie computérisée. Etude expérimentale. J de Radiologie 60:87, 1979.

31. Genant HK, Cann CE, Ettinger B, Gordan GS: Determination of bone mineral loss in the axial skeleton of oophorectomized women using quantitative CT. J Comput Assist Tomogr 6:217, 1982.

32. Cann CE, Genant HK: Cross-sectional studies of vertebral mineral using quantitative CT. J Comput Assist Tomogr 6:216, 1982.

33. Genant HK, Cann CE, Ettinger B, Gordan GS: Quantitative computed tomography of vertebral spongiosa: A sensitive method for detecting early bone loss after oophorectomy. Ann Intern Med 97:799, 1982.

34. Siegelman SS, Zerhouni EA, Leo FP, Khouri NF, Stitik EP: CT of the solitary pulmonary nodule. AJR 135:1, 1980.

35. Cann CE, Gamsu G, Birnberg FA, Webb WR: Quantification of pulmonary calcification using single and dual energy CT. Radiology 145:493, 1982.

36. Gamsu GS, Cann CE, Nicol RF: Calcium quantification in pulmonary nodules using dual-energy CT. Invest Radiol 16:400, 1981.

37. Godwin JD, Speckman JM, Fram EK, Johnson GA, Putman CE, Korobkin M, Breiman RS: Distinguishing benign from malignant pulmonary nodules by computed tomography. Radiology 144:349, 1982.

24 NMR IMAGING OF THE BODY

Peter L. Davis
Albert A. Moss
Alexander R. Margulis
Lawrence E. Crooks
Leon Kaufman

BASIC PRINCIPLES

Nuclear magnetic resonance (NMR) imaging is based on the property of all nuclei with an odd number of particles, protons, neutrons, or both, to act like magnets spinning in random directions. The hydrogen proton has a charge and spin and therefore a magnetic field along the axis of its spin.[1–8] When placed in an externally applied magnetic field, the protons tend to align themselves in the direction of the magnetic field. If the protons are exposed to a radio signal of a specific frequency while in the externally applied magnetic field, they will absorb energy and change the direction of their spins and align themselves against the magnetic field. The extra energy is quickly radiated away as electromagnetic energy of the same frequency as the radiofrequency (RF) source and the protons realign their spins with the external magnetic field. The protons continue to absorb-emit-absorb-emit, i.e., to resonate, as long as the radio waves have the correct energy. The energy (radio signal) that is radiated back by the resonating protons is picked up by an RF coil (antenna) and is the NMR signal that eventually generates a tomographic image.

In order to form an image, the source of the NMR signal must be precisely located within the body. Signal localization is based on the fact that the frequency of the emitted NMR radio signal is proportional to the strength of the magnetic field in which the flipped proton finds itself when it realigns. The imaging concept used is based on the ability to modify the magnetic field so it has a different strength at each position in the body. With the use of gradient magnetic coils, the magnetic field is made to vary slightly in space and those protons realigning in the stronger magnetic field emit NMR radio signals of higher frequencies than those protons realigning in the weaker mag-

1147

netic field. Thus the RF coil receives a composite NMR radio signal consisting of many different frequency components.

A Fourier transformation is performed on the received signal so that the composite radio signal is separated into its different frequency components. The computer in the NMR scanner is programmed to know what frequency corresponds to what magnetic field strength and where that magnetic field strength existed in the body while the gradient coils were turned on. Thus, the computer can match up a frequency component of the received NMR radio signal to the position of the protons in the body that emitted a particular frequency component of the radio signal. The computer then plots the signal intensity of the component and all other components in their proper relative positions. Thus, an image—a map of the NMR signal intensities being emitted by the hydrogen protons in the body—is generated.

In addition to hydrogen density, other physical properties of tissue influence the NMR signal. These properties are called tissue magnetic relaxation times and are a measure of the time it takes a sample to become magnetized or to lose its magnetism along a particular axis. A tissue's relaxation characteristics are relatively complex but have two main components known as the T_1 and T_2 relaxation times.

T_1—also called the thermal, longitudinal, or "spin lattice" relaxation time—is related to the interval it takes a group of protons to align with the magnetic field. Liquids are held by weaker forces than solids, take a shorter time to magnetize, and thus have a shorter T_1 time than solids. Because alignment is dependent on collisions with other molecules in the lattice, T_1 has been referred to as the spin-lattice relaxation time. Liquid molecules collide more frequently than solids, and T_1 is thus long for solids and short for liquids.

The T_2 relaxation time is related to the interval it takes a group of signal-emitting hydrogen protons to lose synchronization after being synchronized by the flipping radio signal. T_2 is termed the "spin-spin" or transverse relaxation time and is a measure of how long the substance holds the temporary transverse magnetism induced by the RF pulse, which is perpendicular to the external magnetic field. Synchronization is lost as a result of small variations of the local magnetic field within the tissue itself. Liquids have weaker internal fields and thus maintain synchronization longer (in seconds). Solids with strong internal fields have short T_2 values (in microseconds). As synchronization is decaying at the rate T_2, the longitudinal component is growing at a rate of T_1. The T_1 and T_2 relaxation times are affected by the physical state of a tissue (temperature and viscosity), its composition, and molecular structure.

IMAGING PROCESS

The T_1 and T_2 relaxation times play an important role in providing contrast between different soft tissues.[9-11] This is because although the hydrogen content of most soft tissues varies over a range of approximately 20 per cent, T_1 and T_2 can vary over a range of 500 per cent. In actual practice, the received NMR signal intensity is a synthesis of the hydrogen concentration and the T_1 and T_2 relaxation times of the hydrogen. How these three components are combined depends on the imaging methods employed.

Basic to an understanding of nuclear magnetic resonance is a knowledge of the mechanism by which different T_1 and T_2 relaxation times translate into image contrast. There are several imaging techniques, each one combining the hydrogen concentration and the T_1 and T_2 effects differently.

SATURATION RECOVERY

In the saturation recovery imaging technique (proton imaging, repeated free induction decay [FID] imaging), the protons in the magnetic field are flipped by an RF pulse at 90° to the static magnetic field.[2-4, 8] Image contrast is dependent on a variety of factors in saturation recovery imaging but depends most strongly on proton density and the T_1 relaxation time of the tissues.

When protons are placed in a magnetic field, they do not align in the direction of the field instantaneously but instead align in an exponential manner. Initially, alignment occurs rapidly, but the rate of alignment gradually decreases the longer the protons are in the magnetic field. The process of proton alignment in a magnetic field can be described by the equation:

$$A = (1 - e^{-b/T_1}) \qquad (24-1)$$

A is the fraction of the protons aligned after being placed in a magnetic field for a specific period of time. T_1 is the T_1 relaxation time of the protons in the tissue, and b is the amount of time the protons have had to align with the magnetic field. Therefore, the protons in tissues with short T_1 times align faster than those with long T_1 times (Fig. 24–1).

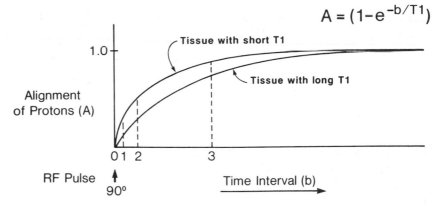

Figure 24–1. Saturation recovery imaging technique. Alignment of protons in magnetic field following 90° radiofrequency (RF) pulse. Alignment is 0 immediately after the RF pulse. $A = 1$ when b is 4 to 5 times the T_1 value of the tissue. Tissue with a short T_1 time aligns more quickly than tissue with a long T_1 time. Contrast between the two tissues varies with time.

Each time the protons are flipped by the 90° RF pulse, they lose all their alignment with the magnetic field and thus b and A become 0 (Fig. 24–2). As time passes and b increases, A also increases as more protons realign with the magnetic field. As a rule, at any particular time b, tissues with different T_1 relaxation times will have different fractions (A) of their protons in alignment with the magnetic field. However, there are two exceptions to this rule. As shown in Figure 24–1, immediately after the protons are flipped, they are totally out of alignment and $b = 0$, $A = 0$; also, when $b = \infty$, $A = 1$, indicating that all protons are now in alignment. For practical purposes, $A = 1$ when b is greater than 4 to 5 times the T_1 value of a tissue.

The intensity (I) of the radio signal received after the protons are flipped is proportional to the total number of protons aligned with the magnetic field just before the 90° pulse. The total number of protons aligned with the field is the fraction of protons in alignment (A) multiplied by the hydrogen density (H) of the tissue. This relationship can be described by the equation:

$$I = k \cdot H \cdot A \qquad (24\text{–}2)$$

where I is the radio signal intensity and k is a proportionality constant. As shown by Equation 24–2, the more protons (H) aligned (A), the more intense the radio signal will be when the protons are flipped. From the relationship of Equation 24–2 to Equation 24–1, it is apparent that

$$I = k \cdot H \cdot A = k \cdot H \cdot (1 - e^{-b/T_1}) \qquad (24\text{–}3)$$

and that as shown in Figure 24–2, a tissue with a short T_1 time will produce a more intense NMR signal than a tissue with a long T_1 time.

The contrast between two tissues is equal to the ratio of the signal intensities, assuming that the hydrogen densities of the two tissues are similar. This assumption is reasonably true for most soft tissues in the body; thus tissue contrast is dependent largely on the ratio of the fraction (A) of protons in each tissue that have aligned prior to being flipped 90° by the RF pulse.

Tissue contrast can be displayed graphically as a ratio of the heights of the exponential curves. In Figure 24–1, for example, the greatest contrast between the two tissues will occur if the protons are flipped at Time 2. At shorter or longer times (Times 1 and 3, respectively), the contrast be-

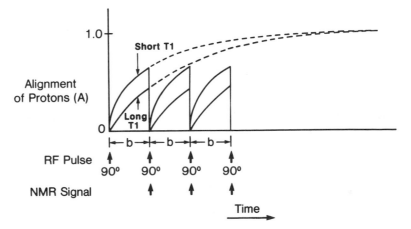

Figure 24–2. Saturation recovery imaging sequence. Alignment of protons following RF pulse drops to 0 just after 90° RF pulse. Alignment of protons increases with time but is different for tissues having unequal T_1 times.

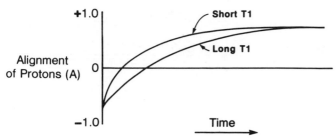

Figure 24–3. Inversion recovery imaging technique. Alignment of protons in magnetic field following 180° RF pulse. Immediately after 180° RF pulse, the maximum number of protons are aligned against the magnetic field, but once flipped, they realign with the magnetic field according to their T_1 times. Tissues with short T_1 values align more rapidly than tissues with long T_1 times.

tween the two tissues will be less. For different tissues having different T_1 times, the time at which maximum contrast will be obtained will be different.

Thus it is clear that NMR imaging employing only a single time, b, will probably not be sufficient to obtain optimum contrast between normal and pathologic tissue in every instance. Because the optimum timing parameters have not yet been determined, a number of NMR images using different adjustments of b are currently obtained. Using the saturation recovery technique, if b is varied, from Time 2 to Time 3 (Fig. 24–1), the signal intensity received for each tissue will be different and thus contrast between tissues changed. The T_1 relaxation time of each tissue can be calculated using a saturation recovery technique by solving Equation 24–3 as b is varied and a different signal intensity is received.

INVERSION RECOVERY

In the saturation recovery technique, when the protons are flipped 90°, they lose their alignment with the magnetic field, thus, the same number of protons are in alignment with the field as opposed to the field-force (net alignment is zero).[2–4]

In the inversion recovery technique, protons are flipped 180° so that there are more protons opposed to the magnetic field than aligned with the field. The maximum number of protons are

aligned against the field immediately after the 180° flip. Once the protons are flipped, they begin to realign with the magnetic field according to their T_1 times (Fig. 24–3) and as follows:

$$A = (1 - 2e^{-b/T_1}) \qquad (24–4)$$

In order to obtain an NMR signal, the protons must undergo a 90° flip in addition to the 180° flip. Thus a complete inversion recovery sequence (Fig. 24–4) consists of a 180° flip, followed by a period of realignment (t_r), then a 90° flip, at which time the NMR signal is received. The protons are then allowed to realign with the external magnetic field before the 180° pulse is repeated. This latter realignment follows Equation 24–1 and may be complete or partial, depending on the amount of time ($b - t_r$) allowed and the T_1 of the tissue.

Contrast between tissues in the inversion recovery images is highly dependent on the time at which the 90° flip is performed. This is due to the fact that the net negative alignment (Fig. 24–5a) that occurs after the 180° pulse generates a positive intensity (Fig. 24–5b). If the 90° flip is performed at Time 1, tissue with a long T_1 will have a higher intensity than tissue with a short T_1 time. If the 90° flip is performed at Time 2, the tissue having a short T_1 will have no intensity and will appear black on the NMR image, thus assur-

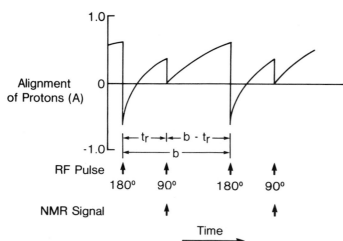

Figure 24–4. Inversion recovery imaging sequence. Complete sequence consists of 180° RF pulse, followed by a period of realignment (t_r) and then a 90° RF pulse at which time the nuclear magnetic resonance (NMR) signal is received. Protons are then allowed to realign before 180° RF pulse is repeated. b = Time between 180° RF pulses.

Figure 24–5. Variation in contrast between tissues using an inversion recovery imaging technique. **a** A net negative alignment of protons occurs immediately after the 180° RF pulse. Tissues with different T_1 times then realign at unequal rates. **b** Intensity of NMR signal. Just after 180° RF pulse (Time 0), the intensity of the NMR signal is positive. If the 90° RF pulse is performed at Time 1, the signal intensity of tissue with long T_1 is greater than tissue with short T_1 time. At Time 2, tissue with a short T_1 will have no signal intensity and appear black on the image, assuring high contrast between tissues. Tissue contrast is less at Time 3, whereas at Time 4 the tissues will have equal intensities and will be indistinguishable. At Times 5, 6, and 7, tissue with a short T_1 time will appear more intense than tissue with a long T_1 time.

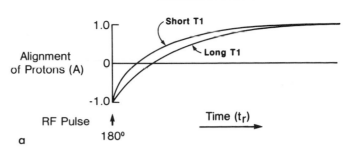

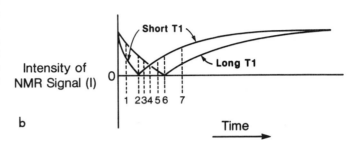

ing high contrast between the two tissues. At Time 3, the long T_1 tissue appears more intense than the short T_1 tissue, but the contrast between the two tissues is less than present at Time 2. At Time 4, both tissues have the same intensity and are indistinguishable. If flipped at time 5, however, the tissue with the short T_1 will now appear more intense than the tissue with a long T_2 time. Images generated at Time 6 will reveal tissue with a long T_1 time to have no intensity, thus assuring high contrast between the two tissues. Images obtained at Time 7 will still demonstrate the tissue having a short T_1 as more intense than tissue with a longer T_1 value; however, the image contrast will be less than at Time 6.

Thus it is evident that image contrast in the inversion recovery technique is strongly dependent on hydrogen density and a tissue's T_1 value and when the 90° flip occurs. The chief advantage of the inversion recovery technique is it provides relatively high contrast images over a narrow range of T_1 relaxation times. As with the saturation recovery technique, the T_1 relaxation time of a tissue can be calculated.

SPIN ECHO

Nuclear magnetic resonance images can also be obtained using a spin echo technique. This method involves an initial 90° flip followed at a later time by a 180° flip.[2–4, 11] The images obtained by the spin echo method are dependent on both the T_1 and T_2 relaxation times of the tissue.

In theory, the NMR radio signal (called the FID signal) decays exponentially following a 90° flip (Fig. 24–6):

$$D = I_0 e^{-a/T_2} \qquad (24–5)$$

In this equation, a is the time since the 90° flip has occurred, D is the amplitude of the NMR radio signal at time a, I_0 is the radio signal's initial value at time $a = 0$, and T_2 is the T_2 relaxation time of the tissue.

The exponential decay of FID signal is shown graphically in Fig. 24–6a. Initially, after a 90° flip, the protons are synchronized and begin emitting radio signals in a synchronized fashion. The frequency of the radio wave generated by each proton at any moment is dependent on the strength of the magnetic field surrounding the proton. Within each tissue are small variations of the local magnetic field owing to tissue structure; those protons in areas having stronger fields will emit radio signals of higher frequencies than those protons in regions of weaker fields. As a result of the inhomogeneity of tissue magnetic fields, the radio signals generated from the two areas will gradually lose synchronization, finally canceling each other so that no signal is received. The loss of synchronization is independent of the realignment of the protons, which is occurring simultaneously.

Loss of synchronization occurs rapidly and, except for pure fluid, is usually more rapid than proton realignment. In theory, it is possible to calculate the T_2 relaxation time of a tissue by meas-

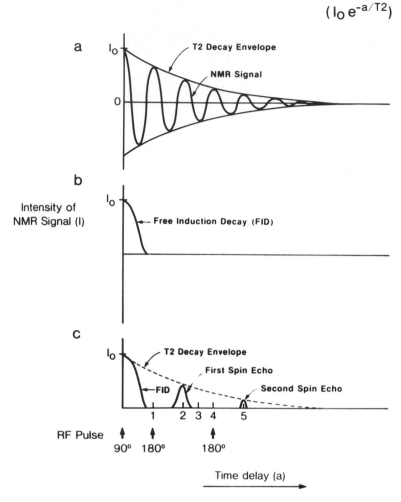

$$(I_0 \, e^{-a/T2})$$

Figure 24–6. Relationship of T_2 decay and NMR signal intensity in spin echo imaging. **a** Exponential decay of free induction decay signal following 90° RF pulse in an ideal uniform magnetic field. **b** Free induction decay in actual nonuniform magnetic field occurs more rapidly than in the ideal uniform field. **c** NMR signal intensity at various intervals following 180° RF pulse (Time 1). At Time 2, a radio signal, first spin echo, is received with an intensity strongly dependent on the tissue's T_2 relaxation time. The intensity of the signal rapidly decays (Time 3). If another 180° RF pulse is performed at Time 4, a second weaker radio signal (second spin echo) is received at Time 5. A tissue's T_2 relaxation time can be calculated by placing the two different intensities from the two spin echo signals into equation 24–5 (see text).

uring its NMR radio signal's decay over time. However, the T_2 relaxation time cannot be calculated by simply measuring the FID signal because nonuniformity of the main magnetic field is usually stronger than the internal tissue field variations. This causes the FID signal to decay more rapidly than it would in a perfectly uniform magnetic field (Fig. 24–6b).

The spin echo technique temporarily corrects for variations of the external magnetic field by performing a 180° proton flip at an interval following the initial 90° flip (Fig. 24–6c, Time 1). With this approach, the relative differences in synchronization losses between protons can be reversed so that after a delay equal to the interval between the 90° and 180° flip, the individual radio signals are again synchronized, and a radio signal—the spin echo—is received (Fig. 24–6c, Time 2). Because this technique corrects only the external field variations, the maximum intensity of the signal received will be strongly dependent on the tissue's T_2 relaxation time.

After the radio signals have become resyn-

chronized, synchronization immediately begins to be lost and the intensity of the radio signal decays (Fig. 24–6c, Time 3). If another 180° flip is performed (Fig. 24–6c, Time 4), the radio signal can be resynchronized and an equal time later (Fig. 24–6c, Time 5) a second spin echo received. In practice, the timing and number of 180° flips are computer controlled. If the two different intensities from the successive spin echo signals are placed into Equation 24–5, the T_2 relaxation time of a tissue can be calculated.

The contrast between two tissues having different T_2 relaxation times is dependent on the time interval between the 90° pulse and occurrence of the spin echo signal. In Figure 24–7 the contrast between tissues having long and short T_2 relaxation times is greater at Time 2 than at Time 1. Although the contrast between tissues using the spin echo technique is strongly dependent on differences in T_2 relaxation times, the T_1 tissue relaxation time also influences final tissue contrast.

In the example shown in Figure 24–7, it was assumed that both tissue signals had the same initial

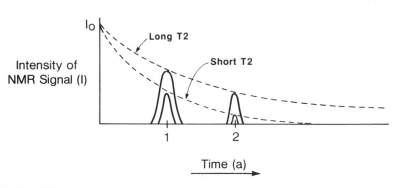

Figure 24–7. Effect of tissue T_2 differences on spin echo signal intensity. Contrast between tissues is dependent on the time interval between the 90° pulse and the time at which spin echo occurs. Contrast is greater at Time 2 than at Time 1, even though signal intensity for both tissues is greater at Time 1.

intensity after the 90° flip. Actually, this assumption is not necessarily true because the intensity of the initial signal is dependent on the percentage of protons aligned with the external magnetic field, which is dependent on the T_1 relaxation times of the tissues. Thus the interrelationship of T_1 and T_2 times to signal intensity is complex (Fig. 24–8). After the initial 90° flip, the FID radio signal occurs; then 180° pulses cause spin echoes to be generated at the same time the protons are realigning. This procedure is then repeated in order that an interrogation at several locations of the signals can be performed, thus generating an image. In addition, repetition permits several signals to be averaged, thus improving the signal-to-noise ratio of the image.

The relationship of T_1 and T_2 relaxation times to tissue contrast using spin echo imaging techniques is demonstrated in Figure 24–9. Following the 90° pulse, the intensity from Tissue A is greater than the intensity from Tissue B (Fig. 24–9A). If Tissue A has a longer T_2 time than Tissue B (Fig. 24–9B), the contrast between tissues will be greater at Time 2 than at Time 1. If Tissue A has a shorter T_2 time than Tissue B (Fig. 24–9C), the contrast can vary drastically, depending upon the time the signal is obtained. For example, at Time 3, Tissue A is more intense than Tissue B; at Time 4, Tissue A has the same intensity as Tissue B; and at Time 5, Tissue A is less intense than Tissue B. Thus contrast between tissues using spin echo techniques is variable, depending upon the timing parameters employed as well as inherent T_1 and T_2 relaxation times.

The intensity equation for the spin echo technique is simply the product of the Equations 24–3 and 24–5:

$$I = kH \ e^{-a/T_2} \ (1 - e^{-b/T_1}) \qquad (24-6)$$

Although the effects of hydrogen density have largely been ignored in this discussion (as shown in Equation 24–6), hydrogen density does affect the intensity and tissue contrast obtained by the spin echo technique.

Currently, the timing parameters we use to

Figure 24–8. Interrelationships of T_1 and T_2 times to signal intensity in spin echo sequence. **a** Alignment of protons (A) is dependent upon T_1 time of tissue. **b** Detailed diagram of events occurring shortly after initial 90° RF pulse. An FID signal occurs after 90° RF pulse, then 180° RF pulses cause spin echo signals to be generated at the same time protons are realigning. The intensity of signal is strongly dependent on the tissue's T_2 time and on the T_1 time of the tissue.

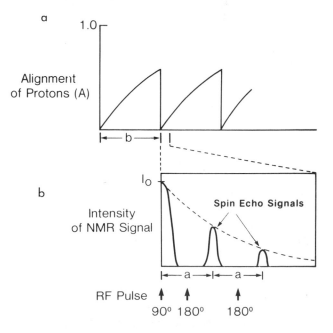

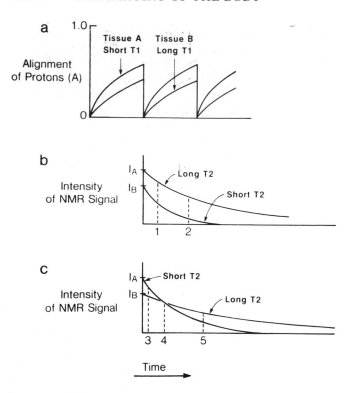

a
1.0

Tissue A Short T1   Tissue B Long T1

Alignment of Protons (A)

0

b
I_A
I_B

Intensity of NMR Signal

Long T2

Short T2

1   2

c
I_A
I_B

Intensity of NMR Signal

Short T2

Long T2

3 4   5

Time

Figure 24–9. Relationship of T_1 and T_2 times to tissue contrast using spin echo imaging techniques. **a** Following the 90° RF pulse, alignment of protons (and signal intensity) will be greater for Tissue A with a short T_1 time than for Tissue B with a long T_1 time. **b** If tissue A has a longer T_2 time, contrast will be greater at Time 2 than at Time 1. **c** If tissue A has a shorter T_2 time, contrast can vary, depending upon time the signal is obtained. At Time 3, Tissue A is more intense than B. At Time 4, the intensities are equal. At Time 5, Tissue A is less intense than B.

generate spin echo images are a pulse echo delay (TE) of 28 or 56 milliseconds and a pulse sequence repetition rate (TR) of 0.5, 1.0, 1.5, or 2.0 seconds. These parameters have proved adequate for obtaining good contrast between most normal and pathologic tissues.

Compared with saturation recovery and inversion recovery techniques, spin echo imaging requires more complex computer hardware and software. In addition, spin echo signal intensities can be 40 to 80 per cent lower than signal intensities using the saturation recovery method; thus, signal-to-noise problems are greater. However, by taking advantage of the T_2 signal decay, greater soft-tissue contrast can be obtained and T_2 times calculated for tissue characterization.

Besides hydrogen density and the T_1 and T_2 relaxation times, a fourth factor, movement, affects the NMR image. Because the NMR process takes a finite period of time (about 50 milliseconds), if the flipped protons move out of the volume element being imaged before that time period, their contribution to the emitted NMR signal is lost. Flowing blood usually demonstrates this effect,[12] and blood vessel lumens usually image with little or no intensity.

Gray Scale of Spin Echo Images

Most of the images presented in this chapter have been obtained using a spin echo imaging technique. Image intensity results from a combination of hydrogen density, the effects of T_1 and T_2 relaxation times, and imager parameters. The gray scale, is, in decreasing intensity, fat, other highly lipid tissues such as brain and spinal cord, other soft tissues, water, bone, cortex, and air. If several images of the same plane are obtained with appropriately different imager parameters, T_1 and T_2 relaxation times can be calculated on a pixel-by-pixel basis for images or on a region-of-interest basis for statistics.

TISSUE CHARACTERIZATION

One of the potential advantages of NMR is the capacity to calculate the T_1 and T_2 relaxation times of tissues and thus provide more precise tissue characterization than possible with computed tomography (CT). Early in vitro work[9] demonstrated that the T_1 times of tumors were longer than most normal tissues, and that in rats most normal tissues and several pathologic tissues, such as hematomas and abscesses, could be characterized by T_1 and T_2 relaxation times.

With measurement of both T_1 and T_2 relaxation times, tissue characterization is more accurate but still not completely specific. This is due to the fact that tumors do not have a narrow range of T_1 and T_2 values. Experimental studies on two implanted tumor models in the rat revealed that the T_1 and T_2 values for hepatomas and mammary adenocarcinomas ranged from near normal to markedly abnormal.[10, 13] Moreover, the T_1 and T_2 values from the tumors overlapped the range of other pathologies. However, by having both T_1 and T_2 values available, the overlap was smaller than if just one relaxation time was available.

Several investigators have measured T_1 and T_2 relaxation times in vivo in humans.[11, 14–19] Doyle and associates[14] measured the T_1 times of normal and pathologic liver tissues and demonstrated the T_1 times of different pathologic tissues overlapped the times of the normal liver. Moss and colleagues[18] reported a wide range of T_1 and T_2 values for hepatic tumors and noted the T_2 relaxation time to vary from being significantly less to significantly more than that of the liver.[18] Distinction between serous cysts and hemorrhagic cysts appears possible by NMR, as does detection of the presence of excessive iron in the liver or bone marrow.[20, 21]

Undoubtedly, refinement in NMR techniques will permit easier and more accurate determinations of tissue relaxation times. Through the use of these measurements, information regarding tissue characterization will be available as an aid to diagnosis. However, it must be understood that the measured T_1 and T_2 values are dependent upon the magnetic field strength employed by a particular NMR imager, thus there are no "absolute" T_1 or T_2 values for particular tissues; and that comparison of T_1 and T_2 values obtained on different NMR systems will be difficult. It remains unclear as to what the ultimate usefulness of these measurements will be, but it is clear that images having strong T_1 or T_2 dependence will be of great importance in clinical diagnosis.

CONTRAST AGENTS

There are essentially two ways to alter a tissue's NMR characteristics. The first requires a change in the hydrogen content of the tissue. This is a relatively difficult feat to accomplish in soft tissues, but it is possible to increase the hydrogen content of the gut by oral administration of mineral oil.

The second requires a change in the T_1 and T_2 relaxation times of the hydrogen already present in the tissue. This can be done by delivering a paramagnetic material to the tissue. A paramagnetic material is any substance that becomes slightly magnetic when placed in a magnetic field thus changing the local magnetic field, and affect-

ing the T_1 and T_2 relaxation times of the nearby hydrogen. Substances under investigation include diatomic oxygen, manganese, and paramagnetic free radicals.[22, 23] It appears manganese will be too toxic for human use and that the most likely substance will be a nitroxyl free radical attached to a safe molecule that localizes in a particular organ or organs in the body.

ARTIFACTS

Subject-dependent artifacts can affect NMR imaging. Although less important than in CT scanning, patient motion will degrade an NMR image. Although some imaging techniques are more immune to motion than others, any significant motion will result in a general loss of signal; this will result in poorer images. The presence of any magnetic material within the body will create image artifacts because of the distortion of magnetic field uniformity the magnetic material produces. Most surgical clips and prostheses are nonmagnetic and do not cause artifacts on NMR scans, but artifacts can arise from surgical wires and dental bridgework, which is magnetic. Any high NMR intensity source near the RF coil will distort the image. This most commonly occurs when a patient comes into direct contact with the RF coil, causing very high intensities to be received from the subcutaneous fat or bone marrow. Repositioning the patient or compensating electronically will alleviate this artifact.

BODY IMAGING

CARDIOVASCULAR SYSTEM

The NMR appearance of blood depends upon the imaging techniques employed, on the velocity and direction of flow, and on the T_1 and T_2 values of blood.[12] In the spin echo images shown in this chapter, blood flowing at 15 to 25 cm/second emits almost no NMR signal and thus appears black on spin echo and inversion recovery images. Thus blood vessels are depicted as tubular black structures that are easily detected against adjacent soft tissues, which produce an NMR signal. Since NMR signal intensity increases linearly as flow diminishes, when blood flow becomes slow (1 to 5 cm/second), the intensity of signal from the blood increases in such a way that it changes from black to gray. When the flow rate is very slow or when flow is stopped, the signal from the blood becomes intense (white).[12]

The major vascular structures of the neck (Fig.

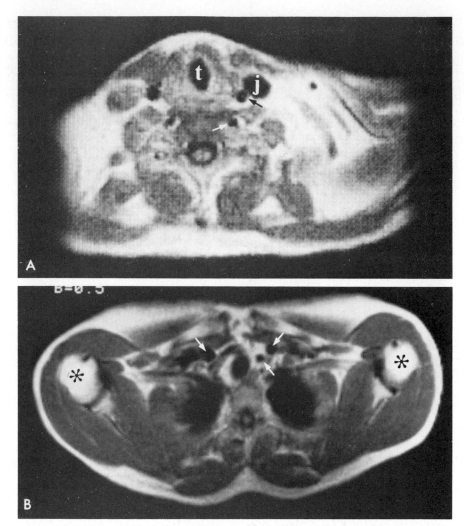

Figure 24–10. A Transverse spin echo NMR image through neck at level of larynx. The internal jugular vein (j), common carotid artery (black arrow), and vertebral artery (white arrow) are seen as low-intensity structures caused by rapid blood flow. t = Trachea. **B** Transverse spin echo image through the shoulders of a normal man. The great vessels of the neck (arrows) are seen; the fatty marrow (asterisks) within the humeral head appears as a high-intensity structure. No streak artifacts are generated by the humeral heads.

24–10), thorax, abdomen (Fig. 24–11), pelvis, and extremities are readily imaged by NMR techniques. Atherosclerotic plaques in the carotid aorta (Fig. 24–12) and femoral arteries (Fig. 24–13) can be seen, possibly because of their high lipid and cholesterol content, but the sensitivity of the NMR method is still undetermined.

Without the administration of contrast material, vascular abnormalities, such as a persistent left inferior vena cava, can be distinguished from para-aortic masses. The intimal flap in a dissecting thoracic or abdominal aortic aneurysm can be directly imaged (Fig. 24–14) and measurements made as to the size and location of aneurysms. In patients with aortic dissections, differences in flow between the true and false lumen may be de-

tected by differences in the signal intensity between the lumens.

It is possible to obtain excellent cardiac images using both gated and nongated cardiac studies.[11, 24–26] Gated techniques produce the best images, permitting identification of all four cardiac chambers and occasionally the mitral and tricuspid valves. The chamber sizes can be measured at various points through the cardiac cycle and physiologic measurements such as stroke volume and wall motion obtained. Even without gating, surprisingly good NMR images are obtainable.[24, 27] This results from the fact that the heart spends most of its cycle in diastole, and during the short systole, the heart is moving quickly and thus emits a weak signal. Therefore, the ungated

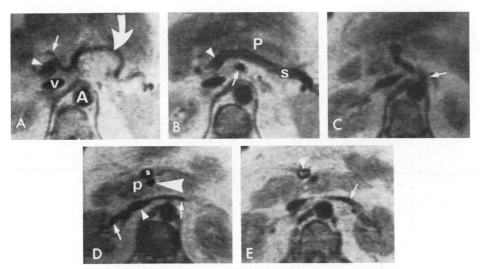

Figure 24–11. Abdominal vascular anatomy on spin echo NMR images. **A** The splenic (curved arrow) and hepatic (arrow) branches of the celiac artery are shown just anterior to the aorta (A). The portal vein (arrowhead) is seen anterior to the inferior vena cava (v). **B** The splenic vein (S) courses from the spleen to join the superior mesenteric vein (arrowhead) to form the portal vein. Arrow = Superior mesenteric artery; P = pancreas. **C** The origin of the superior mesenteric artery (arrow) is clearly shown. **D** The right and left renal veins (arrows) are shown joining the inferior vena cava (small arrowhead). p = Pancreatic head; S = superior mesenteric vein; large arrowhead = superior mesenteric artery. **E** The left renal vein (arrow) is seen draining the left kidney. The superior mesenteric vein (arrowhead) has a high intensity center probably due to slow flow.

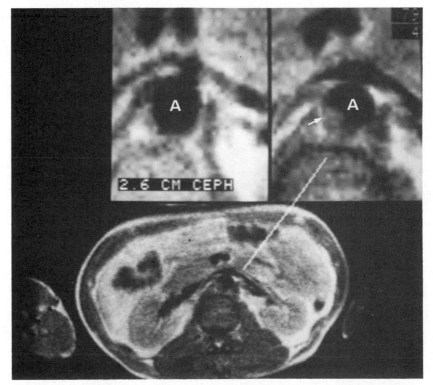

Figure 24–12. Transverse spin echo NMR image through the level of the kidneys. The renal veins are seen entering the inferior vena cava. Anteriorly the superior mesenteric vein and artery are seen as dark structures. In the upper right magnification view, the aorta (A) is eccentrically narrowed by an atherosclerotic plaque (arrow), which is seen as a high-intensity lesion in the lumen of the aorta. The magnification view obtained 2.6 cm more cephalad revealed the lumen of the aorta to be normal at this level.

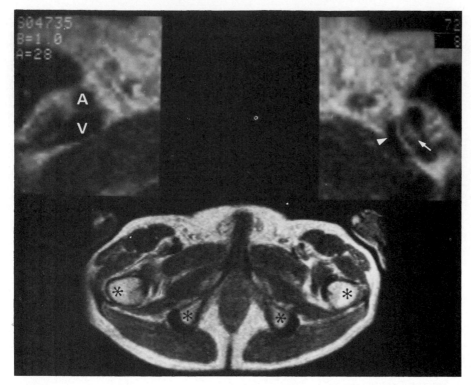

Figure 24–13. Transverse spin echo NMR images through the lower pelvis of an individual with documented atherosclerotic vascular disease. The marrow cavity (asterisks) in the femoral shaft and ischial tuberosities appear as high-intensity tissues. The inserts are magnified images of the femoral arteries and veins. The right femoral artery (A) and right femoral vein (V) appear as dark, rounded structures having a low intensity. The left femoral vein (arrowhead) is compressed by a distorted femoral artery, containing a high-intensity lesion (arrow) proven to be an atherosclerotic plaque.

cardiac NMR image most closely resembles an image of the heart in diastole.

Native coronary arteries are occasionally detectable on current NMR scanners. Coronary artery bypass grafts (Fig. 24–15) that are patent are seen as round structures having a dark lumen, indicating blood is flowing rapidly through the graft.[27]

CHEST

In normal subjects, the vascular structures, mediastinal contents, and chest wall are well delineated (Fig. 24–16).[11, 17, 24, 25, 28] The ascending and descending aorta, arch vessels, and systemic venous system of the thorax—including the subclavian veins, brachiocephalic veins and vena cava—are demonstrated without contrast material. The walls of the aorta and great vessels are visible, but in normal individuals no signal is evident within these vessels. The ascending portion of the arch of the azygos vein is evident in about 50 per cent of subjects.[29]

The trachea, main bronchi, and intermediate

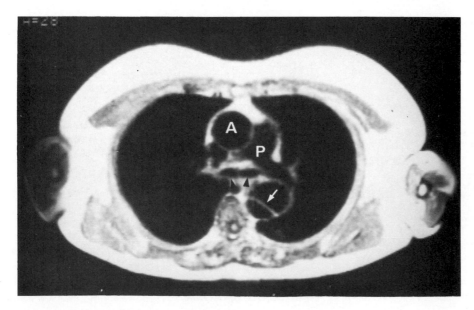

Figure 24–14. Transverse spin echo NMR image through the chest of a woman with a dissecting aortic aneurysm. The tissue flap (arrow) is seen between the true and false lumens in the descending aorta. Anteriorly the ascending aorta (A) and pulmonary artery (P) bifurcation are seen. At this level, the trachea is seen bifurcating into the main bronchi (arrowheads). (From Herkens RJ, Higgins CB, Hricak H, Lipton MJ, Crooks LE, Lanzer P, Botvinick E, Brundage B, Sheldon PE, Kaufman L: Nuclear magnetic resonance imaging of the cardiovascular system: Normal and pathologic findings. Radiology 147:749, 1983.)

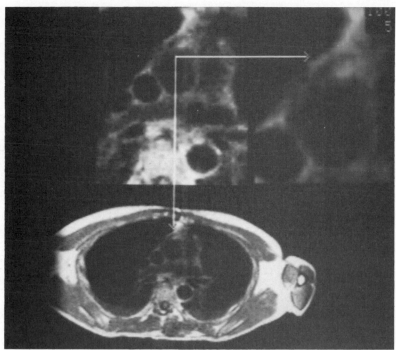

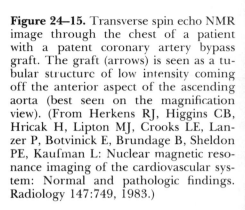

Figure 24–15. Transverse spin echo NMR image through the chest of a patient with a patent coronary artery bypass graft. The graft (arrows) is seen as a tubular structure of low intensity coming off the anterior aspect of the ascending aorta (best seen on the magnification view). (From Herkens RJ, Higgins CB, Hricak H, Lipton MJ, Crooks LE, Lanzer P, Botvinick E, Brundage B, Sheldon PE, Kaufman L: Nuclear magnetic resonance imaging of the cardiovascular system: Normal and pathologic findings. Radiology 147:749, 1983.)

bronchi are demonstrated, but only rarely is a segmental bronchus visualized. The pulmonary circulation appears similar to the systemic circulation, with only the walls of the vessels being demonstrated. No signal is seen within the pulmonary artery or veins. The main pulmonary artery, left and right pulmonary arteries, right anterior trunk, and descending left pulmonary artery are all well seen on spin echo images, the black image of the vascular lumen contrasted against the intensely white signal from the mediastinal fat (Fig. 24–14). Pulmonary vessels beyond the hila are not well visualized. The fine detail of the lung parenchyma is not well delineated because of a combination of low hydrogen density in the lung and respiratory excursion during the imaging period. However, streak artifacts, commonly present on CT scans, do not occur with NMR techniques, even at the level of the hila and diaphragm.

Normally, the only visible mediastinal structures are the walls of vessels and airways and mediastinal fat. Mediastinal masses due to lymphadenopathy or direct invasion of the mediastinum

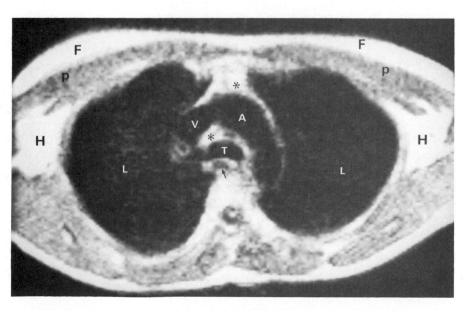

Figure 24–16. Spin echo NMR image at level of aortic arch (A). The superior vena cava (V), tracheal bifurcation (T), pectoralis major muscles (p), subcutaneous fat (F), air in the esophagus (arrow), mediastinal fat (asterisks), and marrow in humeral heads (H) are clearly shown.

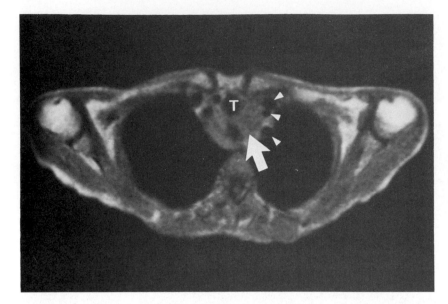

Figure 24–17. Squamous cell carcinoma. Transverse spin echo NMR image through upper chest and mediastinum. A mediastinal tumor (arrow) is demonstrated as a mass having an intensity greater than flowing blood but less than fat. The tumor displaced but does not invade adjacent vessels (arrowheads). T = Trachea.

by paramediastinal neoplasms are well demonstrated (Fig. 24–17). Nodal masses can be identified in the subcarinal, pretracheal, paratracheal, retrotracheal, and prevascular spaces because the T_1 values of tumor masses and lymphadenopathy are longer than the T_1 value of mediastinal fat (Fig. 24–18). However, when longer pulse sequence intervals are employed, the contrast between the mediastinal fat and tumor is decreased.

Thus NMR images using short pulse sequence intervals appear to provide optimal tumor-fat contrast. Measurement of the T_2 relaxation times of tumors and fat have not revealed any significant difference.[25] Overlap has also been found between the T_1 and T_2 values of various tumors, and a specific tissue diagnosis, therefore, cannot be made solely on the calculated tissue relaxation times.

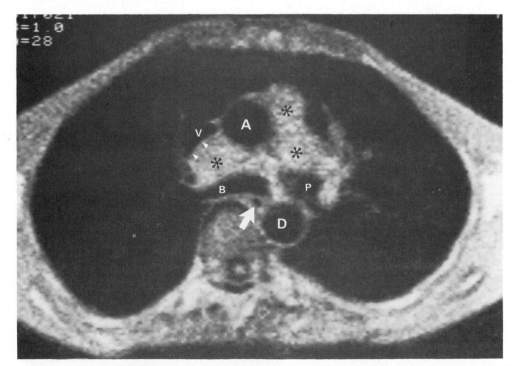

Figure 24–18. Extensive mediastinal adenopathy from bronchogenic carcinoma. Spin echo image demonstrates compression (arrowheads) of the superior vena cava without contrast material. Tumor (asterisks) is shown to involve the mediastinum diffusely. A = Aortic root; D = descending aorta; B = right main bronchus; P = left pulmonary artery; arrow = air in the esophagus.

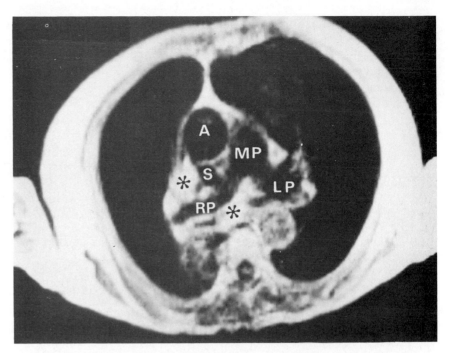

Figure 24–19. Squamous cell carcinoma involving right hilum and mediastinum. The tumor (asterisks) wraps around the right pulmonary artery (RP) and extends into the mediastinum. The tumor (asterisks) MP = main pulmonary artery; LP = left pulmonary artery; S = displaced superior vena cava.

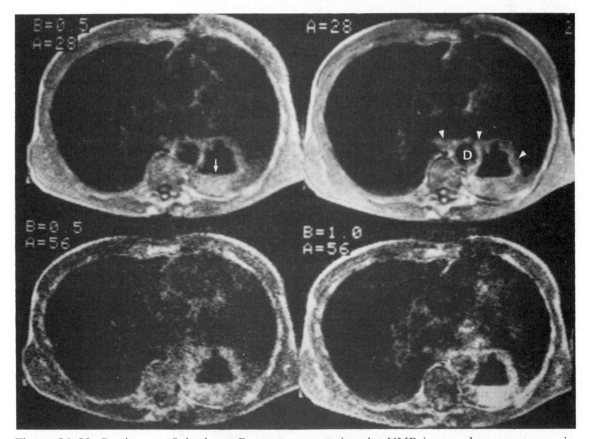

Figure 24–20. Carcinoma of the lung. Four transverse spin echo NMR images demonstrate an air-fluid level (arrow) within the tumor mass. The tumor (arrowheads) has extended around the descending aorta (D) to invade the mediastinum. The intensity of the tumor is greatest on the 1000/56 image; spatial resolution is greatest on the 500/28 image. A = interval between application of RF pulse and reception of a signal (in milliseconds); B = time interval between successive RF pulses (in seconds).

The pulmonary hilum is a complex image of overlapping vessels and airways. High-resolution CT scans provide more information than conventional tomography, but often intravenous contrast material must be administered as a bolus injection to permit distinction of vascular from soft-tissue masses. The absence of a signal from blood on NMR images simplifies the hila to vascular and bronchial outlines surrounded by a small amount of fat. Thus on NMR images hilar masses can easily be distinguished from blood vessels because of differences in their T_1 values or signal intensities (Figs. 24–18 and 24–19). Distinguishing between parahilar masses and collapsed consolidated lung does not appear easy, since the T_1 and T_2 values for tumor have been similar to those for consolidated or collapsed lung tissue.

Parenchymal lung tumors (Fig. 24–20) and nodules as small as 1.5 cm in diameter have been demonstrated on NMR spin echo images. Because no signal is obtained from normal lung tissue, it is probable that NMR will be capable of detecting most pulmonary nodules as masses having a moderate signal intensity. However, the respiratory motion resulting from long data acquisition times, the spatial resolution of NMR images, and the in-

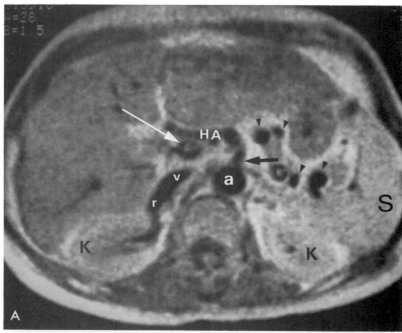

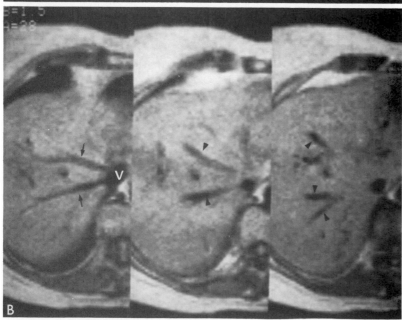

Figure 24–21. Normal liver anatomy. **A** Spin echo image demonstrates the celiac axis (black arrow) arising from the aorta (a) and the hepatic artery (HA). The splenic artery (arrowheads) is tortuous and courses in and out of the image plane. Right renal vein (r), inferior vena cava (v) and portal vein (white arrow) are displayed. The liver is slightly less intense than the spleen (S) or kidneys (K). Slow flow is seen in the portal vein. **B** Three contiguous images through the liver. The hepatic veins (arrows) are seen to enter the inferior vena cava (V) on the most cephalad image. On the other two images, branches (arrowheads) of the hepatic veins are clearly seen without contrast material.

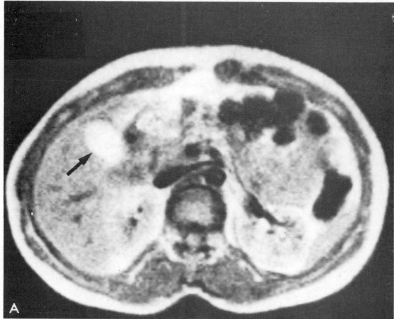

Figure 24–22. A Transverse spin echo NMR image through the gallbladder (arrow) of a woman who has been fasting for 20 hours. The gallbladder contents have a high intensity. **B** Four spin echo images obtained with different timing parameters through the gallbladder (G) in a nonfasting patient. The bile has a moderately low intensity, and layers (arrowheads) on top of gallstones (arrow), which have a very low intensity. By changing the timing parameters, the relative contrast between bile, gallstones, and surrounding liver is shown to vary considerably. A parapelvic cyst (C) is present in the right kidney. (From Hricak H, Filly RA, Margulis AR, Moon KL, Crooks LE, Kaufman L: Works in progress: Nuclear magnetic resonance imaging of the Gallbladder. Radiology 147:481, 1983.)

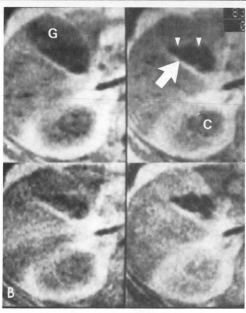

ability of NMR images to detect calcium are limiting factors.

ABDOMEN

Nuclear magnetic resonance imaging of the abdomen has proven capable of accurately displaying both normal anatomy and a variety of organ pathology.[8, 11, 17–20, 28, 30–34] All solid organs (liver, spleen, kidney, pancreas, adrenal glands, and musculature) are readily demonstrated as structures having a low NMR signal and being surrounded by fat, which has an intense signal. However, the normal gastrointestinal tract remains difficult to image because of peristalsis. Although intestinal peristalsis does not produce streak arti-

facts, because of signal loss the margins of the gut are blurred and ill defined. Glucagon injection may permit improved gastrointestinal tract imaging, but optimal imaging will probably not be achieved until an oral NMR contrast agent is developed.

Liver and Gallbladder

The liver and its contents are well delineated by NMR imaging. Normal hepatic vascular structures are particularly well delineated (Fig. 24–21), and the biliary systems can be differentiated from the vascular system by varying imaging techniques.[11, 14, 17, 18, 28, 30, 33, 34] Hricak and associates[35] demonstrated the gallbladder to appear as either

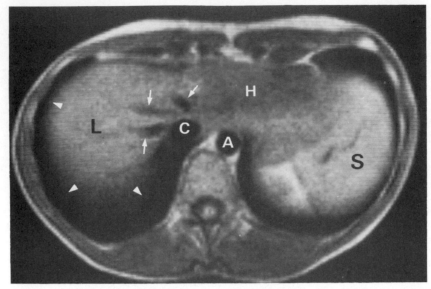

Figure 24–23. Normal liver. NMR spin echo image through the upper portion of the liver (L). Although the edges of the diaphragm (arrowheads) are ill defined, there are no streak artifacts. The aorta (A), inferior vena cava (C), right, middle, and left hepatic veins (arrows), spleen (S), and base of heart (H) are clearly shown.

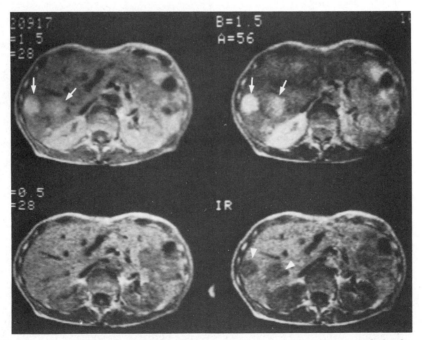

Figure 24–24. Four transverse NMR images through the liver. The upper and the lower left images were obtained using spin echo techniques with different timing parameters. The lower right is an inversion recovery image. The upper two spin echo images demonstrate the metastases as masses (arrows) of increased intensity. The metastases become isointense with normal liver in the lower left spin echo image. The lesions appear as areas of decreased intensity (arrowhead) in the inversion recovery image. Contrast between tumor and liver is greatest in the spin echo image (upper right), having a timing parameter of 1500/56.

a high- or low-intensity organ. Gallbladder contents were found to have a high intensity after fasting (concentrated bile) (Fig. 24–22A) and low intensity after eating (fresh bile) on spin echo images (Fig. 24–22B). Following stimulation of gallbladder contraction, fresh bile was seen to layer on top of concentrated bile. When patients are unable to concentrate their bile because of previous disease, bile had a low intensity even after fasting. Gallstones are also detectable by NMR and image as gallbladder filling defects, which have lower intensity than bile (Fig. 24–22B).[35]

The normal liver is readily demonstrated as an organ of homogeneous moderate intensity in the right upper abdomen (Fig. 24–21). Hepatic vasculature is well demonstrated (Figs. 24–21 and 24–23) without contrast media, and hepatic size and volume are readily calculated.

Tumors, both primary and metastatic, have been detected by NMR (Fig. 24–24),[11, 14, 17, 18, 28, 32–34, 36] but optimum imaging parameters have not as yet been determined. Young's group[17] reported inversion recovery images to show much greater soft-tissue contrast than saturation recovery images and reported inversion recovery images provided the best tumor-liver contrast differ-

ence. Haaga and associates[36] compared hepatic saturation recovery, inversion-recovery, and calculated T_1 images. Moss's group[18] evaluated primary and metastatic hepatic tumors using spin echo and inversion recovery techniques and compared the results with those of CT. Both NMR and CT techniques demonstrated a similar number of lesions, with some tumors being better displayed by NMR and others by CT. Spin echo techniques better demonstrated some tumors, whereas inversion recovery techniques appeared to give better display in others.

Primary liver tumors were found to have long T_1 values and were best visualized with spin echo techniques using a long interval between excitations or inversion recovery images.[18, 36] Most hepatomas showed a higher intensity than normal liver (Fig. 24–25) when the spin echo technique was used with long intervals between excitations. Distinction of hepatomas from surrounding normal liver was less apparent using spin echo images with short intervals (less than 1.0 seconds) between excitations. Hepatomas image as masses having a lower intensity than normal liver on inversion recovery scans. Nuclear magnetic resonance imaging is of particular value in demon-

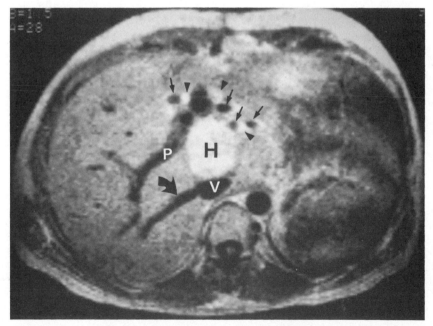

Figure 24–25. Hepatoma. Transverse spin echo image through the liver demonstrates a hepatoma (H) as a mass of increased intensity in the caudate lobe. Particularly well defined is the displacement but lack of invasion of the portal vein (P), hepatic vein (curved arrow) and inferior vena cava (V). Several small, round structures (arrows) in the porta hepatis represent metallic clips that give no NMR signal. The adjacent high-intensity circles (arrowheads) are artifacts generated by the magnetic clips.

strating internal structure within hepatomas, displaying the margin of tumors, and in depicting the relationship of hepatic vasculature to the malignancy. Both T_1 and T_2 relaxation times vary among hepatomas in different patients, among different regions of a single hepatoma, and among multifocal hepatomas in individual patients. The T_1 values vary to a greater extent than T_2 values.

Metastatic tumors are readily detected by spin echo and inversion recovery NMR scanning techniques without the use of intravenous contrast media. Most metastases appear as masses of low intensity on inversion recovery scans and as masses having a greater or lower intensity than normal liver on spin echo NMR images (Fig. 24–24). As in primary liver tumors, metastatic tumors are usually best demonstrated on spin echo imagings with long intervals between excitations (Fig. 24–24). Analysis of the intensities of tumors reveals a wide range of intensities for the same type of tumor in different individuals, among various tumors, and even within different parts of the same tumor. The T_1 and T_2 relaxation times vary more in metastatic disease than in hepatomas, with calculated T_2 relaxation times varying more than T_1 values.

Although the average calculated T_1 and T_2 relaxation times of both primary and metastatic hepatic tumors differ from those of normal liver, there is sufficient overlap between values so that a single T_1 or T_2 calculation does not appear to be specific for a particular hepatic neoplasm. Distinction between benign and malignant hepatic tumors also appears difficult, since hepatic adenoma (Fig. 24–26) appears similar to a hepatoma or to metastatic foci.

Although metabolic liver disease has not been widely studied by NMR, in patients with thalassemia major and transfusion-induced hemachromatosis, the liver has a strikingly low intensity on spin echo images (Fig. 24–27).[21] The marked low intensity of the liver appears to be due to the excessive hepatic iron stores that alter the relaxation times of the hepatic tissue.[21] In a patient with von Gierke's disease, the liver and kidneys appeared to be of slightly higher intensity (Fig. 24–26). Cirrhosis has been reported to prolong T_1 relaxation time, resulting in the liver's having a decreased intensity on inversion recovery images.[14, 17] Biliary cirrhosis with an elevated hepatic copper produced a liver having a very short T_1 relaxation time, thus appearing unusually intense,[14] but no abnormality in T_1 time was found in patients with steatosis[17] or Wilson's disease.[14]

Spleen

The spleen appears as a homogeneous structure having an NMR signal usually slightly more intense than the liver using spin echo techniques (Figs. 24–21A and 24–23) and less intense on in-

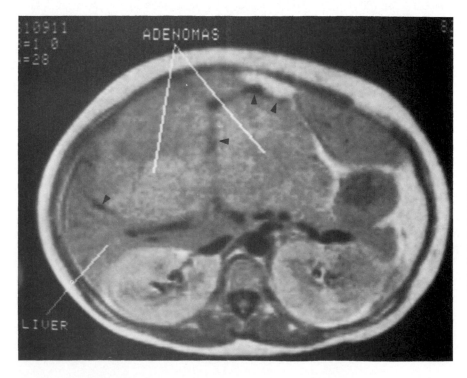

Figure 24–26. Hepatic adenomas. Two hepatic adenomas are demonstrated as masses having a slightly greater intensity than normal liver parenchyma. A low-intensity band (arrowheads) partially surrounding the adenomas is present but the exact nature of this structure is unclear. The patient has glycogen storage disease, which has thickened the renal cortex and has resulted in the liver and renal cortex having a slightly greater intensity than normal.

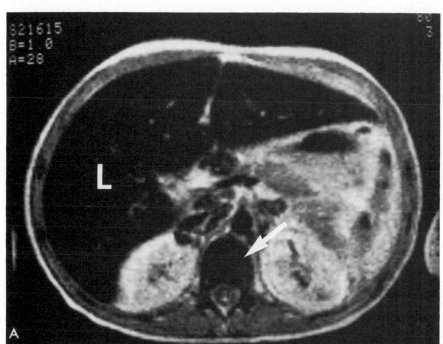

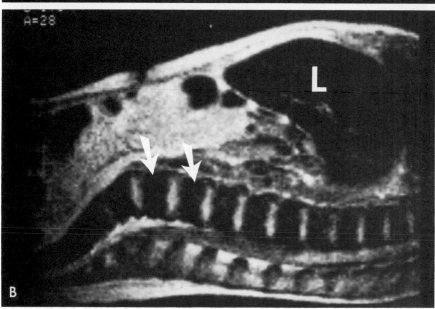

Figure 24–27. Transfusion-induced hemochromatosis in a child with thalassemia major. **A** Transverse spin echo NMR image shows the liver (L) with an extremely low intensity produced by its high iron content. The marrow space of the spine (arrow) also has excessive iron deposition. **B** Midsagittal NMR image. The bone marrow (arrows) of the entire spine is abnormally dark because of its high iron content. L = Liver.

version recovery scans. The spleen is readily demonstrated on NMR, since it is surrounded by retroperitoneal and intra-abdominal fat, which have a very intense signal. As in the liver, splenic vessels are demonstrable without contrast injection.

The NMR appearance of splenic abnormalities has not been fully described. A splenic metastasis producing a low-intensity mass and a pheochromocytoma partially occluding the venous drainage of a portion of the spleen resulted in the affected portion of the spleen having a prolonged T_1 relaxation time (Fig. 24–28).[37]

Pancreas

Although Smith's group[19] did not visualize the normal pancreas, this organ can be routinely imaged as a structure of medium intensity on high-resolution NMR scans (Fig. 24–29). However, of all the abdominal organs, the pancreas appears to be the most difficult to completely image by NMR. When the pancreas is completely surrounded by contrasting tissue such as fat, vascular structures, and/or gas in the stomach and duodenum, it is particularly well delineated (Figs. 24–

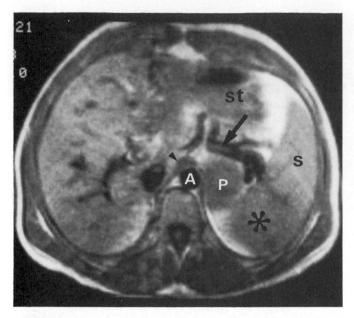

Figure 24–28. Pheochromocytoma. Spin echo image reveals a left adrenal pheochromocytoma (P) as a homogeneous hypointense mass between the spleen (S) and aorta (A). The posterior portion of the spleen (asterisk) has a decreased intensity secondary to congestion owing to the tumor's partially occluding splenic venous flow. Slow flow is shown in the splenic vein by the intense signal (arrow) with its lumen. st = Stomach; arrowhead = right diaphragmatic crura. (From Moon KL Jr, Hricak H, Crooks LE, Gooding CA, Moss AA, Engelstad, BL, Kaufman L: Nuclear magnetic resonance imaging of the adrenal gland: A pulmonary report. Radiology 147:155, 1983.)

11 and 24–29). However, when there is little peripancreatic fat, no gas in the duodenum or loops of small intestine adjacent to the tail of the pancreas, the parenchyma of the pancreas is poorly imaged. Despite these difficulties, NMR superbly delineates the splenic artery and vein, superior mesenteric artery and vein, and the portal venous confluence.

Pancreatic carcinomas larger than 3 cm produce focal mass lesions that have different intensity values than surrounding normal pancreas (Figs. 24–30, 24–31 and 24–32),[11, 17, 19] and the relationship of the pancreatic neoplasm to sur-

rounding vascular structures is clearly shown. However, no documentation is available concerning detection of small (less than 3 cm) tumors, infiltrating lesions, or benign pancreatic neoplasms. Pancreatic cancers have longer T_1 values than the normal pancreas, and pancreatitis has been reported to increase T_1 but to a lesser extent than either a pancreatic pseudocyst or abscess.[17, 19]

Kidneys

The kidneys are clearly delineated as organs having a medium intensity on NMR images (Figs.

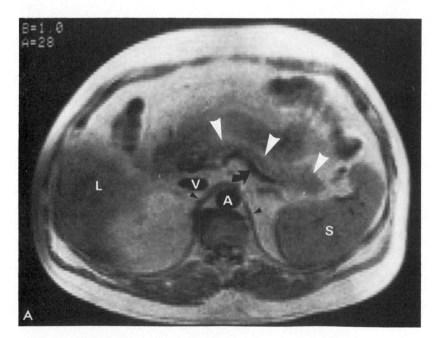

Figure 24–29. Normal pancreas, spin echo images. **A** The body and tail of the pancreas (large arrowheads) are seen anterior to the splenic vein (curved arrow). The aorta (A), vena cava (V), crura of the diaphragm (small arrowheads), spleen, and liver (L) are also demonstrated.

Illustration continued on opposite page

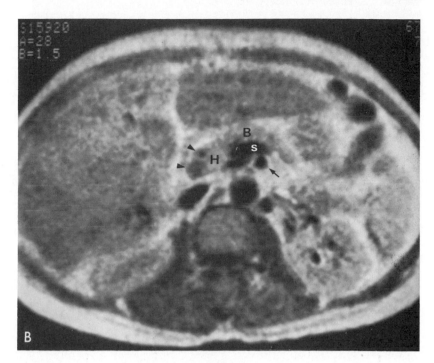

Figure 24–29 *Continued* **B** The head of the pancreas (H) is demonstrated adjacent to the fluid-filled duodenum (arrowheads). The splenic vein (S) arches over the superior mesenteric artery (arrow). Just anterior to the splenic vein, the body of the pancreas (B) is clearly shown.

24–32 and 24–33).[11, 17, 20, 28, 38] On spin echo images, the outer renal margin is particularly well displayed, being contrasted against the perirenal fat, which has a very high intensity. The renal cortex and medulla can be separated without intravenous contrast, as can the renal vasculature and collecting system (Figs. 24–32 and 24–33). The ability to obtain direct sagittal and coronal images is useful in separating the liver from the upper pole of the right kidney and/or in distinguishing adrenal from renal masses.

Nuclear magnetic resonance imaging can accurately differentiate between solid and cystic masses.[20, 36, 37] Simple renal cysts image as homogeneous, low-intensity masses with no internal structure (Figs. 24–22*B* and 24–34 through 24–36). Simple cysts have a sharp interface with renal parenchyma, and the wall of the cyst is not identifiable. The T_1 values of cysts are typically longer than 2 seconds and the T_2 values greater than 200 milliseconds.

Hemorrhagic renal cysts appear as high-inten-

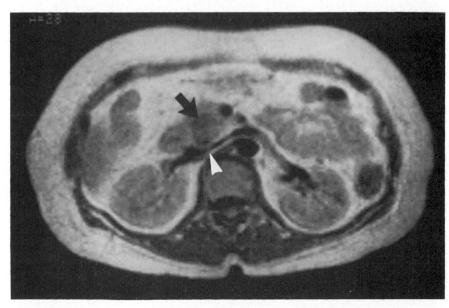

Figure 24–30. Pancreatic carcinoma. A small pancreatic carcinoma (arrow) is demonstrated as an area of decreased intensity in the head of the pancreas. The tumor is displacing but not invading the left renal vein (arrowhead).

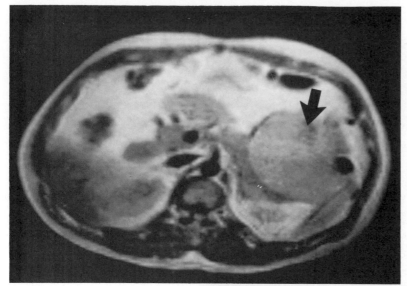

Figure 24–31. Malignant pancreatic islet cell carcinoma. A transverse spin echo NMR image clearly demonstrates the large pancreatic tumor (arrow) arising in the tail of the pancreas. The tumor appears well encapsulated and has a slightly greater intensity than the normal pancreas.

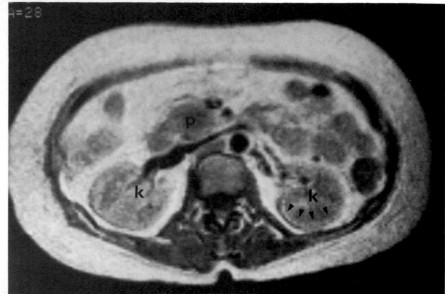

Figure 24–32. Normal kidneys. NMR spin echo image demonstrates kidneys (k) as organs having a moderate intensity. The renal cortex (arrowheads) can be clearly separated from the renal medulla without contrast material. A small pancreatic carcinoma (p) is present in the head of the pancreas.

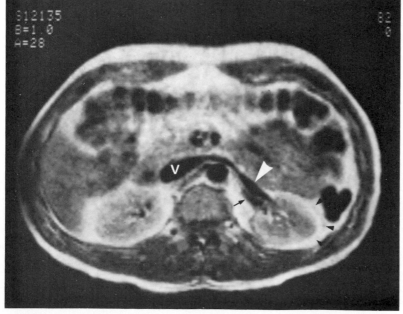

Figure 24–33. Normal kidneys. Spin echo image demonstrating left renal vein (large arrowhead), left renal artery (arrow), and the inferior vena cava (V). Gerota's fascia (small arrowheads) is clearly shown separating perirenal from pararenal fat.

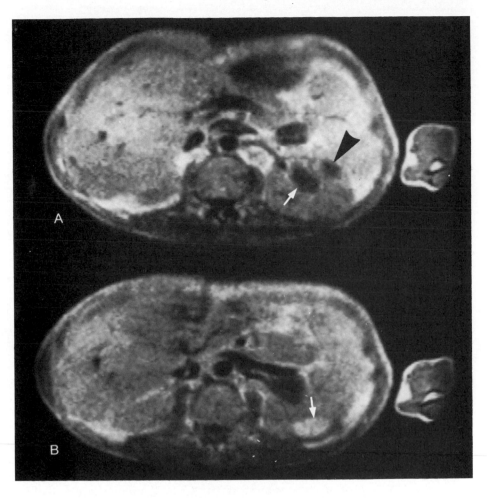

Figure 24–34. Abnormal left kidney, simple and hemorrhagic cysts. **A** Spin echo image reveals hydronephrosis (arrow) and simple cortical cyst (arrowhead). Both the dilated collecting system and renal cyst have a very low intensity. **B** Spin echo image at a different level. A cyst (arrow) is seen in the posterior portion of the kidney, which has a very high intensity. A hemorrhagic cyst was found at surgery.

sity masses, having shorter T_1 and T_2 values (Fig. 24–34B and 24–36).[20] Calcification in the wall of a cyst is poorly demonstrated by NMR but can be suggested when a thick, low-intensity peripheral margin surrounds the renal cyst. Obstructed and/or dilated intrarenal and extrarenal collecting structures have an NMR appearance similar to that of simple renal cysts on spin echo images (Figs. 24–34, and 24–37).

The NMR appearance of renal cell carcinoma is variable, the NMR intensity of tumors ranging from hyperintense to isointense to hypointense,

Figure 24–35. Bilateral parapelvic cysts and gallstones. The parapelvic cysts (arrows) have a low intensity, no internal structure, and a sharp interface with the adjacent renal parenchyma. Arrowheads = gallstones layering in the gallbladder.

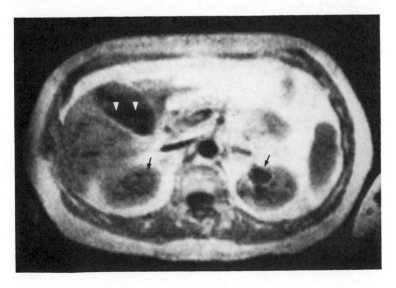

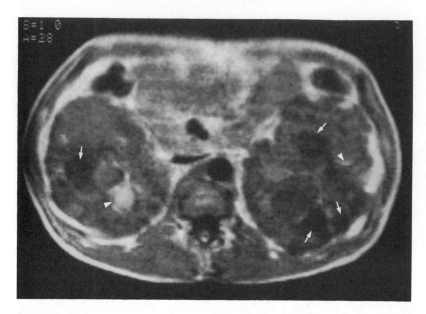

Figure 24–36. Polycystic kidneys. A spin echo image demonstrates enlarged kidneys, which contain cysts of various sizes and intensities. Simple cysts (arrows) appear hypointense, whereas cysts with recent hemorrhage are hyperintense (arrowheads.)

compared with normal renal parenchyma (Fig. 24–38). Regions of inhomogeneity, representing areas of tumor necrosis, are often present and a low-intensity line interposed between the tumor and normal renal parenchyma has been shown pathologically to be a tumor pseudocapsule.[20]

The T_1 values for renal cell carcinoma have ranged from 1 to 1.6 seconds (mean 1.3 seconds), with T_2 values ranging from 55 to 107 milliseconds (mean 76).[20] The T_1 value of renal carcinoma is higher than normal parenchyma, and T_2 values are similar or higher than those of adjacent renal parenchyma. Nuclear magnetic resonance imaging has been particularly valuable in staging

renal cell carcinoma because it can readily and accurately assess tumor extension into the parinephric space, renal vessels, and inferior vena cava (Fig. 24–38B).

The NMR appearance of renal angiomyolipoma has been shown to vary, depending on the imaging parameters employed.[20] It appeared as a slightly heterogeneous high-intensity mass that was difficult to distinguish from adjacent perirenal fat on a spin echo image with a pulse sequence interval (TR) of 500 milliseconds and an echo delay (TE) time of 28 milliseconds but readily apparent as a low-intensity mass when the echo delay time was prolonged to 56 milliseconds.

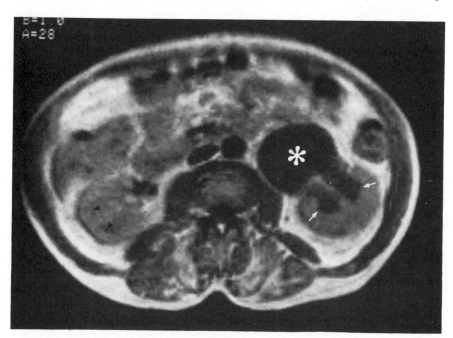

Figure 24–37. Hydronephrotic left kidney. The dilated extrarenal pelvis (asterisk) and intrarenal collecting system (arrows) are well demonstrated and have an intensity similar to simple renal cysts. The cortical medullary demarcation (arrowheads) seen in the right kidney is lost in the hydronephrotic kidney. (From Hricak H, Crooks L, Sheldon P, Kaufman L: Nuclear magnetic resonance imaging of the kidney. Radiology 146:425, 1983.)

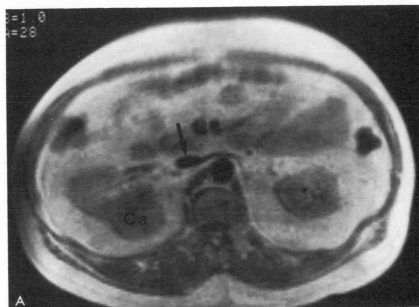

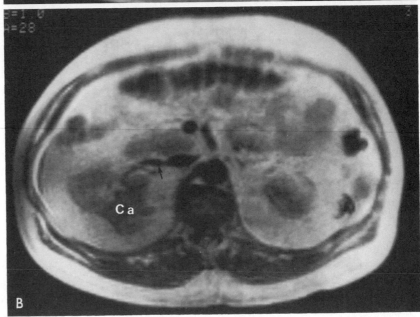

Figure 24–38. Renal cell carcinoma. **A** Spin echo image demonstrates right renal cell carcinoma (Ca) as a slightly hypointense mass originating from the posterior aspect of the kidney. The inferior vena cava (arrow) appears normal. **B** Image at a more cephalad level again demonstrates the carcinoma (Ca) and reveals the right renal vein (arrow) to be patent and free of tumor. (From Hricak H, Williams RD, Moon KL Jr, Moss AA, Alpers C, Crooks LE, Kaufman L: Nuclear magnetic imaging of the kidney. Radiology 147:765, 1983.)

Renal contusion produced a localized area of low intensity and a renal abscess an inhomogeneous mass of lower intensity than normal parenchyma.[20]

The size of the kidneys is easily measured by NMR, and alterations in renal contour readily demonstrated. In chronic pyelonephritis, cortical width is thinned and diminutive kidneys are seen in chronic glomerulonephritis. In several diseases, including acute glomerulonephritis and hydronephrosis, the separation between cortex and medulla is lost. In glycogen storage disease, the kidneys may be enlarged and have a higher intensity than normal.[20]

Adrenal Glands

Normal-sized adrenal glands are usually well demonstrated on NMR images as a linear, inverted triangle or as Y-shaped structures of relatively homogeneous low intensity surrounded by high intensity retroperitoneal fat (Fig. 24–39).[11, 17, 37] Moon and others[37] detected 36 of 36 (100 per cent) of normal left and 30 of 36 (83 per cent) of normal right adrenal glands. The adrenal gland generally has a lower intensity than the liver, a feature that facilitates delineation of the right adrenal gland in thin people. A mean T_1 value of 335 milliseconds and a T_2 value of 59 were re-

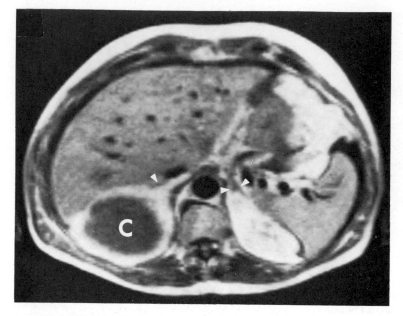

Figure 24–39. Normal adrenal glands. Spin echo image demonstrating normal adrenal glands (arrowheads) as linear-shaped structures surrounded by retroperitoneal fat. A right renal cyst (C) is also present. (From Hricak H, Williams RD, Moon KL Jr, Moss AA, Alpers C, Crooks LE, Kaufman L: Nuclear magnetic resonance imaging of the kidney: Renal masses. Radiology 147:765, 1983.)

ported by Moon,[37] but accurate measurements of T_1 and T_2 values were difficult due to the small size of the normal glands.

On spin echo images, the adrenal cortex appears slightly more intense than the medulla, the differentiation probably being due to the higher lipid content of the adrenal cortex. A high lipid content would be expected to shorten the T_1 and lengthen the T_2 values of the cortex relative to the medulla, both of which would tend to produce a higher intensity signal from the cortex.

Nuclear magnetic resonance imaging of adrenal abnormalities appears comparable with CT scanning except for the smallest lesions.[37] Adrenal metastases (Fig. 24–40) and primary adrenal tumors (see Fig. 24–28) are shown as masses of lower intensity that are either homogeneous or contain foci of different intensities. Adrenal hyperplasia produces enlargement of both glands with maintenance of the basic shape of the adrenal glands. Although insufficient data is available to determine whether tissue relaxation values (T_1, T_2) will be sufficiently precise to permit distinction between various adrenal tumors, it is probable that there will be overlap of T_1 and T_2 values in benign and malignant adrenal disease.

PELVIS

The pelvis is particularly well displayed by NMR because the absence of movement and en-

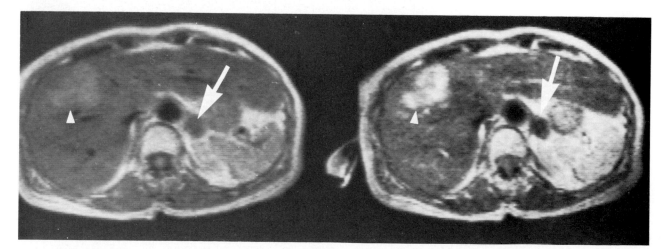

Figure 24–40. Adrenal cyst and hepatic metastases. The adrenal cyst (arrow) produces a hypointense adrenal mass having sharp borders. Metastatic colon carcinoma is present in the liver (arrowhead). (From Moon LL Jr, Hricak H, Crooks LE, Gooding CA, Moss AA, Engelstad BL, Kaufman L: Nuclear magnetic resonance imaging of the adrenal gland: A preliminary report. Radiology 147:155, 1983.)

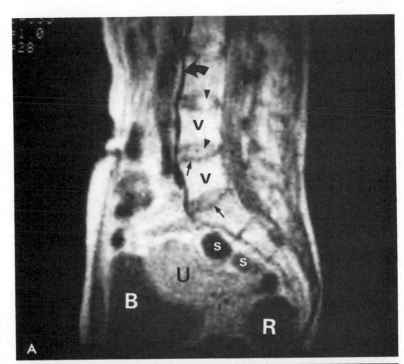

Figure 24–41. Normal pelvic anatomy, direct sagittal NMR spin echo images. **A** Female pelvis. The uterus (U) is demonstrated posterior and superior to the bladder (B). The vertebral bodies (V) containing marrow give an intense signal. The annulus fibrosis (arrow) has a lower intensity than the nucleus pulposis (arrowhead) in the disc interspace. R = Rectum; s = sigmoid colon; curved arrow = longitudinal ligament. **B** Male pelvis. The relationships of the prostate (P), bladder (B), rectum (R), and sigmoid colon (S) are clearly depicted.

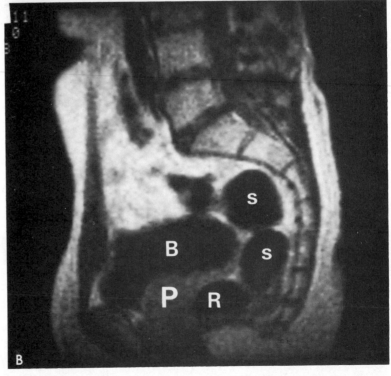

casement of soft-tissue elements by bone and fat make it an ideal region to image.[40] In addition to axial images, direct coronal and sagittal NMR images of the pelvis are very useful for displaying the anatomic relationships between various pelvic organs (Figs. 24–41 and 24–42).

In men, tumors of the bladder and prostate and evaluation of involvement of the seminal vesicles by neoplasm can be seen to unprecedented advantage.[40] Prostatic hypertrophy can be identified (Fig. 24–43) and it may be possible to distinguish prostatic carcinoma (Fig. 24–44) from adjacent benign prostatic hypertrophy. Invasion of tumor into the seminal vesicles is shown by loss of

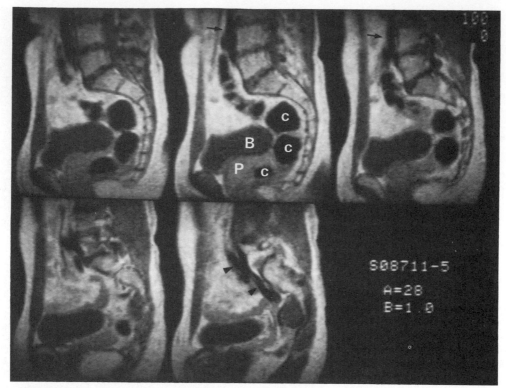

Figure 24–42. Five contiguous sagittal NMR images through the pelvis of a normal man. The bladder (B) is seen cephalic to the prostate (P). The course of the sigmoid colon (c) is well delineated. In the upper row of images, the abdominal aorta (arrow) is first seen on left as a tubular structure, which then divides as the images proceed to the right. In the lower row, the iliac artery and vein (arrow-heads) are apparent as dark tubular structures.

normal surrounding fat and demonstration of a tumor mass invading the seminal vesicle.

In women, tumors of the bladder, ovary, uterus and vagina are accurately displayed. However, it may be in pregnancy that NMR, with its lack of ionizing radiation will have its greatest impact.

Smith and associates[41] studied the uterus in pregnant women prior to abortion. The detail and amount of information obtained indicated that NMR may rival ultrasound when the long-term biologic effects of NMR have been studied sufficiently to the satisfaction of regulatory agencies.

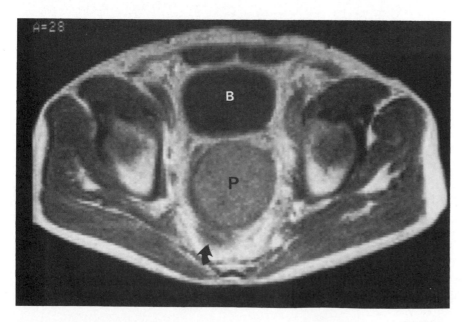

Figure 24–43. Prostatic hypertrophy. A transverse spin echo image demonstrates an enlarged but homogeneous prostate (P) of intermediate intensity posterior to the bladder (B) and anterior to the rectum (arrow).

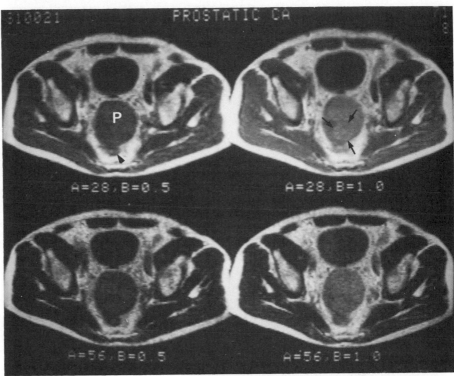

Figure 24–44. Prostatic carcinoma and prostatic hypertrophy. Four spin echo images obtained using different imaging parameters. The enlarged prostate (P) appears as an oval mass between the bladder and compressed rectum (arrowhead). By varying the imager parameters, the contrast between the different tissues changes and a small foci of prostatic carcinoma (arrows) is identified as a prostatic mass having a slightly higher intensity.

SPINE AND MUSCULOSKELETAL SYSTEM

In the neck, the major muscles, outlined by fat, are all readily identified. The carotid artery and internal jugular veins can be imaged, and the spinal cord is clearly delineated in the spinal canal (Fig. 24–45). The base of the neck, an area difficult to image by CT because of artifacts generated from the shoulders, is demonstrated without artifacts (Fig. 24–10). Tumors of the neck encroaching upon the great vessels are clearly shown, the contrast between normal and abnormal tissues and vascular structures being excellent (Fig. 24–46).

The spinal column can be imaged directly in the transverse[47] (axial) or sagittal planes. Disc material, vertebral body cortex and medullary cavity, epidural fat and vessels, thecal sac, lumbar spinal cord, and nerve roots are all well seen in the axial images.

Axial and sagittal images through the intervertebral disc demonstrate a moderately intense central portion (nucleus pulposus) surrounded by a ring of lower intensity (annular fibrosa) (Figs. 24–41 and 24–47).[42] The bony cortex of the vertebral bodies and ligamentous structures closely applied to the cortex have a low intensity, whereas the medullary cavity is of relatively high intensity. Epidural fat is readily identified, even when present in small amounts, because of its high signal in-

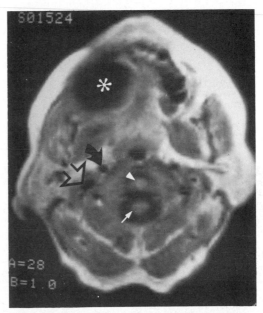

Figure 24–45. Normal anatomy. Transverse spin echo image at the level of the maxillary alveolar ridge. The dark circle (asterisk) anteriorly is an artifact resulting from magnetic material in the patient's denture, disturbing the homogeneity of the magnetic field. Posteriorly the spinal cord (arrow) is seen surrounded by low-intensity spinal fluid, just posterior to the odontoid process (arrowhead), which appears bright because of its marrow content. The internal carotid artery (curved arrow) and internal jugular vein (open arrow) are clearly shown.

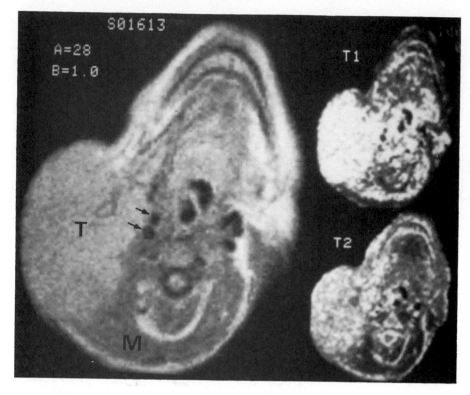

Figure 24–46. Squamous cell carcinoma of the neck. The tumor (T) is clearly shown as a mass of greater intensity than surrounding musculature (M) but less than adjacent fat. The mass is displacing the internal carotid artery and vein (arrows). On the T_1 and T_2 relaxation time images, the tumor appears intense, indicating long T_1 and T_2 relaxation times.

tensity compared with that of surrounding tissues. Epidural fat deposits are symmetrical in normal patients. In the upper lumbar region, the spinal cord is visible as a relatively high-intensity structure surrounded by low-intensity cerebrospinal fluid. The thecal sac and nerve roots are seen as round low-intensity structures highlighted by high-intensity epidural and paraspinous fat. The longitudinal ligaments, intervertebral discs, spinal cord, and nerve roots traversing the neural foramina are well demonstrated on direct sagittal images (Fig. 24–41).

Moderate-sized disc herniations are demonstrated by NMR as masses protruding into the thecal sac nerve root. The signal intensity of the abnormal disc is lower than normal and appears

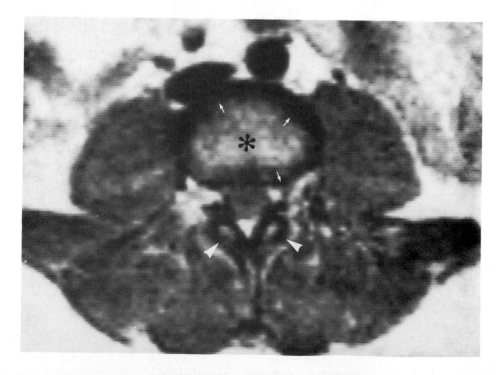

Figure 24–47. Normal lumbosacral spine. Spin echo NMR image obtained through L4–5 intervertebral disc. Disc material has a high-intensity center (asterisk) and a low-intensity outer ring (arrows). Cortical bone in the posterior elements is black (arrowheads). The thecal sac and L4 nerve roots are outlined by high-intensity epidural fat.

Figure 24–48. Disc herniation. Axial spin echo image of lumbosacral spine at L5–S1 level disc herniation is demonstrated as a mass (arrow) of intermediate intensity in the anterior portion of the spinal canal, which impinges on the thecal sac (S) and the right S1 nerve root. The epidural fat is asymmetric, and the right nerve root and thecal sac are displaced from their normal positions. (From Moon KL Jr, Genant HK, Helms CA, Chafety NI, Crooks LE, Kaufman L: Musculoskeletal applications of nuclear magnetic resonance. Radiology 147:161, 1983.)

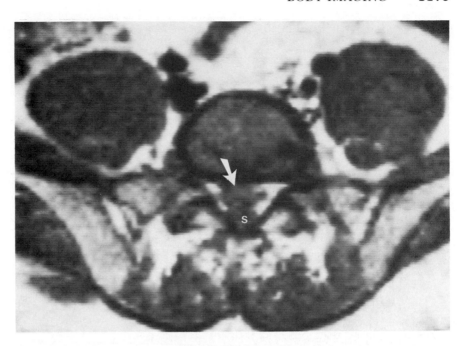

to be markedly diminished following chymopapain injection (Fig. 24–48). In evaluating the postoperative spine, NMR can easily distinguish among fatty, vascular, and fibrotic tissue and is not affected by vascular clips or residual contrast material.

Metastatic tumors involving the spine are well delineated by NMR (Fig. 24–49). The metastases have an overall lower signal intensity than that of adjacent normal medullary bone. The cortical margin can be seen to be destroyed, and when present, extrusion into adjacent structures can be shown (Fig. 24–49). Brady and co-workers[43] reported similar findings in patients with a giant cell tumor of the upper extremities.

Soft-tissue tumors such as hemangiomas and liposarcomas appear to be better delineated on NMR than on CT. Nuclear magnetic resonance imaging is capable of assessing vascular supply and to some extent blood flow through soft tissues without a contrast injection.

As in the spine, the bony cortex of the appendicular skeleton, as a result of its low hydrogen content, produces a very low NMR signal. The cortex thus appears as a dark, black line surrounding the medullary cavity, which has an intense signal because of its high fat and protein content.[42, 43] Compared with the normal hip joint, femoral heads in patients with avascular necrosis have revealed a significant decrease in signal intensity in the superior aspect of the medullary space.[42]

Examination of the normal knee joint has shown NMR capable of imaging the muscles, ligaments, tendons, and blood vessels as well as the surrounding bony structures.[42] Tendons have a lower signal intensity than muscle, thus permitting discrimination between the two. Cruciate ligaments are seen as low-intensity structures outlined by fat in the intercondylar space. Meniscal

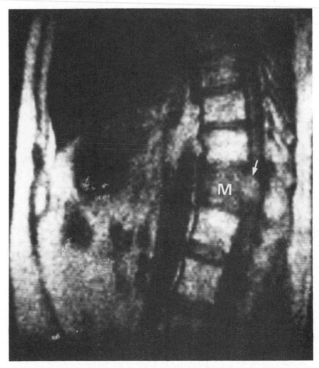

Figure 24–49. Vertebral body metastasis. Sagittal spin echo image demonstrates metastatic renal cell carcinoma to the T_{11} vertebral body (M). The cortex of the posterior aspect of the vertebral body is destroyed, and the tumor extends into the spinal canal (arrow), compressing the spinal cord. (From Moon KL Jr, Genant HK, Helms CA, Chafety NI, Crooks LE, Kaufman L: Musculoskeletal applications of nuclear magnetic resonance. Radiology 147:161, 1983.)

cartilage has not been well shown on NMR images.

BREAST

Imaging of the breast by NMR has proved feasible.[44–46] The breast with extensive fatty replacement has a short T_1 value, whereas tumors have been shown to have prolonged T_1 values.[45] T_1 values for mammary dysplasia have extended over a wide range on saturation recovery images[45] and have tended to overlap those of tumors. However, benign breast cysts are clearly distinguished from solid abnormalities by their long T_1 values, and NMR thus appears to have great potential as a nonionizing method of screening for breast malignancy.

SAFETY OF NMR IMAGING

Because NMR uses no ionizing radiation, it is potentially a harmless method of obtaining high-resolution cross-sectional tomographic images. Experiments to date[47–50] have confirmed that using currently available instruments NMR is harmless.

Schwartz and Crooks[47] and Wolf and others[48] reported negative effects of NMR exposure on chromosome aberrations, sister chromatid exchanges, and the inhibition of DNA synthesis, all indicators of genetic damage. Exposure levels used in these NMR studies were greater than those utilized in clinical situations and did not induce any detectable mutagenic or cytotoxic effect.

Budinger[49] studied the thresholds for health effects for static magnetic fields, changing magnetic fields and RF heating. Static magnetic fields have no harmful effects at magnetic fields below 2 tesla (T). Induced internal electric currents are produced from superimposition of rapidly changing magnetic fields on the main static field. These electric currents appear harmless if the maximum amplitude of the sinusoidally switching field is below 50 gauss, a level not approached in current NMR imagers. No significant tissue heating was found from implanted small surgical chips during greater exposures than employed clinically.[50] The heating effects of large metallic implants have not been widely studied, but a rise of 1.3 to 1.7°C was found in an experimental situation in which the prostheses were totally surrounded by a conducting solution.[50] The heating of larger metallic prostheses and rods does not appear to be a problem in clinical NMR imaging because they are not totally surrounded by a conducting solution.

Based on evidence to date, NMR appears completely harmless except in patients with ferromagnetic surgical clips or implanted electronic devices that would be disturbed by the large magnetic field, by the rapid change of the varying magnetic fields, or by the RF signal. Most surgical clips are nonmagnetic and will present no problems; however, a few, including a few aneurysmal vascular clips, are slightly ferromagnetic and can be pulled or torqued by the magnetic field.

REFERENCES

1. Lauterbur PC: Image formation by induced local interactions: Examples employing NMR. Nature 242:190, 1973.
2. Gore JC, Emery EW, Orr JS, Doyle FH: Medical nuclear magnetic resonance imaging: I. Physical principles. Invest Radiol 16:269, 1981.
3. Bradley WG, Tosteson H: Basic principles of NMR. In Kaufman L, Crooks LE, Margulis AR (eds): Nuclear Magnetic Resonance in Medicine. Tokyo, Kgaku-Shoin, 1981, pp 11–29.
4. Pykett IL, Newhouse JH, Buonanno FS, Brady TJ, Goldman MR, Kistler JP, Pohost GM: Principles of nuclear magnetic resonance in aging. Radiology 143:157, 1982.
5. Pykett IL: NMR imaging in medicine. Scientific American 246:78, 1982.
6. Shepp LA: Computerized tomography and nuclear magnetic resonance. J Comput Assist Tomogr 4:94, 1980.
7. Louis AK: Optimal sampling in nuclear magnetic resonance (NMR) tomography. J Comput Assist Tomogr 6:334, 1982.
8. James AE Jr, Partain CL, Holland GN, Gore FD, Harms SE, Price RR: Nuclear magnetic resonance imaging: The current state. AJR 138:201, 1981.
9. Herfkens R, Davis PL, Crooks LE, Kaufman L, Price D, Miller T, Margulis AR, Watts J, Hoenninger J, Arakawa M, McRee R: NMR imaging of the abnormal live rat and correlation with tissue characteristics. Radiology 141:211, 1981.
10. Davis PL, Kaufman L, Crooks LE, Miller TR: Detectability of hepatomas in rat livers by nuclear magnetic resonance imaging. Invest Radiol 16:354, 1981.
11. Crooks L, Arakawa M, Hoenninger J, Watts J, McRee R, Kaufman L, Davis PL, Margulis AR, DeGroot J: NMR whole body imager operating at 3.5 kGauss. Radiology 143:169, 1982.
12. Kaufman L, Crooks LE, Sheldon PE, Rowan W: Evaluation of NMR imaging for detection and quantification of obstructions in vessels. Invest Radiol 17:554, 1982.
13. Davis PL, Sheldon P, Kaufman L, Crooks L, Margulis AR, Muller T, Watts J, Arakawa M, Hoenninger J: Nuclear magnetic resonance imaging of mammary adenocarcinomas in the rat. Cancer 51:433, 1983.
14. Doyle FH, Pennock JM, Banks LM, McDonnell MJ,, Bydder GM, Steiner RE, Young IR, Clarke GJ, Pasmore T, Gilderdale DJ: Nuclear magnetic resonance imaging of the liver: Initial experience. AJR:138:193, 1982.
15. Bydder GM, Steiner RE, Young IR, Hall AS, Thomas DJ,

Marshall J, Pallis CA, Legg NJ: Clinical NMR imaging of the brain: 140 cases. AJR 139:215, 1982.

16. Hutchinson JMS, Smith FW: Human NMR imaging. In Kaufman L, Crooks LE, Margulis AR (eds): Nuclear Magnetic Resonance Imaging in Medicine. Tokyo, Igaku-Shoin, 1981, pp 101–127.

17. Young IR, Bailes DR, Burl M, Collins AG, Smith DT, McDonnell MJ, Orr JS, Banks LM, Bydder GM, Greenspan RH, Steiner RE: Initial clinical evaluation of a whole body nuclear magnetic resonance (NMR) tomograph. J Comput Assist Tomogr 6:1, 1982.

18. Moss AA, Davis PL, Goldberg HI, Margulis AR, Stark D, Crooks L, Kaufman L: NMR imaging of hepatic tumors: Evaluation of various imaging techniques. Presented at First Annual Meeting of Nuclear Magnetic Resonance in Medicine, Boston, Mass., Aug. 16–18, 1982.

19. Smith RW, Reid A, Hutchinson JMS, Mallard JR: Nuclear magnetic resonance imaging of the pancreas. Radiology 142:677, 1982.

20. Hricak H, Williams R, Moon KL Jr, Moss AA, Alpers C, Crooks LE, Kaufman L: NMR imaging of the kidney: Renal masses. Radiology. 147:765, 1983.

21. Brasch RC, Wesbey G, Gooding CA, Kerper MA: NMR imaging of depositional iron in transfusion hemosiderosis. Presented at Works-in-Progress Session, Radiologic Society of North America, Chicago, December 1, 1982.

22. Brasch RC: Concepts of contrast enhancement for nuclear magnetic resonance imaging: What works and why. In Moss AA (ed): NMR, Interventional Radiology and Diagnostic Imaging Modalities. San Francisco, University of California Press, 1983, pp 57–67.

23. Brady TJ, Goldman MR, Pykett IL, Kistler JP, Newhouse JH, Burt CT, Hinshaw WS, Pohost GM: Proton nuclear magnetic resonance imaging of regionally ischemic canine hearts: Effect of paramagnetic proton signal enhancement. Radiology 144:343, 1982.

24. Hawkes RC, Holland GN, Moore WS, Rolback EJ, Worthington BS: Nuclear magnetic resonance (NMR) tomography of the normal heart. J Comput Assist Tomogr 5:605, 1981.

25. Gamsu G, Webb WR, Sheldon P, Kaufman L, Crooks LE, Brinberg FA, Goodman P, Hinchcliffe WA, Hedgecock M: Nuclear magnetic resonance imaging of the thorax. Radiology 147:473, 1983.

26. Heneghan MA, Biancaniello TM, Heidelberger E, Peterson SB, Marsh MJ, Lauterbur PC: Nuclear magnetic resonance zeugmatographic imaging of the heart: Application to the study of ventricular septal defect. Radiology 143:183, 1982.

27. Kaufman L, Crooks LE, Sheldon P, Hricak H, Herfkens R, Banks W: The potential impact of nuclear magnetic resonance imaging on cardiovascular diagnosis. Circulation 67:251, 1983.

28. Alfidi RF, Haaga JR, Yousef SJ, Bryan PJ, Fletcher BD, LiPuma JP, Morrison SC, Kaufman B, Richey JB, Hinshaw WS, Kramer DM, Yeung HN, Cohen AM, Butler HE, Ament AE, Lieberman JM: Preliminary experimental results in humans and animals with a superconducting whole-body, nuclear magnetic resonance scanner. Radiology 143:175, 1981.

29. Gamsu G, Webb WR: Nuclear magnetic resonance imaging of the lungs and mediastinum. In Moss AA (ed): NMR, Interventional Radiology and Diagnostic Imaging Modalities. San Francisco, University of California Press, 1983, pp 45–53.

30. Hinshaw WS, Andrew ER, Bottomley PA, Holland GN, Moore WS, Worthington BS: Display of cross sectional anatomy by nuclear magnetic resonance imaging. Br J Radiol 51:273, 1978.

31. Partain CL, James AE Jr, Watson JT, Price RR, Coulam CM, Rollo RD: Nuclear magnetic resonance and computed tomography: Comparison of normal body images. Radiology 136:767, 1980.

32. Edelstein WA, Hutchinson JMS, Smith FW, Mallard J, Johnson G, Redpath TW: Human whole-body NMR tomographic imaging: Normal sections. Br J Radiol 54:149, 1981.

33. Smith FW, Mallard JR, Reid A, Hutchinson JMS: Nuclear magnetic imaging in liver disease. Lancet 1:963, 1981.

34. Margulis AR, Moss AA, Crooks LE, Kaufman L: NMR imaging of tumors of the liver. Semin Roentgenol 18:123, 1983.

35. Hricak H, Filly RA, Margulis AR, Moon KL, Crooks LE, Kaufman L, Moon K: Nuclear magnetic resonance imaging of the gallbladder. Radiology 147:481, 1983.

36. Haaga JR, Alfidi RJ, LiPuma JP, Bryan PJ, El Yousef SJ: NMR imaging of the liver. Presented at the 68th Meeting of the Radiologic Society of North America, Chicago, December 1, 1982.

37. Moon KL Jr, Hricak H, Crooks LE, Gooding CA, Moss AA, Engelstad BL, Kaufman L: Nuclear magnetic resonance imaging of the adrenal glands: A preliminary report. Radiology 147:155, 1983.

38. Hricak H, Crooks L, Sheldon P, Kaufman L: NMR imaging of the kidney. Radiology 146: 425, 1983.

39. Smith FW, Hutchison JM, Mallard JR: Renal cyst or tumor—differentiation by whole body nuclear magnetic resonance imaging. Diagn Imaging 50:61, 1981.

40. Hricak H, Spring DB, Kaufman L, Williams L, Crooks L: Anatomy and pathology of the male pelvis as imaged by NMR. Journal of Magnetic Resonance in Medicine (in press).

41. Smith FW: Clinical imaging at Aberdeen. Presented Society of Magnetic Resonance in Medicine, Boston, Aug. 16–18, 1982.

42. Genant HK, Moon KL Jr, Helms CA, Chafetz NI: Nuclear magnetic resonance imaging of the musculoskeletal system. In Moss AA (ed): NMR, Interventional Radiology and Diagnostic Imaging. San Francisco, University of California Press, 1983, pp 73–84.

43. Brady TJ, Gebbhardt MC, Pykett IL, Buonanno FS, Newhouse JH, Burt CT, Smith RJ, Manken HJ, Kistler JP, Goldman MR, Hinshaw WS, Pohost GM: NMR imaging of forearms in healthy volunteers and patients with Grantcell tumors of bone. Radiology 144:549, 1982.

44. Mansfield P, Morris PG, Ordidge R, Coupland RE, Bishop HM, Blamey RW: Carcinoma of the breast imaged by nuclear magnetic resonance (NMR). Br J Radiol 52:242, 1979.

45. Ross RJ, Thompson JS, Kim K, Bailey RA: Nuclear magnetic resonance imaging and evaluation of human breast tissue: Preliminary clinical trials. Radiology 143:195, 1982.

46. Alfidi R: NMR: Current concepts and applications. Presented at the 6th Annual Meeting Society of Computed Body Tomography, San Diego, March 3, 1983.

47. Schwartz JL, Crooks LE: NMR imaging produces no observable mutations or cytotoxicity in mammalian cells. AJR 139:583, 1982.

48. Wolf S, Crooks LE, Brown P, Howard R, Painter RB: Tests for DNA and chromosomal damage induced by nuclear magnetic resonance imaging. Radiology 136:707, 1980.

49. Budinger TF: Nuclear magnetic resonance (NMR): in vivo studies: Known thresholds for health effects. J Comput Assist Tomogr 5:800, 1981.

50. Davis PL, Crooks L, Arakawa M, McRee R, Kaufman L, Margulis AR: Potential hazards in NMR imaging: Heating effects of changing magnetic fields and RF fields on small metallic implants. AJR 137:857, 1981.

INDEX

Note: Page numbers in *italics* refer to illustrations; page numbers followed by (t) refer to tables.